PRIMER ON THE RHEUMATIC DISEASES

EDITION

11

PRIMER ON THE RHEUMATIC DISEASES

EDITION

11

John H. Klippel, MD, EDITOR

Cornelia M. Weyand, MD, PhD, ASSOCIATE EDITOR
Robert L. Wortmann, MD, ASSOCIATE EDITOR

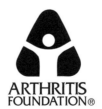

ARTHRITIS FOUNDATION®

Published by the Arthritis Foundation
1330 West Peachtree Street
Atlanta, Georgia 30309

LIBRARY OF CONGRESS CATALOGING-IN-PUBLICATION DATA

Primer on the rheumatic diseases / editor, John H. Klippel;
  associate editors, Cornelia M. Weyand, Robert L. Wortmann.
  – 11th ed.
      p.   cm.
   Includes bibliographical references and index.
   ISBN 0-912423-16-1 (pbk. : alk. paper)
   1. Rheumatism. 2. Arthritis. I. Klippel, John H. II. Weyand,
  Cornelia M. III. Wortmann, Robert.
   [DNLM: 1. Arthritis. 2. Rheumatic Diseases.   WE 344 P953 1997]
  RC927.P67 1997
  616.7'23--dc21
DNLM/DLC
for Library of Congress   97-25311
                                                              CIP

ARTHRITIS
FOUNDATION®

PUBLISHER: William M. Otto, *Group Vice President, Publications*
MANAGING EDITOR: Elizabeth E. Axtell, *Director, Professional Publications*
PRODUCTION DIRECTOR: Elizabeth Compton, *Director of Production, Publications*
ART DIRECTOR: Jennifer L. Rogers, *Art Director, Publications*
EDITORIAL CONTRIBUTORS: Katie Baer, Cynthia Bertelsen, Daphna Gregg,
                        Cynthia Kahn, Shelly Morrow, Emily Simerly

ISBN: 0-912423-16-1

CONTRIBUTORS

The following people contributed to this edition of the *Primer on the Rheumatic Diseases* by writing or revising chapters and sections for the publication of the eleventh edition. Credits for illustrations are given in figure legends.

Steven B. Abramson, MD
Graciela S. Alarcón, MD, MPH
Ronald J. Anderson, MD
William P. Arend, MD
Frank C. Arnett, MD
John P. Atkinson, MD
W. Timothy Ballard, MD
Thomas Bardin, MD
Thomas G. Benedek, MD
Bengt-Åke Bengtsson, MD, PhD
Gene V. Ball, MD
Joseph J. Biundo, Jr., MD
Warren D. Blackburn, Jr., MD
David G. Borenstein, MD
Adele L. Boskey, PhD
Dimitrios T. Boumpas, MD
Laurence A. Bradley, PhD
Peter Brooks, MD
Joseph A. Buckwalter, MD
Ken J. Bulpitt, MD
Joel Buxbaum, MD
Joseph M. Cash, MD
John E. Castaldo, MD
Peter F.M. Choong, MD
Leslie J. Crofford, MD
Thomas R. Cupps, MD
Paul E. DiCorleto, PhD
Paul Dieppe, MD
Dennis Dykstra, MD, PhD
N. Lawrence Edwards, MD
Keith B. Elkon, MD
John M. Esdail, MD, MPH
Rose S. Fife, MD
Robert I. Fox, MD, PhD
Bruce Freundlich, MD
Allan Gibofsky, MD
Gary S. Gilkeson, MD
Dafna D. Gladman, MD
Mary B. Goldring, PhD
Duncan A. Gordon, MD

Jorg J. Goronzy, MD, PhD
Peter K. Gregersen, MD
Valee Harisdankul, MD, PhD
E. Nigel Harris, MD
Peter Hasselbacher, MD
David B. Hellman, MD
Marc C. Hochberg, MD, MPH
Gary S. Hoffman, MD
William A. Horton, MD
Gene C. Hunder, MD
Robert W. Ike, MD
Robert D. Inman, MD
John Kehrl, MD
Muhammad Asim Khan, MD
Farrah Kheradmand, MD
John H. Klippel, MD
Warren Knudson, PhD
William J. Koopman, MD
Klaus E. Kuettner, PhD
Nancy E. Lane, MD
Thomas J.A. Lehman, MD
Lawrence Leventhal, MD
Matthew H. Liang, MD, MPH
M. Kathryn Liszewski
Daniel J. Lovell, MD, MPH
James L. McGuire, MD
Maren Lawson Mahowald, MD
Carlo L. Mainardi, MD
Michael J. Maricic, MD
Manuel Martinez–Lavin, MD
Tom Mason, MD
Eric L. Matteson, MD
Larry W. Moreland, MD
Stanley J. Naides, MD
Gerald T. Nepom, MD, PhD
José Ochoa, MD
J. Desmond O'Duffy, MB
Nancy J. Olsen, MD
John J. O'Shea, MD
Stephen A. Paget, MD

Richard S. Panush, MD
Harold E. Paulus, MD
Robert S. Pinals, MD
David S. Pisetsky, MD, PhD
Parks W. Pratt, MD
Douglas J. Pritchard, MD
Reed Edwin Pyeritz, MD, PhD
Morris Reichlin, MD
James L. Reinertsen, MD
Christopher T. Ritchlin, MD
Laura Robbins, DSW, MSW
M.G. Rock, MD
Ann K. Rosenthal, MD
Lawrence M. Ryan, MD
Eric S. Schned, MD
H. Ralph Schumacher, MD
William W. Scott, Jr., MD
Robert H. Shmerling, MD
Leonard H. Sigal, MD
Peter A. Simkin, MD
Robert W. Simms, MD
Lee S. Simon, MD
Virginia D. Steen, MD
Ioannis O. Tassiulas, MD
Joel D. Taurog, MD
Robert A. Terkeltaub, MD
Murray B. Urowitz, MD
Ronald F. Van Vollenhoven, MD, PhD
Cornelia M. Weyand, MD, PhD
Zena Werb, PhD
Victoria P. Werth, MD
Barbara White, MD
Fredrick M. Wigley, MD
Ronald L. Wilder, MD, PhD
Dorothy Woodward Wortmann, MD
Robert L. Wortmann, MD
Steven R. Ytterberg, MD
John B. Zabriskie, MD

ARTHRITIS FOUNDATION EDITORIAL BOARD

TABLE OF CONTENTS

FOREWORD

Publication of this eleventh edition of the *Primer on the Rheumatic Diseases* represents the Arthritis Foundation's ongoing commitment to educating health professionals about the rheumatic diseases. Of all the Foundation's educational tools for health professionals, the Arthritis Foundation is especially proud of its role in publishing the *Primer on the Rheumatic Diseases.* The *Primer* has set the standard for similar publications in other diseases. It is recognized as a concise, authoritative, and timely summary of what physicians and students need to know about the rheumatic diseases. The Foundation hopes that the *Primer* will inspire students to undertake the care of people with arthritis and that the *Primer* will enable physicians in all fields and in all countries to better understand and manage patients with rheumatic diseases, thus fulfilling the mission of the Arthritis Foundation to better the lives of people with arthritis.

The Arthritis Foundation, publisher of this *Primer,* was founded in 1948 under the name Arthritis and Rheumatism Foundation by an organization of rheumatologists for the purpose of raising funds to support education and research programs. Since then, our name was changed to Arthritis Foundation and our purpose has expanded so that our current mission is to "support research to find the cure for and prevention of arthritis and to improve the quality of life for those affected by arthritis."

Supporting research remains a primary goal of the Foundation. In 1997 the Foundation will spend approximately $17 million to fund the work of postdoctoral fellows, new investigators, biomedical and clinical researchers, and health sciences researchers. The financial commitment by the Arthritis Foundation will increase dramatically by the year 2000.

The effort to improve the quality of life for people with arthritis involves many activities both for patients and the people who care for them. To educate physicians, allied health professionals, and medical students, the Arthritis Foundation offers not only this *Primer*, but the *Bulletin on the Rheumatic Diseases,* videotapes, multimedia resources, and Continuing Medical Education symposia.

Through its 150 service points and by means of cooperative agreements with other agencies, the Arthritis Foundation provides programs and services for people with arthritis to help improve the quality of their lives. These programs include exercise classes and videotapes, advocacy programs, self-help courses, and support groups. Educational materials including books, pamphlets, brochures, videotapes, and audiotapes are also available for people with arthritis and their families. The American Juvenile Arthritis Organization, a council of the Arthritis Foundation, provides other materials and programs designed with special attention to the needs of children with arthritis and their parents.

Very importantly, the Arthritis Foundation seeks to increase the awareness of arthritis as a serious health problem and to dispel the belief that little can be done to help people with arthritis or related diseases. Today, much can be done to help people with all types of arthritis. Disability as an outcome of disease can have profound economic and social costs, and disability from many types of arthritis can be prevented. The Arthritis Foundation is working to convey that message to the public, to healthcare professionals, and to all levels of government. The Foundation advocates increased funding for research in arthritis and related diseases through the National Institute of Arthritis and Musculoskeletal and Skin Diseases, which it was instrumental in founding, and through other government agencies such as the Centers for Disease Control and Prevention. The Arthritis Foundation works to improve access to medical care including specialized care, long-term care, rehabilitation, and other needs for people with arthritis and related diseases.

DOYT CONN, MD
Senior Vice President, Medical Affairs
Arthritis Foundation

INTRODUCTION

The publication of a new *Primer* is cause for celebration and some reflection. The *Primer* has always served an important role in the education of students of the rheumatic diseases, including medical students, residents, clinicians, and academics, who welcome an opportunity to begin their learning or brush up their knowledge on rheumatic diseases. Each of the editors remembers the impact of learning about rheumatic diseases as medical students by reading the *Primer*. As a second year medical student at the University of Cincinnati, I distinctly remember Dr. Evelyn Hess giving me and every other student a copy of the sixth edition of the *Primer* (1). The range of clinical disorders of rheumatology and the science behind it fascinated me and I recall being struck by both how much and how little was actually known as to what causes rheumatic illnesses and how to treat them. In no small part that gift of the *Primer* started me on a path that I still find myself.

The *Primer* evolved from several publications of the American Committee for the Control of Rheumatism – What is Rheumatism? in 1928, Rheumatism Primer: Chronic Arthritis in 1932; and Primer on Rheumatism: Chronic Arthritis in 1934 (2). This latter work, generally considered the first edition of the *Primer*, consisted of a 52-page brochure that was prepared for distribution in connection with a scientific exhibit on arthritis at the Annual Convention of the American Medical Association held in Cleveland, Ohio. A revision, the Primer on Arthritis, was published in the *Journal of the American Medical Association* in 1942 (3) as were editions that appeared in 1949 (third), 1953 (fourth), 1959 (fifth), 1964 (sixth), and 1973 (seventh) (1, 4–7). The Arthritis Foundation has published all subsequent editions, which appeared in 1983 (eighth), 1988 (ninth), and 1993 (tenth) as well as the current (eleventh) edition (8–11).

The purpose of this *Primer* remains the same as that of all previous editions – to provide a thorough yet concise description of the current science, diagnosis, clinical consequences, and principles of management of the rheumatic diseases. This edition of the *Primer* has a number of new features that give it a different look. It is noticeably bigger than previous editions as a result of expansion of the science sections, which reflects the impact of molecular biology, as well as the addition of a number of new clinical chapters. There are many new, first-time *Primer* authors, each experts in their field and highly respected and capable educators. Finally, the appendices have been expanded to include new and revised criteria, practice guidelines for rheumatic disease diagnosis and management, CD markers and genomic loci of relevance to rheumatology, and drugs commonly used to treat rheumatic diseases.

Thanks go to many people who have worked tirelessly for the past 3 years to make the *Primer* possible. First to the Associate Editors Connie Weyand and Bob Wortmann and their assistants Toni Higgins and Suzanne Godley for their help in the planning, organization, editing, and proofing of the chapters – the *Primer* would not have been possible without them. The editorial team wishes to express its sincere thanks to the contributing authors for sharing their expertise, adhering to deadlines, and their understanding and patience in having to deal with the inevitable changes and suggestions offered by the editors. Last but certainly not least, we are all extremely grateful to Beth Axtell and the entire staff at the Arthritis Foundation who coordinated virtually all phases of the *Primer's* development, rewrote and polished countless chapters to make them readable, and deserve all of the credit for the design of the new *Primer*.

The release of this eleventh edition of the *Primer* marks the Arthritis Foundation's 50th year of helping people with arthritis and related conditions and educating the many healthcare professionals who care for them. The editors, contributors, and staff of the Arthritis Foundation sincerely hope that it contributes to the education of individuals wanting to learn more about the rheumatic diseases and perhaps to generate new ideas that will provide a better understanding of the causes of rheumatic illness that lead to improvements in the care of patients who suffer from these disorders.

JOHN H. KLIPPEL, MD
Editor

1. Decker JL, Bollet AJ, Duff IF, et al: Primer on the rheumatic diseases. JAMA 190:127-140, 425-444, 509-530, 741-751, 1964
2. Benedek TG: A century of American rheumatology. Ann Intern Med 106:304-312, 1982
3. Jordan EP, Bauer W, Boots RH, et al: Primer on arthritis. JAMA 119:1089-1104, 1942
4. McEwen C, Bunim JJ, Freyberg RH, et al: Primer on the rheumatic diseases. JAMA 139 :1068-1076, 1139-1146, 1268-1273, 1949
5. Ragan C, Feldman HA, Clark WS, et al: Primer on the rheumatic diseases. JAMA 152:323-331, 405-414, 522-531, 1953
6. Crain DC, Epstein W, Howell D, et al : Primer on the rheumatic diseases. JAMA 171:1205-1220, 1345-1356, 1680-1691, 1959
7. Rodnan GP, Schumacher HR, Zvaifler NJ: Primer on the rheumatic diseases. JAMA 224:661-812, 1973
8. Rodnan GP, Schumacher HR, Zvaifler NJ: Primer on the Rheumatic Diseases. Atlanta, Arthritis Foundation, 1983
9. Schumacher HR, Klippel JH, Robinson DR: Primer on the Rheumatic Diseases. Atlanta, Arthritis Foundation, 1988
10. Schumacher HR, Klippel JH, Koopman WJ: Primer on the Rheumatic Diseases. Atlanta, Arthritis Foundation, 1993
11. Klippel JH, Weyand CM, Wortmann RL: Primer on the Rheumatic Diseases. Atlanta, Arthritis Foundation, 1997

Recognition of rheumatic diseases 2400 years ago is suggested by the fact that 18 of the aphorisms of Hippocrates refer at least in part to joint ailments, with five of these pertaining to gout. The term *rheuma* was introduced in about the first century AD, its meaning resembling the Hippocratic *catarrhos*. Both terms indicated a substance that flows. They were conceived to be derived from *phlegm,* one of the four primary humors, and were believed to originate in the brain. Various ailments were caused, depending on the site where the flow stopped. An example of the association of rheuma with arthritis was conceived by Andrew Boord. To paraphrase: The rheumatic humor, produced in the head, is viscous. Descending from the head to the inferior parts it causes many infirmities. If it, in contrast to the coleric humor, causes joint disease, the affected parts become swollen and red, with engorged vessels (1547, London).

The concept of rheumatism as a systemic musculoskeletal syndrome was introduced by Guillaume Baillou (Ballonius; 1558–1616) in a work not published until 1642. He claimed that "what arthritis is in a joint that is exactly what rheumatism is in the whole body." He explained the pathogenesis picturesquely in that ". . . one may designate the condition we are considering inexactly as rheumatism, better as a sort of precipitation like a seasickness of the vessels (which vomit), until better terms offer themselves" (1). The term *rheumatologist* was coined as recently as 1940 by Bernard Comroe. Curiously, at least in print it preceded *rheumatology,* which was introduced in the textbook edited by Joseph L. Hollander in 1949.

Ancient descriptions of diseases rarely permit a specific modern diagnosis. For centuries *gout* and *gouty diathesis* were used as nonspecifically as *arthritis* is used today. Thomas Sydenham, who was himself beset by gout, began the process of identifying discrete diseases from the mix of rheumatism. Sydenham distinguished an acute febrile polyarthritis ". . . chiefly attacking the young and vigorous" from gout. Most of his description is compatible with acute rheumatic fever, but it also alludes to a chronic phase in which the patient may become ". . . a cripple to the day of his death and wholly lose the use of his limbs whilst the knuckles of his fingers shall become knotty and protuberant . . ."—possibly rheumatoid arthritis. In addition to his portrayals of gout (1683) and acute rheumatism (1685), Sydenham described St. Vitus' dance (Sydenham's chorea, 1686), and in his discussion of *Hysteric Diseases* (1684) may have described fibromyalgia.

Some authors at the beginning of the 19th century realized how little progress had been made in distinguishing specific diseases. For example, William Heberden (1802, London) wrote: "The rheumatism is a common name for many aches and pains, which have yet no peculiar appellation, though owing to very different causes. It is besides often hard to be distinguished from some, which have a certain name and class assigned them. . . ."

GOUT

Gutta in medieval medicine was a synonym for the Greek *podagra.* It meant a drop resulting from "a defluxion of the humors." *Podagra* was employed if the foot was affected, *gonagra* if the knee, *chiagra* if the wrist, and so forth. Little of significance was learned about gout between the 4th century BC and the end of the 18th century. Two concepts prevailed throughout these millennia: that the disease occurred predominantly in sexually mature men, as pointed out by Hippocrates, and that gustatory and sexual excesses predisposed to acute attacks. A huge folklore derived from these beliefs.

Antonj van Leeuwenhoek described the microscopic appearance of urate crystals from a tophus (1634, Delft). More than a century later, Carl W. Scheele, a Swedish pharmacist, demonstrated a hitherto unknown organic acid, originally called lithic acid, in urinary calculi (1776). In 1797 at Cambridge, William H. Wollaston reported that the principal constituent of tophi is "a neutral compound consisting of lithic acid and mineral alkali." The substance was renamed *acide ourique* by the French chemist, Antoine de Fourcroy, who also found it to be a constituent of normal urine (1798, Paris).

Half a century passed before uric acid was more convincingly related to gout. Alfred B. Garrod devised a quantitative gravimetric assay that could detect uric acid in hyperuricemic states such as gout and uremia (1847, London). Because of its difficulty, the procedure was not adopted. A qualitative test he devised in 1854, in which uric acid precipitated on a thread, gained some use, and Garrod's experiments led him to suggest: "Might it not, in doubtful cases, be possible to determine the nature of the affection from an examination of the blood?"

Garrod also demonstrated urate in subcutaneous tissue and articular cartilage in gout. He hypothesized that gout might result either from a loss of renal excretory capacity or from increased formation of uric acid, concepts proven correct a century after the 1859 publication of his monograph on gout. In 1876 Garrod postulated that acute gout results from the precipitation of sodium urate in a joint or adjacent tissue. This was demonstrated directly in 1962 following intra-articular injection of monosodium urate by Hollander and McCarty, and Seegmiller and collaborators (2).

Beginning in 1870, with the first methods devised by Ernest L. Salkowski, a German biochemist, numerous gravimetric assays of urinary uric acid were developed. However, the first technique that was sufficiently sensitive and practical to be applied to blood was colorimetric, one of several eventually devised by Otto Folin (1912, Boston). Folin's first method yielded results which were about one-half of the actual values, but by 1938 sensitivity had been improved to the extent that the sex-related difference in the mean serum uric acid content was established (Bernard M. Jacobson, Boston). Further analytical specificity and sensitivity were obtained with the enzymatic spectrophotometric technique developed by Praetorius and Poulsen (1949-1953, Copenhagen).

RHEUMATIC FEVER

Although Hippocrates mentioned an acute, migratory arthritis of young people, and Sydenham may have recognized the disease (1665, see above), nothing further was added until David Dundas (1808, London) published a description of heart failure in patients with "acute rheumatism." This also contained the first use of the term *rheumatic fever*. He concluded that "this [heart disease] is always the consequence of or connected with, rheumatic affection, [and] points out the necessity of attending to the translation of rheumatism to the chest. . . . "

Both Matthew Baillie and William C. Wells credited David Pitcairn, another London physician, for first having noted ". . . that persons subject to rheumatism were attacked more frequently than others with symptoms of an organic disease of the heart." (1788, unpublished). Baillie mentioned in his pathology text "an ossification or thickening of some heart valves" in patients who had acute rheumatism. Wells confirmed the clinical findings of Dundas and added the description of subcutaneous nodules. Although René T. Laennec (1819, Paris) had recognized cardiac murmurs, James Hope (1831, London) correctly explained their origin. Jean Baptiste Bouillaud (1840, Paris) concluded that "in the great majority of cases of acute articular rheumatism with fever, there exists in a variable degree a rheumatism of the serofibrinous tissue of the heart . . . ," an observation that became known as the *law of coincidence*. Angel Money (1883, London) noted the myocardial granuloma that was described in greater detail by Ludwig Aschoff (1904, Marburg). The *Aschoff nodule* came to be considered diagnostic of rheumatic carditis (3).

Chorea, derived from the Greek for dance, was introduced as a medical term by Paracelsus (1493-1541, Switzerland). In 1686 Sydenham, using the designation St. Vitus' dance, described the type of chorea that is now associated with his name. Richard Bright (1831, London) appears to have been the first to associate this behavior with rheumatic fever, a suggestion that George Sée (1850, Paris) substantiated with an epidemiologic study (4).

James K. Fowler (1880, London) reported that tonsillitis is a common precursor of rheumatic fever. Although Frederick J. Poynton and Alexander Pain (1900, London) isolated a streptococcus from the tonsils of a patient with rheumatic fever, this was only one of several bacteria implicated as pathogens. Homer F. Swift (1928, New York) advanced the hypothesis that rheumatic fever results from the development of hypersensitivity to streptococci, but he considered nonhemolytic strains to be the most likely pathogens. The epidemiologic studies of Alvin F. Coburn in New York and William R. Collis in London, both published in 1931, led to the definite identification of beta-hemolytic streptococcus as the causative organism. The first evidence to support the concept of an immune pathogenesis of rheumatic fever was the discovery of antistreptolysins by Edgar W. Todd (1932, London) (5).

RHEUMATOID ARTHRITIS

The appearance and distribution of lesions in ancient skeletons suggests that rheumatoid arthritis (RA) may have existed in North America 3000 years ago (6). However, the first clinical description of RA usually is credited to Augustin-Jacob Landré-Beauvais (1880, Paris) who described nine women who had a disease he considered to be a variant of gout and therefore called *goutte asthenique primitive*. He believed that a "primary weakness" predisposed the disease to develop and that it was associated with poverty, while true gout occurred generally in robust, affluent persons. While RA may once have been less common, it undoubtedly has existed for centuries, being misdiagnosed as some variety of "rheumatism."

Rheumatoid arthritis was more clearly described by Benjamin C. Brodie (1819, London). He stressed its typically slow progression and pointed out that not only joints, but bursae and tendon sheaths may be affected. His most important contribution was to recognize that the disease begins as a synovitis that may lead to destruction of articular cartilage. Rheumatoid nodules were described by Robert Adams (1857, Dublin) (3).

Jean-Martin Charcot (1867, Paris) made practical clinical distinctions among gout, rheumatic fever, RA, and osteoarthritis, but felt that "it is quite impossible to make an actual distinction between the various forms of rheumatism, but on the contrary, it is frequently possible to show that they all proceed from one and the same cause." He perpetuated Landré-Beauvais' sociologic error, but seems to have recognized that RA is not rare: "While gout is almost unknown in the Salpetriere, chronic rheumatism is, on the contrary, one of the commonest infirmities in this institution; and indeed, this disease prevails among women and among the least favored classes of society."

A.B. Garrod coined the term *rheumatoid arthritis* in 1858. He later explained ". . . that the majority of cases then called 'rheumatic gout' were related neither to true gout nor true rheumatism, and that they had an independent pathology . . . ; if such is the case, the term 'rheumatic gout' was doubly wrong . . . I propose the name of 'rheumatoid arthritis'—a name which does not imply any error, but assumes the disease to be an arthritic or joint disease having some external characters of rheumatism. . . . *Arthritis deformans* [Rudolf Virchow (1869, Berlin)] has been applied to the malady, and this again is not an erroneous name, though in the earlier stages of the disease it is by no means a characteristic one. The term *rheumatic arthritis* is nearly . . . as bad as that of *rheumatic gout*, as it implies the existence of one error instead of two. . . . " Nosologic conflicts continued even after the British Ministry of Health adopted rheumatoid arthritis as the official designation in 1922, a step the American College of Rheumatology (formerly the American Rheumatism Association) did not take until 1941.

The first roentgenogram of joints affected by RA was published by Gilbert A. Bannatyne (1896, Bath). Joel E. Goldthwait (1904, Boston) proposed the first American classification of arthritides and included the roentgenographic appearance among the criteria to differentiate atrophic (rheumatoid) arthritis from hypertrophic (osteo) arthritis. In 1909, Edward Nichols and Frank Richardson differentiated proliferative arthritis, which begins with synovitis and affects articular cartilage secondarily, from degenerative arthritis, in which the primary lesion is in articular cartilage. However, they did not correlate these pathologic observations with either RA or osteoarthritis (1,7).

The discovery of *rheumatoid factor* ultimately began with the hypothesis popularized by Frank Billings (1912, Chicago) that RA is a response to various chronic focal infections. Following research stimulated by this hypothesis, Russell L. Cecil et al (1927, New York) concluded that RA "is a streptococcal infection, caused in a large proportion of cases by a biologically specific strain of this organism." The nonspecificity of this finding was demonstrated by Martin H. Dawson (1932, New York), who was unable to confirm the bacteriologic findings, but showed that rheumatoid sera agglutinated suspensions of various bacteria.

While studying complement fixation, Erik Waaler (1940, Oslo) observed that sheep erythrocytes incubated with rabbit anti-sheep cell serum were agglutinated by some rheumatoid sera. In 1947 this observation was unknown in the laboratory of Harry M. Rose in New York, where serologic studies of Q fever were being conducted. A technician with RA used her own serum in a control test and found that it agglutinated sheep erythrocytes in high titer. This serendipitous observation led Rose and Charles A. Ragan to develop the sensitized sheep erythrocyte agglutination reaction as a diagnostic procedure. The most widely used variation, employing a suspension of polystyrene latex particle coated with human gamma globulin, was described by Jacques M. Singer and Charles M. Plotz (1956, New York) (8). Positive reactions have proven to be more useful in predicting a relatively poor prognosis than as a diagnostic tool.

Amyloidosis as a complication of definite RA was reported in 1933 by M.A. Hardgrove (Rochester, MN). First reports of other important associations are Felty's syndrome (leukopenia and splenomegaly) by Arthur R. Felty (1934, Baltimore), and Caplan's syndrome (rheumatoid pneumoconiosis) by Anthony Caplan (1953, Cardiff, Wales) (9).

JUVENILE CHRONIC POLYARTHRITIS

The report by George F. Still (1897, London) concerning "a form of chronic joint disease in children" was antedated by several brief descriptions, but his was the first detailed investigation. Still described 12 children with polyarthritis that he believed should be distinguished from RA and 6 other children whose disease was clinically indistinguishable from the disease in adults. Distinctive findings in the former group included lymphadenopathy and splenomegaly, the frequent occurrence of pericarditis, and an unusual predilection for involvement of the cervical spine. Still also pointed out the febrile component of the disease and the tendency toward growth retardation. The characteristic rash was not described until 1933 by Harold E. Boldero. Eric L. Bywaters (1971, London) first reported the occurrence of this form of polyarthritis in adulthood (10).

ANKYLOSING SPONDYLITIS

Several clinical and osteologic descriptions of ankylosing spondylitis were published prior to the 1890s. However, interest in this disease was stimulated by a series of articles by Vladimir von Bechterew (1893-1899, St. Petersburg, Russia). The first cases he described were a woman and two of her daughters, and he hypothesized that the principal etiologic factors were a hereditary predisposition and post-traumatic encephalopathy. Adolf Strümpell (1897, Erlangen) and Pierre Marie (1898, Paris) disagreed. They considered spondylitis to be a rheumatic disease, probably distinct from RA in which neither trauma nor heredity were of pathogenic importance. The male predominance of the disease was recognized in 1901 and proposed as a differentiating criterion from spondylitis deformans (degenerative spondylosis) by F. Glaser (Berlin).

A case of iritis with an arthropathy that probably was

ankylosing spondylitis was described in 1861 by James Jackson in Boston. The association was mentioned by Bechterew (1893), but iritis as a manifestation of ankylosing spondylitis was first suggested by E. Kunz and E. Kraupa, German ophthalmologists, in 1933. The initial study of heart disease in ankylosing spondylitis included six cases of aortic insufficiency, but this was attributed to rheumatic fever (l. Bernstein and O.J. Bloch, 1949, Oslo). The association between this arthropathy and aortic insufficiency was noticed serendipitously when the first 100 patients with aortic insufficiency into whom Charles A. Hufnagel (1956, Washington, DC) had inserted a prosthetic aortic valve were reviewed. Five were found to have ankylosing spondylitis, a frequency that was recognized to far exceed chance. Peter Kulka et al (1957, Boston) differentiated this form of aortic insufficiency pathologically from that of rheumatic fever. Despite numerous publications dealing with roentgenographic findings in ankylosing spondylitis, the characteristic obliteration of the sacroiliac joints was not reported until 1934 (Walter Krebs, Aachen).

Epidemiologic evidence of a heritable predisposition to the development of ankylosing spondylitis led Lee Schlosstein et al (Los Angeles) and Derek Brewerton et al (London) to study the HLA antigen distribution in patients with this disease. Each reported in 1973 that 88% and 96%, respectively, of their subjects carried the antigen now designated HLA–B27, which normally occurs in 4% to 8% of the white population. The discovery of such a strong association stimulated numerous studies of the relationship between histocompatibility antigens and the various rheumatic diseases. The decision of the American College of Rheumatology in 1963 to adopt the term ankylosing spondylitis in preference to rheumatoid spondylitis has been supported by the differences in HLA phenotypes in cases of RA and spondylitis (11).

OSTEOARTHRITIS

The term osteoarthritis (OA) was introduced by John K. Spender (1886, Bath) in preference to rheumatoid arthritis and not to designate the condition to which it is now applied (12). The modern usage and the clinical differentiation from RA were introduced by Archibald E. Garrod (1907, London). Aside from the older age at onset of OA, Garrod was impressed by an even stronger female preponderance than he found with RA, as well as a heritable tendency. However, he was unable to make consistent distinctions. William Heberden (1802, posthumous) identified Heberden's nodes, differentiating them from tophi. Garrod related these nodes to OA. Charles J. Bouchard (1884, Paris) described nodes adjacent to the proximal interphalangeal joints that are identical to those Heberden had described distally. Robert M. Stecher (1944, Cleveland) demonstrated the strong female preponderance of and genetic predisposition to the digital nodes, but questioned their relationship with other characteristics of OA. "Osteoarthritis" has been recognized to be an imprecise diagnosis as variants such as "generalized" osteoarthritis (Jonas H. Kellgren, 1952, Manchester, UK) and "inflammatory" or "erosive" osteoarthritis (Darrell C. Crain, 1961, Washington, DC) have been described.

LUPUS ERYTHEMATOSUS

Ferdinand von Hebra (1845, Vienna) described an eruption that occurs ". . . mainly on the face, on the cheeks and nose in a distribution not dissimilar to a butterfly." Lupus *erythemateux* was introduced by Pierre A. Cazenave (1851, Paris) to identify a skin disease that probably was discoid lupus erythematosus. Although Moritz Kaposi described cases with fever and pneumonia, he also used *lupus erythematosus* to designate the cutaneous findings and not to identify a multisystem disease (1872, Vienna). Several visceral manifestations subsequently recognized to belong to lupus erythematosus were described by William Osler (1895-1904, Baltimore) under the name *exudative erythema*. Photosensitivity was noted by Erwin Pulay (1921, Vienna). Emanuel Libman and Benjamin Sacks added nonrheumatic verrucous endocarditis to the syndrome (1923, New York). The characteristic "wire loop" glomerular lesion was pointed out in 1935 by George Baehr et al (New York) (13).

In 1948 Malcolm M. Hargraves (Rochester, MN) described the *LE cell* which he observed in marrow aspirates from several cases of acute systemic lupus erythematosus. Soon thereafter, John H. Haserick (Cleveland) found that the LE cell may be induced by a serum factor, and in 1950 Hargraves demonstrated LE cell formation in peripheral blood. Efforts to elucidate their cytogenesis led to the observation by Peter A. Miescher and M. Fauconnet (1956, Lausanne) that the LE cell-inducing factor can be absorbed from serum by exposure to isolated cell nuclei. Therefore, they suggested that this factor was an antinuclear antibody. A method to detect antinuclear antibodies by labeling with fluorescent anti-human globulin subsequently was described by George J. Friou et al (1958, West Haven, CT) (14).

The term *diffuse collagen disease* was introduced by Paul Klemperer (1942, New York). Based on pathologic studies of systemic lupus erythematosus and scleroderma, he concluded that the most prominent abnormalities occur in the collagenous fibers and ground substance of connective tissue. Klemperer built on the work of Fritz Klinge (1927-1934, Leipzig), who had concluded from his pathologic research that some of the manifestations of rheumatic fever and RA may reflect a disturbance in the connective tissues. The concept of *collagen diseases* gained rapid acceptance, even though the number of diseases it encompassed remained in dispute. Following the suggestion of William E. Ehrich (1952, Philadelphia), the term *connective tissue disease* gradually replaced *collagen disease* in usage (15).

SYSTEMIC SCLEROSIS

Hippocrates commented, "In those persons in whom the skin is stretched, parched and hard, the disease terminates without sweats," (aphorism V:71). However, the earliest definite descriptions of scleroderma were published by W.D. Chowne (1842, London), pertaining to a child, and in an adult by James Startin (1846, London). Several cases were described by French clinicians in 1847, and Elie Gintrac (Bordeaux) suggested the designation *sclerodermie*.

Maurice Raynaud (1862, Paris) described the vasospastic phenomenon that bears his name. He commented on its occurrence in a patient with scleroderma in 1863, and Jonathan Hutchinson (1899, London) pointed out that this is a consistent association. Heinrich Auspitz described death due to renal failure in scleroderma (1862, Vienna), but this was considered a chance association until 1952 (H.C. Moor and H.L. Sheehan, Liverpool). Albercht von Notthafft (1899, Munich) described parenchymatous and vascular pulmonary fibrosis, and Salomon Ehrmann (1903, Vienna) suggested that

dysphagia was due to the occurrence of the same process in the esophagus as in the skin. George Thibierge and Raymond J. Weissenbach (1910, Paris) associated the development of calcinosis with scleroderma. To this were added Raynaud's phenomenon, esophageal dysfunction, and telangiectasias in a case reported by Prosser Thomas (1942, London). The acronym CRST (later CREST) was coined for this syndrome by Richard H. Winterbauer (1964, Baltimore). Despite several descriptions of myocardial fibrosis, beginning with that by Carl F. Westphal (1876, Berlin), this form of cardiac involvement only became recognized as a manifestation of scleroderma following publication of the work of Soma Weiss et al (1943, Boston). Due to the extensive visceral involvement in this disease, R.H. Goetz (1945, Capetown) proposed *progressive systemic sclerosis* as more descriptive than scleroderma. Because the disease may stabilize, the modifier "progressive" has recently been discarded (16,17).

POLYMYOSITIS/DERMATOMYOSITIS

Introduction of the term *polymyositis* is credited to Ernst L. Wagner (1886, Leipzig), although a definite case had been described by Potain (1875, Paris). Heinrich Unverricht (1891, Estonia) coined the term *dermatomyositis* in describing a case. An association between dermatomyositis and cancer was first suggested by Rudolf Bezecny (1935, Prague). A patient who underwent resection of an ovarian carcinoma experienced regression of her skin lesions within a few days, despite peritoneal metastases, and the myopathy improved during subsequent roentgen therapy. The feasibility of evaluating disease activity biochemically was first demonstrated by R.G. Siekert and G.A. Fleisher (1956, Rochester, MN) who measured serum glutamic oxalacetic transaminase (18).

POLYARTERITIDES

From the earliest descriptions of polyarteritis to the present, both the etiologies and classifications that may be valid on clinical or pathologic groups have remained in dispute. The first characteristic lesion was described in a general pathologic study of arterial aneurysms by Karl Rokitansky (1852, Vienna) and re-examined microscopically by Hans Eppinger (1887, Graz). Adolf Kussmaul and Rudolf Maier (1866, Freiburg) published one case with a complete autopsy. They called the disease *periarteritis nodosa* because of the presence of aneurysmal dilatations in most of the medium- and smaller-sized arteries. Enrico Ferrari (1903, Trieste) preferred the term *polyarteritis nodosa* in describing a patient who had severe arteritis without aneurysms.

Giant cell arteritis was described by Jonathan Hutchinson in 1890 and rediscovered by Bayard T. Horton et al (1934, Rochester, MN) as arteritis of the temporal vessels. The association between this arteritis and *polymyalgia rheumatica* was suggested by J.W. Paulley (1956, Ipswich). The latter ailment had been described by William Bruce, a Scottish physician, in 1888 and rediscovered by L. Bagratuni (1953, Oxford). The term was introduced by Stuart Barber (1957, Manchester).

Other distinctive forms of arteritis include one that affects branches of the aortic arch (M. Takayasu, 1908, Tokyo); another primarily involving the respiratory tract and kidneys, first described by Heinz Klinger (1931, Berlin) and in greater detail by Friedrich Wegener (1936, 1939, Breslau), now called *Wegener's granulomatosis*; and *allergic granulomatosis*, a variant characterized by bronchospasm and eosinophilia, differentiated by Jacob Churg and Lotte Strauss (1951, New York) (19).

GONOCOCCAL ARTHRITIS AND REITER'S DISEASE

The early histories of gonococcal arthritis and of Reiter's disease must be considered together because, before the discovery of the gonococcus by Albert Neisser (1879, Breslau), it would have been impossible to differentiate the two diseases. An association between arthritis and urethritis (blennorrhagia) was first described by Francis X. Swediaur (1784, Paris). When Luigi Petrone (1883, Bologna) demonstrated gonococci in the urethral exudates and synovial fluid of two men, the disease was well known. The culture of gonococci from synovial fluid was first accomplished by Heinrich Höck (1893, Vienna) in an infant and in an adult by Neisser a year later. The unity of gonococcal urethritis and arthritis was proven by Ernst Finger (1894, Vienna). A culture made from synovial fluid obtained from a patient with gonococcal arthritis was inoculated into the urethra of a man who then developed typical gonorrhea.

A clue that some early descriptions of arthritis with urethritis did not represent gonococcal disease was the recurrence of arthritis and/or ocular inflammation with urethritis following totally asymptomatic intervals. The first such case report probably was that of Thomas Whateley (1801, London). Benjamin Brodie, beginning in 1818, described several men with recurrent episodes of urethritis, conjunctivitis, and arthritis. One had nine attacks in 20 years. Adolf Vossius (1904), a German ophthalmologist, reported the first case that began with bacillary dysentery. In 1916 Noel Fiessinger and Edgar Leroy published a report concerning dysentery among French troops, incidentally providing a brief description of a "conjunctivo-urethro-synovial syndrome," of which they had seen four cases. One week later Hans Reiter published his first report about the disease with which his name has become associated. His patient, a German officer on the Balkan front, developed urethritis, conjunctivitis, and a febrile polyarthritis after a bout of dysentery (20).

Emil Vidal (1893, Paris) described a man who had suffered two bouts of recurrent gonorrheal arthritis. The term *keratoderma blennorhagicum* was introduced by Anatole M. Chauffard and Georges Froin in describing such a case. Despite little evidence in support of gonococcal etiology, Wiedmann (1934, Vienna) was the first to suggest that *keratoderma blennorhagicum* was a manifestation of Reiter's disease.

RHEUMATOLOGY AS A MEDICAL SPECIALTY

Organization of the specialty of rheumatology in the United States began in 1928 when the American Committee for the Control of Rheumatism was founded (21). This was enlarged in 1934 into the American Association for the Study and Control of Rheumatic Diseases. It was renamed the American Rheumatism Association in 1937, and the American College of Rheumatology in 1988. The first certifying examination in rheumatology was administered in 1972.

THOMAS G. BENEDEK, MD

1. Parish LC: An historical approach to the nomenclature of rheumatoid arthritis. Arthritis Rheum 6:138-158, 1963
2. Rodnan GP: Early theories concerning etiology and pathogenesis of the gout. Arthritis Rheum 8:599-609, 1965
3. Benedek TG: Subcutaneous nodules and the differentiation of rheumatoid arthritis from rheumatic fever. Semin Arthritis Rheum 13:305-321, 1984
4. Schechter DC: St. Vitus dance and rheumatic disease. NY St J Med 75:1094-1102, 1975
5. Murphy GE: The evolution of our knowledge of rheumatic fever. Bull Hist Med 14:123-147, 1943
6. Rothschild BM, Woods RJ: Symmetrical erosive disease in Archaic Indians: the origin of rheumatoid arthritis in the New World? Semin Arthritis Rheum 19:278-284, 1990
7. Short CL: Rheumatoid arthritis: historical aspects. J Chron Dis 10:367-387, 1959
8. Fraser KJ: The Waller-Rose test: anatomy of the eponym. Semin Arthritis Rheum 18:61-71, 1988
9. Benedek TG: Rheumatoid pneumoconiosis. Am J Med 55:515-524, 1973
10. Baum J, Baum ER: George Frederic Still and his account of childhood arthritis—a reappraisal. Am J Dis Child 132:192-194, 1978
11. Spencer DG, Sturrock RD, Buchanan WW: Ankylosing spondylitis: yesterday and today. Med hist 24:60-69, 1980
12. Waldron HA: Prevalence and distribution of osteoarthritis in a population from Georgia and early Victorian London. Ann Rheum Dis 50:301-307, 1991
13. Smith CD, Cyr M: The history of lupus erythematosus from Hippocrates to Osler. Rheum Dis Clin North Am 14:1-14, 1988
14. Hargraves MM: Discovery of the LE cell and its morphology. Mayo Clin proc 44: 579-599, 1969
15. Bywaters EG: The historical evolution of the concept of connective tissue disease. Scand J Rheumatol 5 (suppl 12):11-29, 1976
16. Rodnan GP, Benedek TG: An historical account of the study of progressive systemic sclerosis (diffuse scleroderma). Ann Intern Med 57: 305-319, 1962
17. Benedek TG, Rodnan GP: The early history and nomenclature of scleroderma and of its differentiation from sclerema neonatorum and scleredema. Semin Arthritis Rheum 12:52-67, 1982
18. Pearson CM: Polymyositis. Ann Rev Med 17:63-82, 1966
19. Lie JT: Vasculitis, 1815 to 1991: classification and diagnostic specificity. J Rheumatol 19:83-89, 1992
20. Benedek TG: The first reports of Dr. Hans Reiter on Reiter's disease. J Alb Einstein Med Cent 17:100-105, 1969
21. Benedek TG: A century of American rheumatology. Ann Intern Med 106: 304-312, 1987

THE SOCIAL AND ECONOMIC CONSEQUENCES OF RHEUMATIC DISEASE

2

Most common rheumatic diseases are characterized by chronic pain and progressive physical impairment of joints and soft tissues. They are costly to individuals, families, and society in both economic and social terms. Clinicians and other care providers must understand national economic costs, individual and family expenses, and social consequences of the rheumatic diseases so they may be able to respond to these challenges.

THE NATIONAL ECONOMIC IMPACT

Economic costs of illness are usually divided into two broad components. *Direct costs* are dollars spent to treat the illness. *Indirect costs* are those due to lost productivity as a result of morbidity or mortality. Indirect costs include wages lost when people must leave the work force or reduce hours, implied wages of homemakers who can no longer function in that role, and loss of nonwork activities (expressed as value placed on those activities). In general, lost wages are the most accurately estimated and commonly measured indirect costs.

In comprehensive studies of the national cost of illness, Rice and colleagues conservatively estimated that in 1980 the economic impact of musculoskeletal diseases (excluding gout, osteoporosis, and fractures) was $21 billion, close to 1% of the gross national product (GNP) (1). In 1988, the estimated total cost had risen to 2.5% of the GNP (2). Approximately half of the total costs were direct and the other half were indirect costs, mainly lost wages. Much of the explosive growth in costs is the result of aging of the population and longer duration of disease, both of which are due to decreased mortality rates. As baby boomers continue to age over the next two or three decades, these costs will undoubtedly surge.

The total costs in 1992 dollars of all musculoskeletal conditions and the contribution of all forms of arthritis are shown in Table 2-1. Although direct medical costs of arthritis—more than $15 billion—are substantial, indirect costs due to work

(Table 2-1)
Total, direct, and indirect costs of all musculoskeletal conditions and all forms of arthritis in billions of 1992 dollars*

Condition	Direct Costs	Indirect Costs	Total Costs
All musculo-skeletal conditions	72.3 (48.4%)	77.1 (51.6%)	149.4
All forms of arthritis	15.2 (23.5%)	49.6 (76.5%)	64.8

* Adapted from Yelin and Callahan (5), with permission.

loss are far greater—almost $50 billion. They would be even greater if nonwork losses could be more easily calculated for elderly people and homemaking women, populations disproportionately represented in arthritic diseases.

The overall costs of osteoporosis are also very high and are projected to rise rapidly in the future (3). The burden of osteoporosis comes largely from fractures of the hip and spine. Most of the costs are due to hospitalization for hip fractures and placement in long-term health facilities. In 1988 the total cost of osteoporosis in the United States was $10 billion (4).

Persons with arthritis have high rates of medical care utilization. For example, patients with rheumatoid arthritis (RA) and no comorbidity made 7.8 visits to physicians each year (during the study years 1984 to 1986), more than double the 3.8 visits made per year by all persons in the United States (5). The hospitalization rate for RA patients was double that of the general population. Increased rates of physician visits and hospitalization were also seen in osteoarthritis (OA).

Musculoskeletal diseases accounted for about 10% of the 37 million operations performed in the United States in 1985 (6). In that year, about 300,000 total hip and knee surgeries were performed, and the number may have doubled over the past decade. Most of these operations were for arthritis. The total cost of joint replacement surgeries, including hospital and physician charges, was estimated at about $4 billion and may account for almost one-fifth of all costs for treating musculoskeletal disorders.

WORK DISABILITY

Work disability is the prime contributor to indirect costs of arthritis. It has been shown that work disability develops quickly in persons with RA. Permanent articular damage occurs within 2 years of disease onset in 50% of patients. This is followed by significant functional decline and is reflected in work disability: fewer than 50% of RA patients younger than age 65 years who are working at disease onset are still working 10 years later (7).

A number of studies have demonstrated that clinicians are able to predict functional status and work disability in persons with RA with reasonable accuracy. There is debate whether functional and social indicators or clinical measures are better predictors.

Functional status at baseline, which can be measured by physical tests and questionnaires, correlates with status 9 years later, despite interim fluctuations (8). Other studies have found that social characteristics of the patient, work attitudes, qualities of the work structure, and control over pace and activity of work are more important in predicting whether patients with RA stay employed than traditional measures of disease activity, such as radiographic changes or erythrocyte sedimentation rate.

On the other hand, it was recently shown that the risk of disability over 5 years in a group of patients with a mean time from diagnosis of 8.7 years was predicted more by clinical status at study entry (such as number of deformed or acutely inflamed joints) than by work structure (such as complexity of work tasks) (9).

It seems appropriate that beginning early in the disease course clinicians should pay close attention to clinical, psychologic, and functional parameters, such as workplace characteristics and overall functional status (perhaps with the regular use of functional assessment questionnaires), as well as disease severity. By attending to these areas clinicians may more effectively provide counsel and summon appropriate resources to help keep the patient functional and employed.

ECONOMIC COSTS TO INDIVIDUALS AND FAMILIES

Behind the staggering national costs of rheumatic diseases are the painful costs to individuals. Costs have been estimated for several specific diseases.

In one study, RA patients had a 50% drop in earnings over 9 years, which accounted for a decrease from 69% to 32% of the family income (10). In a national survey, men with symmetric polyarthritis (a surrogate for RA) had half the earnings of men with no arthritis, and women had only one-fourth the earnings of women with no arthritis (11).

In a population-based study of persons with OA, average per capita costs were substantial (12). Direct charges for OA and nonarthritis cohorts were $2043 and $1591, respectively; much of the excess cost was due to comorbid conditions. Indirect expenditures and work disability were higher in the OA group as well: 10% of OA patients reduced work hours and 13.7% retired early, only 1.7% of nonarthritis cohorts worked less and 3.4% retired early.

In a Canadian study, the average annual cost to a person with systemic lupus erythematosus (SLE) was $13,094 (Canadian dollars) (13). Direct medical costs accounted for almost one-half of the total and lost wages for the other half.

Juvenile rheumatoid arthritis (JRA) can be costly and stressful to families. Annual average total direct costs for a child with JRA were $7900 in a 1992 study (14) (Table 2-2).

(Table 2-2)
Direct and family costs for juvenile rehumatoid arthritis

Cost Type	Annualized Mean Cost ($)
Direct costs	
Inpatient medical	1717
Outpatient medical	5700
Nonmedical (eg, transportation, meals)	488
Total	7905
Family costs	
Out-of-pocket medical	708
Salary loss	328
Nonmedical expenses	488
Total	1524

* Adapted from Allaire et al (14), with permission.

Indirect costs incurred by families and paid out-of-pocket averaged $1500, or 5% of family income. Evidence suggests that effects of JRA have long-term economic consequences into adult life for some individuals as well, with lower rates of employment and higher rates of disability.

ACTIVITY LIMITATIONS CAUSED BY ARTHRITIS

Although arthritis seriously impairs work ability and decreases individual and household incomes, the major personal impact involves other facets of life. It is much more difficult, if not impossible, to assign monetary values to these limitations.

Several surveys have looked at nonmonetary impacts of musculoskeletal conditions. In overall terms, these are called *limitations in activities*. Using data from the 1984 National Health Interview Study, it was estimated that 2.8% of the 37.9 million people (15% of the U.S. population) with self-reported arthritis limit their activities because of arthritis (15). Arthritis is the predominant reason for limited activities in the elderly. Fibrositis and SLE have also been shown to result in higher rates of disability.

Two types of disability can result from arthritis. *Physical disability* refers to basic musculoskeletal functions such as bending, lifting, walking, and grasping. *Social disability* refers to higher level social tasks like eating, dressing, going shopping, and interacting with other people. Arthritis first causes physical dysfunctions, which lead to social dysfunctions.

IMPACT ON DAILY LIFE

Research has attempted to measure certain aspects of social disability. Social disability includes 1) basic personal care tasks, called *activities of daily living (ADL)*, such as grooming, toileting, and eating; 2) household tasks, called *instrumental activities of daily living (IADL)*, such as shopping, paying bills, and doing housework; and 3) *discretionary activities of daily living*, such as hobbies and civic activities.

Numerous studies on the impact of RA on daily life have consistently shown high levels of impaired physical and social functioning; these impairments begin early, within 2 years of disease onset (11,16). People with RA go out less frequently to shop or to the supermarket, have more difficulty getting in and out of cars, and spend less time with hobbies like sewing and gardening than people without arthritis. Women with RA have more problems with many aspects of homemaking, including making beds and preparing meals. Many people require adaptations in the home (such as shower, toilet, faucet, and kitchen alterations) and car (such as power steering).

It is clear that arthritis, especially RA, is associated with an increased incidence of psychologic distress. Psychologic stressors, especially depression, are associated with limitations of life activities, particularly social activities. The inability to perform valued activities and lack of independence may be the prime causes of depression and frustration in many people. The psychologic construct *helplessness* (the belief that one is unable to exert some control over his or her symptoms) appears to be as important as disease severity in how patients assess their own health status.

Clinicians often overlook the impact of arthritis on family members, but these effects can be serious and may merit intervention. The main caregiver's life can be significantly altered, requiring a need to change employment status or to hire help. The impact on the family may not correlate with severity of disability of the patient. Rather, the impact depends more on how well the patient adjusts to and copes with the disease and the willingness of family members to be supportive.

Arthritis can strain marriages. Although it is not clear that divorce is more common in RA families, rates of remarriage after divorce are probably lower. Sexual problems are common because of pain, fatigue, depression, reduced joint mobility, reduced sex drive, and fewer opportunities for sex. Clinicians may not fully appreciate these problems if they are reticent about discussing the subject or unaware of the problem. Many patients report difficulty in communicating about sexual problems with their doctor and may also be reluctant to discuss these problems with a sex counselor.

The effect on the children of patients with RA is uncertain. In some cases, children may feel anger and guilt and some express resentment that their parent is ill. On the other hand, most children are cognizant of their parent's pain and limitations. Many report a nurturing attitude toward the parent, and in some cases family ties are bound closer.

Children with arthritis may experience a unique set of social consequences. Studies vary with respect to the frequency and degree of maladjustment that children experience due to arthritis. Some children have substantial behavioral and psychologic problems, including loss of self-esteem, dependency, depression, and concern with body image (17). Both disease severity and other social or familial issues may play a role in these problems. For example, maternal self-esteem, depression in parents, chronic family difficulties and stress, and lower educational attainment may contribute negatively to a child's adjustment. Social competence may suffer for several reasons, including diminished participation in sports and other physical activities and well-meaning over-protection by parents, who underestimate their child's abilities and may restrict their activities.

The social consequences of osteoporotic fractures are borne largely by the elderly. Loss of independence is the major and most dreaded consequence of fractures. Disability rates after hip fractures can be very high; in a recent study, only 38% of elderly highly functioning people who sustained a hip fracture were able to transfer between chair and bed independently, and only 17% could walk alone 6 months after a hip fracture (18). Hip fracture survivors are more likely to have trouble grocery shopping, housekeeping, climbing stairs, and walking. Women with vertebral osteoporotic fractures also have high rates of functional limitation with carrying, lifting, walking, doing housework, and shopping. Loss of social and leisure activities such as travel or dancing are also common.

THE CLINICIAN'S ROLE

The ultimate goals of the physicians, nurses, and other health professionals involved in treating persons with rheumatic diseases are to relieve pain and physical symptoms, assuage psychologic distress, improve physical functioning, and generally aid in the well-being of the patient. Equally important, however, are interventions to prevent and ameliorate socioeconomic problems. Indeed, a majority of the costs, both economic and social, are due to lost function rather than direct medical costs. Until a cure for the many types of arthritis is found or far more effective thera-

pies to prevent joint damage and physical disability are developed, patients will continue to suffer severe, premature economic and social dislocations that will seriously affect their lives. Indeed, as the population ages, society can expect that these impacts will mushroom.

How can physicians and other providers help ameliorate some of these problems faced by patients with arthritis? They must become much more knowledgeable about and familiar with these socioeconomic issues. They must accept that intervening in these areas is extremely important. They should inquire about problems prospectively and frequently, especially because many patients are reluctant to mention these issues. They should be assertive in educating patients, family, and employers about arthritis, its course, and its consequences. Finally, they need to educate payors, health policy officials, and society about the seriousness and impact of musculoskeletal disorders.

Physicians should not rely solely on their own skills and services. There is substantial evidence that nonphysician health professionals are underutilized (10). Social workers can explore personal and family financial concerns and provide assistance. Human resource personnel, occupational therapists, rehabilitation specialists, and physical therapists might assist in modifying work requirements and settings. Mental health professionals should be used in some settings for psychologic problems and marital difficulties. Sex counselors can be helpful.

Providers can and should avail themselves of functional assessment instruments that have been validated and found practical for use in clinical environments (19,20). For example, the Health Assessment Questionnaire and the Arthritis Impact Measurement Scales are helpful in assessing physical functioning, pain, and psychosocial dimensions in adults with RA; instruments for assessing status in JRA, SLE, and fibromyalgia have also been developed. Longitudinal follow-up and a graphic display of numerical scores for individuals can greatly assist the physician in prioritizing and recommending interventions.

In counseling adults with RA and children with JRA about work opportunities, providers should stress autonomy and ability to control or influence work structure, such as flexibility in hours and physical demands. Since patients rate their loss of independence more highly than pain as a stressor in rheumatic diseases, concentration on measures to improve self-efficacy, coping skills, and independence may be more valuable than medications. Physicians might be more aggressive in encouraging patients to use aids and devices such as canes, electric wheelchairs, home modifications, and driving accommodations.

Good clinicians can have a significant impact on the social and economic consequences of rheumatic diseases, if they know as much as possible about these issues and if they apply what they learn to their daily practice.

ERIC S. SCHNED, MD
JAMES L. REINERTSEN, MD

1. Rice D, Hodgson T, Kopstein A: The economic costs of illness: a replication and update. Health Care Financing Review 7:61-80,1985
2. Rice D: Cost of musculoskeletal conditions. In Praemer A, Furner S, Rice D (eds): Musculoskeletal Conditions in the United States. Chicago, American Academy of Orthopedic Surgeons,1992
3. Barrett-Connor E: The economic and human costs of osteoporotic fracture. Am J Med 98(Suppl 2A):2A-35-2A-75,1995
4. Peck WA, Riggs BL, Bell NH: Research directions in osteoporosis. Am J Med 84:275-282,1988

5. Yelin E, Callahan LF: The economic cost and social and psychological impact of musculoskeletal conditions. Arthritis Rheum 38:1351-1362,1995

6. Felts W, Yelin E: The economic impact of the rheumatic diseases in the United States. J Rheumatol 16:867-884,1989

7. Pincus T, Callahan LF: What is the natural history of rheumatoid arthritis? Rheum Dis Clin North Am 119:123-151, 1993

8. Pincus T, Callahan LF: Rheumatology function tests: grip strength, walking time, button test, and questionnaires document and predict long-term morbidity and mortality in rheumatoid arthritis. J Rheumatol 19:1051-1057,1992

9. Reisine S, McQuillan J, Fifield J: Predictors of work disability in rheumatoid arthritis patients. Arthritis Rheum 38:1630-1637,1995

10. Meenan RF, Yelin EH, Nevitt M, Epstein WV: The impact of chronic disease. Arthritis Rheum 24:544-549,1981

11. Mitchell JM, Burkhauser RV, Pincus T: The importance of age, education, and comorbidity in the substantial earnings losses of individuals with symmetric polyarthritis. Arthritis Rheum 31:348-357,1988

12. Gabriel SE, Crowson CS, O'Fallon WM: Cost of osteoarthritis: estimates from a geographically defined population. J Rheumatol 22 (Suppl 43):23-25,1995

13. Clarke AE, Esdaile JM, Bloch DA, LaCaille D, Danoff DS, Fries JF: A Canadian study of the total medical costs for patients with systemic lupus erythematosus and the predictors of costs. Arthritis Rheum 36:1548-1559,1993

14. Allaire SH, DeNardo BS, Szer JS, Meenan RF, Schaller JG: The economic impacts of juvenile rheumatoid arthritis. J Rheumatol 19:952-955,1992

15. Centers for Disease Control and Prevention: Arthritis prevalence and activity limitations, United States, 1990. MMWR 43:433-438,1991

16. Eberhardt K, Larrson B-M, Nived K: Early RA - some social, economical, and psychological aspects. Scand J Rheumatol 22:119-123,1993

17. Daltroy LH, Larson MG, Eaton HM, et al: Psychosocial adjustment in juvenile arthritis. J Pediatr Psychol 17:277-289,1992

18. Cooney LM, Marottoli RA: Functional decline following hip fracture. In Christianson C, Riis BJ (eds): Fourth International Symposium on Osteoporosis and Consensus Development Conference, Hong Kong, 1993

19. Wolfe F, Pincus T: Standard self-report questionnaires in routine clinical and research practice: an opportunity for patients and rheumatologists. J Rheumatol 18:643-646,1991

20. Felson DT, Anderson JJ, Boers M: The American College of Rheumatology core set of disease activity measures to be used in rheumatoid arthritis clinical trials. Arthritis Rheum 36:729-740,1993

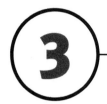

THE MUSCULOSKELETAL SYSTEM
A. JOINTS

Human bones join with each other in a variety of ways to serve the functional requirements of the musculoskeletal system. Foremost among these needs is that of purposeful motion. From the digital dexterity of the accomplished musician to the raw power of the world-class weight lifter, the activities of the human body depend on effective interaction between normal joints and the neuromuscular units that drive them. These same elements also interact reflexively to distribute mechanical stresses among the tissues of the joint. Muscles, tendons, ligaments, cartilage, and bone all do their share to ensure smooth functioning of the human machine. In this role, the supporting elements both unite the abutting bones and position cartilage in optimal relationships for low-friction load-bearing.

CLASSIFICATION

Differing designs of human joints have usually been classified according to a scheme based on histologic features and usual range of motion. *Synarthrosis* describes the suture lines of the skull where adjoining cranial plates are separated only by thin fibrous tissues that interlock to prevent detectable motion but still allow orderly growth. When cranial growth ceases, synarthrodial joints have no further role, and they regularly close.

In *amphiarthroses*, adjacent bones are bound by flexible fibrocartilage that permits modest motion. In the pubic symphysis and in a portion of the sacroiliac joint, amphiarthroses permit minor rotational motion of the pelvic bones. Between the vertebral bodies, the intervertebral disc has developed into a more mobile, highly specialized amphiarthrodial articulation.

Diarthroses are the most mobile joints and are by far the most common articular pattern. Because these joints possess a synovial membrane and contain synovial fluid, diarthrodial joints are more commonly referred to as synovial joints. These joints provide the focus for the remainder of this section.

Synovial joints are further subclassified according to shape: ball and socket (hip), hinge (interphalangeal), saddle (first carpometacarpal), and plane (patellofemoral) joints. These widely varying configurations reflect the fact that form parallels function in the design of diarthrodial joints. In every case, a well-lubricated bearing develops from essentially congruent cartilaginous surfaces that slide freely against each other. The direction and the extent of the permitted motion are defined by the shape and the size of the opposing surfaces (Fig. 3A-1). Within these limitations, a wide variety of designs permit motion in flexion (bending), extension (straightening), abduction (moving away from the midline), adduction (moving toward the midline), and rotation. Individual joints can thus act in one (humero-ulnar joint), two (wrist), or even three (shoulder) axes of motion.

ARTICULAR TISSUES

Synovial joints are surrounded by a capsule that defines the boundary between articular and periarticular tissues. The capsule varies in thickness; in some areas the capsule is an inapparent membrane, and in others it is a strong ligamentous band. For example, a reinforced capsular plate serves as an effective check to prevent hyperextension of most hinge joints. Over the extensor aspects of the same joints, the capsule is a much less consequential structure. Reinforcing the capsule are additional ligaments that are sometimes extracapsular. Further periarticular support is provided by the tendons of muscles acting across the joint. Capsule, ligaments, and tendons all are formed primarily from bundles of type I collagen fibers aligned with the axis of tensile stress (1).

The synovial intima comprises the lining tissue, one to three cells deep, that covers all intracapsular structures other than the contact areas of cartilage (2). This highly flexible, well-lubricated lining is normally collapsed upon itself and upon articular cartilage to minimize the volume of the joint space it encloses. When opened, most normal human joints reveal moist, tacky synovial and cartilaginous surfaces, but contain no obvious pool of synovial fluid.

The synovial lining cells reside in a matrix rich in collagen fibrils and proteoglycans. In most areas, the cells do not abut

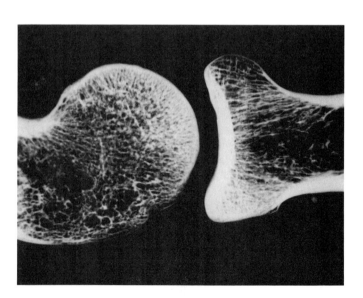

(Figure 3A-1)
Radiograph of a 3-mm sagittal slab through an extended elbow joint. The convex distal humerus has a thin subchondral plate and honeycombed underlying trabeculation, whereas the concave, proximal radius has a thick subchondral plate over coarse, vertical trabecular bone. Comparable convex-concave differences are regularly seen in other large joints. Reprinted from Simkin et al (7) with permission.

directly but are separated by interstitium. The principal cells of the normal synovium come in two forms: type A and type B (Fig. 3A-2). The monocyte-derived type A cell resembles a macrophage in its high content of cytoplasmic organelles, which include lysosomes, smooth-walled vacuoles, and micropinocytotic vesicles. In contrast, the fibroblast-derived type B cell has fewer organelles and a more extensive endoplasmic reticulum. A number of other cells are sometimes seen in normal synovial tissue, including apparent antigen-processing cells with a dendritic configuration, mast cells, and occasional white blood cells.

The synovial lining is supported by a rich bed of fenestrated microvessels (Fig. 3A-3), which, for the most part, lie among the lining cells, close to the surface of the joint space (3). These vessels are terminal branches of an arterial plexus that also supports the capsule and the juxta-articular bone. In addition, synovial tissue includes a generous complement of lymphatic vessels and nerve fibers. The innervation derives from the nerve roots supplying each of the muscles that cross the joint.

The synovial intima overlies a spectrum of matrices ranging from fibrous capsule, to loose areolar connective tissue, to organized structures composed mainly of fat. The latter structures take the form of fat pads, which serve as flexible, space-occupying structures to accommodate changes in geometry during articular motion. In other locations, solid fibrocartilaginous structures play a somewhat similar role. The best examples of these structures are found in the knees, where the medial and lateral menisci help to preserve alignment and distribute loads (4).

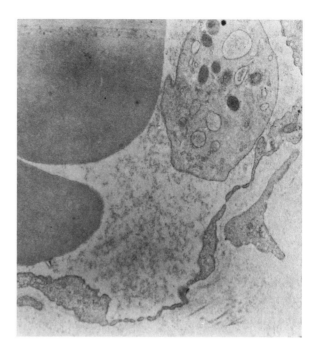

(Figure 3A-3)
Higher magnification electron micrograph of a synovial vessel shows red cells and a platelet in the lumen. The endothelium has fenestrations closed by diaphragms. Courtesy of Dr. HR Schumacher.

STRESS DISTRIBUTION

In active motion, substantial loading forces cross each normal joint. If these forces exceed the inherent limits of a tissue, the structure will fracture or fail. Normal joints distribute these forces, thus minimizing the likelihood of failure in one component. The greatest share of loading energy is taken up within the muscles and tendons crossing each joint. Effective reflexes normally ensure that impact forces are delivered to flexed joints, which bend further under an acute load in a response of the extensor muscles known as *eccentric contraction*. Most people are familiar with the surprise of finding one more step than expected when descending a flight of stairs. The sudden jolt of that moment results from landing on a hip and knee that have not flexed in anticipation of the impact. Appropriate flexion of these joints distributes the stress in time by prolonging the deceleration of landing and in space by loading a larger surface area of each convex joint member as it slides within the embrace of its concave mate.

Loading stress that is not absorbed by surrounding muscles, tendons, and ligaments has a direct impact on the opposing articular cartilages and their underlying trabecular bone. The firm, resilient articular cartilage has viscoelastic properties that allow it to serve as a hydraulic shock absorber analogous to those found in an automobile (5). Despite these desirable characteristics, this tissue is so thin that most loading energy is transmitted through the cartilage into bone (6).

Immediately beneath the cartilage is a continuous plate of subchondral bone supported by a complex meshwork of underlying trabeculae. In convex members—for example, the femoral and humeral heads—this plate is a thin shell supported by a honeycombed structure of interconnecting bony chambers. In contrast, the opposing concave acetabulum and the glenoid fossa have much thicker subchondral plates supported by a coarser and more open framework of

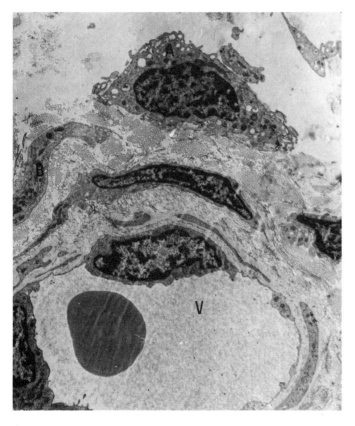

(Figure 3A-2)
Electron micrograph of synovial intima showing both type A and type B lining cells within a well-organized synovial matrix. V indicates a superficial synovial vessel. Courtesy of Dr. HR Schumacher.

trabecular struts (7). This structural difference in bone is matched by a corresponding difference in the thickness of overlying cartilage. In cartilage, however, the thicker layer is on the convex side, whereas the thinner layer is on the concave side and tends to have more of a fibrous than a hyaline composition. These differences in structure provide for stiff concave joint members in opposition to more flexible convex mates. The clinical significance of these structural and functional differences can be seen in patterns of injury where overwhelming stresses regularly explode the stiff, concave side but do not crush its more flexible convex opponent. Similarly, raised subchondral pressures in loaded convex bones may play a role in their special vulnerability to osteonecrosis (8).

STABILITY

A number of factors interact to confer joint stability, while simultaneously permitting motion. First among these is the simple shape of the component parts. In the hip, for example, the articular members are configured and positioned so that normal loading enhances the closeness of fit, and weight bearing drives the femoral head into its acetabular socket.

Ligaments provide a second major stabilizing influence, as they guide and align normal joints through their range of motion. An excellent example is the pair of collateral ligaments along each side of interphalangeal joints. These strong, relatively inelastic structures restrict articular motion to flexion and extension. In addition, the broad, ligamentous posterior capsule serves as a check that prevents hyperextension.

Within the axes of motion, however, more flexible constraints are required. This need is met by muscles and tendons. Muscular stabilization is perhaps most obvious in the shoulder, which is the quintessential polyaxial joint. The rotator cuff muscles approximate and stabilize the articular surfaces of the shoulder, and larger muscles with better leverage provide the power for effective shoulder motion (9).

Synovial fluid contributes significant stabilizing effects as an adhesive seal that freely permits sliding motion between cartilaginous surfaces, but effectively resists distracting forces. This property is most easily demonstrated in small articulations such as the metacarpophalangeal joints. There, the common phenomenon of "knuckle cracking" reflects the fracture of this adhesive bond. Secondary cavitation within the joint space causes a radiologically obvious bubble of gas that requires up to 30 minutes to dissolve before the bond can be reestablished and the joint can be "cracked" again (10). This adhesive property depends on the normally thin film of synovial fluid between all intra-articular structures. When this film enlarges as a pathologic effusion, the stabilizing properties are lost.

The intra-articular pressure is about –4 mmHg in a normal resting knee. This pressure falls when the quadriceps muscle contracts. The difference between atmospheric pressure on overlying tissues and subatmospheric pressures within the joint helps to hold the joint members together, thus providing a stabilizing force. In a pathologic effusion, however, the resting pressure is higher than the atmospheric pressure, and it rises when surrounding muscles contract. Thus, reversal of the normal pressure gradient is an additional destabilizing factor in joints with effusions (11).

LUBRICATION

Synovial joints act as mechanical bearings that facilitate the work of the musculoskeletal machine. As such, normal joints are remarkably effective with coefficients of friction lower than those obtainable with industrial journal bearings. Furthermore, the constant process of renewal and restoration ensures that living articular tissues have a durability far superior to that of any artificial bearing. It is thus axiomatic that no arthroplastic implant can equal the performance of a normal human joint.

The mechanics of normal joint lubrication have provided a productive focus of investigation beginning with the unique structure of the bearing surface. Articular cartilage is elastic, fluid-filled, and backed by a relatively impervious layer of calcified cartilage and bone. Consequently, load-induced compression of cartilage can be expected to force interstitial fluid to flow laterally within the tissue and surface through adjacent cartilage. As that area, in turn, becomes load-bearing, it is partially protected by the newly expressed fluid above it. This is a special form of *hydrodynamic lubrication,* so-called because the dynamic motion of the load-bearing areas produces an aqueous layer that separates and thus protects the contact points (5).

Boundary layer lubrication is the second major mechanism considered important in the low-friction characteristics of normal joints. Here, the critical factor is a small glycoprotein called *lubricin.* The lubricating properties of this synovium-derived molecule are highly specific and depend on its ability to bind to articular cartilage, where it is thought to retain a protective layer of water molecules. Lubricin is not effective in artificial systems and thus does not lubricate artificial joints (12).

Other possible lubricating mechanisms remain under investigation. However, it is interesting that hyaluronic acid, the molecule that makes synovial fluid viscous (*synovia* is Latin meaning "like egg white") has largely been excluded as a lubricant of the cartilage-on-cartilage bearing. Instead, hyaluronic acid lubricates a quite different site of surface contact—that of synovium on cartilage. The well-vascularized, well-innervated synovium must alternately contract and then expand to cover nonloaded cartilage surfaces as each joint moves through its normal range of motion. This process must proceed freely. Were synovial tissue to be pinched, there would be immediate pain, intra-articular bleeding, and inevitable functional compromise. The rarity of these problems testifies to the effectiveness of hyaluronate-mediated synovial lubrication.

SYNOVIAL FLUID

In normal human joints, a thin film of synovial fluid covers the surfaces of synovium and cartilage within the joint space. Only in disease does the volume of this fluid increase to produce a clinically apparent effusion that may be aspirated easily for study. For this reason, most knowledge of human synovial fluid comes not from normal subjects but from patients with joint disease. Because of the clinical frequency, volume, and accessibility of knee effusions, our knowledge is further limited to findings in that joint.

In the synovium, as in all tissues, essential nutrients are delivered and metabolic by-products are cleared by perfusion of the local vasculature. Synovial microvessels contain fenestrations that facilitate diffusion-based exchange between plasma and the surrounding interstitium. Free diffusion provides full equilibration of small solutes between plasma and the immediate interstitial space. Further diffusion extends this equilibration process to include all other intracapsular spaces, including the synovial fluid and the interstitial fluid of cartilage. Synovial plasma flow and the narrow diffusion path between synovial lining cells provide the principal limitations on exchange rates between plasma and synovial fluid (13).

This process is clinically relevant to the transport of therapeutic agents in inflamed synovial joints. Many investigators have made serial observations of drug concentrations in plasma and synovial fluid after oral and intravenous administration. Predictably, plasma levels exceed those in synovial fluid during the early phases of absorption and distribution. This gradient reverses during the subsequent period of elimination when intrasynovial levels exceed those of plasma. These patterns reflect passive diffusion alone, the delays in equilibration primarily reflect effusion volume, and no therapeutic agent is known to be transported into or selectively retained within the joint space (14).

Metabolic evidence of ischemia provides a second instance in which the delivery and removal of small solutes becomes clinically relevant. In normal joints and in most pathologic effusions, essentially full equilibration exists between plasma and synovial fluid. The gradients that drive net delivery of nutrients (glucose and oxygen) or removal of wastes (lactate and carbon dioxide) are too small to be detected. In some cases, however, the synovial microvascular supply is unable to meet local metabolic demand, and significant gradients develop. In these joints, the synovial fluid reveals a low oxygen pressure (PO_2), low glucose, low pH, high lactate, and high carbon dioxide pressure (PCO_2). These fluids are found regularly in septic arthritis, often in rheumatoid arthritis, and occasionally in other kinds of synovitis. These findings presumably reflect both the increased metabolic demand of hyperplastic tissue and an impaired microvascular response. Consistent with this interpretation is the finding that ischemic rheumatoid joints are colder than are joints containing synovial fluid in full equilibration with plasma (15). Like other peripheral tissues, joints normally have temperatures lower than that of the body's core. The knee, for example, has a normal intra-articular temperature of 32°C. With acute local inflammation, articular blood flow increases and the temperature approaches 37°C. As rheumatoid synovitis persists, however, microcirculatory compromise may cause the temperature to fall as the tissues become ischemic.

The clinical implications of local ischemia remain under investigation. For example, decreased synovial fluid pH was found to correlate strongly with radiographic evidence of joint damage in rheumatoid knees (16). Other work has shown that transient increases in intrasynovial pressure may exert a tamponade effect on the synovial vasculature. This finding has led to the suggestion that normal use of swollen joints may create a cycle of ischemia and reperfusion that leads to release of toxic oxygen radicals, which damage tissues (17).

Because normal articular cartilage has no microvascular supply of its own, it is at risk in ischemic joints. In articular cartilage, the normal process of diffusion is supplemented

by the convection induced by cyclic compression and release during joint use. In immature joints, the same pumping process promotes exchange of small molecules with the interstitial fluid of underlying trabecular bone. In adults, however, this potential route of supply is considered unlikely, and all exchange of solutes may occur through synovial fluid. As a result, normal chondrocytes may be farther from their supporting microvasculature than any other cells in the body. The vulnerability of this extended supply line is clearly shown in synovial ischemia.

Normal plasma proteins also enter synovial fluid passively. In contrast to small molecules, however, protein concentrations remain substantially lower in synovial fluid than in plasma. In aspirates from normal knees, the total protein is only 1.3 gm/dl, a value roughly 20% of that in normal plasma (18). Moreover, the distribution of intrasynovial proteins differs from that found in plasma. Large proteins such as IgM and 2-macroglobulin are underrepresented, whereas smaller proteins are present in relatively higher concentrations. The mechanism determining this pattern is reasonably well understood.

The microvascular endothelium provides the major barrier limiting the escape of plasma proteins into the surrounding synovial interstitium. The protein path (or paths) across the endothelium is not yet clear; conflicting experimental evidence supports the fenestrae, intercellular junctions, and cytoplasmic vesicles as the predominant sites of plasma protein escape. What does seem clear is that protein transport is inversely related to molecular size, which means that smaller proteins enter the joint space at rates proportionately faster than those of large proteins.

In contrast, proteins leave synovial fluid through lymphatic vessels, a process that is not size-selective. Protein clearance may vary with joint disease. In particular, removal of proteins is significantly more rapid in joints affected by rheumatoid arthritis than in osteoarthritis (19). Thus, in all joints, the continuing, passive transport of plasma proteins involves synovial delivery in the microvasculature, size-dependent transport across the endothelium, and ultimate lymphatic return to plasma.

The intrasynovial concentration of any protein represents the net contributions of plasma concentration, synovial blood flow, microvascular permeability, and lymphatic removal. In addition, specific proteins may be produced or consumed within the joint space. For example, lubricin is normally synthesized within synovial cells and released into synovial fluid where it facilitates boundary layer lubrication of the cartilage-on-cartilage bearing. In disease, additional proteins may be synthesized (eg, IgG rheumatoid factor in rheumatoid arthritis) or released from inflammatory cells or articular tissues (20). In contrast, intra-articular proteins may be depleted by local consumption, as are complement components in rheumatoid disease.

Synovial fluid protein concentrations vary little between highly inflamed rheumatoid joints and modestly involved osteoarthritic articulations. Microvascular permeability to protein, however, is more than twice as great in RA as in osteoarthritis. This marked difference in permeability leads to only a minimal increase in protein concentration, because the enhanced ingress of proteins is largely offset by a comparable rise in lymphatic egress. These findings illustrate the fact that synovial microvascular permeability cannot be evaluated from protein concentrations unless the kinetics of delivery or removal are assessed concurrently.

PETER A. SIMKIN, MD

1. Amiel D, Frank C, Harwood, et al: Tendons and ligaments: a morphological and biochemical comparison. J Orthop Res 1:257-265, 1984

2. Henderson B, Edwards JCW: The Synovial Lining in Health and Disease. London, Chapman and Hall, 1987

3. Knight AD, Levick JR: Morphometry of the ultrastructure of the blood-joint barrier in the rabbit knee. Q J Exper Physiol 69:271-288, 1984

4. Thompson WO, Thaete FL, Fu FH, Dye SF: Tibial meniscal dynamics using three-dimensional reconstruction of magnetic resonance images. Am J Sports Med 19:210-215, 1991

5. Mow VC, Roth V, Armstrong CG: Biomechanics of joint cartilage. In Frankel VH, Nordin M (eds): Basic Biomechanics of the Skeletal System. Philadelphia, Lea & Febiger, 1980, pp 61-86

6. Radin EL: Mechanics of joint degeneration. Radin EL, Simon SR, Rose RM, Paul IL (eds): Practical Biomechanics for the Orthopedic Surgeon. New York, John Wiley & Sons, 1979

7. Simkin PA, Graney DO, Fiechtner JJ: Roman arches, human joints, and disease: differences between convex and concave sides of joints. Arthritis Rheum 23:1308-1311, 1980

8. Downey DJ, Simkin PA, Taggart R: The effect of compressive loading on intraosseous pressure in the femoral head in vitro. J Bone Joint Surg 70A:871-877, 1988

9. Jobe CM: Gross anatomy of the shoulder. In Rockwood CA, Matsen, FA (eds): The Shoulder. Philadelphia, WB Saunders, 1990

10. Unsworth A, Dowson D, Wright V: "Cracking joints" a bioengineering study of cavitation in the metacarpophalangeal joint. Ann Rheum Dis 30:348-358, 1971

11. Levick JR: Joint pressure-volume studies: Their importance, design and interpretation. J Rheumatol 10:353-357, 1983

12. Swann DA, Silver FH, Slayter HS, et al: The molecular structure and lubricating activity of lubricin isolated from bovine and human synovial fluids. Biochem J 225:195-201, 1985

13. Levick JR: Blood flow and mass transport in synovial joints. In Renkin EM, Michel CC (eds): Handbook of Physiology: Vol. IV. Microcirculation, Part 2. Bethesda, MD, American Physiological Society, 1984, pp 917-947

14. Simkin PA, Wu MP, Foster DM: Articular pharmacokinetics of protein-bound antirheumatic agents. Clin Pharmacokinet 25:342-350, 1993

15. Wallis WJ, Simkin PA, Nelp WB: Low synovial clearance of iodide provides evidence of hypoperfusion in chronic rheumatoid synovitis. Arthritis Rheum 28:1096-1104, 1985

16. Geborek P, Saxne T, Pettersson H, Wollheim F: Synovial fluid acidosis correlates with radiological joint destruction in rheumatoid arthritis knee joints. J Rheumatol 16:468-472, 1989

17. Stevens CR, Williams RB, Farrell AJ, Blake DR: Hypoxia and inflammatory synovitis: observations annd speculations. Ann Rheum Dis 50:124-132, 1991

18. Weinberger A, Simkin PA: Plasma proteins in synovial fluids of normal human joints. Semin Arthritis Rheum 19:66-76, 1989

19. Wallis WJ, Simkin PA, Nelp WB: Protein traffic in human synovial effusions. Arthritis Rheum 30:57-63, 1987

20. Simkin PA, Bassett JE: Cartilage matrix molecules in serum and synovial fluid. Curr Opin Rheumatol 7:346-351, 1995

B. ARTICULAR CARTILAGE

Articular cartilage is a specialized connective tissue that covers the weight-bearing surfaces of articulating (diarthrodial) joints. Its extracellular matrix is composed of an extensive network of collagen fibrils that confers tensile strength and an interlocking mesh of proteoglycans that provides compressive stiffness through the ability to absorb and extrude water. Lubrication by synovial fluid provides frictionless movement of the articulating cartilage surfaces. Chondrocytes comprise the single cellular component of adult hyaline articular cartilage and are responsible for synthesizing and maintaining the highly specialized cartilage matrix macromolecules.

CARTILAGE STRUCTURE

The unique structural properties and biochemical components of diarthrodial joints make them extraordinarily durable load-bearing devices (1). The principal role for the cartilage layer is to reduce friction in the joint and absorb the shock associated with locomotion. The articular cartilage is bathed in synovial fluid, a lubricant that also serves as a source of nutrition for the chondrocytes within the articular cartilage. Articular cartilage contains more than 70% water. Over 90% of its dry weight consists of two components, type II collagen and aggrecan, the aggregating large proteoglycan (2,3). However, several "minor" collagens and small proteoglycans also appear to play a role in cartilage matrix organization (4-6). The physical properties of articular cartilage are determined by the unique fibrillar collagen network interspersed with proteoglycan aggregates that bestow tensile strength and resilience. The proteoglycans are associated with large quantities of water bound to the hydrophilic glycosaminoglycan chains. This cartilaginous extracellular matrix, with its tightly bound water, provides a high degree of resistance to deformation by compressive forces. The capac-

ity to resist compressive forces is associated with the ability to extrude water as the cartilage compresses. Once the compression is released, the proteoglycans contain sufficient fixed charge, now depleted of balancing counter-ions that were removed with the water, to osmotically reabsorb the water and small solutes into the matrix. The articular cartilage then rebounds to its original dimensions.

Normal articular cartilage is white and appears translucent. It is an avascular tissue that is nourished by diffusion from the vasculature of the subchondral bone, as well as from the synovial fluid. Cartilage is rather hypocellular compared with other tissues, since chondrocytes comprise only 1% to 2% of the total volume (7). Despite its thinness (7 mm or less) and apparent homogeneity, mature hyaline articular cartilage is a heterogeneous tissue with four distinct regions: the superficial tangential (or gliding) zone, the middle (or transitional) zone, the deep (or radial) zone, and the calcified cartilage zone located immediately below the tidemark and above the subchondral bone. In the superficial zone, the chondrocytes are flattened and the matrix is composed of thin collagen fibrils in tangential array associated with a high concentration of the small proteoglycan decorin and a low concentration of aggrecan. The middle zone, comprising 40% to 60% of the cartilage weight, consists of rounded chondrocytes surrounded by radial bundles of thick collagen fibrils. In the deep zone, the chondrocytes are frequently grouped in clusters and resemble the hypertrophic chondrocytes of the growth plate. In this region, the collagen bundles are the thickest and are arranged in a radial fashion. Cell density progressively decreases from the surface; cell density in the deep zone is one-half to one-third of that in the superficial zone. The concentration of collagen relative to proteoglycan also decreases progressively from the superficial to deep zones, and the proportion of proteoglycan increases to 50%

(Table 3B-1)

Extracellular matrix components of cartilage

Molecule	Size and Structure	Function and Location
Collagen		
Type II	$[\alpha1(II)]_3$	Tensile strength Major collagen of fibrils in cartilage
Type IX	$\alpha1(IX)\alpha2(IX)\alpha3$ (IX); single CS or DS chain	Regulates fibril size, interactions On surface of fibrils
Type XI	$\alpha1(XI)\alpha2(XI)$ $\alpha3(XI)$	Unknown Within collagen fibril, pericellular
Type VI	$\alpha1(V1)\alpha2(VI)\alpha3$ (VI); microfibrils	Linkage between collagen fibrils and cell surfaces?
Type X	$[\alpha1(X)]_3$	Unknown Developing hypertrophic cartilage and deep calcified zone in adult
Type XII	$[\alpha1(XII)]_3$	Unknown Minor component
Type XIV	$[\alpha1(XIV)]_3$	Unknown Minor component
Type II collagen C-propeptide (CP-II; chondrocalcin)	3×35 kD chains	Binds calcium In calcifying sites
Proteoglycans		
Aggrecan	300 kD core protein with CS and KS side chains (76.3 kD)	Compressive stiffness
Biglycan (PG-S1)	38 kD core protein with two DS chains (76 kD)	Unknown
Decorin (PG-S2)	36.5 kD core protein with one CS or DS side chain	Modulates collagen fibril formation

Molecule	Size and Structure	Function and Location
Fibromodulin	4 N-linked KS chains (58 kD)	Modulates collagen fibril formation
Other Molecules		
Hyaluronic acid (HA)	1000–3000 kD	Retention of aggrecan within matrix
Link protein	38.6 kD	Stabilizes attachment of aggrecan to HA via G1 domain
Anchorin II	34 kD; integral membrane protein	Binds type II collagen and calcium
Syndecan	Integral membrane protein with extracellular HS/CS side chains	Cell-matrix interactions Binds HA
CD44	Integral membrane protein with extracellular HS/CS side chains	Cell-matrix interactions Binds HA
Fibronectin	Dimer of 220 kD subunits	Cell attachment via RGD sequence Binding to collagen and GAGs
Tenascin	Six 200-kD subunits forming hexabrachion structure	Associated with chondrogenesis
Thrombospondin	Three 138-kD subunits	Calcium-binding
Cartilage oligomeric matrix protein	550 kD; five 110-kD subunits	Calcium-binding

of the dry weight in the deep zone. The calcified zone is formed as a result of endochondral ossification and persists as the growth plate is resorbed. The calcified zone serves as an important mechanical buffer between the uncalcified articular cartilage and the subchondral bone.

CARTILAGE MATRIX COMPOSITION

The extracellular matrix components synthesized by chondrocytes include highly cross-linked fibrils of triple helical type II collagen molecules that interact with other cartilage-specific collagens types IX and XI, aggrecan, small proteoglycans such as biglycan and decorin, and other specific and nonspecific matrix proteins (Table 3B-1) (2–4). These organic constituents represent only about 20% of the wet weight. Water and inorganic salts comprise most of the remaining cartilage tissue. Water content is 75% to 80% of the wet weight in the superficial zone and progressively decreases to between 65% and 70% with increasing depth. Col-

lagen, primarily type II, accounts for about 15% to 25% of the wet weight and about half of the dry weight, except in the superficial zone where it represents most of the dry weight. Proteoglycans, primarily aggrecan, account for up to 10% of the wet weight and about 25% of the dry weight. The highly cross-linked type II collagen fibrils form a systematically oriented fibrous network that entraps the highly negatively charged proteoglycan aggregates. The importance of these structural proteins may be observed in heritable disorders, such as chondrodysplasias, or in transgenic animals where mutations in cartilage-specific collagen genes or in genes that affect sulfation of aggrecan result in cartilage abnormalities (8,9).

The Collagens of Articular Cartilage

Type II collagen fibrils are composed of 300-nm tropocollagen molecules of three identical alpha chains, $[\alpha1(II)]_3$, arranged in a triple helix. These molecules are assembled to form fibrils in a quarter-stagger array that is observed by electron microscopy (3). The type II procollagen precursor contains nonhelical amino- and carboxyl-terminal propeptides that are required for correct alignment of the procollagen molecules during fibril assembly and are then removed by specific proteinases. Chondrocalcin, a carboxyl propeptide, remains transiently within the cartilage matrix after cleavage and has been proposed to play a role in mineralization as a calcium-binding protein. The type II collagen in articular cartilage is a product of alternative splicing and lacks a 69-amino acid, cysteine-rich domain of the amino-terminal propeptide encoded by exon 2 in the human type II collagen gene (COL2A1) (10) (Fig. 3B-1). This domain is found in the amino propeptides of other interstitial collagen types and is speculated to play a feedback inhibitory role in collagen biosynthesis. The type IIA procollagen that contains this domain is expressed by interstitial prechondrocytes during development, but not by fully differentiated chondrocytes.

Although collagen types VI, IX, XI, XII, and XIV are quantitatively minor components, they may have important structural and functional properties (3,5,6). Types IX and XI are relatively specific to cartilage, whereas types VI, XII, and XIV are widely distributed in other connective tissues. Type VI collagen, which is present in cartilage as microfibrils in very small quantities localized around the chondrocytes, may play a role in cell attachment. Type IX collagen is both a proteoglycan and a collagen, as it contains a chondroitin sulfate (CS) chain attachment site in one of the noncollagen domains. The helical domains of the type IX collagen molecule form covalent cross-links with type II collagen telopeptides and are observed in the electron microscope to "decorate" the surface of the type II collagen fibrils. It has been suggested that type IX collagen functions as a structural intermediate between type II collagen fibers and the proteoglycan aggregates, thereby serving to enhance the mechanical stability of the fibril network and resist the swelling pressure of the entrapped proteoglycans. Destruction of type IX collagen may accelerate cartilage degradation and loss of function. The α3 chain of type XI collagen has the same primary sequence as the α1(II) chain, and the heterotrimeric type XI collagen molecule is probably located in the same fibril as type II collagen. The recently discovered nonfibrillar collagens XII and XIV, which are structurally related to type IX collagen, modulate the packing of collagen fibers in collagen gel contraction assays in vitro (11). Type X collagen is not present in normal adult articular cartilage, but it is transiently expressed in mature hypertrophic chondrocytes during calcification at the growth plate in growing animals and during certain stages of osteoarthritis (12).

The Proteoglycans of Articular Cartilage

The large aggregating proteoglycan, or aggrecan, consists of a core protein of 225–250 kD with covalently attached side chains of glycosaminoglycans (GAGs), including approxi-

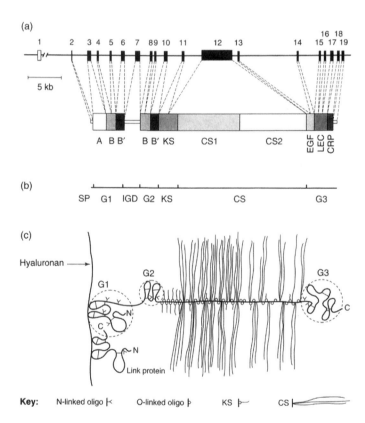

(Figure 3B-1)
Diagram of the COL2A1 gene, types IIA and IIB procollagen mRNAs, and types IIA and IIB procollagens. In the COL2A1 gene, exons are indicated as boxes. Oligonucleotide probes specific for types IIA and IIB procollagen mRNAs are indicated by bars above the mRNAs. In the procollagen molecules, SP = the signal peptide; NH2 = the amino-terminal propeptide; TP = the telopeptide, Gly-X-Y = the triple helical domain; COOH = the carboxy-terminal propeptide; straight lines = triple helical regions; curved lines = globular portions of the protein. In the type 11A procollagen, ↑= differentially spliced domain. Reprinted from Sandell et al (10) with permission.

(Figure 3B-2)
Schematic representation of aggrecan and its domains aligned with the genomic map of the human gene encoding aggrecan. The coding exons (filled bars), noncoding exon 1 (open bar), and introns (line) are shown in (a) and aligned with domains of the core protein and the aggrecan proteoglycan in (b) and (c), respectively. Interaction of the Gl domain with link protein and hyaluronan is indicated in (c), as are a few N- and O-linked oligosaccharides. CS = chondroitin sulfate domain; EGF = epidermal growth factor like-domain; IGD = interglobular domain; KS = keratan sulfate domain; LEC = lectin-like domain. Reprinted from Vertel (9) with permission.

mately 100 CS chains, 30 keratan sulfate (KS) chains, and shorter N- and O-linked oligosaccharides (1,2,9). Link protein, a small glycoprotein, stabilizes the noncovalent linkage between aggrecan and hyaluronic acid (HA; also called hyaluronan) to form the proteoglycan aggregate that may contain as many as 100 aggrecan monomers (Fig. 3B-2). The G1 and G2 N-terminal globular domains of aggrecan and its C-terminal G3 domain have distinct structural properties that function as integral parts of the aggrecan core protein and as cleavage products that accumulate with age or in osteoarthritis. The G1 domain and link protein share sequence homology with the immunoglobulin superfamily. The interaction between these and hyaluronic acid may function in cell adhesion and immune recognition. The G2 domain is separated from G1 by a linear interglobular domain and has two proteoglycan tandem repeats, but it does not bind to HA and has no known function. The G3 domain contains sequence homologies to epidermal growth factor, lectin, and complement regulatory protein, and it participates in growth regulation, cell recognition, intracellular trafficking, and the recognition, assembly, and stabilization of the extracellular matrix. About half of the aggrecan molecules in adult cartilage lack the G3 domain, probably due to proteolytic cleavage during matrix turnover.

The nonaggregating small proteoglycans are not specific to cartilage but are quite abundant; they are thought to serve important roles in cartilage matrix structure (4). These leucine-rich proteoglycans include biglycan (PG-S1), decorin (PG-S2), and fibromodulin (a 59-kD protein) and have structurally related core proteins. Biglycan has two GAG chains, either CS or dermatan sulfate (DS) or both, attached near the N-terminus through two closely spaced serine–glycine dipeptides. Decorin contains only one CS-GAG or DS-GAG chain. Fibromodulin contains several sulfated tyrosine residues in the N-terminus and KS chains linked to the central domain of the core protein. Both decorin and fibromodulin bind to collagen fibrils and influence fibrillogenesis. Both biglycan and decorin bind transforming growth factor-β. Biglycan does not bind to fibril-forming collagens, and its function is as yet unknown.

Other Matrix Proteins

Several other cartilage-specific and nonspecific noncollagenous matrix proteins may play important roles in determining cartilage matrix integrity (4). Anchorin II is a 34-kD integral chondrocyte membrane protein that binds type II collagen and shares extensive homology with the calcium-binding proteins calpactin and lipocortin. Other integral membrane proteins are the cell-surface proteoglycans syndecan and CD44. Both can bind HA through heparan sulfate–CS side chains attached to the extracellular domains.

Several cell adhesion proteins are present in cartilage, including fibronectin, tenascin, and thrombospondin. In other tissues these proteins mediate cell–matrix interactions through binding to cell-surface integrins and syndecan. Whether they have specific roles in cartilage is unknown. Alternative splicing of fibronectin and tenascin mRNAs give rise to different protein products at different stages of chondrocyte differentiation. These serve specific functions in cartilage development and repair. Thrombospondin, a calcium-binding trimeric molecule of 420 kD that was first described in platelets, is a minor cartilage constituent. Cartilage oligomeric matrix protein (COMP), a member of the thrombospondin family, is a disulfide-bonded pentameric 550-kD calcium-binding protein that is found only in cartilage. It constitutes approximately 10% of the noncollagenous, nonproteoglycan protein in normal adult cartilage where its half-life is 48-72 hours, and it is enriched in chondrocyte membrane fractions. COMP is not to be confused with cartilage matrix protein, which is expressed at certain stages of development and is present in tracheal, but not adult articular, cartilage. Synthesis or release of these proteins or fragments is often increased in cartilage that is undergoing repair (4).

Chondrocytes

The chondrocytes in adult articular cartilage are terminally differentiated cells that are interspersed in the cartilage matrix in distinct chondrocyte lacunae. The chondrocytes and the surrounding dense extracellular matrix form a functional unit termed a *chondron* (1). While chondrocytes are biosynthetically active in growing animals, their capacity to replace lost collagen is limited in mature articular cartilage. Only proteoglycan aggregates appear to be continuously synthesized. Normally, chondrocytes are in a homeostatic state. In fact, because of their relatively quiescent nature, adult chondrocytes were once thought to be metabolically inactive. But chondrocytes are now known to be capable of responding to biochemical, structural, and physical stimuli and are able to synthesize various enzymes, enzyme inhibitors, growth factors, and cytokines, as well as all the matrix components described above (13). Unfortunately, adult chondrocytes have a limited repair capacity and may replace damaged or aging articular cartilage with type I collagen-containing fibrotic tissue. Cultured chondrocytes have served as useful models for studying the mechanisms controlling synthesis of cartilage matrix proteins (13). Recent advances in studies of gene expression during development also have increased our understanding of cartilage repair mechanisms in the adult (14).

CARTILAGE MATRIX TURNOVER, DEGRADATION, AND REPAIR

In normal adult articular cartilage, turnover of extracellular matrix components is slow compared with many other connective tissues, and the capacity for repair is limited. The turnover rate of collagen is very slow, except in pericellular sites where there is evidence for ongoing type II cleavage (1). The proteoglycans, particularly the small sulfated GAG components that are more susceptible to enzymatic degradation, are continually resynthesized. Major changes in the structure and content of the components of the proteoglycan aggregates have been demonstrated in human articular cartilage with increasing age. Although the total content of sulfated GAGs does not change significantly with age, notable changes include increased KS associated with decreased CS, decreased size of proteoglycan aggregates, increased amounts of free binding region (G1 or G1 plus G2 together with the KS-rich region and proteolytically cleaved link protein), and increased content of hyaluronan of shorter chain length (15).

IMMUNOLOGIC MARKERS OF CARTILAGE MATRIX DEGRADATION AND TURNOVER

With increasing knowledge of the composition and metabolism of cartilage matrix, new markers have emerged and assays have been developed that have the potential to serve as diagnostic tools for assessing joint damage in arthritis. Since cartilage has a number of components that undergo changes during joint disease, specific antibodies have been developed and used to study altered cartilage metabolism (1,16). Monoclonal antibodies have been developed that recognize products of proteoglycan or collagen degradation (catabolic epitopes) or synthesis of newly synthesized matrix components (anabolic neo-epitopes) that represent attempts to repair the damaged matrix. For example, different monoclonal antibodies can distinguish subtle biochemical differences in CS-GAG or KS-GAG chains that result from degraded versus newly synthesized proteoglycans. Other antibodies that have proved useful as research or diagnostic tools include those that recognize specific proteinase cleavage sites in the aggrecan core protein, the HA binding region (G1 domain), and a CS epitope in the G3 domain. Such epitopes can be detected in the synovial fluids and sera of patients with osteoarthritis and rheumatoid arthritis, and the synovial fluid-to-serum ratio can be useful as a diagnostic indicator. For example, COMP is released in reactive arthritis, and high serum levels in early rheumatoid arthritis can distinguish an aggressive, destructive form of the disease. Similarly, the synthesis of type II collagen can be monitored by measuring the carboxyl-terminal propeptide, CPII or chondrocalcin, and urinary excretion of pyridinoline and hydroxypyridinoline cross-links may indicate collagen degradation. The use of such assays as research tools has generated considerable interest in their further development for use in clinical practice.

MARY B. GOLDRING, PhD

1. Poole AR: Cartilage in health and disease. In McCarty DJ, Koopman WP (eds): Arthritis and Allied Conditions: A Textbook of Rheumatology. Philadelphia, Lea and Febiger, 1993, pp 279-333

2. Hardingham TE, Fosang AJ: Proteoglycans: many forms and many functions. FASEB J 6:861-870, 1992

3. Mayne R, Brewton RG: Extracellular matrix of cartilage. In Woessner JF, Jr, Howell DS (eds): Collagen, Joint Cartilage Degradation: Basic and Clinical Aspects. New York, Marcel Dekker, Inc., 1993, pp 81-108

4. Heinegard DK, Rosa-Pimentel: Cartilage matrix proteins. In Kuettner KE, Schleyerbach R, Peyron JG, Hascall VC (eds): Articular Cartilage and Osteoarthritis. New York, Raven Press, 1992, pp 95-111

5. Jacenko O, Olsen BR, LuValle P: Organization and regulation of collagen genes. Crit Rev Eukaryotic Gene Exp 1:327-353, 1991

6. Eyre DR, Wu J-J, Woods P: Cartilage-specific collagens. In Kuettner KE, Schleyerbach R, Peyron JG, Hascall VC (eds): Structural Studies, Articular Cartilage and Osteoarthritis. New York, Raven Press, 1992, pp 119-130

7. Stockwell RA, Meachim G: The chondrocytes. In Freeman MAR (ed): Adult Articular Cartilage. Tunbridge Wells, England, Pitman Medical, 1979, pp 69-144

8. Jacenko O, Olsen BR, Warman ML: Of mice and men: heritable skeletal disorders. Am J Hum Genet 54:163-168, 1994

9. Vertel BM: The ins and outs of aggrecan. Trends Cell Biol 5:458-464, 1995

10. Sandell LJ, Morris N, Robbins JR, Goldring MB: Alternatively spliced type II procollagen mRNAs define a distinct population of cells during vertebral development: Differential expression of the amino-propeptide. J Cell Biol 114:1307-1319, 1991

11. Nishiyama T, McDonough AM, Bruns RR, Burgeson RE: Type XII and XIV collagens mediate interactions between banded collagen fibers in vitro and may mediate extracellular matrix deformability. J Biol Chem 269:28193-28199, 1994

12. von der Mark K, Kirsch T, Aigner T, Reichenberger E, Nerlich A, Weseloh G, Stös H: The fate of chondrocytes in osteoarthritic cartilage: Regeneration, dedifferentiation, or hypertrophy? In Kuettner K, Schleyerback R, Peyron JG, Hascall VC (eds): Articular Cartilage and Osteoarthritis. New York, Raven Press,1992, pp 221-233

13. Goldring MB: Degradation of articular cartilage in culture: Regulatory factors. In Woessner JF, Jr, Howell DS (eds): Joint Cartilage Degradation: Basic and Clinical Aspects. New York, Marcel Dekker, Inc,1993, pp 281-345

14. DeCrombrugghe B, Horton WA, Olsen BR, Ramirez F (eds): Molecular and developmental biology of cartilage. Ann NY Acad Sci 785:1-361, 1996

15. Bayliss MT: Metabolism of animal and human osteoarthritic cartilage. In Kuettner KE, Schleyerbach R, Peyron JG, Hascall VC (eds): Articular Cartilage and Osteoarthritis. New York, Raven Press,1992, pp 487-498

16. Caterson BC, Hughes CE, Johnstone B, Mort JS: Immunological markers of cartilage proteoglycan metabolism in animal and human osteoarthritis. In Kuettner KE, Schleyerbach R, Peyron JG, Hascall VC (eds): Articular Cartilage and Osteoarthritis. New York, Raven Press,1992, pp 415-427

C. BONE

Bone is a composite tissue consisting of mineral, matrix, cells, and water (Fig. 3C-1). The mineral is an analog of the naturally occurring crystalline calcium phosphate, hydroxyapatite $(Ca_5(PO_4)_3(OH))$. Physiologic mineral crystals, as distinct from geologic apatites, are very small and imperfect, containing fewer hydroxyl groups and many impurities such as carbonate, fluoride, acid phosphate, magnesium, and citrate. The small size of the crystals makes them ideally suited for their function in mineral ion homeostasis, because smaller crystals generally dissolve before larger crystals. Hydroxyapatite crystals also form in tissues that are not normally calcified, for example, in atherosclerotic plaque, soft tissues of some patients with abnormally high circulating calcium or phosphate, and articular cartilage of some patients with degenerative joint diseases (1). These abnormal tissues generally appear distinct from bone because of the larger size of the crystals and the nature of the matrices upon which the crystals are deposited.

STRUCTURE AND FUNCTION

In addition to serving as a source for calcium, magnesium, and phosphate ions, the mineral crystals in bone provide strength and rigidity to the matrix upon which they are deposited. The second major function of bone is mechanical. Bone provides protection for internal organs and facilitates mobility. The bone matrix is essentially type I collagen. The

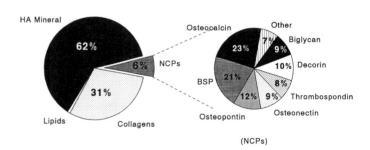

(Figure 3C-1)
Typical composition of adult human trabecular bone. Components of the pie chart on the left reflect the weight percent apatite (HA mineral), lipids, collagens, and noncollagenous proteins (NCPs) found in bone. The pie chart on the right shows the relative (weight percent) distribution of the major types of noncollagenous proteins. BSP = bone sialoprotein.

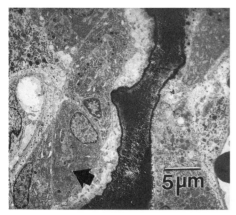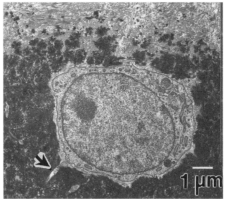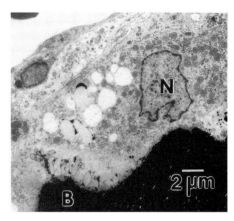

(Figure 3C-2)
Electron micrographs showing **Left:** *osteoblasts,* **Center:** *osteocytes, and* **Right:** *osteoclasts in normal rat bone. Note the abundant rough endoplasmic reticulum (arrow) in the osteoblast, a cell actively involved in matrix deposition. The osteocyte, which shows less synthetic activity, is almost entirely engulfed in electron-dense mineral but is connected to other cells by long channels known as canaliculi (arrow). The osteoclast is a larger cell, often with multiple nuclei (N), which attaches to the bone surface (B), and pumps out protons to dissolve mineral. Courtesy of S.B. Doty, Hospital for Special Surgery, NY.*

collagen fibrils are arranged in the extracellular matrix in patterns related to the function of the tissue in which they are found. The unique triple helical structure of collagen provides strength and flexibility to most of the connective tissues (2). The mineral crystals add extra rigidity to the collagen fibers. Collagen is stabilized by cross-links formed post-translationally in the extracellular matrix. The nature of these cross-links differs in the mineralized and nonmineralized connective tissues (3). Analyses of the cross-links that stabilize bone collagen, as opposed to skin and tendon collagen, provide a useful marker for diseases such as osteoporosis in which breakdown of the matrix is increased (4). In addition to collagen, about 5% of the extracellular matrix of bone is made up of noncollagenous proteins. These proteins play crucial roles in mineral homeostasis, bone metabolism, bone formation, and bone turnover (5,6).

The metabolism, formation, and turnover of bone is governed by cells. Bone has three cell types: osteoblasts, osteocytes, and osteoclasts (Fig. 3C-2). Osteoblasts and osteocytes are derived from the mesenchymal cell lineage and appear to be closely related. Osteoblasts synthesize the bone matrix, while osteocytes, which are enmeshed in an existing bone matrix, appear to be more important in conveying nutrition and information throughout bone. Osteoclasts, multinucleated giant cells believed to be of macrophage origin, are responsible for removing bone. In normal tissues, the functions of osteoblasts and osteoclasts are coupled such that signals from one affect the other (7). The distribution of these bone cells and their relative activities vary with type of bone, age, and disease state. Similarly, distributions of mineral and matrix proteins differ in various bones, and these also change with disease and age.

BONE FORMATION

Bone formation occurs through two distinct processes: endochondral ossification, in which bone replaces a cartilage model, and intramembranous ossification, in which bone forms directly. During embryonic development, the long bones are formed by the former process and the bones of the skull by the latter.

During endochondral ossification, mesenchymal cells differentiate into chondrocytes. These chondrocytes produce a cartilage anlage that is modified to facilitate mineralization, vascular invasion, and replacement by bone. As they mature, chondrocytes change shape and switch from making collagens found in all cartilage (type II and IX) to type X collagen, a form unique to the "hypertrophic" chondrocytes at the interface of cartilage and bone. Although the precise function of type X collagen is not known, defects in its production have been found in several families with various forms of spondylepiphyseal dysplasias, a disease characterized by extreme curvature of the spine (kyphosis), implying that type X collagen has a role in stabilizing the endochondral structure (8). Transgenic mice expressing an abnormal type X collagen develop lymphocytopenia in addition to

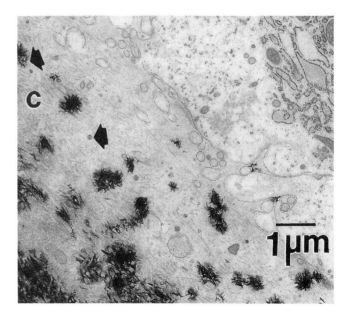

(Figure 3C-3)
Electron micrograph illustrating collagen (c) and matrix vesicle (arrows) mediated calcification in rat periosteal bone. Courtesy of S.B. Doty, Hospital for Special Surgery, NY.

(Table 3C-1)

Hormones and growth factors regulating bone formation*

Factor	Target Cells and Tissue[†]	Effect
Parathyroid hormone	Kidney and bone	Stimulates 1,25D formation and osteoclastic activity; increases circulating calcium concentrations
Calcitonin	Bone osteoclasts	Inhibits action of osteoclasts; lowers circulating calcium concentrations
Vitamin D (1,25D)	Bone osteoblasts	Stimulates collagen, osteopontin, and osteocalcin synthesis; stimulates differentiation; increases circulating calcium concentrations
	Bone osteoclasts	Stimulates activity of osteoclasts
	Kidney	Stimulates calcium retention
	Intestine	Stimulates calcium absorption
Estrogen	Bone	Stimulates formation of calcitonin receptors, inhibiting resorption
Prostaglandins	Osteoclasts	Stimulates resorption and formation
Bone morphogenetic protein	Mesenchyme	Stimulates cartilage protein and bone matrix formation; stimulates replication
TGFβ	Osteoblasts, chondrocytes	Stimulates differentiation
IL-1, IL-3, IL-6, IL-11	Marrow, osteoclasts	Stimulate osteoclast formation
TNFα, GMCSF	Osteoclasts	Stimulates bone resorption
Leukemic inhibitory factor	Osteoblasts, osteoclasts, marrow	Stimulates osteoblast and osteoclast formation

* IL = interleukin; TGF = transforming growth factor; TNF = tumor necrosis factor; GMCSF = granulocyte–macrophage colony-stimulating factor.
[†]Although these factors have effects in other tissues, only those related to bone metabolism are listed.

skeletal kyphosis (9), indicating that type X collagen may have some other, yet-to-be determined function in immunoregulation in addition to preparing the calcifying cartilage matrix for bone formation.

A second alteration that occurs in the cartilaginous matrix as it matures and prepares for calcification is a modification of proteoglycan structure. Several different types of proteoglycans are present in the developing epiphyseal plate. The large chondroitin sulfate/keratan sulfate molecules (*aggrecan*) associate with hyaluronic acid (*hyaluronan*) to form high-molecular weight, space-filling molecules (*aggregates*) that expand to 50 times their volume. The related nonaggregating molecules found in a variety of connective tissues (*versican*) and a unique but related nonaggregating molecule (*epiphysican*) may have similar functions. In addition, there is a smaller dermatan sulfate-containing molecule with only one glycosaminoglycan chain, called *decorin,* that trims the surface of collagen fibrils, and *biglycan,* a related molecule with two component glycosaminoglycan chains per core protein. Chondroitin sulfate analogs of these dermatan sulfate proteoglycans are found in bone and tendon. The large cartilage proteoglycans (aggrecan and its aggregates and versican) function to keep the matrix hydrated and prevent calcification. The smaller proteoglycans are believed to regulate collagen fibril formation and, because of their ability to bind growth factors, to play a key role in cartilage metabolism. Aggrecan and proteoglycan aggregates in solution are effective inhibitors of mineral crystal growth and formation, a finding that may explain the observation that in severe osteoarthritis, calcification occurs around chondrocytes where the proteoglycans have been degraded. As the hypertrophic cartilage is modified, mineralization commences. Initial calcification in cartilage occurs in association with both collagen and extracellular membrane-bound bodies known as *matrix vesicles* (Fig. 3C-3). These vesicles are enriched in en-

zymes that facilitate both the transport of calcium and phosphate ions needed for mineralization into the vesicle and the degradation of the matrix around the vesicle. These vesicles thus provide a protected environment in which ions can accumulate and in which initial mineral deposition can occur in the absence of inhibitors. Mineral crystals break through the vesicles and may fuse with collagen-based mineral as cartilage calcification proceeds (10).

Vascular invasion of the calcified cartilage mediated by growth factors and replacement of the underlying matrix by one containing type I collagen results in the replacement of the calcified cartilage by bone. Osteoblasts produce this bone, sequentially laying down an underlying fibrous network (consisting of fibronectin and vitronectin), type I collagen, and a variety of matrix proteins. Mineral deposition then occurs by processes described below. Once the bone is formed, it remains in a dynamic state, remodeling to provide maximum strength with minimum mass (Wolff's law), to allow growth, and to provide a source of mineral ion homeostasis. The remodeling processes (formation and resorption) are linked so that factors produced by bone-forming cells (osteoblasts) activate remodeling cells (osteoclasts) and vice versa (7). Table 3C-1 provides a partial list of the hormones and growth factors implicated in the regulation of the bone-forming and bone-resorbing cells. The receptors for many of these factors have been identified. Many of these receptors activate kinases, which in turn activate DNA-regulating proteins altering protein synthesis or enzymes that modulate matrix proteins.

ADELE L. BOSKEY, PhD

1. Boskey AL, Vigorita V, Bullough PG: Calcium-acidic phospholipid-phosphate complexes: promoter of mineralization common to pathologic hydroxyapatite-containing calcifications. Am J Pathol 133:22-29, 1988

2. Lees S, Hanson D, Page E, Mook HA: Comparison of dosage-dependent effects of ß-aminopropionitrile, sodium fluoride, and hydrocortisone on selected physical properties of cortical bone. J Bone Miner Res 9:1377-1389, 1994

3. Yamauchi M, Katz EP, Otsubo K, Teraoka K, Mechanic GL: Cross-linking and stereospecific structure of collagen in mineralized skeletal tissues. Connect Tissue Res 21:159-169, 1989

4. Eyre D: New biomarkers of bone resorption. J Clin Endocrin Metab 74:470A-470C, 1992

5. Boskey AL: Mineral-matrix interactions in bone and cartilage. Clin Orthopaed 281:244- 274, 1992

6. Roach HJ: Why does bone matrix contain non-collagenous proteins? The possible roles of osteocalcin, osteonectin, osteopontin, and bone sialoprotein in mineralization and resorption. Cell Biol Int 18:617-628, 1994

7. Manalagos SC, Jilka RL: Bone marrow, cytokines, and bone remodeling: emerging insights into the pathophysiology of osteoporosis. N Engl J Med 332:305-311, 1995

8. Jacenko O, Olsen BR, LuValle P: Organization and regulation of collagen genes. Crit Rev Eukaryot Gene Expe 1:327-353, 1991

9. Jacenko O, LuValle PA, Olsen BR: Spondyloepiphyseal dysplasia in mice carrying a dominant negative mutation in a matrix protein specific for carti-lage-to-bone transition. Nature 365:56-61, 1993

10. Christoffersen J, Landis WJ: A contribution with review to the description of mineralization of bone and other calcified tissues in vivo. Anat Rec 230:435-450, 1991

D. SKELETAL MUSCLE

MORPHOLOGY

Skeletal muscles are organs that contract for the purpose of generating force and movement in specific directions. Most skeletal muscles are connected at each end to bone by tendons. Skeletal muscle is composed of cells termed *fibers* that are structured in a highly ordered fashion (1). Fibers are anatomically grouped in fascicles so that different fibers within a fascicle are innervated by different motor neurons. The parallel arrangements of fascicles between the tendinous ends of muscles allow for the force of contraction to be additive. Functionally, muscle fibers are grouped in motor units that consist of a lower motor neuron originating in a spinal cord anterior horn cell and the muscle fibers it innervates. All muscle fibers within a motor unit are of the same type. Individual human muscles are heterogeneous with regard to fiber type.

Muscle fibers vary with respect to their metabolism and response to stimuli and may be typed accordingly. A variety of fiber-type classifications have emerged based on different biochemical and physiologic properties (2,3). For most purposes, fibers are divided among three types. Type 1 fibers, also called slow twitch oxidative (SO) fibers, respond to electrical stimulation more slowly with a moderate contractile intensity and are fatigue-resistant with repeated stimulation. Type 1 cells have greater numbers of mitochondria and higher lipid content. In contrast, type 2b fibers, known as fast twitch glycolytic (FG) fibers, respond more rapidly with greater force of contraction but fatigue rapidly. These fibers have higher activities of myophosphorylase and myoadenylate deaminase and more glycogen. Type 2a fibers, termed fast twitch oxidative glycolytic (FOG), have properties that are intermediate between those of type 1 and 2b. A type 2c fiber is included in some classification schemes and is believed to represent an undifferentiated cell. The characteristics of each fiber type are originally determined during development and are maintained through interaction with the motor neuron through which it is innervated. Fiber type specificity and distribution can be altered by reinnervation with a different type of motor neuron, physical training, or disease processes (4,5).

Each muscle fiber is an elongated multinucleated cell surrounded by a plasma membrane, termed the *sarcolemma*. Fibers contain contractile proteins (actin, troponin, tropomyosin and myosin) termed myofilaments (Fig. 3D-1). The myofilaments are bathed in cytosol, termed *sarcoplasm*, and organized within fibrils, which are enveloped by the sarcoplasmic reticulum. Communication between the sarcolemma and sarcoplasmic reticulum is provided through a network of pores and channels called the *T-tubule system.*

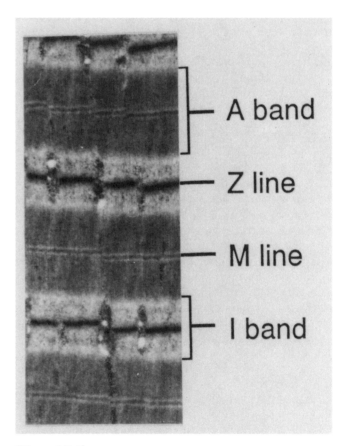

(Figure 3D-1)

The varying refractile indices of the myofilaments give skeletal muscle its characteristic ultrastructural cross-striated appearance. The functional contractile unit of the fiber is the sarcomere, defined as the area between two Z lines. Z lines transect the fibrils and connect the actin filaments. The A band is composed of the thick myofilaments (myosin) and the M line is due to the bulges in the middle of the myosin filaments. In cross-section, each myosin filament is surrounded by six actin filaments in a hexagonal pattern. At rest, the I band is the area occupied by the thin filaments (actin, troponin, and tropomyosin) not overlapped by myosin. With contraction, cross-bridges form between actin and myosin, Z lines move toward the M line, and I bands become smaller.

CONTRACTION AND RELAXATION

Muscle contraction requires shortening of myofilaments located within muscle fibers. Contraction can result from electrical, chemical, or physical stimulation that initiates the orderly transmission of an action potential along the sarcolemma, then through the T-tubule system to the sarcoplasmic reticulum. As a result, calcium is released into the sarcoplasm. As sarcoplasmic calcium concentrations increase, actin is released from an inhibited state allowing actin myosin cross-linkage and shortening of the myofilaments. Shortening continues until calcium is actively pumped back into the sarcoplasmic reticulum, breaking the cross-linkages and allowing relaxation.

Both contraction and relaxation are active processes and require normal levels of electrolytes and adenosine triphosphate (ATP). Sodium, potassium, calcium, and magnesium are critical to the function of three ATPase proteins that must work effectively for normal fiber contraction and relaxation. Sodium-potassium ATPase activity maintains normal polarity of the sarcolemma. The ATPase that controls actin myosin cross-linking is magnesium-dependent. A calcium-dependent ATPase pumps calcium from the sarcoplasm into the sarcoplasmic reticulum permitting relaxation. Phosphorus levels are also critical, because phosphorus is the ion that forms the high energy bonds of ATP, the substrate for the three enzymes.

ENERGY METABOLISM

Energy required for the contraction and relaxation of muscle is derived from the hydrolysis of ATP. Skeletal muscle uses fatty acids and carbohydrates to produce ATP (6,7), with several pathways used to produce energy from each source. The importance of a particular pathway varies with the level of exertion and nutritional status of the individual. Working in concert, these pathways maintain intracellular ATP concentrations at constant levels under most conditions and restore them to normal levels if vigorous activity or hypoxia cause ATP concentrations to fall.

Free fatty acids provide the major source of ATP during fasting intervals, at rest, and for muscle activities of low intensity and long duration. They must enter mitochondria to be processed for energy (8). To enter mitochondria, long-chain fatty acids combine with the carrier molecule carnitine (9) and transfer across the mitochondrial membrane by a process that is catalyzed by two enzymes found on the inner membrane, carnitine palmitoyltransferase (CPT) I and CPT II (10). Once in the mitochondria, fatty acid and carnitine separate. Two carbon fragments of acetylCoA are split off the fatty acid by the process of β-oxidation. These are metabolized sequentially by the tricarboxylic acid cycle and oxidative phosphorylation. By this metabolic route, one molecule of palmitate results in the net gain of 131 molecules of ATP.

Glycogen, the major storage form of carbohydrate, can be metabolized aerobically or anaerobically but provides the primary source of ATP when physical activity is intense or when anaerobic conditions exist. Under such conditions, glycogen is mobilized to form glucose-6-phosphate by the process of glycogenolysis, a process initiated by the activity of myophosphorylase (11). Glucose-6-phosphate is metabolized through the glycolytic pathway to lactate. Under aerobic conditions, this pathway produces pyruvate, which can enter the tricarboxylic acid cycle. The aerobic metabolism of one molecule of glucose nets 38 molecules of ATP, whereas the anaerobic processing results in the generation of only two molecules of ATP.

At rest, oxidative metabolism produces excess amounts of ATP, but intracellular levels of ATP remain constant. Creatine phosphokinase (CK) activity plays a pivotal role in maintaining constant intracellular ATP concentrations, functioning to buffer changes in cytosolic levels. Creatine phosphokinase catalyzes the reversible transphosphorylation of creatine and adenine nucleotides. At rest, the terminal phosphate of ATP is transferred to creatine, forming creatine phosphate and ADP. The creatine phosphate acts as a reservoir of high energy phosphates. With muscle activity and ATP hydrolysis, CK catalyzes the transfer of those phosphates to adenosine diphosphate, rapidly restoring ATP levels to normal. The enzyme—along with its products, creatine and creatine phosphate—also serves as a shuttle mechanism for energy transport between mitochondria, where ATP is generated by oxidative metabolism, and the myofibrils, where ATP is consumed in the active processes of muscle contraction and relaxation (12).

The CK buffering system maintains ATP concentrations at usual levels during exercise until creatine phosphate concentrations are depleted by 50%. If activity continues, ATP concentrations fall and the purine nucleotide cycle begins to play a pivotal role. This tends to occur when glycolysis becomes the major route for ATP generation (13). The first step of the purine nucleotide cycle is conversion of adenosine monophosphate (AMP) to inosine monophosphate (IMP) by myoadenylate deaminase with the generation of ammonia. Both IMP and ammonia stimulate glycolytic activity. As ATP concentrations fall, IMP concentrations rise stoichiometrically. This process continues until muscle activity decreases and recovery can occur. During recovery, oxidative pathways resume a major functional role and AMP is regenerated from IMP by a two-step process with the liberation of fumarate (14). Fumarate is converted to malate, which enters mitochondria and participates as an intermediate in the tricarboxylic acid cycle. The higher concentrations of malate thus act to "drive" the cycle causing efficient regeneration of ATP by oxidative phosphorylation.

ROBERT L. WORTMANN, MD

1. Craig R: The structure of the contractile filaments. In Engel AG, Banker BQ (eds): Myology, lst ed. New York, McGraw-Hill Book Company, 1986, pp 73-124

2. Tunell GL, Hart MN: Simultaneous determination of skeletal muscle fiber types I, IIA, and IIB by histochemistry. Arch Neurol 34:171-176, 1977

3. Pette D, Staron RS: Molecular basis of the phenotypic characteristics of mammalian muscle fibers. Ciba Found Symp 138:22-32, 1988

4. Haggmark T, Eriksson F, Jansson E: Muscle fiber type changes in human skeletal muscle after injuries and immobilization. Orthopedics 9:181-185, 1986

5. Edstrom L, Grimby L: Effect of exercise on the motor unit. Muscle & Nerve 9:104-126, 1986

6. Hochachka PW: Fuels and pathways as designed systems for support of muscle work. J Exp Biol 115:149-164, 1985

7. Layzer RB: How muscles use fuel. N Engl J Med 324:411-412, 1991

8. Lee CP, Schatz G, Dallner G (eds): Mitochondria and Microsomes. Reading, MA: Addison-Wesley, 1981

9. Robouche CJ, Paulson DJ: Carnitine metabolism and function in humans. Ann Rev Nutr 6:41-66, 1986

10. Zierz S, Engel AG: Regulatory properties of a carnitine palmitoyltransferase in human skeletal muscle. Eur J Biochem 149:207-214, 1986

11. Brown DH: Glycogen metabolism and glycolysis in muscle. In Engel AG, Banker BQ (eds): Myology, 1st ed. New York, McGraw-Hill Book Company, 1986, pp 673-698

12. Erikson-Viitanen S, Geiger P, Yang WCT, et al: The creatine-creatine phos-

phate shuttle for energy transport-compartmentation of creatine phosphokinase in muscle. Adv Exp Med Biol 151:115-125, 1982

13. Wy T-FL, Davis EJ: Regulation of glycolytic flux in an energetically controlled cell-free system: The effects of adenine nucleotide ratios, inorganic
phosphate, pH, and citrate. Arch Biochem Biophys 209:85-99, 1981

14. Aragon JJ, Lowenstein JM: The purine nucleotide cycle: Comparison of
the levels of citric acid intermediators with the operation of the purine
nucleotide cycle in rat skeletal muscle during exercise and recovery from exercise. Eur J Biochem 110:371-377, 1980

E. VASCULAR ENDOTHELIUM

The entire circulatory system is lined by a continuous, sin-
gle-cell-thick membrane—the vascular endothelium. Originally, this monolayer of endothelial cells was viewed simply
as a passive permeability barrier; however, in recent years,
the endothelial lining has been shown to be a multifunc-
tional organ. The endothelium is strategically situated to
monitor systemic and locally generated stimuli and to alter
its functional state. Changes in endothelial structure and
function, provoked by pathophysiologic stimuli, can result
in localized, acute and chronic, alterations in the interactions
among the endothelium, the cellular and macromolecular
components of circulating blood, and the underlying tissue.
These alterations include enhanced permeability to (and
subsequent oxidative modification of) plasma lipoproteins;
hyperadhesiveness for blood leukocytes; and functional imbalances in local pro- and antithrombotic factors, growth
stimulators, growth inhibitors, and vasoactive (dilator, con-
strictor) substances. These manifestations, collectively
termed *endothelial dysfunction,* participate in the initiation,
progression, and clinical complications of various forms of
inflammatory and degenerative rheumatic diseases.

ANATOMY AND FUNCTION OF NORMAL ENDOTHELIUM

By virtue of its anatomic location, vascular endothelium
provides a biologically significant interface that defines intra-
and extravascular compartments, serves as a selective permeability barrier, and provides a continuous nonthrombogenic
lining for the cardiovascular system. Its location is also a key
factor in dynamic, reciprocal interactions with other cells,
both in the circulating blood and the surrounding tissue, and
in its ability to monitor, integrate, and transduce blood-borne
signals, thus making it a type of sensory organ (1). This
sensor–transducer function is facilitated by the surfaces of
endothelial cells: the clearly definable "apical" or luminal
surface faces the blood stream, and the "basal" or abluminal
surface is in contact with the subendothelial connective tissues. Each surface is outfitted with a distinct complement of
functional molecules, including enzymes and receptors.

The endothelial surface area covers several thousand
square meters (2). Therefore, it can function as an immense
catalytic surface, a highly selective binding surface, or a relatively nonspecific adsorptive surface. These activities are
especially enhanced in the microcirculation where the endothelial surface area–blood volume ratio is maximal. The
realization that the walls of blood vessels actively participate in the biochemical reactions of blood constituents is a
significant conceptual advance (1). In addition, key surface-
related functions of vascular endothelium can be dynami-
cally altered, thus rendering the endothelial surface an important site of physiologic regulation and pathologic
alteration (3–6).

Another relevant aspect of endothelial organization is its
regional specialization. The vascular endothelium exhibits
site-to-site variations that may have important physiologic
and pathophysiologic implications. These differences are
manifested in properties such as permeability to macromolecules, secretion of biosynthetic products, and responsiveness to various exogenous mediators (2). Dramatic changes
occur in endothelial permeability in response to various
physiologic and pathophysiologic stimuli. For example, histamine and other acute inflammatory mediators act directly
on microvascular endothelial cells to stimulate the opening
of their intercellular junctions, thus permitting rapid flux of
blood products into the extravascular space (7). Thrombin
and certain other mediators also appear to induce a pericellular leakage via a similar mechanism.

Blood does not clot on a healthy endothelial surface because endothelial cells synthesize a unique arachidonate
metabolite prostacyclin that is an extraordinarily potent inhibitor of platelet aggregation. The endothelium also plays a
pivotal role in the coagulation and fibrinolytic system (8).
Several of the body's natural anticoagulant mechanisms are
endothelial-associated (9). These include the heparin–
antithrombin mechanism, the protein C-thrombomodulin
mechanism, and the tissue plasminogen activator mechanism. The dysfunctional endothelial cell also appears capable of active prothrombotic behavior. It synthesizes adhesive
cofactors for platelets, such as von Willebrand factor, fibronectin, and thrombospondin; procoagulant components,
such as factor V; and an inhibitor of the fibrinolytic pathway
plasminogen activator inhibitor-1, which reduces the rate of
fibrin breakdown. Thus, the endothelial cell appears capable
of playing a number of roles, both "pro" and "anti" hemo-
static/thrombotic.

Maintenance of cardiovascular tone was viewed solely as
a function of the vascular smooth-muscle cell responding to
nerve stimulation or circulating hormones until the discovery of endothelium-derived relaxing factor (EDRF). The elucidation of the chemical nature of EDRF as endogenous nitric oxide, its metabolic pathway of generation, and its
mechanism of action in vasodilation has added greatly to
our understanding of the role of cell–cell interactions in regulating vascular tone (10). A number of endothelial-derived
substances that have vasoconstrictor activity balance the
action of nitric oxide and prostacyclin, which are potent va-
sorelaxors. These include angiotensin II, generated at the
endothelial surface by angiotensin-converting enzyme;
platelet-derived growth factor, which is secreted by endothelial cells and can act as an agonist of smooth-muscle
contraction; and endothelin-1, a unique vasoconstrictor substance (11).

The vascular endothelial lining is also the source of a wide
variety of cytokines, growth factors, and growth inhibitors

that act locally to influence the behavior of adjacent vascular cells and interacting blood elements. This makes the endothelium a special kind of endocrine organ that can secrete its hormones in a paracrine (acting on neighbors) or even an autocrine (acting on self) fashion.

THE DYSFUNCTIONAL OR ACTIVATED ENDOTHELIUM

Injury to, or activation of, the endothelium may lead to the induction of genes that are suppressed under physiologic rather than pathologic conditions and/or the halting of expression of "beneficial" genes (3-6). As depicted in Fig. 3E-1, specific endothelial cell functions that may be directly relevant to chronic inflammatory responses and their clinical sequelae include the expression of leukocyte binding sites on the endothelial cell surface, the altered production of paracrine growth factors, chemoattractants and vasoreactive molecules, the ability to oxidize low-density lipoprotein (LDL) and respond to oxidized lipids and lipoproteins, the ability to express pro- rather than anticoagulant activities, and the modulation of plasma component levels within the surrounding tissue through changes in permeability function (6).

The factors that alter endothelial gene expression during inflammation are likely multiple. Leading candidates include local cytokines or proteases, viral infection, and free radicals and oxidized lipids.

Expression of Leukocyte Adhesion Molecules

The molecular interactions between blood-borne leukocytes and the endothelium play pivotal roles in inflammation. Leukocytes can produce paracrine growth factors and cytokines, generate cytotoxic factors for neighboring cells, and cause degradation of local connective tissue. The first step in leukocyte recruitment into the subendothelial space is the attachment of this blood-borne cell to the endothelium. A normal, healthy endothelium does not bind leukocytes. However, neutrophils, monocytes, and lymphocytes bind avidly to newly expressed leukocyte adhesion molecules on the endothelial surface in response to activating

agents such as interleukin-1, tumor necrosis factor α, lipopolysaccharide, oxidized lipids, or many other agents and conditions (12,13).

The process of leukocyte attachment to the endothelium and subsequent diapedesis involves the sequential involvement of various adhesion molecules and chemokines (14,15). The endothelium and the leukocytes play an active role in the process, which includes an initial rolling or tethering event (selectins), a signaling process (chemokines), a strong attachment step (the immunoglobulin family members), and transendothelial cell migration of the leukocyte.

Growth Factor Production by the Activated Endothelium

The activated endothelium is a potential source of growth factor(s) for neighboring smooth-muscle cells and fibroblasts. Platelet-derived growth factor (PDGF), a mitogen that has been implicated in atherosclerotic plaque development, is expressed by endothelial cells. Substantial evidence correlates PDGF expression by endothelial cells with dysfunction and vascular disease (16). The most effective inducer of PDGF production by endothelial cells is the coagulation system protease α-thrombin, which acts both transcriptionally and post-translationally to cause the release of PDGF (17). The endothelium is also known to produce other growth factors in addition to PDGF, including insulin-like growth factor-1, which can modulate gene expression and augment proliferation of neighboring connective tissue cells (18). The endothelium is also a well-recognized source of basic fibroblast growth factor, as well as the pluripotent growth factor/ growth inhibitor, transforming growth factor β (TGF-β). The two factors are interconnected in production since basic FGF has been found to induce activation of latent TGF-β in endothelial cell cultures by increasing plasminogen activator activity (19).

PAUL E. DICORLETO, PhD

1. Gimbrone MA Jr: Vascular endothelium: nature's blood-compatible container. Ann NY Acad Sci 516:5-11, 1987
2. Fishman AP: Endothelium: a distributed organ of diverse capabilities. Ann NY Acad Sci 401:1-8, 1982
3. DiCorleto PE, Chisolm GM: Participation of the endothelium in the development of the atherosclerotic plaque. Prog Lipid Res 25:365-374, 1986
4. Pober JS, Cotran RC: Cytokines and endothelial cell biology. Physiol Rev 70:427-451, 1990
5. Gerritsen ME, Bloor CM: Endothelial cell gene expression in response to injury. FASEB J 7:523-532, 1993
6. DiCorleto PE, Soyombo AA: The role of the endothelium in atherogenesis. Curr Opinions in Lipidol 4:364-372, 1993
7. Svensjo E, Joyner WL: The effects of intermittent and continuous stimulation of microvessels in the cheek pouch of hamsters with histamine and bradykinin on the development of venular leaky sites. Microcirc Endothelium Lymphatics 1:381-396, 1984
8. Rosenberg RD, Rosenberg JS: Natural anticoagulant mechanisms. J Clin Invest 74:1-6, 1984
9. Esmon CT: The regulation of natural anticoagulant pathways. Science 235:1348-1352, 1987
10. Dinerman JL, Lowenstein CJ, Snyder SH: Molecular mechanisms of nitric oxide regulation: potential relevance to cardiovascular disease (mini-review). Circ Res 73:217, 1993
11. Masaki T: Role of endothelin in mechanisms of local blood pressure control. J Hypertension 8(Suppl 7):S107, 1990
12. Faruqi RM, DiCorleto PE: Mechanisms of monocyte recruitment and accumulation. Br Heart J 69:S19-S29, 1993
13. Bevilacqua MP: Endothelial-leukocyte adhesion molecules. Ann Rev Immunol 11:767-804, 1993
14. Springer TA: Traffic signals for lymphocyte recirculation and leukocyte emigration: the multistep paradigm. Cell 6:301-314, 1994

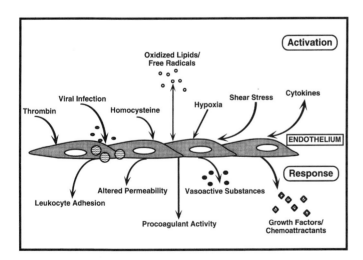

(Figure 3E-1)
Generation of a dysfunctional endothelium. A variety of stimulatory or injury-provoking agents have been implicated in the process of endothelial cell activation. Many of the responses of the endothelium are associated with the progression of vascular disease and inflammation (6).

15. Butcher EC: Leukocyte-endothelial cell recognition: three (or more) steps to specificity and diversity. Cell 67:1033-1036, 1991

16. DiCorleto PE, Fox P: Growth factor production by endothelial cells. In Ryan U (ed): Endothelial Cells, vol. 2. Boca Raton, CRC Press, 1988, pp 51-61

17. Soyombo AA, DiCorleto PE: Stable expression of human platelet-derived growth factor B chain by bovine aortic endothelial cells: cell-association and selective proteolytic cleavage by thrombin. J Biol Chem 269:17734-17740, 1994

18. Taylor WR, Nerem RM, Alexander RW: Polarized secretion of IGF-I and IGF-I binding protein activity by cultured aortic endothelial cells. J Cell Physiol 154:139-142, 1993

19. Flaumenhaft R, Abe M, Mignatti P, Rifkin DB: Basic fibroblast growth factor-induced activation of latent transforming growth factor-β in endothelial cells: regulation of plasminogen activator activity. J Cell Biol 118:901-909, 1992

F. PERIPHERAL NERVES

GENERAL STRUCTURE

The peripheral nervous system is functionally organized into motor, sensory, and autonomic components. *Motor* nerve fibers emerge from anterior horn cell bodies in the neuraxis to innervate extrafusal and intrafusal striated muscle fibers. The cell bodies of bipolar primary *sensory* neurons in dorsal root or cranial nerve ganglia give rise to fibers that innervate sensory receptors in skin, muscle, and deep tissues. Preganglionic sympathetic *autonomic* nerve cell bodies reside in the intermediolateral gray columns of the thoracic and first and second lumbar segments of the spinal cord. Their nerve fibers emerge with ventral roots and enter the sympathetic chain as white rami to synapse with sympathetic ganglion cells. These give rise to unmyelinated axons, which emerge through gray rami and innervate sweat glands and smooth muscle of blood vessels, hair follicles, and other effector organs. Preganglionic neurons of the parasympathetic system reside in the brainstem, integrating functions of cranial nerves Ill, VII, IX, and X and in the S2 through S4 segments of the spinal cord.

Peripheral nerve trunks are composed of tiny nerve fascicles, defined by perineurium, bound together through a connective epineurium. They are vascularized through an anastomotic network of longitudinal and segmental small arteries which ultimately form an endoneurial plexus of capillaries (1,2). Small-vessel occlusive disease with resultant damage to peripheral nerves most commonly occurs at the level of the epineurial arterioles.

NERVE FIBER POPULATIONS, ROLES, AND VULNERABILITY

Most peripheral nerves contain mixtures of myelinated and unmyelinated fibers. Nothing in the fiber structure distinguishes sensory from motor myelinated fibers or autonomic fibers. In nerves to human skin, unmyelinated fibers are the most abundant. Most nerves contain two populations of myelinated fibers and one of unmyelinated fibers. Nerve conduction velocity is a function of axonal diameter (and degree of myelination), a feature that is reflected in the compound nerve action potential (NAP). The different potentials are conformed through more or less synchronous conduction along nerve fibers of the different populations (3).

The components in the sensory NAP include A-alpha (30–72 meters per second), A-delta (4–30 meters per second) (4), and C (0.4–2 meters per second). In human nerves, only the fastest component of the sensory NAP can be comfortably recorded through the skin with surface electrodes (5). All three components can only be recorded in vivo through microneurography or in vitro following nerve biopsy (6). In nerves to skin, the large-diameter myelinated fibers connect with low-threshold mechanoreceptor units (RA, SA-1, SA-11) while A-delta fibers connect with cold units and with nociceptive units for sharp, "first" pain. Within the unmyelinated sensory population are represented two categories of afferent cutaneous units: the high-threshold nociceptive units for dull, "second" (C-type) pain, and units for warmth (7). In nerves to muscle, the largest diameter myelinated fibers are proprioceptive spindle afferents, whereas the smallest are the fusimotor fibers destined for the end plates of intrafusal muscle. Unmyelinated fibers connected to muscle are sympathetic efferent or sensory afferent; the latter are concerned with pain, rather than with thermal sensation.

Diseases causing selective loss of unmyelinated fibers abolish C-type pain and itch and warmth sensations and also cause dysautonomia (8). Conversely, selective block of myelinated fiber activity causes paralysis and sensory loss, except for warmth and C-type pain (9,10). Acute local nerve lesions caused by mechanical trauma tend to affect all nerve fiber types. Neurapraxia from acute local nerve compression is an exception in that it may cause a specific pathologic lesion with conduction block of large-diameter myelinated fibers only (11).

DEGENERATION AND REGENERATION

The *axoplasm* contains specialized organelles that play key roles as conduits for subcellular particle movements (12). Cellulifugal flow of axonal contents from the neuronal perikaryon is essential for maturation, maintenance, and regeneration of distal nerve fibers. In addition to the anterograde trophic influences of the cell bodies upon nerve fibers, satellite Schwann cells, and effector organs, axoplasmic transport is also channeled in a retrograde manner, allowing the periphery to feed back to the soma.

Defects in neuronal synthesis or axoplasmic transport cause disintegration of fibers and decay of target organs. The worst example is Wallerian degeneration from anatomic interruption of the axon, which leads to resorption of axons and myelin in the distal stump and denervation atrophy of target organs. In a large number of neurologic diseases, the structural nerve fiber collapse follows a "dying-back" pattern (13). It is attributable to defective synthesis or flow of trophic material. Such a pattern explains distal emphasis of weakness, wasting, sensory loss, and reflex change.

In general, regeneration of an axon involves a number of steps, including: 1) synthesis of new structural material; 2) its transport down the axon; 3) elongation of the new sprouts (at about 1 mm per day) consequent to locomotion of the growth cone and insertion of new material at the tip;

4) guidance of the sprouts to a peripheral target to re-establish a functional connection; and 5) myelination and maturation in diameter.

DEMYELINATION AND REMYELINATION

There is a single kind of Schwann cell, and yet axons may be myelinated or unmyelinated, depending upon the message given by the axon to its satellite cell. The internode (or segment) is that section of a nerve fiber subserved by a single Schwann cell, bounded by nodes of Ranvier. External to Schwann cell plasma membrane lies a continuous basement membrane (basal lamina) sleeve to which some collagen is intimately attached.

The myelin sheath is a compound unit membrane appendage and arises after cytoplasmic resorption of a Schwann cell process that has wrapped about an axon (14,15). The concentric lamellae of the myelin spiral have a periodicity of 150–180 Å between *major dense lines.* These are separated by a less-electron dense *intraperiod line.* Myelin proteins and lipids are immunogenic and may play a role in experimental allergic neuritis in animals and in idiopathic inflammatory demyelinating neuropathy in humans (16).

THE EXCITABLE MEMBRANE

The unit membrane enveloping the axon is specialized to generate all-or-nothing action potentials in response to adequate excitation. The resting membrane potential is generated largely by selective permeability: various species of ions (chiefly sodium, potassium, chloride, and large-protein anions) are unequally distributed across the plasma membrane. This electrically excitable membrane contains ion-specific, voltage-dependent channels through which ions can move to generate action potentials. These channels may be opened or closed, depending on the electrical potential across the membrane.

After a few milliseconds, sodium influx is interrupted by voltage-dependent closure of sodium channels. During this same period, voltage-regulated potassium channels open. This allows for rapid efflux of positive charges, which repolarize the membrane potential down toward its original potassium (resting) equilibrium potential. The system then remains refractory for 2–4 msec, because sodium inactivation gates remain shut until the membrane fully repolarizes. This absolute refractory period sets the limit for the maximum firing rates of nerve fibers.

Decreased membrane excitability may result from deviations in the resting membrane potential due to abnormal ionic concentration. It may also result from blocking activation of sodium channels, for example, by certain specific neurotoxins or by local anesthetic drugs. Spontaneous impulse generation from nerve fibers may produce a variety of abnormal sensory phenomena, including paresthesia and pain.

Pathologically, conduction of the action potential is slowed along thin regenerated axons. Nerve conduction is also slowed in partially demyelinated axons. Slowing of conduction in demyelinated axons may reflect either abnormally delayed "saltation" or the development of internodal voltage-dependent channels and continuous conduction, as occurs normally in unmyelinated fibers (17–19). Conduction of the action potential may be completely blocked in severe demyelination. A few layers of remyelination may transform conduction block into slowed conduction and hence restore strength to a nerve–muscle system. Patchy demyelination affecting many nerve fibers slows conduction to different extents. Functions requiring synchronous conduction of nerve volleys, such as tendon reflexes and vibration sense, are then selectively disturbed.

PERIPHERAL NEUROPATHY

Peripheral nerve disorders may be broadly categorized into two groups based on their clinical extent: polyneuropathy and mononeuropathy. Polyneuropathies are diffuse disorders presenting as various combinations of muscle weakness (with or without wasting), areflexia, and sensory and autonomic disturbance occurring in a distal-greater-than-proximal distribution that is usually rather symmetrical and affects the feet and legs before the hands and arms. Polyneuropathies may be genetically inherited or acquired from a host of metabolic, toxic, infectious, or nutritional insults. Polyneuropathies can be subclassified as primarily due to axonal degeneration or demyelination. Useful insights into the kind of pathology affecting nerve fibers can be derived from measurements of nerve conduction velocity (20).

Mononeuropathies may occur from acute or chronic mechanical compression (entrapment/ischemia), neoplastic infiltration, or granulomatous disease. Multifocal motor neuropathy may be diagnostically proved, but a genuinely pure motor neuron syndrome of a subacute or chronic nature is rarely due to polyneuropathy and often proves to be a form of anterior horn cell disease.

Paresthesias and sensory loss in a stocking-glove distribution are common symptoms of polyneuropathy. On examination, weakness is greater in a distal distribution in most forms of polyneuropathy, and is usually seen in the feet before the hands. There are notable exceptions to this rule, however. Cranial nerve involvement in polyneuropathy is uncommon. Muscle wasting is not to be expected in pure demyelinating neuropathy or in axonal neuropathies of recent onset. Intact tendon (stretch) reflexes require the normal functioning of spindle afferent nerve fibers, alpha motor neuron fibers to extrafusal muscle, and gamma motor neuron output for appropriate tuning of the intrafusal spindle apparatus. In polyneuropathy, reflexes are lost or diminished in keeping with an axonal dying-back pattern of sensorimotor dysfunction or in keeping with desynchronization of the nerve volleys from demyelination. Brisk reflexes in the setting of a polyneuropathy should suggest concurrent damage of spinal cord and peripheral nerves. Joint deformity might be a consequence of peripheral neuropathy. Indeed, Charcot joints, thought to result from loss of joint nociception, can be a dramatic manifestation of chronic sensory neuropathies, such as diabetic neuropathy and Charcot–Marie–Tooth disease.

JOHN E. CASTALDO, MD
JOSÉ OCHOA, MD

1. Adams WE: The blood supply of nerves. 1. Historical review. J Anat 76:323-341, 1942

2. Sunderland S: Nerve and Nerve Injuries. New York, Churchill Livingstone, 1978

3. Erlanger J, Gasser HS: The compound nature of the action current of nerve as disclosed by the cathode ray oscillograph. Am J Physiol 70:624-666, 1924

4. Burgess PR, Perl ER: Cutaneous mechanoreceptors and noci-receptors. In Iggo A (ed): Handbook of Sensory Physiology, vol. 2. Berlin, Springer Verlag, 1973, pp 29-78

5. Dawson GD: The relative excitability and conduction velocity of sensory and motor nerve fibers in man. J Physiol 131:436-451, 1956

6. Lambert EH, Dyck PJ: Compound action potentials of sural nerve in vitro in peripheral neuropathy. In Dyck PJ, Thomas PK, Lambert EH (eds): Peripheral Neuropathy. Philadelphia, WB Saunders, 1975, pp 427-441

7. Vallbo AB, Hagbarth K-E, Torebjörk HE, Wallin BG: Somatosensory, proprioceptive, and sympathetic activity in human PC peripheral nerves. Physiol Rev 59:919-957, 1979

8. Dyck JP, Lambert EH: Dissociated sensation in amyloidosis. Arch Neurol 20:490-507, 1969

9. Lewis T, Pickering GW, Rothschild P: Centripetal paralysis arising out of arrested blood flow to the limb, including notes on a form of tingling. Heart 16:1-32, 1931

10. Kugelberg E: Accommodation in human nerves. Acta Physiol Scand 8(Suppl 24):1-105, 1944

11. Ochoa J, Fowler TJ, Gilliatt RW: Anatomical changes in peripheral nerves compressed by pneumatic tourniquet. J Anat 113:433-455, 1972

12. Tsukita S, Ishikawa H: The cytoskeleton in myelinated axons: serial section study. Biomed Res 2:424, 1981

13. Cavanagh JB: The significance of the "dying-back" process in experimental and human neurological disease. Int Rev Exp Pathol 3:219-267, 1964

14. Geren BB: The formation from the Schwann cell surface of myelin in the peripheral nerves of chick embryos. Exp Cell Res 7:558-562, 1954

15. Robertson JD: The ultrastructure of adult vertebrate peripheral myelinated nerve fiber in relation to myelinogenesis. J Biophys Biochem Cytol 1:271-278, 1955

16. Waksman BH, Adams RD: Allergic neuritis: an experimental disease of rabbits induced by the injection of peripheral nervous tissue and adjuvant. J Exp Med 102:213-236, 1955

17. Rasminsky M: Physiology of conduction in demyelinated axons. In Waxen SAG (ed): Physiology and Pathobiology of Axons. New York, Raven Press, 1978, pp 361-376

18. Bostock H, Sears TA: The internodal axon membrane: electrical excitability and continuous conduction in segmental demyelination. J Physiol 280:273-301, 1978

19. Bostock H: Conduction changes in mammalian axons following experimental demyelination. In Culp WJ, Ochoa J (eds): Abnormal Nerves and Muscles as Impulse Generators. New York, Oxford University Press, 1982, pp 236-252

20. Gilliatt RW: Nerve conduction in human and experimental neuropathies. Proc Royal Soc Med 59:989-993,1966

STRUCTURE

A. COLLAGEN AND ELASTIN

COLLAGENS

The extracellular matrix consists of highly organized tissue-specific arrangements of collagens, elastins, proteoglycans, and other glycoproteins. Collagen is the most abundant component of the extracellular matrix and, in fact, is the most abundant protein in the body, comprising over 20% of lean body mass. It is the structural foundation of connective tissues; its characteristic triple helical rods confer strength to tissues by their molecular organization into fibrils or networks. In the organs and tissues comprising the musculoskeletal system (ie, tendons, cartilage, bone, fascia) collagen fibrils organize in such a way as to maximize the resistance of tissues to physical forces. In other tissues such as basement membrane, the collagen framework contributes to more specialized functions such as filtration and cell adhesion.

Collagen Structure

All collagens are defined by certain structural features. All collagen molecules are trimers consisting of three polypeptides designated alpha chains. These trimers can consist of three identical alpha chains (homotrimers) or different alpha chains (heterotrimers). A significant portion of the trimeric molecule is organized into a right-handed helix formed by the characteristic primary structure in which every third residue is a glycine, which is sufficiently small to fit into the restricted space at the center of the helix. Thus, the primary structure of the helical region of an alpha chain can be depicted as (Gly-X-Y)n. A characteristic property of collagen is its resistance to degradation by nonspecific proteinases. This trait is specific to the helical domains, whereas the nonhelical extensions and interruptions tend to be proteinase sensitive. Helical regions of collagen require the action of specific collagenases for proteolysis.

The helical regions are enriched with proline and its hydroxylated form, hydroxyproline. These two amino acids combined account for approximately 25% of the amino acids. Proline commonly occupies the X position, while hydroxyproline is frequently found in the Y position. These ring amino acids are essential for the formation and integrity of the helix and maintain the alpha chains in an extended position. Other amino acids are represented in the helical regions except for tyrosine and tryptophan. Disulfide bridges between alpha chains occur in certain collagens and exist in the carboxy-terminal noncollagenous domain (telopeptide) of type I collagen. The presence of lysine and its hydroxylated form, hydroxylysine, is also important in the structure of collagen molecules, because these residues form the basis for oxidative cross-links between alpha chains and between collagen molecules. As collagen becomes more cross-linked, it becomes more resistant to degradation.

Deviations from the (Gly-X-Y)n structure of alpha chains occur in virtually all collagen chains. In fibrillar collagens (types I, II, III, V, and XI), nonhelical or noncollagenous sequences are found in amino-terminal and carboxy-terminal domains. These terminal nonhelical domains are important in molecular assembly and perhaps in the association with cells or other matrix proteins. In fibrillar collagens, most of the terminal nonhelical domains are cleaved from the molecule upon secretion as procollagen and fibrillogenesis, resulting in molecules with a large rigid, helical region (Fig. 4A-1). In other collagen species (types IV, VII, IX, XII, etc.), interruptions in this sequence motif occur within the alpha chains separating helical domains, allowing the molecule to bend or to interact with other molecules.

Classification of Collagens

The isolation, identification, and characterization of collagens have evolved technically from direct tissue extraction through cell culture isolation of secreted collagen to the identification of cDNAs and mRNAs encoding collagens. To date, at least 18 collagen types have been identified representing the products of at least 30 genes (1,2). To add to this complexity, some collagen genes contain alternate promoters, and alternative splicing has been described. Because some of these collagens have been isolated only at the DNA level, it is likely that some of these designations represent collagenous proteins that are not extracellular matrix components. In addition to the structural characteristics defined above, it is generally accepted that the protein should be a component of the extracellular matrix before it can be classified as a collagen. It has been known for some time that certain nonmatrix proteins not classified as collagens contain collagenous domains, such as acetylcholinesterase and C1q. Evidence suggests that several of the more recently identified collagens may be cell membrane components (types XIII and XVII) (3), raising the question whether they should be considered collagens.

The general convention regarding nomenclature of collagens is that the trimeric collagen molecule is designated by a roman numeral assigned in the order of discovery. The constituent alpha chains are numbered with Arabic numer-

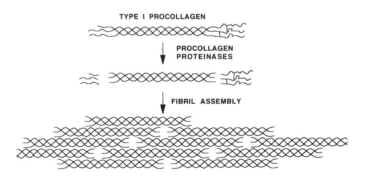

(Figure 4A-1)
Extracellular processing of type I collagen. Type I collagen is secreted from the cell with amino- and carboxy-terminal extensions or propeptides. Specific peptidases cleave the propeptides resulting in a marked reduction in solubility. The central, helical region retains short, nonhelical sequences and assembles in a near-quarter stagger fashion into fibrils. The other fibrillar collagens are similarly processed.

als and a suffix of the roman numeral corresponding to the collagen type. Thus, type I collagen consists of two α1 chains or α1(I) and one α2 chain or α2(I), and its molecular constitution would be defined as [α1(I)2 α2(I)]. The homotrimeric type II collagen would be described as [α1 (II)]3. The nomenclature of the genes encoding for these alpha chains follows a similar convention; the gene is designated as COLXAY where X is the collagen type represented by the roman numeral and Y being the alpha chain represented by the Arabic numeral.

There have been several attempts to classify collagens according to structural characteristics and function. The task is difficult as several collagens are unique and defy classification. Thus, the classification in Table 4A-1 includes only those proteins that are relatively well-characterized and are extracellular matrix components.

Fibrillar Collagens

The major identifiable structure in tissue associated with collagen is the cross-striated fibril. Fibrillar collagens (types I, II, III, V, and XI) are classified as such because of their association with these fibrillar tissue structures or their tendency in vitro to aggregate into striated fibrils. The fibrillar collagens share certain structural characteristics. Each alpha chain has a major helical domain without interruption that consists of approximately 1000 amino acid residues. Nonhelical domains (telopeptides) extend both termini, the carboxy-terminal telopeptide being somewhat conserved whereas the

(Table 4A-1)
Classification of collagens*

Collagen Type	Composition	Distribution
Fibrillar Collagens		
I	[α1(I)]2, α2(I)	Bone, tendon, skin, cornea, etc.
II	[α1(II)]3	Hyaline cartilage, vitreous
III	[α1(III)]3	Blood vessels, gut, skin
V	[α1(V)]2, α2(V)	Bone, skin, cornea, etc.
XI	α1(XI), α2(XI), α3(XI)	Hyaline cartilage
FACIT Collagens		
IX	α1(IX), α2(IX), α3(IX)	Hyaline cartilage, vitreous
XII	α1(XII)3	Skin, tendon
XIV	α1(XIV)3	Similar to type I
Other Collagens		
IV	[α1(IV)]2, α2(IV) also α3-6(IV)	Basement membranes
VI	α1(VI), α2(VI), α3(VI)	Skin, cartilage, etc.
VII	α1(VII)3	Anchoring fibrils
VIII	[α1(VIII)]2, α2(VII)	Descemet's membrane, endothelial cells
X	α1(X)3	Growth plate cartilage

*FACIT = Fibril-associated collagens with interrupted triple helices

amino-terminal telopeptide is variable. These terminal extensions are processed by partial cleavage by specific peptidases during synthesis, secretion, and assembly.

Type I collagen is the major fibrillar collagen in the body and is found primarily in bone, tendon, ligament, skin, and fascia. It is classically found in a heterotrimeric form, although homotrimers of the α1(I) chain have been described but their function is not known. Type II collagen is the major fibrillar collagen of articular cartilage and the vitreous of the eye. This collagen is enriched in hydroxylysine, is more highly glycosylated than type I collagen, and is less readily degraded by collagenases. Alternative splicing of transcripts results in different molecular forms, which have been found in tissue. Type III collagen is a homotrimer (α1(III))3 found in blood vessels, skin, and synovial tissue, but not in bone. This collagen contains interchain disulfide bonds within the helical domain. Type V collagen consists of two different alpha chains, α1(V) and α2(V), and is found as a heterotrimer with two alpha 1 chains or as homotrimers of either chain. It is found in most of the same tissues as type I collagen. Type XI collagen is analogous to type V collagen, but is found in articular cartilage and the ocular vitreous along with type II collagen. It consists of heterotrimers of three different chains, α1, α2, and α3.

Pure preparations of types I and III collagen studied in vitro have been found to aggregate into typical-looking collagen fibrils, which led to the widespread belief that tissue fibrils consisted of a single collagen type. Recent studies, however, have demonstrated that both interstitial fibrils in type I collagen-rich tissues and cartilage collagen fibrils are heterotypic. For example, cartilage fibrils contain types II and XI collagen and are associated on the fibrillar surface with collagen type IX. A similar observation has been made regarding the co-localization of collagen types I and V and the association of types XII or XIV.

Gene mutations have been identified that result in underproduction of types I, II, and III collagen in tissues. Relative underproduction of type I collagen is associated with osteogenesis imperfecta, which is characterized by brittle bones or skeletal deformities, thin blue sclerae, and abnormal tooth development. Similarly, underproduction of type II collagen results in chondrodysplasia, including Stickler's syndrome. Type IV Ehlers-Danlos' syndrome, which is characterized by loose joints and rupture of bowel and major blood vessels, is associated with mutations in the α1(III) collagen gene.

Fibril-Associated Collagens with Interrupted Triple Helices (FACIT)

This category of collagens is characterized by alternating noncollagenous (NC) domains and helical (COL) domains. Although FACIT collagens do not form fibrils independently, they are associated with the major fibrils comprising types I and II collagen. Hence the designation *Fibril-Associated Collagens with Interrupted Triple Helices*. The best studied of these collagens is type IX, which is found in articular cartilage in association with the striated collagen. Type IX collagen is a heterotrimer composed of three different chains (α1, α2, and α3) and contains two collagenous domains that associate with the striated fibril and covalently with type II collagen. A noncollagenous domain separates these two collagenous domains from a third collagenous domain, providing ample flexibility that allows the third domain to extend into the interfibrillar space. A large, highly charged N-terminal noncollagenous domain (NC4) is presumed to interact with other matrix components. The α2(XI) chain contains a large glycosaminoglycan, the function of which is unknown. Fig. 4A-2 depicts the molecular structure of type IX collagen and its relationship with type II collagen fibrils and may serve as a model for the other FACIT collagen.

Types XII and XIV collagen have primary structures similar to that of type IX and are associated with type I collagen fibrils in the same relationship that type IX is associated with type II collagen fibrils. Type XII collagen is a homotrimer with only two collagenous domains and three noncollagenous domains.

Basement Membrane Collagen

Basement membrane is a highly specialized connective tissue composed of unique connective tissue proteins, including laminin, nidogen, entactin, and type IV collagen. The foundation for basement membranes is a delicate network formed by the assembly of type IV collagen molecules. Type IV collagen is a complex protein with long alpha chains (150 kD), two large terminal noncollagenous domains rich in cysteine and disulfide bridges, and multiple interruptions of the helical sequence. The major species of type IV collagen is a heterotrimer consisting of two α1(IV) chains and one α2(IV) chain, although several forms of type IV collagen must exist because six distinct alpha chains have been identified. Unlike the fibrillar collagens, type IV collagen assembles into three-dimensional networks (Fig. 4A-3). Four amino-terminal domains associate into the proteinase-resistant 7s domain, and the four extending large carboxy-terminal noncollagenous (NC1) domains associate tail-to-tail with other type IV collagen tetrad. Side-to-side association of collagen molecules provides a three-dimensional network presumably important in the filtration function of basement membranes (4). Fig. 4A-3 depicts the assembly of type IV collagen networks.

The type IV collagen molecule contains the antigen associated with autoantibodies in Goodpasture's syndrome. Specifically, the putative antigen is contained within the NC1 domain of the α3(IV) chain. Furthermore, mutations in

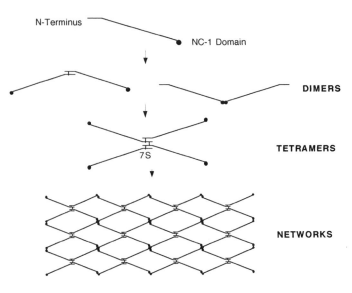

(Figure 4A-3)
Assembly of basement membrane (type IV) collagen into networks. The native type IV collagen molecule has multiple interruptions and imperfections in the helical sequences resulting in flexible regions. Assembly of type IV collagen is by dimerization through "tail-to-tail" interaction between two C-terminal noncollagenous domains (NC-1) and by tetramer-formation through N-terminal interactions. Cross-link formation in the N-terminal region results in a proteinase-resistant region known as 7S collagen. Networks then form resembling "chicken wire" in a two-dimensional orientation. Side-to-side interactions between molecules and networks result in a three-dimensional network.

the α5(IV) collagen gene have been associated with a form of Alport's syndrome characterized by hereditary nephritis and deafness.

Other Collagens

Type VI collagen is widely distributed in cartilage, skin, blood vessels, and other interstitial tissues. Three alpha chains have been identified, and the native molecule is probably a heterotrimer, more than two-thirds of which is noncollagenous in nature since it is formed by two large terminal nonhelical domains. Type VI collagen is the major component of beaded filaments seen in a variety of tissues by electron microscopy. Fig. 4A-4 shows how type VI collagen molecules assemble into dimers and tetramers in a head-to-toe fashion and polymerize to form beaded filaments.

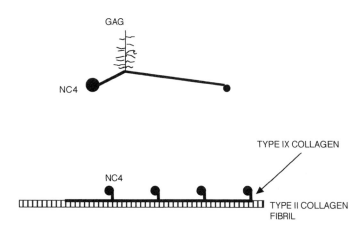

(Figure 4A-2)
Type IX collagen and its relation to type II collagen fibrils. The molecular structure of type IX collagen is displayed with its characteristic "kink" near the carboxy terminus, a large, C-terminal noncollagenous domain, and a proteoglycan component of the α2(IX) chain at the kink region. This collagen associates with type II collagen fibrils with the NC4 domain exposed on the fibril surface. Other FACIT collagens probably interact with other fibrils in a similar manner.

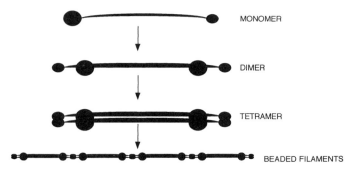

(Figure 4A-4)
Type VI collagen assembly and formation of beaded filaments. The native type VI collagen molecule contains a central helical region and two large terminal globular domains. Dimers form by anti-parallel association of two type VI collagen molecules and side-to-side association of dimers forms tetramers that then associate end-to-end to form beaded filaments found in many tissues.

Type VII collagen is a long-chain homotrimeric molecule. It is the largest collagen described to date. Type VII collagen is the major component of anchoring fibrils and is found exclusively in association with these structures. The molecule contains a complex, trident-like, carboxy-terminal, noncollagenous domain; the fibrils are formed by antiparallel dimerization through the association of two amino-terminal noncollagenous domains that are stabilized through cross-link formation. Mutations of type VII collagen are associated with a dystrophic form of epidermolysis bullosa.

Types VIII and X collagen are often classified as short-chain collagens because of the striking sequence homology between their respective alpha chains; however, their tissue distributions are quite different. These collagens are about half the length of interstitial collagens and consist of a single collagenous domain flanked by two noncollagenous domains. Type VIII collagen is a poorly understood protein that was originally found in endothelial cell cultures and subsequently in other tissues, including Descemet's membrane. It is a heterotrimer and its distribution in Descemet's membrane corresponds to a hexagonal lattice array. Type X collagen is a short-chain homotrimer found exclusively in hypertrophic cartilage which may play a role in enchondral ossification.

Recent investigations at the DNA level have identified several genes encoding collagenous proteins. Although these proteins have been assigned collagen type numbers, their presence in the tissues as matrix constituents and their role in biology have yet to be clarified. Two of these putative collagens, types XIII and XVII, are associated with the cell membrane. At least two other membrane components, macrophage scavenger receptor and C1q, possess collagenous sequences. Therefore, it is possible that types XIII and XVII collagens are related to these receptor proteins. Type XVI collagen resembles a FACIT collagen, but its role requires further clarification. Types XV and XVIII collagen are homologous proteins found in several tissues, but their roles are not clear (3).

Collagen Biosynthesis, Post-translational Modifications, and Processing

The process of collagen biosynthesis and ultimate incorporation as a structural element in the extracellular matrix is a complex series of intracellular and extracellular events, each of which is essential to molecular assembly. Understanding of synthesis and processing of collagen is derived largely from studies of the major fibrillar collagens, especially type I collagen. Thus, post-translational modifications of the nascent collagen chains and processing of the triple helix relate specifically to the formation of collagen fibrils. Although certain of the specific processes (eg, prolyl hydroxylation) are involved in the biosynthesis of all collagens, other molecular modifications (eg, procollagen processing and cross-link formation) may not be as relevant to the assembly of nonfibrillar collagens.

The transcription of collagen genes and translation of collagen mRNA proceeds in a manner similar to the expression of other genes. The nascent pro-alpha chains of the major fibrillar collagens are approximately 150,000 kD, considerably longer than the alpha chains found in mature collagen fibrils (95,000 kD). Disulfide bonds form between the carboxy-terminal nonhelical extensions of three alpha chains, which enable their folding into a triple helix. Hydroxylation of proline (which is dependent on ascorbate, iron, and α-ketoglutarate-dependent) is essential to helix formation.

Collagen comprised of under-hydroxylated proline residues form poor helices. Proline hydroxylase catalyzes the hydroxylation of approximately one-half the propyl residues, and the molecule folds in its wake. In addition to proline, several lysine residues are also hydroxylated and certain hydroxylysines are glycosylated. The hydroxylation and glycosylation of lysine is essential for the formation of inter- and intramolecular cross-links.

These procollagen molecules are transported to the extracellular space where specific procollagen peptidases cleave the amino- and carboxy-terminal propeptides to form the native collagen molecule. These proteolytic steps result in a reduction in the solubility of collagen, and the helices spontaneously assemble into fibrils in a near-quarter stagger fashion (Fig. 4A-1). Intramolecular cross-links form to stabilize the fibrils. It is now clear that these collagen fibrils are heterotypic containing or associating with other collagen types. The process by which types V, XI, IX, XII, and other collagens are incorporated into fibrils is not well understood. Co-translational events and post-translational modification of collagen are summarized in Table 4A-2.

Type IV collagen, in contrast to the fibrillar collagens, organizes into networks that form the structural foundation for basement membranes. The biosynthesis of type IV collagen has been studied and is similar to that of the fibrillar collagens, except that extracellular proteolytic processing does not occur. Instead, intact procollagen chains fold intracellularly into triple helices, which are secreted, and assemble in a network fashion. These networks form through the tail-to-tail (C-termini) formation of dimers and the head-to-head (N-termini) formation of tetrameres (Fig. 4A-2). Side-to-side association extends the network into a three dimensional structure (5).

Collagen Gene Structure and Regulation

At least 25 genes encoding collagen α chains have been identified. The genes encoding fibrillar collagen (COL1A1, COL1A2, COL2A1, and COL3A1) have multiple short coding regions (exons) between which are large noncoding introns. Most of the exons measure 54 base pairs or multiples of 54 bases, suggesting that the ancestral collagen gene encoded 9 amino acids or three Gly-X-Y triplets. Furthermore,

(Table 4A-2)
Post-transcriptional events and post-translational modification of collagen

Events	Enzymes and Co-factors
Intracellular events	
Proline hydroxylation	Prolyl hydroxylase, ascorbate, iron, α-ketoglutarate
Lysine hydroxylation	Lysyl hydroxylase
Glycosylation of hydroxylysines	Galactosyl transferase and glucosyl transferase
C-terminal disulfide bridge formation and helical assembly	
Secretion	
Extracellular events	
Cleavage of N- and C-termini	Procollagen N-peptidase and C-peptidase
Cross-link formation	Lysyl oxidase, copper
Fibrillogenesis	

the fibrillar collagen genes each contain 52–54 exons. Other collagen genes differ significantly from this motif.

Most understanding of collagen gene regulation is derived from extensive studies of type I collagen gene expression. The synthesis of type I collagen requires the coordinate expression of two genes encoding α chains. The expression of type I collagen is tissue-specific (skin, bone, etc.) and must be under tight regulatory control. Regulatory functions are associated with both cis-regulatory elements and trans-acting factors.

Major regulatory elements have been identified in the 5′ flanking or promoter region. The promoter region contains both positive and negative elements, including a CCAAT motif that interacts with a specific binding protein and induces transcription. Binding sites for ubiquitous transcription factors have been found in the promoter region and in the first intron. The role of these elements and the interaction between DNA binding proteins in the 5′ flanking region, as well as the putative regulatory elements in the first intron, appear to be quite complex and remain to be clarified.

Factors that Modulate Collagen Gene Expression

A variety of substances have been identified as extracellular signals that influence the expression of collagen genes. These include cytokines, growth factors, hormones, and other compounds present in the cellular milieu in both physiologic and pathologic conditions. A partial list of these factors is listed in Table 4A-3.

The amino propeptides of types I and III collagen have been shown to inhibit collagen gene expression in vitro, which may play a major role in normal growth and remodeling as a negative feedback mechanism. Transforming growth factor β (TGF-β) is thought to be important in modulating collagen gene expression in pathologic states. This cytokine stimulates excess matrix deposition in vivo and in vitro. It stimulates collagen synthesis by increasing the transcription rate and by stabilizing mRNA. Interferon gamma, another inflammatory cytokine, has exactly the opposite effect and may be considered counter-regulatory to TGF-β. (See references 5 and 6 for reviews of this subject.)

(Table 4A-3)
*Factors that regulate collagen gene expression**

Factors that increase collagen production
  Transforming growth factor-β
  Interleukin 1
  Interleukin 4
  Insulin-like growth factor
  Ascorbate
  Insulin
  Bradykinin
  Products of lipid peroxidation
Factors that decrease collagen production
  Procollagen propeptides
  Glucocorticoids
  γ Interferon
Factors that increase cAMP (PGE$_2$)
  Retinoic acid
  Epidermal growth factor

---

*cAMP = cyclic adenosine monophosphate; PGE = prostaglandin E.

Collagen Degradation

The helical structure of collagens confers a resistance to general proteolysis. Thus, collagens with large, central, uninterrupted triple helical domains were thought to be proteinase resistant until the characterization of vertebrate collagenase, which makes a single cleavage through the triple helices of types I, II, and III collagen. It is now known that vertebrate collagenase is a metalloproteinase and belongs to a class known as the matrix metalloproteinases. This family consists of at least nine distinct enzymes, each capable of degrading one or more components of the extracellular matrix.

ELASTIN AND ELASTIC FIBERS

Elastic fibers provide resiliency and elasticity to tissues and are particularly rich in ligaments, large blood vessels, lung, skin, and certain specialized connective tissues such as the ocular zonule. There are two components to the elastic fibers: an amorphous element composed mainly of the protein tropoelastin and a microfibrillar element composed of fibrillin and other proteins.

Tropoelastin is a single polypeptide with a molecular weight of 72,000 and a unique amino acid composition. The protein consists of hydrophobic domains made primarily of glycine, valine, proline, and alanine alternating with hydrophilic regions rich in lysine residues. The structure of the gene encoding for elastin mirrors this domain structure as the hydrophilic domains and hydrophobic regions are encoded by different exons (reviewed in reference 7).

The lysyl residues of elastin are virtually all enzymatically oxidized through the action of lysyl oxidase, a copper-dependent enzyme found in elastic fibers. These residues form interchain and intrachain cross-links including desmosine and isodesmosine. The resulting network of elastic fibers in tissue is resistant to extraction, boiling, and proteolysis by nonspecific proteinases. Specific elastases are required for enzymatic degradation of elastin.

The human gene encoding the elastin protein consists of 34 exons. Alternative splicing appears to occur commonly with transcription, resulting in a variety of species of elastin whose roles are unknown. The expression of the elastin gene is up-regulated by TGF-β and down-regulated by TNF-α and vitamin D$_3$.

The major protein of the microfibrillar element is a 360-kD glycoprotein known as fibrillin. At least two fibrillins have been identified and are of interest to rheumatologists. Marfan's syndrome has been associated with mutations in fibrillin 1. Manifestations of Marfan's syndrome include abnormalities of tissues rich in elastic fibrils such as ligaments (loose-jointedness), large blood vessels (aortic aneurysms), and ocular zonule (lens subluxation). A gene encoding fibrillin has been linked to congenital contractual arachnodactyly.

CARLO L. MAINARDI, MD

1. van Der Rest M, Garrone R: Collagen family of proteins. FASEB J 5:2814-2823, 1991

2. Burgeson RE, Nimni ME: Collagen types: molecular structure and tissue distribution. Clin Orthop 282:250-272, 1992

3. Pihlajaniemi T, Rehn M: Two new collagen subgroups: membrane-associated collagens and types XV and XVIII. Prog Nucleic Acid Res Mol Biol 50:225-262, 1995

4. Kuhn K: Basement membrane (type IV) collagen. Matrix Biol 14:439-445, 1995

5. Varga J, Jiminez SA: Modulation of collagen gene expression: its relation to fibrosis in systemic sclerosis and other disorders. Ann Intern Med 122:60-62, 1995

6. Rossert JA, Garrett LA: Regulation of type I collagen synthesis. Kidney Int 59(Suppl):S34-S38, 1995

7. Christiano AM, Uitto J: Molecular pathology of the elastic fiber. J Invest Derm 103 (Suppl 5):53s-56s, 1994

B. PROTEOGLYCANS

The proteoglycans are a diverse group of uniquely gly-cosylated proteins that are ubiquitous in the body and most abundant in the extracellular matrix of connective tissues. Like glycoproteins, proteoglycans often contain both N-linked and O-linked oligosaccharides. However, the ad-dition of one or more sulfated glycosaminoglycan side chains to the protein core distinguishes this group of com-plex glycoconjugates as proteoglycans. Glycosaminoglycans are linear anionic polysaccharides with repeating disaccha-ride units containing a hexosamine residue and usually, but not always, a hexuronic acid residue. Proteoglycans display a broad diversity of structures and sizes that are well corre-lated with their vast array of functions within tissues. How-ever, one functional property common to all proteoglycans is the capacity to provide a high-density source of fixed neg-ative charges within the extracellular matrix. In some tissues such as cartilage, proteoglycans are also highly concentrated (to about 100 mg/ml) and are compressed within the matrix to approximately 20% of their maximum extended volume (1). This compression of negatively charged molecules, en-trapped within a collagen network and not freely mobile, provides the osmotic pressure needed to withstand physio-logic loads that can reach 100 to 200 atmospheres within mil-liseconds upon standing (eg, in articular cartilage of the lower extremities). Particular functional attributes of proteo-glycans may reside in the glycosaminoglycan structure or in the core protein. At present, 20 separate genes have been identified that code for proteins and have the capacity to carry one or more glycosaminoglycan side chains (Table 4B-1). Once the nucleic acid sequence of a proteoglycan core protein gene product has been described and documented, the core proteins are often given functional names such as *aggrecan*, *decorin*, and *lumican* (2). However, it should be noted that any given proteoglycan found within a tissue may be the product of extensive post-transcriptional modi-fications, including alternative splicing or the use of differ-ent start sites of a particular core protein mRNA, followed by variations in glycosaminoglycan type and structure as well as selective proteolytic processing that occurs post-translationally (3). Thus, for some proteoglycans, no simple nomenclature is adequate, and often a combination nomen-clature of named core protein plus glycosaminoglycan type or tissue type of origin is often used (eg, chondroitin sulfate decorin and corneal decorin).

GLYCOSAMINOGLYCANS

The glycosaminoglycan side chains found on a particular core protein are commonly divided into three basic groups: *chondroitins, heparins,* and *keratan sulfates.* The chondroitins contain a linear (ie, nonbranching), repeating, N-acetyl-galactosamine-glucuronic acid disaccharide structure com-monly sulfated at the 4 or 6 position of the hexosamine residue to yield chondroitin-4-sulfate (chondroitin sulfate A) or chondroitin-6-sulfate (chondroitin sulfate C). Postsynthe-sis epimerization of glucuronic acid residues of chondroitin-4-sulfate to iduronic acid yields the dermatan sulfate (chon-droitin sulfate B). It should be noted that many of the chondroitin glycosaminoglycans exist as composite poly-

(Table 4B-1)

Summary of proteoglycan properties*

Proteoglycan	Interacts with:	Glycosamin-oglycan	Predominant Tissue Localization
Aggrecan	Hyaluronan	CS/KS	Load-bear-ing tissues (eg, carti-lage, aorta, disc, ten-don)
Versican	Hyaluronan	CS	Ubiquitous, fibrous
Decorin	Collagen types I and II	CS or DS	Ubiquitous
Biglycan	Collagen type VI	CS or DS	Ubiquitous
Fibromodulin	Collagen types I and II	KS	Ubiquitous
Collagen IX	Collagen type II	CS	Cartilage
Syndecan-1	Cell membranes	HS/CS	Epithelial cells
Syndecan-2 (fibroglycan)	Cell membranes	HS/CS	Ubiquitous
Syndecan-3 (N-syndecan)	Cell membranes	HS/CS	Ubiquitous
Syndecan-4 (ryudocan or amphi-glycan)	Cell membranes	HS/CS	Ubiquitous
Glypican	Cell membranes via glycosyl phosphati-dylinositol	HS	Ubiquitous
Serglycin	—	Heparin	Mast cells
Perlecan	Basement membranes	HS	Basement membranes

*Other proteoglycans include: lumican; betaglycan; thrombomodulin; CD44; neurocan; brevican; BEHAB; and osteoadherin.
CS = chondroitin sulfate; DS = dermatan sulfate; KS = keratan sulfate; HS = heparan sulfate.

mers containing hybrid regions along the polysaccharide chain of nonsulfated, 4-sulfated, 6-sulfated, or iduronic acid–containing disaccharides (2). Although known to exist and to be highly regulated by cells, the specific function(s) of these composite glycosaminoglycan structures is incom-pletely understood. The length of chondroitin glycosamino-glycan chains vary, but are seldom more than 200–250 disaccharides (100,000 Da). Keratan sulfates are generally shorter glycosaminoglycans (20–40 disaccharide units) con-taining repeating galactose, N-acetylglucosamine disaccha-ride units that primarily contain sulfate residues at the 6-po-sition of the galactose, the N-acetylglucosamine, or both. The ends of keratan sulfate chains may also be capped by sialic acid residues (2). With such structures, keratan sulfates have been suggested to represent an evolutionary link between glycoproteins and proteoglycans. The heparin glycosaminoglycans exhibit a basic repeating glucuronic acid-N-acetylglucosamine disaccharide structure; however, the presence of alternating α- and β-glycosidic linkages differentiates heparins from all other glycosaminoglycans that are typically all β-linkages. This feature is important because many enzymes that degrade glycosaminoglycans typically have strict specificities for either α- or β-glycosidic linkages. The basic heparin sequence is subsequently sulfated and modified following polymerization. The modifications of heparin glycosaminoglycans are more extensive and specific than those of any other in this family. Examples include unique patterns of sulfation of the uronic acid and hexosamine hydroxyl group, N-deacetylation followed by N-sulfation of the hexosamines, and epimerization of particular glucuronic acid residues to iduronic acid. The degree of modification is sufficient to embed information and specificity within the polysaccharide structure. Historically, the less-modified heparin glycosaminoglycans are termed *heparan sulfates* and the more "mature" glycosaminoglycans, *heparins*.

Heparin as well as chondroitin glycosaminoglycans are linked via an O-glycosidic bond to a core protein via a common tetrasaccharide linkage unit: xylosyl-galactose-galactose-glucuronic acid (2). The linkage region is added to the core protein co-translationally via interaction of the reducing end of the xylose with the hydroxyl of a serine residue of the core protein. A predominant consensus sequence of serine followed immediately by glycine is required for xylosylation of the core protein. Keratan sulfate is attached to core proteins via two modes: a branched hexasaccharide linkage unit O-linked to serine residues, or a branched oligosaccharide linkage unit N-linked to asparagine residues. Keratan sulfate in cartilage is generally attached via O-glycosidic linkages and in cornea via N-glycosylamine linkages.

Another member of the family of glycosaminoglycans is the macromolecule *hyaluronan*. Hyaluronan has a β-linked, repeating glucuronic acid-N-acetylglucosamine disaccharide structure and thus is similar to the glycosaminoglycans described above. However, hyaluronan is not associated with a core protein, is not substituted with sulfate, and exists as a linear nonbranching polymer about 150 times longer than any other glycosaminoglycan with a molecular mass up to 6×10^6 Daltons, ~13,700 disaccharides (Fig. 4B-1). Also, unlike the other glycosaminoglycans, which are synthesized predominately within the Golgi apparatus, hyaluronan is synthesized via a synthase complex within the plasma membrane (4). Thus, it is not surprising that hyaluronan is also the only glycosaminoglycan synthesized by prokaryotes. In some tissues or at specific developmental stages, hyaluronan functions as an independent glycosaminoglycan, but in many tissues it functions as the backbone of a tightly bound supramolecular complex, the proteoglycan aggregate.

PROTEOGLYCANS THAT INTERACT WITH HYALURONAN

Upon secretion into the extracellular matrix, several proteoglycans self-assemble into larger supramolecular structures by binding to filaments of hyaluronan (Fig. 4B-2). All

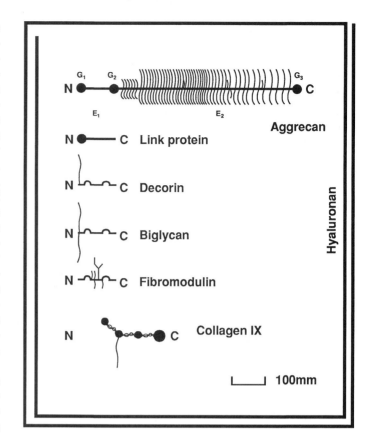

(Figure 4B-1)
Structure of some common proteoglycans. Some of the prototypical proteoglycans found in the extracellular matrix of many connective tissues are depicted at approximate scale for each of the molecules at full extension. Note the length of the hyaluronan that nearly twice frames the other macromolecules. The structural domains of the aggrecan core protein (G_1, G_2, G_3, E_1, and E_2) are also depicted. Courtesy of P.J. Roughley; adapted with permission.

proteoglycans within this group possess a tandem repeat structure within their core protein at the amino-terminal region that is responsible for the specific high-affinity binding to the hyaluronan filament (5,6). Included in this proteoglycan tandem repeat (PTR) family are the proteoglycans *aggrecan, versican, brevican, neurocan, CD44,* and *brain-enriched hyaluronan-binding protein (BEHAP)* (6,7). Aggrecan is by far the best documented, and its structure may be used as the prototype for the PTR family. Aggrecan is the predominant proteoglycan in cartilage, comprising about 90% of the proteoglycan mass in articular cartilage (1,6). Human aggrecan contains a protein core (M_r 254 kD) encoded by 19 exons, with each exon essentially defining a particular protein domain (8). The aggrecan core protein is substituted with two types of glycosaminoglycans, keratan sulfate and chondroitin sulfate, which together comprise 90% of the total mass of the macromolecule (complete aggrecan monomer shown in Fig. 4B-1 = $1 - 5 \times 10^6$ Daltons). Aggrecan core proteins can be separated into five functional units: three globular (G_1, G_2, and G_3) and two extended interglobular (E_1 and E_2) domains (Fig. 4B-1). The glycosaminoglycans are clustered primarily in two regions, both within the E_2 domain. The largest (about 260 nm long), termed the *chondroitin sulfate–rich region,* contains all the chondroitin sulfate chains (more than 100 chains) and some of the keratan sulfate (about 15–25 chains). This distal portion of the E_2 domain is

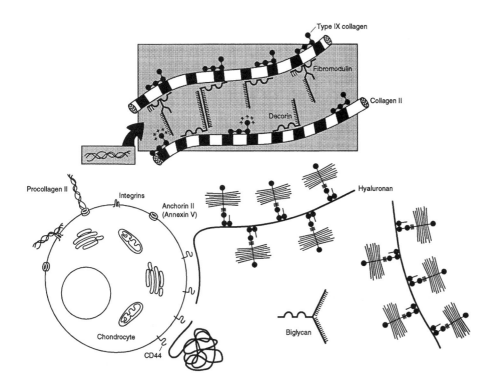

(Figure 4B-2)
Major proteoglycans of articular cartilage and some of their possible multiple interactions. Supramolecular aggregates composed of aggrecan and link protein bound to hyaluronan are shown. Some aggregates, especially within the pericellular matrix, are bound to the chondrocyte cell surface via interaction of the central hyaluronan filament with CD44. Other aggregates are presumably self-containing within the extensive extracellular matrix. The specific location of biglycan is not shown but is thought to be predominately localized within the pericellular matrix. Collagen IX, decorin, and fibromodulin are shown decorating the surface of collagen II fibers and illustrate possible proposed interactions. Also shown are other cell-surface receptors such as anchorin II and integrins that, along with CD44, may participate in cellular recognition of changes in matrix composition or biomechanical stimuli. Adapted from Kuettner (1) with permission.

encoded by a single large exon (exon 12). The second glycosaminoglycan attachment region is the keratan sulfate-rich region located in the proximal portion of the E_2 domain near the G_2 domain and before the chondroitin sulfate-rich region. This smaller attachment region is encoded by exon 11 and a small portion of the 5′ end of exon 12 (8).

The carboxyl-terminal globular domain (G_3) of the aggrecan core protein, encoded by exons 13-18, exhibits three structural motifs: an epidermal growth factor (EGF)-like domain, a lectin-like domain, and a complement regulatory protein (CRP)-like domain. The presence of the G_3 globular domain is highly variable in mature aggrecan due to alternative splicing and proteolytic processing (6,8,9). Only about one-third of the aggrecan molecules isolated from adult cartilage actually contains an intact G_3 domain (1). Many functions related to the homology of these subdomains with other proteins (EGF, hepatic cell-surface lectins, or CRP) have been suggested. However, no conclusive data show that the aggrecan G_3 domain participates in any of these functions. Some data suggest that the G_3 domain plays a more important role in facilitating the secretion of aggrecan (5).

The first globular domain of aggrecan (G_1) at the amino-terminal region is responsible for the binding of aggrecan to hyaluronan. The G_1 domain has a molecular mass of 38 kD and is composed of three subdomains that are encoded by exons 3, 4, and 5 (8). Aggrecan molecules bind to hyaluronan to form aggregates once they are secreted into the extracellular matrix. These aggregates are further stabilized by an accessory protein called *link protein* (Figs. 4B-1 and 4B-2). Link proteins are not proteoglycans, but they exhibit a protein structure highly homologous to aggrecan G_1: a PTR double loop and a structural motif similar to an immunoglobulin (Ig) fold are present on the amino-terminal end of this protein (9). Thus, aggrecan and link protein both belong to the Ig superfamily of proteins. The PTR double loop structure of the G_1 domain and link protein interacts reversibly with five consecutive hyaluronan disaccharide re-

peat units. In addition, aggrecan and link protein interact specifically with each other (mediated via the two common Ig fold parts of the two molecules) forming a ternary complex with hyaluronan (6). Link protein and aggrecan independently exhibit a strong binding affinity for hyaluronan in the range of 10^{-9} M. Together, the affinity of the ternary complex is essentially nondissociable. Thus, both hyaluronan and link protein are required for the stabilization of the aggregate. Only one link protein molecule is present at each hyaluronan-aggrecan linkage site. As many as 200 aggrecan molecules can bind to one single filament of a hyaluronan molecule to form supramolecular structures in the range of 5×10^7 to 5×10^8 Daltons. On electron microscopy, these aggregates are longer than 8 μm (1).

Little is known about the functions of the G_2 domain of aggrecan. It contains a PTR motif with considerable homology to the double loop structure found in the G_1 domain and link protein, yet it does not have the ability to bind to hyaluronan or link protein. Unlike the G_1 domain and link protein, the G_2 does not contain the third Ig-fold loop. Improper folding of the G_2 PTR due to O-glycosylation and the presence of keratan sulfate substitution within the G_2 domain are believed to be responsible for the inability of G_2 to bind to hyaluronan (6).

Other members of the PTR family of proteoglycans have core protein structures homologous to aggrecan. Whereas aggrecan is the predominant proteoglycan of cartilage and other load-bearing tissues, versican is the predominant PTR proteoglycan in most other soft connective tissues (eg, dermis, mesentery, etc). The core protein of versican is similar to that of aggrecan except it contains only two globular domains, one at each terminal of the protein (analogous to aggrecan G_1 and G_3) and fewer consensus sequences for glycosaminoglycan attachment. Thus, by bearing fewer glycosaminoglycans, versican may satisfy a space-filling role in tissues, but not the role of proteoglycans as a source of high-fixed charge density required to compensate for cyclic loading as in aggrecan-rich tissues such as cartilage.

Some of the most recently described members of the PTR family, neurocan, brevican, and BEHAP, are present within the extracellular matrix of neuronal tissues (7). Other central nervous system PTR proteoglycans, *glial hyaluronan-binding protein* and *hyaluronectin,* are related to or derivatives of versican. The lymphocyte homing receptor CD44 is also included in the PTR family, even though it contains only one half of the PTR structural motif (ie, one loop). CD44 is considered a part-time proteoglycan because its substitution with glycosaminoglycan varies, depending on cell type as well as cell state (3,5). Changes in cellular state also appear to regulate whether CD44 becomes substituted with heparan sulfate or chondroitin sulfate. The role of CD44 as a proteoglycan is not clear. However, on many cells CD44 serves a more important function (with or without a glycosaminoglycan side chain) as a plasma membrane intercalated hyaluronan receptor (10). For example, on chondrocytes CD44 serves to anchor a substantial portion of aggrecan molecules within the pericellular matrix, which is itself tethered to hyaluronan (Fig. 4B-2) (11). COS cells transiently transfected with pCD44 gained the capacity to assemble chondrocyte-like pericellular matrices in the presence of added hyaluronan and aggrecan (12). As discussed below, CD44 may also participate in the receptor-mediated catabolism of hyaluronan (13).

PROTEOGLYCANS THAT INTERACT WITH COLLAGEN

Collagen fibers are a predominant component of all connective tissues, forming a three-dimensional network that bestows, as well as limits, tissue shape and integrity. In many tissues, the collagen fibers are complemented by a distinct family of proteoglycans that form tight associations with collagen upon their secretion into the extracellular space. The small proteoglycans *decorin* and *fibromodulin* are the most notable members of this family (3,14). Decorin carries predominantly one dermatan sulfate chain located at its amino-terminus (except in bone, where the chain is not epimerized and is thus expressed as chondroitin sulfate), whereas fibromodulin carries up to four keratan sulfate chains within the central portion of its protein core (Fig. 4B-1). The lack of dermatan or chondroitin sulfate substitution by fibromodulin may be due to the presence of several tyrosine sulfate residues at its amino-terminal end on the fibromodulin core protein (14). Both have been shown to bind (or "decorate") the surface of collagen fibers at specific intervals along the fiber. However, the binding sites on the collagen fiber for each of the two proteoglycans are distinct. The exact function of these proteoglycans is not known. Both have the capacity to inhibit fibrillogenesis in vitro and may therefore regulate collagen fiber diameter. It has also been suggested that these proteoglycans may maintain proper spacing between collagen fibrils as well as regulate hydration and movement of molecules within this domain (3,14). The dermatan sulfate glycosaminoglycan present on decorin has the capacity for chain-to-chain self-association and may thus form bridges between decorins on adjacent collagen fibers (Fig. 4B-2) (15). It has also been suggested that the negatively charged glycosaminoglycan chains on either decorin or fibromodulin may form tight interactions with the highly basic NC4 globular domain of type IX collagen that also decorates the surface of some collagen fibers (Fig. 4B-2). Type IX collagen has a non-triple helical portion allowing a kink in the otherwise linear molecule that extends the NC4 away from the surface of the fibril (1). This conformation would further facilitate interactions with adjacent acidic structures. Interestingly, type IX collagen is itself a proteoglycan, often carrying a chondroitin sulfate chain attached to the NC3 domain of the α2(IX) chain. The function of this substitution is not clear.

The core proteins of decorin and fibromodulin, although the product of separate genes, are highly homologous. The presence of 10–11 hydrophobic, adjacent, leucine-rich repeat sequences of 23–24 amino acids each, as well as conserved disulfate-bonded loop structures, delineate these two proteoglycans as members of a common family of leucine-rich proteoglycans (6,9,14). Several other proteoglycans belong to this family including biglycan (containing two dermatan sulfate chains) and the proteoglycans lumican and osteoadherin. Although biglycan does not associate with fiber-forming collagens (ie, types I and II), it does display affinity for type VI collagen. In addition to collagen, members of this leucine-rich family of proteoglycans have also shown to bind other matrix macromolecules such as fibronectin and growth factors such as transforming growth factor beta (TGF-β) (16). Thus, these proteoglycans may play a multifaceted role of cross-linking collagen lattices or anchoring other components of the extracellular matrix onto collagen (14).

CELL-SURFACE PROTEOGLYCANS

While proteoglycans are commonly viewed as components of the extracellular matrix, some proteoglycans are never secreted and upon synthesis remain closely associated with the cellular plasma membrane. The proteoglycans that predominate at the cell surface fall into one of two groups: the transmembrane proteoglycans represented by the *syndecan* family and *glypican,* a proteoglycan tethered to the cell surface via a phosphatidylinositol linkage (3,17). These two proteoglycan groups, in different combinations and subtypes, are essentially ubiquitous to all cell types (ie, not selectively associated with the plasma membranes of connective tissue cells). For example, it was recently demonstrated that human articular chondrocytes express mRNA for syndecan-4, syndecan-2, betaglycan, and glypican but little mRNA for syndecan-1 (18). All members of the syndecan family have homologous core protein structures that include a C-terminal cytoplasmic domain, a hydrophobic transmembrane domain, and a large N-terminal extracellular domain that bears the glycosaminoglycan chains. Another unique feature of the syndecan core protein family is the presence of a protease-sensitive site within the proximal portion of the extracellular domain close to the plasma membrane. It has been suggested that the presence of this site permits rapid regulation of proteoglycan-related functions via proteolytic shedding of the extracellular domain. The syndecan core protein may carry two or more heparan sulfate chains, alone or in combination with chondroitin sulfate (17). The heparan sulfate is typically located on the distal end of the molecule, and the chondroitin sulfate chains are more centrally located along the extracellular domain. The proteoglycan glypican also provides for the regulated expression of heparan sulfate chains at the cell surface. Glypican is one of several cell-surface proteins that do not exhibit hydrophobic transmembrane domains but become anchored to the plasma via covalent linkage to a glycosyl phosphotidylinositol attachment site, a process called *glypiation* (17). As with the syndecans, it is thought that glypican can be shed rapidly via the action of particular phospholipases.

The presence of glycosaminoglycans localized directly on the cell surface provides cells with an exquisite means for controlling the local cell environment. This may involve all purported functions of glycosaminoglycans including regulation of local hydration and molecular movement, binding of basic growth factors and cytokines, and binding to other matrix components as well as to adjacent cell-surface heparan sulfate receptors. In fact, the binding of other extracellular matrix components (eg, fibronectin, laminin, and collagen) by cell-surface–associated glycosaminoglycans may serve to classify these proteoglycans as matrix receptors. It is thus not surprising that cell-surface heparan sulfates are found to participate prominently in many cell–cell and cell–matrix interactions. The presence of heparan sulfate proteoglycans on the surface of vasculature lining endothelial cells may also serve to provide other functions specific for heparin and heparan sulfates, such as binding to antithrombin III and binding to lipoprotein lipase (17). The more acute anticoagulation properties of the mature mast cell are met by a different heparin- bearing proteoglycan, *serglycin*, the core protein of which contains numerous serine/glycine repeats located within the central portion of the molecule (2,3). Although substituted with heparin side chains, serglycin is not a membrane-bound proteoglycan. During resting states, serglycin exists as an intracellular proteoglycan within storage granules. Interestingly, other hematopoietic cells that are related to mast cells express the same serglycin core protein, but substitute the core with chondroitin sulfate rather than heparin chains (3).

Several other proteoglycans are also known to associate with cell surfaces, but it is the core proteins that are thought to play a major functional role in many of these molecules. For example, the core protein of *betaglycan* is the type III TGF-β receptor (3). Other cell-surface proteins such as *thrombomodulin, transferrin receptor,* and the hyaluronan receptor *CD44* may also exist as proteoglycans (5). However, in these cases the presence of "part-time" glycosaminoglycan substitution may serve to modulate the intrinsic function of the core protein.

PROTEOGLYCAN METABOLISM

Under physiologic conditions, cells regulate a dynamic metabolic steady state in which anabolism (synthesis of matrix macromolecules) is balanced by catabolism (degradation and loss from the matrix) (1). Different tissues use different methods to maintain this delicate balance. However, the maintenance of proteoglycans within cartilage is often a useful paradigm because of the relative isolation of the tissue in terms of its metabolism. Cartilage proteoglycans are regulated, for all intents and purposes, solely by the resident chondrocytes. As in all tissues, anabolism in chondrocytes is regulated by cellular responses to biomechanical stimuli as well as a capacity of the cells to "sense" changes in the composition of their extracellular matrix. The mechanism of these two cellular responses is not clear, but is likely mediated via cell-surface receptors such as *anchorin CII* (annexin V), CD44, and a variety of integrins (Fig. 4B-2) (1,10). Like other types of cells, chondrocytes are also responsive to a variety of cellular mediators including inflammatory mediators such as tumor-necrosis factor alpha (TNF-α), interferon gamma (IFN-γ), and the interleukins (IL) including IL-1 , IL-1α, and IL-6; peptide growth factors such as epidermal growth factor, fibroblast growth factors, platelet-derived growth factors, TGF-α, TGF-β, and other members of the TGF-β superfamily including bone morphogenic proteins (BMPs); bacterial lipopolysaccharides; some retinoids; and degraded portions of matrix macromolecules such as fibronectin fragments (1). These mediators are often bipolar, affecting both anabolism and catabolism. In general, it can

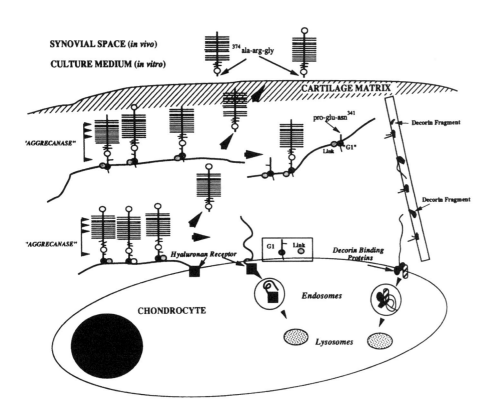

(Figure 4B-3)
Summary of catabolic events thought to occur in the turnover of proteoglycan within articular cartilage tissue. Shown is a postulated scheme for the catabolism of proteoglycans within articular cartilage. Aggrecans, as well as other matrix proteoglycans, are first cleaved at critical sites along their core protein (eg, between G_1 and G_2 of aggrecan) by matrix metalloproteinases (MMPs). Depicted here is putative action by the MMP termed aggrecanase *although action by other MMPs has also been postulated. Hyaluronan, possibly still retaining remnants of aggrecan and link protein, is then internalized via interaction with a hyaluronan receptor such as CD44 (13). Courtesy of A. Plaas and J. Sandy; reproduced with permission.*

be stated that cytokines released by inflammatory cells stimulate cartilage catabolism and inhibit its anabolism, whereas peptide growth factors promote cartilage anabolism and inhibit catabolism (1).

The normal catabolic mechanisms controlled by the chondrocytes are very conservative. Little is known about the turnover of decorin, biglycan, and fibromodulin, which are proteoglycans that associate with collagen. As for aggrecan, in vitro explant culture studies of human articular cartilage suggest that 25 days is the average half-life of newly synthesized aggrecan within tissue (1). It is noteworthy that a comparable half-life (13–25 days) of newly synthesized aggrecan was observed in explant studies on bovine articular cartilage (19). Furthermore, the half-life of newly synthesized hyaluronan was shown to be nearly equivalent to aggrecan, even though the two molecules are believed to be processed via different mechanisms. In general, aggrecan catabolism is thought to occur primarily extracellularly and involve the proteolytic cleavage between the G_1 and G_2 domains of the core protein, resulting in degradation products that are rapidly lost from the cartilage matrix (Fig. 4B-3) (20). The primary proteolytic enzymes responsible for the extracellular cleavage of proteoglycans (as well as other matrix proteins) are the matrix metalloproteases characterized by a bound Zn^{2+} at their active site and a requirement for calcium (1). Extracellular catabolism of hyaluronan has never been demonstrated in cartilage or other tissues; however, accumulating evidence suggests that turnover is primarily intracellular following endocytosis by hyaluronan receptors such as CD44 (13). One unfortunate outcome of cartilage degradation is the exposure of released matrix components, such as aggrecan, to the immune system. Aggrecan and other matrix proteins within healthy cartilage are normally not subjected to immune surveillance, making them potential antigenic determinants upon their release. Thus, molecules such as collagen type II and aggrecan are considered potential causal factors in human rheumatoid joint diseases (21).

WARREN KNUDSON, PhD
KLAUS E. KUETTNER, PhD

1. Kuettner KE: Osteoarthritis: cartilage integrity and homeostasis. In Klippel JH, Dieppe PA (eds): Rheumatology. St. Louis, MO, Mosby Year Book Europe Limited, 1994, pp 6.1-6.16

2. Wight TN, Heinegard DK, Hascall VC: Proteoglycans structure and function. In Hay ED (ed): Cell Biology of the Extracellular Matrix, 2nd ed. New York, Plenum Press, 1991, pp 45-78

3. Roughley PJ, Poole AR: Proteoglycans. In Schumacher HR, Klippel JH, Koopman WJ (eds): Primer on the Rheumatic Diseases, 10th ed. Atlanta, Arthritis Foundation, 1993, pp 23-27

4. Laurent TC, Fraser RE: Hyaluronan. FASEB J 6:2397-2404, 1992

5. Hardingham TE, Fosang AJ: Proteoglycans: many forms and many functions. FASEB J 6:861-870, 1992

6. Neame PJ: Extracellular matrix of cartilage: proteoglycans. In Woessner JF, Howell DS (eds): Joint Cartilage Degradation. New York, Marcel Dekker, 1993, pp 109-138

7. Jaworski DM, Kelly GM, Hockfield S: BEHAB, a new member of the proteoglycan tandem repeat family of hyaluronan-binding proteins that is restricted to the brain. J Cell Biol 125:495-509, 1995

8. Valhmu WB, Palmer GD, Rivers PA, Ebara S, Cheng JF, Fischer S, Ratcliffe A: Structure of the human aggrecan gene: exon-intron organization and association with the protein domains. Biochem J 309:535-542, 1995

9. Sandell LJ, Chansky H, Zamparo O, Hering TM: Molecular biology of cartilage proteoglycans and link protein. In Kuettner KE, Goldberg VM (eds): Osteoarthritic Disorders. Rosemont, IL, American Academy of Orthopaedic Surgeons, 1995, pp 117-130

10. Knudson CB, Knudson W: Hyaluronan-binding proteins in development, tissue homeostasis and disease. FASEB J 7:1233-1241, 1993

11. Knudson CB: Hyaluronan receptor-directed assembly of chondrocyte pericellular matrix. J Cell Biol 120:825-834, 1993

12. Knudson W, Bartnik E, Knudson CB: Assembly of pericellular matrices by COS-7 cells transfected with CD44 homing receptor genes. Proc Natl Acad Sci USA 90:4003-4007, 1993

13. Chow G, Knudson CB, Homandberg G, Knudson W: Increased CD44 expression in bovine articular chondrocytes by catabolic cellular mediators. J Biol Chem 270:27734-27741, 1995

14. Heinegard D, Lorenzo P, Sommarin Y: Articular cartilage matrix proteins. In Kuettner KE, Goldberg VM (eds): Osteoarthritic Disorders. Rosemont, IL, American Academy of Orthopaedic Surgeons, 1995, pp 229-237

15. Scott JE: Supramolecular organization of extracellular matrix glycosaminoglycans, in vitro and in the tissues. FASEB J 6:2639-2645, 1992

16. Hildebrand A, Romaris M, Rasmussen LM, Heinegard D, Twardzik DR, Border WA, Rouslahti E: Interaction of the small interstitial proteoglycans biglycan: decorin and fibromodulin with transforming growth factor β. Biochem J 302:527-534, 1994

17. David G: Integral membrane heparan sulfate proteoglycans. FASEB J 7:1023-1030, 1993

18. Grover J, Roughley PJ: Expression of cell-surface proteoglycan mRNA by human articular chondrocytes. Biochem J 309:963-968, 1995

19. Morales TI, Hascall VC: Correlated metabolism of proteoglycans and hyaluronic acid in bovine cartilage organ cultures. J Biol Chem 263:3632-3638, 1988

20. Plaas AHK, Sandy JD: Proteoglycan anabolism and catabolism in articular cartilage. In Kuettner KE, Goldberg VM (eds): Osteoarthritic Disorders. Rosemont, IL, American Academy of Orthopaedic Surgeons, 1995, pp 103-116

21. Glant TT, Mikecz K, Thonar JMA, Kuettner KE: Immune responses to cartilage proteoglycans in inflammatory animal models and human diseases. In Woessner JF, Howell DS (eds): Joint Cartilage Degradation. New York, Marcel Dekker, 1993, pp 435-473

5

MEDIATORS OF INFLAMMATION, TISSUE DESTRUCTION, AND REPAIR

A. CELLULAR CONSTITUENTS

Inflammation may be simply defined as the local reaction of tissue to injury. Depending on the cause, damaged tissue is infiltrated by both neutrophils and macrophages, accompanied by fluid and exuded proteins. The cellular constituents of the inflammatory response play an important role in clearing debris from injured sites and in promoting tissue repair. Phagocytic cells in particular are essential for the removal of foreign or dead particulate matter at sites of tissue injury. In addition, inflammatory mediators released by phagocytes, such as degradative enzymes and the free radicals superoxide anion and nitric oxide, contribute to the capacity of these cells to degrade macromolecules within exudative effusions.

In autoimmune diseases, the normal function of phagocytic cells (ie, microbial killing, tissue repair) is subverted: cells are activated by complement components, immune complexes, and other stimuli in the apparent absence of invading microorganisms. This chapter focuses on the pathogenic mechanisms by which inflammatory cells are activated to promote tissue injury in rheumatic disease.

NEUTROPHILS

Neutrophils, together with monocyte/macrophages, are the body's "professional phagocytes." While in the circulation neutrophils are maintained in a resting state, with their wide array of cytoxic mediators either stored in cytoplasmic granules or separated into plasma membrane and cytosolic compartments. Activation of the cell may be triggered by the engagement of particles, such as invading microorganisms, or in response to soluble stimuli that engage specific cell-surface receptors (Fig. 5A-1).

Chemotaxis

In inflammation, the initial step of neutrophil activation requires movement toward a target. Such directed migration, or *chemotaxis*, occurs along a chemical gradient originating at the target. Well-described chemoattractants include bacterial products such as formulated peptides and activated complement components such as C5a. These chemoattractants interact with specific surface receptors that have seven hydrophobic transmembrane domains and are linked to GTP-binding proteins (1).

Phagocytosis

Following directed migration along a chemoattractant gradient, phagocytosis is initiated by the attachment or binding of target particles to the neutrophil surface. Attachment is followed by enclosure of the particle within a plasma membrane pouch. Upon closure, this pouch becomes a vacuole in the cytoplasm, and is termed a *phagosome*. In most instances, soon after particle ingestion, primary or secondary lysosomes fuse with the phagosome, which are then termed *phagolysosomes*. Fusion of the respective membranes permits entry of lysosomal contents into the phagosome and the shielded enzymatic degradation of ingested material, an important aspect of the scavenging function of both neutrophils and macrophages. Thus, phagocytosis can deliver a microbial prey to a sequestered compartment in which the noxious action of host cytotoxins (eg, degradative enzymes) can be confined.

Macrophages and neutrophils "recognize" certain serum-derived molecules called antibodies and complement components (originally called opsonins, from the Greek "to pre-

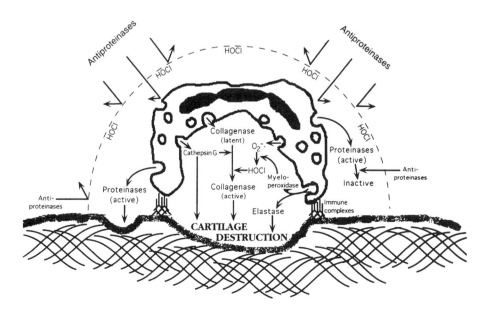

(Figure 5A-1)
A model for mechanisms of antiproteinase defense and cartilage destruction by neutrophils in rheumatoid arthritis. Fc receptors of neutrophils engage immune complexes associated with or embedded in articular cartilage. Neutrophil activation following Fc receptor engagement results in the release of latent and active proteinases and the products of NAPDH oxidase into the space between the neutrophil and cartilage, where they are protected from antiproteinase, leading to destruction of cartilage by proteinases specific for collagen or proteoglycan. Proteinases released into the adjacent synovial fluid may be inactivated by antiproteinases or protected from inactivation by neutrophil-derived HOCl.

pare food for"). These molecules bind to bacteria, cells, or other surfaces and increase the efficiency of phagocytosis. It should be emphasized that the phagocytes recognize antibody- or complement-coated particles because they have surface receptors for immunoglobulin and for the C3 fragments C3b and iC3b. Using this strategy, phagocytes can consume a wide variety of different particles, since the stimulus to phagocytosis depends not upon the characteristics of the organism, but rather upon recognition of the two major opsonins by specific cell-surface receptors.

Phagocytic cells express receptors for the complement fragment C3b (receptor designated CR1) and its inactivated cleavage product iC3b (receptor designated CR3, or CD11b/CD18). Both CR1 and CD11b/CD18 play important roles in the clearance of particles, such as opsonized bacteria, to which C3b or iC3b are bound. This clearance mechanism is also essential for the removal of immune complexes, which covalently bind C3b and iC3b (2). CD11b/CD18 is also the major neutrophil adhesion molecule responsible for adherence to vascular endothelium and to other neutrophils (Fig. 5A-2). CD11b/CD18 is also required for normal phagocytosis, aggregation, adhesion, and chemotaxis. Intercellular adhesion molecule-1 (ICAM-1), expressed on resting and activated endothelial cells, has been identified as a ligand for the CD18 integrins. Interaction between CD18 and ICAM-1 together with the ligation of selectin molecules with their carbohydrate counterreceptors, modulates both the adhesion of neutrophils to vascular endothelium and their egress to the extravascular space (3). It has been shown in diseases such as systemic lupus erythematosus (SLE), characterized by circulating immune complexes and complement activa-

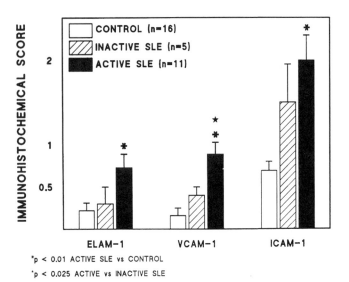

*p < 0.01 ACTIVE SLE vs CONTROL
*p < 0.025 ACTIVE vs INACTIVE SLE

(Figure 5A-3)
Systemic lupus erythematous (SLE) disease exacerbation is accompanied by endothelial cell up-regulation of three adhesion molecules: E-selectin (ELAM-1), vascular cell adhesion molecule 1 (VCAM-1), and intercellular adhesion molecule-1 (ICAM-1). The mean expression of all three adhesion molecules is significantly greater in patients with active SLE versus healthy controls as well as patients with inactive SLE. Reprinted from Belmont et al (4) with permission .

tion, that there is upregulation of endothelial cell adhesion molecules, indicating activation (Fig. 5A-3)(4).

Neutrophils, monocytes/macrophages, platelets, B lymphocytes, and natural killer cells all express receptors for im-

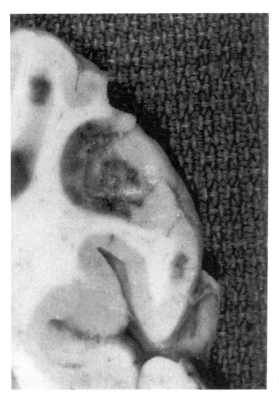

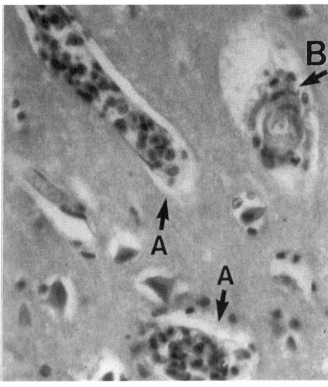

(Figure 5A-2)
*Brain tissue obtained postmortem from a patient with fatal exacerbation of neuropsychiatric lupus without antiphospholipid antibodies. **Left panel:** The frontal lobe reveals numerous small cortical infarcts. **Right panel:** High magnification reveals leukothrombosis, with leukocytes adherent to each other and to vascular endothelium, leading to occlusion of small blood vessels by leukocyte aggregates (A), as well as fibrin thrombi involving other vessels (B). Reprinted from Belmont et al (4) with permission.*

mune complexes. There are three types of receptors for multimeric IgG that bind these complexes via their Fc fragments; these receptors are termed FcRI, II, and III. FcγR polymorphisms affect phagocytic function and may therefore contribute to disease susceptibility factors in the development of autoimmunity (5,6).

Release of Toxic Proteolytic Enzymes

Neutrophils contain two morphologically distinct granules (specific and azurophilic) that contain proteases, which under normal circumstances are sequestered within the granule and the phagolysosome, presenting no threat to the host. However the extracellular release of granule contents may promote inflammation and damage at tissue sites. Phagocytosis is not necessary for neutrophil degranulation, which may be provoked by soluble stimuli (eg, C5a, interleukin-8, and immune complexes). Degranulation is augmented when neutrophils encounter stimuli deposited on a surface; lysosomal release unfolds by a process of reverse endocytosis, or what has been called "frustrated phagocytosis." This exuberant release of lysosomal enzymes from neutrophils may be relevant to the pathogenesis of tissue injury in diseases characterized by the deposition of immune complexes on cell surfaces or on such extracellular surfaces as vascular basement membranes or articular cartilage, as in rheumatoid arthritis (Fig. 5A-1) (7).

In glomerulonephritis, neutrophil-derived proteases can be demonstrated in urine and are involved in the degradation of the extracellular matrix proteins of the glomerular basement membrane and mesangium (8). In addition to proteases, neutrophils also release cationic proteins with bactericidal activity, such as lysozyme, bactericidal/permeability increasing factor and the defensins, which increase glomerular permeability by neutralizing the anionic components of the glomerular basement membrane.

Production of Toxic Oxygen Radicals

When phagocytic leukocytes are activated, molecular oxygen consumption by the leukocyte is increased. Most of this oxygen is transformed directly into superoxide anion radicals, which are significant mediators of inflammation that cause tissue injury and irreversible modification of macromolecules (Table 5A-1) (9).

(Table 5A-1)
Potential effects of oxygen-free radicals

On cells
    Killing of microbes (eg, viruses, bacteria, fungi, protozoa)
    Injury of tumor cells
    Stimulation of secretion by platelets, mast cells, endothelial cells, glomerular cells
    Mutagenesis of bacteria and mammalian cells
    Tumor promotion and carcinogenesis
On extracellular products
    Generation of chemotactic lipids from arachidonate
    Activation of leukocyte collagenase and gelatinase
    Inactivation of chemotactic leukotrienes, chemotactic peptides, α-1-antiprotease, met-enkephalin, leukocyte hydrolases, and bacterial toxins

---

Some of the toxic oxygen metabolites produced by neutrophils are generated by the myeloperoxidase–hydrogen peroxide–halide system. Myeloperoxidase is a highly cationic enzyme present in the azurophilic granules that catalyzes the reaction of hydrogen peroxide with a halide such as chloride to form hypohalous acids (eg, hypochlorous acid). These products are capable of killing a variety of microorganisms and are cytotoxic to host cells (8).

MACROPHAGES

Macrophages/monocytes play an important role in immune-mediated tissue injury, particularly in nephritis (10). These cells express the three major classes of Fc receptors as well as β1, β2, and β3 integrins, which facilitate phagocytosis of opsonized particles, intercellular adhesion, and adhesion to extracellular matrix proteins. Monocytes are recruited into tissues from the circulation in response to chemotactic factors such as C5a, interleukin-8 (IL-8), transforming growth factor beta (TGF-β), fragments of collagen, and fibronectin, which are produced at inflammatory sites. Recruitment requires the expression of adhesion molecules on activated vascular endothelium (eg, ICAM-1, VCAM-1), which are recognized by counter-ligands of the circulating monocyte (eg, LFA-1, VLA-4). When monocytes emigrate into tissues they can be transformed into activated macrophages following exposure to cytokines such as interferon gamma (IFN-γ), IL-1, and tumor necrosis factor (TNF). Macrophage activation results in increased cell size, increased synthesis of proteolytic enzymes, and secretion of a variety of inflammatory products (Table 5A-2).

Release of Inflammatory Mediators and Proteases

Macrophages secrete up to 100 substances, ranging from free radicals such as superoxide anion to large macromolecules such as fibronectin (9). Some products are secreted in response to inflammatory stimuli, while others are constitutively released (Table 5A-2). When stimulated by exposure to immune complexes, endotoxin, IL-1, or C3b-coated particles, macrophages and monocytes exhibit a procoagulant activity. The procoagulant products include tissue factor (identified as a receptor for factor VII), factor X activator, prothrombin activator, and vitamin K-dependent clotting factors II, VII, IX, and X. Monocytes in patients with rheumatic disease display increased procoagulant activity, which may contribute to fibrin deposition at sites of inflammation and has been implicated in crescent formation in glomerulonephritis.

Production of Cytokines

As shown in Table 5A-2, macrophages also secrete a variety of polypeptide hormones that regulate immune function and inflammation as well as wound healing and repair. Macrophages, for example, produce three cytokines, IL-1α, IL-1β, and TNF-α, that not only have overlapping functions but are also capable of inducing each others' release by macrophages themselves (9). Macrophages also produce the cytokine neutrophil–activating peptide-1/IL-8, a potent neutrophil chemoattractant. The production of IL-8, induced by IL-1α, IL-1β, and TNF-α, has been described in a variety of tissues, including alveolar macrophages, renal mesangial cells, and psoriatic skin lesions. IL-8 is now known to be a member of a family of macrophage inflammatory proteins (MIPs) or chemokines. In addition to IL-8, the superfamily of

(Table 5A-2)
Secretory products of mononuclear phagocytes

Polypeptide hormones
    Interleukin 1-α and 1-β
    Tumor necrosis factor-α (cachectin)
    Interferon-α
    Interferon-γ
    Platelet-derived growth factor(s)
    Transforming growth factor-β
    β-Endorphin
Complement components
    Classical pathway: C1, C4, C2, C3, C5
    Alternative pathway: factor B, factor D, properdin
Coagulation factors
    Intrinsic pathway: factors IX, X, V, prothrombin
    Extrinsic pathway: factor VII
    Surface activities: tissue factor, prothrombinase
    Prothrombolytic activity: plasminogen activator
        inhibitors, plasmin inhibitors
Bioactive lipids
    Cyclooxygenase products: prostaglandin E_2,
        prostaglandin F_{2a}, prostacyclin, thromboxane
    Lipo-oxygenase products: monohydroxyeicosatetraenoic
        acids, dihydroxyeicosatetraenoic acids, leukotrienes B4,
        C, D, E
    Platelet-activating factors (1 O-alkyl-2-acetyl-*sn*-glyceryl-
        3-phosphorylcholine)
Reactive oxygen intermediates (eg, superoxide anion)
Reactive nitrogen intermediates (eg, nitric oxide)
Chemokines (eg, IL-8)

---

chemokines include MCP-1, MCP-2, MCP-3, RANTES, MIP-1 alpha, and MIP-1 beta, which act on monocytes but not neutrophils and have additional activities toward basophil and eosinophil granulocytes and T lymphocytes (11).

Production of Arachidonate-Derived Mediators of Inflammation

In addition to the capacity to secrete biologically diverse active proteins, monocytes and macrophages are significant sources of lipid mediators of inflammation that are derived from arachidonic acid. Arachidonic acid is metabolized via two distinct enzymatic pathways, the cyclooxygenase pathway and the lipoxygenase pathway, generating prostaglandins and leukotrienes, respectively.

Prostaglandin G/H synthase, or cyclooxygenase, is the initial enzyme in the prostaglandin pathway and is the target enzyme for inactivation by nonsteroidal anti-inflammatory drugs. There are two isoforms of this enzyme, which, although products of two distinct genes, are highly homologous. Despite the structural homology, these genes are under separate control. The first gene identified, COX_1, appears to be constitutively expressed in a variety of cells. Expression of COX_2 may be restricted to inflammatory cells, is induced by a variety of cytokines and growth factors, and is inhibited by dexamethasone (reviewed in reference 12). Arachidonic acid is also metabolized by the lipoxygenase pathway of enzyme activation, which generates such mediators of acute inflammation as leukotriene (LT) B4, the sulfidopeptide LTs C4, D4, and E4, and the lipoxins (LX) A4 and B4 (13).

Nitric Oxide as a Modulator of Inflammation

Macrophages are also among the cellular sources of reactive nitrogen intermediates such as nitric oxide. Nitric oxide, although originally identified as a product of endothelial cells (which is why it is also called endothelium-derived relaxation factor), is now recognized as a highly reactive molecule with diverse biologic functions. The exposure of macrophages to cytokines (eg, IL-1β, IFN-γ) markedly increases nitric oxide production. Activities of nitric oxide that may be important in the inflammatory response include vasodilation and the capacity to react with superoxide anion to form toxic peroxynitrite compounds. The inhibition of nitric oxide synthesis has recently been demonstrated to reduce the severity of disease in streptococcal cell wall–induced arthritis in Lewis rats (14). In human arthritis, the production of nitric oxide by both synovial macrophages and articular chondrocytes has been demonstrated in both rheumatoid arthritis and osteoarthritis (15–17).

PLATELETS
Platelets as Inflammatory Cells

Platelets, which are derived from marrow megakaryocytes, are involved in hemostasis, wound healing, and cellular responses to injury. In addition to its important hemostatic function, the platelet may also act as an inflammatory effector cell. For example, platelets: 1) display chemotaxis to a variety of stimuli including platelet-activating factor (PAF) and collagen fragments; 2) endocytose immune complexes via Fc receptors; 3) release inflammatory mediators upon activation and aggregation; 4) are activated by phlogistic agents (such as complement-activation products); 5) play a role in animal models of inflammatory disease; and 6) have been identified in localization and activation at tissue injury sites in human inflammatory diseases. There is evidence for platelet activation in immunologically mediated diseases such as asthma, cold urticaria, scleroderma, and systemic lupus erythematosus (SLE) (18).

Normal adhesion to extracellular matrix proteins requires von Willebrand factor, which binds to the platelet surface glycoprotein gpIb and serves as a molecular bridge between platelets and subendothelial collagen. Following adhesion, platelets release granular contents that promote clotting and platelet aggregation. During this process, activated platelets release a variety of both protein and lipid-derived mediators with inflammatory potential, factors with chemotactic, proliferative, thrombogenic, and proteolytic activity (Table 5A-2). Stimuli that activate platelet adhesion and degranulation also trigger the release of arachidonic acid from the membrane. This initiates the synthesis of thromboxane A_2 (TXA$_2$) and 12-hydroxytetraenoic acid (12-HETE). TXA$_2$ promotes platelet aggregation and vasoconstriction; 12-HETE activates neutrophils and macrophages.

Products released from platelets, which may promote local inflammation, are classified according to their intracellular granule of origin. Dense granules release ADP, which activates platelet fibrinogen-binding sites of the β3 integrin gpIIb/IIIa, and serotonin, a potent vasoconstrictor. Alpha granule components include platelet factor 4 and beta-thromboglobulin, which have been reported to activate both mononuclear and polymorphonuclear leukocytes. Alpha granules are also the source of platelet-derived growth factor, which stimulates proliferation of smooth muscle cells and fibroblasts; thrombospondin, which promotes neutrophil adherence to blood vessel walls; factor VIII:VWF; factor V; fibrinogen; and fibronectin.

Platelets in Glomerulonephritis

Platelets have been identified in the glomeruli of patients with SLE nephritis and are believed to play a particularly important role in this disorder (19). Urinary thromboxane levels are elevated in patients with active lupus nephritis, a finding that has several implications. First, it is a sign of abnormal platelet aggregation in the microvasculature with the potential for thrombosis and endothelial injury. Second, the vasoconstrictive properties of TXA_2 would be expected to decrease glomerular filtration rate (GFR) and renal blood flow (RBF). Third, the release of growth factors and other mediators by activated platelets could aggravate the proliferative glomerular lesion. Recent studies of the administration of specific TXA_2 antagonists have shown promise in improving both GFR and RBF in SLE nephritis (20).

Platelets may aggravate immune injury in glomerulonephritis via several mechanisms, including promoting thrombosis, reducing GFR through the production of thromboxane and other vasoactive substances, and releasing products that activate macrophages, neutrophils, and glomerular mesangial cells (8).

STEVEN B. ABRAMSON, MD

1. Snyderman R, Uhing RJ: Chemoattractant stimulus-response coupling. In Goldstein IM, Snyderman R (eds): Inflammation: Basic Principles and Clinical Correlates. New York, Raven Press, 1992, p 421

2. Schifferli JA, Ng YC, Peters DK: The role of complement and its receptor in the elimination of immune complexes. N Engl J Med 315:488-495, 1986

3. Lawrence MB, Springer TA: Leukocytes role on a selection of physiologic flow rates: Distinction from and prerequisite for adhesion through integrins. Cell 65:859-873, 1991

4. Belmont HM, Abramson SB, Lie JT: Pathology and pathogenesis of vascular injury in systemic lupus erythematosus: Interactions of inflammatory cells and activated endothelium. Arthritis Rheum 39:9-22, 1996

5. Salmon JE, Edberg JC, Brogle NL, Kimberly RP: Allelic polymorphisms of human Fc receptor IIA and Fc receptor IIIB: Independent mechanisms for differences in human phagocyte function. J Clin Invest 89:1274-1281, 1992

6. van de Winkel J, Capel P: Human IgG Fc receptor heterogeneity: Molecular aspects, clinical implications. Immunol Today 14:215-221, 1993

7. Pillinger MH, Abramson SB: The neutrophil in rheumatoid arthritis. Rheum Dis Clin North Amer 21:691-714, 1995

8. Johnson RJ, Lovett D, Lehrer RI, Couser WG, Klebanoff SJ: Role of oxidants and proteases in glomerular injury. Kidney Int 45:352-359, 1994

9. Nathan CF: Secretory products of macrophages. J Clin Invest 79:319-326, 1987

10. Nikolic-Paterson DJ, Lan HY, Hill PA, Atkins RC: Macrophages in renal injury. Kidney Int 45:S79-S82, 1994

11. Schall TJ, Bacon KB: Chemokines, leukocyte trafficking and inflammation. Curr Opin Immunol 6:865-873, 1994

12. Baird NR, Morrison AR: Amplification of the arachidonic acid cascade: implications for pharmacologic intervention. Amer J Kidney Dis 21:557-564, 1993

13. Hamberg M, Samuelsson B: Prostaglandin endoperoxides. Novel transformations of arachidonic acid in human platelets. Proc Natl Acad Sci USA 71:3400-3404, 1974

14. McCartney-Francis N, Allen JB, Mizel DE, Albina JE, Xie QW, Nathan CF, Wahl SM: Suppression of arthritis by an inhibitor of nitric oxide synthase. J Exp Med 178:749-754, 1993

15. Amin AR, Di Cesare PE, Vyas P, Attur M, Tzeng E, Billiar TR, Stuchin SA, Abramson SB: The expression and regulation of nitric oxide synthase in human osteoarthritis-affected chondrocytes: Evidence for up-regulated neuronal nitric oxide synthase. J Exp Med 182:2097-2102, 1995

16. Sakurai H, Kohsaka H, Liu M-F, Higashiyama H, Hirata Y, Kanno K, Saito I, Miyasaka N: Nitric oxide production and inducible nitric oxide synthase expression in inflammatory arthritides. J Clin Invest 96:2357-2363, 1996

17. Clancy RM, Abramson SB: Nitric oxide: A novel mediator of inflammation. Soc Exp Biol Med 93-101, 1995

18. Ginsberg MH: Role of platelets in inflammation and rheumatic disease. Adv Inflamm Res 2:53-71, 1986

19. Johnson RJ: Platelets in inflammatory glomerular injury. Seminars Nephrol 11:276-284, 1991

20. Pierucci A, Simonetti BM, Pecci G: Improvement in renal function with selective thromboxane antagonism in lupus nephritis. N Engl J Med 320:421-425, 1989

B. GROWTH FACTORS AND CYTOKINES

Cytokines are small molecular-weight proteins that mediate communication between cells. The generic term "cytokines" includes colony-stimulating factors, growth factors, interleukins, and interferons. The terminology of these molecules is confusing because it is largely on a historical rather than a functional basis. For example, some interleukins primarily serve to regulate cell growth and differentiation, whereas some growth factors have other major properties.

Cytokines carry out their functions largely in the immediate pericellular environment, either in an autocrine fashion, influencing the same cell that produced the cytokine, or in a paracrine fashion, influencing adjacent cells. Cytokines bind to specific plasma membrane receptors on target cells. Secondary messenger pathways or other intracellular mechanisms are subsequently activated that lead to alterations in transcription and production of proteins.

Cytokines are involved as mediator molecules in normal biologic processes. These physiologic functions include growth and differentiation of hematopoietic, lymphoid, and mesenchymal cells, as well as orchestration of host defense mechanisms. Multiple cytokines operate as a network in a redundant, overlapping, and synergistic fashion. However, the cytokine network is largely self-regulating. Pathophysiologic consequences may result from the unregulated action or inappropriate production of particular cytokines.

This chapter reviews information about cytokines and uses arbitrary groupings based upon primary functions. These categorizations include colony-stimulating factors, growth and differentiation factors, immunoregulatory cytokines, and pro-inflammatory cytokines. These groupings are summarized in Table 5B-1. This chapter also emphasizes the relevance of each cytokine to the function of lymphoid and inflammatory cells, particularly their possible role in rheumatic diseases. Last, the self-regulatory nature of the cytokine network is discussed in a review of mechanisms that inhibit the effects of cytokines.

COLONY-STIMULATING FACTORS

Colony-stimulating factors (CSFs) and related molecules function primarily as hematopoietic growth factors (1). However, this group of cytokines also demonstrates profound effects on mature lymphocytes, neutrophils, monocytes, and macrophages. It is in these latter effects where CSFs may play significant roles in rheumatic diseases.

Granulocyte-macrophage CSF (GM-CSF) and interleukin-3 (IL-3) potentiate the growth of numerous early bone marrow precursor cells, whereas erythropoietin influences only erythroid precursor cells. Each of these factors is preceded in its actions by other stem-cell growth and differentiation factors. The effects of GM-CSF and IL-3 are also enhanced by the presence of IL-1 and IL-6. In contrast, granulocyte CSF

(Table 5B-1)
Functional classification of cytokines

Colony-stimulating factors (CSFs)
    GM-CSF (granulocyte-macrophage CSF)
    G-CSF (granulocyte CSF)
    M-CSF (macrophage CSF or CSF-1)
    IL-3 (interleukin-3)
    Erythropoietin
Growth and differentiation factors
    PDGF (platelet-derived growth factor)
    EGF (epidermal growth factor)
    FGF (fibroblast growth factor)
    TGF-β (transforming growth factor β)
Immunoregulatory cytokines
    IFN-γ (interferon γ)
    IL (interleukin) 2, 4, 5, 7, and 9-16
Pro-inflammatory cytokines
    TNF-α (tumor necrosis factor α)
    IL-1 (interleukin-1)
    IL-6 (interleukin-6)
    IL-8 (interleukin-8)

(G-CSF) influences the growth and function of mature neutrophils, while macrophage CSF (M-CSF) serves the same role for monocytes and macrophages. GM-CSF, G-CSF, and M-CSF are all produced by monocytes, fibroblasts, and endothelial cells; in addition, GM-CSF is produced by T lymphocytes.

In addition to its effects as a growth factor, GM-CSF influences the function of mature cells of the granulocytic and monocytic lineages. GM-CSF primes neutrophils, eosinophils, and basophils to respond to triggering agents with enhanced chemotaxis, oxygen radical production, and phagocytosis. In addition, GM-CSF enhances eosinophil cytotoxicity and stimulates basophil release of histamine. These multiple effects of GM-CSF all serve to heighten the inflammatory response in acute rheumatic diseases.

GM-CSF also influences diverse functions of monocytes and macrophages, leading to enhanced ability of these cells to present antigen and induce an immune response. These functions include increased expression of membrane-bound IL-1α and of class II molecules of the major histocompatibility complex (MHC). Monocytes differentiated in the presence of GM-CSF produce more IL-1 receptor antagonist (IL-1Ra), thus possibly leading to an inhibition of IL-1 effects. These properties of GM-CSF illustrate an essential principle of cytokine biology: a single cytokine may simultaneously exhibit both activating and suppressive effects.

The possible role of GM-CSF in rheumatic diseases is best illustrated by rheumatoid arthritis (RA). This is the only human disease in which both GM-CSF protein and mRNA are known to be localized in the damaged tissue. GM-CSF is also present in RA synovial fluids. The enhanced expression of class II MHC molecules observed on macrophages from RA synovial tissue may be secondary to the effects of GM-CSF.

IL-1 and tumor necrosis factor alpha (TNF-α) stimulate monocytes, fibroblasts, and endothelial cells to produce more GM-CSF. Some investigators believe that chronic inflammation and tissue destruction in some patients with RA

may result from a cytokine-mediated self-perpetuating cycle without a significant component of continuous T-cell activation.

GROWTH AND DIFFERENTIATION FACTORS

A number of cytokines exhibit as their major property a growth enhancement of specific cell types. These cytokines include platelet-derived growth factor (PDGF), epidermal growth factor (EGF), fibroblast growth factor (FGF), and transforming growth factor beta (TGF-β). Other cytokines are also growth-promoting, such as the CSFs and many of the interleukins.

PDGF is primarily a product of platelets but also is produced by macrophages, endothelial cells, and other cells (2). There are three different forms of PDGF and two different PDGF receptors. The biologic properties exhibited by PDGF vary with both the form synthesized by a particular cell and the predominant receptor expressed on a target cell. EGF is found throughout the body and is a potent angiogenic factor, as is FGF (3). Two main forms of FGF exist, although many structural variants have been described (4). Both EGF and FGF induce the growth and proliferation of a variety of mesenchymal and epithelial cells.

The marked proliferation of synovial fibroblasts that occurs in RA synovium is probably secondary to the effects of PDGF, EGF, and FGF. Tissue fibrosis present in other diseases, such as scleroderma, may also be due in part to PDGF, EGF, and FGF. The greatly enhanced growth of new capillaries that characterizes synovitis in RA is likely a result of multiple factors including FGF, IL-8, TNF-α, and vascular endothelial growth factor (VEGF). These growth factors are all present in synovial fluid of RA patients and are produced by synovial macrophages.

The last and most important growth factor to be discussed, TGF-β, has both potent pro- and anti-inflammatory effects (5). TGF-β exhibits many biologic properties, but its most important effects in rheumatic diseases include recruitment of monocytes into tissues, dampening of lymphocyte and macrophage functions, and stimulation of tissue fibrosis. More than any other cytokine, TGF-β exemplifies the apparent paradox of simultaneously enhancing inflammatory responses and promoting repair. In general, TGF-β is stimulatory toward resting or immature cells and when confined to local environments, but is inhibitory toward differentiated cells and when present systemically.

TGF-β is the major member of a family of molecules that may serve important roles in embryogenesis of mesenchymal tissues. Many cells in the adult contain mRNA for TGF-β, but macrophages and platelets are the main sources of protein. TGF-β is released in a latent form and must be activated in tissues, presumably by proteases.

The presence of other cytokines in a particular tissue also may influence whether TGF-β enhances or inhibits growth and differentiation in fibroblasts. For example, TGF-β and EGF together may suppress the growth of particular types of fibroblasts, while the combination of PDGF and TGF-β stimulates their growth. The enhancing effects of TGF-β on cell growth may be mediated through inducing PDGF production. TGF-β induces production of collagen and fibronectin in fibroblasts; however, interferon gamma (IFN-γ) and TNF-α both oppose this effect on collagen synthesis. In the presence of PDGF, EGF, and FGF, TGF-β also inhibits fibroblast production of collagenase and other neutral proteases while enhancing production of inhibitors of these enzymes.

TGF-β is thought to be responsible, at least in part, for tissue fibrosis in a variety of human diseases including scleroderma, pulmonary fibrosis, and chronic glomerulonephritis. Infiltrating monocytes in skin and organ lesions in scleroderma contain TGF-β mRNA. TGF-β protein has been found in skin lesions adjacent to fibroblasts and areas of fibrosis. The observation that IFN-γ inhibits TGF-β–induced collagen production by fibroblasts in vitro has given rise to clinical trials of IFN-γ in scleroderma patients.

Lastly, TGF-β exhibits potent effects on both monocytes and lymphocytes. TGF-β is the strongest known chemotactic agent for monocytes. In addition, TGF-β enhances expression of Fc receptor III on these cells but may block production of cytokines. It may promote inflammation; injection of TGF-β into rat joints leads to an influx of monocytes with swelling, redness, and eventual hyperplasia of synovial fibroblasts. However, the net effects of TGF-β on macrophage function are suppressive and include a decrease in HLA-DR expression and a deactivation of H_2O_2 production. Overall, TGF-β is thought to call monocytes into an acutely inflamed tissue, contribute to fibroblast proliferation, and then promote fibrosis.

TGF-β exhibits immunosuppressive effects on B cells, T cells, and natural killer (NK) cells. TGF-β inhibits IL-1–induced T-cell proliferation, B-cell growth, and immunoglobulin (Ig) production after stimulation by IL-2 and IL-4. IFN-γ–induced NK-cell function is opposed by TGF-β. The immunosuppression that occurs in streptococcal cell-wall–induced arthritis in rats is thought to be secondary to TGF-β, and a similar situation may be present in the joints of patients with RA.

Thus, growth and differentiation factors may be primarily responsible for fibroblast proliferation and angiogenesis in many human chronic inflammatory diseases. In addition, TGF-β may be involved in enhancing acute inflammatory events. It should be emphasized that these net biologic effects are secondary to multiple cytokines acting in both synergistic and opposing fashions. In addition, the state of differentiation of potential target cells for growth factors influences the resultant biologic response.

IMMUNOREGULATORY CYTOKINES

Interleukins 2, 4, 5, 7, 9, 10, and 11 and IFN-γ are all produced by T-cell subsets during an immune response and exert effects primarily on that response. In addition, IL-4, IL-10, and IFN-γ exhibit important effects on monocytes and macrophages. Other recently described immunoregulatory cytokines include interleukins 12 through 16.

T helper (Th) cells are divided into two subsets: Th1 cells produce IFN-γ, TNF-α, and IL-1, and Th2 cells secrete IL-4, IL-5, and IL-10. In part, these cytokines function to regulate differentiation of T-cell subsets. Th1-cell differentiation is enhanced by IFN-γ and IL-12, the latter cytokine produced primarily by macrophages and NK cells. However, Th1-cell differentiation is suppressed by IL-4 and IL-10. In contrast, Th2-cell differentiation is enhanced by IL-4 and inhibited by IFN-γ and IL-12.

Macrophage presentation of processed antigen in complex with a class II MHC molecule stimulates IL-2 production by CD4 helper T cells. IL-2 then binds to a specific two-chain receptor on target cells in the immediate micro-environment. IL-2 induces a clonal expansion of T cells, enhances B-cell growth, augments NK cell function, and activates macrophages.

IL-2 production was originally thought to be deficient in patients with autoimmune diseases such as RA and systemic lupus erythematosus (SLE) (6). However, these observations may represent an in vitro artifact, and IL-2 production actually may be excessive in these diseases in vivo. The administration of monoclonal antibodies to the IL-2 receptor ameliorates collagen-induced arthritis and lupus in mice. This observation argues for the probable importance of IL-2–driven T-cell responses in the counterpart human diseases of RA and SLE.

Soluble IL-2 receptors are found in the circulation of many patients with autoimmune, chronic inflammatory, or neoplastic diseases (7). These receptors are probably released by activated T cells, and their circulating levels correlate with clinical disease activity in some diseases including SLE.

In addition to Th2 cells, mast cells also produce IL-4 (8). IL-4 exerts a major influence on B cells through enhancing IgG_1 and IgE production, inducing the expression of Fc receptors for IgE, and stimulating the expression of class II MHC molecules. IL-4 exhibits both stimulatory and suppressive effects on mononuclear phagocytes, again illustrating the principle that a single cytokine may produce mixed or opposing consequences. IL-4 enhances the ability of these cells to present antigen by inducing the expression of class II MHC molecules. Paradoxically, IL-4 directly inhibits monocyte production of IL-1, IL-6, and TNF-α at the level of transcription; these effects of IL-4 are potentially quite anti-inflammatory. IL-10 and IL-13 function similarly to IL-4 in suppressing monocyte function (9,10). In addition, IL-4 alters the pattern of expression of adhesion molecules on endothelial cells to decrease neutrophil attachment but enhance lymphocyte migration into tissues. Although not yet directly proved, IL-4 may influence the function of many immune and inflammatory cells in human rheumatic diseases.

Interleukins 5, 7, 9, 11, 14, 15, and 16 function primarily as growth and differentiation factors. IL-5 is produced by T cells and enhances the immune response through effects on both T and B cells. IL-5 increases IL-2 receptor expression on these cells and promotes antibody secretion by B cells. In addition, IL-5 is the most active known cytokine on eosinophils, inducing chemotaxis, enhancing growth, and stimulating superoxide production. IL-14 is a potent growth factor for B cells.

Interleukins 7, 9, 11, 15, and 16 are primarily growth factors for T lymphocytes. IL-7 and 11 are synthesized by bone marrow stromal cells and exhibit additional effects on B cells and hematopoietic cells. IL-7 is a requisite factor for IL-1–induced thymocyte proliferation. These cytokines influence the function of other cells in addition to T lymphocytes. IL-9 induces proliferation of mast cells; IL-11 synergizes with IL-3 stimulation of megakaryocytes; IL-11, along with IL-1 and IL-6, induces the hepatic synthesis of acute-phase proteins; and IL-11 enhances antigen-specific B-cell responses. IL-15 shares biologic properties with IL-2 and is present in high concentrations in RA joints, where it may be responsible for attracting and activating T cells. IL-16 is a chemoattractant for CD4 T cells.

Unlike IL-2, most immunoregulatory cytokines have not been directly incriminated in pathophysiologic events in rheumatic diseases. However, these cytokines are indirectly involved through their effects on T lymphocytes and other cells. Endogenous IL-4 and IL-5 may play a role in asthma, and endogenous IL-10 and IL-13 may dampen synovitis in RA.

IFN-γ is produced simultaneously with IL-2 by antigen-stimulated T cells. A major function of IFN-γ is to enhance antigen presentation by stimulating the expression of MHC class I and II molecules on macrophages, endothelial cells, fibroblasts, and other more tissue-specific cells. IFN-γ is also a potent activator of macrophages, cytotoxic T cells, and NK cells. In addition, IFN-γ stimulates antibody production by B cells but, paradoxically, opposes the effects of IL-4 on these cells. This represents an example of self-regulation of the cytokine network through opposing effects.

IFN-γ may be relevant to many human autoimmune diseases, particularly SLE and RA. In SLE, the poor production of IFN-γ by T cells in vitro and the weak response to IFN-γ may reflect cells exhausted by intense IFN-γ effects in vivo, similar to IL-2. In RA, IFN-γ potentially could antagonize the stimulatory effects of TNF-α on many functions of synovial fibroblasts. IFN-γ production is probably deficient in the rheumatoid synovium, predisposing to unregulated TNF-α effects. However, the therapeutic administration of IFN-γ in RA patients appears not to offer more than moderate benefit.

Thus, the immunoregulatory cytokines may be important in rheumatic disease, both for their effects on immune cells and on macrophages. The possibility of manipulating this group of cytokines for therapeutic advantage has yet to be completely explored.

PRO-INFLAMMATORY CYTOKINES

The last group of cytokines to be discussed includes TNF-α and interleukins 1, 6, and 8. The functions of these molecules in normal physiology remain unclear, but an understanding of their possible role as inadvertent mediators of inflammation and tissue necrosis continues to grow. TNF-α and IL-1 are usually produced together and may act separately or together in different diseases. Clarifying the independent contribution of TNF-α and IL-1 to pathophysiologic events is made more difficult by the fact that each cytokine can induce production of itself and of the other.

TNF-α and TNF-β are related molecules that share the same receptors on plasma membranes of target cells (11). TNF-α structurally resembles a transmembrane molecule, and 1%–2% of TNF-α produced resides in the plasma membrane. TNF-α is produced by monocytes, macrophages, lymphocytes, and a variety of transformed cell lines. TNF-α production is stimulated by endotoxin, viruses, and other cytokines.

Two different TNF-α receptors are present on a variety of target cells. The extracellular portions of both TNF-α receptors can be cleaved, probably by proteases, releasing soluble receptors. Endogenously produced soluble TNF receptors may possibly function as regulators of extracellular TNF-α effects.

TNF-α exhibits many biologic properties that may be relevant to rheumatic diseases. Along with IL-1, TNF-α induces collagenase and prostaglandin E_2 (PGE_2) production in synovial fibroblasts. TNF-α is present in RA synovial tissues and may be an important inducer of IL-1 in this disease. TNF-α also may induce muscle breakdown and has been associated with the cachexia of congestive heart failure and other chronic diseases. In addition, TNF-α may play pathophysiologic roles in sepsis syndrome and in acute respiratory distress syndrome.

IL-1 is a family of three known molecules: IL-1 receptor antagonist (IL-1Ra), IL-1α, and IL-1β. These latter two family members bind to the same receptors and produce the same biologic responses (12). IL-1α, and IL-1β are primarily products of monocytes and macrophages but may also be produced by endothelial cells, epithelial cells, fibroblasts, activated T cells, and numerous other cells. In humans, IL-1β is the major extracellular product, whereas IL-1α remains primarily membrane-bound.

Two different IL-1 receptors exist: type I IL-1 receptors are present on T cells, endothelial cells, and fibroblasts, and type II IL-1 receptors predominate on B cells, monocytes, and neutrophils (13). Only type I IL-1 receptors are functionally active, whereas type II IL-1 receptors are not capable of inducing intracellular signals. Target cells are exquisitely sensitive to small concentrations of IL-1; occupancy of only 1%–2% of available type I IL-1 receptors stimulates a cell to display complete biologic responses. The expression of IL-1 type I receptors can be down-regulated by TGF-β, partially explaining the immunosuppressive properties of this cytokine.

IL-1 exhibits both systemic and local biologic effects in acute and chronic inflammatory diseases. Some systemic effects of IL-1 include fever, muscle breakdown, and, like IL-6 and IL-11, induction of acute-phase proteins in the liver. The local effects of IL-1 are best summarized by describing its purported role in RA (14). Early in the disease process, IL-1 may enhance expression of adhesion molecules on endothelial cells and induce chemotaxis of neutrophils, monocytes, and lymphocytes. Furthermore, IL-1 may contribute to tissue destruction in the rheumatoid joint through inducing PGE_2 and collagenase production by synovial fibroblasts and by chondrocytes present in the articular cartilage. IL-1 may exert similar effects on fibroblasts in other immune and inflammatory diseases, producing tissue damage in lungs, kidneys, or other organs.

IL-6 and IL-8 also play important roles in acute inflammatory diseases. IL-6 is produced by many cells, including synovial cells stimulated by IL-1 or TNF-α. The major functions of IL-6 are probably to induce hepatic synthesis of acute-phase proteins and to enhance Ig synthesis by B cells (15). High levels of IL-6 are present in inflammatory synovial fluids, and IL-6 is present in fibroblasts found in the synovium of RA patients. However, in RA, IL-6 does not induce collagenase and PGE_2 production by synovial fibroblasts and may actually enhance synthesis of a collagenase inhibitor. IL-6 may be primarily responsible for the hypergammaglobulinemia that characterizes many chronic inflammatory diseases.

IL-8 is one member of a family of chemotactic peptides (16). TNF-α and IL-1 stimulate IL-8 production by monocytes, macrophages, endothelial cells, fibroblasts, and other cells. IL-8 is an extremely potent chemotactic factor for neutrophils and may be responsible for attracting these cells into the joint in RA, gout, and other forms of inflammatory arthritis. In addition, IL-8 enhances other neutrophil properties including expression of adhesion molecules, generation of oxygen radicals, and release of lysosomal enzymes. Thus, IL-8 may contribute to rheumatic diseases by calling neutrophils into sites of acute inflammation and by activating these cells into an enhanced destructive profile.

REGULATION OF CYTOKINE EFFECTS

As emphasized throughout this chapter, the cytokine network functions in a self-regulatory fashion. Five different mechanisms regulate the actions of cytokines: specific receptor antagonists, soluble cytokine receptors, opposing actions of different cytokines, antibodies to cytokines, and protein binding of cytokines.

A specific receptor antagonist of IL-1 was originally described in the supernatants of monocytes cultured on adherent IgG and in the urine of febrile patients (17). Recombinant IL-1Ra has been studied in experimental models of disease in animals and in human diseases. IL-1Ra is structurally related to IL-1 and binds to both types of human IL-1 receptors on a variety of target cells without inducing discernable biologic responses. IL-1Ra represents the first known naturally occurring molecule that functions as a specific receptor antagonist.

A secreted form of IL-1Ra is produced by monocytes, macrophages, and neutrophils. An intracellular variant of IL-1Ra, which lacks the structural characteristics that lead to secretion, is produced by keratinocytes and other epithelial cells. Alveolar and synovial macrophages secrete little IL-1β, but synthesize large amounts of IL-1Ra, particularly under the influence of GM-CSF. Thus, IL-1Ra is a major product of tissue macrophages and may offer significant antagonism to IL-1 in the pericellular microenvironment of inflammatory tissues.

IL-1Ra has been extensively evaluated in vitro and in vivo, and this molecule blocks the inflammatory effects of IL-1 in every system evaluated (17). Most importantly, IL-1Ra does not affect normal T- or B-cell responses in vitro or in vivo, suggesting that IL-1 is not required for these responses. IL-1Ra has shown beneficial effects in many animal and in vitro models of human disease, including RA, septic shock, graft-versus-host disease, inflammatory bowel disease, chronic myelogenous leukemia, diabetes mellitus, and asthma. However, very high concentrations of IL-1Ra are required to block the effects of IL-1 in vivo. IL-1Ra was found not to be effective for treating patients with sepsis syndrome. Clinical trials in other human diseases are in progress.

Soluble cytokine receptors offer another possible mechanism of interference in vivo by binding cytokines in solution and blocking their interaction with target cells (18). A truncated form of the type I IL-1 receptor was genetically engineered, but it was not effective as a therapeutic agent in rheumatoid arthritis. Both types of TNF receptors occur in soluble forms and may be effective in blocking TNF effects in vitro and in vivo. Other soluble cytokine receptors have been described, but their in vivo relevance remains unclear.

Numerous examples have been given throughout this chapter of the opposing action of different cytokines. TGF-β has some opposing effects to IL-1 and TNF-α, whereas some effects of TGF-β are opposed by IFN-γ and TNF-α. Last, both IL-4 and IL-10 block monocyte production of IL-1, TNF-α, IL-6, and other cytokines. Whether these opposing biologic effects of cytokines can be utilized in the treatment of human diseases has not yet been determined.

Antibodies to many cytokines have been described in the serum of normal individuals, including antibodies to IL-1α (but not IL-1β), TNF-α, and IL-6 (19). These antibodies appear to block the biologic effects of some cytokines, but their in vivo relevance has not been established. Monoclonal antibodies to TNF-α are being evaluated as a therapeutic agent in sepsis syndrome, RA, and other human diseases. Multiple cytokines bind to α2-macroglobulin (α₂M) in circulation; however, many of these cytokines still retain partial or full biologic activities. Thus, protein binding of cytokines as a mechanism to inhibit the effects of cytokines in vivo has not been proved. These and other approaches to inhibiting the effects of cytokines in human diseases have recently been reviewed (20).

CONCLUSION

The field of cytokine biology is in its infancy. New cytokines continue to be discovered, and existing cytokines are found to possess previously unrecognized biologic properties. Cytokines do not exist solely to cause human diseases; rather, they are mediators of normal cellular events. Particular cytokines may cause unwanted consequences in human disease because they are produced in excess or because their effects are unregulated. Interference with cytokine actions may offer therapeutic efficacy in human diseases, possibly when used in conjunction with other established clinical approaches.

WILLIAM P. AREND, MD

1. Lieschke GJ, Burgess AW: Granulocyte colony-stimulating factor and granulocyte-macrophage colony-stimulating factor. New Engl J Med 327:28-35 and 99-106, 1992

2. Raines EW, Bowen-Pope DF, Ross R: Platelet-derived growth factors. In Sporn MB, Roberts AB (eds): Peptide Growth Factors and Their Receptors I. Berlin, Springer-Verlag, 1990

3. Carpenter C, Wahl MI: The epidermal growth factor family. In Sporn MB, Roberts AB (eds): Peptide Growth Factors and Their Receptors I. Berlin, Springer-Verlag, 1990

4. Baird A, Pöhlen P: Fibroblast growth factors. In Sporn MB, Roberts AB (eds.): Peptide Growth Factors and Their Receptors I. Berlin, Springer-Verlag, 1990

5. McCartney-Francis NL, Wahl SM: Transforming growth factor : a matter of life and death. J Leuk Biol 55:401-409, 1994

6. Kroemer G, Wick G: The role of interleukin 2 in autoimmunity. Immunol Today 10:246-251, 1989

7. Rubin LA, Nelson DL: The soluble IL-2 receptor: biology, function and clinical application. Ann Intern Med 113:619-627, 1990

8. Paul WE: Interleukin-4: a prototypic immunoregulatory lymphokine. Blood 77:1859-1870, 1991

9. Mosmann TR: Properties and functions of interleukin 10. Adv Immunol 56:1-26, 1994

10. Zurawski G, de Vries JE: Interleukin 13, an interleukin 4-like cytokine that acts on monocytes and B cells, but not on T cells. Immunol Today 15:19-26, 1994

11. Vassalli P: The pathophysiology of tumor necrosis factors. Ann Rev Immunol 10:411-452, 1992

12. Dinarello CA: Interleukin-1 and its biologically related cytokines. Adv Immunol 44:153-205, 1989

13. Sims JE, Giri JG, Dower SK: The two interleukin-1 receptors play different roles in IL-1 actions. Clin Immunol Immunopathol 72:9-14, 1994

14. Arend WP, Dayer J-M: Inhibition of the production and effects of IL-1 and TNF-α in rheumatoid arthritis. Arthritis Rheum 38:151-160, 1995

15. Akira S, Taga T, Kishimoto T: Interleukin 6 in biology and medicine. Adv Immunol 54:1-78, 1993

16. Oppenheim JJ, Zachariae COC, Mukaida N, Matsushima K: Properties of the novel proinflammatory supergene "intracrine" cytokine family. Ann Rev Immunol 9:617-648, 1991

17. Arend WP: IL-1 receptor antagonist. Adv Immunol 54:167-227, 1993

18. Fernandez-Botran R: Soluble cytokine receptors: their role in immunoregulation. FASEB J 5:2567-2574, 1991

19. Bendtzen K, Svenson M, Jonsson V, Hippe E: Autoantibodies to cytokines: friends or foes? Immunol Today 11:167-169, 1990

20. Arend WP: Inhibiting the effects of cytokines in human diseases. Adv Int Med 40:365-394, 1995

The complement system consists of at least 30 proteins that provide an innate defense against microbes and a "complement" to humoral immunity. It accomplishes this task by 1) depositing on pathologic targets and 2) promoting inflammation. Much of the early reaction sequence behaves as a biologic cascade in which, by limited proteolysis, one component activates the next, causing a rapid and robust amplification of the system. Because of its pro-inflammatory and injurious capabilities, nearly half of complement proteins are regulators.

In antibody-mediated autoimmune syndromes, complement components unwittingly serve as misguided missiles contributing to host tissue damage. Many rheumatic diseases are also mediated by immune complexes (IC) that deposit in tissue. The complement system is critical to the normal processing of IC, but it can produce damage if complexes inappropriately lodge in tissues such as the kidney. Deficiencies of components predispose the host to infectious and rheumatic diseases. For these reasons, complement measurements facilitate the diagnosis and management of rheumatic diseases.

COMPLEMENT DISCOVERY AND FUNCTION

An ancestral version of the complement system emerged more than 600 million years ago as a host defense system, predating antibody and T-cell–dependent immunity. Complement systems similar to those of mammals have been found in birds, reptiles, amphibians, and fish. Complement was identified in the 1890s as a heat-labile fraction in serum that assisted (complemented) a heat-stable fraction (antibody) to produce bacterial lysis. In the 1950s, a second pathway of complement activation was discovered that provided natural (innate) immunity. This system, the alternative pathway, was capable of identifying and destroying foreign elements independent of antibody. Recently the so-called "lectin pathway" has been described. It is similar to the activation scheme of the classical pathway except that antibody is not required. Instead, mannose-binding protein (MBP) and related proteins bind to sugar residues on the surface of a pathogen and then cause complement activation via the classical pathway.

The complement system consists of plasma and membrane proteins (1). The latter are synthesized in the liver as well as locally by cells such as monocytes/macrophages and fibroblasts.

Following activation, the complement system acts in two major ways (Fig. 5C-1): it modifies membranes and promotes inflammation.

Membrane Modification

Activated complement components deposit in large amounts on microbes and unwanted materials (such as immune aggregates). For example, several million activated fragments can attach to a bacterial surface in less than 5 minutes. The most critical function of these deposited complement proteins is to coat or *opsonize* the particle. Receptors on peripheral blood cells recognize these as ligands, subse-

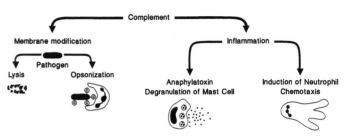

Complement Pathway

(Figure 5C-1)
The primary function of complement is to disrupt the membranes of pathogens by lysis or to coat their surfaces with complement components (opsonization) that facilitate their removal. Additionally, complement promotes inflammation by causing mast cells and basophils to "fire" and by attracting phagocytic cells to an area of inflammation.

quently binding to and then ingesting the complement-coated materials. Additionally, the membranes of some microorganisms are disrupted by the terminal complement components that cause osmotic lysis.

Promotion of Inflammation by Cell Activation

During complement activation, mediators are released whose purpose is to elicit a local inflammatory reaction. These fragments (eg, C3a, C5a) are termed *anaphylatoxins* because in excessive amounts, they may induce a reaction resembling anaphylaxis. By binding to cellular receptors at the site of complement activation, they trigger release of mediators (eg, histamine) that promote smooth-muscle contraction and dilation of blood vessels. Additionally, C5a serves as a chemotactic factor attracting phagocytic cells to an inflammatory locus.

NOMENCLATURE

Traditionally the complement system has been divided into two branches—the alternative pathway and the classical pathway. However, as mentioned, the newly discovered lectin pathway also can initiate the classical pathway. These pathways merge at the step of C3 activation and proceed to a common lytic pathway termed the *membrane attack complex* (MAC) (Fig. 5C-2). Nomenclature for the complement system is as follows: some serum components are identified by capital letters (factor B, D, and P of the alternative pathway) or numbers (C1–C4 for the classical pathway and C5–C9 for the MAC). Upon proteolytic activation, a smaller fragment may be liberated and is designated by a small "a" ("C3a" or "Ba"). The remaining, larger fragment attaches to a substrate and is noted with a "b," as in C3b or Bb. Inactivation produces further breakdown products designated by suffixes, such as when C3b is cleaved into C3c and C3d fragments.

CLASSICAL PATHWAY

Four concepts facilitate an understanding of the classical pathway: attachment, activation, amplification, and attack.

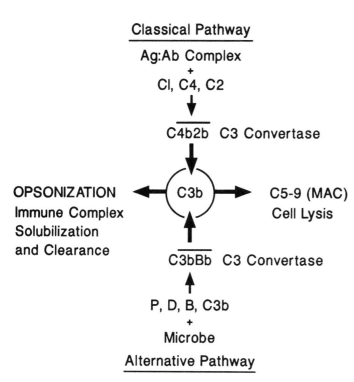

Classical Pathway

Ag:Ab Complex
+
Cl, C4, C2

C4b2b C3 Convertase

OPSONIZATION — C3b — C5-9 (MAC)
Immune Complex Cell Lysis
Solubilization
and Clearance

C3bBb C3 Convertase

P, D, B, C3b
+
Microbe

Alternative Pathway

(Figure 5C-2)
Simplified scheme of complement activation emphasizing the central role of C3b. Generation of C3b by the C3 convertases is the major physiologic goal of complement activation. C3b (and its fragments) are ligands for receptors on immune cells. C3b also serves as the gateway to the membrane attack complex (MAC).

Attachment

The classical cascade is activated by the binding of the C1q subcomponent of C1 to the Fc portion of an antibody in an antigen-antibody (Ag-Ab) complex. C1q is part of a large calcium-dependent complex termed *C1* that also includes the tetramer C1s-C1r-C1r-C1s. IgM and IgG subclasses 1 and 3 activate complement, but not IgA, IgD, or IgE.

Activation

After binding the C1q portion to Ab, the serine protease C1r undergoes an autoactivation cleavage process and then cleaves the serine protease, C1s. C1s, in turn, cleaves C4 and C2. Large fragments derived from C4 (C4b) and C2 (C2b) assemble on the target surface forming the enzymatic C3 convertase, C4b2b. C4 possesses a remarkable post-translational thioester modification that, when cleaved, allows C4b to covalently attach to a foreign particle by forming ester or amide linkages. C3 also possesses this feature, usually binding to a substrate via an ester linkage.

Amplification

Each activated C1 generates many C4b and C2b fragments. Most C4b fragments serve as opsonins while some bind C2b to form C3 convertases. Each C3 convertase can rapidly generate many activated C3 molecules. In a study quantitating classical pathway–mediated activation on nucleated cells, after Ab affixed to cellular membrane antigens, 2.4×10^6 C4 molecules and 0.67×10^6 C2 molecules subsequently attached to form C3 convertases (2). Within 5 minutes, 2.1×10^7 molecules of C3b were deposited. Finally, approximately 1×10^6 MACs were formed. Concomitantly, the

anaphylatoxins C3a and C4a are generated equal to the number of C3b and C4b fragments formed.

Attack

Most C3b fragments deposited on targets serve as opsonins (ligands) for C3b receptors. A smaller percentage of C3b fragments covalently bind to C4b in the C4b2b enzymatic complex (C3 convertase) generating the C5 convertase, C4b2b3b. C5 is the substrate for this trimeric enzymatic complex. Generation of C5b leads to the subsequent formation of the MAC (C5b + C6 + C7 + C8 + multiple C9). After C5 cleavage, the assembly of the MAC occurs via protein–protein interactions (ie, no proteolysis is involved) (3).

ALTERNATIVE PATHWAY

Although Ab binding to Ag initiates the classical cascade, the alternative pathway has no such requirement for Ab. A small amount of auto-activated C3 (so-called "C3 tickover") is always present in the system so that if it encounters a foreign surface, C3 quickly engages the alternative pathway. Although, this is a "shot-gun" approach to host defense, it nonetheless provides an important surveillance role in the nonimmune host (ie, provides innate immunity). Amplification occurs in the presence of foreign material. A feedback loop or auto-amplification pathway develops on the foreign material. C3b covalently attaches to the foreign particle and then binds factor B. The latter undergoes proteolytic cleavage mediated by factor D to produce the fragments Bb and Ba. The alternative pathway C3 convertase, C3bBb, is stabilized by properdin (P). As the convertase cleaves more C3 to C3b, a feedback/amplification loop is set in motion, resulting in the deposition of large amounts of C3b. The alternative pathway may also engage the MAC. In this case, the C5 convertase is C3bBbC3bP.

Lectins are carbohydrate-binding proteins. They were initially described in the 1890s as proteins capable of agglutinating red blood cells. Recently they have been found to be an important part of the innate immune system. In particular, MBP is a serum protein that preferentially binds to a specific type of N-linked bi-antennary complex type oligosaccharide. This subtle, yet specific recognition of a foreign natural carbohydrate allows MBP to attack the pathogen.

MBP has a structure resembling C1q in that it is an oligomer with an N-terminal collagenous domain and a globular C-terminal domain. The main difference is that the C-terminus of MBP possesses a carbohydrate-recognition domain, whereas C1q has an immunoglobulin-binding domain. Similar to C1q, MBP may activate C1r and C1s in order to cleave C4 and C2. Also, a receptor (termed the collection receptor) binds to MBP complexed with a pathogen to assist in clearing the complex. Thus, MBP, like antibody, acts as an opsonin. Similar to the alternative pathway, the lectin pathway does not require prior contact with the pathogen and thus is part of innate immunity.

COMPLEMENT RECEPTORS

The complement system exerts much of its effector function via receptors. C3a and C5a mediate vasodilation and chemotaxis through interaction with C3a and C5a receptors on basophils, leukocytes, and mast cells (4). The larger opsonic polypeptide fragments, including C3b and C4b, mediate clearance of IC and bacteria through complement receptor type one (CR1). Further degradation of C3b leads to the formation of iC3b and C3dg, which interact with two other complement receptors, CR3 and CR2, respectively.

CR1 plays as an important role in IC clearance. The majority of CR1 in the peripheral blood is found on erythrocytes, where it binds C3b/C4b-coated IC for processing and transport to the liver or spleen (5). The IC are transferred from the erythrocyte to tissue macrophages, allowing the erythrocyte to return to the circulation. CR1 on granulocytes and monocytes promotes IC adherence and phagocytosis, while on lymphocytes CR1 facilitates trapping of such IC in lymphoid organs.

CONTROL OF THE COMPLEMENT SYSTEM

Unregulated, the complement system would fire to exhaustion, a point well-illustrated by inborn errors of regulatory proteins. Checks and balances occur at each major step in the pathway (6). This regulation prevents excessive activation on one target, fluid-phase activation (ie, no target), and activation on self (ie, inappropriate target). In the early phase of the classical pathway, C1 inhibitor prevents excessive activation on one target and fluid-phase C1 activation. The convertase steps of both pathways are monitored by a family of proteins that includes the membrane proteins decay-accelerating factor (DAF, also known as CD55) and membrane cofactor protein (MCP, also known as CD46), as well as serum components C4-binding protein (C4bp) and factor H. These proteins function in two ways: by disassembling the convertases (decay accelerating activity), and by facilitating their proteolytic inactivation (cofactor activity) in collaboration with the serine protease factor I. The terminal components, MAC, are also regulated by both serum and cell-anchored proteins. CD59 inhibits the MAC from fully assembling on host tissue, while vitronectin (S-protein) controls fluid-phase MAC. As a result, complement attack is focused on foreign surfaces (which usually lack complement regulators) and held in check on host cells and in body fluids. Interestingly, a number of microorganisms "capture" complement regulatory molecules or have evolved their own in order to subvert the system (7).

COMPLEMENT AND RHEUMATIC DISEASE
Immune Complex Diseases

The pathophysiologic history of many inflammatory diseases includes the synthesis of autoantibodies and/or the presence of excessive quantities of IC. For example, if the host synthesizes an antibody reacting with a self-antigen or an erythrocyte, antibody will bind to this autoantigen and activate the complement cascade. Thus, just the complement system may destroy a microbe, it may lyse an erythrocyte, phagocytose a platelet, or disrupt a basement membrane. Further, some types of IC lodge in tissues, activate complement, and cause synovitis, vasculitis, dermatitis, and glomerulonephritis.

Complement Deficiency

Although rare, inherited deficiencies of complement components predispose to bacterial infections and/or immune-complex excess syndromes such as systemic lupus erythematosus (SLE) (Table 5C-1) (8). Deficiencies are inherited autosomal codominant (recessive) traits, except those of C1 inhibitor (autosomal dominant) and properdin (X-linked).

Acquired complement deficiency may result from excessive consumption, as is the case for SLE. Acquired decreases

(Table 5C-1)
Inherited complement deficiencies

Components	Associated Illness
C1q, C1r, C1s, C4*, C2	SLE, glomerulonephritis, vasculitic syndromes
C3	Pyogenic infections, SLE
C5–8	*Neisseria* infections
D and Properdin	*Neisseria meningitides* infections
C1 Inhibitor	Hereditary angioedema
DAF and CD59	Paroxysmal nocturnal hemglobinuria
Factors H and I	Pyogenic infections, urticaria, glomerulonephritis, (secondary deficiency of C3)

* C4 consists of two subtypes termed C4A and C4B that are more than 99% homologous. The few amino acid differences lead to functional consequences, ie, C4A more efficiently forms amide linkages with substrates, whereas C4B more efficiently forms ester bonds. The C4 genes are tandemly arranged on chromosome 6 in the major histocompatibility locus. The C4A deficiency in SLE is usually found as part of the HLA complex containing B8 and DR3. About 10%–15% of white SLE patients are homozygous for C4A deficiency.

secondary to classical pathway activation (ie, C1–9) are observed in >50% of SLE patients. Generally, the more active the disease, the more likely complement levels will be low; this is particularly true for lupus nephritis. Additionally, an acquired deficiency of CR1 on erythrocytes also may be present, resulting in diminished ability to eliminate IC. The presence of antibody to native DNA coupled with low serum complement levels is highly specific for the diagnosis of SLE.

A C3 deficiency state is acquired when an autoimmune antibody is made against a C3 convertase. The autoantibody is called the "C3 nephritic factor" if against the alternative pathway convertase, or a "C4 nephritic factor" if against the classical pathway convertase. The autoantibody stabilizes the convertase causing excessive C3 cleavage, which produces a secondary deficiency of C3. These patients are predominantly children who may present with glomerulonephritis, partial lipodystrophy, or frequent infections with encapsulated bacteria.

COMPLEMENT MEASUREMENT

Complement can be assessed by either functional or antigenic assays. Generally used in clinical practice are the total hemolytic complement assay (THC, CH_{50}), which measures activation of the entire classical pathway, and immunoassays for C3 and C4 (9). The THC is based on the ability of the test serum to lyse sheep erythrocytes optimally sensitized with rabbit antibody. All nine components of the classical pathway (ie, C1–9) are required for a normal THC value. A THC of 200 means that at a dilution of 1:200, the tested serum lysed 50% of the Ab-coated sheep erythrocytes. THC is a useful screening tool for detecting the homozygous deficiency of complement proteins because a deficiency of any one of C1–9 components will lower the THC.

Assays for C4 and C3 also are widely available. They are usually measured in nephelometric immunoassays, which

(Table 5C-2)
Interpretation of results of complement determinations

Patient	THC (units/ml)	C4 (mg/dl)	C3 (mg/ml)	Interpretation*
–	150–200	16–48	100–180	Normal ranges
1	300	50	200	Acute phase response
2	100	10	80	CP activation
3	<10	30	140	Inherited deficiency or in vitro activation†
4	75	30	50	AP activation

* CP and AP refer to the classical and alternative pathways.
† In vitro activation is more common than an inherited deficiency state. The lack of activity (<10 THC) in the setting of normal C4 and C3 antigenic levels suggests improperly handled sample, cold activation (such as by cryoglobulins), or homozygous component deficiency (most commonly C2 with a lupus-like presentation or one of the MAC proteins if *Neisseria* infection coexists).

detect changes in the intensity of light scatter as complement proteins interact with specific antibodies. The assays are useful in following the course of patients undergoing treatment who initially present with low levels. Table 5C-2 provides examples of serum complement test results and their interpretation.

Becoming more widely available are tests for the detection of activation or cleavage products such the anaphylatoxins (C3a, C5a); the cleavage peptides released from C4 (C4d), C3 (C3d), or factor B (Bb); and neoantigens produced by activation fragments. Their clinical utility relates to the fact that they are dynamic activation parameters reflecting ongoing turnover of the system, and are not affected by partial inherited deficiencies or alterations in synthetic rate. However, they are not widely available, generally are more costly, and are not necessary in most clinical situations.

THERAPEUTIC IMPLICATIONS OF COMPLEMENT

Study of the complement system has undergone a renaissance over the past decade. Much of this revival relates to the discovery and characterization of the membrane regulatory and receptor proteins. The cloning of components permits their genetic manipulation for therapeutic intervention. For example, by liberating the cell-anchored regulators from their membrane tethering, soluble versions are being developed and tested for their ability to inhibit complement activation. Such engineering already has led to developing a soluble version of CR1 (10). Experimental infusion of soluble CR1 blocks several types of inflammatory and vasculitic destructive processes that are complement-dependent. Surprisingly, complement inhibition by soluble CR1 also reduced infarct size in two animal model systems of myocardial infarction and in several other models of reperfusion injury. These remarkable results suggest that the complement system also plays a role in removing dead and dying tissue. Unfortunately, at present there is no commercially available inhibitor of the complement system.

Another potential use of complement regulatory proteins is in xenotransplantation (11). Normally, transplantation of a nonhuman organ into a human results in rapid rejection of the organ, largely due to complement activation. However, organs from transgenic pigs that express human complement regulatory proteins are being developed. Such organs should be "protected" and resistant to the acute rejection mediated by complement.

SUMMARY

The complement system provides natural immunity against microbes and complements the antibody-mediated system. It promotes the inflammatory process by activating cells and assists the host in the handling of IC. In disease states (especially those with autoantibodies and excessive IC formation), complement contributes to tissue destruction. The critical functions of complement are highlighted by diseases such as hereditary angioedema and SLE that develop due to inherited deficiencies. Tight control of this system is a necessity indicated by the fact that nearly half of complement components serve a role in regulation.

M. KATHRYN LISZEWSKI
JOHN P. ATKINSON, MD

1. Liszewski MK, Atkinson JP: The complement system. In Paul WE (ed): Fundamental Immunology. New York: Raven Press, 1993, 917-939.
2. Ollert MW, Kadlec JV, David K, Petrella EC, Bredehorst R, Vogel C-W: Antibody-mediated complement activation on nucleated cells: a quantitative analysis of the individual reaction steps. J Immunol 153:2213-2221, 1994.
3. Morgan BP: Effects of the membrane attack complex of complement on nucleated cells. Curr Top Microbiol Immunol 178:115-140, 1992.
4. Hugli TE: Biochemistry and biology of anaphylatoxins. Complement 3:11-127, 1986.
5. Hebert LA, Cosio FG: The erythrocyte-immune complex-glomerulonephritis connection in man. Kidney Int 31:877-885, 1987.
6. Liszewski MK, Farries TC, Lublin DM, Rooney IA, Atkinson JP: Control of the complement system. Adv Immunol 61:201-283, 1995.
7. Cooper NR: Complement evasion strategies of microorganisms. Immunol Today 12:327-331, 1991.
8. Densen P: Human complement deficiency states and infection. In Whaley K, Loos M, Weiler JM (eds): Complement in Health and Disease. Boston: Kluwer, 1993, 173-197
9. Morgan BP: Complement measurement and potential for therapeutic manipulation. In Morgan BP (ed): Complement: Clinical Aspects and Relevance to Disease. New York: Academic Press, 1990, 193-208
10. Moore FD Jr: Therapeutic regulation of the complement system in acute injury states. Adv Immunol 56:267-299, 1994
11. Cozzi E, White DJG: The generation of transgenic pigs as potential organ donors for humans. Nature Med 1:964-966, 1995

Maintenance of tissue homeostasis requires a dynamic and reciprocal dialogue between the cell and the surrounding tissue extracellular matrix (ECM). In pathologic states such as inflammation and rheumatic diseases, this intricate balance of ECM synthesis and degradation by proteinases is disturbed. In the past few years, development of targeted gene expression or disruption of proteinases and their inhibitors has increased our knowledge of the biochemical and biological aspects of these molecules.

EXTRACELLULAR MATRIX-DEGRADING PROTEINASES

Proteinases are mediators of ECM degradation necessary for normal processes such as wound healing, embryonic implantation, and reproductive tissue remodeling during and after pregnancy, as well as for pathological processes such as lung fibrosis, chronic inflammation, osteoarthritis, atherosclerosis, and tumor invasion. There are four classes of proteinases: two active at acid pH (aspartic and cysteine proteinases), and two active at neutral pH (serine and matrix metalloproteinases) (Tables 5D-1 and 5D-2). Proteinases can be derived from virtually all mammalian cell types, including inflammatory cells, epithelial cells, and stromal cells. Specific proteinases are regulated by factors such as cytokines, growth factors, and ECM molecules (1).

Aspartic Proteinases

Aspartic proteinases have a catalytic motif that includes an essential aspartic acid residue. Two of the most prominent aspartic proteinases acting at acid pH are cathepsin D and cathepsin E, enzymes in the same multigene family as pepsin, renin, and HIV protease (reviewed in Werb and Alexander [1]). Cathepsin D is found in the endosomes and lysosomes of most cells, including fibroblasts; however, its activity is higher in phagocytic cells, such as macrophages, and is increased by connective tissue activation. It functions primarily in intralysosomal protein degradation and may be involved in degradation of antigens for presentation. Under inflammatory conditions and during periods of rapid ECM destruction, cathepsin D is secreted extracellularly by macrophages and connective tissue cells, mostly as the proenzyme. A surprising biologic function of cathepsin D was recently discovered by targeted gene disruption of this enzyme (2). Transgenic mice deficient for the lysosomal enzyme cathepsin D exhibited progressive atrophy followed by necrosis of intestinal mucosa, as well as profound destruction of thymus and spleen with fulminant loss of T and B cells.

Cathepsin E functions as a homodimer, consisting of two monomers linked by an intermolecular disulfide bond. Cathepsin E has been localized to endocytotic vacuoles in the ruffled border membrane of active osteoclasts in the physiologic bone modeling process. In active bone remodeling, cathepsin E is involved both in the extracellular degradation of bone organic matrix in the closed extracellular acidic environment and in the intracellular breakdown of ingested substances (3). Cathepsin E is elevated in the brains of patients with Alzheimer's disease, suggesting a role for this enzyme in neurodegradation of Alzheimer-type dementia (4).

Aspartic proteinases have few natural inhibitors. However, the microbial inhibitor pepstatin and its derivatives are effective inhibitors in experimental systems.

Cysteine Proteinases

Cysteine proteinases consist of a large family of enzymes that show significant sequence homology. They are evolutionarily related to papain and have catalytic sites that require cysteine and histidine residues (1). The three most prominent cysteine proteinases, cathepsins B, K(Os), and L, have been associated with inflammatory reactions and with osteoclasts in bone. In human tissues, the cysteine proteinases with greatest activity against collagens and proteoglycans are cathepsins L and N. Cysteine proteinases are inactivated by thiol-blocking reagents in general, but more selective inhibitors usable in biologic systems are leupeptin, E-64, and certain fluoromethyl and chloromethyl ketones. The natural inhibitors in plasma are α_1-cysteine proteinase inhibitor and α_2-macroglobulin (5). In an in vitro model of bone resorption, the addition of parathyroid hormone, $1\alpha,25\text{-}(OH)_2D3$, or tumor necrosis factor α markedly enhanced secretion of procathepsin L. The direct biologic significance of this finding was observed in pit formation in bone, which was inhibited by a cathepsin L inhibitor (5). Inhibitors of these cysteine proteinases reduce parathyroid hormone-induced bone resorption in vivo (5). The importance of cathepsin K in osteoclast function has been underscored by the finding that in pyknodysostosis, the cathepsin K gene has mutations (6).

Interleukin-1β–converting enzyme (ICE) and its relatives are cytoplasmic enzymes that participate in protein processing and have key functions in the cell death program of apoptosis (7). ICE is essential for the processing and secretion of the cytokine interleukin-1β. ICE and its family members are also critical in the cleavage of intracellular proteins during programmed cell death of lymphocytes and other cells. Degradation of nuclear proteins by ICE family proteinases may generate certain autoantigens seen in systemic lupus erythematosus. The ICE proteinases are inhibited by specific serpin-like inhibitors from viruses, for example crmA from cowpox virus, that help the virus evade the host response to kill the infected cell by apoptosis. Mammalian counterparts of this serpin have not yet been identified.

Serine Proteinases

The serine proteinase family is a large family of enzymes, the majority of which are structurally related to trypsin. A smaller subset of distinct proteinases related to subtilisin include the furin family of enzymes, which are involved in processing cell surface and secreted proteins and hormones. These proteinases, with a catalytically essential serine residue at their active site, are most active at neutral pH. Their physiologic importance is reflected by the fact that serine proteinase inhibitors represent 10% of all plasma proteins. The serine proteinases include many of the proteins of the cascades of coagulation, fibrinolysis, complement, and kinins in the plasma, such as thrombin, plasmin, Cls, Clr,

(Table 5D-1)

*Secreted aspartic, cysteine, and serine proteinase families and relevant biologic functions**

Class	Enzyme	Primary Substrate	Primary Location	Transgenic Mice and Other Disease Models
Aspartic	Cathepsin D	Elastin	Macrophages	Atrophy of ileal mucosa, loss of T and B cells
	Cathepsin E	Bone matrix	Osteoclasts, cerebral cortex	Bone remodeling, Alzheimer-type dementia
Cysteine	Cathepsin B	Proteoglycan, collagen type I, fibronectin		Lung cancer
	Cathepsin L	Proteoglycan, fibronectin		Breast cancer
	ICE	Interleukin-1	Monocytes	
Serine	Plasmin	Fibrin, proteoglycan, collagen types III and IV, fibronectin, laminin		Atherosclerosis, fibrin deposition
	Kallikrein	Plasminogen		
	Thrombin	Fibrinogen	Platelets	
	Urokinase	Fibronectin, plasminogen	Endothelial cells	
	Plasminogen activator			
	Tissue-type plasminogen activator	Fibronectin, plasminogen	Endothelial cells	
	PMN elastase	Elastin, collagen types I and IV, heparan sulfate proteoglycan, laminin	PMN	Wegener's granulomatosis
	Cathepsin G	Cartilage proteoglycan, fibronectin		
	Mast cell chymases	Cartilage proteoglycan, heparan sulfate proteoglycan	Mast cells	Asthma
	Mast cell tryptases		Mast cells	Asthma
	Granzyme B	Intracellular	Cytotoxic T cells	Induces apoptosis

* ICE = interleukin-1-β-converting enzyme; PMN = polymorphonuclear leukocytes.

and kallikrein, as well as trypsin, chymotrypsin, and elastase from the exocrine pancreas. Plasmin and the plasminogen activators–ie, plasma kallikrein, tissue kallikreins, and the serine proteinases from the granules of polymorphonuclear leukocytes (PMN)–cytotoxic T cells, and mast cells play a role in tissue degradation.

Plasmin

Plasmin is a broad-spectrum serine proteinase that is converted from the inactive circulating precursor form plasminogen to the catalytically active form by the plasminogen activators. Plasmin is also a potent activator of most matrix metalloproteinases by promoting cleavage of the latent propeptides to active molecules (1). Plasmin primarily mediates the degradation of provisional and rapidly remodeling matrices such as fibrin and fibronectin, whereas it does not cleave interstitial collagens. Mice with null mutations in their plasminogen gene have severe wound healing deficits owing to the massive accumulation of fibrin (8).

Plasminogen activators

The two physiologic plasminogen activators, tissue-type plasminogen activator (tPA) and urokinase-type plasminogen activator (uPA), are products of separate genes with different chromosomal locations that activate the proenzyme plasminogen to plasmin (9). Plasma kallikrein also has plasminogen-activating activity. The binding and activation of uPA on the cell surface via uPA-specific receptors provides a mechanism for localizing proteolytic activity in the microenvironment below the cell (9). This directional proteolysis is an essential part of such diverse biologic phenomena as angiogenesis, ovulation, embryonic implantation, and wound healing. Intravenous injection of recombinant tPA is widely used in medical practice to achieve thrombolytic

(Table 5D-2)

Matrix metalloproteinase (MMP) family of proteinase enzymes and relevant biological functions

Enzyme	MMP Nomenclature	Other Names	Substrate
Gelatinases			
Gelatinase A	MMP-2	72-kD gelatinase, type IV collagenase	Denatured collagen and native collagen types I, IV, V, VII, X
Gelatinase B	MMP-9	92-kD gelatinase	Elastin, fibronectin
Collagenases			
Collagenase-1	MMP-1	Fibroblast-type, interstitial collagenase	Collagen types I, II, III, VII, VIII, X
Collagenase-2	MMP-8	PMN-type	Collagen types I, III
Collagenase-3	MMP-13	Osteoblast-type	Collagen types I, III
Stromelysins			
Stromelysin-1	MMP-3	Transin	Cartilage proteoglycans, fibronectin, laminin, collagen types IV, IX, X
Stromelysin-2	MMP-10	Transin-2	Elastin, α_1-proteinase inhibitor
Stromelysin-3	MMP-11		
Metalloelastase	MMP-12	Macrophage elastase	Proteoglycan, elastin, α_1-proteinase inhibitor, fibronectin
Matrilysin	MMP-7	Pump-1	Fibronectin, cartilage proteoglycan, laminin, collagen type IV
Membrane-type MMP			
MT-MMP-1	MMP-14		Progelatinase A
MT-MMP-2	MMP-15		
MT-MMP	MMP-16		

canalization of occluded arteries in acute ischemic myocardial infarction. tPA primarily removes fibrin from intravascular clots, whereas uPA has a lower affinity for fibrin. Therefore, the role of uPA in thrombolysis was not well understood until recently, when the physiologic loss of plasminogen activator gene function was addressed in a study of uPA- and tPA-targeted gene disruption (9). Macrophages in transgenic mice lacking the uPA gene were incapable of fibrin lysis, although invasion of macrophages into the peritoneal cavity was not altered. Doubly deficient (uPA and tPA) knockout mice survived embryonic development but had retarded postnatal growth, reduced fertility, and a shortened life span.

Leukocyte elastase

The PMN elastase is present in the azurophil granules of PMN and monocytes as a precursor containing two additional amino acid residues (GlyGlu) compared with the active form, as is also true for cathepsin G (1). It degrades cartilage proteoglycan by removing the hyaluronic acid–binding region and then fragmenting the glycosaminoglycan attachment region. Elastin, the cross-linked structural protein important for the elastic strength of the arterial walls, lung, joint capsule, and skin, is degraded by PMN elastase. The PMN elastase also actively degrades fibronectin, laminin, proteoglycans, and type IV collagen of basement membranes, making it highly destructive to ECM. Extracellular activity of PMN elastase is controlled by α_1-proteinase inhibitor and α_2-macroglobulin. Antineutrophil cytoplasmic antibodies (ANCA) are autoantibodies against the proteinase found in the azurophilic granules of PMN. Clinically, detection of ANCA levels in the serum has be-

come a valuable tool in the diagnosis of patients suspected of having vasculitis such as Wegener's granulomatosis.

Cathepsin G

Cathepsin G is a chymotrypsin enzyme of PMN that is structurally related to the chymases of mast cell granules. The action of cathepsin G on cartilage proteoglycan is somewhat more restricted than that of PMN elastase, and the enzyme has little or no action on elastin or type I collagen (1). Cathepsin G is effective in solubilizing collagen from cartilage and may generate physiologically active products from complement components. Physiologic inhibitors of cathepsin G include the plasma proteins α_1-antichymotrypsin, α_1-proteinase inhibitor, and α_2-macroglobulin. Cathepsin G is an activator of metalloproteinases.

Metalloproteinases

The matrix metalloproteinases (MMP) constitute a closely related group of zinc-dependent enzymes that degrade ECM macromolecules at neutral pH. These enzymes are fundamentally responsible for many diverse biologic functions of the cell, including cell migration, proliferation, wound healing, tumor invasion, and metastasis. The MMP gene family consists of a number of well-characterized proteinases in human tissue that have been cloned and show significant sequence homology. The MMP are classified into four major subclasses: collagenases, gelatinases, stromelysins, and a new subclass, membrane-type MMP (MT-MMP) (Table 5D-2). All MMP share several common properties and are inactivated by tissue inhibitors of metalloproteinases (TIMP), EDTA, and zinc-chelating agents such as 1,10-phenanthroline. The primary sequence of MMP consists of activation, catalytic zinc-binding, hemopexin/vitronectin homology, and transmembrane domains (10).

Collagenases

There are three distinct collagenases, enzymes that are able to cleave the triple helical backbone of fibrillar collagens. Interstitial collagenase (also called MMP-1) is specific for collagen as substrate and cleaves all three chains of the triple helix at one susceptible point, between residues 775 and 776 of the α(I) chain. The bonds cleaved are between residues of glycine and isoleucine of collagens of type I, II, and III (12). Collagenase-1 also cleaves collagens of type VII and VIII and makes two cleavages in collagen type X, but it does not degrade basement membrane collagen type IV or types V or VI collagen. Interstitial collagenase is produced by a wide variety of cells, including macrophages, fibroblasts, synovial cells, chondrocytes, and endothelial cells (13).

Polymorphonuclear leukocytes have collagenase-2, a proteinase that has a sequence different from that produced by cells of tissues such as the synovium, although it is closely related. The PMN collagenase (also called MMP-8), which is about 75 kD, is stored in tertiary granules of PMN and secreted rapidly in response to chemotactic and other stimuli (12). Collagenase-2 degrades type I collagen more readily than type III collagen and prefers collagen in solution to fibrillar collagen. The PMN collagenase is present in much smaller amounts in the cells than are elastase and cathepsin G, and its significance in collagen degradation remains to be determined.

Osteoblasts and osteosarcoma cells from rats, mice, and humans express collagenase-3 (MMP-13), an enzyme that degrades triple helical collagens but has a sequence as distinct from interstitial and PMN collagenases as from the stromelysins (11). Its physiologic role in collagen turnover has yet to be elucidated.

Collagenases and the other mammalian MMP are commonly found in culture and tissues in inactive proenzyme form. The procollagenases of about 55 kD are activated by a multi-enzyme cascade and a cysteine switch mechanism to active forms of about 45 kD (11,12).

Most of the inhibitory capacity of plasma and rheumatoid synovial fluid for collagenase is due to α_2-macroglobulin, which reacts more slowly with PMN collagenase than with interstitial collagenase from other cells (12). Although plasma concentrations of MMP appear to be controlled by α_2-macroglobulin, the primary tissue inhibitor is TIMP-1, a glycoprotein of about 28 kD. TIMP-1, unlike α_2-macroglobulin, can enter the interstitial spaces such as cartilage matrix and forms tight complexes with all members of the MMP family. Two other members of the TIMP family, TIMP-2 and TIMP-3, also inhibit collagenase (14).

Stromelysins

Several distinct genes with stromelysin-type function in humans have been identified. Stromelysin-1 (also called proteoglycanase, MMP-3, transin, or neutral proteinase) is the primary MMP, other than collagenase, and is produced as a proenzyme of about 51 kD that is activated to forms of 41 kD and further degraded to active enzymes of 21–25 kD. Stromelysin-1 has a wide variety of connective tissue and plasma protein substrates, including proteoglycans, some collagen types (IV, V, VII, and IX), denatured type I collagen, laminin, fibronectin, elastin, α_1-proteinase inhibitor, im-

munoglobulins, and substance P. In addition, it has a significant function in the multi-enzyme cascade involved in activating procollagenase (12,13,14).

Stromelysin-1 is inhibited by α_2-macroglobulin and TIMP-1. Stromelysin-1 is produced by the same range of cells as collagenase-1. Although it is frequently synthesized and secreted in coordination with both collagenase-1 and stromelysin-1, it may be independently regulated in human fibroblasts, chondrocytes, and macrophages.

A second enzyme closely related to stromelysin-1 is stromelysin-2 (also called MMP-10 or transin-2), which has been cloned and characterized (10, 11). It has nearly identical substrate specificity with stromelysin-1 (nearly 80%), but very distinct regulation with predominant expression in epithelial cells. Dermal fibroblasts isolated from patients with scleroderma, an autoimmune disorder in which excessive ECM is collected in skin and lungs, produce less stromelysin-1 than do normal dermal fibroblasts (15,16). Thus, abnormalities in the production of matrix enzymes appear to play a part in the pathogenesis of systemic sclerosis.

Matrilysin (also known as Pump-1, punctuated metalloproteinase, small uterine metalloproteinase, or MMP-7) was initially described as a truncated cDNA with the pro-enzyme activation, catalytic, and zinc-binding sequences of MMP, but lacking the hemopexin domain found in all other members of the family (1,10,11). It is clearly a stromelysin-like enzyme with substrate specificity like that of stromelysin, able to degrade fibronectin, proteoglycans, and gelatin. It also is a co-activator of collagenase. Matrilysin is expressed in involuting uterus and certain tumors and is induced in fibroblasts by concanavalin A.

A fourth member of the stromelysin subclass is metalloelastase (MMP-12). Although its pro-enzyme form is about 50 kD, stimulated macrophages secrete this MMP in a 21-kD form that degrades elastin, proteoglycan, type IV collagen, fibronectin, and serpin serine proteinase inhibitors, including α_1-proteinase inhibitor (1). Because this enzyme is produced by macrophage-like cells of the synovial lining, it has the potential to contribute to tissue damage. In mice with a null mutation in the gene for this enzyme, macrophage-mediated ECM degradation is inhibited, and macrophages fail to enter the peritoneal cavity in response to inflammatory stimuli (10).

Another member of the MMP family, stromelysin-3, was cloned as a stromal gene induced in human breast carcinoma (11,16,17). Although it is in the same size class and general domain structure of stromelysins and collagenases, it is distantly related to both (about 40% sequence identity). It has one feature in common with MT-MMP: a dibasic sequence at the cleavage site of its propeptide that is cleaved by intracellular prohormone processing enzymes of the furin family (11,16). Its only documented substrate is 1-proteinase inhibitor. Because it is also associated with apoptosis and is expressed in human embryonic fibroblasts after treatment with growth factors or phorbol esters, stromelysin-3 may have significance in inflammatory diseases.

Gelatinases

The gelatinase subfamily of MMP consists of two members that differ in size. The gelatin-degrading proteinase of 72 kD (also called gelatinase A, MMP-2, or type IV collagenase) that is secreted by many cells in culture, including fibroblasts, has been characterized as an enzyme that degrades type IV collagen (10–12,16,17). The 72-kD gelatinase shows sequence homology with collagenase and stromelysin and even more so with the 92-kD gelatinase (10,11,18). The size difference compared to collagenase is due to an additional domain homologous with the collagen-binding domain of fibronectin, which is inserted next to the zinc- binding pocket of the active site. It too requires proteolytic cleavage for activation and is inhibited by TIMP-1 and TIMP-2. The 72-kD gelatinase in pro-enzyme form binds one molecule of TIMP-2 (19). A second molecule is required to inhibit the activated enzyme. The TIMP-2 bound to the pro-enzyme may stabilize it against auto-activation. In addition to denatured collagen and type IV collagen, it has significant proteolytic activity against fibronectin and collagen types V, VII, and X but not against collagen types I and VI (11,17,18). Gelatinase A has also been shown to cleave plasminogen to give rise to the anti-angiogenic peptide (angiostatin).

The 92-kD gelatinase (also called gelatinase B, type V collagenase, or MMP-9) is a major secretion product of stimulated PMN, macrophages, and osteoclasts (10,11). In PMN this gelatinase is present in tertiary granules that are secreted in response to chemotactic stimuli. In sequence it is related to the 72-kD gelatinase, which is characterized by a domain closely related to the binding sequence of fibronectin. It also has a sequence related to the non-helical C-terminal domain of $\alpha_2(V)$ collagen.

Like other MMP, the 92-kD gelatinase is a pro-enzyme that requires limited proteolytic cleavage for activation. However, the plasminogen activator—plasmin cascade does not activate this enzyme. The active forms of this gelatinase cleave denatured collagens, fibronectin, elastin, and collagens of type IV, V, VII, and XI (10,11). It is inhibited by TIMP-1 and, in parallel with 72-kD gelatinase and TIMP-2, the pro-enzyme form of the 92-kD enzyme binds one molecule of TIMP-1, requiring a second molecule for inhibiting the activated form. It does not cross-react immunologically with the 72-kD gelatinase.

Membrane-type matrix metalloproteinases

MT–MMP-1 (MMP-14) was the first reported member of the growing family of membrane-bound metalloproteinases with a C-terminus transmembrane domain (16,18). MT–MMP-1 is expressed on the surface of invasive lung tumor cells, where it primarily activates stromal progelatinase A. Thus by activating gelatinase A, MT–MMP is an essential component of ECM degradation in the immediate vicinity of invasive tumor cells (16, 18). At least two other members of the family have been cloned recently. MT–MMP is present on the surface in an active form that is inhibited by TIMP-2. Like stromelysin-3, these enzymes have a dibasic insert region at the propeptide cleavage site, suggesting that they are activated intracellularly during transport through the secretory pathway.

REGULATION OF ECM DEGRADATION

Uncontrolled activation of proteinases can result in a complete collapse of the ECM framework around cells and tissues. Therefore, it is not surprising that the activity of proteinases is tightly controlled at multiple levels of regulation. The three major mechanisms for regulating ECM degradation in eukaryotic systems are transcriptional regulation at the gene level, activation of latent proenzyme forms, and inhibition of active enzymes by TIMP.

Transcriptional regulation of proteinases is a first level of regulation of the destructive ECM-degrading enzymes. Many of the members of the MMP gene family, such as gelatinase A and B, share identical substrate specificity, but they respond to different cytokines at the transcriptional level. Gelatinase B is strongly responsive to growth factors, whereas gelatinase A production appears to be repressed (10).

The molecular basis of photo-aging lies in transcriptional regulation of MMP by solar ultraviolet irradiation (UVB). In human skin, in vivo exposure to UVB induces a marked increase in several MMP, including interstitial collagenase, 92-kD gelatinase, and stromelysin-1. Interestingly, all-transretinoic acid, which is a known inhibitor of the early-response genes, that is applied before irradiation with UVB significantly reduces MMP induction (20). Collagenase-1 and stromelysin-1 expression increase during fibroblast aging and in response to stress in culture. With increasing age, stromelysin-1 can be extracted from human cartilage (21). The fragments of fibronectin produced by plasmin and MMP may also amplify MMP expression by acting as agonistic ligands for the fibronectin receptor (22). This may play an important role in osteoarthritis because of the increase in fibronectin in cartilage. Whereas fibroblast collagenase production is tightly regulated at the transcriptional level, PMN-type collagenase is preformed and released instantly from storage granules of triggered PMN. In PMN, exposure to phorbol diester results in a one-time immediate release of all enzymes stored. In fibroblasts, exposure to inductive agents such as phorbol diesters results in an 8- to 10-hour delay in production of collagenase, but this protein synthesis is sustained for several days (12).

Tissue inhibitors of metalloproteinases are a gene family consisting of TIMP-1, -2, and -3. All TIMPs most likely exert similar degrees of MMP inhibition. However, regulation of TIMP at the gene level or the diverse C-terminus protein structure can result in different biologic functions attributable to each member of the TIMP family. For example, bone has the highest concentration of TIMP-1, which may interact with active gelatinase B, thereby forming a complex that inhibits active MMP-9. In inflammation, however, release of the serine proteinase neutrophil elastase results in binding to the TIMP–MMP-9 complex, thus inactivating TIMP. Inhibition of TIMP regulatory action renders the MMP-9 proenzyme a target molecule for activation by nearby pro-inflammatory proteinases (23).

TIMP-3 is found exclusively in the ECM of many cultured human cell lines and shares significant homology with TIMP-1. However, mutations in the TIMP-3 gene have been linked to a familial cause of blindness known as Sorsby's fundus dystrophy.

CONTROL OF PROTEINASE ACTIVATION

Most proteinases are present in tissues as pro-enzymes. Activation of the cysteine and serine tissue proteinases, such as uPA and PMN elastase, is as key to tissue turnover as is activation of MMP.

Activation of pro-enzyme forms provides the second level of regulation, which involves a complex series of negative- and positive-feedback loops. An excellent example of such tightly regulated mechanisms is the interaction of the serine proteinase plasmin and the metalloproteinases stromelysin-1 and collagenase-1. In this system, activation of plasmin by uPA or tPA results in activation of a downstream molecule, namely, stromelysin-1, which then activates the latent enzyme procollagenase. Acting in a positive-feedback loop, activation of procollagenase in turn is known to produce a 5- to 10-fold increase in stromelysin proteolytic activity (12,17).

It has been appreciated for many years that MMP is activated by multiple pathways (reviewed in references 11, 12, 17). There is a pathway involving initial cleavage by a proteinase such as trypsin (for collagenase-1) between amino acid residues 81 and 82, followed by a concentration-independent autocatalysis. Collagenase-1 is activated in the absence of stromelysin-1; however, stromelysin-1 and -2, matrilysin, or small forms of collagenase are required for the full activation of procollagenase by trypsin (15). Stromelysin-1 is activated by the proteinases that activate collagenase, as well as by mast cell tryptase, PMN elastase, and cathepsin G. In vivo, the generation of plasmin by uPA or tPA is likely to be a significant activation mechanism for collagenase and stromelysin (1). The mechanism of activation of the 72-kD and 92-kD gelatinases in vivo is just beginning to be elucidated. Plasmin does not activate these enzymes (12,24); however, the PMN serine proteinases cathepsin G and elastase can activate the 72-kD gelatinase. The MT–MMP functions as a membrane-bound activating system for the 72-kD gelatinase. The presence of a single component of an activation system at the plasma membrane effectively localizes degradation to the immediate vicinity of the cell surface (17). TIMP-2 also regulates activation of the 72 kD gelatinase by a mechanism involved in controlling autocatalytic activation (11,12).

The degradation of ECM macromolecules is mediated by the availability of active proteolytic enzymes in the presence of large amounts of proteinase inhibitors from plasma and local tissue sources. These inhibitors serve to control cascade activation reactions and limit proteolysis to areas where the enzyme-inhibitor balance is in favor of the enzyme. Tissues such as cartilage that are resistant to degradation and invasion by synovial pannus and blood vessels are rich in inhibitors such as TIMP-1 and TIMP-2 (11,25). The regulatory mechanisms involved in ECM degradation are complicated and involve a fine balance between proteolytic enzyme and inhibitor activity (1). Growth regulatory peptide factors such as transforming growth factor-β, platelet-derived growth factor, and cytokines are regulators of ECM synthesis, proteinase, and inhibitor expression (Fig. 5D-1). However, their precise role in the fine control of matrix degradation remains to be elucidated.

FARRAH KHERADMAND, MD
ZENA WERB, PhD

1. Werb Z, Alexander CM: Proteinases and matrix degradation. In Kelley WN, Harris ED, Ruddy S, Sledge CB (eds): Textbook of Rheumatology, 4th edition. WB Saunders Co., Philadelphia, PA. 248-268, 1992

2. Saftig P, Hetman M, Schmahl W, et al: Mice deficient for the lysosomal proteinase cathepsin D exhibit progressive atrophy of the intestinal mucosa and profound destruction of lymphoid cells. EMBO J 14:3599-3608, 1995

3. Yoshimine Y, Tsukuba T, Isobe R, et al: Specific immunocytochemical localization of cathepsin E at the ruffled border membrane of active osteoclasts. Cell Tissue Res 281:85-91, 1995

4. Bernstein HG, Wiederanders B: An immunohistochemical study of cathepsin E in Alzheimer- type dementia brains. Brain Res 667:287-290, 1994

5. Kakegawa H, Tagami K, Ohba Y, Sumitani K, Kawata T, Katunuma N: Secretion and processing mechanisms of procathepsin L in bone resorption. Febs Lett 370:78-82, 1995

6. Gelb B, Shi G-P, Chapman HA, Desnick RJ: Pycnodysostosis, a lysosomal disease caused by cathepsin K deficiency. Science 273:1236-1238, 1996

7. Singer II, Scott S, Chin J, et al: The interleukin-1b-converting enzyme (ICE) is localized on the external cell surface membrane and in the cytoplasmic ground substance of human monocytes by immuno-electron microscopy. J Exp Med 182:1447-1459, 1995

8. Romer J, Buggeth A, Pyke C, Lund LR, Flick MJ, Degen JL, Dano K: Impaired wound healing in mice with a disrupted plasminogen gene. Nature Med 2:287-292, 1996

9. Carmeliet P, Schoonjans L, Kieckens L, et al: Physiological consequences of loss of plasminogen activator gene function in mice. Nature 368:419-424, 1994

10. Birkedal-Hansen H: Proteolytic remodeling of extracellular matrix. Curr Opin Cell Biol 7:728- 735, 1995

11. Coussens LM, Werb Z: Matrix metalloproteinase expression and neoplasia. Chemistry & Biol 3:895-904, 1996

12. Birkedal-Hansen H, Moore WG, Bodden MK, et al: Matrix metalloproteinases: a review. Crit Rev Oral Biol Med. 4:197-250, 1993

13. Werb Z: The biological role of metalloproteinases and their inhibitors. In Kuettner KE, Schleyerbach R, Peyron JG, Hascall VC (eds): Articular Cartilage and Osteoarthritis. Raven Press, New York. 295-304, 1991

14. Murphy G, Cockett MI, Stephens PE, Smith BJ, Docherty AJ: Stromelysin is an activator of procollagenase. A study with natural and recombinant enzymes. Biochem J 248:265-268, 1987

15. Bou GG, Osman J, Atherton A, et al: Expression of ectopeptidases in scleroderma. Ann Rheum Dis 54:111-116, 1995

16. Alexander CM, Werb Z: Proteinases and extracellular matrix remodeling. Curr Opin Cell Biol 1:974-982, 1989

17. Crawford HC, Matrisian LM: Tumor and stromal expression of matrix metalloproteinases and their role in tumor progression. Invasion Metastasis 14:234-245, 1994

18. Sato H, Takino T, Okada Y, et al: A matrix metalloproteinase expressed on the surface of invasive tumour cells. Nature 370:61-65, 1994

19. Stetler SW, Krutzsch HC, Liotta LA: Tissue inhibitor of metalloproteinase (TIMP-2). A new member of the metalloproteinase inhibitor family. J Biol Chem 264:17374-17378, 1989

20. Fisher GJ, Datta SC, Talwar HS, Wang ZQ, Varani J, Kang S, Voorhees JJ: Molecular basis of sun-induced premature skin ageing and retinoid antagonism. Nature 379:335-339, 1996

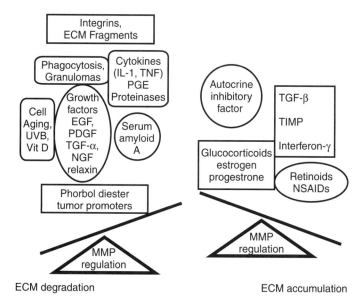

(Figure 5D-1)

Regulation of metalloproteinase expression and its net effect on ECM. Regulation of MMP expression at the level of gene expression controls an intricate balance of ECM degradation or accumulation. Stimulatory factors (left) result in synthesis and secretion of MMP, whereas inhibitory factors (right) downregulate MMP synthesis and/or inactivate the enzymes, leading to ECM accumulation. EGF = epidermal growth factor; IL = interleukin; NGF = nerve growth factor; NSAIDs = nonsteroidal anti-inflammatory drugs; PDGF = platelet-derived growth factor; PGE = prostaglandin E; TGF = transforming growth factor; TIMP = tissue inhibitor of metalloproteinases; TNF = tumor necrosis factor; UVB = ultraviolet B; Vit D = 1,25-dihydroxy vitamin D.

21. Gunja SZ, Nagase H, Woessner JJ: Purification of the neutral proteogly-can-degrading metalloproteinase from human articular cartilage tissue and its identification as stromelysin matrix metalloproteinase-3. Biochem J 258:115-119, 1989

22. Tremble P, Chiquet ER, Werb Z: The extracellular matrix ligands fibronectin and tenascin collaborate in regulating collagenase gene expression in fibroblasts. Mol Biol Cell 5:439-453, 1994

23. Rice A, Banda MJ: Neutrophil elastase processing of gelatinase A is mediated by extracellular matrix. Biochemistry 34:9249-9256, 1995

24. Behrendtsen O, Alexander CM, Werb Z: Metalloproteinases mediate extracellular matrix degradation by cells from mouse blastocyst outgrowths. Development 114:447-456, 1992

25. Moses MA, Sudhalter J, Langer R: Identification of an inhibitor of neovascularization from cartilage. Science 248:1408-1410, 1990

E. ARACHIDONIC ACID DERIVATIVES, KININS, CLOTTING FACTORS, AMINES, NITRIC OXIDE, AND REACTIVE OXYGEN SPECIES

The immune system utilizes a cascade of soluble inflammatory mediators to generate and enhance an immune response. Included within this spectrum are cytokines, chemokines, and surface receptor ligands, which are discussed in detail in this chapter. Prostaglandins, leukotrienes, kinins, thromboxanes, nitric oxide, and reactive oxygen species are also important mediators in the immune response, more specifically in localized inflammation. In addition to their common role in inflammation, some of these molecules are linked by common derivation from arachidonic acid (ie, prostaglandins, lipoxins, and leukotrienes) and production of some is induced by similar mechanisms (ie, prostaglandins, reactive oxygen species, and nitric oxide). Significant advances in understanding the function of prostaglandins and their receptors have recently been reported. The recently discovered role of nitric oxide in inflammation and the immune system in humans is still being defined.

Because of their important role in inflammation, these molecules are receiving ever-increasing attention as potential targets of therapy to block inflammation in a variety of disease states. All of these molecules have normal physiologic roles; only when inappropriately expressed or overexpressed in disease do they become targets for therapeutic intervention.

PROSTAGLANDINS

Prostaglandins were initially identified by the ability of prostatic secretions to stimulate uterine contraction, hence the name. The active component of prostatic secretions was found to be lipid-based, and subsequently similar compounds with diverse activities were isolated from a variety of tissues.

Prostaglandins are derived primarily from arachidonic acid stored in the cellular membrane of all cells in the membrane phospholipids phosphatidylinositol and phosphatidylcholine (1). Arachidonic acid is released from membrane phospholipids primarily via the enzyme phospholipase A_2; phospholipase C_2 may also release arachidonic acid from the cell membrane (Fig. 5E-1). Release of arachidonic acid is a key rate-determining step of prostaglandin synthesis. A natural inhibitor of phospholipase A_2 is lipomodulin; one of the anti-inflammatory properties of corticosteroids is stimulating lipomodulin synthesis.

Once released, arachidonic acid can be either directly oxidized or converted via a number of biochemical pathways to prostaglandins, thromboxanes, or leukotrienes. Tissue type, enzyme concentrations, and cytokine milieu, among other factors, determine the metabolic pathway to which available arachidonic acid is directed.

Prostaglandins (PGs) derived from arachidonic acid are produced through a series of biosynthetic pathways. The initial enzyme is cyclooxygenase (COX), which is also called prostaglandin endoperoxide synthase (PGHS). Recently, two different cyclo-oxygenases have been identified: COX_1 ($PGHS_1$) and COX_2 ($PGHS_2$). COX_1 and COX_2 are derived from two genes on different chromosomes, although the genes share significant similarities in sequence and structure (2). However, they differ in cellular location and stimulus for production. COX_1 is primarily cytoplasmic and is constitutively produced, suggesting that prostaglandins produced by this enzyme play a key homeostatic role in gastric mucosal protection, renal hemodynamics, and platelet thrombogenesis. COX_1 messenger RNA is relatively long-lived and stable, allowing long-term and rapid transcription.

In contrast, COX_2 is localized to the nuclear envelope and is induced in fibroblasts, endothelial cells, and macrophages by cytokines, mitogens, and tumor promoters. COX_2 is not present in any resting cells other than the brain; its role in the brain is unknown. Prostaglandins produced by COX_2 likely play a key role in the immune response, both normally and in autoimmune disorders. Currently available nonsteroidal anti-inflammatory drugs (NSAIDs) inhibit both COX_1 and COX_2; inhibition of COX_1 produces the most notable side effects of NSAIDs (ie, gastric ulceration and renal insufficiency). Selective COX_2 inhibitors are currently undergoing therapeutic trials for the treatment of inflammatory diseases. Animal studies of these agents suggest they are effective with less gastrointestinal and renal toxicity than currently available NSAIDs.

Recently, through genetic manipulation, knockout mice have been produced that lack either a functional COX_1 or COX_2 gene (3,4). The phenotype of the mice was not what was expected, however. COX_1-deficient mice were predicted to have developmental abnormalities, susceptibility to gastric ulcerations, and renal hemodynamic abnormalities. Surprisingly, the mice appear normal and do not develop gastric ulcerations. Indeed, when given indomethacin, they had fewer ulcers than mice with normal COX_1 expression. COX_2 expression was not up-regulated in these mice. Because a total lack of gastric prostaglandin production is not pro-

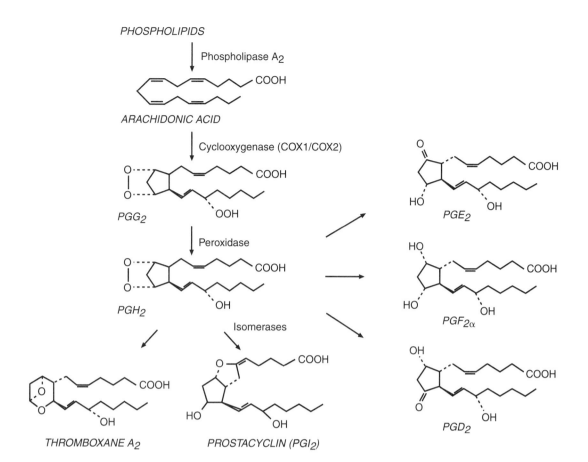

(Figure 5E-1)

Synthesis of prostaglandins (PG) and thromboxane A₂. Reprinted from Robinson DR: Lipid mediators of inflammation. In Zvaifler N (ed): Rheumatic Disease Clinics of North America. Philadelphia, WB Saunders, 1987, pp 385-405, with permission.

ulcerogenic, a rethinking of the role of gastric prostaglandins in mucosal protection seems necessary. COX_1-deficient mice, when bred to each other, conceive and sustain a normal pregnancy, but all pups are stillborn. Thus COX_1 expression does appear necessary for successful parturition.

Alternatively, COX_2-deficient mice died at an early age. Necropsy revealed the mice had poorly developed kidneys with glomerular agenesis. The few properly formed glomeruli were hypertrophied. Unexpectedly, COX_2-deficient mice were just as susceptible to induction of inflammation as normal litter mates; COX_1-deficient mice, however, developed milder inflammation, less often. These results suggest that COX_2 is necessary for normal kidney morphogenesis, yet is not necessary for the early inflammatory response. The constitutive expression of COX_1 makes it readily available for prostaglandin production during the acute inflammatory response. Chronic inflammation likely requires COX_2 expression. These studies point out the differences between acute pharmacologic blockade of an inflammatory mediator and the long-term genetic absence of the mediator.

Cyclo-oxygenases catalyze two sequential reactions: arachidonic acid is initially oxygenated to yield the first prostaglandin structure PGG_2 (Fig. 5E-1), a short-lived intermediate that is rapidly reduced by cyclooxygenase to PGH_2. Both of these reactions require heme as a cofactor. The reduction step can be accelerated for COX_2 by the presence of

lipid hydroperoxides formed by inflammatory cells such as polymorphonucleocytes (PMNs) and macrophages. PGH_2 is then converted by various isomerases to the biologically active PGs: PGD_2, PGI_2, PGE_2, and $PGF_{2\alpha}$. Thromboxane A_2 (TXA_2) is also produced via isomerization of PGH_2. Which PG is produced depends on tissue type, as tissues produce different isomerases. Prostaglandins can act in an autocrine, paracrine, or endocrine manner. They are relatively short-lived as active compounds, being rapidly converted enzymatically to biologically inactive keto-derivatives that accumulate in the blood prior to urinary excretion.

The biologic effect of prostaglandins depends on their interactions with their receptors and the relative amounts of the types of prostaglandins produced (5). Seven surface receptors for prostaglandins are known; each is a member of the family of receptors with 7 membrane-spanning domains that interact with G proteins for intracellular signal transduction. Three different PGE_2 receptors have been isolated, and PGD_2, PGI_2, $PGF_{2\alpha}$, and TXA_2 each have a currently known receptor. All these receptors are expressed on smooth muscle, although the type of receptor expressed varies in different organs. Stimulation of the primary PGE_2 receptor, the PGI_2 receptor, and the PGD_2 receptor leads to smooth-muscle relaxation through the release of intracellular cAMP (cyclic 3′, 5′-adenosine monophosphate). The other two PGE_2 receptors, the $PGF_{2\alpha}$ receptor, and the TXA_2 receptor initiate smooth-muscle contraction through the release of intracellular calcium.

Two receptors expressed on platelets also have opposing actions: PGI_2 inhibits platelet aggregation, whereas the TXA_2 induces platelet aggregation. One PGE_2 receptor (EP_2), which is expressed on PMNs and lymphocytes, modulates many of the prostaglandin effects in immunity. Two of the PGE_2, $PGF_{2\alpha}$ and TXA_2 receptors, are expressed in the kidney. Stimulation of these receptors affects glomerular filtration and distal tubular water absorption. A confounding factor is that most receptors can be stimulated by most prostaglandins; the receptors merely differ in the relative amounts of individual prostaglandins needed for stimulation. Thus, if PGI_2 is present in large amounts in a tissue with PGE_2 receptors, a PGE_2-like response will occur. The controls of receptor production are currently being delineated. Specific blocking of PG receptors is a likely strategy for future pharmacologic interventions.

Overall, PGE_2 and PGI_2 are pro-inflammatory, leading to vasodilation and increased vascular permeability. PGE_2 also induces T-cell migration and production of metalloproteinases. These two PGs also stimulate osteoclast bone resorption, suggesting a role for prostaglandins in inflammatory bone erosions. In contrast, the direct effects of PGE_2 and PGI_2 on inflammatory cells are inhibitory. PGE_2 inhibits T-cell responses in vitro, thus decreasing IL-2 production. B-cell maturation is also blocked by PGE_2. Indeed, thromboxane and prostaglandin receptors were recently demonstrated in the thymus. Recent data suggest that prostaglandins and thromboxanes play a key role in thymic T-cell development and selection. PGE_2 appears to protect a developing T cell from negative selection.

THROMBOXANE

As described earlier, TXA_2 is derived from arachidonic acid through the same biosynthetic pathways as the prostaglandins, with the initial steps catalyzed by the cyclooxygenases. Subsequently, thromboxane synthase converts PGH_2 to TXA_2 (Fig. 5E-1). Thromboxane A_2 differs from the prostaglandins in having a 6-carbon primary ring rather than the 5-member ring that characterizes prostaglandins.

The thromboxane receptor is found in the kidney, on epithelial cells, on platelets, and on smooth muscles of the arterial system, venous system, and pulmonary airways. Stimulation of TXA_2 receptors results in smooth-muscle contraction, platelet aggregation, increased intestinal secretion, and increased glomerular filtration.

Thromboxane A_2 recently has been shown to be a key mediator in inflammatory renal disease and in asthma (5, 6). Levels of thromboxane are elevated in murine lupus models. High levels of TXA_2 in the kidney result in intense vasoconstriction, platelet aggregation, mesangial cell contraction, and increased production of extracellular matrix leading to decreased renal function (5). Blocking TXA_2 synthesis results in both short-term and long-term improvement in renal function and survival in lupus mice. Disease is not totally inhibited, however, as mice in which TXA_2 synthesis is blocked later develop renal disease and die. Thus TXA_2 plays a role, but is not the sole inflammatory mediator in lupus nephritis.

TXA_2 and leukotrienes are also important in asthma. Healthy individuals who inhale preparations containing TXA_2 develop bronchoconstriction and increased airway secretions. Metabolites of TXA_2 (TXB_2) are increased in the blood, urine, and bronchioalveolar lavage fluids of patients with asthma. Agents that block either TXA_2 production or the TXA_2 receptor are effective for treating bronchoconstriction in humans and animals. Indeed, blocking TXA_2 alone is effective therapy, even when leukotriene levels remain high. It is very likely that inhibitors of TXA_2 will quickly become part of the treatment regimen for asthma. Other uses for TXA_2 inhibitors remain to be defined.

Physiologically, TXA_2 also appears to be important in thymic development because it induces cell death in developing thymocytes, indicating a role in negative selection. PGE_2 inhibits TXA_2-induced cell death. Thus, production of eicosanoids by thymic epithelial cells and expression of eicosanoid receptors by developing thymocytes appear important in positive and negative selection of T cells and the resultant T-cell repertoire.

LEUKOTRIENES

Like prostaglandins, leukotrienes (LTs) are produced primarily from arachidonic acid released from phospholipids in the cellular membrane by phospholipase A_2 (7). Specific cellular signals lead to translocation of the phospholipase–arachidonic acid complex to the nuclear membrane. The same signals also cause the enzyme 5-lipoxygenase (5-LO) to migrate from the cytoplasm to the nuclear membrane (Fig. 5E-2). A protein called 5-lipoxygenase–activating protein (FLAP) facilitates the transfer of arachidonic acid from phospholipase A_2 to 5-LO. In the test tube, 5-LO alone can convert arachidonic acid to leukotrienes; in the cell, however, FLAP is necessary for the series of reactions that convert arachidonic acid to leukotrienes.

Arachidonic acid is converted by 5-LO to 5-hydroperoxyeicosa-tetranoic acid (5-HPETE) by a dioxygenase reaction. 5-HPETE is subsequently transformed to LTA_4 via dehydrase activity. LTA_4 then enters divergent pathways: LTA_4 hydrolase converts LTA_4 to LTB_4 by the addition of H_2O, or alternatively, LTC_4 synthetase with the addition of a glutathione transforms LTA_4 to LTC_4. By the action of gamma-glutamyl transferase, LAC_4 is converted to LTD_4, and removal of the terminal glycine by dipeptidase produces LTE_4. LTC_4, LTD_4, and LTE_4 are commonly referred to as the *peptide leukotrienes;* they make up the majority of the biologic activity in SRS-A (the slow-reacting substance of anaphylaxis).

The peptide leukotrienes have significant biologic effects including constriction of respiratory, gastrointestinal, and vascular smooth muscle. Other actions include increasing vascular permeability, constricting mesangial cells, stimulating bronchial mucus secretion, inhibiting ciliary function, and enhancing mucosal edema. These agents also enhance the responsiveness of the airway to other bronchoconstrictors.

The primary action of LTB_4 is to accentuate PMN function. It is a potent chemoattractant for PMNs and results in degranulation and release of active oxygen species and proteolytic enzymes. LTB_4 also has effects on lymphocytes, enhancing the effects of gamma interferon on activating classical cell-mediated pathways, inhibiting apoptosis of thymic T cells, and inducing differentiation of resting B cells. LTB_4 also enhances proliferation and synthetic responses of B cells.

Receptors for leukotrienes are also of the 7-domain transmembrane motif with signaling through G proteins. Specific receptors for LTB_4 and LTC_4 have been isolated. These receptors are located at the sites these compounds are active:

(Figure 5E-2)

Synthesis of leukotrienes. Reprinted from Robinson DR: Lipid mediators of inflammation. In Zvaifler N (ed): Rheumatic Disease Clinics of North America. Philadelphia, WB Saunders, 1987, pp 385-405, with permission.

LTB_4 receptors are on PMNs and lymphocytes, while LTC_4 receptors are found in respiratory, gastrointestinal, and vascular epithelia.

Leukotrienes are postulated to be key mediators in a number of diseases including asthma, psoriasis, allergic rhinitis, rheumatoid arthritis, inflammatory bowel disease, and gout. In each of these diseases, elevated levels of leukotrienes have been demonstrated at sites of disease activity. Most of the currently available pharmacologic agents are 5-LO antagonists. The most extensive experience with these agents is in asthma where 5-LO inhibitors are effective in preventing and treating bronchospasm. These effects appear additive to the action of β-adrenergic agents. 5-LO inhibitors will likely become part of the treatment regimen for asthma in addition to other agents that block leukotriene production such as antagonists of FLAP, LTC_4 synthetase, and LTC_4 receptors.

Therapeutic trials of leukotriene inhibitors in other diseases have not been as promising. Trials in psoriasis, rheumatoid arthritis, and inflammatory bowel disease produced minimal, if any, improvement. In some of these trials, inhibition of 5-LO activity was incomplete, suggesting that more effective 5-LO inhibition may subsequently prove useful in these diseases. Specific inhibitors of LTB_4 versus LTC_4 production may also prove therapeutically useful.

LIPOXINS

Lipoxins (LXs) are a group of compounds related to leukotrienes in that they are derived from arachidonic acid through lipoxygenase activity (8). The lipoxygenases 12-LO and 15-LO are involved in lipoxin formation, producing 12- or 15-HPETE. Through a series of reactions the lipoxins LXA_4 and LXB_4 are formed. These molecules are primarily vasodilatory and immunomodulatory. Elevated levels of lipoxins are found in inflammatory lesions including some forms of inflammatory arthritis and glomerulonephritis. These compounds are produced primarily by PMNs and platelets. A lack of specific inhibitors of lipoxin formation limits the understanding of their true biologic functions in normal immunity or in autoimmune diseases.

KININS

Kinins are a group of proteins activated in a sequence similar to the coagulation cascade. Tissue and plasma prekallikreins are cleaved via trauma, immunologic signals, or plasmin, which produces activated kallikrein. Plasma kallikrein then acts on high-molecular weight kininogen to produce bradykinin, a biologically active nonapeptide. Tissue kallikrein cleaves low-molecular weight kininogen to release kallidin, which has many of the same properties of bradykinin (Fig. 5E-3). The ability to produce kinins is ubiquitous throughout body tissues. Specific receptors for bradykinin have been isolated. These receptors vary in what tissues they are expressed (9).

The kinins have a wide spectrum of biologic activities. They stimulate smooth-muscle contraction and bronchospasm, increase vascular permeability, mediate pain and vasodilation, and induce hypotension. At an inflammatory site, kinins enhance the release of phospholipids, freeing arachidonic acid for the production of prostaglandins and leukotrienes. Kinins also stimulate the production of platelet-activating factor. Thus kinins act as pro-inflammatory agents and are present in increased concentrations in the rheumatoid joint. Specific inhibitors of bradykinin have been developed that block the development of inflammation in animal models. Such agents, given either systemically or locally, may be beneficial in treating inflammatory lesions.

Natural inhibitors of bradykinin are dipeptidases. One, kininase II, is identical to angiotensin-converting enzyme (ACE). ACE inhibitors block the function of kininase II. In clinical situations where bradykinin is overproduced, ACE inhibitors may accentuate the clinical syndrome by blocking the metabolic breakdown of bradykinin (ie, enhance vasodilatation, hypotension, and increased vascular permeability).

COAGULATION SYSTEM

The coagulation system is also intricately involved in inflammation. Fibrin is a prominent component of any inflammatory reaction, indicating that activation of the coagulation system is integral to the immune response. Components of the coagulation system and the fibrinolytic system can become proinflammatory by their activation of other factors. Hageman factor is able to activate the kinin system. Certain fibrin split products are potent chemoattractants for PMNs. Plasmin is capable of cleaving the complement component C3. Thus the coagulation system can be a potent proinflammatory cascade (10).

Much of the damage done by inflammation is secondary to the scarring and fibrosis that follows an acute inflammatory response. Fibrin again plays a key role in the early component of this scarring. Certain inflammatory diseases in animals have been treated successfully with heparin, but it is not clear if therapeutic benefits are secondary to anticoagulation or other effects of heparin. There are no convincing data that anticoagulation is useful for treating inflammatory diseases in humans, however.

VASOACTIVE AMINES

Some low-molecular weight amines have potent inflammatory effects. The role of histamine in the allergic response is well known. Histamine is stored in mast cell granules and released by activating signals such as IgE binding to antigen. Histamine then binds to cellular receptors, resulting in the clinical effects of vasodilation, increased vascular permeability, bronchoconstriction, and increased mucus production.

Serotonin is noted for its role in depression, but it also plays a role in inflammation. Outside the central nervous system, it is stored primarily in dense body granules of platelets. Serotonin causes vasoconstriction, increased vascular permeability, and enhanced fibrosis. Blocking serotonin can cause fibrotic changes, as exemplified by the infrequent side effect of retroperitoneal fibrosis by the drug methysergide maleate (Sansert), which is used to treat severe vascular headaches.

Another amine with biologic activity is adenosine, recently notable as an agent for blocking tachyarrhythmias. Accumulation of adenosine and its resulting toxic effects on lymphocytes is the proximate cause of combined immunodeficiency due to adenosine deaminase deficiency.

Although adenosine has also been known for many years to have anti-inflammatory effects at the site of its release, interest has grown recently because there is now evidence that the effects of methotrexate may be mediated by adenosine (11). In therapeutic doses, methotrexate promotes accumulation of the compound 5-aminoimidazole-4-carboxamide ribonucleotide (AICAR), which enhances local release of adenosine. The addition of adenosine deaminase breaks down adenosine and abrogates the anti-inflammatory actions of methotrexate. Other methods of increasing local adenosine release may be of use in the treatment of inflammatory diseases.

NITRIC OXIDE

Investigating the role of nitric oxide in health and disease has created an explosion of research over the past few years. Although a gas and closely related, nitric oxide and its properties are distinct from the laughing gas, nitrous oxide. Interest in nitric oxide began when it was identified as the endothelial-derived relaxation factor (EDRF). Subsequently,

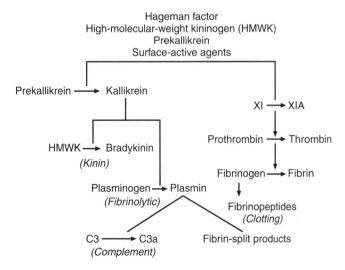

(Figure 5E-3)
Kinins and the coagulation system. Reprinted from Cotran et al (10), with permission.

nitric oxide was shown to play a key role in cell-mediated immunity and also to serve as a neurotransmitter. Almost daily, new actions of nitric oxide are described.

Nitric oxide is derived from the amino acid arginine through the activity of the enzyme nitric oxide synthase (NOS) (Fig. 5E-4). There are at least three forms of NOS derived from three separate genes. Two forms of NOS (endothelial and neuronal) are constitutively expressed and are dependent on calcium and calmodulin. Both forms produce the nitric oxide that is responsible for maintaining vascular tone and neurotransmission. In the vascular system, nitric oxide is a potent vasodilator and is the active moiety of sodium nitroprusside and nitroglycerin (12).

The third NOS gene produces an inducible form termed iNOS, which is primarily found in immune cells, most notably macrophages and macrophage-derived cells. In addition, iNOS is present in endothelial cells, some neuronal cells, PMNs, lymphocytes, and natural killer cells. Nitric oxide produced by immune cells participates in killing intracellular pathogens and certain tumors. A key role of nitric oxide in autoimmunity was demonstrated in animal models of arthritis, diabetes, multiple sclerosis, and SLE. Blocking the production of nitric oxide with arginine analogs such as N-monomethyl arginine (NMMA) prevented or treated autoimmune disease in these animals (13).

The role of nitric oxide in human disease is not as clear as in murine disease, however. Unlike macrophages from rodents, human macrophages cannot be stimulated to produce nitric oxide by immune mediators such as cytokines or endotoxin. Recent studies, however, provide evidence that nitric oxide is overproduced in human autoimmune diseases. Elevated serum levels of nitric oxide metabolites are present in patients with RA and SLE. Peripheral blood monocytes and synovial cells from RA patients demonstrate increased levels of iNOS compared with controls.

Nitric oxide can cause direct tissue injury by interfering with the function of enzymes in the respiratory burst chain. It can also interact with superoxide to form peroxynitrite, a highly toxic compound that can nitrosylate proteins and alter their function. In addition to these direct actions on tissues, nitric oxide apparently has other functions in immunity. It blocks apoptosis of B lymphocytes, participates in maintaining viral latency, and alters the ratio of Th1 to Th2 cells.

Currently, a number of pharmaceutical companies are searching for suitable compounds for human use that block nitric oxide production by iNOS. Nonspecific blockers of NOS such as NMMA will likely have significant central nervous system and vascular side effects with long-term use. Due to its apparent role in autoimmune tissue damage, nitric oxide remains a leading target for therapy in a number of diseases.

REACTIVE OXYGEN SPECIES

Oxygen is an unusual molecule. Because it possesses two unpaired electrons, oxygen is easily converted to reactive and toxic species by the simple addition or subtraction of electrons. The addition of one electron to oxygen forms the superoxide radical $O2^-$, whereas subtracting the two electrons via superoxide dismutase (SOD) forms hydrogen peroxide H_2O_2. Another reduction product of oxygen is the hydroxyl radical $\cdot OH$, formed by the reaction of hydrogen peroxide with iron (Fenton reaction).

Oxygen radicals appear to be important in the ability of PMNs to kill bacteria and other pathogens. Indeed, a defect in the generation of superoxide by PMNs is the underlying pathogenesis of chronic granulomatous disease. Confirmation of this point was recently derived from knockout mice in which a subunit of cytochrome b oxidase was inactivated. PMNs from these mice could not produce superoxide, and the mice were susceptible to staphylococcal and fungal infections.

Although increased levels of reactive oxygen species have been found in autoimmune diseases, whether they play a key role in these diseases remains unclear (14). The use of the superoxide knockout mice as well as SOD knockout mice may provide insight into the role of oxygen radicals in disease. Agents that prevent oxygen radical production or quench them after they are produced are being actively studied.

GARY S. GILKESON, MD

1. O'Neill C: The biochemistry of prostaglandins: a primer. Aust NZ Obstet Gynecol 34:332-337, 1994

2. Goetzl EJ, Songzhu AN, Smith WL: Specificity of expression and effects of eicosanoid mediators in normal physiology and human diseases. FASEB J 9:1051-1058, 1995

3. Langenbach R, Morham SG, Tiano HF, Loftin CD, Ghanayem BI, Chulada PC, Mahler JF, Lee CA, Goulding EH, Kluckman KD, Kim HS, Smithies O: Prostaglandin synthase I gene disruption in mice reduces arachidonic acid induced inflammation and indomethacin-induced gastric ulceration. Cell 83:483-492, 1995

4. Morham SG, Langenbach R, Loftin C, Tiano HF, Vouloumanos N, Jennette JC, Mahler JF, Kluckman KD, Leford A, Lee CA, Smithies O: Postaglandin synthase 2 gene disruption causes severe renal pathology in the mouse. Cell 83:473-482, 1995

5. Salvati P, Lamberti E, Ferrario R, Ferrario RG, Scampini G, Pugliese F, Barsotti P, Patrono C: Long term thromboxane-synthase inhibition prolongs survival in murine lupus nephritis. Kidney Int 47:1168-1175, 1995

6. Obata T, Yamashita N, Nakagawa T: Leukotriene and thromboxane antagonists. Clin Rev Allergy Immunol 12:79-93, 1994

7. Harris RR, Carter GW, Bell RL, Moore JL, Brooks DW: Clinical activity of leukotriene inhibitors. Int J Immunopharmac 17:147-156, 1995

8. Serhan CN: Lipoxin biosynthesis and its impact in inflammatory and vascular events. Biochimica et Biophysica Acta 1212:1-25, 1994

9. Sharma JN, Buchanan WW: Pathogenic responses of bradykinin system in chronic inflammatory rheumatoid disease. Exp Toxic Pathol 46:421-433, 1994

10. Cotran RS, Kumar V, Robbins SL: Inflammation and repair. In Cotran RS, Kumar V, Robbins SL (ed): Robbins Pathologic Basis of Disease, 4th ed. Philadelphia, WB Saunders, 1989, pp 39-86

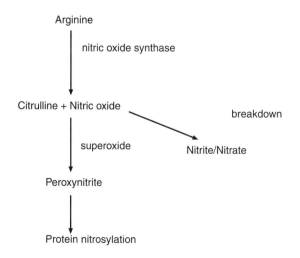

(Figure 5E-4)

Nitric oxide synthesis and metabolism.

11. Cronstein BN, Naime D, Ostad E: The antiinflammatory mechanism of methotrexate: increased adenosine release at inflamed sites diminishes leukocyte accumulation in an in vivo model of inflammation. J Clin Invest 92:2675-2687, 1993

12. Nathan CF: Nitric oxide as a secretory product of mammalian cells. FASEB J 6:3051-3064, 1992

13. Weinberg J, Pisetsky D, Seldin M, Misukonis M, Pippen A, Ruiz P, Wood E, Granger D, Gilkeson G: The role of nitric oxide in the pathogenesis of spontaneous murine autoimmune disease. J Exp Med 179:651-660, 1994

14. Greenwald RA: Oxygen radicals, inflammation, and arthritis: pathophysiological consideration and implications for treatment. Sem Arthritis Rheum 20:219-240, 1991

6

IMMUNITY
A. IMPACT OF MOLECULAR BIOLOGY ON RHEUMATIC DISEASE

Clinicians recognize and treat signs and symptoms of rheumatic diseases using traditional clinical tools of history and physical examination, laboratory and imaging studies, and clinical response to antirheumatic therapies. Underlying the clinical disease is a complex web of interactions on a molecular scale, namely, the genetic and molecular events that cause and accelerate disease and those that can stop it. This chapter will briefly outline concepts underlying the application of molecular medicine to rheumatic diseases in the areas of diagnosis, prognosis, and therapeutics (Table 6A-1).

MOLECULAR DIAGNOSTICS

A good illustration of the impact of molecular biology in the rheumatic diseases is in the area of diagnostics. Autoantibody specificity, genetic defects, and susceptibility genes provide significant new information to improve the specificity of clinical diagnosis. For example, autoantibodies (that is, antibodies against normal self-tissues) are a common feature of many rheumatic diseases. The response is very complex and heterogeneous, targeting many different molecules in a variety of cell types. When analyzed by morphologic criteria such as antinuclear antibodies, which are defined as antibodies that stain nuclear structures, there is a great deal of overlap among different diagnostic categories, because different antibodies stain similar-looking structures. A significant advance has come in recent years from the molecular cloning of many of the target molecules, which are the self-antigens for the autoantibody responses. Thus, for example, individual molecular members of the ribonuclear protein complexes within the nucleus and various other DNA binding proteins are now recognized as distinct targets of specific autoantibodies. In many cases, knowing these detailed specificities improves the diagnostic specificity and helps identify distinct clinical subsets of systemic

sclerosis, myositis, systemic lupus erythematosus (SLE), and other autoimmune disorders (1).

SUSCEPTIBILITY GENES

The ability to clone genes that encode autoantigens has brought a welcome degree of clarity to one of the more puzzling manifestations of rheumatic disease, namely the spectrum of autoantibodies produced. Molecular cloning of genes that cause or predispose to disease has the potential for even more dramatic impact on diagnosis.

Some rheumatic diseases, although rare, are monogenic—that is, a single gene defect appears to account for the clinical manifestations. For example, some forms of osteoarthritis result from an inherited defect in the collagen gene itself (2,3). However, most of the genetic predispositions to rheumatic diseases such as rheumatoid arthritis (RA) and SLE appear to be multigenic—that is, a combination of several genes, each contributing a degree of susceptibility, is responsible for the clinical manifestations.

How susceptibility genes influence predisposition and clinical diagnosis in multigenic disorders is illustrated in Fig. 6A-1. The figure is adapted from a mouse model of SLE in which four different genes were postulated to contribute to disease pathogenesis (4). Individuals with zero or one susceptibility gene have little chance of developing disease, whereas individuals with three or four genes have a very high likelihood of developing disease. Individuals with two genes have an intermediate probability of clinical disease.

In addition to the simple quantitative relationship, the model also incorporates two other concepts that serve as paradigms for human multigenic rheumatic diseases. First, within a set of different susceptibility genes, some of these

(Table 6A-1)
Areas of application of molecular biology to rheumatic diseases

Diagnosis
    Autoantibody specificity
    Genetic defects
    Susceptibility genes
Prognosis
    Stratification
    Clinical heterogeneity
    Disease progression
Response to therapy
Design of therapeutics
    Animal models
    Molecular mechanisms

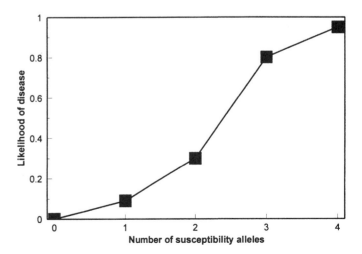

(Figure 6A-1)
Influence of susceptibility genes on the development of multigenic disorders.

genes predispose to specific physiologic or pathologic abnormalities, such as antinuclear antibodies, and others correlate with specific clinical signs and symptoms, such as nephritis or hematologic involvement. Thus, the heterogeneity of clinical manifestations for some of the autoimmune diseases may be an inherent property of the precise genetic array in each individual patient. Second, individuals with any two, three, or four susceptibility genes have the same probability of disease as other individuals with some other combination of susceptibility genes, *even if the specific sets of genes in these individuals are not the same.* In other words, an individual with susceptibility genes 1, 2, and 3 may have the same likelihood of disease as an individual with susceptibility genes 2, 3, and 4, suggesting that there is some sort of cumulative threshold achieved through the expression of multiple susceptibility genes.

In multigenic diseases, each susceptibility gene contributes an increased element of disease risk. The research challenge is to assess at what point a genetic combination in an individual patient crosses a threshold for clinical diagnosis. A great deal of research work at the present time is going into identifying these susceptibility genes, with a view toward early assessment of risk and accurate diagnosis of the preclinical autoimmune state. At the moment, there are no multigenic rheumatic diseases where enough is known about the individual susceptibility genes to predict accurately a diagnosis in a presymptomatic individual.

MOLECULAR PROGNOSIS

In the future, it may be possible to use molecular tools and tests to determine more accurately the disease prognosis in an individual patient. The use of molecular markers has the potential to stratify patients, for example, along a scale from mild to severe disease, according to a variety of characteristics. Potentially even more useful is that, in a clinically heterogeneous disease, discrete clinical subtypes may correspond to distinct molecular markers. Thus, molecular testing as part of the early assessment of patients with rheumatic disease may be useful for stratification, clinical heterogeneity, and disease progression prognosis. The best example of this in rheumatology is adult rheumatoid arthritis. Roughly half of all patients with RA are likely to progress toward severe crippling forms of the disease with multiple joint erosions over time. Other patients with a similar diagnosis have a more benign form of the disease with few, if any, joint erosions and little permanent damage to the joints. Interestingly, one of the best clinical predictors to distinguish between these groups of patients is a molecular marker for genes that helps trigger the autoimmune response. Specific human leukocyte antigen (HLA) genes are highly associated with the severe erosive forms of RA. HLA typing at the time of initial diagnosis can be used to help assess the likely disease progression in the individual patient (5–9).

The HLA genes associated with RA are but one example of immune response genes involved in disease. The complex interplay between genes of the immune system is expressed in lymphocytes, macrophages, and synovial cells, all of which participate in the early and progressive inflammatory response. Some of these genes encode cytokines (see Chapter 5B), which are soluble mediators of inflammation and immune regulation, and some encode the more specific members of the immune recognition cascade, including T-

cell receptors for antigen, HLA molecules, and autoantigens themselves. As each of these molecular participants are cloned, new methods for monitoring disease activity will follow. Several new molecular markers have already been identified that can be detected and measured in samples from patients' blood or synovium (7,10–12). Indeed, a major emphasis in clinical research is to identify combinations of these specific molecular markers that can serve as reliable measures of clinical course.

RESPONSE TO THERAPY

With many of the rheumatic diseases, it is often weeks or months after initiation of a therapy before clinical improvement can be assessed. More immediate and accurate tools are needed, and the molecular markers that measure disease activity have an important role in this regard. Although measures such as the erythrocyte sedimentation rate and C-reactive protein are general nonspecific surrogates for inflammatory reactions, it is likely that more sensitive and specific molecular markers will be developed for routine clinical use.

The discovery of new molecular markers of disease activity will likely be identified in the course of studies of pathogenic mechanisms. For example, RNA from synovial tissues of RA patients with active disease will be compared with RNA from quiescent, noninvolved tissues. Since mRNA in these tissue samples includes the spectrum of genes encoding molecular signals and mediators of disease, a direct comparison of the mRNA between affected and uninvolved tissues will identify a set of genes that are activated in RA. Several technical procedures are now readily available to perform this kind of direct mRNA analysis, and in the next few years, these research techniques will probably be adapted for the clinical setting, making it practical to use molecular markers to evaluate disease status.

NEW THERAPEUTIC APPROACHES

Molecular biology holds great promise for the development of new scientifically based approaches to therapy for the rheumatic diseases. All of the biologic mediators of disease—cytokines, cytokine receptors, antigen receptors, and differentiation markers on lymphocytes—are potentially new and effective targets for therapy. As each potential target is cloned, it can be studied in isolation and used for the rational design of therapeutic agents to block, antagonize, decoy, mimic, or otherwise interfere with the function of the target molecule.

Strategies that might be used to construct such molecularly designed biologic modifiers are illustrated in Fig. 6A-2. A simple three-cell model for immunologic interactions in autoimmunity is outlined, in which host tissue, antigen-presenting cells, and T lymphocytes directly interact through a number of key soluble mediators, cell-surface molecules, and other signals. Pro-inflammatory and pro-autoimmune mediators between the antigen-presenting cell and the tissue cells include cytokines, growth factors, proteases, and protease inhibitors, each of which is a potential target for immunomodulation. Signals between the antigen-presenting cells and T lymphocytes include some of the same cytokines, but also specific genetically controlled activation signals mediated by cell-surface molecules. Thus, anti-HLA compounds, anti-T cell compounds, and molecular mechanisms for targeting specific T-cell molecules, such

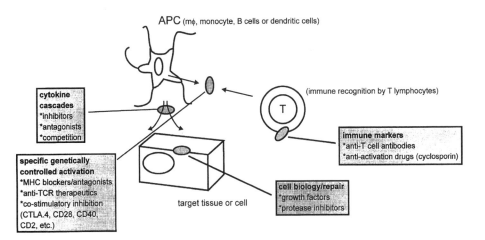

APC (mφ, monocyte, B cells or dendritic cells)

cytokine cascades
*inhibitors
*antagonists
*competition

(immune recognition by T lymphocytes)

T

immune markers
*anti-T cell antibodies
*anti-activation drugs (cyclosporin)

specific genetically controlled activation
*MHC blockers/antagonists
*anti-TCR therapeutics
*co-stimulatory inhibition (CTLA.4, CD28, CD40, CD2, etc.)

target tissue or cell

cell biology/repair
*growth factors
*protease inhibitors

(Figure 6A-2)
Molecular events in the pathogenesis of rheumatic diseases create potential therapeutic targets.

as the antigen-specific T-cell receptor and co-stimulator molecules, are designed to interfere at this step of interaction. Each of these interactions corresponds to several downstream biochemical and metabolic effects, such as intracellular signaling and gene activation, which are also prime targets for rationally designed therapeutics.

In practice, tools of molecular biology are used to genetically engineer soluble forms of the target molecules (or their respective receptors and ligands) and to create and express large quantities of these molecules, forming a new category of biotherapeutics that is just beginning to be applied in the rheumatic diseases. There is little doubt that major expansion in this area in the next few years will introduce new therapeutic tools for the clinical practitioner (13,14).

ANIMAL MODELS

Along with the expansion of new molecular therapeutics, molecularly sophisticated animal models of rheumatic disease have been developed. The introduction of genes into the germ lines of host animals (ie, transgenic mice) has been used to create animal models of human rheumatic disease, which will permit faster and more extensive analysis of disease mechanisms and provide a nonhuman host for initial testing of new therapeutics. Indeed, the question "what causes rheumatic diseases?" will likely be answered when a set of specific genes implicated in the cause and progression of human disease is transferred to a normal animal and reproduces the clinical syndrome.

SUMMARY

The fundamental pathway of molecular biology from gene to RNA to protein is recapitulated in the clinical applications of molecular biology in rheumatic disease. Examples include analyzing germline genes to detect a person's predisposition to disease and to assess disease prognosis for patients; and analyzing RNA transcripts from expressed genes that reflect disease activity and classifications of disease heterogeneity, as well as functioning as markers for response to therapy. Molecular design and engineering of pharmacologic antagonists for immune receptors and mediators of disease constitute a new and rapidly expanding area of molecular medicine.

GERALD T. NEPOM, MD, PhD

1. Elkon KB: Systemic lupus erythematosis: autoantibodies in SLE. In Klippel JH, Dieppe PA (eds): Rheumatology, St. Louis, Mosby, 1994, Section 6, pp 4.1-4.10

2. Bleasel JF, Holderbaum D, Haqqi TM, Moskowitz RW: Clinical correlations of osteoarthritis associated with single base mutations in the type II procollagen gene. J Rheumatol (Suppl) 43:34-36, 1995

3. Williams CJ, Jimenez SA: Heritable diseases of cartilage caused by mutations in collagen genes. J Rheumatol 43(Suppl):28-33, 1995

4. Morel L, Rudofsky UH, Longmate JA, Schiffenbauer J, Wakeland EK: Polygenic control of susceptibility to murine systemic lupus erythematosus. Immunity 1:219-229, 1994

5. Weyand CM, McCarthy TG, Goronzy JJ: Correlations between disease phenotype and genetic heterogeneity in rheumatoid arthritis. J Clin Invest 95:2120-2126, 1995

6. Combe B, Eliaou J-F, Daures J-P, Meyer O, Clot J, Sany J: Prognostic factors in rheumatoid arthritis. Comparative study of two subsets of patients according to severity of articular damage. Br J Rheumatol 34:529-534, 1995

7. MacGregor A, Ollier W, Thomson W, Jawaheer D, Silman A: HLA-DRB1*0401/0404 genotype and rheumatoid arthritis: Increased association in men, young age at onset, and disease severity. J Rheumatol 22:1032-1036, 1995

8. Nepom GT, Nepom BS: Prediction of susceptibility to rheumatoid arthritis by human leukocyte antigen genotyping. In Nepom GT (ed): Rheumatic Disease Clinics of North America, 18th ed. Philadelphia, W.B. Saunders Company, 1992, pp 785-792

9. Nepom GT, Gersuk V, Nepom BS: Prognostic implications of HLA genotyping in the early assessment of patients with rheumatoid arthritis. J Rheumatol 23: 5-9 (suppl 44), 1996.

10. Kinne RW, Boehm S, Iftner T, Aigner T, Vornehm S, Weseloh G, Bravo R, Emmrich F, Kroczek RA: Synovial fibroblast-like cells strongly express jun-B and C-fos proto-oncogenes in rheumatoid- and osteoarthritis. Scand J Rheumatol 101(Suppl):121-125, 1995

11. Kriegsmann J, Keyszer GM, Geiler T, Brauer R, Gay RE, Gay S: Expression of vascular cell adhesion molecule-1 mRNA and protein in rheumatoid synovium demonstrated by in situ hybridization and immunohistochemistry. Lab Invest 72:209-214, 1995

12. Li Y, Sun GR, Tumang JR, Crow MK, Friedman SM: CDR3 sequence motifs shared by oligoclonal rheumatoid arthritis synovial T cells. Evidence for an antigen-driven response. J Clin Invest 94:2525-2531, 1994

13. Moreland LW, Heck LW, Koopman WJ: Biologic agents for treating rheumatoid arthritis. Arthritis Rheum 40:397-409, 1997

14. Maini RN, Brennan FM, Williams R, Chu CQ, Cope AP, Gibbons D, Elliott M, Feldmann M: TNF-alpha in rheumatoid arthritis and prospects of anti-TNF therapy. Clin Exp Rheumatol 8(Suppl):S173-S175, 1993

B. MOLECULAR AND CELLULAR BASIS OF IMMUNITY

Despite the gaps in our understanding of the pathogenesis of rheumatic diseases, knowledge of the basic science that underlies the immune response has become extraordinarily sophisticated. There are now numerous examples (albeit for the most part in animal models) in which mutation of a single gene leads to immunologic disease. Perhaps the surprise is that so many different genetic lesions lead to autoimmune disease. This chapter briefly reviews the important features of the immune system, including some of its most critical molecules, and the principles that relate to the pathogenesis of immune-mediated diseases.

OVERVIEW OF THE IMMUNE SYSTEM

The immune system, a coordinated response of highly antigen-specific cells with nonspecific inflammatory cells and soluble factors, evolved to protect the body from infectious microorganisms. It is typically divided into *natural (nonspecific) immunity* and *acquired (specific) immunity*. The natural immune response consists of barriers such as skin and mucosa, phagocytic cells of the myelomonocytic lineage, and serum constituents such as complement. The cells that contribute to acquired immunity include *T and B lymphocytes*. Natural killer (NK) cells are another lymphocyte subset, but they do not have specific antigen receptors like T and B cells (1). *Antigen-presenting cells (APC)* are also key constituents of acquired immunity.

The acquired immune response is further divided into humoral and cell-mediated immunity. *Humoral immunity* principally consists of the B-cell and immunoglobulin (Ig) response, whereas *cell-mediated immunity* refers to the T-cell and APC-dependent response.

Although useful conceptually, the division of the immune response between natural versus acquired immunity and humoral versus cellular immunity is somewhat arbitrary. Not only do T cells (cell-mediated immunity) regulate immunoglobulin production by B cells (humoral immunity), but T cells (specific immunity) also secrete cytokines that recruit inflammatory cells of the myelomonocytic lineage (natural immunity). It is important to appreciate this coordination of responses in considering the pathogenesis and treatment of immunologic diseases.

Lymphocytes and mononuclear phagocytes are derived from hematopoietic stem cells. Embryonically, stem cells arise from the fetal yolk sac and populate the bone marrow, spleen, and liver. In the adult, bone marrow is the predominant source of lymphocytic and myelomonocytic progenitor cells. Lymphoid organs include the thymus, spleen, and lymph nodes. In the thymus, immature T cells develop into mature T lymphocytes, whereas B lymphocytes develop within the bone marrow. The spleen and lymph nodes are sites where B-cell differentiation occurs and T and B cells engage antigen. Antigen presentation to T cells occurs here, as do B–T-cell interactions. The spleen, the major site where lymphocytes encounter blood-borne antigen, also clears the circulation of senescent red blood cells and foreign substances. Lymph-borne antigen is also first encountered in the lymph nodes.

ANTIGENS, ANTIGEN-PRESENTING CELLS, AND MHC MOLECULES

A fundamentally important concept in immunology is that of antigenicity. Simply speaking, an antigen is a substance that generates an immune response. Lymphocytes recognize antigen by virtue of clonally specific antigen receptors. These receptors are immunoglobulin-like molecules located in the plasma membranes of T cells and B cells. Although T and B cells use a similar strategy to produce these extraordinary receptors, they "see" antigen very differently. B cells recognize soluble peptides, proteins, nucleic acids, polysaccharides, lipids, and small synthetic molecules. These antigens bind directly to the *B-cell antigen receptor (BCR)*, a membrane-associated form of immunoglobulin. Consequently, B cells have no need for antigen-presenting cells (Fig. 6B-1).

In contrast, T cells need antigen to be presented—that is, the *T-cell antigen receptor (TCR)* recognizes peptide fragments only when they are bound to *major histocompatibility complex (MHC) molecules*. An exception to this rule appears to be γδ T cells (2), a subset comprising less than 5% of peripheral blood T cells. Although some γδ cells respond to peptide antigens, others recognize nonpeptide antigen such as prenyl pyrophosphate derivatives of mycobacteria (3).

There are two types of MHC molecules, class I and class II. The three-dimensional structure of both classes creates a cleft, or groove, in which peptides are bound and can be recognized by T cells. MHC molecules, therefore, are antigen-presenting molecules for T cells (4). The association of peptides with MHC molecules is determined by primary and secondary structures of both molecules. Each MHC molecule binds a single peptide, but the pool of MHC molecules produced can bind an array of different peptides. Thus, MHC molecules are important determinants in controlling the immune response to protein antigens and, not surprisingly, certain MHC alleles correlate with susceptibility to autoimmune disease. However, the types of antigens that class I and class II molecules bind are quite distinct.

The primary function of MHC class I molecules is to present endogenous peptides. Class I molecules are expressed on nearly all cells and consist of two subunits. The α chain of class I proteins, encoded by genes within the HLA locus (HLA-A, -B, and-C), associates with a non–MHC-encoded protein, β_2 microglobulin. Class I molecules bind fragments of proteins that are degraded within the cell, including peptides derived from pathogens such as viruses, as well as normal cellular proteins. Cytosolic proteins are degraded in the proteasome and transferred to the endoplasmic reticulum by peptide transporter molecules (TAPs), which are also encoded within the MHC locus. There the MHC class I molecules are synthesized and assembled. The nascent MHC molecules associate with peptides and translocate to the plasma membrane where they can be recognized by T cells. Class I molecules bind peptides that are 9 to 11 amino acids in length. The T-cell accessory molecule, CD8, binds to class I molecules in a region distinct from the TCR; thus *CD8-*

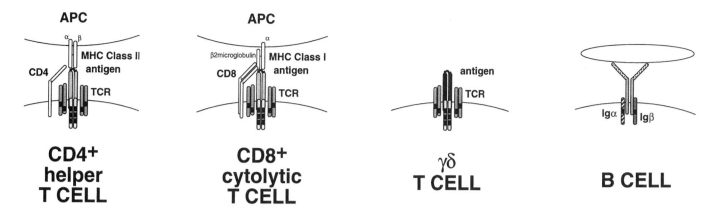

(Figure 6B-1)

Antigen recognition by T cells versus B cells. The CD4 molecule is a co-receptor for major histocompatibility complex (MHC) class II molecules. Thus CD4 or helper T cells recognize processed peptide antigen presented by class II molecules, which are expressed only on specialized cells. The CD8 molecule is a co-receptor for class I molecules, so CD8 T cells recognize peptide antigens presented by cells expressing class I molecules, which are present on most cells. In contrast, γδ T cells do not express either CD4 or CD8 and, unlike αβ T cells, can also recognize nonpeptide antigens. B cells recognize many different types of soluble antigens in their native state and thus do not require antigen presentation. The black boxes indicate immune tyrosine-based activation (ITAM) motifs.

expressing T cells are class I-restricted. Because of their ability to bind MHC, the CD8 and CD4 molecules are called *co-receptors.* When CD8 T cells are activated, they become cytotoxic T lymphocytes and are important in controlling viral infections by destroying virally infected cells.

The primary function of class II molecules is to present exogenous peptides. Class II molecules are composed of two chains that are products of different MHC genes (HLA-DR, -DQ, and -DP). Only B cells, macrophages, dendritic cells, activated T cells, and activated endothelial cells express class II molecules. Bone marrow-derived dendritic cells, which are present in lymph nodes and the spleen, are extremely efficient APCs.

Antigen processing by class II-expressing APCs occurs in three steps: extracellular antigens are ingested, internalized, and proteolyzed. MHC class II molecules are synthesized and assembled, but they are prevented from binding endogenous peptide antigens because the class II complex associates with a molecule termed the invariant chain. In the appropriate intracellular compartment, however, the invariant chain dissociates and allows processed extracellularly derived antigen to bind to class II molecules, thus enabling the presentation of these antigens to T cells. Class II molecules bind peptides that range from 10 to 30 amino acids in length. The CD4 molecule binds MHC class II molecules, and therefore *CD4-expressing or helper T cells are class II-restricted.* Helper T cells, which comprise about 60% of total T cells, are key immunoregulatory cells that control cellular and humoral immune responses.

RECOGNITION OF ANTIGEN BY T CELLS

The TCR complex is composed of both antigen-recognition and signal-transducing subunits. Four TCR genes encode the subunits responsible for antigen recognition: α, β, γ, and δ (5). These genes are members of the Ig gene superfamily and are similar to Ig genes. TCR genes undergo DNA rearrangement of variable (V), diversity (D), joining (J), and constant (C) region segments (Fig. 6B-2). This recombination of gene segments is generated by the action of a number of enzymes, including the recombinase activating genes

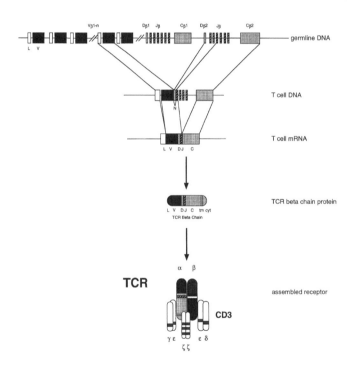

(Figure 6B-2)

Processes that generate a T-cell receptor. DNA is in the germline configuration in T-cell precursors. During T-cell development in the thymus, the T-cell receptor (TCR) gene segments rearrange in a specific order bringing variable (V), diversity (D), joining (J), and constant (C) segments into proximity to generate functional receptor genes. Random nucleotide additions (N) are inserted by terminal deoxytransferase. The β locus has 75 V, two D, 10 or 12 J, and two C segments. The α gene has 50 V, no D, 70 J, and one C segments. The δ gene, which is embedded within the α gene, has four V, two D, three J, and one C segments, whereas the γ locus has eight V, five J, and two C segments. After DNA rearrangement, mRNA is produced and spliced to form the mature RNA. After transcription, the receptor subunit associates with another subunit that is also the product of a gene rearrangement plus invariant chains. This process occurs in the endoplasmic reticulum, and the receptor complex is transported to the cell surface.

RAG-1 and RAG-2. The rearranged gene is then transcribed and translated to produce a protein subunit. Two of these subunits combine to form two types of heterodimeric receptors, αβ and γδ receptors, that function as the antigen recognition unit. The majority of T cells in peripheral blood, lymph nodes, and spleen have αβ receptors. The V region gene segments are highly polymorphic. Diversity can be further increased by recombinant assembly of the different V D J segments and insertion of random nucleotides at the junctions by the enzyme terminal deoxytransferase. Thus, an individual has the genetic capacity of producing a vast number of T-cell clones with specific antigen receptors—potentially about 10^{16} αβ T-cell receptors. TCR genes show allelic exclusion; that is, if one chromosome undergoes rearrangement and produces a functional receptor chain, the genes on the other chromosome are prevented from rearranging. Hence, each T-cell clone expresses only one antigen receptor, and antigen-specific T cells develop in unimmunized or naive individuals independent of exposure to antigen. Subsequent, antigen exposure leads to *clonal selection* or expansion of lymphocytes with the appropriate antigen receptors. Clonal selection improves the efficiency of the immune response and produces immunologic memory.

TCR αβ or γδ subunits provide an elegant solution to the problem of antigen recognition, but these subunits do not transmit activation signals. Instead, the antigen-recognizing subunits associate with signaling subunits called *invariant chains* because they are not polymorphic. The invariant subunits include the CD3 family of molecules (γ, δ, ε) and the ζ chain, which can exist as either a homodimer (ζ-ζ) or a heterodimer (ζ-η), the η chain being an alternatively spliced form of ζ. The stoichiometry of the TCR most likely is TCRαβ/CD3γδε₂ζ₂.

TCR Signal Transduction

In response to recognition of foreign antigen by the antigen-recognition subunits, the first known biochemical event is phosphorylation of the invariant chains on tyrosine residues by protein tyrosine kinases (PTK) (6). Upon recognition of antigen–MHC complex, Lck, a PTK that binds CD4 and CB8 molecules, is brought into the TCR complex where it phosphorylates the invariant chains. Fyn, another PTK, is associated with the TCR complex and also phosphorylates the invariant chains. In addition to PTKs, a protein tyrosine phosphatase, CD45, is also critical for TCR signaling. The phosphorylated sites on CD3 γ, δ, ε, and ζ subunits are termed *ITAMs* (immune tyrosine-based activation motifs) (7). Other receptors including the B-cell and Fc receptors also have ITAMs (8). ITAM motifs are composed of 17 amino acids with a duplicated sequence: tyrosine, X, X, leucine (X denotes any amino acid). ITAMs are docking sites for proteins with SH2 (src homology 2) domains that bind phosphotyrosine. Such proteins include another PTK, ZAP-70 (zeta-associated protein of 70 kD) (9), SHC, and phosphatidylinositol-phospholipase Cγ (PLCγ). Deficiency of Zap-70 causes severe combined immunodeficiency (SCID). SHC, an adapter protein, leads to the activation of a cascade of serine–threonine kinases by activating the GTP binding protein ras. Activation of PLCγ cleaves phosphatidylinositol bisphosphate (PIP₂) to produce diacylglycerol, which activates protein kinase C. PLCγ also cleaves PIP₂ to produce inositol triphosphate, which releases intracellular calcium. The presence of calcium in the cell activates calcineurin, a phosphatase that dephosphorylates the transcription factor NFAT (nuclear factor of activated T cells), an action that is blocked by the immunosuppressive drugs cyclosporin A and FK506 (10). Transcription factors are key regulatory proteins that modulate gene expression. Factors such

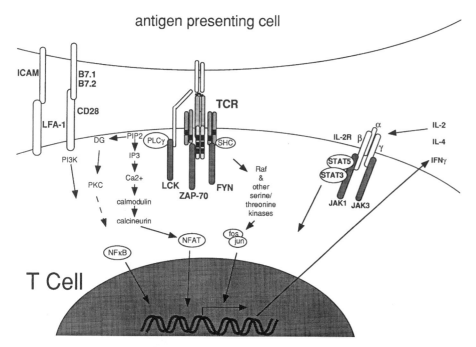

(Figure 6B-3)

T-cell activation. Upon encountering foreign antigen in association with the major histocompatibility complex (MHC), CD4 or CD8 is brought into proximity of the T-cell receptor (TCR) complex along with the protein tyrosine kinase Lck, which phosphorylates the TCR invariant subunits on immune tyrosine-based activation motif (ITAM) sites (shown as black boxes on the receptor subunits). This forms a site that can be bound by SHC-containing enzymes such as ZAP-70 and PLCγ, which activates serine/threonine kinase and raises intracellular calcium (Ca²⁺) levels. These signals regulate the function of transcription factors such as nuclear factor of activated T cells (NFAT), NFκB, Fos, and Jun. These factors, in turn, regulate the expression of T-cell activation genes such as interleukin-2 (IL-2) and the IL-2Rα subunit. IL-2 is secreted and activates T cells through its receptor, which interacts with the tyrosine kinases, JAK3 and JAK1. These kinases then activate STATs, a class of transcription factors. Also shown are adhesion molecules (ICAM and LFA-1 [CD11a/CD18]) and the important costimulatory molecule CD28. IP3, PI3K, and PIP2 are phosphorylated derivatives of a phospholipid component of the plasma membrane. Other abbreviations are diacylglycerol (DG) and protein kinase C (PKC).

as NFκ B, Fos, and Jun as well as NFAT up-regulate transcription of genes that encode cytokines, receptors (including cytokine receptors), and other genes.

Occupancy of the T-cell receptor alone, however, does not lead to T-cell activation, since the perturbation of other surface molecules is necessary (Fig. 6B-3). These molecules include *co-stimulatory molecules* such as CD28 and *adhesion molecules* (CD11a/CD18, CD2, and others). TCR stimulation in the absence of a CD28-mediated signal can lead to a state of anergy, or unresponsiveness. Interestingly, interference of CD28 signaling in murine lupus ameliorates autoimmune disease in mice (11). The counter receptors for CD28 are B7-1 and B7-2. In addition, another molecule, CTLA-4, also binds B7-1 and B7-2. Unlike CD28, which provides costimulatory signals, CTLA-4 functions to downregulate the immune response. This is illustrated by CTLA-4 knockout mice, which develop lethal lymphoproliferative disease.

T-cell Development

Precursor T cells originate in the bone marrow where their TCR genes have yet to rearrange, and they do not express CD4 or CD8. These cells migrate to the thymus where they differentiate into mature T cells that express TCR and either CD4 or CD8. Of considerable interest is that the vast majority of T cells entering the thymus die there. To survive, T cells must have produced TCRs that recognize self-MHC molecules, a process termed *positive selection* (12). While some TCRs recognize self-MHC molecules and self-peptides with high affinity, these potentially autoreactive clones are eliminated (*negative selection* or clonal deletion) (13). This is one mechanism that is believed to achieve tolerance to self and is termed *central tolerance*. There are other mechanisms for achieving tolerance outside the thymus and this is termed *peripheral tolerance*. Much of the T-cell death that occurs in the thymus is due to programmed cell death (*apoptosis*).

IMMUNOGLOBULINS AND B CELLS

Immunoglobulin molecules, inserted into the membrane of a B lymphocyte, are responsible for the ability of B cells to recognize antigen (Fig. 6B-1). In addition, Ig secreted by terminally differentiated B lymphocytes, called plasma cells, assists in the clearance of pathogenic organisms. Ig molecules are composed of two types of polypeptides, light and heavy chains (14). There are two *Ig light (L) chain* classes (isotypes), κ and λ, and nine distinct *Ig heavy (H) chain* isotypes (Table 6B-1). The H chain isotypes correspond with the five different classes of immunoglobulins—γ, α, μ, δ, and ε for IgG, IgA, IgM, IgD, and IgE, respectively—and the subclasses of IgG (γ1, γ2, γ3, and γ4) and IgA (α1 and α2). For example, an IgG1 molecule contains two identical Igγ1 chains and two identical L chains (either κ or λ) bound together by noncovalent and disulfide bonds. In contrast, most IgM and many IgA molecules are higher order multimers of H and L chains interconnected via interdisulfide bonds and a unique protein called a J chain. IgA often functions at epithelial surfaces and, when secreted through the epithelium, is associated with a secretory fragment.

Each H and L chain has a variable and a constant region. Many of the effector functions of Ig, such as binding to complement and Fc receptors, depend upon the constant region of H chain isotype, while the antigen-binding capability of Ig resides in the variable regions of both the H and L chains. Because each developing B cell has the genetic potential for assembling an antigen-receptor complex of a unique specificity, the sum of the specificities is vast and is called the B-cell repertoire. Similar to the T-cell repertoire, the B-cell repertoire is diversified by using different V genes, imprecise joining of different D and J segments, and diversification of N segments (nucleotide insertions). In addition, the B-cell repertoire is capable of somatic hypermutation.

B-Cell Development

B-cell lymphopoiesis begins in the fetal liver and later switches to the bone marrow. While conventional B cells (B-2) are continuously generated in the adult bone marrow, B-1 (formerly called CD5) B cells are predominantly produced early in ontogeny. Two major events occur in B-cell development: the rearrangement and expression of Ig genes. All the H chain genes are on chromosome 14. Their successful rearrangement requires the joining of a J_H segment, a D_H segment, and a V_H region (Fig. 6B-4). B-cell precursors first assemble $D_H J_H$ rearrangements, and after V_H is successfully joined to $D_H J_H$, heavy chain rearrangements cease. B-cell precursors that have not initiated Ig rearrangement or with only DJ rearrangements are termed pro-B cells, while those

(Table 6B-1)
Human immunoglobulin classes (heavy chain isotypes)

	IgM	IgD	IgG1	IgG2	IgG3	IgG4	IgA1	IgA2	IgE
H chain	μ	δ	γ1	γ2	γ3	γ4	α1	α2	ε
Molecular weight (kD)	900	180	150	150	150	150	160–350	160–350	190
Serum concentration (mg %)	100	3	900	300	100	50	300	50	0.001
Complement fixation by classical pathway	+++	−	++	+	+++	−	−	−	−
Placental transfer	−	−	+	+	+	+	−	−	−
Plasma half life (days)	5	3	21	20	7	21	6	6	2
$(H_2L_2)_n$, n=	5	1	1	1	1	1	1,2	1,2	1
Number of domains per heavy chain	5	5	4	4	4	4	4	4	5
Carbohydrate (%)	12	12	3	3	3	3	9	9	12

(Figure 6B-4)

Genetic organization and rearrangement of immunoglobulin heavy chain genes. Shown is a simplified version of the portion of chromosome 14 containing the immunoglobulin heavy chain variable region and constant region genes. A: Genomic organization found in all cells except committed B cells. B: Initial rearrangement produces the D-J joining, which results from deletion of the DNA enclosed in the dashed box in A. The junction between D and J regions includes additional random necleotides constituting an N region. C: The next step in rearrangement is V-D-J joining, which results from the deletion of the DNA enclosed in dashed box in B. A B cell expressing the rearrangement gene shown in C might express IgM with the V_{H2} variable region. D: Such a B cell could then undergo an isotype switch by deleting the DNA shown in the dashed box in C to express IgGl with the same V_{H2} variable region.

that have rearranged, transcribed, and translated an H chain are pre-B cells. The translated μ chains in pre-B cells are intracellular, with the exception of small amounts found on the plasma membrane in conjunction with surrogate light chain (derived from the λ5 and V pre-β gene products). Together the heavy chain and the surrogate light chain form the pre-B-cell receptor complex. Likely an external ligand engages this complex signaling the pre-B cell to rearrange one of its L chains. The κ and λ loci are on chromosomes 2 and 22, respectively. Their rearrangement requires a VJ joint. Once a B-cell precursor successfully rearranges an H and L gene, the process stops and the cell expresses surface Ig; it is now termed an immature B cell. Many precursor cells fail to make successful rearrangements or to express a functional pre-B-cell receptor and die in situ via apoptosis.

The protein RAG-2 is required for rearrangement of the Ig and for the TCR loci. The lack of RAG-2 results in the absence of mature lymphocytes. In general, any mutation that impairs H chain rearrangement or expression will block B-cell development (15). In addition, the cytokine interleukin (IL)-7, the kinase Syk, the cell-survival gene *bcl-x,* and the transcription factors E2A, EBF, and BSAP all have critical roles in B-cell development, as does the Bruton tyrosine kinase (BTK) gene. Mutations in the BTK gene cause Bruton's X-linked agammaglobulinemia, a disease characterized by impaired B-cell development (16).

B-Cell Activation

Once a B-cell precursor expresses surface Ig, it can respond to exogenous and self-antigens. However, the binding of antigens to the BCR on immature B cells does not trigger cellular activation, but a cellular response leading to *self-tolerance.* Multivalent self-antigens such as double-stranded DNA induce programmed cell death, while oligovalent self-antigens render immature B cells refractory to further stimulation. Such a cell may escape anergy by rearranging another light chain Ig gene, changing its BCR specificity, and losing its self-reactivity, a process called *receptor editing.*

Mature B cells with nonself-reactive BCRs enter secondary lymphoid tissues such as spleen or lymph nodes where they may encounter foreign antigens. B-cell antigens

are broadly divided into *thymus-dependent (TD)* and *thymus-independent (TI)* antigens. TD antigens are largely soluble protein antigens that require MHC class II-restricted T-cell help for antibody production, whereas TI antigens do not require such help. TI antigens are often multivalent and poorly degraded in vivo; bacterial polysaccharides are examples of these antigens. In general, TI responses generate poor immunologic memory, induce minimal germinal center formation, and trigger IgG2 secretion (17). The B cells responding to TI antigens have a distinct phenotype and localize in the marginal zone of the spleen. The dependence on these splenic B cells for responses to TI antigens may account for the poor responses to polysaccharide antigens seen in splenectomized individuals and in infants (the marginal zone B cells do not mature until about 2 years of age). Coupling polysaccharides to a carrier protein produces an effective infant vaccine, since the conjugate triggers a TD response.

The BCR has a dual role: 1) it binds and internalizes antigen for processing into peptides that assemble with class II molecules for presentation to CD4 T cells, and 2) it activates the antigen-recognizing B cell (18). The signal transducing capability of the BCR lies not with surface Ig but with two associated transmembrane proteins: Ig-α and Ig-β. Similar to the TCR-associated molecules, their intracellular domains contain ITAM motifs. Ig-α/Ig-β heterodimers couple the BCR to the Src-related kinases Lyn, Blk, and Fyn, and the ZAP-70-related tyrosine kinase Syk. The B-cell transmembrane proteins CD19 and CD22 modulate BCR signaling. Although the ligands for CD19 and CD22 are unknown, their intracellular portions also associate with tyrosine kinases. In Lyn-deficient mice, defective B-cell clonal expansion and terminal differentiation occur, as does a failure to eliminate autoreactive B cells. The Syk and the Src-related kinases phosphorylate other downstream effectors, thus activating the B cell and increasing the membrane levels of the T-cell co-stimulatory ligands B7-1 and B7-2 needed for B–T-cell collaboration.

B-Cell Differentiation

Exposure to a TD antigen triggers two pathways of B-cell differentiation: the extrafollicular pathway, which leads to early antibody production, and the germinal center pathway, which leads to germinal center formation, immunologic memory, and the generation of plasma-cell precursors (19). In the spleen, antigen-activated B cells migrate to T-cell–rich zones in the periarteriolar lymphoid sheath searching for T-cell help. Failure to find it likely results in anergy, but successful B–T-cell collaboration produces short-lived oligoclonal proliferative foci (each derived from several B cells). Many of the B cells in these foci secrete IgM and undergo *isotype switching*, a DNA splicing event that exchanges the heavy chain constant regions of an Ig gene, while the VDJ gene segments remain the same. By this mechanism, IgM antibodies of a given antigen specificity can be converted to IgG or IgE. These events are dependent upon direct co-stimulatory signals, CD40 and CD40L interactions, and cytokines such as IL-2, IL-4, IL-6, and IL-10 (20). Antibody affinity may also be altered by the introduction of mutations in variable gene segments, a process known as *somatic mutation.*

Some B cells migrate from these proliferative foci to primary follicles and enter the germinal center pathway. Within a primary follicle, an oligoclonal expansion of B cells forms the dark zone. Eventually these cells migrate into a region called the light zone, where they interact with helper T cells and follicular dendritic cells that have trapped and localized antigen on their surfaces. Here, B cells that possess high-affinity BCRs are selected to survive, whereas those that do not, die. B cells in which somatic mutations generated an autoreactive BCR are also eliminated. Rescue signals induce the survival genes *bcl-x* and *bcl-2*, resulting in the persistence of the selected cells. B7-1, CD19, CD40 on B cells, and CD40L on activated T cells have critical roles in germinal center formation. Individuals with the X-linked hyper IgM syndrome do not express functional CD40L following T-cell activation, which underscores the importance of CD40L. Consequently, B cells do not form germinal centers, and their Ig genes are unable to undergo class switching (16). CD40 and CD40L are members of the tumor necrosis factor α (TNF-α) family.

Passage through the germinal center leads to the formation of memory B cells or plasma-cell precursors; few antibody-secreting cells remain within the germinal center. Cytokines and CD40L influence this decision; IL-2, IL-10, and IL-6 promote differentiation into plasma cells, while CD40/CD40L interactions promote memory-cell formation and inhibit plasma-cell generation. Cytokines also contribute to isotype switching. IL-4 enhances switching to IgE and IgG4; IL-10 to IgG1, IgG3, and IgA; and transforming growth factor β (TGF-β) to IgA (20).

Plasma cells secrete large amounts of Ig, but they are short-lived cells that need constant replenishment to sustain high antibody levels. Plasma cells lose their membrane Ig and many of the markers that identify B cells, although they express high levels of CD38. Memory B cells are long-lived cells that contain somatically mutated V genes and are morphologically distinct from naive B cells. They can be rapidly re-stimulated to generate a secondary antibody response. Together, the extrafollicular and germinal center pathways of B-cell differentiation lead to a coordinated humoral response that provides the very rapid production of low-affinity antibodies, the subsequent production of high-affinity antibodies, and the potential for a rapid amnestic response.

IMMUNOREGULATION AND CYTOKINES

The ability of the immune system to mount a response is regulated at many levels. MHC and TCR molecules determine which antigens will be recognized. In addition, other factors influence the immune response, including the nature of antigen, the route of exposure, and the quantity of antigen. Co-administration of an adjuvant increases the immunogenicity of a substance because adjuvants activate antigen-presenting cells and other nonspecific cellular components. A major immunoregulatory mechanism is the production by lymphoid and nonlymphoid cells of a large number of cytokines. Many cytokines mediate natural immunity and inflammation and are of great importance in the pathogenesis of rheumatic disease. For example, IL-1 and TNF are major mediators of inflammation and tissue injury; interfering with the action of TNF-α is one strategy for treating rheumatoid arthritis (21). Other cytokines are critically important in hematopoiesis, and several are widely used clinically (eg, erythropoietin and granulocyte colony stimulating factor). However, only those cytokines with important immunoregulatory activities (22) will be reviewed here.

Th1 and Th2

CD4 or helper T cells differentiate to one of two phenotypes (23): T helper 1 (Th1) and T helper 2 (Th2) cells. Th1 cells produce IL-2 and IFN-γ, promoting a cell-mediated response. IL-2, an autocrine T-cell growth factor, is important in determining the magnitude of T-cell and NK-cell responses. IL-15 has similar effects as it binds the IL-2R β and γ subunits. However, IL-15 is produced by nonlymphoid cells and may be of importance in immunologically mediated diseases. IFN-γ activates macrophages, enhances their ability to kill microorganisms, up-regulates class II expression, and suppresses Th2 responses. IL-12 is a key inducer of Th1 differentiation and is produced by B cells and monocytes in response to pathogenic organisms. It also enhances T- and NK-cell cytolytic activity and induces IFN-γ secretion.

In contrast, Th2 cells produce IL-4, IL-5, IL-9, and IL-10 and thus promote humoral or allergic responses. IL-4 is a major regulator of allergic responses. It inhibits macrophage activation, blocks the effects of IFN-γ, is a growth factor for mast cells, and is required for class switching of B cells to produce IgE. IL-4 is also a major factor that influences Th2 differentiation of naive helper T cells. IL-5 promotes the growth, differentiation, and activation of eosinophils, whereas IL-9 supports growth of T cells and bone marrow-derived mast-cell precursors. In contradistinction to IFN-γ, IL-10 inhibits macrophage antigen presentation and decreases expression of class II molecules. The importance of IL-10 as an endogenous inhibitor of cell-mediated immunity is underscored by the finding that IL-10 knockout mice develop autoimmune disease (24).

Precisely how Th1 versus Th2 differentiation occurs is not fully understood, but cytokines themselves, especially IL-12 and IL-4, are clearly important in the outcome. IL-7 is essential for T- and B-cell development.

Many, but not all, cytokines bind to receptors that are members of the hematopoietic cytokine receptor superfamily. A family of cytoplasmic PTKs known as Janus kinases (JAKs) is particularly important for signaling by these receptors. JAKs bind to cytokine receptors, become activated following cytokine binding, and phosphorylate the receptor (25). Different JAKs are activated by different cytokines. The importance of this family is supported by the demonstration that patients who lack JAK3 are immunodeficient. JAK3 binds to the cytokine subunit γc that is a component of the receptors for IL-2, IL-4, IL-7, IL-9, and IL-15, all of which activate JAK3. Deficiency of either γc or JAK3 leads to the same phenotype of severe combined immunodeficiency.

An important class of substrate for the JAKs is the STAT (signal transducers and activators of transcription) family of transcription factors. Having SH2 domains, STATs bind the phosphorylated cytokine receptor, become phosphorylated by the JAKs, and then translocate to the nucleus where they regulate gene expression. Different cytokine receptors recruit and activate different members of the STAT family. The importance of STAT molecules in the immune response is underscored by the recent generation of STAT knockout mice. Mice deficient in STAT4, which is activated by IL-12, have impaired Th1 differentiation; whereas mice deficient in STAT6, which is activated by IL-4, have impaired Th2 responses.

Turning the Immune Response Off

A key feature of the immune response is that it is self-limited. Two key cytokines that function to down-regulate the immune response are IL-10 and TGF-β1. TGF-β1 knockout mice die of overwhelming immunologic disease (26) characterized by lymphoid and mononuclear infiltration of the heart, lung, and other tissues. Like patients with Sjögren's syndrome, these mice also develop salivary gland infiltrates, pseudolymphoma, and anti-dsDNA, anti-ssDNA, and anti-Sm ribonucleoprotein antibodies (27). IL-10 knockout mice also have autoimmune disease.

Another important mechanism that dampens the immune response is mediated by the Fas molecule, which induces T cells to undergo apoptosis. The importance of this molecule is illustrated by the discovery of Fas gene mutations in both mice and humans that cause severe lymphoproliferative disease associated with autoimmunity, which in humans is called autoimmune lymphoproliferative syndrome (28). FAS-dependent apoptosis is one mechanism of achieving peripheral tolerance. The effect of the CTLA-4 counter receptor has been discussed previously.

THE IMMUNE RESPONSE TO PATHOGENIC ORGANISMS

Different types of infectious organisms elicit different types of immune responses. Even though these mechanisms evolved to protect the host, tissue injury and disease often occur as a consequence of host response. Indeed, it is well established that through a variety of immunologic and inflammatory mechanisms, some rheumatologic diseases are triggered by infectious agents.

A major host response to endotoxins such as lipopolysaccharide, produced by Gram-negative bacteria, is the production of cytokines such as TNF by macrophages, vascular endothelium, and other cells. A severe consequence of this response is septic shock. Staphylococci, in contrast, produce enterotoxins that are the most potent natural T-cell mitogens. The enterotoxins bind TCR variable regions (Vβ) and class II molecules, thereby activating T cells, which can result in toxic shock syndrome characterized by fever, exfoliative skin disease, disseminated intravascular coagulation, and cardiovascular shock.

The immune response to extracellular bacteria is largely humoral. Toxins are neutralized by antibody, and organisms are either lysed by complement or opsonized with antibody and complement and then phagocytosed. An exaggerated response can also lead to disease in the host, such as post-streptococcal glomerulonephritis, in which the profuse production and deposition of antigen–antibody (immune) complexes leads to kidney damage.

Cell-mediated immunity is the primary defense against intracellular pathogens like *Mycobacteria.* Antigen-specific T cells recognize foreign peptides presented by APCs. The T cells proliferate and secrete cytokines that activate endothelial cells, resulting in the recruitment and activation of other leukocytes. Monocytes are recruited, differentiate to macrophages, and kill the microorganisms. With chronic stimulation, however, macrophages fuse to generate multinucleate giant cells that can participate in granuloma formation. Fibrin is also deposited, causing tissue induration. This response is termed delayed-type hypersensitivity (DTH). The immune response may then subside without permanent damage to the host tissue, although this is not always the case. Cell-mediated immunity to intracellular organisms such as *M. tuberculosis* can cause significant tissue destruction and fibrosis. Granulomatous diseases such as sarcoidosis and Wegener's granulomatosis may be due to a cell-mediated response to an unknown organism.

Immunity to viruses is mediated by interferon α/β (natural immunity) and the production of specific antibodies (acquired immunity). Immune complex disease can occur as a consequence of viral infection (eg, hepatitis B infection and arteritis). The cellular response to virus is mediated by CD8 T cells that recognize viral peptides in association with class I molecules. These T cells can destroy virally infected cells, a process termed *cell-mediated cytotoxicity.* In addition, NK cells lyse virally infected cells.

The Th2 response, characterized by production of IL-4 and IL-5 and subsequent eosinophilia, is key to the immune response to parasitic infestations. The importance of this response is demonstrated by IL-4 knockout mice, which rapidly succumb to certain parasitic infestations.

IMMUNOPATHOLOGY

The pathogenesis of rheumatologic diseases is not fully understood, but, nonetheless, it is useful to characterize diseases based on their predominant immunopathologic lesion. Although this classification is useful conceptually, it is important to keep in mind two facts: 1) the components of the immune system are interdependent, and 2) similar immunopathologic abnormalities may arise by different mechanisms.

Diseases Caused by Antibodies

Immediate hypersensitivity (type I hypersensitivity) is due to the production of IgE that binds to Fc receptors on mast cells and basophils. Antigen cross-linking of receptor-bound IgE triggers the release of histamine and the production of pro-inflammatory lipid mediators and cytokines. The inflammatory component (late-phase response) is clinically important in diseases such as asthma. Allergic rhinitis and anaphylaxis are other examples of immediate hypersensitivity disease.

Antibodies against circulating or fixed cells (type II hypersensitivity) are involved in the pathogenesis of a variety of diseases including autoimmune hemolytic anemia, autoimmune thrombocytopenia, Goodpasture's syndrome, pemphigus, pemphigoid, pernicious anemia, myasthenia gravis, and Graves' disease. Pathogenic antibodies cause tissue damage by a variety of mechanisms including lysis by complement and phagocytosis of opsonized cells. In addition, inflammatory cells are recruited to tissues by antibody deposition and complement activation. Finally, antibodies bind to receptors and alter cellular function without damaging the cells. Antibodies can be present but may not be involved in disease pathogenesis, as is likely the case in rheumatoid arthritis.

In immune complex disease (type III hypersensitivity), antibody and antigen form complexes that activate complement. These complexes are normally cleared by macrophages in the spleen and elsewhere. However, immune complexes may be deposited in other organs and tissues such as the kidney, skin, and serosal surfaces. A number of factors influence immune complex deposition including physicochemical properties, anatomic site of deposition, local tissue response (eg, local production of cytokines), and the host's ability to clear the complexes. Examples of immune complex disease include systemic lupus erythematosus, polyarteritis nodosa, and poststreptococcal glomerulonephritis.

Diseases Caused by T Cells

In a number of animal models and human diseases, T cells have a pathogenic role. The mechanisms of T-cell–mediated tissue injury include DTH and direct lysis by cytolytic (CD8) T cells. Contact dermatitis is a typical DTH process. In addition, T cells play a role in the pathogenesis of insulin-dependent diabetes mellitus, experimental allergic encephalomyelitis (a mouse model for multiple sclerosis), myasthenia gravis, and Graves' disease.

Although it is useful to classify diseases according to B- or T-cell involvement, there is a great deal of overlap. For example, B-cell antibody production (the mediator of types I, II, and III hypersensitivity) is regulated to a great extent by T cells. Thus T cells may have a major pathogenic role in these diseases.

SUMMARY

The human immune response is composed of highly antigen-specific elements that trigger the recruitment of cells and secretion of factors that nonspecifically induce inflammation. Ordinarily, this orchestrated process efficiently rids the host of pathogenic organisms, but not always. Immune-mediated tissue injury can occur as part of the normal response. Moreover, dysregulation of immune/inflammatory homeostasis at any one of many steps can lead to autoimmune disease. Hormonal and environmental factors also influence the immune and inflammatory responses.

The molecular basis of autoimmune disease in humans is probably heterogenous—that is, a variety of mutations or polymorphisms in an array of separate genes contribute to disease susceptibility. Although this makes the study of the pathogenesis of rheumatologic diseases extraordinarily

complex, it also provides many distinct avenues for therapeutic intervention.

JOHN J. O'SHEA, MD
JOHN KEHRL, MD

1. Yokoyama WM, Daniels BF, Seaman WE, Hunziker R, Margulies DH, Smith HR: A family of murine NK cell receptors specific for target cell MHC class I molecules. Semin Immunol 7:89-101, 1995

2. Haas WP, Pereira P, Tonegawa S: Gamma/delta cells. Ann Rev Immunol 11:637-685, 1993

3. Tanaka Y, Morita CT, Tanaka Y, Nieves E, Brenner MB, Bloom BR: Natural and synthetic non-peptide antigens recognized by human gamma delta T cells. Nature 375:155-158, 1995

4. Germain RN, Margulies DH: The biochemistry and cell biology of antigen processing and presentation. Ann Rev Immunol 11:403-450 1993

5. Abbas AK, Lichtman AH, Pober JS (eds): Cellular and Molecular Immunology, 2nd ed. Philadelphia, WB Saunders, 1994

6. Samelson LE, Donovan JA, Isakov N, Ota Y, Wange RL: Signal transduction mediated by the T-cell antigen receptor. Ann NY Acad Sci 766:157-172, 1995

7. Cambier JC: Antigen and Fc receptor signaling: the awesome power of the immunoreceptor tyrosine-based activation motif (ITAM). J Immunol 155:3281-3285, 1995

8. Keegan AD, Paul WE: Multichain immune recognition receptors: similarities in structure and signaling pathways. Immunol Today 13:63-68, 1992

9. Chan AC, Desai DM, Weiss A: The role of protein tyrosine kinases and protein tyrosine phosphatases in T cell antigen receptor signal transduction. Annu Rev Immunol 12:555-592, 1994

10. Bierer BE: Biology of cyclosporin A and FK506. Prog Clin Biol Res 390:203-223, 1994

11. Finck BK, Linsley PS, Wofsy D: Treatment of murine lupus with CTLA4Ig. Science 265:1225-1227, 1994

12. von Boehmer H, Kisielow P: Self-nonself discrimination by T cells. Science 248:1369-1373, 1990

13. Ramsdell F, Fowlkes BJ: Clonal deletion versus clonal anergy: the role of the thymus in inducing self tolerance. Science 248:1342-1348, 1990

14. Max EE: Immunoglobulins: molecular genetics in fundamental immunology. In Paul WE (ed): Fundamental Immunology. New York, Raven Press, 1993

15. Loffert D, Schaal S, Ehlich A, Hardy RR, Aon YR, Muller W, Rajewsky K: Early B-cell development in the mouse: insights from mutations introduced by gene targeting. Immunol Rev 137:135-153, 1994

16. Puck JM: Molecular and genetic basis of X-linked immunodeficiency disorders. J Clin Immunol 14:81-89, 1994

17. Mond JJ, Lees A, Snapper CM: T cell-independent antigens type 2. Annu Rev Immunol 13:655-692, 1995

18. Gold MR, DeFranco AL: Biochemistry of B lymphocyte activation. Adv Immunol 55:221-295, 1994

19. MacLennan ICM: Germinal centers. Annu Rev Immunol 12:117-139, 1994

20. Banchereau J, Biere F, Liu YJ, Rousset F: Molecular control of B lymphocyte growth and differentiation. Stem Cells 12:278-288, 1994

21. Feldmann M, Brennan FM, Elliott MJ, Williams RO, Maini RN: TNF alpha is an effective therapeutic target for rheumatoid arthritis. Ann N Y Acad Sci 766:272-278, 1995

22. Paul WE, Seder RA: Lymphocyte responses and cytokines. Cell 76:241-251, 1994

23. O'Garra A, Murphy K: Role of cytokines in determining T-lymphocyte function. Curr Opin Immunol 3:458-466, 1994

24. Rennick D, Davidson N, Berg D: Interleukin-10 gene knock-out mice: a model of chronic inflammation. Clin Immunol Immunopathol 76(3 Pt 2):S174-S178, 1995

25. Johnston JA, Bacon C, Riedy MC, O'Shea JJ: Signaling by the IL-2 and related receptors: JAKs, STATs and relationship to immunodeficiency. J Leuk Biol 60:441-452, 1996

26. Schull MM, Ormsby I, Kier AB, et al: Targeted disruption of the mouse transforming growth factor beta-1 gene results in multifocal inflammatory disease. Nature 359:693-699, 1992

27. Dang H, Geiser AG, Letterio JJ, Nakabayashi T, Kong L, Fernandes G, Talal N: SLE- like autoantibodies and Sjögren's syndome-like lymphoproliferation in TGF-beta knockout mice. J Immunol 155:3205-3212, 1995

28. Fisher GH, Rosenberg FJ, Straus SE, et al: Dominant interfering Fas gene mutations impair apoptosis in a human autoimmune lymphoproliferative syndrome. Cell 81:935-946, 1995

C. IMMUNOGENETICS

Inherited traits account for a large portion of the variation between individuals in human populations. This phenotypic diversity extends to differences in immune responsiveness and explains, for example, why some individuals respond poorly to immunization against hepatitis B, while others mount a vigorous antibody response (1). The most important genes that determine individual immune response patterns are located within the major histocompatibility complex (MHC) on chromosome 6; they encode the human leukocyte antigens (HLA), often referred to as HLA molecules or MHC antigens. In addition to influencing immune response differences among normal individuals, certain variants of HLA molecules are also associated with susceptibility to a variety of rheumatic diseases.

HLA MOLECULES AND ANTIGEN PRESENTATION

In general, purified T cells are unable to recognize and respond to antigens in their native configuration. Rather, T-cell recognition of foreign antigens requires a complex series of biochemical and cellular interactions that are often summarized by the term *antigen presentation*. The presentation of exogenous soluble antigens to CD4 T cells involves a number of steps: 1) the antigen is endocytized by an antigen-presenting cell (usually a monocyte/macrophage or B cell); 2) the antigen is processed into small peptide fragments by proteolytic cleavage; 3) peptide antigen fragments are loaded onto an HLA class II molecule in an endosomal compartment; 4) the HLA–peptide complex is transported to the cell's surface; and 5) the peptide–HLA complex on the cell surface is recognized by a specific T-cell receptor on the surface of the responding T cell (Fig. 6C-1). The exact geometry of how the T-cell receptor contacts the HLA–peptide complex has not been established. However, it is clear that T-cell recognition is directly influenced by the structure of both the antigenic peptide and the HLA molecule itself. Thus, a different HLA molecule (perhaps present on the antigen-presenting cells of another person) will not successfully present the same peptide antigen to the same T cell. This requirement for a specific HLA molecule is referred to as *MHC-restricted T-cell recognition*. The structural diversity of HLA molecules between different individuals in the population is also the primary means by which the T-cell arm of the immune system distinguishes "self" from "nonself" tissues.

THE STRUCTURE OF HLA MOLECULES

Given the central role of MHC molecules in antigen presentation to T cells, their structure is clearly of great interest. Fig. 6C-2 shows a schematic representation of the two major classes of HLA molecules, class I and class II. Table 6C-1 summarizes their essential structural and functional features. Both class I and class II molecules are cell-surface glycoproteins, anchored to the membrane by hydrophobic transmembrane segments. HLA class I molecules are distributed widely on most somatic cells, with the major exception being red blood cells. In contrast, class II molecules

have a much more restricted tissue distribution; they are generally found only on "professional" antigen-presenting cells, such as monocytes, Macrophages, B cells, and dendritic cells, although HLA class II expression can be induced on other cells by inflammatory cytokines such as gamma interferon. In addition, HLA class I and class II molecules present antigenic peptides to distinct T-cell subsets: HLA class I molecules generally present endogenously derived antigens (such as viral antigens, as well as self antigens) to CD8 T cells, whereas HLA class II molecules are predominantly involved in the presentation of exogenous antigens to CD4 T cells. Consistent with this difference in the source of antigen, the antigen-processing pathways for HLA class I and class II molecules are also different: peptides are loaded onto class I molecules shortly after they are synthesized in the endoplasmic reticulum, whereas peptide loading of class II molecules occurs in an endosomal compartment.

The three-dimensional structure of an HLA class I molecule was determined in 1987 by Bjorkman (2). This observation was arguably the most important event in immunology during the 1980s. The structure is shown in Fig. 6C-3. The most essential feature is the presence of a peptide-binding cleft at the membrane distal end of the molecule. In the case of class I, this cleft will accommodate a peptide of approximately 8–9 amino acids in length. It has been shown

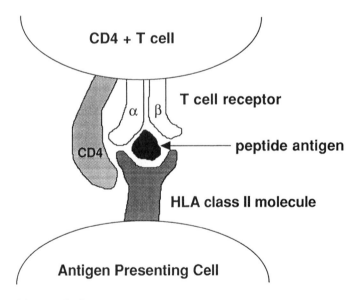

(Figure 6C-1)
Schematic representation of major histocompatibility complex restricted CD4+ T-cell recognition. This recognition event takes place at the cell surface after the antigen has been internalized and "processed" into peptide fragments by the antigen presenting cell (see text). A trimolecular complex of T-cell receptor, peptide antigen, and human leukocyte antigen (HLA) molecule is formed during antigen specific T-cell recognition. The topographic details of this interaction are unknown, but it is probable that the T-cell receptor makes direct contact with both the HLA molecule and its bound peptide antigen. In addition, accessory molecules, such as CD4, make direct contact with the HLA class II molecule. In the case of CD8+ T cells, HLA class I molecules present the bound peptide antigen for T-cell receptor recognition, in an analogous interaction to the one shown here.

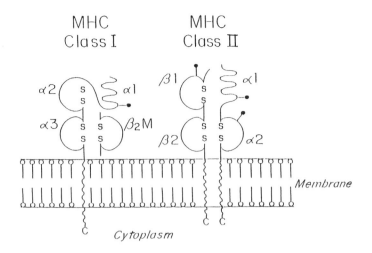

(Figure 6C-2)
A schematic comparison of the structural features of major histocompatibility complex (MHC) class I and class II molecules. MHC class I molecules are anchored in the membrane by a single transmembrane segment contained in the 45 kD α chain. The MHC class I α chain is noncovalently associated with β2 microglobulin (12 kD). There are four external domains, three of which contain intramolecular disulfide bonds, as indicated. In contrast, MHC class II molecules consist of noncovalently associated α (32 kD) and β (28 kD) chains, both of which are anchored within the membrane. The overall domain organization of the two molecules is highly similar, however. Glycosylation sites on both molecules are indicated.

that a wide variety of such peptides can be bound in the cleft of any given HLA molecule, although different HLA molecules may bind somewhat different groups of peptide antigens. Recently, the structure of HLA class II molecules has been shown to be quite similar to that of class I, including the presence of a prominent peptide binding cleft (3). However, class II molecules appear to bind substantially longer antigenic peptides, commonly in the 12–19 amino acid range.

HLA MOLECULES GENE ENCODING

The student of the MHC must inevitably confront the bewildering array of different genes and alleles that are encoded within this gene cluster. (See Table 6C-2 for definitions of the terminology used in this discussion.) A map of the MHC is given in Fig. 6C-4. The first thing to notice is that the HLA class I and class II genes are encoded in separate but adjacent regions. At least six different genes are found in the class I region. Only three of these (HLA-A, -B, and -C) are

(Table 6C-1)
Comparison of the structural and functional features of HLA class I and class II molecules

	HLA Class I	HLA Class II
Structure	44-kD α chain 12-kD β₂ micro- globulin	32-kD α chain 28-kD β chain
Major polymorphic loci	HLA-A, B, C	HLA-DR, DQ, DP
Tissue distribution	All somatic cells except red blood cells and trophoblasts	Antigen-presenting cells, some T cells; inducible on other cell types
Source of antigen	Cytoplasmic, such as endogenous viral antigens	Exogenous soluble protein antigens
Site of peptide loading onto HLA	Endoplasmic reticulum	Endosomes
Size of antigenic peptides	8–9 amino acids	12–19 amino acids
Type of T-cell recognition	CD8 T cells (effector/cytotoxic)	CD4 T cells (helper or effector)

substantially polymorphic in the population, and the HLA-B locus is of most interest for the rheumatic diseases, because it encodes the HLA-B27 alleles. The β₂ microglobulin molecule, which forms part of the HLA class I heterodimer (Fig. 6C-2, Table 6C-1), is not encoded within the MHC, but rather on chromosome 15 (also see Appendix IV).

The HLA class II region lies approximately 1 million base pairs centromeric to class I, and encodes the HLA-DR, -DQ, and -DP molecules. Most rheumatic diseases are associated with allelic variants at one or more of these loci. The situation is further complicated because the gene organization of the class II region differs among different haplotypes. Thus, as shown in the boxed inset, haplotypes that encode DR8 have only one DRB gene (DRB1), whereas other haplotypes may have as many as four DRB loci.

Within the class II region, the HLA-DR and -DQ loci have been the most thoroughly studied; alleles at these loci are generally the most strongly associated with rheumatic diseases. HLA class II molecules are composed of α and β chains (Fig. 6C-2, Table 6C-1), both of which are encoded in the same region (Fig. 6C-4). In the case of HLA-DR, only one α chain gene exists (DRA), and this gene does not vary substantially in structure in different individuals (ie, it is not polymorphic). The invariant DR α chain may pair with one or more DR β chains, depending on the number of DRB genes present on the haplotype. In the DQ subregion are two α and two β chain genes. However, only one pair is expressed (the DQA1 and DQB1 genes), and, therefore, each haplotype encodes only one functional DQ heterodimer.

HLA MOLECULES ARE HIGHLY POLYMORPHIC

The structural complexity of the MHC relates not only to the large number of genes encoded within the complex, but also to the fact that many variants, or alleles, of these genes are found in the human population. Genes with this property are referred to as *polymorphic*. The formal definition of polymorphism is given in Table 6C-2, and generally refers to a situation in which two or more alleles exist in the population, the most common of which does not exceed a frequency of 98%. The HLA genes are the most polymorphic loci known in humans (4). For example, in the case of the HLA-B locus, nearly 100 different alleles have been described, and it is rare for any one of those alleles to exceed a

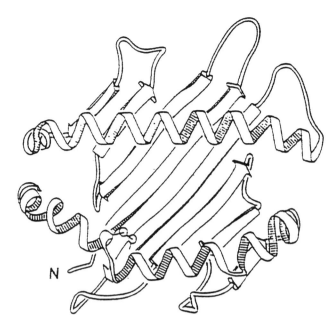

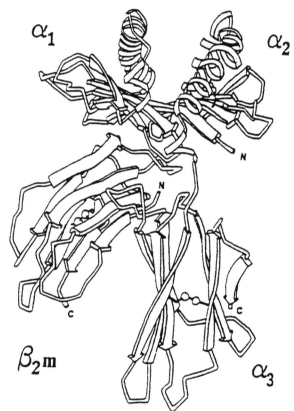

(Figure 6C-3A,B)

Three-dimensional structure of a human leukocyte antigen (HLA) class I molecule, based on the X crystallographic analysis of Bjorkman (2). A side view is shown on top. A peptide binding cleft is formed by the α1 and α2 domains at the top of the molecule. The α3 and β2 microglobulin domains are similar in structure to immunoglobulin domains, and essentially act as a platform on which the peptide binding cleft rests, as well as providing contact sites for the CD8 molecule during CD8+ T-cell recognition. A top view of the empty peptide binding cleft is shown on the bottom. This "T-cell view" of the major histocompatibility complex molecule would normally include a peptide bound within the cleft. Note the disulfide bond that connects the a helix of the α2 domain with the floor of the cleft. Recent studies indicate that the HLA class II molecule has a very similar structure. Reprinted from Bjorkman et al (2) with permission.

(Table 6C-2)
Common genetic terminology

Gene	A segment of DNA containing information required for the production of a polypepetide chain (protein)
Locus	The position on a chromosone where the gene for a trait is located
Allele	One of several alternative forms of a gene at a given locus
Haplotype	A group of linked genes or alleles located close together in a chromosomal region
Genotype	The genetic constitution of an individual; may also refer to the specific alleles at a given locus
Phenotype	A characteristic of an individual produced by the interaction of particular genes (or alleles) with the environment
Polymorphism	Refers to the frequency distribution of alleles in populations; polymorphism exists when there are two or more alleles in the population, and the less frequent allele is found in at least 2% of the population
Homologous	Corresponding or alike in structure or organization
Allotype *	An inherited alternative form of a gene (allele) or protein
Isotype†	Homologous, but non-allelic, forms of genes or proteins; different isotypes are encoded at distinct loci

*Allo (from the Greek **Allos,** "other") = same species, different individual.
† Iso (from Greek **iso,** "equal") = similar.

frequency of 50%, even in an ethnically homogeneous population.

Sequence analysis of many HLA genes has revealed that numerous nucleotide differences may be found when different HLA alleles are compared. An example of this is shown in Fig. 6C-5, where the sequences of several DR4 alleles are compared with each other and with DR10. Note that DR10 (DRB1*1001) differs from the three DR4 alleles by anywhere from 11 to 13 amino acids. In contrast, the DR4 alleles differ from one another by only 1 to 3 amino acids. Nevertheless, even these relatively minor amino acid changes among DR4 alleles can have a major impact on antigen presentation and T-cell recognition, as well as susceptibility to rheumatic disease (5). The reason is because the overwhelming majority of these differences are clustered within the region of the DRB1 gene, which encodes the peptide-binding cleft (Fig. 6C-3). Thus in the course of evolution, there has been a selection for individual variation in a region of the HLA molecule that is directly involved in antigen presentation to T cells. It is presumed that this diversity has been driven by the selective advantage of having several different types of HLA alleles with which to present the diverse array of antigens present in the environment.

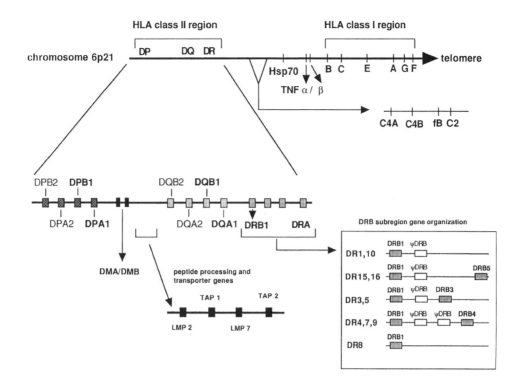

(Figure 6C-4)

Map of the human major histocompatibility complex (MHC). The human leukocyte antigen (HLA) class I and class II molecules are encoded in distinct regions of the MHC, distinguish the DR4 alleles from DR10. In contrast, within the DR4 group, a small number of amino acid differences distinguish these closely related alleles. Nevertheless, these few amino acid changes can lead to functional differences in antigen presentation, and in disease susceptibility (5,7,12).

HLA ASSOCIATION WITH RHEUMATIC DISEASES

Although genes within the MHC are clearly involved in predisposing to the development of many rheumatic diseases, the inheritance of these genes does not give rise to disease in most people. Part of the reason for this may be that several other genes are also required in order to develop the illness. However, even if an individual were to inherit all of the relevant genes, he or she would not develop the disease in most cases. The most direct demonstration comes from studies that found identical (monozygotic) twins are con-

cordant for diseases such as systemic lupus erythematosus and rheumatoid arthritis (RA) only 15%–30% of the time—meaning that when one monozygotic twin has RA, there is still only a 15%–30% chance that the genetically identical co-twin will also get the illness. Thus, the relationship between genetics and autoimmune disease is complex, and, clearly, there are factors other than inheritance that influence disease expression (6). Some of the most common associations are shown in Table 6C-3.

A consideration of HLA–disease association data should include an understanding of the strengths and weaknesses of this approach to genetic analysis. First, since this type of data depends on statistical analysis, false-positive results can and do occur. This can be due to chance or to poor study design, in particular the failure to match disease and control groups for ethnicity or other relevant parameters. Thus, it is important to repeat genetic studies in many different populations before drawing firm conclusions, as has been done for most of the common rheumatic diseases associated with HLA. Second, a positive association between a disease and an HLA allele does not mean that the HLA allele itself is the risk factor. Positive HLA association only indicates that some gene(s) in the HLA region confer(s) risk for disease, because genes within the HLA complex tend to be inherited as a unit and are frequently found together as groups of alleles, even in unrelated individuals. This phenomenon is referred to as *linkage disequilibrium*. As a result, a positive HLA association may simply reflect the involvement of another gene nearby on the haplotype. This gene may or may not be an HLA gene. Other genes in the MHC (such as genes for complement components, tumor necrosis factor, and antigen-processing molecules) could potentially be involved in predisposing to autoimmunity.

```
                 10         20         30         40         50
DRB1*0401   GDTRPRFLEQ VKHECHFFNG TERVRFLDRY FYHQEEYVRF DSDVGEYRAV
DRB1*0402   ---------- ---------- ---------- ---------- ----------
DRB1*0404   ---------- ---------- ---------- ---------- ----------

DRB1*1001   ---------E --F------- -----L-E-R VHN----A-Y ----------

                 60         70         80         90
DRB1*0401   TELGRPDAEY WNSQKDLLEQ KRAAVDTYCR HNYGVGESFT
DRB1*0402   ---------- ------I--D E--------- ----------
DRB1*0404   ---------- ---------- R--------- ----------

DRB1*1001   ---------- ---------R R--------- ----------
```

(Figure 6C-5)

Representative amino acid sequences from DR4 (top three) and DR10 (bottom) alleles. Only the first domains of these proteins are shown. This segment of these proteins is located within the peptide-binding cleft of the intact human leukocyte antigen (HLA) class II molecule. Note that many amino acid differences distinguish the DR4 alleles from DR10. In contrast, within the DR4 group, a small number of amino acid differences distinguish these closely related alleles. Nevertheless, these few amino acid changes can lead to functional differences in antigen presentation and in disease susceptibility (5,7,12).

(Table 6C-3)
Some common HLA associations with rheumatic and autoimmune diseases

Disease	HLA Allele (Serologically Defined)	Approximate Allele Frequency in White Patients	Approximate Allele Frequency in White Controls	Approximate Relative Risk
Ankylosing spondylitis	B27	90%	8%	90
Reiter's syndrome	B27	70%	8%	40
Spondylitis/inflammatory bowel disease	B27	50%	8%	10
Rheumatoid arthritis	DR4	70%	30%	6
Systemic lupus	DR2	45%	20%	3.5
erythematosus	DR3	50%	25%	3
Multiple sclerosis	DR2	60%	20%	4
Juvenile diabetes	DR3	55%	25%	3
	DR4	75%	30%	6

Despite these caveats, it is widely assumed that HLA polymorphisms themselves are directly involved in conferring susceptibility to at least some autoimmune diseases. Perhaps the strongest evidence for this relates to the HLA–B27-associated diseases (8-10). There is also considerable support for a direct role for HLA-DR polymorphisms in RA, although the mechanism is unclear and this point remains controversial (5,7). If HLA molecules are directly involved in causing these and other diseases, it implies that individual differences in the ability to present specific antigens to T cells are important in the pathogenesis of autoimmunity. It further suggests that allelic variants of other molecules involved in antigen recognition, such the T-cell receptor, might also be involved in susceptibility to autoimmune disease. Some experimental evidence supports this idea (11), and it is likely that future genetic studies will uncover other genetic regions that confer risk for the rheumatic diseases.

Because HLA polymorphisms lack specificity as markers of disease risk (many normal individuals carry the disease-associated alleles), HLA typing has not generally been used for clinical diagnostic purposes. However, recent studies indicate that HLA typing may provide probability information on disease outcome. Thus, certain DR4 alleles associated with RA appear to increase the risk of severe disease in white populations (12). It is unclear whether this applies to all populations of RA patients, and it is premature to base clinical decisions on these findings. Nevertheless, in the future it may be possible to use HLA typing, along with other genetic information, to provide therapies tailored to the immunogenetic makeup of each patient.

PETER K. GREGERSEN, MD

1. Egea E, Iglesias A, Salazar M, et al: The cellular basis for lack of antibody responses to Hepatitis B vaccine in humans. J Exp Med 173:531-538, 1991

2. Bjorkman PJ, Saper MA, Samraoui B, Bennett WS, Strominger JL, Wiley DC: Structure of the human class I histocompatibility antigen, HLA-A2. Nature 329:506-512, 1987

3. Stern LJ, Brown JH, Jardetzky TS, Gorga JC, Urban RG, Strominger JL, Wiley DC: Crystal structure of the human class II MHC protein HLA-DR1 complexed with an influenza peptide. Nature 368:215-221, 1994

4. Bodmer JG, Marsh SGE, Albert E, et al: Nomenclature for factors of the HLA system, 1994. Tissue Antigens 44:1-18, 1994

5. Ollier W, Thompson W: Population genetics of rheumatoid arthritis. Rheum Dis Clinics N Am 18:741-759, 1992

6. Gregersen PK: Discordance for autoimmunity in monozygotic twins: are "identical" twins really identical? Arthritis Rheum 36:1185-1192, 1993

7. Gregersen PK: Genetic analysis of the rheumatic diseases. In Kelley WN, Harris ED, Ruddy S, Sledge CB (eds): Textbook of Rheumatology, 5th Ed. Philadelphia, WB Saunders, pp 209-227, 1996

8. Khan MA, Kellner H: Immunogenetics of spondyloarthropathies. Rheum Dis Clinics N Am 18:837-864, 1992

9. Rubin LA, Amos CI, Wade JA, et al: Investigating the genetic basis for ankylosing spondylitis; linkage studies with the major histocompatibility complex region. Arthritis Rheum 37:1212-1220, 1994

10. Taurog JD, Richardson JA, Croft JT, Simmons WA, Zhou M, Fernandez-Sueiro JL, Balish E, Hammer RE: The germfree state prevents development of gut and joint inflammatory disease in HLA-B27 transgenic rats. J Exp Med 180:2359-2364, 1994

11. McDermott M, Kastner DL, Holloman JD, et al: The role of T cell receptor ß-chain genes in susceptibility to rheumatoid arthritis. Arthritis Rheum 38:91-95, 1995

12. Weyand CM, Hicok KC, Conn DL, Goronzy JJ: The influence of HLA-DRB1 genes on disease severity in rheumatoid arthritis. Ann Intern Med 117:869-879, 1992

D. NEUROENDOCRINE INFLUENCES

Increasing experimental evidence demonstrates bidirectional interactions between the neuroendocrine and immune systems. A large number of shared regulatory mediators (steroid hormones, neuropeptides, cytokines) and receptors provide a molecular basis for the communication between these systems. Functional links between neuroendocrine axes and immune/inflammatory processes will be reviewed, with specific focus on mechanisms by which neuroendocrine systems may impact autoimmune disease.

THE HYPOTHALAMIC–PITUITARY–ADRENAL AXIS

The immune system participates in a regulatory feedback loop with the hypothalamic–pituitary–adrenal (HPA) axis (Fig. 6D-1). The HPA axis is activated by a wide variety of physical and psychological stressors, and products of an activated immune system potently increase HPA axis activity (1). Hypothalamic corticotropin-releasing hormone (CRH)

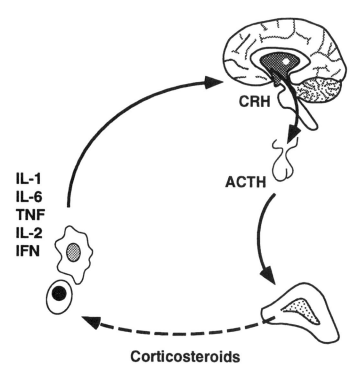

(Figure 6D-1)

The immune–hypothalamic–pituitary–adrenal axis. Activation of the immune system leads to release of cytokines that act to stimulate corticotropin-releasing hormone (CRH) synthesis and release from the paraventricular nucleus of the hypothalamus. CRH stimulates production of adrenocorticotropic hormone (ACTH) by the anterior pituitary, which, in turn, leads to increased corticosteroid production by the adrenal cortex. Corticosteroids are potent inhibitors of many immune and inflammatory processes. This counter-regulatory mechanism prevents excessive or unrestrained amplification of immune and inflammatory processes that themselves may produce injury. IL = interleukin; TNF = tumor necrosis factor; IFN = interferon.

stimulates release of adrenocorticotropic hormone (ACTH) from the anterior pituitary, which results in increased production of cortisol by the adrenal cortex. Corticosteroids are the most potent endogenous inhibitors of immune and inflammatory processes known (2). Because stress-induced elevations of plasma cortisol levels serve to prevent excessive or unrestrained amplification of immune and inflammatory processes that themselves may produce injury, it follows that interruption of this regulatory loop may result in increased susceptibility to, or severity of, autoimmune inflammatory disease.

Cytokine Stimulation

A number of immune and inflammatory mediators stimulate HPA hormone synthesis and secretion. The best characterized of these is interleukin-1 (IL-1), which stimulates secretion of CRH from the hypothalamus (1). IL-1 also stimulates hypothalamic arginine vasopressin (AVP), an adjunctive ACTH secretagogue (1). The precise mechanism by which peripheral IL-1 stimulates the HPA axis via hypothalamic ACTH secretagogues is not understood, but possibilities include IL-1 crossing the blood–brain barrier at relatively permeable sites, alteration of the blood–brain barrier to increase permeability to circulating cytokines during inflammation, or stimulation of a second signal within the central nervous system (3,4). In addition, IL-1 is produced in discrete regions of the central nervous system, including the

hippocampus and hypothalamus, which coordinate the response to stress (4). Finally, IL-1 synergizes with CRH to directly stimulate pituitary production of ACTH (3).

IL-6 is also a potent stimulus for ACTH and cortisol release. Like IL-1, IL-6 is thought to act primarily at the level of CRH and AVP secretion by the hypothalamus (5). After prolonged incubation, however, IL-6 also stimulates release of ACTH by the pituitary and synergizes with ACTH to increase production of cortisol by adrenocortical cells (3). IL-6 is synthesized by adrenal cells themselves after stimulation by IL-1 or ACTH, providing an additional site for regulation of HPA axis hormone production by cytokines (1). Tumor necrosis factor alpha (TNF-α), another of the pro-inflammatory cytokines, acutely stimulates HPA axis activation, while a more delayed HPA-activating potential is manifested by IL-2 and interferon gamma (IFN-γ) (4).

Modulation of Immune and Inflammatory Processes

Corticosteroids inhibit immune and inflammatory responses at multiple levels, including neutrophil and monocyte migration, antigen presentation, lymphocyte proliferation and differentiation, cytokine production by monocytes and certain lymphocyte subtypes, and synthesis of eicosanoids and other lipid mediators (1,2,4). Corticosteroids also appear to regulate thymocyte maturation and differentiation. Thymocytes are more sensitive to the effects of corticosteroids than mature T cells and undergo apoptosis, or programmed cell death, after exposure to corticosteroids. A number of stressors that physiologically increase plasma corticosteroid levels cause thymocyte apoptosis (4). Data are available to support the contention that endogenous corticosteroids are also involved in modulating the activation, expansion, and clonal deletion of peripheral T cells in vivo. Corticosteroids regulate development of T-helper (Th) subtypes, shifting responses from the Th1 to the Th2 type. They also suppress production of Th1 cytokines, IL-2, and IFN-γ, but not Th2 cytokines, such as IL-4. This differential effect on Th1 and Th2 cytokines may be important in the control of immune responses, because Th2 cells antagonize the Th1 subset and may function as suppressor cells in autoimmune disease (1,4).

In addition to the local and systemic effects of corticosteroids on peripheral inflammatory responses, other HPA axis hormones are locally expressed during inflammation. There is evidence for the presence of molecules, such as ACTH, derived from pro-opiomelanocortin in the immune system, which appear to be regulated by immunologic challenge (2,6). The consequences of increased expression of these peptides remain uncertain. In addition, CRH is present in the joints of experimental animals with inflammatory arthritis and patients with rheumatoid arthritis (RA) (7). Though the peripheral effects of CRH are poorly understood, available data suggest that locally expressed CRH may have in vivo immunomodulatory activity (8).

Impaired HPA Axis Activation and Autoimmune Inflammatory Diseases

The concept that impaired neuroendocrine–immune counterregulatory activity might increase susceptibility to, or affect severity of, autoimmune inflammatory diseases is bolstered by observations in experimental animals (Table

(Table 6D-1)

*HPA axis defects in animal models of autoimmune disease**

Strain	Disease Model	HPA Axis Defect
Lewis rat	Rheumatoid arthritis, multiple sclerosis	Blunted CRH to IL-1 and other stressors
NZB/NZW F_1	SLE	Blunted IL-1-stimulated corticosterone
MRL lpr/lpr	SLE	Blunted IL-1 stimulated corticosterone
NOD	Diabetes mellitus	Thymocyte resistance to corticosteroid-induced apoptosis
OS chicken	Hashimoto's thyroiditis	Decreased free corticosterone. Blunted corticosterone response to IL-1
UCD200 chicken	Scleroderma	Adrenal hyporesponsiveness to increased ACTH

*Modified from Wick et al (4) with permission.
HPA = hypothalamic–pituitary–adrenal; IL = interleukin; SLE = systemic lupus erythematosus; ACTH = adrenocorticotropic hormone.

6D-1). Lewis rats are susceptible to a wide range of experimentally induced autoimmune inflammatory diseases that include models for RA and multiple sclerosis. In contrast, Fischer rats are resistant to developing these autoimmune diseases. These rat strains also differ markedly in the severity of the inflammatory response induced by nonspecific irritants. One possible underlying mechanism is that these rat strains display dramatically different HPA axis responses to inflammatory stimuli (1,9,10). Lewis rats exhibit blunted CRH, ACTH, and cortisol secretion in response to many types of stressors, including IL-1, whereas Fischer rats robustly increase these HPA axis hormones. The observations that supplementation with small physiologic doses of corticosteroid profoundly suppresses the severity of inflammation in Lewis rats, and that administration of a glucocorticoid receptor antagonist leads to severe inflammatory disease in Fisher rats, support a critical role for the HPA axis in determining susceptibility to severe disease.

Inbred mouse strains that develop systemic autoimmune disease resembling systemic lupus erythematosus (SLE), including MRL lpr/lpr and NZB/NZW F_1 mice, exhibit blunted IL-1–stimulated corticosterone levels (4). In the nonobese diabetic (NOD) mouse strain, both T and B lymphocytes display extended survival, and thymocytes are relatively resistant to corticosteroid-induced apoptosis (1).

OS chickens are an inbred strain that develop spontaneous autoimmune thyroiditis clinically similar to Hashimoto's thyroiditis. OS chickens have decreased free corticosterone levels due primarily to increased levels of cortisol-binding globulin. They also have blunted corticosterone response to IL-1, similar to the Lewis rat (4). University of California at Davis (UCD) line 200 chickens spontaneously develop systemic inflammatory disease and fibrosis similar to systemic sclerosis. In response to administration of cytokine-containing conditioned media, UCD line 200 chickens display markedly increased ACTH production and normal levels of corticosterone; however, in relation to ACTH levels, these corticosterone levels are relatively blunted, indicating adrenal hyporesponsiveness (4).

The HPA Axis in Human Autoimmune Disease

The discovery of the anti-inflammatory properties of corticosteroids, as well as the dramatic clinical response of patients with RA to administration of corticosteroids, led to the hypothesis that RA develops as a consequence of adrenal insufficiency (11). Evidence, as provided by animal models, has led investigators to re-examine HPA axis function in this disease. RA patients, stratified on the basis of erythrocyte sedimentation rate (ESR), display positive linear correlation between ESR and mean serum cortisol levels. However, patients with mild disease had lower than normal cortisol output, suggesting insufficient adrenal cortisol secretion in this group of patients (1). Since there are inherent difficulties in evaluating the appropriateness of a given level of cortisol for a particular level of ongoing inflammation, RA patients were compared with patients who had osteomyelitis and similarly elevated ESR (12). The patients with RA displayed significantly lower circadian cortisol secretion than those with osteomyelitis, suggesting blunted HPA axis responses for a given level of inflammation. Major surgical stress increased cortisol levels in patients with osteomyelitis and osteoarthritis, but not in those with RA (12). RA patients treated with low-dose corticosteroids demonstrate elevated rather than depressed ACTH levels, suggesting ongoing drive for cortisol production and relative adrenal hyporesponsiveness to ACTH. Evidence of cortisol resistance in peripheral tissues and decreased numbers of glucocorticoid receptors on peripheral mononuclear cells have also been noted in some RA patients (1).

PROLACTIN AND GROWTH HORMONE

Prolactin and growth hormone (GH) are immunostimulatory pituitary hormones (Table 6D-2). Although hypophysectomy leads to profound immunodeficiency and thymic hypoplasia, this can be reversed by prolactin or GH, but not other pituitary hormones. Most data suggest that GH promotes thymocyte proliferation, while prolactin promotes proliferation and differentiation of antigen-specific T cells (13). Bromocriptine, a drug that inhibits pituitary release of prolactin, selectively reduces lymphocyte reactivity in rats. Prolactin stimulates the expression of IL-2 receptors and enhances the IL-2-induced proliferative response of T lymphocytes (13). Both GH and prolactin have cell-surface receptors structurally homologous to the receptor for IL-6 and other cytokines, and these hormone receptors are present on lymphocytes (13,14).

(Table 6D-2)

Selected neuroendocrine hormones and peptides with immunomodulatory effects

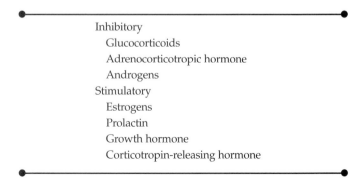

Inhibitory
    Glucocorticoids
    Adrenocorticotropic hormone
    Androgens
Stimulatory
    Estrogens
    Prolactin
    Growth hormone
    Corticotropin-releasing hormone

It has been suggested that expression of autoimmune disease may be modulated by prolactin levels. For example, elevated prolactin levels were found in some patients with SLE and other autoimmune diseases (14). In addition, bromocriptine was shown to ameliorate some types of experimental autoimmune diseases in animals (15).

THE HYPOTHALAMIC—PITUITARY—GONADAL (HPG) AXIS

There is a striking female preponderance of many autoimmune diseases characterized by activation of humoral immunity. Estrogens appear to play an important role in the pathogenesis of SLE, as demonstrated by the observations that disease may begin at the time of menarche, some patients experience exacerbations of symptoms during specific phases of the menstrual cycle or with pregnancy, oral contraceptives or estrogen replacement therapy may exacerbate SLE (although available data to support this view are incomplete), and patients may have disease remission at menopause (1,16,17). Both males and females with SLE have abnormal sex steroid hormone metabolism (1,17). For example, an increase in the activity of the aromatase enzyme, which converts precursor androgens to estrogens, has been reported in SLE patients (1). Klinefelter's syndrome, a condition associated with the XXY genotype and abnormal sexual development, has also been associated with SLE (16).

As in SLE, there is a female preponderance for the development of RA; however, estrogens appear to suppress disease activity (1). For example, oral contraceptives may be protective in RA, patients may experience remission during pregnancy, and there is an increasing incidence with age as estrogen levels fall (18,19). Androgen levels may be important in the pathogenesis of RA since studies have demonstrated low testosterone levels in males with RA and depressed adrenal androgen levels, particularly in premenopausal women (19). These clinical observations support the concept that sex steroids play an important role in expression of autoimmune diseases. However, effects may be variable depending on specific immune mechanisms of disease (18,20).

Sex Steroid Influences on the Immune Response

Underlying the sexual dimorphism in expression of autoimmune diseases, there are clear differences between males and females in immunologic responses (20,21). Estrogens may indirectly influence immune responses through their ability to stimulate prolactin; however, direct sex steroid effects are clearly operative (1). Estrogen receptors are present in lymphoid and thymic tissue, and androgen receptors are present in thymic epithelial cells. Both estrogen and testosterone appear to alter thymocyte development, since castration leads to thymic enlargement, and estrogen and testosterone decrease thymic mass (1). Estrogen stimulates hyperreactivity in humoral immune responses, while testosterone appears to depress humoral immunity (20). For example, females display increased immunoglobulin concentrations and stronger primary and secondary antibody responses to certain infectious agents. Treatment of castrated males with estrogens reproduces hyperactive humoral immune responses. The effects of sex steroid hormones on cellular immune processes are less clear, but it appears that cell-mediated immune responses are more active in females except during pregnancy (21). The effects of female sex on cellular immunity may be independent of sex steroids because estrogens appear to suppress at least some T–cell–dependent immune responses (18).

Sex Steroids in Animal Models of Autoimmune Disease

The role of sex steroids has been intensively investigated in the NZB/NZW F₁ mice, a model for SLE. In these mice, renal disease and autoantibody production progress more rapidly in females. Castration or androgen therapy decreases disease activity in females, while castration or estrogen therapy increases disease activity in males (1,20). Of interest, recent data using the autoimmune-prone MRL +/+ mice demonstrate that estrogens selectively enhance B-cell–mediated humoral immune responses, such as immunoglobulin levels, autoantibody production, and immune-complex glomerulonephritis, while T-cell–mediated immune responses are diminished by estrogens (1).

Animal models of RA demonstrate differences in sexual dimorphism depending on the species and model. Female Lewis rats are more susceptible to streptococcal cell wall arthritis, castration of male Lewis rats leads to female-like disease, and high doses of estrogen increase incidence and severity of disease (20). Female rats are also more susceptible to collagen-induced arthritis, but in mice, collagen-induced arthritis is more severe in males (18,21). In another demonstration of differential effects of estrogen on humoral versus cell-mediated immunity, estrogen treatment suppresses anti-type II collagen T-cell immune responses although stimulating the humoral immune response in collagen-induced arthritis in mice (18). Similar to RA, disease remission occurs during pregnancy in mice with collagen-induced arthritis, although postpartum exacerbation has been described (20).

DEHYDROEPIANDROSTERONE

The adrenal androgens dehydroepiandrosterone (DHEA) and DHEA sulfate (DHEAS) are synthesized under the control of ACTH and other ill-defined factors. The circulating form is the inactive DHEAS. The presence of DHEA sulfatase in lymphoid tissues allows release of the active steroid hormone (1). Levels of DHEAS vary greatly over life cycles and decline with age, which stands in sharp contrast to relatively stable cortisol levels (19). Levels of DHEAS are lower in RA patients than controls, with the difference being greatest in premenopausal women (19), and levels are inversely correlated with disease severity (1). In addition, it has been shown that premenopausal women have decreased serum DHEAS levels prior to the development of RA, suggesting low adrenal androgens as a potential risk factor for RA (19).

LESLIE J. CROFFORD, MD

1. Wilder RL: Neuroendocrine-immune system interactions and autoimmunity. Annu Rev Immunol 13:307-338, 1995

2. Bateman A, Singh A, Kral T, Solomon S: The immune-hypothalamic-pituitary-adrenal axis. Endocrine Rev 10:92-112, 1989

3. Busbridge NJ, Grossman AB: Stress and the single cytokine: interleukin modulation of the pituitary-adrenal axis. Mol Cell Endocrinol 82:209-214, 1991

4. Wick G, Hu Y, Schwarz S, Kroemer G: Immunoendocrine communication via the hypothalamic-pituitary-adrenal axis in autoimmune diseases. Endocrine Rev 14:539-563, 1993

5. Mastorakos G, Weber JS, Magiakou M-A, Gunn H, Chrousos GP: Hypothalamic-pituitary-adrenal axis activation and stimulation of systemic

vasopressin secretion by recombinant interleukin-6 in humans: potential implications for the syndrome of inappropriate vasopressin secretion. J Clin Endocrinol Metab 79:934-939, 1994

6. Blalock JE: A molecular basis for bidirectional communication between the immune and neuroendocrine systems. Physiological Rev 69:1-32, 1989

7. Crofford LJ, Sano H, Karalis K, et al: Corticotropin-releasing hormone in synovial fluids and tissues of patients with rheumatoid arthritis and osteoarthritis. J Immunol 151:1587-1596, 1993

8. Karalis K, Sano H, Redwine J, Listwak S, Wilder RL, Chrousos GP: Autocrine or paracrine inflammatory actions of corticotropin-releasing hormone in vivo. Science 254:421-423, 1991

9. Sternberg EM, Hill JM, Chrousos GP, Kamilaris T, Listwak SJ, Gold PW, Wilder RL: Inflammatory mediator-induced hypothalamic-pituitary-adrenal axis activation is defective in streptococcal cell wall arthritis-susceptible Lewis rats. Proc Natl Acad Sci USA 86:2374-2378, 1989

10. Sternberg EM, Young WS III, Bernardini R, Calogero AE, Chrousos GP, Gold PW, Wilder RL: A central nervous system defect in biosynthesis of corticotropin-releasing hormone is associated with susceptibility to streptococcal cell wall-induced arthritis in Lewis rats. Proc Natl Acad Sci USA 86:4771-4775, 1989

11. Hench PS, Kendall EC, Slocumb LH, Polley HF: The effect of a hormone of the adrenal cortex (17-hydroxy-11-dehydrocorticosterone: compound E) and of pituitary adrenocorticotropic hormone on rheumatoid arthritis. Proc Mayo Clin 24:181-197, 1949

12. Chikanza IC, Petrou P, Kingsley G, Chrousos G, Panayi GS: Defective hypothalamic response to immune and inflammatory stimuli in patients with rheumatoid arthritis. Arthritis Rheum 35:1281-1288, 1992

13. Goetzl EJ, Sreedharan SP: Mediators of communication and adaptation in the neuroendocrine and immune systems. FASEB J 6:2646-2652, 1992

14. Berczi I: Prolactin, pregnancy and autoimmune disease. J Rheumatology 20:1095-1100, 1993

15. Reichlin S: Neuroendocrine-immune interactions. N Engl J Med 329:1246-1253, 1992

16. Lahita RG: The importance of estrogens in systemic lupus erythematosus. Clin Immunol Immunopathol 63:17-18, 1992

17. Homo-Delarche F, Fitzpatrick F, Christeff N, Nunez EA, Back JF, Dardenne M: Sex steroids, glucocorticoids, stress, and autoimmunity. J Steroid Biochem Molec Biol 40:619-637, 1991

18. Holmdahl R: Estrogen exaggerates lupus but suppresses T-cell-dependent autoimmune disease. J Autoimmunity 2:651-656, 1989

19. Masi AT, Feigenbaum SL, Chatterton RT: Hormonal and pregnancy relationships to rheumatoid arthritis: convergent effects with immunologic and microvascular systems. Semin Arthritis Rheum 25:1-27, 1995

20. Schuurs AHWM, Verheul HAM: Effects of gender and sex steroids on the immune response. J Steroid Biochem 35:157-172, 1990

21. Grossman CJ, Roselle GA, Mendenhall CL: Sex steroid regulation of autoimmunity. J Steroid Biochem Molec Biol 40:649-659, 1991

E. AUTOIMMUNITY: SELF VERSUS NONSELF

The fundamental function of the immune system is to protect the individual from infectious organisms (nonself or foreign antigens). Lymphocytes play a key role in this process and are equipped with unique receptors to monitor the antigens to which the individual is exposed. The antigen receptors are transmembrane proteins composed of variable and constant regions located on the cell surface and a small intracellular domain that is necessary for facilitating intracellular signal transduction. To be able to recognize the universe of foreign antigens, T- and B-lymphocyte antigen receptors (TCR and BCR, respectively) are randomly generated. The consequence of this strategy is that lymphocytes with reactivity against self-antigens are also produced and, to allow the host to survive, must be eliminated or held in check.

The concept of immunologic tolerance was evoked to explain the failure of cells of the immune system to react against self-antigens. Although tolerance is usually described in terms of the self–nonself dichotomy, lymphocytes cannot distinguish self from nonself. Rather, the immune system has evolved numerous strategies to ensure that an immune response against self-antigens does not occur. These mechanisms can be broadly classified as central and peripheral tolerance.

CENTRAL TOLERANCE

Billions of lymphocyte progenitor cells are produced by the bone marrow daily. Many of these cells are eliminated due to faulty rearrangement of their antigen receptor genes. For those cells that undergo productive rearrangement of their antigen receptors, the receptor is forced to engage the environment as a test for self-reactivity. Cells that bind to antigen with high affinity at this stage of maturation are deleted by a programmed cell death pathway called *apoptosis*. Many of the principles that control tolerance of immature cells are similar between T and B cells, but there are also some important differences.

T Cells

T-cell maturation in the thymus, which is reviewed in Robey and Fowlkes (1), is conveniently monitored by the display of the coreceptors CD4 and CD8 as well as the TCR and signalling complex, CD3. Pre-T cells entering the cortex of the thymus initially do not express any of these phenotypic markers. As they mature, they express both CD4 and CD8 ("double positive") together with the TCR/CD3 complex and enter the corticomedullary junction. Through the random nature of TCR generation, some of the T cells will engage antigens (either MHC alone or MHC containing a peptide) and some will not. T cells that do not receive any signals through their T-cell receptor die. Those T cells that engage antigen with high affinity are deleted (negative selection). T cells that engage antigen with low affinity are positively selected and mature into either CD4 or CD8 ("single positive") T cells in the thymic medulla. These cells then seed into the periphery to perform their protective function. Kinetic studies in animals suggest that only about 5% of all thymocytes survive the selection process and mature into single-positive T cells.

B Cells

In humans, B cells develop entirely in the bone marrow. The stages of B cell ontogeny—from pro- to pre- to early B to mature B cell—are also marked by phenotypic changes, the most important of which is expression of the BCR for antigen on the cell surface at the early B cell stage of development. Analogous to T-cell ontogeny, large numbers of cells die through faulty rearrangement of receptors in the pro- to pre-B-cell transition.

In early B cells, the BCR is a surface form of IgM (sIgM). As in the case of cortical thymocytes that express TCR, high-affinity interaction with antigen leads to cell death (2). But unlike the TCR, the BCR binds to epitopes on soluble antigens and does not require presentation by MHC molecules. Since IgM is pentavalent, antigens that most efficiently cross-link sIgM (eg, cell-membrane antigens) are usually those that are highly efficient at negative selection. There is no compelling evidence for positive selection of B cells; experiments with transgenic mice suggest B cells that bind to antigen with low affinity or encounter oligovalent antigens that are unable to cross-link sIgM become anergized (3). Anergy refers to functional inactivation of the lymphocyte so that re-exposure of the cell to the antigen in the periphery will result in a failure to produce antibodies. Fully mature B cells express surface IgD as well as IgM through alternative splicing of the pre-mRNA for IgM. Each B cell therefore expresses sIgM and sIgD with the same immunoglobulin variable region but with different constant regions.

Immature lymphoid cells in the central lymphoid organs cannot distinguish self from foreign antigens, as evidenced by the ready ability of animals to be rendered tolerant to foreign antigens by systemic immunization during the neonatal period. Since almost all antigens encountered in the thymus or bone marrow in neonates would be expected to be derived from self-antigens, autoreactive cells that bind to these antigens with high affinity are efficiently deleted or inactivated.

PERIPHERAL TOLERANCE

Lymphocytes in the thymus and the bone marrow are exposed to antigens derived from fixed and circulating cells, as well as from serum components. Tolerance to these self-components are therefore readily induced by the mechanisms described above. However, a number of antigens that are expressed at specialized sites in the body are unlikely to be present in the thymus or bone marrow. Also, "new antigens" are expressed during puberty. The immune system has therefore devised a number of strategies to deal with potentially autoreactive lymphocytes in the periphery.

The Context of Antigen Presentation

Mature T cells require two signals for full activation, one through the antigen receptor and a second through a co-stimulatory pathway (4). The most important co-stimulatory molecules identified so far are CD28 and CTLA-4 on the T cell and their counter-receptor, B7, which is predominantly expressed on activated B cells and macrophages (antigen-presenting cells, or APC). Self-antigens are continuously presented by class I (all nucleated cells) and class II MHC molecules (on specialized APC such as macrophages, B lymphocytes, and dendritic cells) in most organs throughout the body. The requirement for two signals provides a checkpoint to avoid T-cell response to antigen in a noninflammatory setting. Significantly, signalling through the TCR alone is tolerogenic, resulting in anergy of the T cell (Fig. 6E-1A). A more detailed discussion of co-stimulation as it relates to tolerance is presented elsewhere (5).

The immune system has evolved innate responses to bacterial and other pathogens that serve as the second signal. For example, bacterial lipopolysaccharide (LPS) induces profound B-cell and macrophage activation resulting in up-regulation of the key co-stimulatory molecule, B7. This, in turn, activates CD28 resulting in full T-cell activation (Fig. 6E-1B). Since bacterial products are exposed to B and T cells in this inflammatory setting, a powerful immune response is generated to the bacterial antigens. The release of certain cytokines such as interferon gamma also enhances B7 expression and promotes a T-cell response. Some bacterial products such as superantigens are able to induce striking T-cell activation without a need for co-stimulatory molecules.

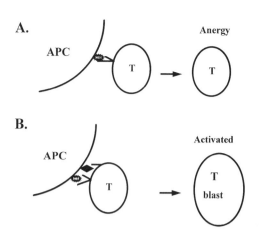

(Figure 6E-1)

The role of co-stimulatory molecules in T cell tolerance or activation. A: If mature T cells engage antigen presented by a B cell, macrophage, or dendritic cell (APC) in the absence of a co-stimulatory molecule, the T cells become anergic. This situation would be most common for the presentation of self-antigens. B: When mature T cells encounter antigen as well as a second signal (B7 on the APC binds CD 28 on the T cell), the T cell becomes fully activated. This situation occurs during infections where bacterial products or the release of cytokines up-regulate B7.

Activation-Induced Cell Death

During the inflammatory response, activated T cells secrete potent pro-inflammatory cytokines and are armed with cytotoxic molecules. They are therefore not only dangerous to pathogens but are also life-threatening to the host, as evidenced by the effects of cytokines released in toxic shock syndrome. To limit the opportunity for lymphocyte reactivity to host antigens, activated cells are deleted by a phenomenon called activation-induced cell death (AICD) (see reference 6 for review). Many of the pathways responsible for AICD have recently been elucidated and involve Fas (APO-1/CD95) and tumor necrosis factor (TNF), both members of the nerve growth factor (NGF) receptor family.

The Fas receptor (FasR) is expressed at low levels on resting T and B lymphocytes (7) and on macrophages (8). When these cells are activated by antigens or cytokines, FasR expression is up-regulated and the FasR signal transduction pathway is facilitated. The Fas ligand (FasL) is expressed predominantly on activated CD4 T helper (Th) Th1 and CD8 T cells. These T-cell subsets are therefore major regulators of AICD through this pathway. FasL-bearing cells are able to induce apoptosis of other activated T cells, B cells, and macrophages (Fig. 6E-2). The Fas pathway is therefore largely responsible for terminating the immune response. The importance of this pathway in eliminating activated lymphocytes is illustrated by the development of systemic autoimmunity similar to systemic lupus erythematosus (SLE) in mice with mutations in the FasR or FasL (7). The receptors for TNF-α are ubiquitously expressed, but TNF-α appears to induce apoptosis predominantly of activated CD8 T cells.

Unlike T cells, activated B cells are subjected to a third round of selection in germinal centers located within the spleen and lymph nodes (9). Here, B cells that have been triggered by antigen undergo somatic hypermutation and are either positively selected (high-affinity clones) or die by apoptosis (low-affinity clones). Since mutations are ran-

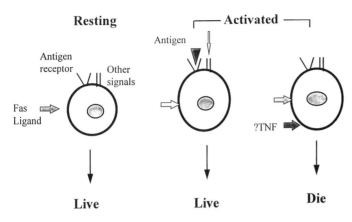

(Figure 6E-2)

*The role of Fas in activation-induced cell death (AICD). Resting lymphocytes **(left panel)** are not susceptible to Fas-mediated apoptosis. Once activated, the Fas signal transduction pathway becomes functional. If, however, the antigen receptor is occupied, the cell is protected from Fas-mediated apoptosis **(center panel).** This mechanism allows the elimination of bystander activated lymphocytes **(right panel)** but also permits clonal expansion of antigen-specific cells. Removal of activated lymphocytes and APC is necessary to avoid autoimmunity.*

domly generated in the variable regions of the immunoglobulin heavy and light chains, it is likely that autoreactive cells are also generated by this mechanism. It is not yet certain how autoreactive B cells are eliminated in this microenvironment.

Apoptosis

Apoptosis is of particular relevance to immunology (10) because tolerance induction (negative selection) of self-reactive T cells in the thymus and B cells in the bone marrow occurs by apoptosis. As in the case of cells dying during embryogenesis, naive mature lymphocytes probably die by a programmed pathway unless they are recruited into the immune response. As discussed above, during the process of AICD, lymphocyte death is also induced by apoptosis by cell-surface ligands such as FasL and TNF. It is important to note that cytotoxic T cells, natural killer (NK) cells, and antibody-dependent cytotoxic cells (ADCC) are, themselves, inducers of apoptosis in their corresponding targets (11). Apoptosis (12) is the form of cell death seen during normal physiologic processes such as embryogenesis and metamorphosis, as well as in certain pathologic conditions such as cancer. The term apoptosis was first applied to the morphologic appearance of these cells as depicted by electron microscopy. In contrast to necrotic cells, apoptotic cells are shrunken, have condensed nuclei, and undergo dissolution by blebbing. The resulting apoptotic bodies are phagocytosed by surrounding cells and rapidly degraded in lysozymes.

An important difference between programmed (apoptotic) versus accidental or toxic (necrotic) death is that programmed cell death results in the ordered fragmentation of the cell. Because apoptosis occurs through complex biochemical pathways, the apoptotic process is usually slow (6–48 hours). Phagocytosis of apoptotic bodies by neighboring cells or professional phagocytes does not activate the engulfing cell and therefore an inflammatory response does not ensue. Although cell death by apoptosis takes hours, removal of apoptotic fragments is so rapid that apoptotic cells

are rarely seen—even in tissues such as the thymus where up to 95% of cells undergo apoptosis.

The mechanisms whereby apoptotic cells are efficiently identified, removed, and degraded are not well understood. Initial studies suggested that a lectin–sugar interaction may be responsible for the clearance of apoptotic thymocytes. More recently, a number of receptors and potential ligands involved in the clearance of apoptotic fragments have been reported (13).

Although the morphologic descriptions of apoptosis were reported more than 30 years ago, the complex biochemical pathways responsible for its regulation have only recently been appreciated. Fas-mediated apoptosis is illustrated in Fig. 6E-3. Cells are first primed by signalling through their antigen, cytokine, or other receptors (stage 1). Cells contact FasL (stage 2), which induces trimerization of the receptor (stage 3). Trimerization of the receptor, in turn, facilitates binding of several Fas signal-transduction proteins, particularly to the death domain (stage 4). A key event is activation of the interleukin-1β-converting enzyme (ICE) family of proteases (now called caspases) (stage 5), which act on nuclear lamins, cytoskeletal structures, and other targets. Numerous changes occur in the cell membrane, including translocation of phosphatidyl serine to the outer layer of the membrane following activation of a lipid scramblase (stage 6). A number of other biochemical events ensue, including

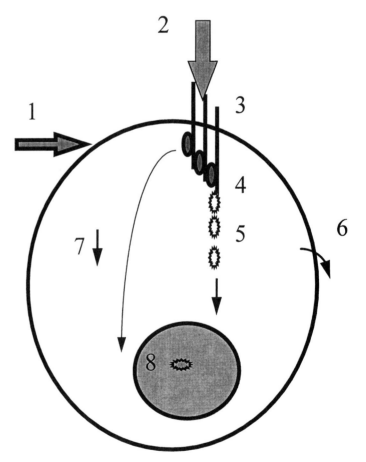

(Figure 6E-3)

The biochemistry of apoptosis. In this example, a lymphocyte is primed (step 1) by engagement of its antigen receptor and/or cytokines. Following exposure to Fas ligand (stage 2), it is induced to undergo apoptosis by ligation of the Fas receptor (stage 3). See text for further details.

sphingomyelinase, protein kinase, and phosphatase activation (stage 7). Within the nucleus, DNase(s) cleave chromatin at the H1 linker region (stage 8), releasing nucleosomes. Although steps 5-8 are shown in Fig. 6E-3 as consecutive, many occur simultaneously.

Several other intracellular proteins regulate apoptosis under certain conditions. The most important proteins identified so far are the *Bcl-2* family, which protects cells from many different inducers of apoptosis. A number of *Bcl-2* family members (see reference 14) have been identified, as well as proteins such as c-myc and p53, which regulate apoptosis under certain conditions. A more detailed discussion is presented elsewhere (15).

AUTOIMMUNITY

Given the sophisticated and overlapping mechanisms to avoid autoimmunity, the primary mechanisms responsible for autoimmune diseases are unclear. While the etiology and pathogenesis of a human systemic autoimmune disease are yet to be resolved, a number of important clues are available from both human and mouse studies.

Autoimmunity by Immunization

In several mouse models of autoimmunity, tolerance can be overcome by immunization with antigen (eg, myelin basic protein in the case of experimental allergic encephalomyelitis and collagen in the case of collagen-induced arthritis) in the presence of an adjuvant. These models illustrate a number of important points: 1) Potentially autoreactive T cells exist in normal subjects. Several scenarios could explain how immunization with a foreign antigen leads to autoimmunity. The immunogen may share sequence similarity with self-antigen (this is obviously the case when mice are immunized with chick collagen and develop autoimmunity against mouse collagen). In this case the immune response is at first focused on the immunogen but then cross-reacts with self-antigen (molecular mimicry). 2) While loss of tolerance is often initiated with foreign antigen, many of these diseases can be induced with self-antigen in the presence of a powerful adjuvant. The adjuvant markedly facilitates the immune response by inducing cytokines and, of particular relevance to the discussion above, by up-regulation of co-stimulatory molecules. Self-antigens are also likely to be presented in this pro-inflammatory context. 3) Autoimmunity is strain dependant, suggesting either that peptide binding to MHC dictates susceptibility to disease or that T-cell autoreactivity might be explained by failure of peptide-specific T cells to be tolerized.

Infection and Initiation of Autoimmunity

Certain diseases considered autoimmune in nature (eg, reactive arthritis) are unequivocally initiated by exposure to bacteria such as *Salmonella*, *Shigella*, and *Yersinia*. Although the mechanisms of inflammation are unclear, the very strong association between HLA-B27 and these diseases suggests the possibility that bacterial peptide antigens presented by MHC class I molecules induce immune responses that cross-react between host and bacterial products. In the setting of co-stimulation, a powerful immune response ensues. This may be another example of molecular mimicry.

Apart from serving as targets of the immune response, infectious organisms can manipulate the immune response in numerous ways. Different viruses have been shown to induce polyclonal B-cell activation, interfere with the complement cascade, modify cytokine expression and receptor function, and inhibit class I expression. A number of viruses subvert the regulation of cell survival and death. Mammalian DNA viruses synthesize proteins including a *Bcl-2* homolog, BHRF (Epstein-Barr virus), and the E1B 19-kD protein (adenovirus) that inhibit cell death. Disruption of apoptotic pathways may predispose to autoimmunity.

Cryptic Epitopes

During central tolerance, T lymphocytes that react with high affinity to peptide antigens are deleted. In most situations, only a very limited number of peptides derived from each protein are presented to T cells. In fact, usually one peptide is "dominant." This dominance is explained by the highly ordered degradation, transport, and binding of peptides to MHC molecules. This being the case, tolerance will only be induced by the dominant, and perhaps subdominant, epitopes. Several studies have suggested that tolerance to a protein antigen may be broken if a new "cryptic" peptide is presented to peripheral T cells (16). Presentation of this cryptic peptide may occur through a variety of mechanisms; for example, binding of antibody or a foreign protein may cause altered processing or intracellular transport of the protein. If this occurs in an inflammatory setting (ie, in the presence of co-stimulatory molecules), a vigorous immune response to self-antigens could occur.

Defined Mutations Predisposing to Autoimmunity

Loss of function mutations of the early complement components (particularly C1q, C2, and C4) predispose to SLE. Although the precise relationship is not understood, loss of complement may either predispose the patient to infections or lead to defective clearance of antigen–antibody complexes. In the case of C1q deficiencies, it appears that no other defects are required since almost all individuals with mutations develop SLE (17).

Three independent autosomal recessive mutations of the Fas receptor or its ligand have arisen in three different mouse strains (7). All of these mice develop massive lymphadenopathy and lupus-like autoimmunity. It is of interest to note the highly variable expression of lupus in terms of severity of disease, organ involvement, and autoantibody production in these strains as well as other normal strains onto which the *lpr* gene mutation has been crossed (18). This variability stresses the importance of background genes in the expression of mutations affecting the same receptor–ligand pair. These findings demonstrate that mutations in apoptosis-inducing molecules or overexpression of molecules that promote lymphocyte survival may result in a lupus-like syndrome.

Autoimmunity could occur in several ways. In the case of Fas pathway mutations, autoimmunity could arise when potentially autoreactive cells emerging from the thymus are activated by self-antigens but fail to be deleted. In either Fas pathway mutations or *Bcl-2* overexpression, cells stimulated by foreign antigen have an increased opportunity to cross-react with self-antigens in the periphery. This event is a significant problem for B cells, which have the opportunity to mutate their antigen receptor toward higher affinity binding for self-antigens in germinal centers. Although Fas mutations have been reported in a small number of humans, Fas expression and function appears to be normal in most patients with SLE (19).

KEITH B. ELKON, MD

1. Robey E, Fowlkes BJ: Selective events in T cell development. Annu Rev Immunol 12:675-705, 1994

2. Nossal GJV: Negative selection of lymphocytes. Cell 76:229, 1994

3. Goodnow CC: Transgenic mice and analysis of B cell tolerance. Ann Rev Immunol 10:489-518, 1992

4. Clark EA, Ledbetter JA: How B and T cells talk to each other. Nature 367:425-428, 1994

5. Matzinger P: Tolerance, danger, and the extended family. Ann Rev Immunol 12:991-1045, 1994

6. Green DR, Scott DW: Activation-induced apoptosis in lymphocytes. Curr Opin Immunol 6:476-487, 1994

7. Nagata S, Golstein P: The Fas death factor. Science 267:1449-1456, 1995

8. Ashany D, Song X, Lacy E, Nikolic-Zugic J, Friedman SM, Elkon KB: Lymphocytes delete activated macrophages through the Fas/APO-1 pathway. Proc Natl Acad Sci USA 92:11225-11229, 1995

9. MacLennan JCM, Liu Y-J, Johnson JD: Maturation and dispersal of B cell clones during T cell-dependent antibody responses. Immunol Rev 126:143-161, 1992

10. Cohen JJ, Duke RC, Fadok VA, Sellins K: Apoptosis and programmed cell death in immunity. Ann Rev Immunol 10:267-293, 1992

11. Henkart PA: Lymphocyte-mediated cytotoxicity: Two pathways and multiple effector molecules. Immunity 1:343-346, 1994

12. Duvall E, Wyllie AH: Death and the cell. Immunol Today 7:115, 1986

13. Savill J, Fadok V, Henson P, Haslett C: Phagocyte recognition of cells undergoing apoptosis. Immunol Today 14:131-136, 1993

14. Oltvai ZN, Korsmeyer SJ: Checkpoints of dueling dimers foil death wishes. Cell 79:189-192, 1994

15. Elkon KB: Apoptosis. In Wallace DJ, Hahn BH (eds): Dubois' Lupus Erythematosus, 5th ed. Baltimore, Williams & Wilkins, 1997, pp133-142

16. Lehmann PV, Forsthuber T, Miller A, Sercarz EE: Spreading of T cell autoimmunity to cryptic determinants of an autoantigen. Nature 358:155-157, 1992

17. Bowness P, Davies KA, Norsworthy PJ, Athanassiou P, Taylor-Weideman J, Borysiewicz LK, Meyer PAR, Walport MJ: Hereditary C1q deficiency and systemic lupus erythematosus. Quart J Med 87:455-464, 1994

18. Cohen PL, Eisenberg RA: lpr and gld: single gene models of systemic autoimmunity and lymphoproliferative disease. Annu Rev Immunol 9:243-269, 1991

19. Mysler E, Bini P, Drappa J, Ramos P, Friedman SM, Krammer PH, Elkon KB: The APO-a/Fas protein in human systemic lupus erythematosus. J Clin Invest 93:1029-1034, 1994

EVALUATION OF THE PATIENT
A. HISTORY AND PHYSICAL EXAMINATION

The practitioner attempting to diagnosis a patient who may have a rheumatic disease must depend upon the information gathered from four sources: medical history, physical examination, medical knowledge base, and diagnostic tests (1–4). Arguably, the medical history is the most important of these four. Indeed, most experienced clinicians can arrive at the correct diagnosis, or at least substantially narrow the possibilities, with several well-phrased questions. The physical examination clarifies the patient's complaint and provides clues about asymptomatic disease manifestations. The greater the knowledge base of the clinician, the more efficient he or she may be in integrating data acquired from other facets of the medical evaluation. Laboratory and radiographic tests help confirm or exclude possible diagnoses, but rarely do they supersede the clinical evaluation.

MEDICAL HISTORY

Several aspects of the medical history are important in all patients and may best be obtained in the initial phases of the interview.

Chief Complaint

Patients should be asked to describe the complaint that prompted them to seek medical care. They should be encouraged to describe the problems in their own words and avoid medical jargon or second-hand discussions of diagnostic tests. If the patient has been referred, the clinician should ascertain the primary question the referring physician wants answered.

Chronology of Illness

Because most rheumatic diseases have characteristic natural histories, patients should be questioned closely about how the problem developed. The most important chronologic question is, "How long have you had this problem?" The answer defines the problem as either acute or chronic, thus eliminating many diagnoses from consideration. Has the problem remitted and then recurred? Have additional areas become symptomatic over time? It is also important to know whether the intensity of symptoms is stable, improving, or worsening over time. For example, gout can be strongly suspected because of its unique chronology. Patients frequently will have had an intensely painful monarticular or oligoarticular arthritis lasting for several days or weeks, which then completely remits with prolonged symptom-free intervals, only to recur.

Demographic Considerations

The patient's age at onset of symptoms is obviously important since some conditions are more common in older people than younger people, or vice versa. Ethnic background occasionally is helpful in the differential diagnosis (eg, familial Mediterranean fever occurs in Sephardic Jews, Armenians, and Turks). Education, financial state, and family resources have a major bearing on the patient's ability to comply with treatment and on the long-term prognosis.

Functional Impact

The clinician should ask if the condition described in the chief complaint limits the patient's ability to work, meet family responsibilities, or enjoy leisure time. This information provides a basis for recommendations regarding assistive devices, application for disability, and the appropriateness of aggressive medical or surgical treatment.

Family History

Patients with fibromyalgia or chronic pain often have a family history of alcoholism, depression, migraine headaches, or panic attacks. Patients with systemic inflammatory disorders may have a family history of an identical or related disorder such as rheumatoid arthritis (RA), systemic lupus erythematosus (SLE), autoimmune thyroid disease, multiple sclerosis, or myasthenia gravis. Other rheumatic diseases that are often genetically linked include early disseminated osteoarthritis (OA) and seronegative spondyloarthropathy.

Review of Systems

Patients should be questioned carefully about symptoms or diagnoses involving other organ systems. In particular, the presence of sicca symptoms, uveitis, pleurisy, chest pain, oral or genital ulcers, urethral or vaginal discharge, skin rash or photosensitivity, hair loss, diarrhea, and dysphagia should be elicited.

SYMPTOMS OF RHEUMATIC DISORDERS
Pain

Many patients use inaccurate anatomical terms to describe the location of pain. It is best to have the patient point directly to the area that hurts. If a patient's description is inadequate, follow-up questions should be directed to determine whether the pain is constant or intermittent, generalized or localized, symmetric or asymmetric. Patients should be asked whether pain is limited to the joints or mostly involves soft tissue structures between joints. If several anatomic areas are painful, the pain may be predominantly distal (as in RA) or proximal (as in fibromyalgia or polymyalgia rheumatica). Does activity improve or worsen the pain? Gentle activity frequently eases the pain of inflammatory disorders but does not usually relieve the pain of OA or fibromyalgia. Does weight-bearing activity aggravate lower extremity pain? If so, this suggests arthritis of major weight-bearing joints.

The time of day when the pain is worse is often important. Patients with inflammatory disorders may have stiffness or pain primarily in the morning that gradually improves with movement during the day. Pain that accelerates during the day and is worse in the evening suggests OA. Night pain is frequently associated with advanced structural damage, such as occurs in end-stage osteoarthritis of the knee, complete rotator cuff tear, and cancer. In contrast, patients with inflammatory disease are rarely awakened by pain. The character of pain may be important as well. Pain associated with numbness occurs in both neurologic disorders and fibromyalgia. Burning pain suggests neurologic impingement. Pain that is clearly brought on with activity and resolves predictably with rest suggests vascular insufficiency or claudication.

Stiffness

Stiffness is a common complaint that can be differentiated from pain. Inflammatory disorders such as RA and polymyalgia rheumatica are marked by prolonged stiffness in the morning (longer than 1 hour) of the involved areas. This stiffness is relieved with activity, but recurs after the patient sits down and subsequently attempts to resume activity (gel phenomenon).

Swelling

Patients who experience pain frequently also report swelling. Close questioning may be necessary to distinguish whether swelling is articular (as in arthritis), is periarticular (as in tenosynovitis and ganglion cysts), involves an entire limb or structure (as in lymphedema), or occurs in other areas (as in lipoma or palpable tumors). Is swelling limited to painful areas, or does it occur elsewhere? Is it intermittent or persistent, symmetric or asymmetric? Finally, is swelling minimal in the morning but worsens during the day (as in dependent edema)?

Weakness

One of the most common complaints of patients with musculoskeletal symptoms is weakness. Patients with generalized weakness should be asked whether there are any specific tasks that they are unable to do because of weakness. Do they have difficulty climbing stairs, arising from a low chair, or performing tasks with arms raised above the head? Patients with difficulty performing any of these tasks may have muscle disease. If the weakness involves one limb without evidence of weakness elsewhere, a neurologic disorder should be strongly suspected. Subjective weakness is a common complaint of patients with systemic illness or fibromyalgia in the absence of muscle disease, thus, the condition must be confirmed with a careful physical examination.

Constitutional Symptoms

The presence or absence of constitutional symptoms is important in the differential diagnosis. Patients with objective fever (temperature higher than 38.5°C) on a persistent basis may have underlying infection, malignancy, or a systemic inflammatory disease such as SLE or vasculitis. In contrast, patients with a chronic pain syndrome such as fibromyalgia frequently complain of "low-grade fevers," but rarely have persistent, objective elevated temperature. Weight loss often accompanies persistent fevers in patients with inflammatory or neoplastic disease, while weight gain is the norm in patients with chronic pain or fibromyalgia.

Sleep

A sleep history is often revealing in evaluating patients with chronic pain. Patients with fibromyalgia and inflammatory diseases frequently have difficulty falling asleep, note that their sleep is fragmented, and wake unrefreshed. Occasionally, a careful sleep history will identify a coexistent disorder (such as sleep apnea, nocturia, or narcolepsy) that may be a contributing factor to the patient's problem.

Raynaud's Phenomenon

The diagnosis of Raynaud's phenomenon is based primarily on the history. Patients who have true Raynaud's phenomenon typically note that, on exposure to cold, their fingers turn white or dusky and become quite painful. Subsequently, the digits may become hyperemic during the recovery phase. In addition, patients may complain of numbness while their digits are underperfused and tingling and burning during the recovery phase. Patients with a history of Raynaud's phenomenon should be evaluated closely for the possibility of coexistent SLE, CREST (calcinosis, Raynaud's phenomenon, esophageal dismotility, sclerodactyly, and telangiectasia) syndrome, Sjögren's syndrome, or systemic sclerosis.

PHYSICAL EXAMINATION

Several factors may have a bearing on the thoroughness of the physical examination in the patient with rheumatic complaints. Clearly, patients with constitutional symptoms or other complaints on history suggestive of systemic disease should undergo a thorough general physical examination. In contrast, a regional examination may be adequate for patients with isolated pain that is limited to specific areas. The general physical examination should focus on physical findings that suggest dysfunction of major organs such as the lungs, heart, liver, and kidneys. Patients with suspected systemic disease should also have a thorough skin, lymph node, neurologic, ophthalmologic, and ears, nose, and throat examination.

Joint Examination

Clinicians should be familiar with the anatomy of the affected area that they are examining. In addition, it is important to be familiar with the distribution of joint involvement in the major rheumatic syndromes. Obvious deformity of a joint suggests advanced damage resulting from the underlying process, particularly if the deformity cannot be reversed with manipulation. Joints should be examined for the presence of subtle swelling and compared with the contralateral joint. There are several causes of joint swelling. Fluid within the joint produces a bulge along the lateral margins of the joint that can be easily depressed, causing the fluid to balloon on the opposite side (bulge sign). Swelling caused by fluid accumulation tends to become firm when the joint is flexed. The synovial tissue that lines joints hypertrophies dramatically in inflammatory arthritis, leading to symmetric swelling that feels spongy but does not balloon. Osteoarthritic joints may appear swollen, but on palpation, it is clear that joint enlargement is due to bony hypertrophy. Swollen joints may feel cool to the touch in both inflammatory and degenerative arthritis, but significant warmth raises the suspicion of underlying infection, crystalline arthropathy, or a severe inflammatory arthritis. If the skin over the joint is red, the probability that the process is infectious or due to crystal deposition increases further. Redness may also be caused by inflammation of periarticular tissues such as bursae, tendon sheaths, and skin.

Symptomatic joints should be examined to determine whether they have normal range of motion. True joint disease tends to limit movement and cause pain with both active and passive motion in all planes. When passive movement of a limb exceeds the limits of active movement, the problem usually does not arise from the joint, but from tendons or muscles. Another test that may isolate the problem to a muscle or tendon is having the patient actively attempt to move the affected joint against sufficient force to prevent actual joint movement. If this maneuver reproduces the pain, adjacent tendinitis or muscle damage should be strongly suspected.

Soft tissues adjacent to a joint should be carefully examined in a manner directed by the anatomy. Soft tissue problems readily identified on physical examination that may produce pain or limit joint movement include ganglion cyst, bursitis, and tenosynovitis.

The pattern of involvement is important in determining the ultimate diagnosis. For example, osteoarthritis characteristically affects scattered distal interphalangeal (DIP) and proximal interphalangeal (PIP) joints of the hands in an asymmetric distribution. In addition, metacarpophalangeal (MCP) joints are usually spared and the carpometacarpal joint at the base of the thumb is frequently involved. Wrists are typically not affected by osteoarthritis. In contrast, RA characteristically involves the wrists, MCP joints, and PIP joints in a symmetric fashion. Other typically involved joints are shown in Fig. 7A-1. Patients with fibromyalgia often complain of pain in several areas and may be convinced that they have arthritis. However, close inspection of their joints fails to demonstrate objective signs of arthritis in symptomatic areas. These patients generally experience their most intense pain in nonarticular regions of the body such as paraspinal, trapezius, and brachioradialis muscles; the greater trochanters; and over the medial fat pads of the knees. Usually the clinician can elicit tenderness or "wincing" when applying modest pressure (just enough to blanch the nail bed of the examiner's finger) to symptomatic areas.

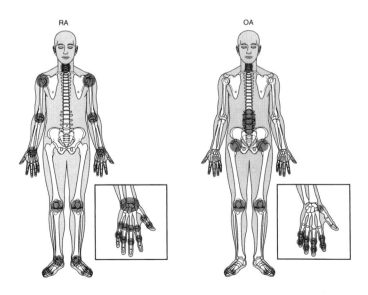

(Figure 7A-1)
Patterns of joint involvement in rheumatoid arthritis (RA) and osteoarthritis (OA).

Hand

Evaluating the hand is one of the most fruitful areas of the physical examination in a patient with polyarticular arthritis or systemic inflammatory disease. Several physical findings in fingertips suggest an underlying inflammatory disease. For example, small infarctions or splinter hemorrhages occur in endocarditis and systemic vasculitis. Characteristics of systemic sclerosis and limited scleroderma include atrophy of the fingertips and nailfold capillary changes, calcific nodules, digital cyanosis, and sclerodactyly (tightening of the skin). Dystrophic nail changes are characteristic of psoriasis, while digital clubbing accompanies chronic cardiac and pulmonary diseases. Bony enlargement or deformities of the DIP joints (Heberden's nodes) are common in OA. PIP joints should be carefully examined for range of motion and for the presence of spongy synovial thickening or bony hypertrophic changes (Bouchard's nodes). Similarly, MCP joints should be examined for bone or hypertrophic changes or synovitis. Always compare joint findings on one hand with those on the other for symmetry. Several other finger deformities are important in the differential diagnosis of arthritis. These include ulnar deviation at MCP joints, palmar subluxation of the MCP joint, swan neck deformity (hyperextension of PIP joint with flexion contracture of DIP joint), boutonnieres deformity (flexion contracture of the PIP joint with hyperextension of the DIP joint), and the Z deformity of the thumb. If these deformities are nonreducible, RA is likely; if they are fully reversible with manipulation, suspect SLE. (Jaccoud's arthropathy).

The two most common inflammatory conditions of the wrists are arthritis and extensor tendon tenosynovitis. Arthritis of the wrist joint is associated with swelling lateral and distal to the radius and ulna and with reduced passive flexion and extension. Extensor tendon tenosynovitis produces swelling that is limited to the tendon sheaths overlying the wrist and hand. The area of swelling may move as fingers are flexed and extended. Ganglion cysts are hard, smooth cystic masses that arise from tendon sheaths or joint capsules at various sites around the wrist. Deformities may be seen in inflammatory arthritis, including volar subluxation of the radiocarpal joint, radial deviation of the wrist, and collapse of the wrist with obvious shortening. Carpal tunnel syndrome is suggested by hand paresthesias, which are reproduced by firm pressure or tapping over the transverse carpal ligament (Tinel's sign) and prolonged wrist flexion (Phalen's sign). Thenar atrophy and sensory loss in the distribution of the medial nerve are late findings. Osteoarthritis usually spares the wrist, except for the first carpometacarpal joint.

Shoulder

Because the shoulder is the most complex joint in the body, clinicians dealing with shoulder complaints should become thoroughly familiar with its anatomy. The humeral head rests on the glenoid fossa, which is quite shallow and thus allows an extremely broad range of motion. Stability does not result from bony encasement, as is the case with the hip joint, but from the joint capsule, surrounding muscles, and tendons. The rotator cuff is a conglomeration of muscles and tendons (supraspinatus, infraspinatus, teres minor, and subscapularis) that collectively lifts and rotates the humerus. Several other muscles are involved in shoulder movement including the deltoid, pectoralis major, teres major, and latissimus dorsi.

The shoulder should be inspected for evidence of erythema and swelling, deformity, and muscle wasting. The clinician should palpate the shoulder to determine if rotator cuff muscles, tendons, or tendon insertion sites are tender. Palpate the biceps tendon in patients with anterior shoulder pain. The cervical and thoracic paraspinal muscles, trapezius muscle, and pectoral muscles may be more diffusely tender in patients with fibromyalgia or myofascial pain. If downward traction on the humerus with the arm relaxed causes a sulcus (hollow) to appear between the humeral head and the lateral acromion, shoulder instability may be present (a common cause of shoulder pain in young athletes).

Most major shoulder syndromes can be diagnosed by examining active range of shoulder movement in all planes, both with and without examiner resistance. The primary movements of the shoulder are abduction, adduction, external rotation, internal rotation, forward flexion, and extension (Fig. 7A-2). Reduction of active range of motion in all planes suggests either glenohumeral joint arthritis or adhesive capsulitis (frozen shoulder). Patients with subacromial bursitis or tendinitis of the rotator cuff muscles (the most common cause of shoulder pain) typically have painless active movement from 0 to 45 degrees, pain with movement from 45 to 120 degrees, then painless movement again through the remainder of the arc from 120 to 180 degrees. Impingement of the subacromial bursa and supraspinatus between the greater tuberosity of the humerus and the acromioclavicular joint and coracoid ligaments is responsible for pain as the shoulder moves through the arc. Reduction of active range of motion in one plane, but not others, suggests nerve or tendon damage.

If active range of motion is not full, the examiner should passively move the shoulder through its range of motion. If passive movement is reduced to a similar degree as active motion, pathology of the glenohumeral joint and/or joint capsule is likely. However, if passive range of motion substantially exceeds active range of motion, the problem most likely is a muscle or tendon problem such as a rotator cuff tear. The presence of a rotator cuff tear can be further con-firmed by the finding of weakness with resisted external rotation or abduction. Significant pain with minimal passive motion of the glenohumeral joint suggests acute synovitis, dislocation, or fracture. Shoulder discomfort without significant physical findings suggests that the pain may be referred from the chest cavity, diaphragm, sternoclavicular joint, or neck.

Spine

The clinician should evaluate patients standing erect, paying particular attention to position of the neck and the contours of the spine (cervical lordosis, thoracic kyphosis, lumbar lordosis). Palpation of the spinous processes and paraspinal muscles should be done to assess for scoliosis and abnormal tenderness or spasm.

Arthritis and inflammatory disease of the spine manifests typically as reduced range of motion. The patient should be asked to rotate, laterally flex (touch ear to shoulder), and flex and extend the neck to the extremes of movement. If movement is limited, ask the patient whether pain restricts movement. Ankylosing spondylitis should be strongly suspected in patients who cannot touch their occiput to the wall while standing erect.

Lumbar flexion is assessed by Schöber's maneuver. A mark is placed at the midline between the "dimples of the pelvis" (at S2) and a second mark is made 10 cm above the first mark. Have the patient bend forward and attempt to touch his or her toes, and then remeasure the distance. Normally, the distance between these points is increased more than 5 cm. In addition, the lumbar curve normally flattens as the patient flexes forward. In ankylosing spondylitis, the lumbar curve is flattened with the patient erect, and Schöber's maneuver reveals minimal, if any, true lumbar flexion as the patient bends forward.

The importance of the neurologic examination in patients with spinal complaints cannot be overstated. It is the clinician's first duty to rule out spinal cord impingement, which is suggested by loss of bladder control, decreased anal sphincter tone, lower extremity weakness, hyper-reflexia, and Babinski's sign. Nerve root impingement is suggested by dermatomal sensory loss, asymmetric reduction of reflexes, or myotomal weakness. Sciatic nerve roots can be stressed by the Lasegue maneuver (straight leg-raising sign). With the patient lying supine, lift the leg with the knee fully extended. Normally, the leg can be raised to 90 degrees without difficulty. If this maneuver is limited, nerve root disease is suggested. Flex the knee to further flex the hip and then straighten the patient's knee again. If this maneuver reproduces the pain, sciatic nerve root irritation (L4-S3) is likely.

Hip

Examination of the hip begins by carefully observing how the patient walks. The most common gait in hip disease is the antalgic gait, in which the patient shortens the time spent bearing weight on the affected side and leans toward the affected side. Patients with chronic hip disease may develop a Trendelenburg gait due to gluteus medius weakness. In this gait, the pelvis drops on the nonaffected side when weight is placed on the affected side.

Palpate the anterior hip joint slightly below the inguinal ligament and lateral to the femoral artery pulse. Tenderness in this area suggests inflammation of the iliopectineal bursa.

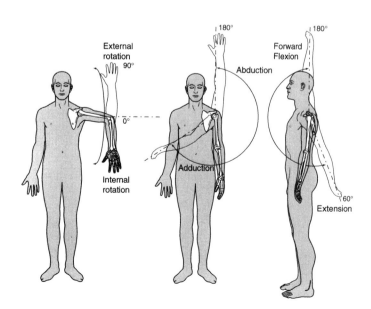

(Figure 7A-2)
Normal shoulder range of motion.

Tenderness over the greater trochanter suggests trochanteric bursitis, one of the most common causes of hip pain.

Range of motion is commonly reduced in patients with arthritis of the hip. Flexion is assessed with the patient supine, knees bent. Normal hip flexion is 90–120 degrees. To assess hip rotation, flex both the hip and knee to 90 degrees, and then place one hand on the knee and the other on the heel. Test internal rotation by rotating the foot laterally (outward) and external rotation by rotating the foot medially (inward). Normal internal rotation is 30–40 degrees and external rotation is 40–60 degrees. Loss of internal rotation is among the earliest physical findings in hip arthritis. Other hip movements that should be tested include extension (normal 10–15 degrees), abduction (normal 30–50 degrees), and adduction (normal approximately 30 degrees). Individuals vary substantially in hip range of motion, however, so it is important to examine both the affected and nonaffected sides.

Knee

Swelling can occur in several extra-articular sites including the anserine bursa (located over the medial aspect of the proximal anterior tibia) and prepatellar bursa (covering the lower half of the patella and upper half of the patellar ligament). Joint swelling is suggested by circumferential swelling centered over the joint line that is easily ballotable. The bulge sign is diagnostic. Other common sites of swelling are the suprapatellar bursa (located superior to the midline of the patella) and popliteal cysts (Baker's cysts), both of which communicate with the knee joint.

Flexion contractures of the knee may be due to either chronic arthritis or hamstring tightness. Collateral ligament stability is tested by flexing the knee to about 20 degrees and applying valgus or varus stress to the tibia with one hand while stabilizing the distal femur with the other hand. The anterior cruciate ligament is best tested at the knee with the patient supine and the knee flexed 20–30 degrees. Grasp the distal femur with one hand and the proximal tibia with the other, and attempt to pull the tibia upward (Lachmann's maneuver). Laxity with this maneuver suggests anterior cruciate instability. Posterior cruciate instability is tested by the posterior drawer test. With the patient supine, both knees flexed 90 degrees, compare the position of the tibias. If the tibia on the affected side is posterior in comparison to the contralateral tibia, and if the deformity can be corrected by pulling the tibia forward, posterior cruciate instability is suggested.

Foot and Ankle

Ankle effusions manifest as anterior swelling along the joint line. Effusions must be differentiated from pitting edema, which may also be prominent posterior to the malleolus. The anterior joint line of the ankle should be palpated for evidence of swelling or tenderness. Ankle dorsiflexion (normal 20 degrees) and plantar flexion (normal 45 degrees) should be tested. Examine the subtalar joint by stabilizing the lower calf and inverting (30 degrees) and everting (20 degrees) the heel.

Pes planus (flat foot), a common cause of foot pain, is best assessed during weight bearing. Painful forefoot deformities such as hammer toes and hallux valgus are easily observable. Note any calluses, which indicate abnormal pressure points between feet and shoes. With the patient

standing, observe the heels for pronation (eversion of the heel) or supination (inversion). Having the patient walk on tiptoes, heels, and outer and inner borders of the feet allows the examiner to assess functional range of motion and muscle power.

Palpate the metatarsophalangeal (MTP) joints, paying attention to deformity, swelling, and tenderness. Marked tenderness localized between the second and third or the third and fourth metatarsal heads suggests Morton's neuroma. A simple screening test for MTP synovitis is to grasp the fore-

(Table 7A-1)
Main features of the GALS screening inspection

Position/Activity	Normal Findings
Gait	Symmetry, smoothness of movement
	Normal stride length
	Normal heel strike, stance, toe off, swing through
	Able to turn quickly
Inspection from behind	Straight spine
	Normal, symmetric paraspinal muscles
	Normal shoulder and gluteal muscle bulk
	Level iliac crests
	No popliteal cysts
	No popliteal swelling
	No hindfoot swelling/deformity
Inspection from the side	Normal cervical and lumbar lordosis
	Normal thoracic kyphosis
"Touch your toes"	Normal lumbar spine (and hip) flexion
Inspection from front	
Arms	
"Place your hands behind your head" (elbows out)	Normal glenohumeral, sternoclavicular, and acromioclavicular joint movement
"Place your hands by your side" (elbows straight)	Full elbow extension
"Place your hands in front" (palms down)	No wrist/finger swelling or deformity
	Able to fully extend fingers
"Turn your hands over"	Normal supination/pronation
	Normal palms
"Make a fist"	Normal grip power
"Place the tip of each finger on the tip of the thumb"	Normal fine precision, pinch
Legs	Normal quadricep bulk/symmetry
	No knee swelling or deformity
	No forefoot/midfoot deformity
	Normal arches
	No abnormal callous formation
Spine	
"Place your ear on your shoulder"	Normal cervical lateral flexion

Modified from Doherty et al (5), with permission.

foot between finger and thumb and squeeze the metatarsal heads. A painful response indicates likely synovitis.

QUICK SCREENING EXAMINATION

The GALS (Gait, Arms, Leg, Spine) locomotor screen is an excellent tool for rapidly determining disability and relevant musculoskeletal disease (5). Patients are asked three basic questions: "Have you any pain or stiffness in your muscles, joints, or back?" "Can you dress yourself completely without any difficulty?" "Can you walk up and down stairs without any difficulty?" Any positive responses are followed with relevant questions.

Next inspect the patient's gait, spine, arms, and legs systematically, first with the patient standing still and then responding to instructions (Table 7A-1). Any abnormalities detected on screening are followed up with a more detailed regional examination. With practice, the examiner can complete the GALS examination in 3 to 4 minutes with most patients.

JOSEPH M. CASH, MD

1. Liang MH, Sturrock: Evaluation of musculoskeletal symptoms. In Klippel JH, Dieppe PA (eds): Practical Rheumatology. London, Mosby, 3-20, 1995
2. Doherty M, Hazleman BL, Hutton CW, et al: Rheumatology Examination and Injection Techniques. London, WB Saunders, 1992
3. Magee DJ: Orthopedic Physical Assessment. Phililadelphia, WB Saunders, 1987
4. Sheon RP, Moskowitz RW, Goldberg VM: Soft Tissue Rheumatic Pain: Recognition, Management, Prevention. Philadelphia, Lea & Febiger, 1987
5. Doherty M, Dacre J, Dieppe P, Snaith M: The GALS locomotor screen. Ann Rheum Dis 51:1165-1169, 1992

B. LABORATORY ASSESSMENT

The laboratory evaluation of patients with rheumatic disease is often informative but rarely definitive (1). Ideally, diagnostic tests should provide clinically useful information and affect management. They should suggest a diagnosis indicating specific rather than symptomatic treatment, help in estimating prognosis, or define response to treatment. Laboratory evaluation in the differential diagnosis of rheumatic complaints is most useful when there is at least a moderate clinical suspicion of a specific disorder as suggested by a constellation of signs and symptoms, occasionally to exclude a condition, or to aid prognosis. In systemic illness, testing is performed to define the extent of disease or detect other organ systems that may be involved. This chapter outlines a strategy for using common laboratory tests in the diagnosis and management of rheumatic disorders (2).

Four characteristics of diagnostic tests help assess their diagnostic utility: sensitivity, specificity, predictive value positive, and predictive value negative (3). *Sensitivity* is the likelihood of a positive test result in a person with a disease. This is also termed the "true positive rate" of a diagnostic test. *Specificity* is the likelihood of a negative test in a patient without disease and is the "true negative rate" of a test. The *predictive value positive* of a test is the probability of a disease if the test is positive; likewise the *predictive value negative* of a test is the probability of a disease being absent if the test is negative. It is possible to calculate the predictive value of a specific test by Bayes' theorem, an equation that utilizes the prevalence of the disease in the population (the pre-test probability of a disease in a given population) and the test's sensitivity and specificity. The prevalence is frequently not known. The relationship is such that the test is most helpful in increasing diagnostic certainty in a given patient when the pre-test likelihood, as judged by the clinician, is moderate.

ACUTE-PHASE REACTANTS

Acute-phase reactants are a heterogeneous group of proteins synthesized in the liver that are rapidly induced in the presence of inflammation or tissue necrosis and that appear to parallel chronic inflammation. They include the coagulation proteins fibrinogen and prothrombin; transport proteins such as haptoglobin, transferrin, and ceruloplasmin; complement components such as C3 and C4; protease inhibitors; and miscellaneous proteins such as albumin, fibronectin, C-reactive protein (CRP), and serum amyloid A-related protein. The tests most commonly used clinically are the erythrocyte sedimentation rate (ESR) and the CRP. C-reactive protein levels respond more rapidly than the ESR to changes in inflammatory activity, and thus CRP is probably a more sensitive early measure of inflammation. However, the ESR takes only 1 hour and requires minimal equipment, whereas the CRP takes a day to perform and requires an enzyme-linked immunosorbent assay (ELISA) or radioimmunodiffusion equipment. The ESR can be high or low in the absence of pathology; it increases with age and anemia and is higher in women than in men. A rough rule of thumb is that the age-adjusted upper limit of normal for an ESR is the age divided by 2 for men. For women, it is the age plus 10 divided by 2.

The ESR is important in the diagnosis of giant cell arteritis (GCA) and polymyalgia rheumatica (PMR), as it is a criterion for the clinical diagnosis of these disorders. However, up to 10% of patients with these diseases may have a normal ESR.

A normal ESR does not sufficiently reduce the probability of crystal-induced or septic arthritis to preclude the need for a synovial fluid examination, nor is it helpful in monitoring disease activity in such patients. The ESR is generally elevated in systemic vasculitis, but is often normal in patients with primary central nervous system angiitis, Henöch-Schönlein purpura, lymphomatoid granulomatosis, and thromboangiitis obliterans.

The ESR is useful for monitoring disease activity of patients with RA and PMR/GCA, but it is less useful in systemic lupus erythematosus (SLE) and spondyloarthropathies (4).

AUTOANTIBODIES

Autoantibodies—immunoglobulins directed against autologous intracellular, cell surface, and extracellular antigens—are seen in a number of rheumatic diseases. The intracellular antigens include nuclear components (antinuclear antibodies) or cytoplasmic components (antineutrophilic cytoplasmic antibodies). Antibodies to cell-surface antigens react with a variety of antigens including HLA molecules. Other antibodies may react with plasma components such as coagulation factors (lupus anticoagulant).

Autoantibodies are detected by a variety of techniques including indirect immunofluorescence, enzyme immunocytochemistry, passive hemagglutination, particle agglutination, immunodiffusion, counter immunoelectrophoresis (CIE), radioimmunoassay (RIA), and ELISA. When autoantibodies are directed against cellular or insoluble extracellular components, indirect immunofluorescence is the method most widely used to screen body fluids for the presence of these antibodies. Autoantibodies directed against soluble components such as coagulation factors, DNA, nuclear protein, and components of complement are assayed by immunodiffusion, CIE, RIA, or ELISA.

The sensitivity of techniques varies considerably. At present there is no standardization of either the assay method or the units in which most autoantibodies are reported. Comparison from one laboratory to another, therefore, is problematic. The detection of many autoantibodies requires sophisticated immunochemistry, which is available primarily in research laboratories. Autoantibodies are present in a small proportion of the normal population, albeit usually in low titer. It is important, therefore, not to assign a rheumatic diagnosis based solely on the finding of an autoantibody.

Antinuclear Antibodies

Testing for antinuclear antibodies (ANA) is useful primarily in the evaluation of suspected SLE, as the test is highly sensitive in this disease. Furthermore, certain ANA subsets such as Sm and double-stranded DNA (dsDNA) are highly specific for SLE. The predictive value of ANA is highest when the titer and pattern are considered in the context of other specific autoantibodies and the clinical presentation. Because the ANA is positive in at least 95% of patients with SLE, a negative test argues strongly against the diagnosis. The pattern of the ANA (diffuse, peripheral, speckled, or nucleolar) correlates with the specific antigen against which the antibody is targeted (5) (Table 7B-1). For example, anti-dsDNA antibodies generally produce a peripheral staining ANA, while anti-Ro antibodies produce a speckled ANA. Although some patterns may add to the specificity of the test, they possess variable, and often limited, sensitivity. When SLE is highly suspected but the ANA is negative, anti-Ro antibody and a CH50 should be ordered, because some "ANA-negative" SLE patients will be anti-Ro–positive and others will be complement-deficient (6,7).

The most important limitation of the ANA test is its lack of specificity. Other rheumatic disorders such as systemic sclerosis, Sjögren's syndrome, and RA are also associated with a positive ANA, although the sensitivity of the test in these diseases is much lower than in SLE (Table 7B-1). Patients without rheumatic disease, including healthy older people, patients with infectious illness, and those taking certain medications (procainamide, hydralazine, phenytoin), may also test positive for ANA. Anti-Sm and anti-dsDNA antibodies are highly specific (although not highly sensitive) for SLE and are subject to variability, depending on the laboratory and the assay technique used.

The prevalence of the conditions associated with ANA in the population for whom the ANA test is ordered affects the utility of the test. For example, if the ANA is routinely ordered for patients with arthralgia or a fever of unknown origin, but no other features to suggest SLE, more false-positive than true-positive results will likely be observed (8). Although false-positive ANAs tend to be in low titer, a significant proportion will be of medium to high titer. Furthermore, a sizeable minority of SLE patients have low-titer ANAs. Thus, the ANA test should be ordered only when the pre-test probability is appreciable, and the result must be interpreted in light of its titer and specific autoantibody profile (9,10).

Antineutrophilic Cytoplasmic Antibodies

Antineutrophilic cytoplasmic antibodies (ANCA) are a family of antibodies first described as a diagnostic test for Wegener's granulomatosis (11). Subsequent studies, however, have demonstrated ANCAs directed against several antigens in a variety of rheumatic and nonrheumatic disorders. Two patterns of ANCA are commonly reported: cytoplasmic staining (c-ANCA) and perinuclear staining (p-ANCA). c-ANCA, an antibody specific for proteinase-3 (PR-3) antigen, is 70%–90% sensitive for active diffuse Wegener's granulomatosis and for crescentic or necrotizing glomerulonephritis. p-ANCA is often attributed to antibody targeting myeloperoxidase (MPO) and most commonly detected in pauci-immune glomerulonephritis, drug-induced lupus, and SLE (11). Non-MPO p-ANCA has recently been reported in inflammatory bowel disease, suggesting that

(Table 7B-1)
Sensitivity of antinuclear antibodies in rheumatic diseases

Disease*	Antinuclear Antibody			Precipitin Panel				
	ANA	Pattern†	Titer	anti-dsDNA	anti-Sm	anti-RNP	anti-Ro	anti-La
SLE	95–99%	P,D,S,N	50%>1:640	20–30%	30%	30–50%	30%	15%
Sjögren's syndrome	75%	D,S	Low	5%	0%	15%	50%	25%
RA	15–35%	D	10%>1:640	<5%	0%	10%	10%	5%
Systemic sclerosis	60–90%	S,N,D	Often high	0%	0%	30%	5%	1%
DILE	100%	D,S	May be high	0%	<5%	<5%	<5%	0%
MCTD	95–99%	S,D	May be high	0%	0%	95%	<5%	<5%
Normal	<5%	D	Rarely>1:80	0%	0%	<5%	<5%	Rare

* SLE = systemic lupus erythematosus; RA = rheumatoid arthritis; DILE = drug-induced lupus erythematosus; MCTD = mixed connective tissue disease.
† P =peripheral; D=diffuse; S=speckled; N=nucleolar; presented in order of decreasing frequency.

ANCA positivity alone is not specific enough to suggest a particular diagnosis. On the other hand, when clinical features are compelling, a high-titer c-ANCA with PR-3 specificity is sufficient for some clinicians to treat patients for Wegener's granulomatosis or "vasculitic" glomerulonephritis without histologic confirmation. The use of ANCA in monitoring disease activity in Wegener's is debated (12). Routinely ordering this test for patients with inflammatory disease of unknown cause or for those unlikely to have vasculitic disease probably yields little useful information.

Myositis-Specific Antibodies

Several myositis-specific antibodies (MSAs) are described, including antisynthetase, antisignal recognition particle (SRP), and anti-Mi-2 antibodies (13,14). Their sensitivity, specificity, and predictive value have not been well studied, but MSAs appear to be useful in defining homogenous subsets of patients with inflammatory myositis. Approximately 50% of patients with idiopathic inflammatory myopathy, including dermatomyositis and polymyositis, have circulating MSAs, whereas these antibodies are much rarer in cancer-associated myositis or myopathy associated with other rheumatic diseases. Moreover, clinical subsets of myositis seem to segregate by the type of antibody: patients with antisynthetase antibodies typically develop Raynaud's phenomenon, arthritis, and interstitial lung disease, with acute onset during the spring and poor prognosis; those with anti-SRP have acute onset in the fall, cardiac involvement, and poor prognosis; patients with anti-Mi-2 have classic dermatomyositis and a good prognosis.

Rheumatoid Factor

Rheumatoid factors (RF) are antibodies directed against the Fc portion of immunoglobulin G (IgG). These autoantibodies appear to be synthesized in response to immunoglobulins that have been conformationally altered after reaction with an antigen. The most common rheumatoid factor is an IgM antibody to IgG. Traditional techniques to detect rheumatoid factor include agglutination of IgG sensitized sheep red blood cells or latex particles coated with human IgG. Results are expressed as the dilution titer at which reactivity is eliminated. Refinements using radioimmunoassays, ELISA, and nephelometric techniques have improved quantitation, reliability, and perhaps sensitivity and specificity.

Rheumatoid factor is among the most frequently ordered tests in the evaluation of patients with arthralgia or suspected rheumatic disease, but its clinical utility is limited (15,16). The test is positive in approximately 75%–90% of patients with RA (sensitivity = 0.75–0.90), but such estimates are derived from highly selected populations such as rheumatology practices or studies establishing criteria for disease; the estimates, therefore, are subject to referral bias (17,18). Other rheumatic diseases may be accompanied by a positive RF, but the sensitivity is even lower. The assay technique used and titer of the RF may alter the sensitivity; however, use of a more sensitive assay or setting a lower cutoff titer for a positive test will make the test less specific.

The RF test has low specificity in nonreferral settings and in the general population. Various nonrheumatic diseases are associated with a positive RF. In the patient with a fever and arthralgia, endocarditis may be a more likely cause of a positive RF than RA. Other rheumatic diseases such as Sjögren's syndrome, SLE, and cryoglobulinemia may have clinical features in common with RA and may also be accompanied by elevated titers of RF. The high specificity reported in referral rheumatology practices may not be observed in patients with weak clinical indications for the test or a high prevalence of confounding diseases. For patients over the age of 75, the reported prevalence of false-positive RF results ranges from 2% to 25% (17,19).

Given the modest sensitivity and specificity of the RF test, the pre-test probability, as estimated by the clinician, in large part determines its usefulness. Even with generous estimates of sensitivity and specificity, the number of false-positive test results is often greater than true-positive results. Therefore the RF should be ordered only for patients with inflammatory joint symptoms or signs suggestive of RA. A positive test result may not affect initial management, even when the result is a true positive. However, some clinicians may prescribe a second-line agent sooner for seropositive RA patients. Population-based studies suggest that, among asymptomatic patients, a positive RF may place the individual at increased risk of developing RA (20). However, the RF performs poorly as a screening test for rheumatoid arthritis due to the high frequency of false-positive results.

Complement

As discussed in Chapter 5C, the complement cascade is a series of over 20 biologically active proteins and inhibitors produced in the liver that comprise 2%–3% of the total plasma protein concentration. Complement activated by the classical pathway is responsible for the lysis of cells coated with antibody directed against cell-surface antigens. Complement may be assayed by techniques that measure the presence of the component or its function. The best screening test for a complement abnormality is the CH50, which is a functional assay of the entire classical pathway. A low level suggests either consumption of complement or a deficiency of one or more components. Complement activation is generally triggered by exposure of the host to a foreign protein, especially when bound to host antibody (immune complex disease). Although the foreign protein is usually unknown in patients with suspected or known rheumatic disease, low complement in such patients may indicate consumption of these proteins.

Conditions characterized by immune complex formation and hypocomplementemia include SLE (especially with nephritis), idiopathic membranoproliferative glomerulonephritis, cryoglobulinemia, chronic infections causing glomerulonephritis or vasculitis, post-streptococcal glomerulonephritis, generalized vasculitis, and serum sickness (21). In SLE nephritis, serial measurement of complement may prove useful for monitoring patients, because complement levels may decrease just before or concomitant with disease flare and return to normal weeks or months later when disease activity diminishes. The correlation of lupus disease activity with complement levels is variable between patients, however, and, thus, complement should be considered in the context of the clinical picture.

Hereditary complement deficiency may cause hypocomplementemia, and, in some instances (especially C2 or C1 component deficiency), SLE or SLE-like illness has been described, often with a negative ANA (7). Thus, for ANA-negative patients in whom the clinical suspicion of SLE is high, a CH50 should be performed along with the anti-Ro antibody. Conditions associated with reduced complement without known immune complex formation include atheromatous embolization, hemolytic uremic syndrome, septic shock, liver failure, severe malnutrition, pancreatitis, severe burns, malaria with hemolysis, and some cases of porphyria.

CIRCULATING IMMUNE COMPLEXES

Circulating immune complexes consisting of an antigen, an antibody, and complement components are believed to play an important role in the pathogenesis of systemic rheumatic diseases such as SLE and vasculitis. Occasionally, low levels of immune complexes may be detected in normal individuals. High concentrations of circulating immune complexes can be seen in active systemic rheumatic diseases, vasculitis, infectious diseases, and some malignancies. In most of these conditions, a clear pathogenic role for the complexes has not been established. Similarly, the clinical utility of this test is unclear. Assays for immune complexes include the Raji cell assay, Clq binding, C1q-precipitin assays, and RIA. Immune complexes may be detected by one assay and not another.

IMMUNOCHEMICAL TESTS

Many rheumatic diseases are thought to be the result of abnormalities of cellular and humoral immunity. However, analysis of lymphocyte phenotypes or electrophoresis of serum proteins are useful only in limited clinical contexts, such as suspected HIV infection, myeloma, or cryoglobulinemia. Otherwise, the information obtained is usually nonspecific and contributes little to a diagnosis.

HLA-B27

The strong association between the HLA-B27 allele and the seronegative spondyloarthropathies makes this genetic marker a potentially useful test in evaluating patients with musculoskeletal symptoms. The diagnostic sensitivity of this test is approximately 95% in ankylosing spondylitis, 80% in Reiter's syndrome, 50% in symptomatic spondylitis associated with inflammatory bowel disease, and 70% in patients with spondylitis and psoriasis. Moreover, patients without rheumatic symptoms who are HLA-B27–positive have an increased relative risk (though low absolute risk) for the development of these associated spondylitides compared with those who are HLA-B27–negative.

The background prevalence of this genetic marker (approximately 6%–10% in white populations) and the fact that only a small minority of HLA-B27–positive individuals will ever develop a spondyloarthropathy limit the utility of the test. For example, even with a sensitivity of 95% and specificity of 94% for ankylosing spondylitis, a patient with a pretest likelihood of 10% has only a 64% chance of having the disease if the test is positive; thus, more than a third of such patients would have positive results without B27-associated disease. When the test is ordered for a patient with low back pain not strongly suggestive of an inflammatory disorder, the test yields more false-positive than true-positive results. In confusing cases, a positive HLA-B27 may provide "soft" evidence that a spondylitis is present; how-ever, significant misclassification will occur if the test is relied on too heavily (22).

ASSESSING ORGAN DAMAGE OR INVOLVEMENT

In patients with systemic rheumatic disorders, extra-articular involvement is often the rule, even in the absence of signs or symptoms. Moreover, the agents used in their treatment may have systemic toxicity. Such involvement can be deduced by appropriate laboratory testing, such as renal or liver function tests, blood counts, muscle enzymes, or urinalysis. For selected patients, more elaborate testing may be indicated, such as a 24-hour urine collection for protein and creatinine clearance or lumbar puncture.

ROBERT H. SHMERLING, MD
MATTHEW H. LIANG, MD, MPH

1. American College of Rheumatology Ad Hoc Committee on Clinical Guidelines: Guidelines for the initial evaluation of the adult patient with acute musculoskeletal symptoms. Arthritis Rheum 39:1-8, 1996

2. ARA Glossary Committee, Dictionary of the Rheumatic Diseases: Vol II: Diagnostic Testing, Contact Associates Int. Ltd. New York, 1985

3. McNeil BJ, Keeler E, Adelstein SJ: Primer on certain elements of medical decision making. New Engl J Med 293:211-215, 1975

4. Sox HC, Jr., Liang MH: The erythrocyte sedimentation rate: Guidelines for rational use. Ann Intern Med 104:515-23, 1986

5. McCarty GA: Autoantibodies and their relation to rheumatic diseases. Med Clin North Am 70:237-61, 1986

6. Atkinson JP: Complement deficiency. Predisposing factor to autoimmune syndromes. Am J Med 85:45-47, 1988

7. Maddison PJ, Provost TT, Reichlin M: Serologic findings in patients with "ANA-negative" systemic lupus erythematosus. Medicine (Baltimore) 60:87-94, 1981

8. Slater CA, Davis RB, Shmerling RH: Antinuclear antibody (ANA) testing: a study of clinical utility. Arch Intern Med 156:1421-1425, 1996

9. Juby A, Johnston C, Davis P: Specificity, sensitivity, and diagnostic predictive value of selected laboratory generated autoantibody profiles in patients with connective tissue diseases. J Rheumatol 18:354-358, 1991

10. Richardson B, Epstein WV: Utility of the fluorescent antinuclear antibody test in a single patient. Ann Intern Med 95:333-338, 1981

11. Kallenberg CG, Brouwer E, Weening JJ, Tervaert JW. Anti-neutrophil cytoplasmic antibodies: current diagnostic and pathophysiological potential. Kidney Int 46:1-15, 1994

12. Rao JK, Weinberger M, Oddone EZ, et al: The role of antineutrophil cytoplasmic antibody (c-ANCA) testing in the diagnosis of Wegener's granulomatosis: a literature review and meta-analysis. Ann Intern Med 123:925-932, 1995

13. Love LA, Leff RL, Fraser DD, Targoff IN, Dalakas M, Plotz PH, Miller FW: A new approach to the classification of idiopathic inflammatory myopathy: Myositis-specific autoantibodies define useful homogeneous patient groups. Medicine 70:360-374, 1991

14. Miller FW: Myositis specific autoantibodies: touchstones for understanding the inflammatory myopathies. JAMA 270:1846-1849, 1993

15. Shmerling RH, Delbanco TL: The rheumatoid factor: An analysis of clinical utility. Am J Med 91:528-534, 1991

16. Lichtenstein MJ, Pincus T: Rheumatoid arthritis identified in population based cross-sectional studies: Low prevalence of rheumatoid factor. J Rheumatol 18:989-993, 1991

17. Wolfe F, Cathey MA, Roberts FK: The latex test revisited: Rheumatoid factor testing in 8,287 rheumatic disease patients. Arthritis Rheum 34:951-960, 1991

18. Arnett FC, Edworthy SM, Bloch DA, et al: The American Rheumatism Association 1987 revised criteria for the classification of rheumatoid arthritis. Arthritis Rheum 31:315-324, 1988

19. Litwin D, Singer JM: Studies of the incidence and significance of antigamma globulin factors in the aging. Arthritis Rheum 8:538-580, 1965

20. Aho K, Heliovaara M, Maatela J, et al: Rheumatoid factors antedating clinical rheumatoid arthritis. J Rheumatol 18:1282-1284, 1991

21. Hebert LA, Cosio FG, Neff JC: Diagnostic significance of hypocomplementemia. Kidney Int 39:811-821, 1991

22. Hawkins BR, Dawkins RL, Christiansen FT, et al: Use of the B27 test in the diagnosis of ankylosing spondylitis: A statistical evaluation. Arthritis Rheum 24:743-746, 1981

C. ARTHROCENTESIS, SYNOVIAL FLUID ANALYSIS, AND SYNOVIAL BIOPSY

Synovial fluid analysis provides unique and valuable information about what is going on inside joints. Together with the medical history, physical examination, and plain radiographs, synovial fluid analysis has a fundamental role in the clinical evaluation of patients with arthritis (1–4). Increasing numbers of formal studies confirm that the findings of synovial fluid analyses frequently alter diagnosis and management decisions (5,6). Technical competence and the ability to interpret the results of analyses are acquired and rewarding skills (7). As with the study of urine, the microscopic analysis of synovial fluid is optimally performed by the physician who is most familiar with the patient.

Because many different laboratory studies can be applied to synovial fluid, it behooves the clinician to be selective about the resources expended and to not use tests of unproven benefit or that are inappropriate in a given situation. Fortunately, much of the most useful information can be provided by the simplest and least expensive tests. Knowledge of what synovial fluid analysis can and cannot tell the clinician is central to the decision to perform arthrocentesis.

ARTHROCENTESIS

Indications

There are a few disorders for which synovial fluid analysis is diagnostic, providing information that is usually not available any other way. Chief among these are infectious and crystal–induced arthritis. In fact, some would argue that the only proper way to confirm these diagnoses is with synovial fluid analysis. It can also suggest or confirm the diagnosis of diseases as disparate as amyloidosis, hypothyroidism, ochronosis, hemochromatosis, systemic lupus erythematosus (SLE), or even simple edema.

Perhaps the most common demand of synovial fluid analysis is to differentiate between inflammatory and non-inflammatory arthritis. This seemingly basic distinction is not always as easy to make clinically as might be believed. The traditional rule of thumb is that a total white blood cell (WBC) count >2000/mm^3 indicates inflammatory arthritis. Thus, one should not uncritically accept a diagnosis of simple osteoarthritis if the WBC is greater than this threshold value, nor a diagnosis of active rheumatoid arthritis (RA) with a lower WBC count.

The coexistence of two or more types of arthritis in a single patient or even in a single joint is not uncommon. Making the correct diagnosis in these situations may be impossible without the aid of synovial fluid analysis, even for experienced clinicians. Rheumatoid arthritis, either active or in complete remission, may coexist with calcium pyrophosphate dihydrate (CPPD) crystal deposition disease, hemarthrosis, infectious arthritis, or secondary OA. Rheumatoid arthritis frequently develops in individuals who have preexisting primary osteoarthritis. Up to 7% of all patients with gout also have chondrocalcinosis. Hemarthrosis and bacterial infection usually occur in joints already damaged by another form of arthritis. Joints previously involved by inflammatory disease of any type can develop secondary degenerative changes.

The most pressing reason to perform synovial fluid analysis is to rule out bacterial infection in severely inflamed joints. There is no other comparably reliable way to differentiate septic arthritis from acute crystal-induced arthritis or from severe flares of idiopathic inflammatory arthritis. Although clinical information may favor another diagnosis, failure to aspirate a severely inflamed joint is to accept some risk of delaying the diagnosis of septic arthritis. The results of synovial fluid analysis dictate the pace of diagnostic and therapeutic intervention. Thus, a WBC >100,000/mm^3 demands that the physician make decisions swiftly because of the likelihood of infectious arthritis with its potential for rapid joint destruction. If the clinical picture is otherwise unthreatening, a WBC <50,000/mm^3 generally permits a more measured approach.

Arthrocentesis may be therapeutic as well as diagnostic. For tense effusions in which the intra-articular pressure is high, removing fluid relieves symptoms and may decrease joint damage (8). Removing the products of inflammation is an important part of treating infectious arthritis.

There are more reasons for performing than for not performing arthrocentesis. It is indicated for all significant undiagnosed arthritis, certainly when a patient's ability to function is altered. Even if the physician is convinced of a diagnosis, arthrocentesis is indicated before embarking on long-term treatment with expensive or toxic drugs. Many physicians would not commit a patient to lifelong urate-lowering drugs without demonstrating urate crystals in fluid (or tophi). Similarly, it is important to confirm the absence of CPPD or urate crystals before committing a patient to second-line agents for suspected RA. Arthrocentesis is also indicated for unusual exacerbations of chronic arthritis. A useful rule of thumb is that if it occurs to the examiner that arthrocentesis might be indicated, it probably is! Don't waste time thinking of reasons not to perform this procedure in a safe and timely way.

Technique

Operators who have received supervised instruction are qualified to handle relatively easy-to-aspirate joints such as the knee, ankle, wrist, and elbow. For less commonly aspirated joints, the advice or participation of an experienced physician who is familiar with the anatomy of the relevant joint is appropriate.

Joints usually have more than one route of entry. The preferred one involves the shortest distance through tissue, and avoids skin lesions, major vessels, tendons, and nerves. Figs. 7C-1 through 7C-5 demonstrate the usual routes of entry.

The patient and physician should both be in comfortable positions. Drapes are not generally necessary. The operator should wear gloves and observe customary precautions against biologic hazards. Great care must be taken with contaminated needles, and fluid should not be transferred in syringes with the needles still attached.

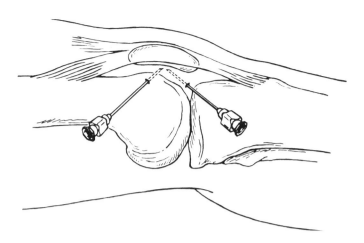

(Figure 7C-1)
Arthrocentesis of the knee. Entry is through the groove between the patella and the femur from either a medial (shown) or lateral approach at the superior third of the patella. Courtesy of David Neustadt.

Anatomic landmarks may be difficult to identify around a swollen joint, but comparison with the contralateral joint is helpful. Immediately before aspiration, the joint should be moved through its passive range of motion to resuspend its particulate contents. The skin should be cleaned of obvious dirt with soap and water. It is not usually necessary to shave the skin. A brief scrub with an alcohol pad, followed by an application of an iodine preparation, provides adequate protection. If desired, the skin can be marked before cleaning or an impression made with a closed retractable pen. To avoid losing the anatomic landmarks, it is best to keep one hand on the joint near the aspiration site to help orient the operator, to position or distract the joint, and to steady the syringe. It is a mistake to clean a vast area and then try to aspirate without such hands-on orientation.

The skin can be infiltrated with lidocaine to decrease the pain of penetration, particularly if the operator anticipates a difficult aspiration. However, this practice increases the materials used, prolongs the procedure, and can, in itself, be painful. Infiltration into the deeper, pain-sensitive structures of the capsule or periosteum risks injecting anesthetic into the joint space and may interfere with the results of the analysis. A simple alternative is to freeze the skin with a

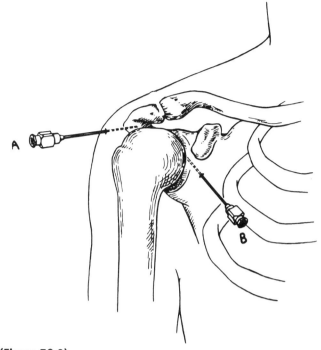

(Figure 7C-3)
Arthrocentesis of the shoulder. Entry may be (A) posterior, 1 inch below the posteriolateral pole of the acromion process, or (B) anterior, just lateral to the coracoid process. Courtesy of David Neustadt.

spray of ethyl chloride immediately before inserting the needle. This reduces the pain and is quite satisfactory for most patients.

It is a mistake to select a small needle with the intention of sparing the patient pain. Viscous fluid full of particulate material flows with difficulty, if at all, through needles smaller

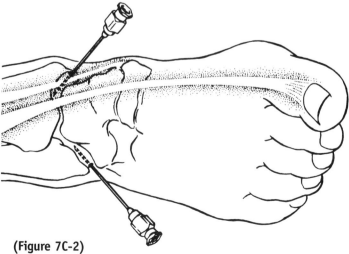

(Figure 7C-2)
Arthrocentesis of the ankle. Entry is anterior to the malleoli (medially or laterally) wherever the joint space can be identified, avoiding the dorsalis pedis artery and major tendons. Courtesy of David Neustadt.

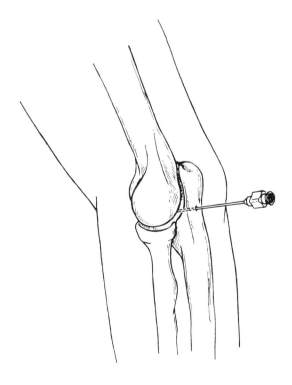

(Figure 7C-4)
Arthrocentesis of the elbow. Entry is lateral through the groove between the olecranon process and lateral epicondyle. Courtesy of David Neustadt.

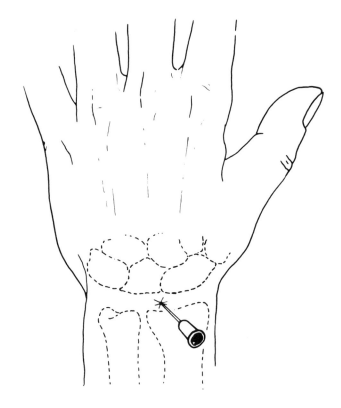

(Figure 7C-5)
Arthrocentesis of the wrist. Entry is on the dorsal aspect at the radio-carpal joint. Courtesy of David Neustadt.

than 20 gauge. In general, an 18- or 19-gauge needle is used for the knee and a 20-gauge needle for smaller joints. The size of the syringe should correlate with the estimated volume of the effusion. Large plastic syringes are hard to manipulate with one hand and can cause unnecessary patient discomfort. Breaking the initial resistance or "bead" of the syringe *before* insertion helps to prevent abrupt movement of the needle afterwards. The skin should be stretched slightly and the needle inserted deftly; gently aspirate and advance the needle until fluid appears in the syringe. If bone is encountered before fluid, the needle may be partially withdrawn and advanced in a different direction. Lateral traction on the skin and deeper tissues by the needle should be avoided. If after a few passes no fluid is obtained, the operator will need to decide whether no effusion was actually present, or whether another site or operator would be more productive.

Fluid frequently stops flowing into the syringe because of inadvertent movement or tissue encroachment onto the needle as the size of the joint space decreases. A slight adjustment of the needle may be in order, if it seems that fluid still remains in the joint space. The needle can also become obstructed. If there is no resistance, a very small volume can be reinjected, which may reestablish flow. For diagnostic aspirations, it is not necessary to remove all the fluid. An entire analysis with culture can be easily performed on 1-5 ml of synovial fluid.

It is best to avoid switching syringes in the middle of the procedure, since this opens the sterile path and increases the possibility of contamination. In addition, removing the needle from the hub may require considerable physical force and cause pain to the patient. If a new syringe must be used (as for injecting corticosteroids), a hemostat or other grasp-ing device to hold the hub steady is helpful. When injecting corticosteroids after arthrocentesis, it is important that the operator know the needle is still in the joint cavity. After the needle is withdrawn, manual pressure on the puncture site will spare the patient a tender bruise and is especially important when repeat aspirations are anticipated (as in infectious arthritis).

Complications

The most serious potential complication of arthrocentesis is iatrogenic infection in a previously sterile joint, but this is a highly unusual event. The likelihood of unsuspected infectious arthritis is many times greater than the estimated iatrogenic infection rate of 1 in 10,000. Often some bleeding occurs at the puncture site and presumably within the joint as well. Anticoagulation therapy by itself is not a contraindication for patients who develop acute arthritis. However, patients with serious coagulation disorders such as hemophilia have major complications from recurrent hemarthrosis. If diagnostic or therapeutic aspiration is necessary in such individuals, prophylactic treatment with the appropriate coagulation factors should be considered.

A potential but unquantifiable complication is direct injury to cartilage by the needle. Should such "divots" be taken, the cartilage will not heal and the area can serve as a nidus for further degenerative changes, particularly in a weight-bearing area of the joint. This possibility can be minimized by 1) not moving the needle from side to side; 2) selecting an aspiration site that will avoid or minimize potential contact with cartilage; 3) aspirating as the needle is advanced so that penetration is not deeper than necessary; and 4) not trying to get every last drop. An occasional patient (or observing companion) experiences a vasovagal episode during or after the procedure. It is best to have patients reclining or seated on an examining table during arthrocentesis and to take care when arising afterwards.

It is important to explain to patients the reasons for recommending arthrocentesis and its possible risks and to document that this has been done. In general, patients should be told that the chances of finding unsuspected infection or useful information far outweigh the very small risk of infection, bleeding, or even pain. Local custom or comfort level may suggest a signed consent form, but not all physicians use one.

SYNOVIAL FLUID TESTS

Historically, synovial fluids were classified according to gross appearance, WBC count, differential cell count, protein, glucose, mucin clot, viscosity, and other parameters. Fluids were classified in numbered groups as normal, noninflammatory, inflammatory, septic, and hemorrhagic. These classifications suffer from a lack of uniform inclusion criteria and terminology, and their diagnostic usefulness is limited because fluids from a single disorder may fall into almost any group. The crucial and correct messages from these older classifications include the following: the importance of differentiating inflammatory from noninflammatory arthritis; attempting to identify a specific cause of the inflammation; and exercising greater vigilance for infectious arthritis when the WBC count is high or the fluid otherwise looks purulent. Rather than assigning an outdated label, management strategies should be based primarily on the leukocyte and differential counts (Table 7C-1).

(Table 7C-1)
*Tests on synovial fluid ***

Always
    Note volume and gross appearance
    Look at wet preparation
    Conduct polarized light examination
    WBC concentration
Usually
    WBC differential count
When indicated by clinical findings
    Culture
    Gram stain
Don't bother
    Viscosity
    Mucin clot
    RBC count
    Protein
    Glucose
    Enzymes
    Complement
    Immune complexes
    Rheumatoid factor or ANA

* WBC = white blood cells; RBC = red blood cells; ANA = antinuclear antibodies

Gross inspection of synovial fluid begins at the time of aspiration. The operator should note whether blood appeared in the syringe only after the aspiration was underway, or whether the fluid was uniformly bloody from the start, indicating prior hemarthrosis (Table 7C-2). After aspiration, the fluid should be transferred to a glass tube anticoagulated with liquid ethylenediaminetetra-acetate (EDTA) or heparin for subsequent inspection, WBC counts, or microscopic and polarized light examination. Powdered anticoagulants of any kind should not be used because undissolved crystals hinder subsequent microscopic examination. When transferring the fluid from the aspirating syringe to a sterile vacuum tube for culture, the operator should use a new sterile needle. In no event should a needle used for transfer or injection of microcrystalline corticosteroids be used to transfer fluid, because this introduces confusing crystals into the fluid. Synovial fluid analysis should be done on the day of aspiration because cell counts and morphology change. Crystals are easily identifiable for a few days, however (9).

Normal and noninflammatory fluids are transparent and yellow or straw-colored, depending on the amount of albumin-bound bilirubin present. Inflammatory fluids are more strongly colored and vary according to the amount of protein, cells, and debris present. A commonly used test for clarity is to determine if newsprint can be read through the glass tube containing the fluid. Inflammatory fluid is usually translucent or opaque, and newsprint cannot be read through it. Cloudiness is not always the result of leukocytes, however, because other particulates can be abundant. Although a grayish or otherwise purulent appearance is cause for concern, there is no discrete gross appearance that distinguishes infected from noninfected fluid. Macroscopic fragments of material suspended in clear fluids can be extracted by pipette for subsequent microscopic inspection (1). Such large particulates provide useful information (Table 7C-3) and are good starting places to look for crystals.

Leukocyte Counts

Total WBC and differential counts should be performed on all synovial fluids removed for diagnostic purposes. The WBC count should be done manually using saline as a diluent. The high viscosity of synovial fluid and its suspended particulates cause artifacts when tested in automated instruments designed to process blood. Acid-containing diluents

(Table 7C-2)
Conditions associated with hemarthrosis

Trauma with or without fracture
Coagulation disorders
    Hemophilia
    von Willebrand's disease
    Anticoagulant therapy
    Other bleeding disorders
Thrombocytopenia
Essential thrombocytosis
Scurvy
Hemangioma or arteriovenous malformation
Pigmented villonodular synovitis
Tumor (metastatic or local)
Ehlers-Danlos syndrome
Pseudoxanthoma elasticum
Sickle cell disease
Following joint surgery
Munchausen's syndrome
Preexisting arthritis with any of the above
Idiopathic

(Table 7C-3)
Particulates in synovial fluid

Cells
Fibrin strands and clumps
Rice bodies
Collagen fibrils
Cartilage fragments
Synovial fragments
Adipose tissue cores from needle puncture
Crystals
    Monosodium urate monohydrate
    Calcium pyrophosphate dihydrate
    Apatite
    Cholesterol
    Calcium oxalate
Lipid globules and crystals
Bacteria and fungi
Amyloid fibrils
Immune complexes
Metal and plastic fragments from prostheses
Parasites
Unrecognizable "junk"

cause mucin to precipitate. Dilute (one-third normal) saline lyses erythrocytes and facilitates counting in the hemocytometer. Red blood cell counts are not helpful.

The absolute leukocyte count is the major discriminating factor between inflammatory and noninflammatory fluid. Additional information is provided by the differential leukocyte count. Traditionally, fluids with a WBC count <2000/mm³ are considered noninflammatory, although such fluids are seen in some patients with systemic inflammatory diseases such as SLE, scleroderma, early or inactive RA, and intercurrent crystal-induced arthritis (10,11). Noninflammatory fluids occur in other disorders besides osteoarthritis, including sickle cell disease, hypertrophic pulmonary osteoarthropathy, hypothyroidism, and amyloidosis.

The standard hemocytometer is not very accurate at low counts. With synovial fluid diluted 1:20 in a WBC pipette, a single cell in the counting chamber represents 200 cells/mm³ of whole fluid. A more meaningful result can be obtained in clear fluids by diluting only 1:10 in the same pipette. An alternative is to add a grain or two of purified hyaluronidase to the whole fluid. This rapidly decreases its viscosity so that undiluted fluid can be placed directly in the hemocytometer chamber and thin smears prepared on glass slides for staining. New approaches using supravital staining are also being investigated. When such special attention is given to fluids with low WBC counts, additional information of clinical usefulness can be obtained. For example, it appears that in uncomplicated osteoarthritis the usual WBC is <1000/mm³ and that fewer than 30% of these are neutrophils (6). Thus, leukocyte counts greater than these values should heighten the suspicion of an intercurrent inflammatory process or spur the examiner to look for crystals with more than the usual diligence.

Although there are other causes of very high WBC counts, fluids with a cell count of >100,000/mm³ should be assumed to be septic until proven otherwise. Even the presence of crystals in such highly inflammatory fluid does not rule out coexisting infection. Fluids with WBC counts between 50,000/mm³ and 100,000/mm³ are problematic (12). Some septic fluids are in this range, and fluids from patients with crystal-induced or idiopathic inflammatory arthritis (such as RA or Reiter's syndrome) are also occasionally >50,000/mm³. Patients with very high WBC counts need to be followed carefully and sometimes treated empirically pending culture results. A repeat aspiration 24 hours later may help clarify the diagnosis.

The differential leukocyte count frequently adds useful information. There are many different types of normal and abnormal resident or transient cell types in synovial fluid. Although special stains can be used to extract more detailed information about the nature of cells within the fluid (6), there is no clinical reason to routinely attempt to differentiate further than neutrophils and mononuclear cells. When, for one reason or another, the amount of fluid is insufficient for cell counts, the differential count alone can provide useful information. A noninflammatory fluid generally has <50% neutrophils. Infected fluids generally have >95% neutrophils, but many crystal-induced effusions also have such a high proportion. Rheumatoid arthritis fluids usually have <90% neutrophils, even when the absolute cell count is very high. As an example of how the differential count might be weighted, a total WBC count of 20,000 with 98% neutrophils without other known cause should still make the physician

consider septic arthritis. This situation can occur in the immunosuppressed patient.

The presence of lupus erythematosus cells in a fresh synovial fluid smear strongly suggests a diagnosis of SLE, although these cells can form in other diseases. Reiter's cells (large histiocytes that have ingested neutrophils or other cells) were originally described in Reiter's syndrome, but they occur frequently in other conditions. In fact, phagocytosis of effete cells by macrophages is the normal and usual physiologic method of removal. Rheumatoid arthritis cells (also called ragocytes) are neutrophils with refractile peripheral inclusions that contain immune complexes and complement. Originally described in RA, cells with this morphology are particularly abundant in seropositive RA but are not considered diagnostic. Sickled red cells indicate the presence of the hemoglobinopathy in either the homozygous or heterozygous state.

Culture

Very turbid fluids or those in which septic arthritis is suspected for other reasons should be sent for culture. It is probably better to err on the side of caution in culturing fluids, but it is not appropriate to culture all fluids. Contamination does occur (6) and can cause unneeded confusion when a patient has a low probability of infection. If the results of the WBC count or differential are truly a surprise, the joint can be re-aspirated promptly for culture. If synovial fluid removed prior to a therapeutic injection of corticosteroids looks unusually turbid, it is better to send the fluid for cell count and culture before injection. It is not necessary to culture routinely for fungal infection or tuberculosis, but in the appropriate clinical situation of refractory monarthritis or oligoarthritis, these studies can be added. In gonococcal disease, the large majority of joint fluid cultures are bacteriologically sterile, although bacterial antigens or products can be demonstrated by special techniques.

Gram stains of synovial fluid should be performed when infection is suspected. Many fluids are so spectacularly positive that little experience is required for interpretation. However, overly thick smears, precipitated stain, pyknotic extracellular or intracellular nuclear material, and debris can create traps for the unwary. False-positive results do occur.

Wet Preparation

All fluids should be examined under a coverslip by routine microscopy for cells and particulate material. Although polarizing light microscopy is the gold standard for identifying crystals (13), the helpfulness of a simple light microscope should not be ignored (14). Unless crystals are very few, they are visible on stained and unstained slides, and at least a preliminary identification based on shape can be made. In fact, refractile CPPD crystals are more easily seen with a good light microscope than a poor polarizing one.

In polarized light microscopy, a crystal is birefringent if it shines white against the dark background produced by two polarizing plates (3). If a first-order red compensating filter is also placed between the polarizing plates, the background becomes reddish. Depending on its orientation in the visual field, a birefringent crystal will appear yellow or blue against a red background. The color of an individual crystal, compared to its orientation with the manufactured intrinsic axis of the filter, determines the direction of birefringence. By convention, the direction of birefringence is designated as either positive or negative. It is important to recognize that the adjectives "positive" and "negative" refer to the *direction* of the birefringence, not to whether the crystal is birefringent at all! A crystal that is not birefringent can have no direction associated with it. Confusion intrinsic to this terminology occasionally appears in reports from clinical laboratories. Because errors are also commonly made determining the direction of birefringence, laboratories attempting this should keep a supply of urate crystals on hand to check the setup of their microscope.

Monosodium urate crystals are needle-shaped or elongated with blunt ends. They are strongly birefringent—brilliantly bright against the dark background. The direction of the birefringence is negative (ie, negatively birefringent). CPPD crystals in the shape of parallelograms or chunky rectangles are more weakly birefringent, and are positively birefringent in compensated polarized light microscopy. Crystals have the same diagnostic significance whether they are intracellular or extracellular, but in general they are easier to find and less likely to be confused with artifacts when they are sought within cells.

The number of different crystals associated with human disease is increasing and includes calcium oxalate in renal failure, protein crystals in dysproteinemic states, cholesterol in chronic inflammatory effusions, and hydroxyapatite. Hydroxyapatite by itself is not detected by polarized light microscopy, but when present in large amounts it is visible as amorphous particulates. Staining of synovial fluid with alizarin red identifies calcium-containing material, which suggests the presence of apatite (2), but this technique has not yet found a place in routine clinical practice. In any event, the significance of apatite in effusions such as in osteoarthritis is not fully understood (13).

A syndrome has been described of acute arthritis associated with intracellular and extracellular positively birefringent spherical inclusions that appear to be lipid in nature (15,16). These structures are shaped like a Maltese cross, and, although not rare, they remain poorly understood. The direction of the birefringence of the circular object is determined by the direction of the yellow and blue arms of the cross seen in compensated polarized microscopy. There are isolated case reports of negatively birefringent spherical forms of apatite (17) and urate, but the significance of these unique observations is unknown. It is helpful to keep samples of known crystal on hand to calibrate the scope and confirm the direction of birefringence.

TESTS OF NO, LIMITED, OR UNCERTAIN VALUE

Glucose and Lactate

Measuring glucose in synovial fluid was traditional, particularly to assist in the diagnosis of septic arthritis. Lactic acid determination served a similar purpose. In severely inflamed joints such as most (but not all) septic joints, glucose is very low and lactic acid is high. The alterations in these metabolites reflect the increased consumption of glucose by articular tissues and a decrease in effective circulation to the synovium, representing a switch to anaerobic metabolism. These changes in joint physiology reflect the *degree* of inflammation in the joint, but not its etiology. In those cases of severe intra-articular inflammation for which the physician needs the most help in ruling against infection, glucose and

lactate measurements are the least useful. Low-to-absent glucose levels can occur in RA and crystal-induced arthritis (18). If glucose measurements are made, it is important to use specimen tubes containing fluoride, since leukocytes convert glucose into lactate acid in vitro. Although the defining clinical studies were performed on fasting patients to allow equilibrium comparison with serum levels, deferring arthrocentesis for this purpose is not appropriate.

Viscosity

Description of synovial fluid viscosity is a time-honored assay. The easiest way to estimate viscosity is to allow a few drops of fluid to drip from the aspirating syringe. A long "string" implies a high viscosity. The traditional reason for estimating viscosity was to differentiate between inflammatory (low viscosity) and noninflammatory fluids. However, when quantitative methods of measuring viscosity are used, the test fails even this simple request. An extremely viscous fluid suggests hypothyroidism or SLE. Synovial fluid has all the potential biohazards of other body fluids, and the estimation of viscosity by manipulating a drop between the fingers is an outdated and completely unnecessary procedure.

Mucin Clot

The mucin clot test estimates the density and friability of the precipitate that forms when synovial fluid is placed in dilute acetic acid. A good or excellent clot implies high-molecular weight hyaluronic acid and normal hyaluronate–protein interactions. A fair or poor clot imputes an inflammatory arthritis. Unfortunately, there are no standard criteria for the performance of the test, and its endpoints are overly subjective. The mucin clot test was once part of the diagnostic criteria for RA, but the best use of the test today is with bloody fluids or fluids of uncertain anatomic origin. The presence of a definite mucin clot suggests only that it is synovial fluid.

Protein

The custom of measuring protein concentration as part of synovial fluid analysis was carried over from evaluating pleural and peritoneal fluids. Although low protein may be useful to differentiate between transudates and exudates in pleural fluid, the equivalent of a joint transudate (edema) is seldom encountered. In any event, there is no useful difference in total protein among any of the major groups of arthritis, including RA and OA. Thus, total protein measurement in synovial fluid is not recommended. The rarely encountered true joint transudate is recognizable by the clinical setting and by the colorless nature of the joint fluid.

Immunologic Tests

Because most synovial fluid immunoglobulin is derived from plasma, any patient with a positive serologic test result may also have a positive result in synovial fluid. Theoretically, seronegative patients could have a positive result in joint fluid as a result of local synthesis of immunoglobulin. Although there may be some research interest in this potential, it is rarely if ever demonstrated and has no clinical value at this time. In fact, because of synovial fluid viscosity and its other physical–chemical properties, the chemical and immunologic protocols now in use for testing serum and plasma do not necessarily apply to synovial fluid.

Measurement of immune complexes and complement proteins in joint tissue and fluids has an important role in research. Low complement levels are common in rheumatoid arthritis because of activation by immune complexes. However, low levels are seen in some patients with crystal-induced arthritis and even with infection. Levels are low in most fluids from SLE patients, but there is no evidence of complement activation to explain this finding. High levels of complement have been described in Reiter's syndrome and psoriatic arthritis, but when corrected for total protein or globulin content, these relative differences disappear. Despite much that has been published about these tests, there is no convincing reason to perform them in a clinical setting.

SYNOVIAL BIOPSY

It is occasionally necessary to obtain a biopsy of the synovial membrane (the connective tissue lining of the joint). In truth, pieces of tissue large enough to examine are commonly found in routine synovial fluid aspirations. Closed (and blind) needle biopsy has always been available to rheumatologists but has not found widespread use (19). With advances in arthroscopic techniques including smaller instruments, guided biopsy through small incisions is possible without the need for open arthrotomy. These tools have been adopted by some rheumatologists (20), but their role in either research or clinical medicine remains to be defined.

It is not possible to enunciate a simple set of guidelines for synovial biopsy. It is usually performed in the setting of chronic nontraumatic synovitis limited to a single or very few joints when a diagnosis is necessary but not otherwise possible. This situation is infrequent in most rheumatologic and general medical practices. Because these cases are usually difficult, consultation with an experienced or specialist physician is advised. The most common indication is to diagnose tuberculous or fungal joint infections, because synovial fluid cultures and smears are often negative. Granulomata in blind biopsies supports a diagnosis of chronic sarcoid arthritis.

Synovial biopsy is not necessary for identifying common bacterial pathogens such as *Staphylococcus*, *Streptococcus*, *Gonococcus*, or gram-negative bacteria. Nor is it indicated for diagnosing RA. The original American Rheumatology Association (now called American College of Rheumatology) criteria for RA included "compatible synovial pathology," but thickening of the synovial cell layer, increased vascularity, fibrin deposition, lymphoid follicles, and infiltration with a variety of chronic inflammatory cells are nonspecific findings.

Biopsy plays an important role in pigmented villonodular synovitis, multiple synovial chondromatoses, and plant-thorn and other foreign body synovitis. Primary or metastatic tumors also occasionally involve the joint. Large tissue samples and biopsy for these disorders is best left in the hands of an operative arthroscopist. Although hemochromatosis, ochronosis, and amyloidosis have distinctive synovial pathology, clinical findings (including synovial fluid analysis) are usually sufficient for diagnosis. There are still some limited but important indications for synovial biopsy. The question is no longer whether the procedure can be easily done but how often it alters diagnosis, patient management, or other outcomes.

PETER HASSELBACHER, MD

1. Hasselbacher P: Synovial fluid analysis. In Utsinger P, Zvaifler N, Ehrlich G (eds): Rheumatoid Arthritis, Etiology, Diagnosis, Management. Philadelphia, JB Lippincott, 1985, pp 193-208

2. Schumacher HR, Jr, Reginato AJ: Atlas of Synovial Fluid Analysis and Crystal Identification. Philadelphia, Lea & Febiger, 1991

3. Gatter RA, Schumacher HR, Jr: A Practical Handbook of Joint Fluid Analysis, 2nd ed. Philadelphia, Lea & Febiger, 1991

4. Shmerling RH: Synovial fluid analysis: a critical reappraisal. Rheum Dis Clin North Am 20:503-512, 1994

5. Eisenberg JM, Schumacher HR, Jr, Davidson PK, Kaufmann L: Usefulness of synovial fluid analysis in the evaluation of joint effusions. Arch Intern Med 144:715-719, 1984

6. Freemont AJ, Denton J, Chuck A, Holt PJ, Davies M: Diagnostic value of synovial fluid microscopy: a reassessment and rationalisation. Ann Rheum Dis 50:101-107, 1991

7. Hasselbacher P: Variation in synovial fluid analysis by hospital laboratories. Arthritis Rheum 30:637-642, 1987

8. James MJ, Cleland LG, Rofe AM, Leslie AL: Intraarticular pressure and the relationship between synovial perfusion and metabolic demand. J Rheumatol 17:521-527, 1990

9. Kerolous G, Clayburne G, Schumacher HR, Jr: Is it mandatory to examine synovial fluids promptly after arthrocentesis? Arthritis Rheum 32:271-278, 1989

10. Pascual E: Persistence of monosodium urate crystals and low-grade inflammation in the synovial fluid of patients with untreated gout. Arthritis Rheum 34:141-145, 1991

11. Louthrenoo W, Sieck M, Clayburne G, Rothfuss S, Schumacher HR, Jr.: Supravital staining of cells in noninflammatory synovial fluids: analysis of the effect of crystals on cell populations. J Rheumatol 18:409-413, 1991

12. Krey P, Bailen D: Synovial fluid leukocytosis: a study of extremes. Am J Med 67:436, 1979

13. Gordon C, Swan A, Dieppe P: Detection of crystals in synovial fluids by light microscopy: sensitivity and reliability. Ann Rheum Dis 48:737-742, 1989

14. Pascual E, Tovar J, Ruiz MT: The ordinary light microscope: an appropriate tool for provisional detection and identification of crystals in synovial fluid. Ann Rheum Dis 48:983-985, 1989

15. Reginato AJ, Schumacher HR, Jr, Allan DA, Rabinowitz JL: Acute monoarthritis associated with lipid liquid crystals. Ann Rheum Dis 44:537-543, 1985

16. Gardner GC, Terkeltaub RA: Acute monoarthritis associated with intracellular positively birefringent Maltese cross appearing spherules. J Rheumatol 16:394-396, 1989

17. Beaudet F, de Medicis R, Magny P, Lussier A: Acute apatite podagra with negative birefringent spherulites in the synovial fluid. J Rheumatol 20:1975-1978, 1993

18. Wheeler AP, Graham BS: Pseudogout presenting with low synovial fluid glucose: identification of crystals by gram stain. Am J Med Sci 289:68-69, 1985

19. Schumacher HR, Jr.: Needle biopsy of the synovial membrane: experience with the Parker-Pearson technique. N Engl J Med 286:416-419, 1972

20. Szachnowski P, Wei N, Arnold W, Cohen L: Complications of office based arthroscopy of the knee. J Rheumatol 22:1722-1725, 1995

D. ARTHROSCOPY

Arthroscopy is an interventional procedure that permits visualization of superficial intra-articular structures (1). The knee is the joint most frequently examined arthroscopically; however, arthroscopes have been placed into nearly all joints, including temporomandibular, interphalangeal, and spinal facet joints. Regardless of the joint examined, the procedure has utility for diagnostic, therapeutic, and research indications.

Examination of cartilage surfaces is best performed by direct arthroscopic visualization. It is considerably superior to plain radiographs and likely better than magnetic resonance imaging (2,3) (Fig. 7D-1). Mechanical abnormalities including meniscal tears, cruciate lesions, cartilage fractures, osteochondritis dessicans, and loose bodies can be readily visualized. Furthermore, visually directed biopsy can be easily performed arthroscopically and is of considerable use in the patient who has an undefined arthritis. Visually directed biopsies allow the clinician to sample several areas of abnormal synovium, making it superior to blind biopsies, since many synovial lesions are patchy in character (Fig. 7D-2). Material obtained at directed biopsies may lead to the diagnosis of indolent infection (tuberculosis or fungi), metabolic abnormalities (ochronosis, hemochromatosis), or neoplasia (pigmented villonodular synovitis, metastatic cancer). Coupled with newer laboratory testing, synovial biopsies may also reveal evidence of infections with organisms responsible for reactive arthritis or Lyme disease.

Therapeutically, arthroscopic interventions have largely replaced open arthrotomy for a number of procedures. Repair of symptomatic meniscal lesions or cruciate ligaments is a common example. Although synovial plicae are frequently seen in normal knees, removal of an inflamed plica occasionally alleviates symptoms in arthritis. In patients with rheumatoid arthritis or other forms of inflammatory arthritis, synovectomy may lead to symptomatic improve-

ment, although it is not yet clear that this will actually modify the disease process. Symptoms of osteoarthritis also improve after arthroscopy and joint lavage. The mechanism of this improvement has not been elucidated. Debridement of abnormal cartilage is still occasionally performed, but whether this procedure is less effective than lavage is not clear. Finally, septic arthritis that has not responded to antibiotics and closed needle drainage can be successfully treated via arthroscopic drainage.

Other joints besides the knee have been subject to arthroscopic therapeutic interventions. Oral surgeons have used arthroscopy to debride and repair the temporomandibular joint. Shoulders, ankles, elbows, and wrists can also be investigated and debrided arthroscopically. In the shoulder, rotator cuff lesions, with or without acromioplasty or lesions of the glenoid labrum, can be performed arthroscopically. Even hips have been entered with extended arthroscopes. Arthroscopic equipment has also been used in treating other musculoskeletal disorders. Carpal tunnel release is such an example: the joint itself is not specifically entered, but arthroscopic equipment produces equivalent results to an open procedure and is less invasive.

Finally, the arthroscope may develop into an indispensable research tool. Direct visualization and grading of cartilage and synovium can be readily accomplished on multiple occasions during a therapeutic trial (4,5). Furthermore, arthroscopic sampling of synovium for ex vivo investigation is a useful mechanism for evaluating therapeutic interventions.

In general, arthroscopic evaluation of a joint is well tolerated. Infection rates are well under 1%, presumably due to the high volume of fluid used for lavage. Effusions are common,

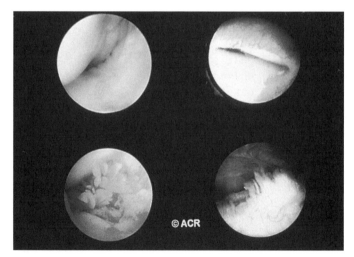

(Figure 7D-2)
Rheumatoid arthritis: synovitis, knees (arthroscopic view). **Upper left:** *This arthroscopic view demonstrates normal articular surfaces and medial meniscus.* **Upper right:** *An example of early rheumatoid arthritis shows the characteristic hyperemic proliferative synovium with normal cartilage.* **Lower right:** *A more advanced hyperemic and villous synovium is seen in the suprapatellar pouch.* **Lower left:** *Edematous hypertrophied villi are characteristic of more advanced rheumatoid arthritis. Reprinted from Clinical Slide Collection on the Rheumatic Diseases, with permission of the American College of Rheumatology.*

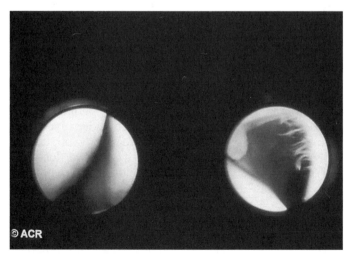

(Figure 7D-1)
Degenerative joint disease: knees (arthroscopic views). **Left:** *This arthroscopic view shows early loss of articular cartilage of the femoral condyle.* **Right:** *There is fibrillation of the patellar cartilage. Reprinted from Clinical Slide Collection on the Rheumatic Diseases, with permission of the American College of Rheumatology.*

particularly in patients who have had therapeutic procedures, but they generally subside without further intervention. Stasis, particularly in conjunction with tourniquets, may lead to venous thrombosis. Other neurovascular or ligamentous complications are infrequent and usually due to extensive tourniquet time or vigorous stress on the joint. Improvements in the instruments have made breakage within the joint rare.

Arthroscopic equipment has continued to evolve. Glass lens systems have been the standard and provide excellent visualization. Their size and flexibility are somewhat limiting, however. Recently, systems have been developed using fiber optic technology, allowing extraordinary flexibility. Using fiber optic technology, arthroscopes with diameters of less than 1 mm have been developed. As might be expected, the field of view of these instruments is smaller than the larger glass lens systems, and visual quality is not as high.

However, joints can be easily visualized with only local anesthesia. As this technology improves, visual quality and perhaps field of view will improve as well.

WARREN D. BLACKBURN, JR., MD

1. Halbrecht JL, Jackson DW: Office arthroscopy: a diagnostic alternative. J Arthroscop Rel Surg 8: 320-326, 1992
2. Fife RS, Brandt KD, Braunstein EM, et al: Relationship between arthroscopic evidence of cartilage damage and radiographic evidence of joint space narrowing in early OA of the knee. Arthritis Rheum 34:377-381, 1991
3. Blackburn WD, Rominger M, Loose L, Bernreuter WK: Arthroscopic evaluation of knee articular cartilage: A comparison with plain radiographs and magnetic resonance imaging. J Rheumatol 21:675-679, 1994
4. Ike RW and O'Rourke KS: Compartment directed physical examination of the knee can predict articular cartilage abnormalities disclosed by needle arthroscopy. Arthritis Rheum 37:917-925, 1995
5. Blackburn WD, Chivers S, and Bernreuter W: Cartilage imaging in osteoarthritis. Seminars Arthritis and Rheum 25:273-281, 1996

E. IMAGING TECHNIQUES

Imaging techniques may aid in making a diagnosis, permit an objective assessment of the severity of disease and its response to treatment, and promote new understanding of the disease process. Imaging modalities that are important in rheumatology include plain radiography, computed radiography (CR), conventional tomography, computed tomography (CT), magnetic resonance imaging (MRI), ultrasound, radionuclide imaging, arthrography, bone densitometry, and angiography.

A basic knowledge of the merits and limitations of these techniques is essential in selecting the most appropriate and cost-effective imaging. This chapter reviews the basic imaging techniques with regard to their spatial and contrast resolution (which determine what structures are well visualized), radiation dose to the patient, availability, interpretational expertise required, and specific uses in assessing musculoskeletal signs and symptoms.

CONVENTIONAL RADIOGRAPHY

The conventional radiographic examination is the starting point for most imaging evaluations in the rheumatic disorders, even when other studies such as MRI are expected to follow. The cost is low and spatial resolution is very high, permitting good visualization of trabecular detail and tiny bone erosions. When necessary, resolution can be further enhanced by magnification techniques and film–screen combinations optimized for detail. However, contrast resolution is poor compared with CT and MRI. This limitation is especially noticeable when trying to evaluate soft tissue. Although plain radiography is a useful tool to assess the effect of a soft tissue mass on nearby bone and to detect calcification within soft tissue, this technique is not suitable for evaluating soft tissue.

Examination of peripheral structures such as the hands and feet delivers a low radiation dose to the patient, and serial studies can be performed without concern about excessive radiation exposure. However, studies of central structures such as the lumbar spine and thick areas of the body expose patients to high radiation doses. Close proximity to the gonads and to bone marrow increases the potential detrimental effects to the patient. Whenever possible, the pelvic region of pregnant or potentially pregnant women should not be exposed to x-rays, and radiation to children should be stringently minimized. When such studies are necessary in these patients, radiation physicists can calculate the minimum radiation dose required for the imaging study. These same basic principles apply to all other x-ray imaging techniques.

Conventional radiography is widely available and convenient. Moreover, a vast fund of knowledge about plain radiographic findings in various rheumatic diseases is available (Figs. 7E-1–3).

COMPUTED RADIOGRAPHY

Computed radiography is a recent innovation for obtaining images that look like conventional radiographs (1). Instead of x-ray film, CR uses a photosensitive phosphor plate to create a digital image, rather than the analog image of conventional radiography. At present, CR images are somewhat higher in cost and lower in resolution than conventional radiographs. However, the resolution is adequate for many routine joint evaluations and can be improved by magnification, if necessary, for special tasks. The radiation dose is slightly lower than for conventional radiography.

Advantages of CR include the ability to manipulate images electronically and to display images in several remote areas simultaneously. Image manipulation permits technically excellent final images to be obtained under adverse circumstances. For this reason, CR is currently popular in emergency departments and intensive care units, locations where it is often difficult to obtain optimal radiographic exposures. The ability to manipulate digital data could also be useful to researchers wishing to make automated measurements on radiographs and to clinicians wishing to send images via the Internet.

The resolution of CR can be improved and conventional high-resolution radiographs can be converted into digital format. CT, MRI, and ultrasound images are acquired in digital form, and all have a similar transport and manipulation capability. Digital images appear to be the future of imaging—once rapid transmission, cost-effective storage, and easy retrieval are realities. Another advantage of this tech-

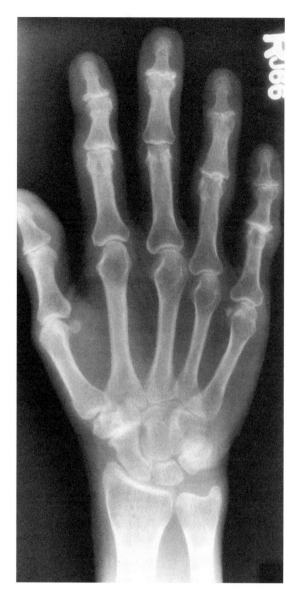

(Figure 7E-1)
Typical plain radiographic findings in osteoarthritis of the hand showing asymmetric joint narrowing with osteophyte formation. The distal interphalangeal joints and first carpometacarpal joint are most commonly involved.

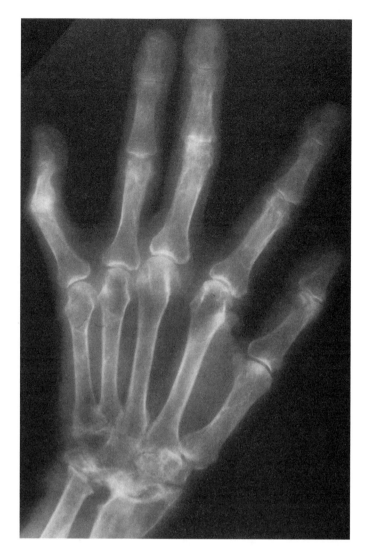

(Figure 7E-2)
Rheumatoid arthritis of the hand showing osteoporosis and severe erosive changes of distal radioulnar, wrist, and intercarpal joints. Some alignment abnormalities of the fingers are present.

nology is the elimination of the "lost" radiograph, a major waste of time and money.

CONVENTIONAL TOMOGRAPHY

Conventional tomography is a technique whereby both the film and the x-ray source are moved during radiographic exposure in such a manner that one plane through the structure of interest remains in focus on the resultant radiograph. This technique and CT are especially useful in areas of complex anatomy and where overlying structures obscure the anatomy.

Tomography is similar in cost to CT. Resolution of bone structures is slightly better than for CT, whereas visualization of soft tissues is much poorer. Sometimes the primary imaging plane for conventional tomography is especially advantageous for demonstrating pathologic features, such as a fracture or other abnormality of the odontoid process of C2 or pseudoarthrosis in a spinal fusion. Where available, conventional tomography is still useful in limited circumstances, but CT has generally replaced this technique. Radi-

ation dose is higher than for an equivalent CT study and should be considered carefully.

COMPUTED TOMOGRAPHY

Although relatively expensive, CT is less costly than MRI. The spatial resolution is better than MRI but inferior to that of conventional radiography. CT demonstrates soft tissue abnormalities far better than conventional radiography but not as well as MRI. CT is widely available, and many physicians are expert in its interpretation.

CT is an excellent technique for evaluating degenerative disc disease of the spine and possible disc herniations in older patients, in whom radiation dose is less critical than in young patients. Bony impingement on the spinal canal and neural foramina is more easily evaluated than with MRI. CT myelography and CT with intravenous contrast enhancement are other tomographic studies used to evaluate disc disease and other spinal diseases. High-quality MRI, if available, is preferred as the second study for investigating disc disease (following plain radiography), but CT is a good alternative and may be useful in circumstances where additional information about osteophytes is important. Else-

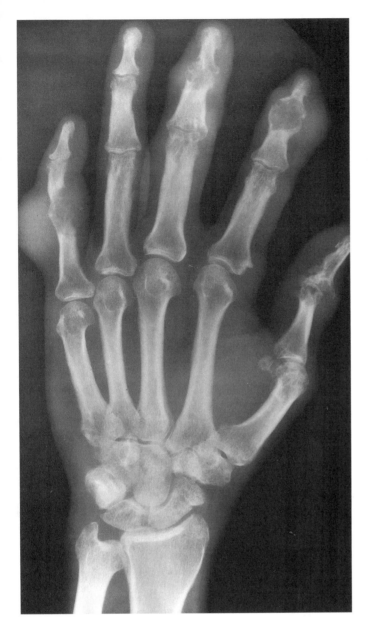

(Figure 7E-3)
Advanced changes of gout in the hand. Note soft tissue masses due to tophi and the large, sharply defined bone erosions, some not immediately at the joint. Scattered distribution of changes is typical.

where in the musculoskeletal system, CT is useful for evaluating structures in areas of complex anatomy where overlying structures obscure the view on conventional radiographs. Examples include tarsal coalitions not visible on plain radiographs (Fig. 7E-4); sacroiliitis, especially that of infectious origin (Fig. 7E-5); and articular collapse of the femoral head following osteonecrosis, indicating the need for joint replacement rather than a core procedure. The sternoclavicular joint, which is notoriously difficult to see on conventional radiography, is quite visible with CT.

The radiation dose from CT is relatively high compared with a single plain radiograph of the same region, but the radiation dose is comparable when several conventional radiographic views of the same area are required. Consequently, the dose is less than for conventional tomography in many circumstances.

If the correct initial data are obtained by appropriately adjusting the location and thickness of the slices, images can be

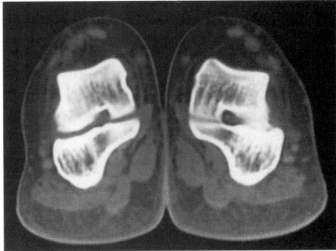

(Figure 7E-4)
Middle-aged woman with rigid flat foot and suspected tarsal coalition. Plain radiographs of the left foot did not demonstrate the coalition. CT scan shows the talocalcaneal coalition on the left, between the sustentaculum of the calcaneus and the talus above.

satisfactorily reconstructed in almost any plane. Three-dimensional images can be obtained, which may aid in evaluating abnormalities of the pelvis and other areas of complex anatomy (2). In spiral CT, the data for many images is acquired during a single breath-hold. This produces better images of joints affected by respiratory motion in the thorax.

Because a number of rheumatologic disorders are associated with pulmonary abnormalities, it is appropriate to note that high-resolution CT of the lung may reveal details of disease not seen on thicker CT slices of the thorax. The demonstration of "ground glass" infiltrates connotes an active process that may respond to treatment (3).

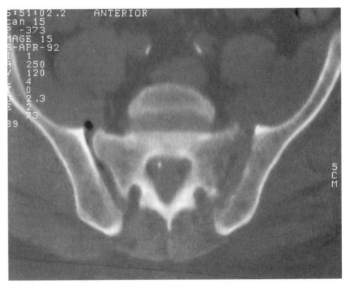

(Figure 7E-5)
A 67-year-old man with diabetes and left hip pain. Plain radiographs demonstrated no abnormalities. CT scan shows marked erosion and widening of the left sacroiliac joint. Blood cultures were positive for Escherichia coli, *and surgical drainage was performed. Note the "vacuum cleft" in the right sacroiliac joint, a common degenerative phenomenon in middle-aged and older persons.*

MAGNETIC RESONANCE IMAGING

MRI has brought huge advances to musculoskeletal imaging because of its ability to image soft tissue structures not visible on conventional radiographs. The technique derives structural information from the density of protons in tissue and the relationship of these protons to their immediate surroundings. It is a complex technique that involves changing the strength and timing of magnetic field gradients, as well as altering radiofrequency pulses and sampling the emitted energy. By altering these factors appropriately, varying amounts of T1 and T2 weighting are imparted to the images. As a result, MRI highlights different types of tissue and metabolic states. Altering these parameters can produce radically different images of the same anatomic site. Because x-ray images, such as CT, map the density of electrons in tissue, these images are often intuitively easier to grasp than are MR images for someone already familiar with conventional radiography.

MRI is relatively more expensive than other imaging studies, largely because of the cost of equipment and the time required to perform the studies. In the future, more attention will probably be given to tailored, limited imaging sequences, which potentially could lower the cost. Newer, faster imaging sequences continue to be developed, which may reduce the time and cost of MRI, as well as provide dynamic studies of joint motion.

MRI is free of the hazards of ionizing radiation, a major advantage in examining central portions of the body where x-ray studies require the highest radiation doses. It has several small hazards of its own, however (4). The strong magnetic field can move metal objects such as surgically implanted vascular clips and foreign metal in the eyes, cause pacemaker malfunction, heat metal objects and produce burns if wire loops are within the magnetic field, and draw metal objects into the magnet. Metallic objects in the vicinity of the magnetic field can also compromise the quality of MRI images, so operators must screen patients and visitors carefully. Patients with claustrophobia may be unable to tolerate being confined during the procedure, a problem also seen with CT, although to a lesser degree. More open configurations for the magnet have been tested to circumvent this problem, but these devices vary in their ability to produce high-quality images. On rare occasions, a patient may experience an unfavorable reaction to gadolinium, a contrast agent used in some MRI studies. Finally, hearing protection should be provided for the patient because application of gradient fields is noisy.

MRI is now widely available, and expertise in its interpretation is growing rapidly. However, studies can vary considerably from one imaging center to another, which can make interpretation of imaging sequences made elsewhere difficult.

Spatial resolution using the latest MRI equipment rivals CT, and the contrast resolution in soft tissues is better than any other modality. Soft tissue joint structures such as the menisci and cruciate ligaments of the knee are clearly demonstrated (Fig. 7E-6). The synovium can be imaged, especially using paramagnetic intravenous contrast agents such as gadolinium. Joint effusions, popliteal cysts, ganglion cysts, meniscal cysts, and bursitis are clearly imaged (Fig. 7E-7), and the integrity of tendons can be assessed (5). MRI is becoming increasingly popular for evaluating ligaments between the carpal bones and the triangular fibrocartilage (6).

Calcifications in the soft tissues are not seen as well as in x-ray images because of their low emitted signal. It was initially supposed that bone, which also emits low signal, might pose a problem, but because of the high-signal bone marrow, MRI is extremely sensitive to subtle bony abnormalities. In fact, microfractures due to trauma or stress—often referred to as bone bruises—were essentially unknown before MRI. Now, recognizing their presence is quite important. For example, much of the pain accompanying some acute meniscal tears may be caused by associated bone bruises. When the bruise heals, the pain disappears, despite the persistent meniscal tear. This finding could have important implications for therapy. It also helps explain why MRI of the knee in older people often reveals asymptomatic meniscal tears. The pattern of bone bruises is also closely related to ligamentous injuries.

Following plain radiography, MRI is an excellent method to study the spine and its contents, such as in cases of suspected disc herniation (Fig. 7E-8), particularly in young patients, because it does not employ ionizing radiation.

MRI is the study of choice for diagnosing osteonecrosis (Fig. 7E-9). Osteonecrosis can mimic other causes of joint pain, especially in the hip. Early in the course of disease, plain radiographs show no abnormalities. MRI is also the best method for evaluating the extent of soft tissue and bone neoplasms and has generally replaced CT in this role (7), although plain radiographs are still the mainstay for diagnosing bone neoplasms. CT may also be useful for identifying

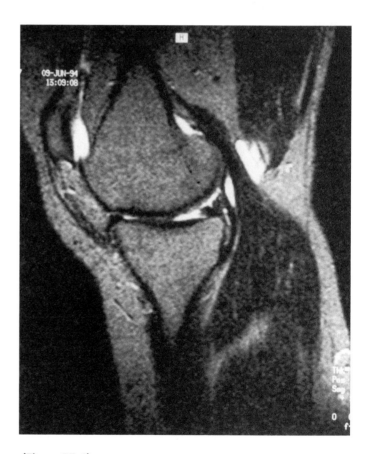

(Figure 7E-6)

A 47-year-old woman with knee pain. Sagittal T2-weighted MRI shows a high-signal joint effusion, a small popliteal cyst, and multiple tears of the posterior horn of the medial meniscus, which normally has a smooth, triangular configuration.

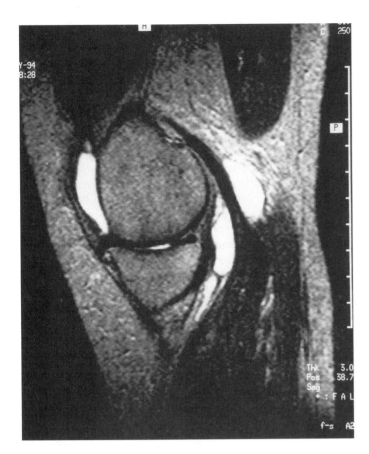

(Figure 7E-7)
A 44-year-old woman with knee pain and swelling. Sagittal T2-weighted MRI shows joint effusion and a popliteal cyst.

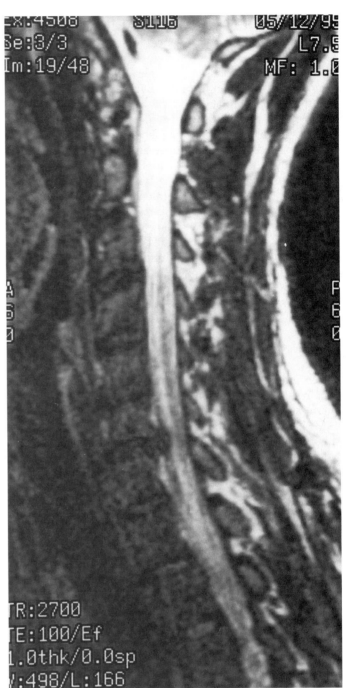

(Figure 7E-8)
A 29-year-old radiology resident experienced sudden neck pain and loss of left arm strength during weight lifting. Sagittal T2-weighted MRI demonstrates a herniated disc at C6-C7 on the left side.

characteristic matrix calcifications that are helpful in diagnosing this type of neoplasm.

MRI is sensitive to the presence of bone infection because of alterations in the marrow signal (8). It is a good choice for evaluating a localized area of suspected osteomyelitis, although radionuclide bone scan is preferred for assessing a multifocal hematogenous process. Small studies have shown variable results for MRI in diagnosing osteomyelitis of the foot in diabetic patients and in differentiating osteomyelitis and neuropathic arthropathy, which is very difficult with other imaging techniques. MRI can also identify soft tissue abscesses.

Muscle abnormalities such as tears and contusions can be identified on MRI. The activity of different muscles during joint motion can be studied by noting signal changes that occur with muscle activity. MRI is the study of choice for evaluating osteochondritis dissecans when information is needed about whether or not a bone fragment is attached.

Alterations in joint cartilage are visible on MRI. Although direct observation with arthroscopy is more sensitive to small superficial changes, refinements are being made constantly that improve the images (9). Certainly MRI provides a useful noninvasive research technique; however, the detection of small abnormalities is clinically useful only if it alters therapy. Medical therapy is usually employed until a joint requires replacement, which can be diagnosed with plain radiographs.

In certain circumstances, MRI is cost effective as the primary method of investigating the knee when internal derangement is suspected, since arthroscopy proves unnecessary in a large percentage of cases (10).

SCINTIGRAPHIC TECHNIQUES

Scintigraphy following intravenous administration of agents such as 99m technetium methylene diphosphonate (^{99m}Tc MDP) for bone scans, ^{99m}Tc sulphur colloid for bone marrow scans, 67 Gallium citrate (^{67}Ga citrate), and leukocytes labeled with 111 Indium (^{111}In-labeled WBCs) are useful for evaluating a variety of musculoskeletal disorders. These studies are similar in cost to CT and deliver a radiation dose similar to a CT scan of the abdomen. Scintigraphy is quite sensitive for detecting many disease processes, and the entire body can be imaged at once. The technique is nonspecific, however, because a number of processes may cause

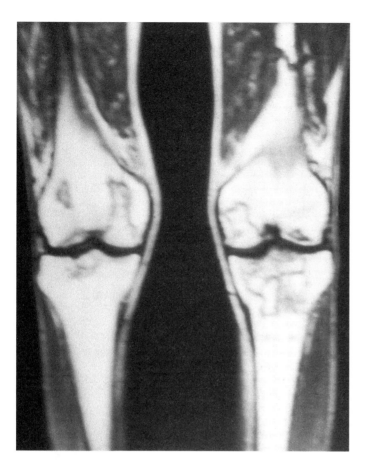

(Figure 7E-9)

Osteonecrosis: knees (MRI). The T1-weighted coronal image of the knees shows geographic, ring-like areas of decreased signal intensity (black) within the femoral condyles and proximal tibias. These areas represent osteonecrosis, which was steroid-induced. The largest area is in the patient's proximal left tibia and extends into the metaphysis. Reprinted from Revised Clinical Slide Collection on the Rheumatic Diseases, with permission of the American College of Rheumatology.

radionuclide accumulation. When areas of increased uptake are detected, additional studies such as radiography are often necessary to add specificity to identify the type of abnormality. In clinical situations where the presence of skeletal disease is uncertain, a bone scan can be useful in excluding disease.

^{99m}Tc MDP, the most commonly used radionuclide, accumulates in areas of bone formation, calcium deposition, and high blood flow. ^{99m}Tc sulphur colloid localizes in the reticuloendothelial system (liver, spleen, and bone marrow). ^{67}Ga citrate accumulates in inflammatory and certain neoplastic processes, and ^{111}In-labeled WBCs localize in inflammatory sites, especially acute inflammatory processes.

The ^{99m}Tc MDP triple-phase bone scan is the study most widely used for early detection of osteomyelitis (11). Images are obtained in the early vascular phase (during bolus injection of the radionuclide), intermediate blood pool phase (5 minutes postinjection), and late bone phase (3 hours postinjection). A fourth phase (24 hours postinjection) can be added to accentuate areas of increased bone uptake, during which time soft tissue background is decreased, although delayed imaging is not widely used because of its inconvenience. If necessary, the specificity of scanning can be increased by also using ^{67}Ga citrate or ^{111}In-labeled WBCs. The ^{111}In-labeled WBC scan is especially useful when osteo-

myelitis is suspected to be superimposed on a healing fracture or surgical incision, since uptake of ^{99m}Tc MDP is increased at these sites. ^{111}In-labeled WBC scans may also be useful in diagnosing osteomyelitis of the foot in people with diabetes. In suspected osteomyelitis of the hematopoietic bone marrow, the combination of ^{99m}Tc MDP and ^{111}In-labeled WBC appears to be an effective diagnostic technique. Spatial localization of bone scans can be improved with single-photon emission computed tomography (SPECT), and radiographs of scan-positive areas can be used to increase specificity.

Joints affected by inflammatory or degenerative arthritis show increased uptake and can map the extent of disease in a single examination. This feature has not proved generally useful, but it can help in certain instances. For example, in a patient with inflammatory arthritis and widespread changes on radiographs, scintigraphy may help locate areas of active inflammation. Bone scans are a reasonable alternative for early detection of osteonecrosis if MRI is not available. Bone scans can also detect stress injuries such as shin splints, tendon avulsions, and stress fractures, which sometimes mimic arthritic complaints (Fig. 7E-10).

ULTRASOUND

Ultrasound provides unique information by creating images based on the location of acoustic interfaces in tissue. It is relatively inexpensive, widely available, and free of the hazards of ionizing radiation. Spatial resolution is similar to CT and MRI, but this depends on the transducer. However, resolution is limited by the depth of tissue being studied; resolution is much higher for superficial structures.

One limitation of ultrasound is dependence on the operator. It is not always possible for one investigator to reproduce the results of another investigator. Because ultrasound lacks a complete cross-section of the body to provide orientation, it may be difficult for individuals who were not actually present during the study to interpret the images.

In some centers ultrasound has proved accurate in detecting rotator cuff tears. It is also excellent for assessing fluid collections such as joint effusions, popliteal cysts, and ganglion cysts, and it can therefore be used to guide aspiration of fluid in joints and elsewhere. Superficially located tendons such as the Achilles tendon and patellar tendon can be studied for tears.

Ultrasound is excellent for differentiating thrombophlebitis from pseudothrombophlebitis. With real-time compression ultrasonography, venous thrombosis and popliteal cysts can be identified (12).

Ultrasound has shown promise in evaluating osteoporosis (13). Sound transmission through bone provides some information about the microtrabecular structure, which relates to bone strength but cannot be assessed directly with radiographic techniques. This information may prove to be complementary to that provided by bone mineral content in evaluating a patient's fracture risk. Ultrasound has been used to assess the surface properties of cartilage (14). In the study of cartilage one must gain access to the joint by an invasive procedure, which greatly limits the appeal of this procedure.

ARTHROGRAPHY

Arthrography involves injecting a contrast agent into the joint, followed by radiography. In conventional arthrogra-

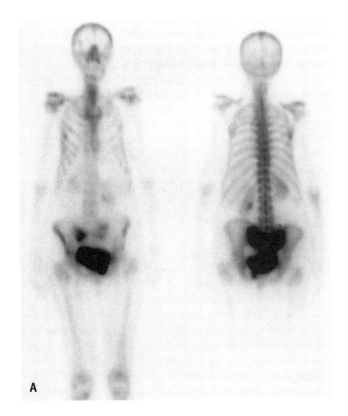

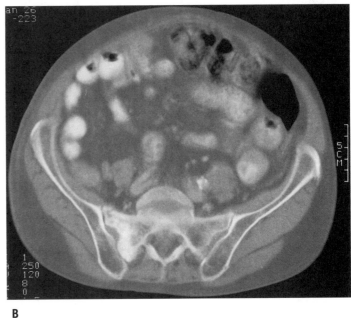

B

A

(Figure 7E-10)

A: An 82-year-old woman with a history of breast cancer and recent onset of lower back pain. Metastases were suspected. ^{99m}Tc MDP bone scan shows increased uptake in the sacrum and right pubic ramus, which are typical of insufficiency fractures. B: CT scan adds specificity to the diagnosis by demonstrating the linear nature of the healing fracture in the sacrum adjacent to the right sacroiliac joint.

phy, the joint cavity is filled with an iodine-containing contrast medium and, sometimes, air. The cost is less than that for CT or MRI, and the procedure can be performed wherever fluoroscopy is available. However, the possibility of introducing bacteria into a joint or encountering reactions to local anesthetic or contrast medium must be considered, although these complications are very rare.

One of the major reasons for developing arthrography was to examine structures within the joint, such as the menisci of the knee, which were not visible on conventional radiographs. Now these structures can be imaged noninvasively by MRI. However, certain important roles remain for arthrography.

Conventional arthrography, using iodine-containing contrast medium, either alone or combined with air, accurately detects full-thickness rotator cuff tears (Fig. 7E-11). CT scanning can be added to the air–contrast arthrogram (CT arthrography), providing an excellent study of the glenoid labrum that is comparable to, or perhaps better than, MRI (15).

Knee arthrography can confirm the diagnosis of a popliteal cyst and permit injection of corticosteroids at the same time. It is an excellent substitute for evaluating the menisci in patients who are claustrophobic or whose size precludes MRI examination (Fig. 7E-12).

Wrist arthrography is excellent for evaluating the integrity of the triangular fibrocartilage, ligaments between the scaphoid and lunate, and ligaments between the lunate and triquetrum (16). Many clinicians prefer arthrography to MRI in this diagnostic situation.

MRI arthrography is performed by distending the shoulder joint with a weak solution of Gadolinium contrast

medium. This technique has been widely studied and probably increases accuracy of diagnosis of glenoid labral tears and rotator cuff tears (17).

Contrast arthrography is used to confirm intra-articular needle location after aspirating synovial fluid from a possibly septic joint. Arthrography is the only reliable way to document the source of the specimen.

BONE DENSITOMETRY

Bone densitometry is used primarily for evaluating osteoporosis. Two precise, accurate, and widely available techniques are dual-energy x-ray absorptiometry (DEXA) and quantitative computed tomography (QCT) (18).

DEXA scans with a narrow x-ray beam that alternates energy (kilovoltage peak; KVP). A sensitive receptor detects the fraction of the x-ray beam that traverses the body, which generates profiles of the amount of radiation that is deflected by the body. Because the absorption characteristics of bone and soft tissue vary at different x-ray energies, the amount of radiation absorbed by bone can be calculated. From this, the amount of bone in the path of the x-ray beam at any point along the scan is determined.

DEXA is relatively inexpensive and delivers very little radiation to the patient. It is thus a good choice for studies that must be repeated. Any part of the body can be studied. Standard values are available for lumbar spine and proximal femur, which are the most widely studied.

QCT scans several lumbar vertebrae while simultaneously scanning a phantom containing different concentrations of bone-equivalent material. A standard curve is constructed from the concentration values versus CT attenuation, and then the bone density at any location scanned is

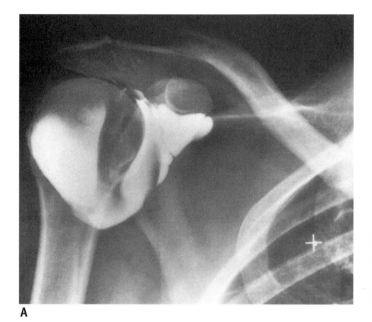

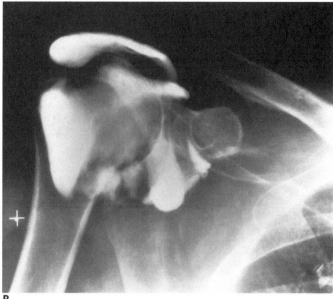

(Figure 7E-11)
A: Single-contrast arthrogram of a normal shoulder. B: Single-contrast shoulder arthrogram of a 66-year-old man with a painful shoulder and history of injury in distant past. Contrast media fills not only the shoulder joint (as in Fig. 11A) but has filled the subdeltoid–subacromial bursa superiorly, a finding diagnostic of full-thickness rotator cuff tear. Interpretation is very straightforward.

determined from the standard curve. The cost of this study is moderate and the radiation dose fairly low, although not as low as that for DEXA. A claimed advantage of this technique is that cancellous bone in the middle of the vertebrae can be evaluated, since overlying cortical bone and posterior

elements of the vertebrae are not measured. The cancellous bone has tremendous surface area and is more rapidly affected during bone loss than is cortical bone.

ANGIOGRAPHY

Angiography is useful in the primary diagnosis of rheumatologic disorders with vascular components. In polyarteritis nodosa, for example, demonstrating multiple small aneurysms of medium-sized visceral arteries is an important feature. In systemic lupus erythematosus, angiography may be valuable in diagnosing central nervous system involvement.

Angiography is more costly than MRI and is an invasive procedure. It should be used only in specific limited circumstances when other modalities will not provide the required diagnostic information.

IMAGING DECISIONS

Almost all imaging should begin with plain radiography, which is frequently all that is required. If more diagnostic information is needed and will alter the clinical actions, MRI is frequently the second imaging study. In many cases, MRI findings must be correlated with plain films, since MRI does not demonstrate calcifications or subtle cortical erosions.

Recent MRI studies continue to demonstrate that many individuals have anatomic abnormalities that are unrelated to symptoms (19). Therefore, clinical and imaging findings must be correlated. Imaging studies should not be obtained unless they have the potential to answer clinically significant questions.

In many cases simple, low-cost imaging may provide all the information necessary for clinical decision-making. If a plain radiograph of the shoulder shows the humeral head subluxed upward, eroding the inferior aspect of the acromion, the clinician can be quite certain, without obtaining an MRI, that the rotator cuff is torn and atrophic (Fig. 7E-

(Figure 7E-12)
A 40-year-old woman, too large to fit in the MRI scanner, was suspected of having a popliteal cyst. Double contrast arthrogram demonstrated a popliteal cyst and also a torn medial meniscus.

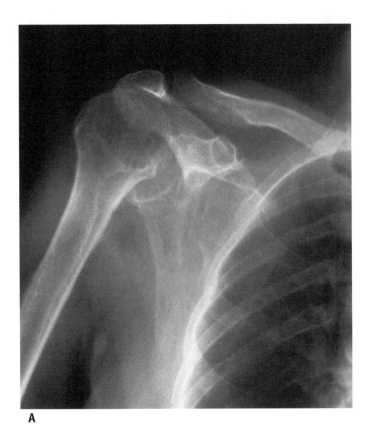

A

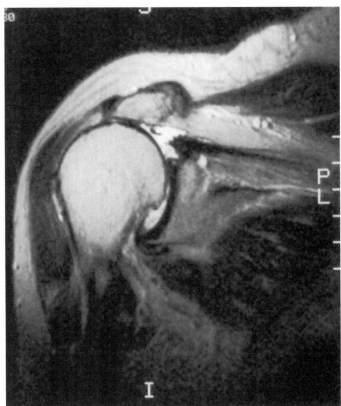

B

(Figure 7E-13)
A: An 80-year-old woman with weakness and pain in the right shoulder. Radiograph shows superior subluxation of the humeral head and markedly decreased space between humeral head and acromion. B: Oblique-coronal T2-weighted MRI shows similar decreased distance between the acromion and humeral head, as well as a complete rotator cuff tear and retraction of the supraspinatus muscle and remaining tendon. MRI findings could have been predicted from the plain radiograph and the clinical history.

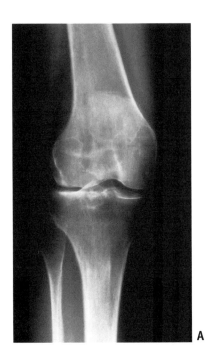

A

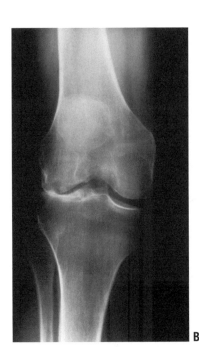

B

(Figure 7E-14)
A: A 60-year-old woman with knee pain. Standing anteroposterior radiograph shows what appears to be minimal narrowing of the cartilage of the lateral compartment of the knee joint. B: Standing posteroanterior flexed view of the same knee shows severe cartilage loss with bone-on-bone contact in the lateral compartment. This view frequently shows cartilage loss not seen on the anteroposterior standing view.

13). Standing anteroposterior and standing flexed posteroanterior radiographs of the knees cannot show the minimal erosions that are visible on MRI, but they do demonstrate when the cartilage is gone (Fig. 7E-14).

Finally, it is critically important for the clinician to work closely with the radiologist to decide exactly what information is needed from an imaging study, and then select the technique that will supply that information. MRI provides such a wealth of information about so many structures that an exhaustive MRI study may be appropriate in a very puzzling joint condition. In other instances, a tailored, abbreviated MRI or a simpler imaging procedure may provide the specific diagnostic information in less time for less money.

WILLIAM W. SCOTT, JR., MD

1. Murphey MD, Quale JL, Martin NL, Bramble JM, Cook LT, Dwyer SJ: Computed radiography in musculoskeletal imaging: state of the art. Am J Roentgenol 158:19-27, 1992

2. Scott WW Jr, Fishman EK, Magid D: Acetabular fractures: optimal imaging. Radiology 165:537-539, 1987

3. Lee JS, June-GI I, Ahn JM, Kim YM, han MC: Fibrosing alveolitis: prognostic implication of ground attenuation of high-resolution CT. Radiology 184:451-454,1992

4. Kanal E, Shellock FG, Talagala L: Safety considerations in MR imaging. Radiology 176:593-606,1990

5. Schweitzer ME, Caccese R, Karasick D, Wapner KL, Mitchell DG: Posterior tibial tendon tears: utility of secondary signs for MR imaging diagnosis. Radiology 188:655-659, 1993

6. Schweitzer ME, Brahme SK, Hodler J, et al: Chronic wrist pain: spin-echo and short tau inversion recovery MR imaging and conventional and MR arthrography. Radiology 182:205-211, 1992

7. Kransdorf MJ, Jelinek JS, Moser RP Jr: Imaging of soft tissue tumors. Radiol Clin North Am 31:359-372,1993

8. Erdman WA, Tamburro F, Jayson HT, Weatherall PT, Ferry KB, Peshock RM: Osteomyelitis: characteristics and pitfalls of diagnosis with MR imaging. Radiology 180: 533-539,1991

9. Broderick LS, Turner DA, Renfrew DL, Schnitzer TJ, Huff JP, Harris C: Severity of articular cartilage abnormality in patients with osteoarthritis: evaluation with fast spin-echo MR vs arthroscopy. Am J Roentgenol 162:99-103,1994

10. Ruwe PA, Wright J, Randall RL, Lynch JK, Jokl P, McCarthy S: Can MR imaging effectively replace diagnostic arthroscopy? Radiology 183:335-339,1992

11. Schauwecker DS: The scintigraphic diagnosis of osteomyelitis. Am J Roentgenol 158:9-18,1992

12. Heijboer H, Buller HR, Lensing AWA, Turpie AGG, Colly LP, Cate JW: A comparison of real-time compression ultrasonography with impedance plethysmography for the diagnosis of deep-vein thrombosis in symptomatic outpatients. N Engl J Med 329:1365-1369,1993

13. Herd RJM, Blake GM, Ramalingam R, Miller CG, Ryan PJ, Fogelman I: Measurements of postmenopausal bone loss with a new contact ultrasound system. Calcif Tissue Int 53:153-157, 1993

14. Adler RS, Dedrick DK, Laing TJ, et al: Quantitative assessment of cartilage surface roughness in osteoarthritis using high frequency ultrasound. Ultrasound Med Biol 18:51-58,1992

15. Stiles RG, Otte MT: Imaging of the shoulder. Radiology 188:603-613,1993

16. Metz VM, Mann FA, Gilula LA: Three-compartment wrist arthrography: correlation of pain site with location of uni- and bidirectional communications. Am J Roentgenol 160:819-822,1993

17. Palmer WE, Brown JH, Rosenthal DI: Labral-ligamentous complex of the shoulder: evaluation with MR arthrography. Radiology 190:645-651,1994

18. Guglielmi G, Grimston SK, Fischer KC, Pacifici R: Osteoporosis: diagnosis with lateral and posteroanterior dual x-ray absorptiometry compared with quantitative CT. Radiology 192:845-850,1994

19. Jensen MC, Brant-Zawadski MN, Obuchowski N, Modic MT, Malkasian D, Ross JS: Magnetic resonance imaging of the lumbar spine in people without back pain. N Engl J Med 331:69-73-1994

SIGNS AND SYMPTOMS OF MUSCULOSKELETAL DISORDERS
A. MONARTICULAR JOINT DISEASE

Pain or swelling of a single joint merits prompt evaluation to identify patients in need of urgent and aggressive care (1). Although there are many minor and easily managed causes of monarthritis, infectious arthritis with its risk of prolonged morbidity (and even mortality, if untreated) requires that this more serious problem always be considered.

The underlying causes of monarthritis are divided into two groups: inflammatory diseases (Table 8A-1) and mechanical or infiltrative disorders (Table 8A-2). Triage into one of these categories is the first step in the differential diagnosis of monarthritis.

DIAGNOSIS OF MONARTICULAR JOINT DISEASE
History

It is important to determine the course and duration of symptoms, although patients frequently have difficulty establishing the exact time of onset and the rate of evolution. Acute problems or sudden onset of monarthritis often require immediate evaluation and therapy. The course of symptoms may provide critical information. Bacterial infection tends to increase in severity until treated. Viral monarthritis often resolves spontaneously. Osteoarthritic symptoms wax and wane with physical activity. Morning stiffness lasting more than an hour suggests an inflammatory disease.

A history of previous episodes provides support for a crystalline or other noninfectious cause. Patients with established rheumatoid arthritis, (RA) who develop a dramatic monarthritis should always be evaluated for septic arthritis or superimposed crystal-associated disease (2). Patients with antecedent joint disease or surgery should raise the clinician's concern about infection. In patients with a prosthesis in the involved joint, loosening of the implant should also be investigated.

Monarticular arthritis is occasionally the first symptom of polyarticular disease such as Reiter's syndrome or other reactive arthritis, inflammatory bowel disease, psoriatic arthritis, or RA. A history of fever, chills, tick bites, sexual risk factors, intravenous drug use, and travel outside the country can contribute clues to infectious causes. Symptoms such as rash, diarrhea, urethritis, or uveitis might suggest reactive arthritis. Weight loss can suggest malignancy or other serious systemic disease.

A history of trauma suggests fracture or an internal derangement, but minor trauma can also precipitate acute gout or psoriatic arthritis, or can introduce infection. Occupations involving repetitive use of the joint favor osteoarthritis. Concurrent illnesses and medication use may also provide important clues; in addition, they can affect test results and influence the choice or outcome of therapy. Because some monarticular diseases are inherited, family history can be helpful.

Physical Examination
The clinician must first distinguish arthritis, which involves the articular space, from problems in periarticular areas, such as a bursitis, tendinitis, or cellulitis. In arthritis, the swelling and tenderness tend to surround the joint. If normal joint motion is retained, true arthritis is unlikely. Painful limitation of motion in all planes usually indicates joint

(Table 8A-1)
Some inflammatory causes of monarthritis

Crystal-induced arthritis
  Monosodium urate (gout)
  Calcium pyrophosphate dihydrate
  Apatite
  Calcium oxalate
  Liquid lipid microspherules
Infectious arthritis
  Bacteria
  Fungi
  Lyme disease or disease due to other spirochetes
  Mycobacteria
  Virus (HIV, hepatitis B, others)
Systemic diseases presenting with monarticular involvement
  Psoriatic arthritis
  Reactive arthritis
  Rheumatoid arthritis
  Systemic lupus erythematosus

(Table 8A-2)
Some noninflammatory causes of monarthritis

Amyloidosis
Osteonecrosis
Benign tumor
  Osteochondroma
  Osteoid osteoma
  Pigmented villonodular synovitis
Fracture
Hemarthrosis
Internal derangement
Malignancy
Osteoarthritis

involvement. Pain limited to one movement or tenderness on only one side of the joint suggests a periarticular problem.

In any patient with acute monarthritis, it is important to look for extra-articular signs that might provide clues to specific causes. For example, mouth ulcers may occur in Behcet's syndrome, Reiter's syndrome, and systemic lupus erythematosus (SLE). Small patches of psoriasis may be found in the anal crease or behind the ears. The keratoderma blennorrhagicum of Reiter's syndrome can be subtle and often affects only the feet. Erythema nodosum may occur in sarcoidosis and inflammatory bowel disease. Skin ulcerations can be a source of infection.

Synovial Fluid Analysis

Arthrocentesis should be performed in almost every patient with monarthritis, and it is obligatory if infection is suspected. Virtually all the important information from synovial fluid analysis is obtained through the gross examination, total leukocyte and differential count, cultures, gram staining, and examination of a wet preparation for crystals and other microscopic abnormalities (3). All these studies can be performed with only 1 to 2 ml of fluid. Even a few drops may be adequate for culture, Gram staining, and wet preparations. Cloudy synovial fluid is likely to be caused by inflammatory arthritis and is confirmed by a leukocyte count. See also Chapter 7C.

Normally, synovial fluid contains fewer than 180 white blood cells (WBC)/mm^3, most of which are mononuclear cells. The fluid is considered to be "noninflammatory" if it contains fewer than 2,000 cells/mm^3, although most samples of synovial fluids from patients with osteoarthritis contain fewer than 500 cells/mm^3. Synovial fluids with a count of more than 2,000 leukocytes/mm^3 indicate an inflammatory process. In general, the leukocyte count and the suspicion of infection should rise at the same rate — the higher the count, the greater the suspicion. Effusions with more than 100,000 leukocytes/mm^3 are considered septic until proved otherwise. However, leukocyte counts vary widely in both sterile and septic inflammatory arthritis. Synovial fluid should be cultured if there is any suggestion of infection. Special stains and cultures for mycobacteria and fungi are sometimes appropriate.

Careful examination for crystals in synovial fluid can establish a diagnosis early and avoid unnecessary hospital admissions for the treatment of suspected infectious arthritis. A tentative diagnosis can be made by standard light microscopy. Monosodium urate crystals are needle shaped, and calcium pyrophosphate dihydrate (CPPD) crystals are usually rods, squares, or rhomboids. Polarized light examination can confirm the nature of these crystals. Individual apatite crystals, which cause acute monarthritis or periarthritis, are visible only on electron microscopy. However, masses of these crystals look like shiny, nonbirefringent clumps that resemble cell debris. Special stains such as alizarin red S can confirm that these clumps are masses of calcium crystals.

The presence of crystals does not exclude infection, however, especially since antecedent joint disease such as gout may increase the likelihood of septic arthritis. Large fat droplets in synovial fluid suggest a bone fracture involving the marrow space. Small lipid droplets may also indicate fracture or pancreatic fat necrosis. Coulter counters sometimes misread these small droplets as leukocytes, thus providing misleading information.

Laboratory Tests

Synovial fluid may be sterile in infectious arthritis. This is especially true for gonococcal arthritis, as only about 25% of patients have positive synovial fluid cultures. For this reason, cultures and Gram stains of blood, skin lesions or ulcers, cervical or urethral swabs, urine, or any other possible sources of microorganisms should be ordered in suspected infectious arthritis. Tests for HIV antibodies and Lyme antibodies may also be appropriate. However, no single serologic test can establish the cause of any arthritis. For example, rheumatoid factor can be positive in many diseases besides RA, including sarcoidosis and subacute bacterial endocarditis. Similarly, an elevated serum uric acid does not mean a patient has gout, and conversely, normal levels are seen during the acute phase of gouty arthritis.

Radiographs

Radiologic findings are typically unremarkable in most patients with acute inflammatory arthritis, other than showing soft-tissue swelling. However, x-ray studies can help exclude some causes and can provide a useful baseline for future comparisons. Radiographs of the involved joint may show fractures, tumors, or signs of antecedent chronic disease such as osteoarthritis. Chondrocalcinosis in the involved joint suggests, but does not prove, that the arthritis is caused by CPPD crystals. Magnetic resonance imaging, although often overused, can localize an infectious or inflammatory process in the joint, its surrounding tissue, or bone. It can also identify meniscal tears and ligament damage (4).

Synovial Biopsy

Needle biopsy of the synovial membrane or a biopsy obtained during arthroscopy may be critical in patients with monarthropathy that remains undiagnosed (5). A culture of synovial tissue may be more informative than a synovial fluid culture in certain settings, such as when gonococcal or mycobacterial disease is suspected or when no fluid is available for culture. Biopsies can identify infiltrative diseases such as amyloidosis, sarcoidosis, pigmented villonodular synovitis, or tumor. The polymerase chain reaction and immunoelectron microscopy may help identify DNA sequences from *Borrelia burgdorferi*, *Neisseria gonorrhoeae*, chlamydia, and ureaplasma (6).

Initial Treatment

Management decisions often must be made before all test results are available. For instance, a patient with synovial fluid indicating a highly inflammatory process, a negative Gram stain, and no obvious cause or source of infection requires antibiotic coverage while testing proceeds. Always obtain several cultures before treatment.

Suspected crystal-induced arthritis in a patient whose course is uncomplicated can be treated with doses of nonsteroidal anti-inflammatory drugs (NSAIDs) near the upper limit of each agent's recommended range, with the dosage tapered as the inflammation subsides. Oral or intravenous colchicine or corticosteroids are also effective in gout and pseudogout. NSAIDs are an acceptable symptomatic treatment in other unexplained inflammatory arthritis. Acetaminophen may be used during the evaluation of non-inflammatory arthritis. However, because NSAIDs and acetaminophen can interrupt fever patterns and delay diagnosis, propoxyphene or codeine might be preferred in some instances. Acutely swollen joints can safely be rested, but should not be casted unless a fracture is proved.

SPECIFIC TYPES OF MONARTHRITIS
Infection
Between 80% and 90% of nongonococcal bacterial infections are monarticular. Most joint infections develop from hematogenous spread. The discovery of a primary site of infection can be an important clue to the infectious agent involved. By far the most common agents are gram-positive aerobes (approximately 80%) (7), with *Staphylococcus aureus* accounting for 60%. Gram-negative bacteria account for 18% of infections, and anaerobes are increasingly common causes as a result of parenteral drug use and the rising number of immunocompromised hosts. Anaerobic infections are also more common in patients who have wounds of an extremity or gastrointestinal cancers.

N. gonorrhoeae is still probably the most common cause of septic arthritis. It is often preceded by a migratory tendinitis or arthritis. Mycobacterial infection may cause monarthritis or may involve several joints. The disease is more likely to be chronic, but acute mycobacterial arthritis has been reported and may even cause podagra (8). Atypical mycobacterial infections can involve the synovium and should be considered in the differential diagnosis, especially in immunocompromised hosts and in patients whose joints have been injected frequently with corticosteroids. Fungal arthritis is usually indolent, but cases of acute monarthritis due to blastomycosis or Candida species have been reported. Acute monarthritis associated with herpes simplex virus, Coxsackie B, HIV, parvovirus, and other viruses has also been described (9,10).

The joint symptoms of Lyme disease range from intermittent arthralgias to chronic monarthritis (most often in the knee) to oligoarthritis. Monarthritis can also be caused by other spirochetes such as *Treponema pallidum.*

Crystal-Induced Arthritis
Gout, which is caused by monosodium urate crystals, is the most common type of inflammatory monarthritis. Typically, gout involves the first metatarsophalangeal (MTP) joint, ankle, midfoot, or knee. However, acute attacks of gout can occur in any joint. Later attacks may be monarticular or polyarticular. Accompanying fever, although less common with monarticular than with polyarticular gout, can mimic infection.

CPPD crystals can cause monarthritis that is clinically indistinguishable from gout and thus is often called pseudogout. Pseudogout is most common in the knee and wrist, but it has been reported in a variety of other joints, including the first MTP joint. Among other crystals known to cause acute monarthritis are apatites, calcium oxalate, and liquid lipid crystals. Apatites have also been recently emphasized as a cause of goutlike podagra.

Osteoarthritis, Osteonecrosis, Trauma, and Foreign Body Reactions
Although osteoarthritis is primarily a chronic and slowly progressive disease, it may present with suddenly worsening pain and swelling in a single joint. New pain in the knee is often due to an effusion as a result of overuse or minor trauma. Spontaneous osteonecrosis, especially of the knee, is seen in elderly patients and can lead to pain in a single joint with or without effusion (11). Trauma to a joint leading to internal derangement, hemarthrosis, or fracture can also lead to monarticular disease. Penetrating injuries from thorns, wood fragments, or other foreign materials can cause monarthritis (12).

Hemarthrosis
The most common causes of hemarthrosis, or bleeding into a joint, are clotting abnormalities due to anticoagulant therapy or congenital disorders such as hemophilia. Hemarthrosis can also result from scurvy. Fracture of the joint should always be considered in patients with hemarthrosis, especially if the synovial fluid is bloody and contains fat.

Systemic Rheumatic Diseases
Many systemic diseases may present as acute monarticular arthritis, but this is decidedly uncommon and should not be emphasized in the differential diagnosis. RA, SLE, arthritis of inflammatory bowel disease, psoriatic arthritis, Behcet's disease, Reiter's syndrome, and other forms of reactive arthritis can all begin as acute monarthritis. Other causes include sarcoidosis, serum sickness, hepatitis, hyperlipidemias, and malignancies. Persistence in evaluating patients for underlying systemic diseases can sometimes lead to an early diagnosis of systemic disease.

In a substantial number of patients with synovial fluid findings indicative of inflammatory arthritis, the cause cannot be determined. Many of these patients have transient monarthritis with no recurrences. Guidelines for the initial evaluation of patients with acute musculoskeletal symptoms have been published and include aspects of evaluation of monarthropathy (13) (see Appendix II).

H. RALPH SCHUMACHER, MD

1. Baker DG, Schumacher HR: Acute monarthritis. N Engl J Med 329:1013-1020, 1993
2. VanLinhoudt D, Schumacher HR: Acute monosynovitis or oligoarthritis in patients with quiescent rheumatoid arthritis. J Clin Rheumatol 1:46-53, 1995
3. Gatter RA, Schumacher HR: Joint aspiration: indications and technique. In Gatter RA, Schumacher HR (eds): A practical handbook of synovial fluid analysis. Philadelphia: Lea & Febiger, 1991, pp 14-23
4. Weissman BN, Hussain S: Magnetic resonance imaging of the knee. Rheum Dis Clin North Am 17:637-68, 1991
5. Schumacher HR, Kulka JP: Needle biopsy of the synovial membrane: experience with the Parker-Pearson technic. N Engl J Med 286:416-19, 1972
6. Rahman MU, Cheema S, Schumacher HR, Hudson AP: Molecular evidence for the presence of chlamydia in the synovium of patients with Reiter's syndrome. Arthritis Rheum 35:521-9, 1992
7. Goldenberg DL, Reed JI: Bacterial arthritis. N Engl J Med 312:764-771, 1985
8. Boulware DW, Lopez M, Gum OB: Tuberculosis podagra. J Rheumatol 12:1022-24, 1985
9. Rivier G, Gerster JC, Terrier P, Cheseaux JJ: Parvovirus B19 associated monarthritis in a 5 year old boy. J Rheumatol 22:766-777, 1995
10. Nussinovitch M, Harel L, Varsano I: Arthritis after mumps and measles vaccination. Arch Dis Childhood 72:348-349, 1995
11. Lotke PA, Ecker ML: Osteonecrosis of the knee. Orthop Clin North Am 16:797-808, 1985
12. Olenginski TP, Bush DC, Harrington TM: Plant thorn synovitis: an uncommon cause of monarthritis. Sem Arth Rheum 21:40-46, 1991
13. American College of Rheumatology Ad Hoc Committee on Clinical Guidelines: Guidelines for the initial evaluation of the adult patient with acute musculoskeletal symptoms. Arthritis Rheum 39:1-8, 1996

B. POLYARTICULAR JOINT DISEASE

A thorough history and physical examination are the most important diagnostic tools in the evaluation of polyarticular joint complaints (1–4) (see Appendix II). Potentially useful information includes preceding illnesses or trauma, prior episodes, and a family history of arthritis or back pain. The pattern and evolution of joint involvement may offer clues. Are large or small joints affected? Is the arthritis limited to just a few joints? Is it symmetrical? Does it involve several joints simultaneously, or does it appear in an additive or migratory fashion? In the additive pattern, new joint involvement occurs at intervals but symptoms persist once the joint is involved; with migratory arthritis, the duration of involvement of each joint is only a few days. What is the pattern of pain? In osteoarthritis, pain is aggravated by use and weight-bearing and is relieved by rest. In inflammatory arthritis, particularly rheumatoid arthritis (RA), symptoms are aggravated by immobility. Is there evidence of systemic disease or other organ involvement?

On physical examination, the presence of soft-tissue swelling and effusion should be noted. These signs usually point toward an inflammatory synovitis—even when redness, warmth, and marked tenderness are absent. However, swelling and effusion may occur in noninflammatory arthritis. If the joints appear normal in patients with widespread pain, nonarticular causes should be considered (eg, fibromyalgia, polymyalgia rheumatica, bone disease, neuropathy). Because joint pain is sometimes the initial manifestation of systemic illnesses, a complete physical examination is appropriate for all patients with polyarthritis. Particular attention should be given to examining the skin for rashes, subcutaneous nodules, and other lesions associated with rheumatic diseases. The musculoskeletal examination should include the spine and muscles, as well as the joints.

Laboratory studies include standard hematologic and biochemical tests; nonspecific indicators of inflammation or dysproteinemia, such as erythrocyte sedimentation rate; antibody tests for exposure to pathogens (eg, group A streptococcus, parvovirus B19, *Borrelia burgdorferi*); and autoantibodies that may be associated with a single condition or limited group of illnesses.

If the diagnosis is uncertain after history, physical examination, and results of standard laboratory tests are evaluated, synovial fluid should always be examined if it is readily obtainable. Synovial fluid analysis must be done immediately on patients who are febrile or acutely ill. The analysis may be diagnostic in patients with bacterial infections or crystal-induced synovitis. In other conditions, it may permit the examiner to classify the arthritis as either inflammatory or noninflammatory.

Imaging studies may yield valuable information in patients with chondrocalcinosis caused by calcium pyrophosphate dihydrate deposition (CPPD) disease, with back pain typical of sacroiliac joint involvement, or erosions typical of rheumatoid arthritis. However, most imaging studies and many laboratory tests are expensive and should not be ordered routinely, nor should imaging include all involved joints. The physician should first outline the differential di-agnosis and estimate the likelihood that a test or study will distinguish between the leading diagnoses or alter the treatment plan.

Biopsy of the synovium or other tissue may be necessary to confirm or establish a diagnosis of rare diseases such as Whipple's disease, vasculitis, mycobacterial arthritis, or fungal infections.

CLASSIFICATION OF POLYARTICULAR JOINT DISEASE

There are two main categories of polyarticular joint disease: inflammatory and noninflammatory. Both groups include conditions with great etiologic and clinical diversity (Table 8B-1). The presence of abnormal findings in another organ system is often valuable in the diagnosis of polyarthropathy, since many of the possible causes involve multiple systems (Table 8B-2).

Polyarticular arthritis can also be grouped by mode of presentation (acute, subacute, chronic), occurrence in different age groups, pattern of joint involvement, or immunogenetic associations. However, not all patients fit the expected profile, and atypical presentations do occur. For example, the onset of RA is typically insidious or subacute and involves multiple small and some large joints, but occasionally its onset is acute and joint involvement is monarticular or oligoarticular. Middle-aged women are affected most often, but RA can occur at any age and also can affect men. The following discussions focus on the most typical presentations of disorders that can cause polyarticular arthritis.

ACUTE INFLAMMATORY POLYARTHRITIS

Patients with acute inflammatory polyarthritis frequently have a high- or low-grade fever (Table 8B-2). *Rheumatic fever* is the prototype in this group. Children are typically affected with migratory arthritis that involves several joints simultaneously but persists in each joint for only a few days. In adults, the arthritis is often additive and of longer duration. Carditis may not be evident initially. Streptococcal pharyngitis preceding the symptoms is commonly asymptomatic, but serologic evidence should be sought in all patient with acute polyarthritis and fever. Fever usually fluctuates without returning to normal for a week or more, but, characteristically, both fever and arthritis respond dramatically to high-dose aspirin therapy.

Septic arthritis generally affects a single joint, but about 20% of adults have two or more large joints involved. Risk factors for polyarthritis include immunosuppression, intravenous drug use, and preexisting joint disease, particularly RA. *Gonococcal* and *meningococcal arthritis* are frequently polyarticular and may even present with a migratory pattern. Typical vesiculopustular skin lesions on an erythematous base provide an important diagnostic clue in gonococcemia. Tenosynovitis in the wrist and ankle extensor tendon sheaths is frequently found. Synovial fluid is usually sterile in polyarticular neisserial infection, but blood cultures may be diagnostic.

In early *Lyme disease,* dissemination of *B. burgdorferi* is often manifested by fever and migratory arthralgia with little

Inflammatory

Crystal-induced arthritis

Infectious arthritis

  Bacterial
    Gonococcal and meningococcal
    Lyme disease
    Bacterial endocarditis
  Viral
  Other infections

Postinfectious or reactive arthritis
  Enteric infection
  Urogenital infection (Reiter's syndrome)
  Rheumatic fever

Other seronegative spondyloarthropathies
  Ankylosing spondylitis
  Psoriatic arthritis
  Inflammatory bowel disease

Rheumatoid arthritis

Inflammatory osteoarthritis

Systemic rheumatic illnesses
  Systemic lupus erythematosus
  Systemic vasculitis
  Systemic sclerosis
  Polymyositis/dermatomyositis
  Still's disease
  Behçet's syndrome
  Relapsing polychondritis

Other systemic illnesses
  Sarcoidosis
  Palindromic rheumatism
  Familial Mediterranean fever
  Malignancy
  Hyperlipoproteinemias
  Whipple's disease

Noninflammatory

Osteoarthritis
  Metabolic/endocrine
  Hemochromatosis
  Acromegaly
  Ochronosis

Hematologic
  Amyloidosis
  Leukemia
  Hemophilia
  Sickle cell disease

Hypertrophic pulmonary osteoarthropathy

or no joint swelling. A persistent oligoarticular arthritis may appear months later.

Bacterial endocarditis may present with fever, back pain, and arthralgia. A minority of patients have large-joint oligoarticular arthritis, usually with sterile synovial fluid cultures. Endocarditis should be suspected in patients with a heart murmur and fever, and confirmed by blood cultures.

Mycobacterial or fungal arthritis is usually monarticular, but occasionally an indolent oligoarthritis occurs.

Acute polyarthritis may be a sequel to *parvovirus B19* and *rubella infection,* especially in young women. Although self-limited, viral arthropathies resemble acute RA, with morning stiffness, symmetric involvement of the hands and wrists, and occasionally a positive test for rheumatoid factor. The typical viral exanthem may be absent, but the diagnosis

should be suspected in patients exposed to one of these viruses, and can be confirmed serologically. A similar arthritis may precede the symptoms of *hepatitis B viral infection* and is often accompanied by an urticarial rash. Several types of arthropathy may occur in patients with *human immunodeficiency virus (HIV) infection,* including acute episodic oligoarthritis and persistent polyarthritis. HIV-induced arthropathies may be related directly to viral infection or to secondary septic or reactive arthritis. *Crystal-induced arthritis* is generally monarticular, but it may present as acute oligoarticular arthritis, often with fever. Typically the joints are warm and erythematous, and swelling extends to the soft tissue well beyond the joint. With both crystal-induced and septic arthritis in large joints of the lower extremity, the patient may be unable to bear weight or may walk with a pronounced limp. Gouty arthritis usually affects the feet, especially the first metatarsophalangeal (MTP) joint, and tophi may be present. In older women with osteoarthritis, gout sometimes presents with acute inflammation in a Heberden's node. Demonstration of crystals in synovial fluid confirms the diagnosis. Radiographs showing chondrocalcinosis support the diagnosis of CPPD disease.

Palindromic rheumatism and *familial Mediterranean fever (FMF)* cause recurrent attacks of acute synovitis or periarticular inflammation, usually in one or two joints, with long symptom-free intervals between attacks. In FMF there is usually a family history of similar attacks starting in childhood; pleuritis and abdominal pain may also occur. Episodic arthritis and periarthritis have also been described in some types of hyperlipoproteinemia.

Acute leukemia in children may cause recurrent acute episodes of arthralgia, arthritis, and bone pain. Acute *sarcoid arthritis* is usually accompanied by fever, erythema nodosum, and hilar adenopathy. Marked periarticular swelling and erythema in both ankles should suggest sarcoid arthritis.

SUBACUTE AND CHRONIC INFLAMMATORY POLYARTHRITIS

Rheumatoid arthritis, the most prominent member of this group, varies in its presentation. Some patients have a symmetric polyarthritis that usually affects small joints, such as metacarpophalangeal and proximal interphalangeal joints of the fingers. Other patients have an additive pattern with a monarticular or oligoarticular onset. Symptoms are increased upon awakening (morning stiffness) or after periods of inactivity. In the early stages, joint tenderness and swelling are the main physical findings, but later, limitation of motion and joint deformity develop. Although subcutaneous nodules develop in less than half of RA patients, their presence may support the diagnosis. About two-thirds to three-fourths of RA patients test positive for rheumatoid factor, including almost all patients with nodules.

Seronegative RA may be difficult to distinguish from some varieties of *seronegative spondyloarthropathy.* This clinically heterogeneous group of disorders includes ankylosing spondylitis, psoriatic arthritis, and reactive arthritis. The spine and sacroiliac joints are frequently involved, and isolated dactylitis (sausage digit) and enthesopathy (pain at sites of tendon or ligament attachment to bone) are common findings. Disease susceptibility is often genetically determined.

Ankylosing spondylitis may present with peripheral joint symptoms, but the axial joints (hips and shoulders espe-

Systemic and organ involvement associated with polyarthropathy

Disorder	Fever	Lungs	Eye	GI system	Heart
			Organ Involvement		
Amyloidosis	-	-	-	X	X
Bacterial arthritis	X	-	-	-	-
Bacterial endocarditis	X	-	-	-	X
Behçet's syndrome	-	-	X	-	-
Crystal-induced arthritis	X	-	-	-	-
Erythema nodosum	X	X	-	-	-
Familial Mediterranean fever	X	X	-	X	-
Hemochromatosis	-	-	-	-	X
Hypertrophic pulmonary arthritis	-	X	-	-	-
Inflammatory bowel disease	X	-	X	X	-
Intestinal bypass surgery	-	-	X	X	X
Juvenile chronic arthritis	-	-	X	-	X
Leukemia	X	-	X	-	-
Lyme disease	X	-	-	-	X
Polymyositis/dermatomyositis	-	X	-	-	X
Reactive arthritis	X	-	X	X	-
Relapsing polychondritis	X	X	X	-	X
Rheumatic fever	X	X	-	-	X
Rheumatoid arthritis	-	X	X	-	X
Sarcoidosis	X	X	X	-	X
Seronegative spondyloarthropathy	-	-	X	X	X
Sjögren's syndrome	-	X	X	-	-
Still's disease	X	X	X	-	X
Systemic lupus erythematosus	X	X	X	X	X
Systemic sclerosis	-	X	-	X	X
Systemic vasculitis	X	X	X	X	X
Viral arthritis	X	-	-	-	-
Whipple's disease	X	X	X	X	X

cially) are more likely to be affected than in early RA, and low back pain is usually present. Like RA, pain and stiffness are prominent after inactivity and improve after movement.

Psoriatic arthritis has several variants, but it is typically oligoarticular at onset and may evolve into a polyarthritis indistinguishable from RA, particularly if the appearance of skin lesions is delayed. Prominent involvement of the distal interphalangeal joints and pitting of the nails supports the diagnosis of psoriatic arthritis.

Reactive arthritis may develop, particularly in HLA-B27 positive individuals, as a postinfectious sterile oligoarthritis following certain enteric or genitourinary infections. In *Reiter's syndrome* (urethritis, conjunctivitis, and arthritis), large joints of the lower extremity are most often involved. Large-joint oligoarthritis may also occur in active *inflammatory bowel disease*, and usually remits when the bowel inflammation is suppressed. In many patients, large effusions are accompanied by little or no pain, particularly in the knees.

Juvenile chronic polyarthritis and *Still's disease* (the adult onset form) also resemble seronegative RA. Polyarthritis is accompanied by systemic signs that resemble an infectious illness, with high spiking fever, neutrophilic leukocytosis, and evanescent macular rash. Many patients also have lymphadenopathy, splenomegaly, and pericarditis. Synovitis may be absent or intermittent initially, but a persistent polyarthritis resembling RA develops in most patients.

Whipple's disease is a chronic infection that may cause both enteritis and oligoarticular or migratory arthritis. Multiple organ involvement may suggest the diagnosis; confirmation is by biopsy of intestinal mucosa or lymph nodes. Intermittent polyarthritis has been described in morbidly obese patients following *intestinal bypass surgery*. Joint symptoms are often accompanied by a variety of skin lesions.

Polyarthritis is a common mode of presentation in *systemic lupus erythematosus (SLE)*. Differentiation from RA may be difficult if nonarticular manifestations of SLE have not yet appeared. The arthritis is variable and may be migratory or intermittent. Morning stiffness is generally not as prominent as in RA. Although hand deformities may develop, they are not accompanied by articular erosions on radiographs. *Drug-induced lupus* presents with a symmetric polyarthritis and frequently with systemic manifestations including low-grade fever and serositis. Many drugs may provoke this reaction, but procainamide is the most common.

Polyarthritis may occur in other systemic rheumatic illnesses, both at presentation and later in the disease course. The presence of extra-articular manifestations can generally help in distinguishing these conditions from RA. For example, Raynaud's phenomenon and skin thickening are usually found in *systemic sclerosis* and *mixed connective tissue disease*. *Polymyositis* and *dermatomyositis* are accompanied by proximal muscle weakness. Patients with systemic vasculitis have characteristic skin lesions, neuropathy, and visceral involvement. *Polymyalgia rheumatica* presents with diffuse pain and morning stiffness, but usually joint pain is most prominent in the axial areas (hips and shoulders) and joint swelling is absent. Small effusions in the knees are often minimally symptomatic and cell counts are lower than in RA.

In *Behçet's syndrome,* recurrent oral and genital ulcerations are often accompanied by skin, eye, and neurologic manifestations. About half of these patients have arthritis at some time during their course. Recurrent oligoarticular arthritis is a frequent early or late finding in *relapsing polychondritis,* but extra-articular manifestations dominate the picture and include inflammation and destruction of cartilaginous tissue in the nose, ears, and upper airway. However, recurrent oligoarticular arthritis is a frequent early or late finding.

NONINFLAMMATORY POLYARTHROPATHY

Osteoarthritis (OA) is characterized by progressive attrition of articular cartilage and new bone formation at the margins of the joint. Typically, pain is aggravated by weight-bearing and motion and is relieved by rest. In more advanced disease, particularly in OA of the hip, there may also be nocturnal pain. Pain is usually much less severe in nonweight-bearing joints. On examination, bony enlargement may be detectable (such as Heberden's and Bouchard's nodes), and crepitus confirms the presence of articular cartilage roughening. Although less prominent than in inflammatory arthritis, synovial effusions may occur, especially in the knees. However, the fluid does not show inflammatory changes. Joint involvement in OA is usually focal rather than generalized; joints frequently involved include the hips, knees, and acromioclavicular, first MTP, first carpometacarpal, and interphalangeal joints. Patients with hand involvement often have a strong family history of OA.

Erosive inflammatory osteoarthritis of the distal and proximal finger joints causes more pain, tenderness, and soft-tissue swelling than does ordinary OA. Patients with this variant also experience more rapid loss of motion and bone erosion, culminating in bony ankylosis. The intermittent signs of inflammation may resemble RA, but erosive inflammatory OA is limited to the fingers.

Primary generalized osteoarthritis is caused by several conditions, some of which may have a genetic basis. The arthritis involves many joints, and often begins at an earlier age than is typical of OA. Several metabolic disorders can cause premature osteoarthritis, including hereditary *CPPD disease.* Patients with this disorder may also have episodes of acute crystal-induced inflammation (pseudogout). *Acromegaly* causes cartilage overgrowth initially, but the late arthropathy resembles generalized OA. In *ochronosis* the enzyme that metabolizes homogentisic acid is absent. Polymers of this tyrosine derivative are deposited in cartilage, which takes on a gray or black discoloration. The pigmentation may also be detected in the ears and sclerae. Polyarthropathy is a common early feature of *hemochromatosis* and typically involves the hands, particularly the metacarpophalangeal joints. This pattern resembles RA rather than OA. Moreover, the presence of mild soft tissue swelling may suggest an inflammatory arthritis. However, examination of the synovial membrane reveals iron deposition rather than inflammatory cells. Elevated iron saturation or ferritin levels support the diagnosis.

Other systemic illnesses may cause noninflammatory arthropathy. *Amyloidosis* due to AL amyloid deposition may be a primary disease or may be secondary to multiple myeloma. Most patients have prominent renal involvement and evidence that other organs are affected. However, arthritis due to amyloid deposits in and around the joints is the main symptom in a minority of patients. Shoulder swelling may be impressive (shoulder-pad sign), and hand swelling and deformity may resemble RA. Monoclonal immunoglobulins or light chains are usually found in the serum or urine. Patients receiving hemodialysis may have amyloid deposits derived from β2-microglobulin in articular tissues, resulting in chronic arthritis and carpal tunnel syndrome.

Hypertrophic pulmonary osteoarthropathy is a syndrome that may be caused by many thoracic or abdominal disorders, but carcinoma of the lung is the most common. The main features are clubbing of the fingers, osteoarticular pain, and radiographic evidence of periosteal new bone formation. Some patients have symmetric joint swelling, warmth, and effusions, suggesting the possibility of RA, but synovial fluid analysis fails to confirm inflammation.

Hemophilia causes recurrent episodes of pain and swelling due to intra-articular and periarticular hemorrhage. The attacks start in childhood and usually affect only one or two joints at a time. In the absence of factor VIII replacement therapy, a deforming polyarthritis may develop. *Sickle cell disease,* which also begins in childhood, often involves bones and joints; monarticular or oligoarticular joint swelling is an occasional finding.

EPIDEMIOLOGY OF POLYARTHRITIS

A patient's age, gender, and race may provide helpful clues in the differential diagnosis of polyarthritis. Young women are the likeliest group to have gonococcal arthritis, parvoviral and rubella arthritis, and SLE. Young men are more likely to develop ankylosing spondylitis, Reiter's syndrome, and HIV-related arthritis. RA and OA of the fingers start most frequently in middle-aged women, whereas gout, hemochromatosis, and polyarteritis nodosum are more common in middle-aged men. Elderly patients are more likely to have generalized osteoarthritis, CPPD disease, and polymyalgia rheumatica. African Americans have a high prevalence of SLE, sarcoidosis, and arthritis due to sickle cell disease, although this group has a decreased prevalence of ankylosing spondylitis and polymyalgia rheumatica. Infectious or postinfectious illnesses are endemic in some regions, such as Lyme disease in the northeastern coastal states and rheumatic fever in various South American and Asian nations. Geographic location and race may be closely intertwined. Behçet's disease occurs much more frequently in Japan and the Eastern Mediterranean than in other parts of the world.

ROBERT S. PINALS, MD

1. Pinals RS: Polyarthritis and fever. N Engl J Med 330:769-774, 1994

2. Liang MH, Sturrock RD: Evaluation of musculoskeletal symptoms, In Klippel JH, Dieppe PA (eds): Rheumatology. London, Mosby-Year Book, 1994, pp 2.1.1-2.1.18

3. Sergent JS: Polyarticular arthritis. In Kelley WN, Harris ED, Ruddy S, Sledge CB (eds): Textbook of Rheumatology. Philadelphia, WB Saunders, 1993, pp 381-388

4. McCarty DJ: Differential diagnosis of arthritis: analysis of signs and symptoms. In McCarty DJ, Koopman WJ (eds): Arthritis and Allied Conditions, 12th ed. Philadelphia, Lea & Febiger, 1993, pp 49-61

C. DIFFUSE PAIN SYNDROMES

Diffuse nonarticular musculoskeletal pain can be divided into acute and chronic entities. Acute pain typically has an obvious precipitating cause—a viral infection or trauma are two common examples. When a patient complains of generalized pain that is chronic, the etiology is usually less apparent. Although patients with chronic pain that present to a rheumatologist often have fibromyalgia syndrome (FMS), the clinician should be flexible, particularly early in the differential diagnosis process.

EVALUATION OF DIFFUSE MUSCULOSKELETAL PAIN

A complete history and thorough physical examination are essential to differentiate the various causes of diffuse pain (Table 8C-1). It is important to make certain that joints or tendons are not involved, even though the pain may appear to be originating from soft tissues. In early rheumatoid arthritis (RA) or the spondyloarthropathies for example, joint inflammation may not be initially obvious, particularly if the joints are not carefully examined. Morning stiffness in RA or accompanying tendinopathy from reactive arthritis may be mistaken for nonarticular disease. It is also crucial to check for evidence of a systemic illness. Connective tissue disease, vasculitis, chronic viral infection, malignancy, and endocrinopathies may all be associated with diffuse pain. In most instances, other clues alert the clinician to these diagnoses. Rashes or skin changes, neurologic findings, sicca symptoms, or renal abnormalities suggest the possibility of connective tissue disease or vasculitis. A predominance of fatigue and viral-like complaints suggest chronic fatigue syndrome. Thyroid disease should be suspected with weight change, strong reaction to ambient temperature, and chronic diarrhea or constipation. Chronic urticaria may signify a systemic mastocytosis with diffuse bone pain.

Diffuse pain can emanate from bones, muscles, or surrounding soft tissue. Bone metastases or multiple myeloma can cause diffuse pain that is usually severe and often associated with weight loss. Osteomalacia with microfractures can present as widespread pain. Polymyositis uncommonly may be accompanied by muscle pain, although weakness almost always predominates. In elderly patients with shoulder and hip girdle pain, polymyalgia rheumatica should be suspected.

Diffuse pain syndromes have recently been associated with exposure to environmental toxins. Ingestion of contaminated L-tryptophan, for example, causes eosinophilia–myalgia syndrome, which is characterized by high eosinophil counts and severe diffuse muscle pain (1). Patients with silicone breast implants may develop diffuse myalgias with pain that tends to abate after removal of the implants (2). It is important, therefore, to obtain a complete history of chemical exposures and prior surgeries.

In the physical examination of patients with diffuse chronic pain, the clinician should pay particular attention to fever, fast or irregular heart rhythms, thyromegaly, proximal muscle weakness, tender or swollen joints or tendons, rashes, neurologic abnormalities, hepatosplenomegaly, and lymphadenopathy. Limited or painful range of motion of the axial skeleton may be evidence of degenerative spine disease or spondyloarthropathy. Examination for tender points should be performed (see below).

Initial laboratory analysis should include a complete blood cell count, urine analysis, erythrocyte sedimentation rate (ESR), and thyroid-stimulating hormone. Other tests such as an antinuclear antibody (ANA), rheumatoid factor, serum complement levels, Lyme titer, Epstein–Barr virus tests, muscle enzymes, radiographs or other imaging studies, or electromyelography are warranted only if the history and examination suggest a particular diagnosis. Rare metabolic causes of diffuse pain such as hyper- or hypoparathyroidism may be discovered by laboratory testing, while

(Table 8C-1)

Diffuse musculoskeletal pain: differential diagnosis

Disorder	Clinical Characteristics	Laboratory Findings*
Rheumatoid arthritis	Joint pain predominance, joint swelling, nodules	Elevated ESR and CRP, positive rheumatoid factor, joint erosions on radiographs
Spondyloarthropathy	Back pain, tendinitis	HLA-B27 positive, radiographic changes
Lyme disease	Endemic area, rash	Positive serologies ELISA, Western blot
Systemic lupus erythematosus	Multisystem disease	Antinuclear antibodies, hypocomplementemia
Vasculitis	Systemic disease	Biopsy findings, antineutrophilic and cytoplasmic antibodies
Polymyositis/ Dermatomyositis	Weakness, rash	CPK/aldolase elevations, EMG abnormalities, biopsy findings
Polymyalgia rheumatica	Elderly, shoulder/ hip girdle pain	Elevated ESR
Eosinophilia-myalgia	L-tryptophan use, skin changes	Eosinophilia
Hyperthyroidism	Heat intolerance, diarrhea, atrial fibrillation	TSH decrease
Hypothyroidism	Cold intolerance, constipation, weight gain	TSH increase
Osteomalacia	Fractures	DEXA scan
Chronic fatigue syndrome	Fatigue predominates	None
Psychogenic rheumatism	Disproportionate pain	None
Silicone implants	Exposure history	None

*ESR = erythrocyte sedimentation rate; CRP = C-reactive protein; ELISA = enzyme-linked immunosorbent assay; CPK = creatine phosphokinase; TSH = thyroid-stimulating hormone; DEXA = dual-energy x-ray absorptiometry

Paget's disease of bone, osteomalacia, or metastatic bone disease may be found on radiographs.

THE FIBROMYALGIA SYNDROME

The fibromyalgia syndrome (FMS) is the most common rheumatic cause of chronic diffuse pain. The most important clinical features of FMS are symptoms of diffuse aching, stiffness, and fatigue coupled with a physical examination that demonstrates multiple tender points in specific areas. Although the pathophysiology has yet to be fully elucidated, FMS does not appear to be an inflammatory process, so the old term "fibrositis" has been abandoned. Patients may have no underlying disease or may have concomitant chronic diseases such as RA, osteoarthritis, Lyme disease, or sleep apnea. In the absence of an underlying condition, FMS is characterized by a strong female predominance (>75% in most series) with a peak incidence at ages 20-60 years old. FMS has been observed in up to 15% of rheumatology patients and about 5% of patients from a general medical practice. It was present in 2% of a random sample of midwestern residents (3).

Clinical Features

Patients with FMS most frequently report diffuse soft tissue pain. The pain is characteristically concentrated in axial locations such as the neck and lower back, with the proximal trapezius muscles commonly involved. Pain is often accompanied by stiffness, which also tends to be generalized and worse in the morning. This morning stiffness may mimic that accompanying RA. The symptoms are chronic but can vary in intensity from day to day. They are commonly exacerbated by various factors, such as moderate physical exercise, inactivity, poor sleep, emotional stress, and humid weather. Exacerbation of an underlying condition such as peripheral arthritis or lower back pain may also aggravate FMS. The pain associated with FMS is comparable in magnitude to that experienced with RA. A recent study demonstrated that FMS has an adverse effect on family income in 65% of patients, compared with 75% of RA patients (4). The consequences of this functional disability on a national scale are likely to be quite costly.

Other problems encountered in association with FMS include irritable bowel syndrome, tension headaches, paresthesias, and the sensation of swollen hands. Irritable bowel syndrome has been documented in up to 50% of cases. The headaches in these patients frequently begin with neck discomfort. Despite the common complaint of paresthesias in the upper extremities, results of nerve conduction studies are usually normal. Examination of the hands usually fails to confirm actual swelling.

Fatigue, which is often prominent in FMS, is frequently due to poor sleep (5). Patients commonly experience nonrestorative or nonrefreshing sleep. The vast majority of patients acknowledge a problem with sleep, although some may actually deny poor sleep. Even patients who do not complain of poor sleep may admit to light sleep, several awakenings at night, or fatigue that begins 30 minutes to several hours after arising in the morning. These complaints are difficult to interpret because they are not uncommon in the general population.

Criteria for the diagnosis of FMS were established by a multicenter trial sponsored by the American College of Rheumatology (ACR; see Appendix I) (6). The proposed criteria consist of widespread pain in combination with tenderness of at least 11 of 18 specific tender point sites (Fig. 8C-1). These criteria were developed after testing multiple variables in a population of FMS patients against matched controls with various rheumatic disorders. While the criteria were able to distinguish between these two groups, no differences were noted among patients who had fibromyalgia, with or without an associated rheumatic disease. Thus, it was suggested that the terms "primary" and "secondary" fibromyalgia should be abandoned. Patients with diffuse musculoskeletal pain and nonrestorative sleep but with fewer tender points may nevertheless have FMS.

On physical examination, tenderness on palpation with a moderate amount of pressure is noted in characteristic locations. However, there is clearly a subjective component to tender point examination. Tender points may be missed when the physician fails to press hard enough or the patient is obese or wearing protective clothing during the examination. Conversely, an examiner who presses too hard may elicit a reaction that is not truly point tenderness. An instrument called a dolorimeter that distributes pressure equally over a discrete point has been helpful in research settings to more objectively study these patients. The technique records the amount of pressure required to produce pain in a given area. Nontender control points (such as mid-forehead and the anterior thigh) should be included in the examination, although they are not included in the ACR criteria. These control points may be useful in distinguishing FMS from a conversion reaction, often referred to as psychogenic rheumatism, in which tenderness may be present virtually everywhere. Recent evidence suggests that FMS patients may have a generalized lowered threshold for pain on palpation, and the so-called control points may also on occasion be tender (7).

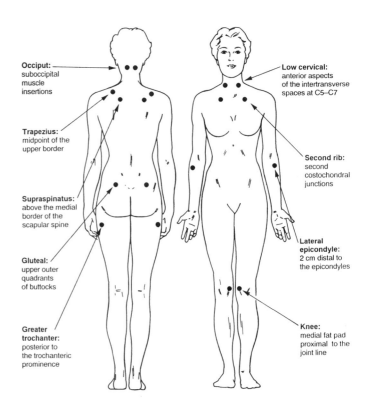

(Figure 8C-1)
Location of the specific tender points in fibromyalgia.

The lack of laboratory and radiographic abnormalities that can be attributed to FMS is conspicuous. The results of screening tests for diffuse pain (listed above) should be normal unless there is an underlying disorder. Radiographs or electromyelograms limited to very symptomatic areas may be useful in selected patients. A sleep study may be appropriate in patients with a history suggestive of particular types of sleep disturbances. Complaints of daytime napping, loud snoring, or spouse-witnessed long respiratory pauses during sleep are suggestive of sleep apnea and may warrant a sleep study.

Because FMS is found in association with a wide variety of conditions, the concomitant diagnosis of this disorder may be obscured by an underlying problem such as RA. Upper torso pain in a patient with RA, for example, may be erroneously attributed to cervical arthritis rather than muscle pain secondary to the poor sleep and FMS associated with RA. Muscular strain of the upper torso from motor vehicle accidents or sports injuries may produce aching and stiffness that simulates FMS with a limited number of tender points. Although FMS may initially be absent following an injury, these limited symptoms may persist causing disturbed sleep, and FMS may develop as a secondary process over time. Conversely, new patients who present with FMS symptoms should be evaluated for an underlying condition. FMS can be associated with arthritis, primary sleep disorders, metabolic disturbances such as hypothyroidism, and infectious processes such as Lyme disease. The diverse nature of these conditions reinforces the concept of FMS as a final common pathway.

It is important to distinguish FMS from more localized musculoskeletal pain, such as myofascial pain syndrome (Table 8C-2). Patients with myofascial pain syndrome typically have a localized unilateral muscular pain that is not associated with generalized aching, stiffness, or fatigue. The condition has an equal gender distribution and usually responds to local therapy such as stretching, heat, and local anesthetic or corticosteroid injections. In these cases, it is important to identify and eliminate activities that aggravate the pain.

The clinician may infrequently encounter a patient whose reports of musculoskeletal pain are so generalized and so amplified that a psychiatric disturbance should be suspected. The term *psychogenic rheumatism* has been applied to patients with this profile. Their complaints appear excessive and are often described in vivid images such as "searing hot

(Table 8C-2)
Differential features of fibromyalgia syndrome (FMS) and myofascial pain syndrome

Feature	FMS	Myofascial Pain
Pain	Diffuse	Local
Fatigue	Common	Uncommon
AM stiffness	Common	Uncommon
Tender points	Diffuse	Local
Treatment	Exercise Sleep medication	Local measures
Prognosis	Tends to be chronic	Resolves with treatment but may recur

knives going through my entire body." Unlike most patients with FMS, these patients have exquisite tenderness over their entire body, which may make examination difficult.

One final entity that bears resemblance to and overlaps with FMS is chronic fatigue syndrome, which is characterized by disabling fatigue of at least 6 months duration, and is usually accompanied by symptoms suggestive of a viral infection (8). Although fatigue predominates, patients frequently complain of generalized musculoskeletal pain and have tender points similar to FMS patients. The overlap of symptoms between these two syndromes is striking. Moreover, many patients with FMS describe viral-like symptoms, including recurrent pharyngitis, adenopathy, and low-grade fevers. Although infectious mononucleosis can on rare occasions lead to persistent fatigue and achiness, there is no evidence that chronic Epstein–Barr virus infection plays a role in FMS. Several infectious agents have been associated with FMS, including *Borrelia burgdorferi* (9), HIV (10), and parvovirus B19 (11).

Pathophysiology and Etiology

The etiology of FMS is unknown. Biopsies of tender points from patients have revealed no clear-cut histologic abnormalities when compared to normal subjects. There are some data to suggest diminished blood flow accompanied by a decrease in high-energy phosphates in these areas, but this has not been confirmed using spectroscopy (12). Decreased cerebral blood flow in the thalamus and caudate nucleus measured by single photon emission computed tomography accompanied by a generalized lower pain threshold has been demonstrated in women with FMS, compared with normal controls (7).

A subset of patients may have various immunologic abnormalities such as dermal–epidermal immune complex deposition, which suggests an autoimmune link. Although early reports suggested an increased incidence of positive antinuclear antibodies in patients with FMS, recent studies have not supported an increase when compared with healthy controls. Endocrine dysfunctions such as abnormalities of the hypophyseal–adrenal axis have been described (13). Increased substance P levels in the cerebral spinal fluid have been found, but levels correlate weakly with tenderness on examination (14). Blood levels of serotonin, an important neurotransmitter in brain centers involved with pain, sleep, and mood, may be decreased.

Due to a paucity of objective findings, patients with FMS are often considered to have a nonorganic basis for their illness. The association of tension headaches, irritable bowel syndrome, and stress-exacerbated symptoms further corroborates the impression of a psychiatric problem. Although there appears to be an increased incidence of prior personal and family history of depression in patients, the majority of patients do not have a primary major depression at the time of diagnosis. The chronic pain component in FMS may make the interpretation of some psychologic testing imprecise. Not uncommonly, FMS patients develop a reactive depression to this chronic, poorly understood, and disabling condition.

Sleep Disturbances

Almost any chronic rheumatologic condition that produces pain may be associated with FMS. The mechanism of this association may be related to a sleep disturbance. It has been documented that some patients with RA and osteoarthritis have fragmented sleep with multiple arousals to lighter sleep stages and actual awakenings associated with movement, presumably secondary to pain. One sleep study found that a group of patients with RA had an average of 3.4 awakenings and 43.2 arousals per hour (15). Despite feeling fatigued during the day, most of these patients were unaware of the frequency of these nocturnal events, which illustrates the lack of sensitivity in obtaining a sleep history.

Primary sleep disturbances such as sleep apnea and nocturnal myoclonus have also been associated with FMS (5). The common link among these conditions appears to be fragmented sleep. In sleep apnea, sleep disruption is caused by either obstruction of the upper airways or decreased respiratory signaling from the central nervous system. Nocturnal myoclonus is manifested by involuntary leg motion during sleep. Arousals and awakenings in both sleep apnea and nocturnal myoclonus occur in a manner analogous to that seen with arthritis. The FMS associated with these conditions tends to dissipate when the underlying problem is treated, and sleep subsequently improves. Conditions associated with sleep disturbance and FMS are listed in Table 8C-3.

Several other findings suggest a link between FMS and a sleep disturbance. About 80% of patients consider their sleep to be nonrestorative (6). Patients may also admit to being light sleepers or waking more than once per night. The fatigue associated with FMS improves with effective therapy, such as medications that enhance the quality of sleep. Moldofsky was able to reproduce the signs and symptoms of FMS in healthy young controls by disrupting nonrapid eye movement (non-REM) stage 3-4 sleep with an auditory stimulus (5). This stage of sleep is characterized by high-amplitude, low-frequency delta waves on electroencephalogram (EEG) recordings. Control subjects deprived of REM sleep did not manifest these symptoms. Delta wave sleep, which is the deepest stage of sleep and the most difficult to awaken a subject from, is more highly preserved in evolution than REM sleep and may therefore have an important restorative function. It had been noted in sleeping FMS patients that the low-frequency EEG waves of stage 3-4 sleep were interrupted by high-frequency alpha waves, which is termed alpha wave intrusion. However, a controlled blinded study of FMS patients, healthy controls, and patients without FMS but with other generalized musculoskeletal pain showed no differences in the amount of alpha wave intrusion (16).

Treatment

The initial aspect of therapy for FMS should include patient education and reassurance. Patients should be informed that it is not a psychiatric disturbance and that it is not a rare disorder. The clinician should stress that FMS is not deforming or life-threatening, and that, although it is frequently a chronic problem, effective treatments are available.

Medications that improve sleep appear to be the most effective pharmacologic intervention. Blinded, short-term, randomized, placebo-controlled studies of amitriptyline (5), cyclobenzaprine, and alprazolam (17) given at bedtime have shown these drugs to be effective in treating FMS. Amitriptyline and cyclobenzaprine appear to become ineffective over a 6-month period, however (18). In general, these medications are helpful in achieving a more restorative sleep, but the dosage and timing are important. Drowsiness and anticholinergic side effects can undermine the positive actions. Tricyclic antidepressants with fewer anticholinergic side effects, such as nortriptyline, appear to be better tolerated, and long-term compliance may be superior. Treatment should be initiated at the lowest available dose of whatever drug is chosen and increased until restorative sleep is achieved or adverse effects are encountered. Medication tends to be more effective if taken 1-2 hours before bedtime. Hypnotic agents such as flurazepam, temazepam, triazolam, and zolpidem are generally less useful, unless the patient has a problem falling asleep. Patients should be assured that once the sleep improves, the pain will dissipate over time.

Nonsteroidal anti-inflammatory drugs (NSAIDs) and corticosteroids have not been effective as single agents. Ibuprofen, however, was found to enhance the efficacy of alprazolam (17). If pain is a factor interfering with quality sleep, a long-acting NSAID can be given at nighttime. Certainly, any coexistent disease should be treated appropriately. For example, using NSAIDs to treat underlying tendinitis or degenerative arthritis may also be beneficial for FMS. Narcotics should be avoided for this chronic process. If narcotics appear necessary to control pain, strong consideration should be given to referring the patient to a pain clinic or obtaining a psychiatric evaluation.

Other forms of therapy include biofeedback, meditation, acupuncture, injection of tender points with local anesthetics or corticosteroids, ultrasound treatments, massage, and exercise. Physical therapists can be quite useful in administering some of these treatments. Aerobic exercise as opposed to simple stretching appears to be more beneficial (19). Heat in the form of whirlpool or ultrasound coupled with electrical stimulation are temporarily beneficial. Daily exercise programs, although often helpful, may exacerbate the condition if performed incorrectly. Thus the clinician should be sensitive to the pace at which patients advance their exercise program. A good rule is to begin exercise at a low intensity,

(Table 8C-3)
Conditions associated with sleep disturbance and fibromyalgia

Symptoms	Diagnoses to Consider
Headaches, rhinitis	Sinusitis
Nocturia	Diabetes mellitus, diuretic use, interstitial cystitis
Dry mouth	Sjögren's syndrome, anticholinergic medications
Snoring, daytime naps	Sleep apnea
Morning leg pain	Nocturnal myoclonus, restless leg syndrome
Morning facial pain	Bruxism, temporomandibular disorder
Joint pain, swelling	Rheumatologic conditions
Shortness of breath	Asthma, coronary heart failure
Awaken for unknown reasons	Spouse snores, pet in room, noises, lights, dry air

concentrating mostly on stretching, and then gradually progress to more strenuous aerobic exercises.

It is important to identify and treat patients who have underlying depression. In these instances, it is preferable to prescribe a tricyclic antidepressant at night rather than a benzodiazepine. Psychiatric consultation should be sought if the situation is unclear, but this is unnecessary for the majority of patients. Secondary depression can be treated by patient education.

Although fibromyalgia is a chronic disorder, a recent community-based study found that one-quarter of patients were in remission at the end of 2 years (20). Patients who are younger and those with less severe presentations tend to have better outcomes. Patients who respond to therapy may nevertheless continue to complain of a lower-level, persistent, but tolerable pain. Medication for the symptoms of FMS may often times be necessary for years.

BRUCE FREUNDLICH, MD
LAWRENCE LEVENTHAL, MD

1. Freundlich B: The eosinophilia myalgia syndrome. In Kelley WN, et al (eds): Textbook of Rheumatology, 4th Edition. Philadelphia, W.B. Saunders Co., 1993

2. Borenstein D: Siliconosis: a spectrum of illness. Semin Arthritis Rheum 24s:1-7, 1994

3. Wolfe F, Ross K, Anderson J, et al: The prevalence and characteristics of fibromyalgia in the general population. Arthritis Rheum 38:19-28, 1995

4. Martinez JE, Ferraz MB, Sato EI, et al: Fibromyalgia versus rheumatoid arthritis: a longitudinal comparison of the quality of life. J Rheumatol 22:270-274, 1995

5. Moldofsky H: Sleep and fibrositis syndrome. Rheum Dis Clin North Am 15:90-103, 1989

6. Wolfe F, Smythe HA, Yunus MB, et al: The American College of Rheumatology 1990 criteria for the classification of fibromyalgia. Report of the multicenter criteria committee. Arthritis Rheum 33:160-172, 1990

7. Mountz JM, Bradley LA, Modell JG, et al: Fibromyalgia in women. Abnormalities of regional cerebral blood flow in the thalamus and the caudate nucleus are associated with low pain threshold levels. Arthritis Rheum 38:926-928, 1995

8. Shafran SD: The chronic fatigue syndrome. Am J Med 90:730-739, 1991

9. Sigal LH: Summary of the first 100 patients seen at a Lyme Disease Referral Center. Am J Med 88:577-581, 1990

10. Medina-Rodriguez F, Guzman C, Jara C, et al: Rheumatic manifestations in human immunodeficiency virus positive and negative individuals. J Rheumatol 20:1880-1884, 1993

11. Leventhal LJ, Naides SJ, Freundlich B: Fibromyalgia and parvovirus infection. Arthritis Rheum 34:1319-1342, 1991

12. Simms RW, Roy SH, Hrovat M. et al: Lack of association between fibromyalgia syndrome and abnormalities in energy muscle metabolism. Arthritis Rheum 37:794-800, 1994

13. Grofford LJ, Pillemer SR, Kalogeras KT, et al: Hypothalamic-pituitary-adrenal axis perturbations in patients with fibromyalgia. Arthritis Rheum 37:1583-1592, 1994

14. Russell IJ, Orr MD, Littman B, et al: Elevated cerebrospinal fluid levels of substance P in patients with the fibromyalgia syndrome. Arthritis Rheum 37:1593-1601, 1994

15. Mahowald MW, Mahowald ML, Bundlie SR, et al: Sleep fragmentation in rheumatoid arthritis. Arthritis Rheum 32:974-983, 1989

16. Leventhal L, Freundlich B, Lewis J, Gillen K, Henry J, Dinges D: Controlled study of alpha NREM sleep in patients with fibromyalgia. J Clin Rheumatol 1:110-113, 1995

17. Russell IJ, Fletcher EM, Michalek JE, et al: Treatment of primary fibrositis/fibromyalgia syndrome with ibuprofen and alprazolam. A double-blind, placebo-controlled study. Arthritis Rheum 35:552-560, 1991

18. Carrette S, Bell MJ, Reynolds WJ, et al: Comparison of amitriptyline, cyclobenzaprine and placebo in the treatment of fibromyalgia: a randomized, double-blind clinical trial. Arthritis Rheum 37:32-40, 1994

19. McCain GA, Bell DA, Mai FM, et al: A controlled study of the effects of a supervised cardiovascular fitness training program on the manifestations of primary fibromyalgia. Arthritis Rheum 31:1135-1141, 1988

20. Granges G, Zilko P, Littlejohn GO: Fibromyalgia syndrome: assessment of severity of the condition 2 years after diagnosis. J Rheumatol 21:523-529, 1994

D. PERIODIC SYNDROMES

Intermittent inflammatory synovitis is a major clinical feature of many rheumatic disorders. Among the conditions in which intermittent joint swelling occurs are systemic lupus erythematosus (SLE), Lyme arthritis, HIV infection, crystal-induced arthritis, Still's disease, sclerosing cholangitis, Whipple's disease, inflammatory bowel disease, and urticaria, angioedema, and other allergic and inflammatory cutaneous disorders. Hydrarthrosis may also be a drug side effect, for example, with pefloxacine (1).

PALINDROMIC RHEUMATISM

The term *palindromic rheumatism* is used to describe patients with recurrent, afebrile episodes of acute arthritis and periarthritis. Derived from the Greek *palindromous,* meaning to "run back," the term reflects the feature of recurrence. The episodes usually last for hours or a few days with complete resolution between intervals (2). Men and women appear to be equally affected, and the onset is typically between the third and sixth decades. The prevalence of palindromic rheumatism is estimated to be roughly one-tenth that of rheumatoid arthritis (RA) (3).

The attacks generally occur without an identified inciting event but have been reported to follow childbirth, vigorous exercise, and infection (2,3). The episodes are irregular and may overlap in individual joints. Virtually any joint may be affected, although involvement of the spine, temporomandibular joint, and sternoclavicular joint is exceedingly rare (Table 8D-1) (4).

Marked soft tissue swelling and even subcutaneous nodules sometimes accompany these episodes. The nodules are usually pea-sized and tend to appear over tendons in the hands or fingers and the thumb pads. Constitutional symptoms are unusual during the attacks, and extra-articular disease is rare.

Laboratory findings are nonspecific. The erythrocyte sedimentation rate (ESR) may be elevated during the attack. Approximately one-third of patients develop rheumatoid factor (RF) and appear to eventually develop RA more frequently than RF-negative patients (3). Antinuclear antibodies are absent (5). The synovium is characterized by a nonspecific inflammatory reaction with thickening of the joint capsule and infiltration of polymorphonuclear cells without eosinophils (2). Perivascular lymphocytes, fibrin and cellular thrombi in synovial blood vessels, and perivascular fibrosis may be seen (6). The subcutaneous nodules may show nonspecific inflammation, but without necrotic zones or areas of central fibrinoid necrosis and palisading mononuclear cells that are typical of rheumatoid nodules (2,7).

(Table 8D-1)

*Distribution of joint involvement in attacks based on a cumulative experience with 227 patients**

Joints Involved	% of Patients	
	Mean	Range
MCP and PIP	91	74–100
Wrists	78	54–82
Knees	64	41–94
Shoulders	65	33–75
Ankles	50	10–67
Feet	43	15–73
Elbows	38	13–60
Hips	17	0–40
Temporomandibular	8	0–28
Spine	4	0–11
Sternoclavicular	2	0–6
Para-articular sites	27	20–29

* Modified from Guerne et al (4) with permission.
MCP = metacarpophalangeal; PIP = proximal interphalangeal.

Although palindromic rheumatism may occur in families, a strong genetic association has not been demonstrated with human leukocyte antigens (HLA) including HLA-DR4 and HLA-DR1 (5,8).

Chronic arthritis indistinguishable from RA develops in approximately one-third to one-half of patients. From a literature review of follow-up ranging from months to 30 years, approximately 48% of patients continued to have palindromic rheumatism, 33% progressed to RA, 4% developed other conditions, and 15% had prolonged remission (4). There are no good markers to predict the disease course.

There are no controlled therapeutic trials of palindromic rheumatism. Nonsteroidal anti-inflammatory drugs (NSAIDs) may be helpful in relieving symptoms (2,3). Prophylactic corticosteroids and colchicine have rarely been helpful in preventing attacks, although intramuscular gold, hydroxychloroquine, and sulfasalazine may be beneficial (4,9).

INTERMITTENT HYDRARTHROSIS

Intermittent hydrarthrosis is a syndrome of episodic attacks of synovitis usually in large joints, most commonly the knees. Typically, attacks occur in one knee at a time, although both knees may be affected simultaneously. The condition usually begins in adolescence but can present up to the fifth decade (10). Both genders are affected equally. The attacks generally last 2–4 days, and joints are normal in the interval. In contrast to palindromic rheumatism, which affects different joints at different times, intermittent hydrarthrosis almost always affects the same few joints.

Laboratory tests are unremarkable, including ESR and rheumatoid factor. Radiographs show no evidence of bony erosion or cartilage loss. No successful treatment for preventing or aborting the attacks has been documented.

FAMILIAL MEDITERRANEAN FEVER

Familial Mediterranean fever (FMF) is an inherited autosomal recessive disorder of unknown pathogenesis. It occurs almost exclusively among people of Mediterranean ancestry, especially non-Ashkenazi Jews, Armenians, Turks, and Levantine Arabs (11). The periodic attacks usually begin in childhood and are accompanied by fever and one or more inflammatory manifestations, including (in order of frequency) peritonitis, arthritis, pleuritis, and erysipelatous rash. Peritonitis may lead to unnecessary surgery for an acute abdominal emergency if FMF is not diagnosed. The attacks usually resolve spontaneously within a few days.

Arthralgias are common in FMF patients. The arthritis generally affects one large joint at a time and is accompanied by acute attacks of pain and swelling that usually subside over 2–3 days, although the attack may last longer, especially if the hip is involved (12). Swelling is modest but pain may be severe. As with most other periodic syndromes, permanent joint damage does not occur.

Laboratory abnormalities include elevated ESR and synovial fluid leukocyte counts during the attacks. Synovial biopsies are unremarkable. Radiographs may reveal nonspecific joint-space narrowing, sclerosis, and osteophyte formation. In chronic cases, periarticular osteopenia may occur.

Patients with FMF lack a protein that inhibits neutrophil chemotaxis by antagonizing the complement-derived inflammatory mediator C5A. The C5A inhibitor has been shown to be lacking in patients' synovial and peritoneal fluids (13). The gene that encodes the inhibitor protein has not been identified.

Poor regulation of other inflammatory substances has also been postulated. Underlying these abnormalities may be a lipocortin deficiency, caused by either an absence of lipocortin or a dysfunctional lipoprotein molecule (14). Lipocortins inhibit phospholipase, which converts phospholipids into arachidonic acid. Any stimulus such as trauma that increases the activity of adenyl cyclase in the absence of lipocortin may produce an attack of fever and pain. This may also be the explanation for the lack of therapeutic response to corticosteroids in these patients (12).

The gene(s) that cause FMF in non-Ashkenazi Jews map to the short arm of chromosome 16 (15). There is a high carrier frequency of the FMF gene(s) that increases the chance of inbred offspring having the disease without being homozygous (15). See Appendix IV.

Glucocorticosteroids are ineffective in preventing or treating the attacks. Prophylactic colchicine at doses of 1.2–1.8 mg/day reduces the frequency of attacks (16) and may delay the onset of amyloidosis, a late complication of FMF and the main cause of death in some groups of patients. Amyloid type AA deposition frequently leads to end-stage renal disease in certain ethnic groups. The therapeutic dosage of colchicine for amyloidosis in FMF patients is greater than 1.5 mg/day, which is said to be effective only in patients with an initial serum creatinine level of less than 1.5 mg/deciliter.

RS3PE SYNDROME

Relapsing seronegative symmetrical synovitis with pitting edema (RS3PE syndrome) is associated with marked joint stiffness and symmetric polysynovitis involving especially the hands and feet (17). The onset is typically abrupt, and profound pitting edema of the hands may lead to carpal tunnel syndrome. Large joint involvement may also occur, but like most periodic syndromes, it is not associated with joint destruction. The incidence of RS3PE is unknown; it is typically seen in patients over the age of 60 and is more common in men (17,18).

The ESR varies from normal to more than 100 mm/hour. Synovial fluid analysis reveals nonspecific inflammation. Rheumatoid factor is negative.

The synovitis and edema respond dramatically to low doses of corticosteroids, usually 5–15 mg of prednisone per day. Symptoms usually resolve within 2–3 months on this treatment. NSAIDs and hydroxychloroquine are also useful (17,18). When treated within the first 6 months, complete remission even after corticosteroid taper is the rule, distinguishing this condition from polymyalgia rheumatica.

Because many of the patients are elderly and have multiple risk factors for long-term steroid therapy, the use of NSAIDs and/or hydroxychloroquine has been advocated as adequate therapy (18). Unlike other periodic syndromes, symptoms frequently do not recur after treatment, but the role of treatment in modifying the natural history is unknown.

Some patients appear to have symptoms of RS3PE as part of a syndrome linked to polymyalgia rheumatica. But unlike polymyalgia rheumatica, RS3PE syndrome may be accompanied by finger, wrist, and elbow contractures. In addition, flares following reduction of corticosteroids in RS3PE are rare (17,18).

HYPERIMMUNOGLOBULIN D AND PERIODIC FEVER SYNDROME

Periodic fever syndrome associated with elevated levels of polyclonal immunoglobulin D was described in 1984 by Van der Meer et al (19). Patients experience recurrent attacks of chills, fever, headaches, lymphadenopathy, abdominal pain, and diarrhea. The episodes can be similar to familial Mediterranean fever. The attacks usually begin within the first 6 months of life, but the first event may occur in patients up to 53 years of age (20). Typically, attacks occur once or twice a month, although they may be less frequent, and may be preceded by viral infection or immunization.

About 80% of patients have polyarthralgias, and about 68% have arthritis with swollen and painful joints (20). Virtually any appendicular joint may be involved, although the large joints are more commonly affected. The arthritis may be symmetric. Arthritis attacks appear to decrease with age.

During the attacks, elevated ESR and leukocytosis may occur. Serologic tests are unrevealing; synovial fluid may reveal a high white blood cell count with predominant polymorphonuclear cells. The joint disease is nondestructive, and there are no specific radiographic changes (20). Treatment with short bursts of high-dose corticosteroids and/or NSAIDs appears effective for managing the symptoms of the attacks, which are usually self-limited. Colchicine may reduce the frequency and intensity of the attacks in a minority of patients; many other therapies including cytotoxic therapies and gammaglobulin have been suggested.

The pathogenesis of periodic fever syndrome is unknown, although type III hypersensitivity reaction with involvement of IgD-containing complexes has been postulated (20).

ERIC L. MATTESON, MD

1. Touzet P, Thibaud D: Hydrarthrosis complicating a treatment with pefloxacine in a 14-year-old adolescent (letter). Arch Fr Pediatr 48:151-152, 1991

2. Hench PS, Rosenberg EF: Palindromic rheumatism. New oft recurring disease of joints (arthritis, periarthritis, paraarthritis) apparently producing no articular residues: report of 34 cases (its relationship to "angroneural arthrosis," "allergic rheumatism" and rheumatoid arthritis). Proc Mayo Clin 16:808, 1941

3. Pasero G, Barbieri P: Palindromic rheumatism: you just have to think about it. Clin Exp Rheumatol 4:197-199, 1986

4. Guerne PA, Weisman MH: Palindromic rheumatism: part of or apart from the spectrum of rheumatoid arthritis. Am J Med 93:451-460, 1992

5. Hannonen P, Mittînen T, Oka M: Palindromic rheumatism: a clinical survey of sixty patients. Scand J Rheumatol 16:413-420, 1987

6. Schumacher HR: Palindromic onset of rheumatoid arthritis. Clinical synovial fluid and biopsy studies. Arthritis Rheum 25:361-369, 1982

7. Schreiber S, Schumacher HR, Cherian PV: Palindromic rheumatism with rheumatoid nodules: a case report with ultrastructural studies. Ann Rheum Dis 45:78-81, 1986

8. Fisher LR, Kirk A, Awad J, Festenstein H, Alouso A, Perry JD, Shipley M: HLA antigens in palindromic rheumatism and palindromic onset rheumatoid arthritis. Br J Rheumatol 25:345-348, 1986

9. Youssef W, Yan A, Russell AS: Palindromic rheumatism: a response to chloroquine. J Rheumatol 18:35-37, 1991

10. Weiner AB, Ghormley RK: Periodic benign synovitis: idiopathic hydrarthrosis. J Bone Joint Surg 38A:1034-1055, 1956

11. Sohar E, Gafni J, Pras M, Heller H: Familial Mediterranean fever: a survey of 470 cases and review of the literature. Am J Med 43:227-253, 1967

12. Garcia-Gonzalez A, Weisman MH: The arthritis of familial Mediterranean fever. Semin Arthritis Rheum 22:139-150, 1992

13. Matzner Y, Ayesh SK, Hochner-Celniker D, Ackerman Z, Ferne M: Proposed mechanism of the inflammatory attacks in familial Mediterranean fever. Arch Intern Med 150:1289-1291, 1990

14. Shohat M, Korenberg JR, Schwabe AD, Rotter JI: Hypothesis: familial Mediterranean fever - a genetic disorder of the lipocortin family? Am J Med Genet 34:163-167, 1989

15. Pras E, Aksentijevich I, Gruberg L, Balow JE Jr, Prosen L, Dean M, Steinberg AD, Pras M, Kastner DL: Mapping of a gene causing familial Mediterranean fever to the short arm of chromosome 16. N Engl J Med 326:1509-1513, 1992

16. Zemer D, Pras M, Sohar E, Modan M, Cabili S, Gafni J: Colchicine in the prevention and treatment of the amyloidosis of familial Mediterranean fever. N Engl J Med 314:1001-1005, 1986

17. McCarty DJ, O'Duffy JD, Pearson L, Hunter JB: Remitting seronegative symmetrical synovitis with pitting edema: RS3PE syndrome. JAMA 254:2763-2767, 1985

18. Bridges AJ, Hickman PL: RS3PE syndrome and polymyalgia rheumatica: distinguishing features. J Rheumatol 18:1764-1765, 1991

19. Van der Meer JWM, Vossen JM, Radl J, Van Nieuwkoop JA, Meijer CJLM, Lobatto S, Van Furth R: Hyperimmunoglobulinemia D and periodic fever. A new syndrome. Lancet 1087-1090, 1984

20. Drenth JPH, Haagsma CJ, Van der Meer JWM: Hyperimmunoglobulinemia D and periodic fever syndrome: the clinical spectrum in a series of 50 patients. Medicine (Baltimore) 73:133-144, 1994

E. DISORDERS OF THE LOW BACK AND NECK

Low-back and neck pain are second only to the common cold as the most common affliction of humans. Approximately 10%–20% of the US population experiences either back or neck pain each year (1). Low-back pain is the fifth most common reason for visiting a physician, according to a National Ambulatory Care Survey (2).

The symptom of axial skeleton pain is associated with a wide variety of mechanical and medical disorders (3,4) (Table 8E-1). Mechanical disorders of the axial skeleton are caused by overuse (muscle strain), trauma (herniated intervertebral disc), or physical deformity of an anatomic structure. Medical disorders that cause spine pain are associated with constitutional symptoms, disease in other organ systems, and inflammatory or infiltrative disease of the axial skeleton. As many as 90% of patients with low-back and neck pain have a mechanical reason for their discomfort. Characteristically, mechanical disorders are exacerbated by certain physical activities and are relieved by others, and most resolve over a short period of time. More than 50% of all patients improve after 1 week, and more than 90% are better at 8 weeks (5).

INITIAL EVALUATION

In the initial evaluation of patients with spinal pain, the physician must separate those individuals with mechanical disorders from those with systemic illnesses. The patient's symptoms and physical signs help differentiate mechanical from systemic causes of axial pain. The initial diagnostic evaluation includes a history and physical examination with complete evaluation of the musculoskeletal system, including palpation of the axial skeleton and assessment of range of motion and alignment of the spine. Neurologic examination to detect evidence of spinal cord, spinal root, or peripheral nerve dysfunction is essential. In most patients, radiographic and laboratory tests are not necessary. Plain radiographs and erythrocyte sedimentation rate (ESR) are most informative in patients who are 50 years or older, who have a history of cancer, or who have constitutional symptoms (6).

The initial evaluation should eliminate the presence of cauda equina syndrome and cervical myelopathy, which are rare conditions that require emergency interventions. *Cauda equina compression* is characterized by low-back pain, bilateral motor weakness of the lower extremities, bilateral sciatica, saddle anesthesia, and bladder or bowel incontinence. The common causes of cauda equina compression include central herniation of an intervertebral disc, epidural abscess or hematoma, and tumor masses. In the cervical spine, myelopathy with long-tract signs (eg, spasticity, clonus, Babinski's sign, incontinence) indicate compression of the spinal cord. The common causes of myelopathy include disc herniation and osteophytic overgrowth. If cauda equina syndrome or cervical myelopathy is suspected, radiographic evaluation is mandatory. Magnetic resonance imaging (MRI) is the most sensitive technique for visualizing the spine. If the clinician's suspicion is confirmed, surgical decompression of the compromised neural elements is indicated (7).

SYSTEMIC DISORDERS

The majority of patients with spinal pain and systemic illnesses can be identified by the presence of one or more of the following: 1) fever or weight loss, 2) pain with recumbency, 3) prolonged morning stiffness, 4) localized bone pain, or 5) visceral pain.

Fever and Weight Loss

In patients with a history of fever or weight loss, frequently spinal pain is caused by an infection or tumor (8). Vertebral osteomyelitis causes pain that is slowly progressive, may be either intermittent or constant, is present at rest, and is exacerbated by motion. Tumor pain progresses more rapidly. Plain radiographs are not informative unless more than 30% of the bone calcium has been lost in the area of the lesion. Bone scintigraphy is a sensitive but nonspecific test for bone lesions. Areas of bony involvement and soft tissue extension are best identified by computed tomography (CT) and MRI, respectively.

Pain with Recumbency

Tumors, benign or malignant, of the spinal column or spinal cord are the prime concern in patients with nocturnal pain or pain on recumbency (9). Compression of neural elements by expanding masses and associated inflammation accounts for the pain. Physical examination demonstrates localized tenderness and, if the spinal cord or roots are compressed, neurologic dysfunction. MRI is the most sensitive method to detect bony abnormalities, spinal cord or root compromise, and soft tissue extension of neoplastic lesions.

Morning Stiffness

Morning stiffness lasting an hour or less is a common symptom of mechanical spinal disorders. In contrast, morning stiffness of the lumbar or cervical spine lasting several hours is a common symptom of seronegative spondyloarthropathy. Bilateral sacroiliac pain is associated with ankylosing spondylitis and enteropathic arthritis, while Reiter's syndrome and psoriatic spondylitis may cause unilateral sacroiliac pain or spondylitis without sacroiliitis. Women with spondyloarthropathy may have neck pain and stiffness with minimal low-back pain. On physical examination, these patients demonstrate stiffness in all planes of spinal motion. Plain radiographs of the lumbosacral spine are helpful for identifying early changes, including loss of lumbar lordosis, joint erosions in the lower one-third of the sacroiliac joints, and squaring of vertebral bodies. More costly radiographic studies are not necessary to identify skeletal abnormalities in patients with spondylitis.

Localized Bone Pain

Spinal pain localized to the midline over osseous structures is associated with disorders that fracture or expand bone. Any systemic process that increases mineral loss from bone (osteoporosis), causes bone necrosis (hemoglobinopathy), or replaces bone cells with inflammatory or neoplastic cells (multiple myeloma) weakens vertebral bone to the point that fracture may occur spontaneously or with

(Table 8E-1)

Disorders of the low back and neck

Mechanical
  Muscle strain
  Herniated intervertebral disc
  Osteoarthritis
  Spinal stenosis
  Spinal stenosis with myelopathy*
  Spondylolysis/spondylolisthesis[†]
  Adult scoliosis[†]
  Whiplash*
Rheumatologic
  Ankylosing spondylitis
  Reiter's syndrome
  Psoriatic arthritis
  Enteropathic arthritis
  Rheumatoid arthritis*
  Diffuse idiopathic skeletal hyperostosis
  Vertebral osteochondritis[†]
  Polymyalgia rheumatica
  Fibromyalgia
  Behçet's syndrome[†]
  Whipple's disease[†]
  Hidradenitis suppurativa[†]
  Osteitis condensans ilii[†]
Endocrinologic/Metabolic
  Osteoporosis
  Osteomalacia
  Parathyroid disease
  Microcrystalline disease
  Ochronosis
  Fluorosis
  Heritable genetic disorders
Neurologic/Psychiatric
  Neuropathic arthropathy
  Neuropathies
    Tumors
    Vasculitis
    Compression
  Psychogenic rheumatism
  Depression
  Malingering
Miscellaneous
  Paget's disease of bone
  Vertebral sarcoidosis
Infectious
  Vertebral osteomyelitis
  Meningitis*
  Discitis
  Pyogenic sacroiliitis[†]

  Herpes zoster
  Lyme disease
Neoplastic/Infiltrative
  Benign tumors
    Osteoid osteoma[†]
    Osteoblastoma
    Osteochondroma
    Giant cell tumor
    Aneurysmal bone cyst
    Hemangioma
    Eosinophilic granuloma
    Gaucher's disease[†]
    Sacroiliac lipoma[†]
  Malignant tumors
    Skeletal metastases
    Multiple myeloma
    Chondrosarcoma
    Chordoma
    Lymphoma[†]
  Intraspinal lesions
    Metastases
    Meningioma
    Vascular malformations
    Gliomas
    Syringomyelia*
Hematologic
  Hemoglobinopathies[†]
  Myelofibrosis[†]
  Mastocytosis[†]
Referred Pain
  Vascular
    Abdominal aorta[†]
    Carotid*
    Thoracic aorta*
  Gastrointestinal
    Pancreas
    Gallbladder
    Intestine
    Esophagus*
Subacute bacterial endocarditis
Retroperitoneal fibrosis
Genitourinary[†]
  Kidney
  Ureter
  Bladder
  Uterus
  Ovary
  Prostate

---

* Neck predominance.
[†] Low back predominance.
Modified from Borenstein et al (3,4), with permission.

minimal trauma. Patients with acute fractures experience sudden onset of local pain. Bone pain may be the initial manifestation of the underlying disorder. On physical examination, palpation of the affected area produces pain. Plain radiographs may reveal alterations but do not show microfractures. Scintigraphy can detect increased bone activity soon after a fracture occurs, and CT scan may identify the abnormality. However, locating the lesion is not sufficient to define the specific cause of bony changes. Laboratory tests, including ESR, serum chemistries, and complete blood cell count, are most helpful in differentiating between metabolic and neoplastic disorders that can cause localized bone pain.

Visceral Pain

Abnormalities in organs that share segmental innervation with part of the axial skeleton can cause referred back pain. Viscerogenic pain may arise from vascular, gastrointestinal, or genitourinary disorders. The duration and sequence of back pain follows the periodicity of the diseased organ. Colicky pain is associated with spasm in hollow structures such as the ureter, colon, and gallbladder. Throbbing pain occurs with vascular lesions. Exertional pain that radiates into the left arm in a C7 distribution may be associated with angina and coronary artery disease (10). Back pain that coincides with a woman's menstrual cycle may be related to endometriosis. Physical examination of the abdomen may reveal tenderness over the diseased organ. Laboratory tests are useful to document the presence of an abnormality in the genitourinary (hematuria) or gastrointestinal (amylase) systems. Radiographic tests are helpful for diagnosing some visceral disorders; for example, CT of the aorta and barium swallow when abdominal aneurysm or esophageal diverticulum are suspected, respectively.

MECHANICAL DISORDERS OF THE LUMBOSACRAL SPINE

Mechanical disorders are the most common causes of low back pain. They include muscle strain, herniated nucleus pulposus, osteoarthritis, spinal stenosis, spondylolisthesis, and adult scoliosis. The clinical characteristics of these disorders are listed in Table 8E-2.

Back Strain

Back strain is preceded by some traumatic event that can range from coughing or sneezing to lifting an object heavier than can be supported by the muscles and ligaments of the lumbosacral spine (11). The typical history of muscle strain is acute back pain that radiates up the ipsilateral paraspinous muscles, across the lumbar area, and sometimes caudally to the buttocks without radiation to the thigh. Physical examination reveals limited range of motion in the lumbar area and paraspinous muscle contraction. No neurologic abnormalities are present on examination. Therapy includes physical activity, nonsteroidal anti-inflammatory drugs (NSAIDs), and muscle relaxants.

Lumbar Disc Herniation

Intervertebral disc herniation causes nerve impingement and inflammation that results in radicular pain (sciatica). Herniation occurs with sudden movement and is frequently associated with heavy lifting. Sciatica is exacerbated by activities that increase intradiskal pressure, such as sitting, bending, or Valsalva maneuver. On physical examination, any movement that creates tension in the affected nerve, such as the straight leg-raising test, elicits radicular pain. Neurologic examination may reveal sensory deficit, asymmetry of reflexes, or motor weakness corresponding to the damaged spinal nerve root and degree of impingement (Table 8E-3). MRI is the best technique to identify the location of disc herniation and nerve impingement (12). Electromyography (EMG) and nerve conduction tests may document abnormal nerve function after impingement has been present for 8 weeks or longer. Therapy for disc herniation includes controlled physical activity, NSAIDs, and epidural corticosteroid injection. For most patients, radicular pain resolves over a 12-week period. Only 5% or less of patients with a herniated disc require surgical decompression.

Lumbosacral Spondylosis

Osteoarthritis of the lumbosacral spine may cause localized low-back pain. The disorder may progress, causing increased narrowing of the spinal canal that results in spinal stenosis and compression of neural elements (lumbosacral spondylosis). The clinical manifestation of spinal stenosis is neurogenic claudication. As the intervertebral

(Table 8E-2)
*Mechanical low-back pain**

	Back Strain	Herniated Disc	Osteoarthritis	Spinal Stenosis	Spondylolisthesis	Adult Scoliosis
Age at onset	20–40	30–50	>50	>60	20–30	20–40
Pain pattern						
Location	Back	Back/leg	Back	Leg	Back	Back
Onset	Acute	Acute	Insidious	Insidious	Insidious	Insidious
Upright	I	D	I	I	I	I
Sitting	D	I	D	D	D	D
Bending	I	I	D	D	I	I
SLR	–	+	–	+(exertion)	–	–
Plain radiograph	–	–	+	+	+	+
CT/Myelogram	–	+	±	+	+	–
MRI	–	+	±	+	±	±

* I = increased; D = decreased; – = normal; + = abnormal; SLR = straight leg-raising; CT = computed tomography; MRI = magnetic resonance imaging.

Vertebra	Pain Distribution	Sensory Loss	Motor Loss	Reflex Loss
L4	Anterior thigh to medial leg	Medial leg to medial malleolus	Anterior tibialis	Patellar
L5	Lateral leg to dorsal foot	Lateral leg to dorsal foot	Extensor hallucis longus	(Posterior tibial)
S1	Lateral foot	Lateral foot, sole	Peroneus longus and brevis	Achilles
C5	Neck to outer shoulder, arm	Shoulder	Deltoid	Biceps, supinator
C6	Outer arm to thumb, index finger	Thumb, index finger	Biceps, wrist extensors	Biceps, supinator
C7	Outer arm to middle finger	Index, middle fingers	Triceps	Triceps
C8	Inner arm to ring, little fingers	Ring, little fingers	Hand muscles	None

disc degenerates, intersegmental instability and approximation of the vertebral bodies shift the compressive forces across the zygapophyseal joints. The transition of these facet joints from nonweight-bearing to weight-bearing joints leads to zygapophyseal osteoarthritis. As a result, patients develop lumbar pain that increases at the end of the day and radiates across the low back. Physical examination reveals that pain worsens with extension of the spine, and no neurologic deficits are present. Pain radiates into the posterior thigh and is exacerbated by ipsilateral bending to the side with the osteoarthritic joints (facet syndrome). Oblique radiographic views of the lumbar spine demonstrate facet joint narrowing, periarticular sclerosis, and osteophytes (13).

Lumbar Spinal Stenosis

Spinal stenosis is secondary to the growth of osteophytes, redundancy of the ligamentum flavum, and posterior bulging of the intervertebral discs. Lumbar stenosis may be located in the center of the canal, the lateral recess, or the intervertebral foramen, and may occur at single or multiple levels. The pattern of radicular pain depends on the location of nerve compression (14). With central canal stenosis, pain in one or both legs occurs with walking. Unlike vascular claudication, leg pain appears after walking variable distances. Individuals with vascular claudication must stop walking to gain relief of pain, whereas those with neurogenic claudication must sit or flex forward, which increases room in the spinal canal and restores blood flow to the spinal roots, to decrease pain.

Lateral stenosis causes unilateral leg pain with standing. Stenosis of the intervertebral foramen causes leg pain that is persistent, regardless of the patient's position. The physical examination may be unrevealing unless the patient exercises to the point of developing symptoms. Sensory, motor, and reflex examination during the episode of pain reveals abnormalities that reverse when the pain disappears. Motor weakness is present in one-third of patients, and one-half have reflex abnormalities. Plain radiographs of the lumbar spine may demonstrate degenerative disc disease with zygapophyseal joint narrowing, even in patients who are asymptomatic. Thus radiographic alterations are significant only if the patient has corresponding symptoms. CT scan identifies zygapophyseal joint disease, trefoil configura-

tion of the spinal canal, and reduced dimensions of the canal. MRI can document the location of neural compression (Fig. 8E-1).

The initial therapy for osteoarthritis and spinal stenosis is NSAIDs and teaching patients appropriate spinal biomechanics. Facet joint injections should be considered for individuals who are resistant to conservative medical therapy. Patients with spinal stenosis may benefit from epidural corticosteroid injections given weekly for 3 weeks. Surgical decompression is reserved for patients who are totally incapacitated by pain. Most patients with spinal stenosis do not require surgery. The first decompression operation for spinal stenosis has the greatest chance for an excellent outcome.

Spondylolisthesis

Spondylolisthesis is the anterior displacement of a vertebral body in relation to the underlying vertebra. Spondylolisthesis is usually secondary to degeneration of intervertebral discs and reorientation of the plane of motion of the zygapophyseal joints. The process may also occur as a developmental abnormality with separation of the pars interarticularis (spondylolysis) (15). Patients with spondylolisthesis complain of low-back pain that is exacerbated with standing and is relieved with rest. Individuals with severe subluxation also have leg pain. Physical examination reveals increased lordosis with a "step off." The neurologic examination reveals no abnormalities. Plain radiographs are adequate to demonstrate the lytic lesions in the pars interarticularis, and lateral views demonstrate the degree of subluxation (Fig. 8E-2). MRI can detect entrapment and direct impingement of spinal nerve roots associated with this disorder. Treatment of spondylolisthesis includes flexion strengthening exercises, NSAIDs, and orthopedic corsets. Fusion surgery is useful for patients with greater that grade II slippage and persistent symptoms of neural compression.

Scoliosis

Scoliosis, a lateral curvature of the spine in excess of 10 degrees, most commonly first begins to develop in adolescent girls (16). In the lumbar spine, a curve greater than 40 degrees generally leads to a constant rate of progression of 1 degree per year. Patients complain of increasing back pain that is relieved with bedrest. Neurologic examination reveals findings of nerve com-

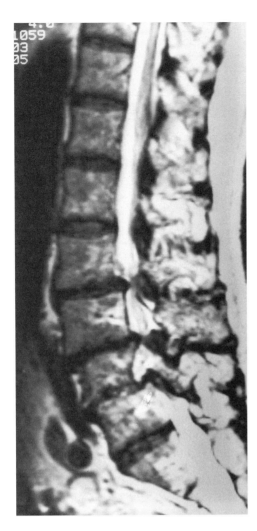

(Figure 8E-1)
T2-weighted sagittal magnetic resonance image (MRI) of the lumbar spine. This 82-year-old man had neurogenic claudication in the right leg after walking one block. MRI reveals severe degenerative disc disease with spinal stenosis at multiple levels in the lower lumbar spine.

pression in more severely affected patients. Plain radiographs allow the clinician to measure the degree of scoliosis by Cobb's method (Fig. 8E-3). In patients with scoliosis of 40 degrees or less, exercises, braces, and NSAIDs are effective in reducing pain and maintaining function. Surgical fusion and placement of Harrington rods are reserved for patients with progressive scoliosis that increases the risk of pulmonary compromise.

MECHANICAL DISORDERS OF THE CERVICAL SPINE

Mechanical disorders of the cervical spine are less common than lumbar spine disorders, tend to be less disabling, and result in fewer physician consultations (Table 8E-4).

Neck Strain

Neck strain causes pain in the middle or lower part of the posterior aspect of the neck. The area of pain may be unilateral or bilateral and may cover a diffuse area. Pain may radiate toward the head and shoulder, sparing the arms. Neck strain, which is rarely associated with a specific trauma, typically is triggered by sleeping in an awkward position, turning the head rapidly, or sneezing. Physical examination reveals local tenderness in the paracervical muscles, decreased range of motion, and loss of cervical lordosis (17). Muscles

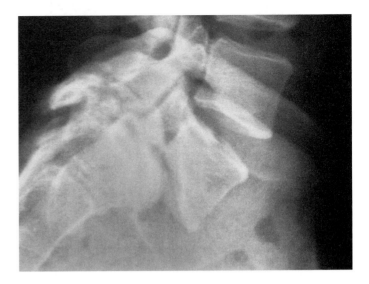

(Figure 8E-2)
Lateral spot view of the lumbosacral spine. A grade II spondylolisthesis is seen with 50% slippage of the vertebral body.

most commonly affected include the sternocleidomastoid and the trapezius. No abnormalities are found on shoulder or neurologic examination, laboratory tests, or radiographic studies. Treatment of neck strain includes controlled physical activity, limited use of cervical orthoses, NSAIDs, and muscle relaxants. Injections of anesthetic and corticosteroid are helpful to decrease local muscle pain, and isometric exercises should be prescribed to maintain muscle strength in

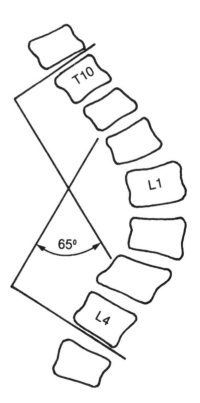

(Figure 8E-3)
Cobb's method for measuring spinal curvature. Lines drawn along the superior end vertebra at the uppermost extension of the vertebra and along the lower border of the inferior end vertebra. The angle formed by the intersecting lines drawn perpendicular to the end plates is Cobb's angle.

	Neck Strain	Herniated Disc	Osteoarthritis	Myelopathy	Whiplash
Age at onset	20–40	30–50	>50	>60	30–40
Pain Pattern					
Location	Neck	Neck/arm	Neck	Arm/leg	Neck
Onset	Acute	Acute	Insidious	Insidious	Acute
Flexion	I	I	D	D	I
Extension	D	I/D	I	I	I
Plain radiograph	–	–	+	+	–
CT/Myelogram	–	+	±	+	–
MRI	–	+	±	+	–

* I = increased; D = decreased; – = normal; + = abnormal; SLR = straight leg-raising; CT = computed tomography; MRI = magnetic resonance imaging.

the neck. Modifications in body mechanics while the patient is at work may help prevent recurrences.

Cervical Disc Herniation

Intervertebral disc herniation in the cervical spine causes radicular pain (brachialgia) that radiates from the shoulder to the forearm and hand. The pain may be so severe that the use of the arm is limited. Neck pain is minimal or absent. Cervical herniation occurs with sudden exertion and is frequently associated with heavy lifting. Physical examination reveals increased radicular pain with any maneuver that narrows the intervertebral foramen and places tension on the affected nerve. Spurling's sign (compression, extension, and lateral flexion of the cervical spine) causes radicular pain. Neurologic examination may reveal sensory deficit, reflex asymmetry, or motor weakness corresponding to the damaged spinal nerve root and degree of impingement (Table 8E-3). MRI is the best technique to identify the location of disc herniation and nerve impingement (18). EMG and nerve conduction tests may document abnormal nerve function. Therapy includes controlled physical activity, cervical orthoses, NSAIDs, and cervical traction. The pain typically subsides within 3 months; only 20% or less of patients require surgical decompression.

Cervical Spondylosis

Osteoarthritis of the cervical spine produces a clinical syndrome similar to that in the lumbosacral spine. As the disc degenerates and the articular structures are brought close together, the cervical spine becomes unstable. Increased instability results in osteophyte formation in the uncovertebral and zygapophyseal joints and local synovial inflammation (cervical spondylosis). Neck pain is diffuse and may radiate to the shoulders, suboccipital areas, interscapular muscles, or anterior chest. Involvement of the sympathetic nervous system may cause blurred vision, vertigo, or tinnitus. Physical examination is unrevealing in most patients, other than midline tenderness. Plain radiographs of the cervical spine are adequate to show intervertebral narrowing and facet joint sclerosis. The presence of abnormalities is necessarily associated with clinical symptoms, however. For example, an MRI study of individuals 40 years of age and older found over one-half had degenerative cervical discs (19).

Conservative therapy is effective for cervical spondylosis. NSAIDs and local injections may diminish neck and referred pain. The appropriate amount of immobilization is controversial, however. The use of cervical orthoses may in-

crease neck stiffness and pain. Patient education should stress the importance of keeping a balance between restricting neck movement with a cervical collar and maintaining neck flexibility with range of motion exercises. Most patients with cervical spondylosis have a relapsing course with recurrent exacerbations of acute neck pain.

Myelopathy

The most serious sequelae of cervical spondylosis is myelopathy. This disorder occurs as a consequence of spinal cord compression by osteophytes, ligamentum flavum, or intervertebral disc (spinal stenosis). Cervical spondylitic myelopathy is the most common cause of spinal cord dysfunction in individuals older than 55 years of age (20). With disc degeneration, osteophytes develop posteriorly and project into the spinal canal, compressing the cord and its vascular supply. Symptoms may occur with or without movement. The size of the spinal canal is the important static component. Stenosis is associated with an anteroposterior diameter of 10 mm or less. Dynamic stenosis, which is secondary to instability, causes compression of the spinal cord with flexion or extension of the neck. Protruding structures that are located anterior to the spinal cord can compress the posterior and lateral columns. Compression of the anterior spinal artery in the lower cervical spine is another mechanism of spinal cord injury. Neck pain is mentioned by only one-third of patients with myelopathy.

Clinical symptoms include a history of peculiar sensations in the hands, associated with weakness and incoordination. In the lower extremities, this disorder can cause gait disturbances, spasticity, leg weakness, and spontaneous leg movements. Older patients may describe leg stiffness, foot shuffling, and a fear of falling. Incontinence is a late manifestation. Physical examination reveals weakness of the appendages in association with spasticity and fasciculations. Sensory deficits include decreased dermatomal sensation and loss of proprioception. Hyperreflexia, clonus, and Babinski's reflex are findings in the lower extremities. Plain radiographs reveal advanced degenerative disease with narrowed disc spaces, osteophytes, facet joint sclerosis, and cervical instability. MRI is the most useful method to detect the extent of spinal cord compression and the effects of compression on the integrity of the cord. Combined CT-myelogram imaging is useful for distinguishing between protruding discs and osteophytes.

Although some patients improve with conservative therapy, progressive myelopathy requires surgery to prevent further cord compression and vascular compromise. Surgical intervention works best before severe neurologic deficits are present.

Whiplash

Cervical hyperextension injuries of the neck are most commonly associated with rear-end collision motor vehicle accidents. Impact from the rear causes acceleration–deceleration injury to the soft tissue structures in the neck. Paracervical muscles (sternocleidomastoid, longus coli) are stretched or torn, and the sympathetic ganglia may be damaged, resulting in Horner's syndrome (ptosis, meiosis, anhydrosis), nausea, or dizziness. Cervical intervertebral disc injuries may also occur.

The symptoms of stiffness and pain with motion are first noticed 12-24 hours after the accident. Headache is a common complaint. Patients may have difficulty swallowing or chewing and may have paresthesias in the arms. Physical examination reveals decreased range of neck motion and persistent paracervical muscle contraction. Neurologic examination is unremarkable, and radiographs do not show soft tissue abnormalities other than loss of cervical lordosis.

Treatment of whiplash includes the use of cervical collars for minimal periods of time (21). Mild analgesics, NSAIDs, and muscle relaxants are prescribed to encourage motion of the neck. Most patients improve after about 4 weeks of therapy. Patients with persistent symptoms for greater than 6 months rarely experience significant improvement.

DAVID G. BORENSTEIN, MD

1. Frymoyer JW, Pope MH, Costanza MC, Rosen JC, Goggin JE, Wilder DG: Epidemiologic studies of low-back pain. Spine 5:419-423, 1980
2. Hart LG, Deyo RA, Cherkin DC: Physician office visits for low back pain: frequency, clinical evaluation, and treatment patterns from a U.S. national survey. Spine 20:11-19, 1995
3. Borenstein DG, Wiesel SW, Boden SD: Low Back Pain: Medical Diagnosis and Comprehensive Management, 2nd ed. Philadelphia, WB Saunders, 1996, pp 182-589
4. Borenstein DG, Wiesel SW, Boden SD: Neck Pain: Medical Diagnosis and Comprehensive Management. Philadelphia, WB Saunders, 1996, pp 161-437
5. Dillane JB, Fry J, Kaiton G: Acute back syndrome: a study from general practice. Br Med J II:82-84, 1966
6. Deyo RA, Rainville J, Kent DL: What can the history and physical examination tell us about low back pain? JAMA 268:760-765, 1992
7. Floman Y, Wiesel SW, Rothman RH: Cauda equina syndrome presenting as a herniated lumbar disk. Clin Orthop 147:234-237, 1980
8. Zimmermann B, Lally EV: Infectious disease of the spine. Semin Spine Surg 7:177-186, 1995
9. Nicholas JJ, Christy WC: Spinal pain made worse by recumbency: a clue to spinal cord tumors. Arch Phys Med Rehabil 67:598-600, 1986
10. Brodsky AE: Cervical angina: a correlative study with emphasis on the use of coronary arteriography. Spine 10:699-709, 1985
11. Cooper RG: Understanding paraspinal muscle dysfunction in low back pain: a way forward. Ann Rheum Dis 52:413-415, 1993
12. Modic MT, Masaryk T, Boumphrey F, Goormastic M, Bell G: Lumbar herniated disk disease and canal stenosis: prospective evaluation by surface coil MR, CT and myelography. Am J Neuroradiol 7:709-717, 1986
13. Pate D, Goobar J, Resnick D, Haghighi P, Sartoris DJ, Pathria MN: Traction osteophytes of the lumbar spine: radiographic-pathologic correlation. Radiology 166:843-846, 1988
14. Moreland LW, Lopez-Mendez A, Alarcon GS: Spinal stenosis: a comprehensive review of the literature. Semin Arthritis Rheum 19:127-149, 1989
15. Frederickson BE, Baker D, McHolick WJ, Yuan HA, Lubicky JP: The natural history of spondylolysis and spondylolisthesis. J Bone Joint Surg 66A:699-707, 1984
16. Perennou D, Marcelli C, Herisson C, Simon L: Adult lumbar scoliosis: epidemiologic aspects in low-back pain population. Spine 19:123-128, 1994
17. Helliwell PS, Evans PF, Wright V: The straight cervical spine: does it indicate muscle spasm? J Bone Joint Surg 76B:103-106, 1994
18. Brown BM, Schwartz RH, Frank E, Blank NK: Preoperative evaluation of cervical radiculopathy and myelopathy by surface-coil MR imaging. Am J Neuroradiol 9:859-866, 1988
19. Lehto IJ, Tertti MO, Komu ME, Paajanen HEK, Tuominen J, Kormano MJ: Age-related MRI changes at 0.1 T in cervical discs in asymptomatic subjects. Neuroradiology 36:49-53, 1994
20. Bernhardt M, Hynes RA, Blume HW, White AA III: Cervical spondylotic myelopathy. J Bone Joint Surg 75A:119-128, 1993
21. Spitzer WO, Skovron ML, Salmi LR, Cassidy JD, Duranceau J, Suissa S, Zeiss E: Scientific monograph of the Quebec Task Force on whiplash-associated disorders: redefining "whiplash" and its management. Spine 20:1S-73S, 1995

F. REGIONAL RHEUMATIC PAIN SYNDROMES

The regional rheumatic pain syndromes, because of their prevalence, complexity, and lack of diagnostic laboratory tests, present a challenge to the clinician. Yet success in diagnosis and treatment is most gratifying. The conditions discussed in this chapter include disorders involving muscles, tendons, entheses, joints, cartilage, ligaments, fascia, bone, and nerve. A working knowledge of regional anatomy and an approach utilizing a regional differential diagnosis will help in obtaining a specific diagnosis (1).

A precise history is needed to identify the conditions present; more than one syndrome can occur concomitantly. A complete neuromusculoskeletal examination should be performed emphasizing careful palpation, passive range of motion (ROM), and active ROM alone and sometimes with resistance. Some guidelines for the management of these conditions are provided in Table 8F-1.

CAUSATIVE FACTORS

Many syndromes of the neuromusculoskeletal system are the result of injury from a specific activity or event, ranging from one episode to repetitive overuse, especially when abnormal body position or mechanics is present. Tendons become less flexible and elastic with aging, making them more susceptible to injury. Also with aging and with disuse atrophy, the muscles become weaker and exhibit less endurance and bulk, resulting in a decreased muscle absorption of mechanical forces otherwise transmitted to joints, tendons, ligaments, and entheses. A musculotendinous unit shortened from lack of stretching is more prone to injury. In addition, genetic predisposition to certain regional syndromes exists, resulting from variations in anatomy and abnormal biomechanics. Systemic inflammatory diseases may have characteristic local manifestations. Unfortunately, causative factor(s) often are not identified.

1. Exclude systemic disease and infection by appropriate methods. Diagnostic aspiration is mandatory in suspected septic bursitis. Gram stain and culture of bursal fluid provide prompt diagnosis of a septic bursitis
2. Teach the patient to recognize and avoid aggravating factors that cause recurrences
3. Instruct the patient in self-help therapy including the daily performance of mobilizing exercises
4. Provide an explanation of the cause of pain, thus alleviating concern for a crippling disease. When the regional rheumatic pain syndrome overlies another rheumatic problem, the clinician must explain the contribution each disorder plays in the symptom complex and then help the patient deal with each one
5. Provide relief from pain with safe analgesics, counterirritants (heat, ice, vapocoolant sprays), and if appropriate, intralesional injection of a local anesthetic or anesthetic with depository corticosteroid agent
6. Provide the patient with an idea of the duration of therapy necessary to restore order to the musculoskeletal system
7. Symptomatic relief often corroborates the diagnosis

GENERAL CONCEPTS OF MANAGEMENT
Drug Therapy

Oral medications, including nonsteroidal anti-inflammatory drugs (NSAIDs) and analgesics, play a role in management of regional musculoskeletal disorders. The NSAIDs help reduce inflammation and pain. For additional pain relief, analgesics such as acetaminophen can be added. Tricyclic antidepressants such as amitriptyline may also be useful in chronic pain and neurogenic or myofascial pain.

Comprehensive management of these regional syndromes should be undertaken rather than relying on oral medications alone. The causative aspects should be evaluated, and activity modification should be advised as needed. Local injections and physical therapy also can be useful components of treatment.

Intralesional Injections

After specific diagnosis of a regional rheumatic pain syndrome, local injection with lidocaine, corticosteroids, or both is often of benefit (2). In fact, the immediate pain relief from a properly directed injection into a tendon sheath, bursa, enthesis, or nerve area, for a specific problem, further validates the diagnosis. Injection of an area of nonspecific muscle tenderness with a corticosteroid preparation should be discouraged.

Basic principles of intralesional injections include aseptic technique and use of small needles (25-gauge $5/8''$ or $1 1/2''$ or a 22-gauge $1 1/2''$). The use of separate syringes for lidocaine and corticosteroid avoids mixing of the two substances, and permits infiltration of lidocaine beginning intracutaneously with a small wheal and continuing to the site of the lesion. This method makes the injection relatively painless. When the needle reaches the desired site, the syringe is changed with the needle left in place, and the corticosteroid is then injected. This technique helps avoid possible subcutaneous and skin atrophy secondary to corticosteroid use. When injecting a tendon sheath, the needle should be placed parallel to the tendon fibers and not into the tendon itself. Using a more water-soluble corticosteroid may lessen the possibility of corticosteroid-induced tendon weakness or post-injection flare in some patients.

Physical Therapy

The goals of therapeutic exercise are to increase flexibility by stretching, increase muscle strength by resistive exercises, and improve muscle endurance by some repetitive regimen. The physician should become knowledgeable about exercise prescriptions for the various conditions (3). For example, older women tend to have tight calf muscles, which predispose to calf cramps, Achilles tendon problems, or other ankle and foot disorders. Tight quadriceps, hamstring, and iliopsoas muscles are related to problems in the low back, hip, and knee regions. Exercises to stretch these muscles can be taught by the physician. Instruction for quadriceps strengthening, especially by straight leg raising from the sitting position, and for pelvic tilt exercise can be given in the office (4).

Heat or cold modalities provide pain relief and muscle relaxation and serve as a prelude to an exercise regimen. They are of doubtful benefit when used alone over an extended period.

DISORDERS OF THE SHOULDER REGION

Shoulder pain is one of the most common musculoskeletal complaints in people over age 40. In younger people athletic injuries are a frequent source of such pain. The shoulder itself is a remarkable ball and socket joint, which allows for considerable motion. This mobility, however, is accompanied by some instability, from which shoulder problems can result. Many shoulder conditions have similar precipitating factors and symptoms, and multiple lesions involving different structures around the joint may be present in the same shoulder. Understanding the anatomy is important to diagnosis and management.

The glenohumeral, acromioclavicular, sternoclavicular, and scapulothoracic joints all work synchronously to achieve the desired motion. Important shoulder ligaments include the acromioclavicular capsular, coracoacromial, coracoclavicular (trapezoid and conoid), coracohumeral, sternoclavicular, and glenohumeral ligaments. The subacromial bursa, which is inferior to the acromion, is contiguous with the subdeltoid bursa and covers the humeral head. Overlying the bursa is the deltoid muscle. The rotator cuff is composed of the tendons of the supraspinatus, infraspinatus, teres minor, and subscapularis muscles and attaches at the humeral tuberosities. The rotator cuff provides internal and external rotation of the shoulder. It also fixes the humeral head in the glenoid fossa during abduction to counteract the pull of the deltoid, which tends to displace the humeral head from the glenoid. The mechanism whereby the deltoid muscle and the downward-acting short rotators combine to produce abduction is called *force-couple*. After 30° of abduction, a constant 1:2 ratio exists between movement of the scapular articulation and the glenohumeral joint, with a combined movement known as *scapulohumeral rhythm*.

Pain may be referred to the shoulder from the cervical region due to cervical spondylosis, from the thorax due to a Pancoast tumor, from the abdomen area secondary to gallbladder or hepatic lesions, or from the diaphragm.

Rotator Cuff Tendinitis

Rotator cuff tendinitis, or impingement syndrome, is the most common cause of shoulder pain. Tendinitis (and not bursitis) is the primary cause of pain but secondary involvement of the subacromial bursa occurs in some cases. The condition may be acute or chronic and may or may not be associated with calcific deposits within the tendon. The key finding is pain in the rotator cuff on active abduction, especially between 60° and 120°, and sometimes when lowering the arm. In more severe cases, however, pain may begin on initial abduction and continue throughout the ROM. In acute tendinitis pain comes on more abruptly and may be excruciating. Such cases tend to occur in younger patients and are more likely to have calcific deposits in the supraspinatus tendon insertion (Fig. 8F-1). The deposits are best seen on the shoulder radiograph in external rotation, appearing round or oval and several centimeters in length. These deposits may resolve spontaneously over a period of time. A true subacromial bursitis may also be present when calcific material ruptures into the bursa.

The more typical chronic rotator cuff tendinitis manifests as an ache in the shoulder, usually over the lateral deltoid, and occurs on various movements, especially on abduction and internal rotation. Other symptoms include difficulty in dressing oneself and night pain due to difficulty in positioning the shoulders. Tenderness on palpation and some loss of motion may be evident on examination. The initial movement to detect rotator cuff tendinitis is to determine whether pain is present on active abduction of the arm in the horizontal position. Passive abduction is then carried out. Usually less pain is present on passive abduction than active abduction. Conversely, pain may be increased on active abduction against resistance. The impingement sign is nearly always positive. This maneuver is performed by the examiner using one hand to raise the patient's arm in forced flexion while the other hand prevents scapular rotation (5). A positive sign occurs if pain develops at or before 180° of forward flexion. Another useful test to confirm rotator cuff disease is the *impingement test,* performed by injecting 2–5 ml of 2% lidocaine into the subacromial bursa. Pain relief on abduction following the injection denotes a positive impingement test. The same test can be used in another way to determine whether apparent shoulder weakness is due to pain. Once pain is eliminated with the injection, the arm is retested for weakness. If the weakness is still present, the result is again considered positive.

The causes of rotator cuff tendinitis are multifactorial, but relative overuse, especially from overhead activity causing impingement of the rotator cuff, is commonly implicated. Compression of the rotator cuff occurs above by the edge and under surface of the anterior third of the acromion and the coracohumeral ligament and below by the humeral head. There is also age-related decrease in vascularity and degeneration of the cuff tendons and reduction of strength of the cuff muscles due to aging or decline in use. Osteophytes on the inferior portion of the acromioclavicular joint or acute trauma to the shoulder region contribute to development of tendinitis. An inflammatory process such as rheumatoid arthritis (RA) can also cause rotator cuff tendinitis independent of impingement.

Treatment consists of rest and modalities such as hot packs, ultrasound, or cold applications, with specific ROM exercises as soon as tolerated. Nonsteroidal antiinflammatory drugs are often beneficial; however, the most frequent treatment is injection of a depot corticosteroid into the subacromial bursa, the floor of which is contiguous with the rotator cuff.

Rotator Cuff Tear

An acute tear of a rotator cuff after trauma is easily recognized. The trauma may be superimposed on an already degenerative and possibly even partially torn cuff. In trauma resulting in a ruptured cuff, especially falls, fractures of the humeral head and dislocation of the joint should also be considered. However, at least one-half of patients with a tear recall no trauma. In these cases, degeneration of the rotator cuff gradually occurs, resulting in a complete tear. Rotator cuff tears are classified as small (1 cm or less), medium (1–3 cm), large (3–5 cm), or massive (>5 cm) (6). Shoulder pain, weakness on abduction, and loss of motion occur in varying degrees, ranging from severe pain and mild weakness to no pain and marked weakness. A positive drop-arm sign with inability to actively maintain 90° of passive shoulder abduction may be present in large or massive tears. Surgical repair is indicated in younger patients.

Less easily diagnosed is the smaller, chronic complete (full thickness) tear of the rotator cuff or a partial (incomplete or non-full thickness) tear. Pain on abduction, night pain, weakness, loss of abduction, and tenderness on palpation can be present in both of these types of tears. A small complete tear, however, can exist despite fairly good abduction. Tears of the rotator cuff may also occur as a result of the chronic inflammation in RA, and is often present with cystic swelling around the shoulder.

The definitive diagnosis of a ruptured rotator cuff is established by an abnormal arthrogram showing a communication between the glenohumeral joint and the subacromial

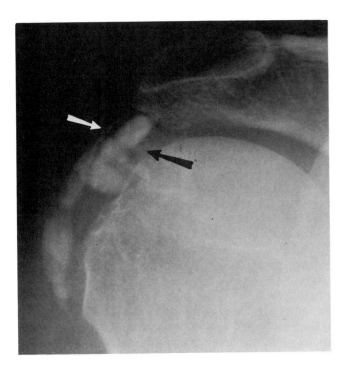

(Figure 8F-1)
Right shoulder of a 44-year-old man illustrating massive calcific deposits in the supraspinatus tendon (white arrow) and subdeltoid bursa (black arrow).

bursa. In a partial tear, in which an intact layer of rotator cuff tissue still separates the joint space from the subacromial bursa, a small ulcer-like crater is seen on the arthrogram. Diagnostic ultrasonography or magnetic resonance imaging (MRI) are also helpful in identifying rotator cuff tears (7). Small complete tears and incomplete tears of the rotator cuff are treated conservatively with rest, physical therapy, and NSAIDs. Although their role has not yet been established by careful studies, subacromial injections of a corticosteroid may relieve pain.

Bicipital Tendinitis

This condition is manifested by pain, most often in the anterior region of the shoulder and occasionally more diffusely. The pain may be acute, but is usually chronic and is related to impingement of the biceps tendon by the acromion. Tenosynovitis of the long head of the biceps is present, and the tendon may be frayed and fibrotic. Palpation over the bicipital groove reveals localized tenderness. The patient's response should be compared with palpation of the opposite side, as this tendon has normal tenderness. Pain may be reproduced over the bicipital tendon in some cases by supination of the forearm against resistance (Yergason's sign), shoulder flexion against resistance (Speed's test), or by extension of the shoulder. Bicipital tendinitis and rotator cuff tendinitis may occur at the same time. Treatment of bicipital tendinitis consists of rest, hot packs, ultrasound, and as pain subsides, passive then active ROM exercises. NSAIDs may be helpful, and occasionally a small amount of corticosteroid carefully injected in the tendon sheath may be of benefit (8).

Subluxation of the bicipital tendon is manifested as pain, with the shoulder going out and then popping back in. Tenderness may be present over the bicipital tendon, and a snap over the tendon may be noted in the shoulder when the arm is passively abducted to 90° and then moved from internal to external rotation and back. Rupture of the biceps tendon occurs at the superior edge of the bicipital groove. Full rupture of the long head of the tendon produces a characteristic bulbous enlargement of the lateral half of the muscle belly. Generally, these two latter conditions of the biceps tendon are treated conservatively.

Adhesive Capsulitis

Known also as *frozen shoulder* or *pericapsulitis,* adhesive capsulitis is associated with generalized pain and tenderness with severe loss of active and passive motion in all planes. It is rare before age 40 and may be secondary to any type of shoulder problem. Muscle atrophy may occur early in the course. Every stiff and painful shoulder, however, is not necessarily adhesive capsulitis. Inflammatory arthritis and diabetes may also be causes of adhesive capsulitis. Additional factors such as immobility, low pain threshold, depression, and neglect or improper initial treatment also favor the development of a frozen shoulder. Many cases, however, are idiopathic. The joint capsule adheres to the anatomic neck, and the axillary fold binds to itself, causing restricted motion. The capsule becomes thickened and contracted.

Arthrography helps confirm this diagnosis by showing a decrease in volume of the shoulder joint capsule with loss of the normal axillary pouch and often the absence of dye in the biceps tendon sheath. The joint may accept as little as

0.5–3.0 ml of dye or occasionally up to 10 ml, whereas a normal shoulder joint has a capacity of 28–35 ml. A frozen shoulder is best treated with a comprehensive program involving NSAIDs and corticosteroid injections into the glenohumeral joint and the subacromial bursa (9). Physical therapy consists of ice packs, ultrasound, transcutaneous electrical nerve stimulation, and gentle ROM exercises—beginning with pendulum exercises and wall climbing with the fingers—and finally active ROM and strengthening exercises. Manipulation under anesthesia may be needed in rare resistant cases.

Suprascapular Neuropathy

The suprascapular nerve, which innervates the supraspinatus and infraspinatus muscles, may be damaged by trauma, overactivity of the shoulder, local ganglion, or a fracture of the scapula. The nerve may be compressed at the suprascapular notch. The condition is marked by weakness on abduction and external rotation. In chronic cases atrophy of the supraspinatus and infraspinatus muscles may be seen. Electrodiagnostic studies help confirm the diagnosis. Treatment generally consists of physical therapy and may include a local corticosteroid injection into the area of the suprascapular notch. In some chronic cases, surgical decompression is needed.

Long Thoracic Nerve Paralysis

Injury to the long thoracic nerve produces weakness of the serratus anterior muscle, resulting in a winged scapula. Pain may be felt along the base of the neck and downward over the scapula and deltoid region, along with fatigue on elevation of the arm. The winging of the scapula becomes apparent when the patient pushes against the wall with arms outstretched. Trauma and diabetes seem to be common causes of this disorder, but it is often idiopathic and usually self-limited.

Brachial Plexopathy

Brachial plexopathy presents with a deep, sharp shoulder pain of rapid onset made worse by abduction and rotation and followed by weakness of the shoulder girdle. An electromyogram helps confirm this diagnosis by demonstrating positive sharp waves and fibrillations in the involved muscles. Recovery may take from one month to several years. Brachial plexopathy can result from trauma, tumor, radiation, inoculation neuritis, diabetes, infection, or median sternotomy done for cardiac surgery, or it can be idiopathic.

Thoracic Outlet Syndrome

The thoracic outlet syndrome includes a constellation of symptoms resulting from compression of the neurovascular bundle, where the brachial plexus and subclavian artery and vein exit beneath the clavicle and subclavius muscle. The neurovascular bundle is bordered below by the first rib, anteriorly by the scalenus anterior muscle, and posteriorly by the scalenus medius muscle. The clinical picture depends on which component is compressed—neural, vascular, or both. Neurologic symptoms predominate in most patients. Pain, paresthesia, and numbness are the principal symptoms, radiating from the neck and shoulder down to the arm and hand, especially distributing to the ring and little fingers. Symptoms are worsened by activity. Weakness and atrophy of intrinsic muscles may be a late finding. Vascular symptoms consist of discoloration, temperature change, pain on use, and Raynaud's phenomenon.

The differential list is large, so the diagnosis is arrived at in part by exclusion. Women outnumber men in incidence. Inquiries about the relationship of symptoms to activities must be made, because shoulder abduction may initiate or worsen symptoms. A careful neurologic examination and evaluation for arterial and venous insufficiency and postural abnormalities should be done. The Adson test, in which the patient holds a deep breath, extends his neck, and then turns his chin toward the side being examined, is positive when the radial pulse becomes extremely weak or disappears. Many normal people have this finding, but if the maneuver reproduces the patient's symptoms, it is more significant. With the hyperabduction maneuver, the radial pulse is monitored when the patient raises an arm above the head. A reduction in the radial pulse strength may indicate arterial compression. Again, this test may be positive in normal people. A chest roentgenogram should be obtained to look for a cervical rib, an elongated transverse process of C7, or healing fractures or exostoses. Because of the difficulty in measuring nerve conduction velocity of the involved nerves, results of these tests have been somewhat inconsistent, but in capable hands they furnish additional supporting information. Somatosensory evoked potentials have also been used successfully. An angiogram or venogram can be obtained in cases of suspected arterial or venous compression.

In general, management of thoracic outlet syndrome is conservative. Good posture is emphasized. Stretching of the scalene and pectoral muscles, together with scapula mobilization and strengthening of the shoulder girdle musculature, is beneficial. A local anesthetic injection into the scalene anticus muscle, if a trigger point is present, may be helpful as well. In resistant or severe cases of thoracic outlet syndrome, the first rib and the scalene muscle may be resected.

DISORDERS OF THE ELBOW REGION
Olecranon Bursitis
The subcutaneous olecranon bursa is frequently involved with bursitis, either secondary to trauma or as an idiopathic condition. The bursa is characteristically swollen and tender on pressure, but pain may be minimal and generally no motion is lost. Aspiration may yield clear or blood-tinged fluid with a low viscosity, or grossly hemorrhagic fluid. Aspiration alone and protection from trauma are generally sufficient to resolve the condition. A small dose of corticosteroid may be injected, but there is a possibility of secondary infection, skin atrophy, or chronic local pain that apparently results from subclinical skin atrophy (10). Inflammatory olecranon bursitis may be due to gout, RA, or calcium pyrophosphate dihydrate deposition disease. Olecranon bursitis has also been seen in uremic patients undergoing hemodialysis. With septic olecranon bursitis, localized erythema is the major clue. Heat, pain, and a positive culture are also frequently present. The condition is treated by aspiration, drainage, and the administration of appropriate antibiotics. Surgical excision is occasionally needed.

Lateral Epicondylitis
Lateral epicondylitis, or tennis elbow, is a common condition in those who overuse their arms. Localized tenderness directly over or slightly anterior to the lateral epicondyle is the hallmark of this disorder. Pain may occur during handshakes, lifting a briefcase, or other similar activities. Probably less than 10% of patients actually acquire lateral epicondylitis through playing tennis; job and recreational activities, including gardening and other athletics, are the usual causes. Pathologically, the condition consists of degeneration of the common extensor tendon, particularly of the extensor carpi radialis brevis tendon. Tendon tears may be the cause of chronic cases.

Treatment is aimed at altering activities and preventing overuse of the forearm musculature. Ice packs, heat, and NSAIDs are of some benefit. A forearm brace can also be used. A local corticosteroid injection with a 25-gauge needle over the lateral epicondyle often produces satisfactory initial relief. Isometric strengthening is important as the initial part of a rehabilitation program.

Evaluation of chronic cases should include a roentgenogram to check for calcification, exostosis, or other bony abnormalities. Entrapment of the radial nerve at the elbow can also cause discomfort and a vague aching at that site. Forced forearm supination against resistance seems to aggravate the symptoms of a neural entrapment more than the symptoms of lateral epicondylitis, in which resisted wrist extension aggravates the pain.

Medial Epicondylitis
Medial epicondylitis, or golfer's elbow, which mainly involves the flexor carpi radialis, is less common and less disabling than lateral epicondylitis. Local pain and tenderness over the medial epicondyle are present, and resistance to wrist flexion exacerbates the pain. Alteration of activities and use of NSAIDs usually alleviate the problem, although occasionally a local corticosteroid injection is required.

Tendinitis of Musculotendinous Insertion of Biceps
Tendinitis of the distal insertion of the biceps (lacertus fibrosus) may cause dull pain throughout the antecubital fossa of the elbow (11). Palpation confirms the source of pain, and mild swelling may be present. Heat, NSAIDs, rest, and occasionally a local injection of corticosteroids generally are beneficial in this self-limiting condition.

Ulnar Nerve Entrapment
Entrapment of the ulnar nerve at the elbow produces numbness and paresthesia of the little finger and adjacent side of the ring finger, as well as aching of the medial aspect of the elbow. Hand clumsiness can be present. Tenderness may be elicited when the ulnar nerve groove, located on the postero-inferior surface of the medial epicondyle, is compressed. The little finger may have decreased sensation and weakness on abduction and flexion. Elevating the hand by resting the forearm on the head for 1 minute may produce paresthesia. In long standing cases, atrophy and weakness of the ulnar intrinsic muscles of the hand occur. A positive Tinel's sign, elicited by tapping the nerve at the elbow, is often present. Similar symptoms may result from subluxation of the nerve.

Ulnar nerve entrapment has many causes, including external compression from occupation, compression during anesthesia, trauma, prolonged bed rest, earlier fractures, and arthritis. A nerve conduction test that shows slowing of ulnar motor and sensory conduction and prolonged proximal latency aids in confirming the diagnosis. Avoiding pressure on the elbow and repetitive elbow flexion may be all that is necessary, but in severe persistent cases, surgical correction is needed.

DISORDERS OF THE WRIST AND HAND

Ganglion

A ganglion is a cystic swelling arising from a joint or tendon sheath that occurs most commonly over the dorsum of the wrist. It is lined with synovia and contains thick jelly-like fluid. Ganglia are generally of unknown cause but may develop secondary to trauma or prolonged wrist extension. Usually, the only symptom is swelling, but occasionally a large ganglion produces discomfort on wrist extension. Treatment, if indicated, consists of aspiration of the fluid, with or without injection of corticosteroid. Use of a splint may help prevent recurrence. In severe cases, the whole ganglion may be removed surgically.

De Quervain's Tenosynovitis

De Quervain's tenosynovitis may result from repetitive activity that involves pinching with the thumb while moving the wrist. It has been reported to occur as a complication of pregnancy, in new mothers, and from repetitive diapering using safety pins. The symptoms are pain, tenderness, and occasionally swelling over the radial styloid. Pathologic findings include inflammation and narrowing of the tendon sheath around the abductor pollicis longus and extensor pollicis brevis. A positive Finkelstein test result is usually seen: pain increases when the thumb is folded across the palm and the fingers are flexed over the thumb as the examiner passively deviates the wrist toward the ulnar side. Treatment involves splinting, local corticosteroid injection, and NSAIDs as indicated. Rarely, surgical removal of inflamed tenosynovium is needed.

Tenosynovitis of the Wrist

Tenosynovitis occurs in other flexor and extensor tendons of the wrist in addition to those involved in De Quervain's tenosynovitis (12). The individual tendons on the extensor side that may be vulnerable are the extensor pollicis longus, extensor indicis proprius, extensor digiti minimi, and extensor carpi ulnaris; and on the flexor side, the flexor carpi radialis, flexor carpi ulnaris, flexor digitorum superficialis, and flexor digitorum profundus.

The findings vary depending on which tendon is involved. Localized pain and tenderness are usually present, and there is sometimes swelling. Pain on resisted movement is often seen. The tenosynovitis may be misinterpreted as arthritis of the wrist.

This problem may be due to repetitive use, a traumatic episode, inflammatory arthritis, or may be idiopathic. The treatment consists of avoiding overuse, splinting, and NSAIDs. A local corticosteroid injection into the tendon sheath, avoiding direct injection into the tendon itself, is usually of benefit.

Pronator Teres Syndrome

An uncommon condition, pronator teres syndrome may be difficult to diagnose because some features are similar to carpal tunnel syndrome. In this case, however, the median nerve is compressed at the level of the pronator teres muscle. The patient may complain of aching in the volar aspect of the forearm, numbness in the thumb and index finger, weakness on gripping with the thumb, and writer's cramp. The most specific finding is tenderness of the proximal part of the pronator teres, which may be aggravated by resistive pronation of the forearm. Pronator compression often produces paresthesia after 30 seconds or less. In some patients, a positive Tinel's sign is found at the proximal edge of the pronator teres. Unlike carpal tunnel syndrome, nocturnal awakening and numbness in the morning are absent. Pronator teres syndrome is thought to result from overuse by repetitive grasping or pronation, trauma, or a space-occupying lesion.

Electrodiagnostic studies may reveal signs of denervation of the forearm muscles supplied by the median nerve but sparing the pronator teres; however, they often fail to localize the lesion. If the condition does not improve with alteration of activities and with time, exploratory surgery may be undertaken to look for fibrous or tendinous bands, or a hypertrophied pronator muscle may be found.

Anterior Interosseous Nerve Syndrome

Compression of the anterior interosseous nerve near its bifurcation from the median nerve produces weakness of the flexor pollicis longus, flexor digitorum profundus, and pronator quadratus muscles. Sensation is not affected, but a person with this syndrome cannot form an "O" with the thumb and index finger, because motion is lost in the interphalangeal (IP) joint of the thumb and the distal interphalangeal (DIP) joint of the index finger. Electromyography may help confirm the diagnosis. Repetitive overuse, trauma, and fibrous bands are the principal causes of this syndrome. Protection from trauma usually results in improvement; if not, surgical exploration may be undertaken.

Radial Nerve Palsy

The most common type of radial nerve palsy is the spiral groove syndrome, or bridegroom palsy, in which the radial nerve is compressed against the humerus. The most prominent feature is a wrist-drop with flexion of the metacarpophalangeal (MCP) joints and adduction of the thumb. Anesthesia in the web space and hypesthesia from the dorsal aspect of the forearm to the thumb, index, and middle fingers may be present. If the radial nerve is compressed more proximally through improper use of crutches or prolonged leaning of the arm over the back of a chair ("Saturday night palsy"), weakness of the triceps and brachioradialis muscles may also occur. Compression injuries generally heal over a period of weeks. Splinting the wrist during this recovery time prevents overstretching of the paralyzed muscles and ligaments. Electrodiagnostic studies are helpful in determining the specific point of compression.

Posterior Interosseous Nerve Syndrome

Posterior interosseous nerve entrapment in the radial tunnel produces discomfort in the proximal lateral portion of the forearm. The fingers cannot be extended at the MCP joints. The posterior interosseous nerve, a branch of the radial nerve, is primarily a motor nerve, so sensory disturbances are rare. Occupational or recreational repetitive activity with forceful supination, wrist extension, or radial deviation against resistance may be a factor. Direct trauma and such nontraumatic conditions as a ganglion also have been implicated. Interestingly, this syndrome has been seen in RA due to synovial compression of the nerve and, therefore, must be distinguished from a ruptured extensor tendon.

Superficial Radial Neuropathy (Cheiralgia Paresthetica)

A lesion of this sensory nerve is more common than previously thought and causes symptoms of a burning or shooting pain and sometimes numbness and tingling over the dorso-radial aspect of the wrist, thumb, and index fingers. Hyperpronation and ulnar wrist flexion may be provocative. Decreased pin prick sensation and a positive Tinel's sign may be seen. Electrodiagnostic studies are helpful in the diagnosis.

Tight wrist restraints from handcuffs or watch bands are well known causes. Trauma to the area, repetitive wrist motion, diabetes, ganglion cyst, venipuncture, and local surgical procedures are other possible etiologies. The neuropathy may resolve with time. Treatment consists of splinting, NSAIDs, local corticosteroid injection, or surgical neurolysis in some cases.

Carpal Tunnel Syndrome

Carpal tunnel syndrome is the most common cause of paresthesias in the hands. The median nerve and flexor tendons pass through a common tunnel at the wrist whose rigid walls are bounded dorsally and on the sides by the carpal bones, and on the volar aspect by the transverse carpal ligament (Fig. 8F-2). Any process encroaching on this tunnel compresses the median nerve, which innervates the thenar muscles (for flexion, opposition, abduction); the radial lumbricales; and the skin of the radial side of the palm, thumb, second and third fingers, and the radial half of the fourth finger.

Symptoms are variable, but episodes of burning pain or tingling in the hand are common, often occurring during the night and relieved by vigorous shaking or movement of the hand. Numbness commonly affects the index and middle fingers, radial side of the ring fingers, and occasionally the thumb. Some patients experience only numbness without much pain. Numbness may also occur with activities such as driving or holding a newspaper or book. The patient may have a sensation of hand swelling when in fact no swelling is visible. Occasionally the pain spreads above the wrist into the forearm or, rarely, even above the elbow and up the arm. Bilateral disease is common.

A positive Tinel's sign or Phalen's sign may be present. Phalen's test is performed by holding the flexed wrists against each other. Loss of sensation may be demonstrated in the index, middle finger, or radial side of the fourth finger. Weakness and atrophy of the muscles of the thenar eminence may gradually appear in chronic cases. Confirmation of the diagnosis can be obtained by demonstrating prolonged distal latency times during electrodiagnostic studies.

A variety of disorders may cause carpal tunnel syndrome, including edema from pregnancy or trauma, osteophytes, ganglia related to tenosynovial sheaths, lipomata, and anomalous muscles, tendons, and blood vessels that compress the median nerve. Carpal tunnel syndrome has been observed in various infections such as tuberculosis, histoplasmosis, sporotrichosis, coccidioidomycosis, and rubella. Rheumatoid arthritis, gout, pseudogout, and other inflammatory diseases of the wrist can cause compression of the median nerve. Amyloid deposits of the primary type or in association with multiple myeloma can occur at this site, and carpal tunnel syndrome may be the initial manifestation of the disease. The syndrome has also been reported to occur in myxedema and acromegaly. In many cases, however, no obvious cause can be found or a nonspecific tenosynovitis is evident. Many idiopathic cases may be due to occupational stress.

In milder cases, splinting the wrist in a neutral position may relieve symptoms. Local injections of corticosteroids into the carpal tunnel area, using a 25-gauge needle, are helpful for nonspecific or inflammatory tenosynovitis. The benefit may be only temporary, depending on the degree of compression and the reversibility of the neural injury. When conservative treatment fails, surgical decompression of the tunnel by release of the transverse carpal ligament and removal of tissue compressing the median nerve is often beneficial. Even with surgery, however, symptoms may sometimes recur.

Ulnar Nerve Entrapment at the Wrist

The ulnar nerve can become entrapped at the wrist proximal to Guyon's canal, in the canal itself, or distal to it (13). Guyon's canal is roughly bounded medially by the pisiform bone, laterally by the hook of the hamate, superiorly by the volar carpal ligament (pisohamate ligament), and inferiorly by the transverse carpal ligament. Because the ulnar nerve, on entering the canal, bifurcates into the superficial and deep branches, the clinical picture may vary, with only sensory, only motor, or both sensory and motor findings.

The complete clinical picture includes pain, numbness, and paresthesias of the hypothenar area, clumsiness, and a weak hand grip, including difficulty using the thumb in a pinching movement. Pressure over the ulnar nerve at the hook of the hamate may cause tingling or pain. Atrophy of the hypothenar and intrinsic muscles can occur. Clawing of ring and little fingers may be seen, resulting from weakness of the third and fourth lumbricales. Loss of sensation occurs over the hypothenar area.

If the superficial branch alone is involved, then only numbness, pain, and loss of sensation occur. Entrapment of the deep branch produces only motor weakness of the ulnar innervated muscles. The sites of motor weakness depend on the exact location of nerve compression; for example, if the

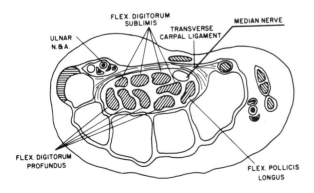

(Figure 8F-2)
Cross section of wrist illustrating the position of the transverse carpal ligament (flexor retinaculum) and the structures occupying the osseous-fibrous carpal tunnel.

compression is more distal, then the hypothenar muscles and intrinsics may be spared, causing weakness and atrophy of only the adductor pollicis, deep head of the flexor pollicis brevis, and first dorsal interosseous muscles. The causes of ulnar neuropathy at the wrist include trauma, ganglia, bicycling, inflammatory arthritis, flexor carpi ulnaris hypertrophy, fractures, neuroma, lipomata, and diabetes.

The diagnosis is assisted by electrodiagnostic studies, indicating a prolonged distal latency of the ulnar nerve at the wrist and denervation of the ulnar innervated muscles. Treatment includes rest from offending activity, splinting, or a local corticosteroid injection; however, surgical exploration and decompression may be necessary.

Volar Flexor Tenosynovitis

Inflammation of the tendon sheaths of the flexor digitorum superficialis and flexor digitorum profundus tendons in the palm is extremely common but often unrecognized. Pain in the palm is felt on finger flexion, but in some cases the pain may radiate to the proximal interphalangeal (PIP) and MCP joints on the dorsal side, thus misleading the examiner. The diagnosis is made by palpation and identification of localized tenderness and swelling of the volar tendon sheaths. The middle and index fingers are most commonly involved, but the ring and little fingers can also be affected. Often a nodule composed of fibrous tissue can be palpated in the palm just proximal to the MCP joint on the volar side. The nodule interferes with the normal tendon gliding and can cause a triggering or locking, which may be intermittent and may produce an uncomfortable sensation. Similar involvement can occur at the flexor tendon of the thumb. Volar tenosynovitis may be part of inflammatory conditions, such as RA, psoriatic arthritis, or apatite crystal deposition disease. It is seen frequently in conjunction with osteoarthritis (OA) of the hands. The most common cause is overuse trauma of the hands from gripping with increased pull on the flexor tendons. Injection of a long-acting steroid into the tendon sheath usually relieves the problem (14), although surgery on the tendon sheath may be needed in unremitting cases.

Infection of the tendon sheaths in the hand requires drainage and antibiotics. People with drug addictions and diabetes may be at increased risk for such infections. Atypical mycobacterium or fungal infections also cause a chronic tenosynovitis in the hands. *Mycobacterium marinum,* which is found in infected fish, barnacles, fish tanks, and swimming pools, is a common culprit (15).

Dupuytren's Contracture

In Dupuytren's contracture a thickening and shortening of the palmar fascia occurs. In established cases the diagnosis is obvious, with typical thick, cord-like superficial fibrous tissue felt in the palm causing a contracture, usually of the ring finger. The fifth, third, and second fingers are involved in decreasing order of frequency. Initially, a mildly tender fibrous nodule in the volar fascia of the palm may be the only finding, leading to a confusion with volar flexor tenosynovitis. Dimpling or puckering of the skin over the involved fascia helps identify the early Dupuytren's contracture. The initial nodules probably result from a contraction of proliferative myofibroblasts. The tendon and tendon sheaths are not implicated, but the dermis is frequently involved, re-

sulting in fixation to the fascia. Progression of the disease varies, ranging from little or no change over many years to rapid progression and complete flexion contracture of one or more digits.

The cause of this condition is unknown, but a hereditary predisposition appears to be present. Some patients also have associated plantar fasciitis, knuckle pads, and fibrosis in the shaft of the penis. The disorder is about five times more frequent in men, occurs predominantly in Caucasians, and is more common in Europe. A gradual increase in incidence of the disease occurs with age. Associations exist between Dupuytren's contracture and chronic alcoholism, epilepsy, and diabetes.

Treatment depends entirely on the severity of the findings. Heat, stretching, ultrasound, and intralesional injection of corticosteroids may be helpful in early stages. When actual contractures occur, surgical intervention may be desirable. Limited fasciectomy is effective in most instances, but more radical procedures, including digital amputation, may rarely be necessary. Palmar fasciotomy is a useful and more benign procedure, but if the disease remains active, recurrence is likely.

DISORDERS OF THE HIP REGION
Trochanteric Bursitis

Although common, trochanteric bursitis frequently goes undiagnosed. It occurs predominantly in middle-aged to elderly people, and somewhat more often in women than men. The main symptom is aching over the trochanteric area and lateral thigh. Walking, various movements, and lying on the involved hip may intensify the pain. Onset may be acute, but more often is gradual with symptoms lasting for months. In chronic cases the patient may fail to adequately locate or describe the pain, or the physician may fail to note the symptoms or interpret them correctly. Occasionally the pain may have a pseudoradiculopathic quality, radiating down the lateral aspect of the thigh. In a few cases the pain is so severe that the patient cannot walk and complains of diffuse pain of the entire thigh.

The best way to diagnose trochanteric bursitis is to palpate over the trochanteric area and elicit point tenderness. In addition to specific pain on deep pressure over the trochanter, other tender points may be noted throughout the lateral aspect of the thigh muscle. Pain may be worse with external rotation and abduction against resistance. Although bursitis is generally considered to be the principal problem, the condition may actually arise at the insertions of the gluteus maximus and gluteus medius tendons. Local trauma and degeneration play a role in the pathogenesis. In some cases calcification of the trochanteric bursa is seen. Conditions that may contribute to trochanteric bursitis, apparently by adding stress to the area, include OA of the lumbar spine or of the hip, leg-length discrepancy, and scoliosis. Treatment consists of local injection of depot corticosteroid using a 22-gauge, 3 1/2" needle to ensure that the bursal area is reached (16). Nonsteroidal anti-inflammatory drugs, weight loss, and strengthening and stretching of the gluteus medius muscle and iliotibial band help in overall management.

Iliopsoas (Iliopectineal) Bursitis

The iliopsoas bursa lies behind the iliopsoas muscle, anterior to the hip joint and lateral to the femoral vessels. It communicates with the hip in 15% of iliopsoas bursitis cases.

When the bursa is involved, groin and anterior thigh pain are present. This pain becomes worse on passive hip hyperextension and sometimes on flexion, especially with resistance. Tenderness is palpable over the involved bursa. The patient may hold the hip in flexion and external rotation to eliminate pain and may limp to prevent hyperextension. The diagnosis is more apparent if a cystic mass, which is present in about 30% of cases, is seen; however, other causes of cystic swelling in the femoral area must be excluded. A bursal mass may cause femoral venous obstruction or femoral nerve compression. As with most bursitis, acute or recurrent trauma and inflammatory conditions like RA may be a cause. The diagnosis is confirmed by plain roentgenogram and injection of a contrast medium into the bursa, or by computed tomography or MRI. Iliopsoas bursitis generally responds to conservative treatment including corticosteroid injections. With recurrent involvement, excision of the bursa may be necessary.

Ischial (Ischiogluteal) Bursitis

Ischial bursitis is caused by trauma or prolonged sitting on hard surfaces, as evidenced by the name, *weaver's bottom.* Pain is often exquisite when sitting or lying down. Because the ischiogluteal bursa is located superficial to the ischial tuberosity and separates the gluteus maximus from the tuberosity, the pain may radiate down the back of the thigh. Point tenderness over the ischial tuberosity is present. Use of cushions and local injection of a corticosteroid are helpful.

Piriformis Syndrome

Piriformis syndrome is not well recognized and incompletely understood, even though it was first described in 1928 (17). The main symptom is pain over the buttocks, often radiating down the back of the leg as in sciatica. A limp may be noted on the involved side. Women are more often affected, and trauma plays a major role. Diagnosis is aided by tenderness of the piriformis muscle on rectal or vaginal examination. Pain is evident on internal rotation of hips against resistance. Pain and weakness have also been noted on resisted abduction and external rotation. A carefully done local injection of lidocaine and corticosteroid into the piriformis muscle may help.

Meralgia Paresthetica

The lateral femoral cutaneous nerve (L2-L3) innervates the anterolateral aspect of the thigh and is a sensory nerve. Compression of the nerve causes a characteristic intermittent burning pain associated with hypesthesia and sometimes with numbness of the anterolateral thigh. Extension and abduction of the thigh or prolonged standing and walking may make symptoms worse, whereas sitting may relieve the pain. Touch and pin-prick sensation over the anterolateral thigh may be decreased. Pain can be elicited by pressing on the inguinal ligament just medial to the anterior superior iliac spine. This syndrome is seen more commonly in people who have diabetes, are pregnant, or are obese. Direct trauma, compression from a corset, or a leg-length discrepancy may also be factors. Nerve conduction velocity studies help confirm the diagnosis. Weight loss, heel correction, and time generally alleviate the problem. Because entrapment of the nerve often occurs just medial to the anterior superior iliac spine, a local injection of a corticosteroid at that site may help.

DISORDERS OF THE KNEE REGION
Popliteal Cysts

Popliteal cysts, also known as *Baker's cysts,* are not uncommon, and the clinician should be well aware of the possibility of dissection or rupture. A cystic swelling with mild or no discomfort may be the only initial finding. With further distention of the cyst, however, a greater awareness and discomfort is experienced, particularly on full flexion or extension. The cyst is best seen when the patient is standing and is examined from behind. Any knee disease having a synovial effusion can be complicated by a popliteal cyst. A naturally occurring communication may exist between the knee joint and the semimembranosus-gastrocnemius bursa, which is located beneath the medial head of the gastrocnemius muscle. A one-way valve-like mechanism between the joint and the bursa is activated by pressure from the knee effusion. An autopsy series has shown that about 40% of the population have a knee joint–bursa communication.

Popliteal cysts are most common secondary to RA, OA, or internal derangements of the knee. There are a few reported cases secondary to gout and Reiter's syndrome. A syndrome mimicking thrombophlebitis may occur, resulting from cyst dissection into the calf or actual rupture of the cyst. Findings include diffuse swelling of the calf, pain, and sometimes erythema and edema of the ankle. An arthrogram of the knee will confirm both the cyst and the possible dissection or rupture. Ultrasound is also useful in making a diagnosis and monitoring the course. History of a knee effusion is often a hint that a dissected Baker's cyst is the cause of the patient's swollen leg. If necessary, a venogram can exclude the possibility of concomitant thrombophlebitis. A cyst related to an inflammatory arthritis is treated by injecting a depot corticosteroid into the knee joint and possibly into the cyst itself, which usually resolves the problem. If the cyst results from OA or an internal derangement of the knee, surgical repair of the underlying joint lesion is usually necessary to prevent recurrence of the cyst.

Anserine Bursitis

Seen predominantly in overweight, middle-aged to elderly women with big legs and OA of the knees, anserine bursitis produces pain and tenderness over the medial aspect of the knee about 2″ below the joint margin. Pain is worsened by climbing stairs. The pes anserinus (Latin for "goose foot") is composed of the conjoined tendons of the sartorius, gracilis, and semitendinosus muscles. The bursa extends between the tendons and the tibial collateral ligament. The diagnosis is made by eliciting exquisite tenderness over the bursa and by relieving pain with a local lidocaine injection. The treatment is rest, stretching of the adductor and quadriceps muscles, and a corticosteroid injection into the bursa.

Anserine bursitis is often overlooked as it frequently occurs concomitantly with OA of the knee, which when present is the assumed cause of pain; however, in some cases of dual involvement, anserine bursitis is the principal source of pain.

No Name, No Fame Bursitis

An unnamed bursa is located between the superficial and deep portions of the medial collateral ligament. When inflamed, pain and point tenderness over the area occur (18). Pain is noted particularly when the knee is flexed at 90°. A local corticosteroid injection into the bursa usually alleviates the symptoms.

Prepatellar Bursitis

Manifested as a swelling superficial to the kneecap, prepatellar bursitis results from trauma such as frequent kneeling, leading to the name "housemaid's knee." The prepatellar bursa lies anterior to the lower half of the patella and upper half of the patellar ligament. The pain is generally slight unless pressure is applied directly over the bursa. The infrapatellar bursa, which lies between the patellar ligament and the tibia, is also subject to trauma and swelling. Chronic prepatellar bursitis can be treated by protecting the knee from the irritating trauma.

Septic prepatellar bursitis should also be considered when swelling is noted in this area. Generally, erythema, heat, and increased tenderness and pain are present. The history may include trauma to the knee with puncture or abrasion of the skin overlying the bursa. The bursal fluid should be aspirated and cultured, and treatment with appropriate antibiotics should be instituted if infection is demonstrated.

Medial Plica Syndrome

A plica is a synovial fold in the knee joint, and infrapatellar, suprapatellar, and medial plicae have been identified. The medial plica can sometimes cause knee symptoms (19). Patella pain may be the predominant complaint, and snapping or clicking of the knee, a sense of instability, and possible pseudolocking of the knee may be seen. The plica become symptomatic through any traumatic or inflammatory event in the knee. Diagnosis and treatment are made by arthroscopy, in which a thickened, inflamed, and occasionally fibrotic medial patella plica, leading to a bowstring process, is seen.

Popliteal Tendinitis

Pain in the posterolateral aspect of the knee may occur secondary to tendinitis of the popliteal tendons (hamstring and popliteus). With the knee flexed at 90°, tenderness on palpation may be found. Straight leg raising with or without palpation may cause pain. Running downhill increases the strain on the popliteus and can lead to tendinitis. Rest and conservative treatment are indicated; occasionally a corticosteroid injection may be beneficial.

Pellegrini–Stieda Syndrome

Pellegrini–Stieda syndrome, which generally occurs in men, is thought to result from trauma and is followed by an asymptomatic period. Later, the symptomatic stage of medial knee pain and progressive restriction of knee movement coincides with the beginning of calcification of the medial collateral ligament, typically appearing as an elongated, amorphous shadow on roentgenogram (20). The pain is self-limited, and improvement usually occurs within several months.

Patellar Tendinitis

Patellar tendinitis, or jumper's knee, is seen predominantly in athletes engaging in repetitive running, jumping, or kicking activities. Pain and tenderness are present over the patellar tendon. Treatment consists of rest, NSAIDs, ice, knee bracing, and stretching and strengthening of the quadriceps and hamstring muscles. Corticosteroid injections are usually contraindicated due to risk of rupture. In some chronic cases surgery is needed.

Rupture of Quadriceps Tendon and Infrapatellar Tendon

When the tendons around the patella rupture, the quadriceps tendon is involved about 50% of the time; otherwise, the infrapatellar tendon is involved. Quadriceps tendon rupture is generally caused by sudden violent contractions of the quadriceps muscle when the knee is flexed. A hemarthrosis of the knee joint may follow. Rupture of the infrapatellar tendon has been associated with a specific episode of trauma, repetitive trauma from sporting activities, and systemic diseases. Patients with chronic renal failure, RA, hyperparathyroidism, gout, and systemic lupus erythematosus patients on steroids have been reported to have spontaneous ruptures of the quadriceps tendon. The patient experiences a sudden sharp pain and cannot extend the leg. Roentgenograms may show a high riding patella. The tendon is generally found to be degenerated, and surgical repair is necessary.

Peroneal Nerve Palsy

In peroneal nerve palsy, a painless foot drop with a steppage gait is usually evident. Pain sensation may be slightly decreased along the lower lateral aspect of the leg and the dorsum of the foot. Direct trauma, fracture of the lower portion of the femur or upper portion of the tibia, compression of the nerve over the head of the fibula, and stretch injuries are all causes of this palsy. Generally, the common peroneal nerve is compressed, affecting the muscles innervated by the superficial peroneal nerve (which supplies the everters), and the deep peroneal nerve (which supplies the dorsiflexors of the foot and toes). An electromyogram is helpful in demonstrating slowing of nerve conduction velocities. Treatment consists of removing the source of compression and use of an ankle–foot orthosis if necessary. Occasionally, surgical exploration is needed.

Patellofemoral Pain Syndrome

This syndrome consists of pain and crepitus in the patellar region (21). Stiffness occurs after prolonged sitting and is alleviated by activity; overactivity involving knee flexion, particularly under loaded conditions such as stair climbing, aggravates the pain. On examination, pain occurs when the patella is compressed against the femoral condyle or when the patella is displaced laterally. Joint effusions are uncommon and usually small. The symptoms of patellofemoral pain syndrome are often bilateral and occur in a young age group. This syndrome may be caused by a variety of patellar problems such as patella alta, abnormal quadriceps angle, and trauma. The term *chondromalacia patellae* has been used for this syndrome, but patellofemoral pain syndrome is preferred by many. Treatment consists of analgesics, NSAIDs, ice, rest, and avoidance of knee overuse. Isometric strengthening exercises for the quadriceps muscles are of benefit. In some patients, however, surgical realignment may be tried.

DISORDERS OF THE ANKLE AND FOOT REGION
Achilles Tendinitis

Usually resulting from trauma, athletic overactivity, or improperly fitting shoes with a stiff heel counter, Achilles tendinitis can also be caused by inflammatory conditions such as ankylosing spondylitis, Reiter's syndrome, gout, RA, and calcium pyrophosphate dihydrate crystal deposition disease. Pain, swelling, and tenderness occur over the Achilles tendon at its attachment and in the area proximal to the attachment. Crepitus on motion and pain on dorsiflexion may be present. Management includes NSAIDs, rest, shoe corrections, heel lift, gentle stretching, and sometimes a splint with slight plantar flexion. The Achilles tendon is vulnerable to rupture, and the tendon itself must not be injected with a corticosteroid.

Retrocalcaneal Bursitis

The retrocalcaneus bursa is located between the posterior surface of the Achilles tendon and the calcaneus. The bursa's anterior wall is fibrocartilage where it attaches to the calcaneus, whereas its posterior wall blends with the epitenon of the Achilles tendon. Manifestations of bursitis include pain at the back of the heel, tenderness of the area anterior to the Achilles tendon, and pain on dorsiflexion. Local swelling is present, with bulging on the medial and lateral aspects of the tendon. Retrocalcaneal bursitis, also called sub-Achilles bursitis, may coexist with Achilles tendinitis; distinguishing the two is sometimes difficult. This condition may be secondary to RA, spondylitis, Reiter's syndrome, gout, or trauma. Treatment consists of administration of NSAIDs, rest, and a local injection of a corticosteroid carefully directed into the bursa.

Subcutaneous Achilles Bursitis

A subcutaneous bursa superficial to the Achilles tendon may become swollen in the absence of systemic disease. This bursitis, known as pump-bumps, is seen predominantly in women and results from pressure of shoes, although it can also result from bony exostoses. Other than relief from shoe pressure, no treatment is indicated.

Plantar Fasciitis (Subcalcaneal Pain Syndrome)

Plantar fasciitis, which is seen primarily in persons between 40 and 60 years of age, is characterized by pain in the plantar area of the heel. The onset may be gradual or may follow some trauma or overuse from some activity, such as athletics, prolonged walking, using improper shoes, or striking the heel with some force. Plantar fasciitis may be idiopathic; it also is likely to be present in younger patients with spondyloarthritis. The pain characteristically occurs in the morning upon arising and is most severe for the first few steps. After an initial improvement, the pain may worsen later in the day, especially after prolonged standing or walking. The pain is burning, aching, and occasionally lancinating. Palpation typically reveals tenderness anteromedially on the medial calcaneal tubercle at the origin of the plantar fascia. Treatment includes relative rest with a reduction in stressful activities, NSAIDs, use of heel pad or heel cup orthoses, arch support, and stretching of the heel cord and plantar fascia. A local corticosteroid injection, using a 25-gauge needle, is often of help.

Achilles Tendon Rupture

Spontaneous rupture of the Achilles tendon is well known and occurs with a sudden onset of pain during forced dorsiflexion. An audible snap may be heard, followed by difficulty in walking and standing on toes. Swelling and edema over the area usually develop. Diagnosis can be made with the Thompson test, in which the patient kneels on a chair with the feet extending over the edge, and the examiner squeezes the calf and pushes toward the knee. Normally this produces plantar flexion, but in a ruptured tendon no plantar flexion occurs. Achilles tendon rupture is generally due to athletic events or trauma from jumps or falls. The tendon is more prone to tear in those having preexisting Achilles tendon disease or in those on corticosteroids. Orthopedic consultation should be obtained, and immobilization or surgery may be selected, depending on the situation.

Tarsal Tunnel Syndrome

In the tarsal tunnel syndrome, the posterior tibial nerve is compressed at or near the flexor retinaculum. Just distally, the nerve divides into the medial plantar, lateral plantar, and posterior calcaneal branches. The flexor retinaculum is located posterior and inferior to the medial malleolus. Numbness, burning pain, and paresthesias of the toes and sole extend proximally to the area over the medial malleolus. Nocturnal exacerbation may be reported. The patient gets some relief by leg, foot, and ankle movements. A positive Tinel's sign may be elicited on percussion posterior to the medial malleolus, and loss of pin-prick and two-point discrimination may be present. Women are more often affected than men. Trauma to the foot, especially fracture, valgus foot deformity, hypermobility, and occupational factors may relate to development of this. An electrodiagnostic test may show prolonged motor and sensory latencies and slowing of the nerve conduction velocities. In addition, a positive tourniquet test and pressure over the flexor retinaculum can induce symptoms. Shoe corrections and steroid injection into the tarsal tunnel may be of benefit, but often surgical decompression is needed.

Posterior Tibial Tendinitis

Pain and tenderness just posterior to the medial malleolus occur in posterior tibial tendinitis. This can be due to trauma, excessive pronation, RA, or spondyloarthropathy. Extension and flexion may be normal, but pain is present on resisted inversion or passive eversion. The discomfort is usually worse after athletic events, and swelling and localized tenderness may be present. Treatment usually includes rest, NSAIDs, and possibly a local injection of corticosteroid. Immobilization with a splint is sometimes needed.

Peroneal Tendon Dislocation and Peroneal Tendinitis

Dislocation of the peroneal tendon may occur from a direct blow, repetitive trauma, or sudden dorsiflexion with eversion. Sometimes a painless snapping noise is heard at the time of dislocation. Other patients report more severe pain and tenderness of the tendon area that lies over the lateral malleolus. The condition may be confused with an acute ankle sprain. Conservative treatment with immobilization is often satisfactory because the peroneal tendon usually reduces spontaneously. If the retinaculum supporting the tendon is ruptured, however, surgical correction may be needed. Peroneal tendinitis can also occur and be manifested as localized tenderness over the lateral malleolus. Conservative treatment is usually indicated.

Hallux Valgus

In hallux valgus, deviation of the large toe lateral to the midline and deviation of the first metatarsal medially occur.

A bunion (adventitious bursa) on the head of the first metatarsophalangeal (MTP) joint may be present, often causing pain, tenderness, and swelling. Hallux valgus is more common in women. It may be caused by a genetic tendency or wearing pointed shoes, or it can be secondary to RA or generalized OA. Stretching of shoes, use of bunion pads, or surgery may be indicated. Metatarsus primus varus, a condition in which the first metatarsal is angulated medially, is seen in association with or secondary to the hallux valgus deformity.

Bunionette

A bunionette, or tailor's bunion, is a prominence of the fifth metatarsal head resulting from the overlying bursa and a localized callus. The fifth metatarsal has a lateral (valgus) deviation.

Hammer Toe

In hammer toe, the PIP joint is flexed and the tip of the toe points downward. The second toe is most commonly involved. Calluses may form at the tip of the toe and over the dorsum of the interphalangeal joint, resulting from pressure against the shoe. Hammer toe may be congenital or acquired secondary to hallux valgus and may result from improper footwear. When the MTP joint is hyperextended, the deformity is known as cocked-up toes. This may be seen in RA.

Morton's Neuroma

Middle-aged women are most frequently affected by Morton's neuroma, an entrapment neuropathy of the interdigital nerve occurring most often between the third and fourth toes. Paresthesia and a burning, aching pain are experienced in the fourth toe. The symptoms are made worse by walking on hard surfaces or wearing tight shoes or high heels. Tenderness may be elicited by palpation between the third and fourth metatarsal heads. Occasionally, a neuroma is seen between the second and third toes. Compression of the interdigital nerve by the transverse metatarsal ligament and possibly by an intermetatarsophalangeal bursa or synovial cyst may be responsible for the entrapment. Treatment usually includes a metatarsal bar or a local steroid injection into the web space. Ultimately, surgical excision of the neuroma and a portion of the nerve may be needed.

Metatarsalgia

Pain arising from the metatarsal heads, known as metatarsalgia, is a symptom resulting from a variety of conditions. Pain on standing and tenderness on palpation of the metatarsal heads are present. Calluses over the metatarsal heads are usually seen. The causes of metatarsalgia are many, including foot strain, high-heeled shoes, everted foot, trauma, sesamoiditis, hallux valgus, arthritis, foot surgery, or a foot with a high longitudinal arch. Flattening of the transverse arch and weakness of the intrinsic muscles occur, resulting in a maldistribution of weight on the forefoot. Treatment is directed at elevating the middle portion of the transverse arch with an orthotic device, strengthening of the intrinsic muscles, weight reduction, and use of metatarsal pads or a metatarsal bar.

Pes Planus

Pes planus, or "flat foot," is often asymptomatic, but may cause fatigue of the foot muscles and aching with intoler-

ance to prolonged walking or standing. There is loss of the longitudinal arch on the medial side and prominence of the navicular and head of the talus (Fig. 8F-3). The calcaneus is everted (valgus), and out-toeing can be seen on ambulation. The tendency for this condition is largely inherited and is seen with generalized hypermobility. A Thomas heel, firm shoes, and grasping exercises to strengthen the intrinsic muscles are helpful. A shoe orthosis may be needed for more cases. The asymptomatic flat foot is left untreated.

Pes Cavus

In contradistinction to pes planus, pes cavus, or claw foot, is characterized by an unusually high medial arch, and in severe cases, a high longitudinal arch, resulting in shortening of the foot. These abnormally high arches further result in shortening of the extensor ligaments, causing dorsiflexion of the PIP joints and plantar flexion of the DIP joints, giving a claw-like appearance to the toes. The plantar fascia may also be contracted. Generally, a tendency to pes cavus is inherited, and in a high percentage of cases an underlying neurologic disorder is present. Although pes cavus can cause foot fatigue, pain, and tenderness over the metatarsal heads with callus formation, it may also be asymptomatic. Calluses generally develop over the dorsum of the toes. Use of metatarsal pads or a bar is helpful, and stretching of the toe extensors is usually prescribed. In severe cases surgical correction may be needed.

Posterior Tibialis Tendon Rupture

The rupture of the posterior tibialis tendon, which is not commonly recognized, is a cause of progressive flat foot (22). It may be caused by trauma, chronic tendon degeneration, or RA. An insidious onset of pain and tenderness may be noted along the course of the tendon just distal to the medial malleolus, along with swelling medial to the hindfoot. The unilateral deformity of hindfoot valgus and forefoot abduction is an important finding. The forefoot abduction can best be seen from behind; more toes are seen from this posi-

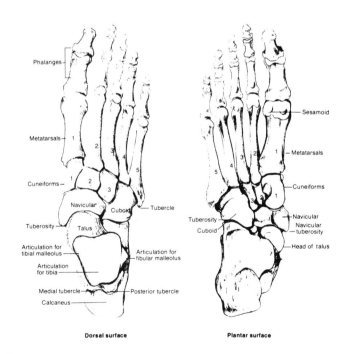

(Figure 8F-3)
Bones of the feet. Courtesy of Dr JJ Calabro.

tion than would be seen normally. The result of the single heel rise test is positive when the patient is unable to rise onto the ball of the affected foot while the contralateral foot is off the floor. Orthopedic consultation should be obtained to determine whether the rupture should be treated conservatively with NSAIDs and casting or with a surgical repair.

DISORDERS OF THE ANTERIOR CHEST WALL

Chest wall pain of a musculoskeletal origin is fairly common. It must be differentiated from chest pain of a cardiac nature, which is the usual main concern, or from pain due to pulmonary or gastrointestinal disease. Pain can also radiate to the chest as a result of cervical or thoracic spine disease. The musculoskeletal syndromes usually associated with chest wall pain are Tietze's syndrome and costochondritis. Both conditions are characterized by tenderness of one or more costal cartilages, and the terms have sometimes been used interchangeably. The two disorders, however, are generally separated by the presence of local swelling in Tietze's syndrome but not in costochondritis (23).

Tietze's syndrome is much less common than costochondritis and is of unknown etiology. Its onset may be gradual or abrupt, with swelling usually occurring in the second or third costal cartilage. Pain, which ranges from mild to severe, may radiate to the shoulder and be aggravated by coughing, sneezing, inspiration, or by various movements affecting the chest wall. Tenderness is elicited on palpation, and approximately 80% of patients have a single site.

Costochondritis is more common and is associated with pain and tenderness of the chest wall, without swelling. Tenderness is often present over more than one costochondral junction, and palpation should duplicate the described pain. In one study of 100 patients with noncardiac chest pain, 69% were found to have local tenderness on palpation and in 16%, the palpation elicited the typical pain (24). Other names attached to costochondritis include anterior wall syndrome, costosternal syndrome, parasternal chondrodynia, and chest wall syndrome. Some individuals with chest wall pain are found to have fibromyalgia or localized myofascial pain. Chest wall pain can also complicate heart or lung disease, so its presence does not exclude more serious problems.

Xiphoid cartilage syndrome or xiphoidalgia, also known as hypersensitive xiphoid or *xiphodynia*, is characterized by pain over the xiphoid area and tenderness on palpation. Pain may be intermittent and brought on by overeating and various twisting movements.

These three conditions are often self-limiting. Treatment consists of reassurance, heat, stretching of chest wall muscles, or local injections of lidocaine, corticosteroid, or both.

In addition, a number of other disorders may produce chest wall pain. Sternocostoclavicular hyperostosis is manifested by a painful swelling of the clavicles, sternum, or ribs and may be relapsing. It is associated with an elevated erythrocyte sedimentation rate, pustules on the palms and soles, and progression to ossification of the chest wall lesions. Condensing osteitis of clavicles is a rare, benign condition of unknown etiology, occurring primarily in women of child-bearing age. It is characterized by sclerosis of the medial ends of the clavicles without involvement of the sternoclavicular joints. Pain and local tenderness are present.

Any condition involving the sternoclavicular joint, including spondyloarthropathy, OA, and infection, can cause chest wall pain. Stress fracture of the ribs, cough fracture, herpes zoster of the thorax, and intercostobrachial nerve entrapment are other causes of chest pain.

Thorough palpation of the chest wall must be done including the sternoclavicular joint, costochondral junctions, sternum, and chest wall muscles. Maneuvers such as crossed-chest adduction of the arm and backward extension of the arm from 90% of abduction help in elucidating whether chest pain is of a musculoskeletal origin. Imaging studies may include plain roentgenogram of the ribs, special roentgenogram of the sternoclavicular joint, tomogram, and bone scan. A computed tomography scan or MRI provide the most detail of the sternoclavicular joint.

JOSEPH J. BIUNDO, JR, MD

1. Shoen RP, Moskowitz RW, Goldberg VM: Soft Tissue Rheumatic Pain: Recognition, Management, Prevention. Philadelphia, Lea & Febiger, 1988

2. Petri M, Dobrow R, Neiman R, et al: Randomized double-blind placebo controlled study of the treatment of the painful shoulder. Arthritis Rheum 30:1040-1045, 1987

3. Kisner C, Colby LA: Therapeutic Exercise: Foundations and Techniques, 2nd ed., Philadelphia, FA Davis, 1990

4. Biundo JJ, Hughes GM: Rheumatoid arthritis rehabilitation: practical guidelines, Part I. J Musculoskeletal Med 8(8):85-96, 1991

5. Neer CR: Impingement lesions. Clin Orthop 173:70-77, 1983

6. Post M, Silver R, Singh M: Rotator cuff tear: diagnosis and treatment. Clin Orthop Rel Res 173:78-91, 1983

7. Crass JR, Craig EV, Thompson RC, et al: Ultrasonography of the rotator cuff: surgical correlation. J Clin Ultrasound 12:487-492, 1984

8. Neviaser RJ: Lesions of the biceps and tendinitis of the shoulder. Orthop Clin N Am 11:343-348, 1980

9. Steinbrocker O, Arojyros TG: Frozen shoulder: treatment by local injections of depot corticosteroids. Arch Phys Med Rehab 55:209-213, 1974

10. Weinstein PS, Canoso JJ, Wohlgethan JR: Long-term follow up of corticosteroid injection for traumatic olecranon bursitis. Ann Rheum Dis 43:44-46, 1984

11. Cyriax J: Diagnosis of soft tissue lesions, Textbook of Orthopaedic Medicine, Vol. 1. London, Bailliere Tindall, 1982, pp 173

12. Stern PJ: Tendinitis, overuse syndromes, and tendon injuries. Hand Clinics 6(3):467-475, 1990

13. Wu JS, Morris JD, Hogan GR: Ulnar neuropathy at the wrist: Case report and review of the literature. Arch Phys Med Rehabil 66:785-788, 1985

14. Anderson B, Kaye S: Treatment of flexor tenosynovitis of the hand ("trigger finger") with corticosteroids. Ann Intern Med 151:153-156, 1991

15. Williams CS, Riordan DC: Mycobacterium mariunum infections of the hand. J Bone Joint Surg 55A:1042-1050, 1973

16. Ege Rasmussen KJ, Farro N: Trochanteric bursitis, treatment by corticosteroid injection. Scand J Rheumatol 14:417-420, 1985

17. Wyant GM: Chronic pain syndromes and their treatment. III. The piriformis syndrome. Can Anaesth Soc J 26:305-308, 1979

18. Stuttle FL: The no-name and no-fame bursa. Clin Orthop 15:197-199, 1959

19. Galloway MT, Jokl P: Patella plica syndrome. Ann Sports Med 5:38-41, 1990

20. O'Donoghue DH: Treatment of Injuries to Athletes, 4th ed. Philadelphia, WB Saunders, 1984, pp 509-510

21. Cox JS: Chondromalacia of the patella: a review of update - Part 1. Comtemp Orthop 6:17-31, 1983

22. Rosenberg ZS, Cheung Y, Jahss MH, et al: Rupture of posterior tibial tendon: CT and MR imaging with surgical correlation. Radiology 169:229-235, 1988

23. Calabro JJ: Costochondritis. N Engl J Med 296:946-947, 1977

24. Wise CM, Semble L, Dalton CB: Musculoskeletal chest wall syndromes in patients with noncardiac chest pain: a study of 100 patients. Arch Phys Med Rehabil 72:147-149, 1992

G. SPORTS AND OCCUPATIONAL INJURIES

Musculoskeletal injuries occurring at the workplace and in athletic pursuits continue to increase in number and severity in the United States, with significant socioeconomic, physical, and psychologic ramifications. The workplace has evolved in the last decade to accommodate high-tech computerized instruments that have replaced some physically demanding occupations but have also introduced a new spectrum of physical disabilities. At the same time, workplace demographics have changed to include an ever-increasing number of women, senior citizens, and disabled individuals.

Individual and team-oriented athletic activity has increased exponentially over the past two decades, largely as a product of the society becoming sensitized to the benefits of physical fitness. It is currently estimated that 30 million people participate in some form of organized sport annually in this country (1). Countless millions more are involved in nonorganized sports and may have the same propensity to physical injury. Approximately 25% of high-school athletes will sustain an injury at some time. Direct costs of such injuries exceed $250 million per year (1). Recognizing the impact on fiscal health care dollars and on physical well-being, a federal initiative entitled Health 2000 will stimulate injury prevention research in sports with the goal of increasing overall health, fitness, pleasure, and relaxation. To this end, conditioning and warm-up exercises have assumed greater priority, as have modifications to equipment and the physical environment in which sports are played. Similarly, the field of ergonomics has evolved to modify the workplace to the benefit of the employee.

Despite these initiatives, injuries will continue to occur. These can be acute, occurring at a specific time and place, or chronic, due to repetitive microtrauma. Injuries to the musculoskeletal system include those to bone, ligaments, muscle and tendon, and joints.

SPORTS INJURIES
Bone Injuries

Although considerably less common than injuries to soft tissue, bone injuries have increased over the past decade because more people are engaging in inherently more dangerous sports such as motorcross, hang-gliding, cycling, and snowmobiling. The spectrum of bone injuries encompasses contusion, stress fracture, avulsive injury, and fracture, including growth-plate injuries in the skeletally immature adolescent.

Contusions to bone generally occur upon direct impact with another player, a surface, or an object in the playing field. Bone contusion can also occur indirectly when a ligament injury produces laxity of the contiguous joint, allowing excessive contact between joint surfaces. Such an indirect insult is commonly seen with an acute anterior cruciate ligament injury that allows the tibia to rotate and translate excessively on the femur with subsequent impaction between the joint surfaces. Direct injuries tend to occur in subcutaneous locations such as the distal and proximal fibula, femoral condyles at the knee, patella, condyles of the distal humerus, and styloid of the radius. The player presents with

an acute onset of pain in the vicinity of the contact, which may be obvious due to an abrasion, laceration, ecchymosis, or hematoma. Palpation directly over the area elicits discomfort but no evident underlying bone defect. Examination of the contiguous joint reveals no evidence of an effusion or ligament disruption, and, although somewhat uncomfortable, full motion is usually possible. After excluding associated ligament and osseous injuries with radiographs, local treatment includes ice, elevation, and a local compressive dressing, and encouraging the patient to maintain and promote motion. The patient can gradually return to activities.

Stress fractures are incomplete fractures brought about by prolonged repetitive strains on normal bone from periarticular muscle contractions that exceed the bone's ability to withstand such forces. These fractures are distinguished from pathologic fractures due to osteoporosis, Paget's disease, hyperparathyroidism, or malignancy. Stress fractures can occur when an athlete suddenly changes activity, training, or equipment including footwear (2). Some athletes are predisposed because of developmental or congenital abnormalities such as genu varum and hindfoot or forefoot varum, all of which place greater stresses on the compressive side of the bones of the lower extremity. The most common sites of stress fractures include the metatarsals, calcaneus, tibia, fibula, and femoral neck. The patient presents with localized pain and is often unable to place full weight or hop on the involved limb. For subcutaneous areas such as the fibula, tibia, calcaneus, and metatarsals, there is localized tenderness, swelling, and, if callus has already developed, a local deformity of bone. Unlike other areas, the hip cannot be effectively palpated, and the clinician must rely on imaging to make the diagnosis. Plain radiographic evidence of injury is not present for at least 2 weeks and even as long as several months after symptom onset. Periosteal reaction, callus, and a linear sclerotic line will usually confirm the diagnosis. Bone scintigraphy often allows diagnosis in the early stages, and magnetic resonance imaging (MRI) for proximal femoral stress fracture can determine whether the injury was caused by tension or compression and whether the fracture pattern is complete or incomplete.

Treatment involves discontinuing the physical activity, adopting other means of aerobic exercise while protecting the limb, and modified weight bearing. Once radiographic and clinical examination show that union is secure, the patient may return to the activity with a modified program while addressing any predisposing factors to avoid refracture.

Proximal femoral neck stress fractures are unique (3). The inferior neck stress or compressive fracture generally heals with the previously described recommendations. However, the superior neck or vertically oriented fracture on the tensile side of the femoral neck has a propensity for completing the fracture and displacing. Most patients with this complication require surgical stabilization to minimize the possibility of displacement, osteonecrosis, or malunion.

Avulsive injuries of the lower extremity are unique to adolescent athletes (4). This injury is a counterpart to the muscle tendon strain or disruption that occurs in the adult athlete. The avulsive injury involves secondary growth centers (apophyses) and causes the cartilaginous growth plate to separate from the underlying bone. These injuries may occur before ossification of the secondary growth center, and therefore may not be immediately evident on radiographs. The injury is a result of a sudden contracture of the muscle attached to the apophysis while the extremity is forced in the opposite direction, which suddenly and violently increases the length of the muscle–tendon unit. The most common sites of involvement are the ischial apophysis (hamstring origin), lesser trochanteric apophysis (iliopsoas insertion), anterior-superior iliac spine apophysis (sartorius origin), and anterior-inferior iliac spine apophysis (rectus femoris origin). Displacement of the avulsed segment is minimized due to the extensive periosteal and perichondral insertion.

The patient presents with severe sudden onset of pain at the site of the injury, inability to actively resist stretching of the involved muscle, ecchymosis and swelling at the avulsed site, and inability to place full weight on the involved extremity. The treatment of these conditions is directed toward minimizing any further displacement of the apophysis. Immediate treatment should be given in the following sequence: analgesic, ice, protected weight bearing, and positioning the extremity to relax the involved muscle. After the acute pain has resolved, active excursion of the muscle is encouraged, progressing to recruiting muscles in close proximity. Resistive exercises can be initiated when active motion has returned fully. Patients can resume sports activities when full motion and muscle power is restored, which generally takes up to 6 weeks.

Definitive fractures of long bones, pelvis, and spine are rare among athletes. They are usually associated with high-speed motorized sporting activity or falls from heights (5). The patient presents with pain, inability to move the extremity, deformity, and crepitation at the fracture site at examination. Local ecchymosis and swelling are often evident in subcutaneous locations such as the ankle and the forearm, but these signs may be absent in fractures of the thigh, spine, and pelvis. Most of these injuries are treated at trauma centers and necessitate either closed reduction and immobilization or open reduction and internal fixation, depending on the nature of the injury. Growth-plate injuries through epiphyses occur in skeletally immature adolescents (6). These injuries are often missed and assumed to be ligament injuries, because the physical findings are similar, including instability to the contiguous joint. However, recognizing the skeletally immature status of the patient and the possibility of apophyseal injury should prompt stress views, which can often delineate the nature of the growth-plate injury. These injuries can be devastating because of the associated interruption of growth and maturation of the limb.

Muscle and Tendon Injuries

Since most sports require sudden, powerful, and repetitive muscle contractions, injuries to muscles and tendons are common in athletes. These injuries include muscle cramps, exercise-induced muscle soreness, contusion, strains, lacerations, and compartment syndromes.

Although the exact mechanism of *muscle cramps* is not well understood, the physical findings are uniformly similar (7). The patient experiences sudden onset of discomfort, muscle spasm with visible fasciculations, pain on palpation, and involuntary movement of contiguous joints. Muscle cramps more commonly involve the lower extremity than the upper limbs. Onset is generally due to sudden contracture of an already shortened muscle. It may occur in perfectly healthy young athletes and in those who have a significant electrolyte imbalance with alterations in serum sodium, calcium, or magnesium. The cramp can be aborted by forcefully stretching the muscle or by activating antagonistic muscles. Muscle excitability and fasciculations can last for several days, well after the process has largely been reversed.

Exercise-induced muscle soreness is experienced by most, if not all, athletes who start or resume a particularly demanding physical activity. Acute pain during exercise is likely the product of lactic acid accumulation within the muscle. Although unpleasant, it is not usually associated with any visible or palpable muscle spasm and usually resolves shortly after the person ceases activity. In contrast, delayed muscle soreness 1 or even 2 days after the activity is likely a product of microtears within the muscle. Local pain with contraction or stretching of the muscle is typical. Applying ice and a compressive bandage may assist in resolving the discomfort. Graduated return to physical activity after the acute phase is recommended. Recurrence may be avoided by adopting less aggressive training techniques (7).

Direct muscle injury is common in contact sports (8) such as rugger, football, hockey, and basketball. The most frequently injured site is the anterior thigh from contact with instruments, equipment, or an opposition player. The injury is heralded by swelling, sometimes ecchymosis, and pain with any active or passive movement of the muscle. Largely as a result of documenting these injuries in military recruits (9), contusions are graded according to severity of the disability, which depends primarily on the degree of pain and swelling immediately after the injury. For example, a grade I quadriceps contusion is that in which knee flexion can readily be accomplished beyond 90 degrees, grade II is flexion from 45 to 90 degrees, and grade III is less than 45 degrees of active flexion. The disability is minimized by applying ice immediately, elevating the limb, using a compressive dressing, and starting active movement early. It also prevents myositis ossificans, which is ossification of the hematoma in muscle that can be seen radiographically approximately 2–3 weeks after the injury. Myositis ossificans can prolong both disability and discomfort. Myositis ossificans evolves through an inflammation phase during which fibroblasts mature into chondrocytes then ultimately into immature bone. With resolution of the acute inflammation, the newly developed bone matures histologically and radiographically. In spite of the presence of a sizable bulk of bone in the muscle, rarely does it cause sufficient symptoms to warrant surgical elusion. Physical therapy with passive assisted motion or with constant passive motion machines has been associated with the development of myositis ossificans. Recent studies suggest that immobilizing the contused muscle in a maximum stretch position serves to reduce disability and return motion rapidly (10).

Lacerations to the muscle–tendon unit is an unusual event in sport. On rare occasions it has occurred in ice hockey, where a sharp skate blade partially or totally transected a muscle. More commonly, *tendon disruption* occurs from sudden, violent contraction of a muscle against sudden resistance. Common tendon injuries in the senior athlete involve the Achilles, quadriceps, or patellar tendon or the long head of the biceps at the shoulder or radial tuberosity. With the exception of the proximal biceps, rupture of these tendons is disabling and requires surgical repair. Achilles tendon rupture is most common in racquet sports and basketball, where sudden deceleration on the court produces such tension in the tendon as to rupture several centimeters from the bony insertion. The athlete experiences immediate pain and is unable to put full weight on the lower limb. Findings on physical examination are ecchymoses on the distal posterior aspect of the calf and an obvious palpable deformity, positive Thompson's sign, inability to plantar flex the foot with any power, and on rare occasions, decreased sensation of the sural nerve dermatome. Similarly, athletes who experience quadriceps or patellar tendon disruptions lose the extensor mechanism and are unable to walk. Disruptions of the biceps tendon causes swelling and ecchymosis at the site. If proximal disruption occurs, the muscle portion of the biceps migrates distally, causing the muscle to bulge markedly. If a tear occurs at the radial styloid insertion, the muscle migrates proximally, which is more disabling than proximal tears because it interferes more with elbow flexion and supination.

Compartment syndrome is characterized by a pathologic increase in the interstitial pressure within an anatomically confined muscle compartment, thereby interfering with neurovascular innervation, which can lead to myonecrosis. The sudden increase in intracompartmental pressure can be caused by hemorrhage or by intracellular or even extracellular edema. Although rare (11), acute compartment syndrome has been seen in motorcross and snowmobile participants who strike their calf on a solid object, causing hemorrhage. The clinical presentation includes an inordinate amount of pain (particularly on active and passive stretching of muscles within the compartment), paresthesias in the distribution of nerves coursing through the compartment, and a definitive and marked increase in resistance to palpation. The pulses may be intact distally and not diminished. Diagnosis is confirmed by measuring the intracompartmental pressure. Pressure in excess of 30–40 mmHg or within 30 mm of the diastolic pressure is indicative of evolving or actual compartment syndrome and the need for emergent fasciotomy.

Chronic exertional compartment syndromes are more common and are generally seen among long-distance runners. Pain is isolated to the anterior or lateral compartment and begins early in the athlete's training program. It can be a difficult diagnosis to make and to differentiate from stress fractures, shin splints, popliteal entrapment syndrome, and other conditions remote from the calf such as piriformis syndrome. The diagnosis is suggested by intracompartmental pressure elevations above normal during exercise and a slow return to resting levels at the conclusion of exercise. Once confirmed, it may be necessary to perform fasciotomy.

With the increasing presence of senior athletes in sports has come an exponential increase in chronic overuse syndromes (12). These injuries are a result of repetitive demands on muscle and tendon that eclipse the adaptive and healing capabilities of these structures. The pain associated with this phenomenon can occur after or during exercise, with or without alterations in performance level. The evolution of this process follows three stages, characterized by inflam-

mation and edema, progressing to scarring, and then thickening and fibrosis within the tendon. If medical intervention or modification in activity is not initiated, continued embarrassment to the tendon can result in partial or complete rupture. Several classic examples of repetitive overuse tendinitis can be cited. Throwing sports, overhead activity on a repetitive basis, and maldirected weightlifting can contribute to impingement syndrome of the shoulder, one of the more common overuse injuries. Other examples are deltoid tendinitis at its insertion on the mid to upper humerus, common extensor muscle originating from the lateral epicondyle of the elbow, and Achilles tendon insertion on the calcaneus. Patients with overuse syndromes universally complain of pain when performing their activities and have localized discomfort, sometimes manifest crepitation, and may even have palpable thickness of the tendons as a result of edema and inflammation. Treatment consists of ice, modification of activities, nonsteroidal anti-inflammatory drugs, ultrasound treatment, and gentle eccentric stretching of the musculotendinous units. Modification of training or performance may minimize further insult (Table 8G-1). For those who have progressed to partial or full thickness tears, surgical reconstruction may be necessary to restore normal power and motion.

Injuries to Ligaments and Capsule

Joints are supported and stabilized by the congruency of the articulating surfaces. The shoulder, hip, and knee are further reinforced by fibrocartilage extensions of the articulating segments in the form of a labrum or menisci. Additionally, there are well-defined ligaments that minimize excursion of the articulating segments in certain planes of movement. One or all of these structures can be injured by force applied either to the joint directly or to the bone in such a way that increases the distance between the articulating surfaces and overcomes the ability of ligaments to resist such forces. The degree of injury depends on the magnitude and direction of the force, the position of the joint at the time of injury, and the speed at which the force was applied.

Ligament injuries are classified according to the extent of tear and degree of laxity, which can usually be determined by a thorough clinical examination (Table 8G-2). Ligament injuries of the knee are common in athletes because this joint

(Table 8G-1)
*Chronic overuse syndrome**

Grade	Symptoms	Treatment
I	Pain after activity only	Ice
II	Pain during and after activity, but no significant interference with performance	Ice and 10%–25% decrease in activity
III	Pain during and after activity with interference with performance	Ice, 25%–75% decrease in activity, and NSAIDs
IV	Constant pain that interferes with activities of daily living	Ice, complete rest of involved area, and NSAIDs

* NSAIDs = nonsteroidal anti-inflammatory drugs.

(Table 8G-2)

Classification and treatment of ligament tears

	1st Degree	2nd Degree	3rd Degree
Injury	Minimal tear	Partial tear	Complete tear
Laxity	None	Mild to moderate	Unstable
Treatment	Ice with rehabilitation and supportive care	Ice, muscle rehabilitation, functional bracing, and possible cast	Ice, splint, and possible surgery
Prognosis	Excellent	Good	Variable

is the most vulnerable part of the anatomy in most contact sports. Knee injuries are also likely to be the most disabling if ligament tears are missed or misdiagnosed, because chronic instability precipitates further intra-articular damage in the form of meniscal tears, chondral contusions and disruptions, and possibly premature degenerative arthritis. Knee ligament injuries should be diagnosed early and appropriate treatment initiated to minimize the sequelae. Varus or valgus force jeopardizes the lateral or medial collateral ligament, respectively. Likewise, anterior or posterior force may injure the anterior or posterior cruciate. It is rare that force is applied in an isolated, unidirectional manner. Generally, the force includes a significant rotational element that contributes to a combination of ligament injuries or ligament and meniscal pathology.

Most athletes who sustain ligament injuries cannot continue to practice or play (13). They feel a tearing sensation or a "pop" that may be heard even by people nearby, suggesting complete ligament disruption or significant bony injury. The patient has difficulty standing on the injured leg and often needs support. Acute swelling within the knee suggests intra-articular hemorrhage and the strong probability of cruciate ligament injury. Effusions that occur 24–36 hours after injury suggest meniscal tears without concomitant ligament injury.

Initial assessment of the patient should include a thorough neurovascular examination distal to the injury, evaluation of the injured limb's orientation compared with the uninvolved limb, and the extent of effusion. The orientation of the patella relative to the underlying femur should be assessed because ligament injuries and patellofemoral dislocations may occur together. Active and passive range of motion should be assessed. A knee that cannot be flexed passively or extended beyond the resting flexed position suggests the presence of a displaced bucket-handle tear of the meniscus. Similarly, a knee that is "locked" in full extension and has what appears to be a soft mechanical block suggests displaced meniscal pathology, a loose fragment, or a torn anterior cruciate that has fallen between the articulating segments. Assessment of the knee should include varus/valgus stressing in extension and in 30 degrees of flexion to determine the integrity of the collateral ligaments. Assessment of the anterior cruciate ligament should include the Lachman's test, anterior drawer test at 70–90 degrees of flexion, and the pivot shift test. Maximum flexion with rotation may elicit discomfort or a classic clicking sound, which are associated with a positive McMurray's sign for meniscal pathology. Pain elicited by palpation along either joint line

suggests meniscal tears, and pain at the condylar insertion and origin of the collateral ligaments suggests injury to these structures.

Radiographs may show an avulsive injury of the collateral or cruciate ligaments, osteocartilaginous loose bodies within the knee joint, or previously undiagnosed osteochondritis dissecans. A flake of bone from the lateral tibial condyle (Segond's sign) is pathognomonic for an associated anterior cruciate injury. In the presence of acute hemarthrosis and pain, it may be initially impossible to ascertain the extent of ligament and associated injuries. By applying a knee immobilizer and initiating protective ambulation, the clinician can further evaluate the knee after it becomes less irritable. It may also be necessary to order magnetic resonance imaging to determine the full extent of injury and develop a more effective treatment plan.

Most grade I and grade II isolated ligament injuries can be treated with ice, compressive bandage, protected ambulation, and functional bracing, as necessary, followed by early return of motion and resuming routine activities. Grade III isolated medial collateral ligament injuries can generally be treated conservatively in a similar manner. Ligaments will heal more rapidly if joint movement is initiated early rather than keeping the knee immobilized.

The treatment of isolated anterior cruciate ligament injuries depends on the patient's age and anticipated future physical activities (13). It may be appropriate to initiate rehabilitation as described above, incorporate closed kinetic chain exercises early to compensate for the cruciate deficiency, and have the patient wear a brace during athletic activities. Active individuals may elect to have anterior cruciate ligament reconstruction surgery. Multiligament injuries or anterior cruciate injuries associated with significant meniscal pathology are best treated by surgical reconstruction.

Another common site for ligament injury is the anterior lateral aspect of the ankle. An inversion plantar-flexed position of the foot with sudden weight bearing principally injures the anterior talofibular ligament and less often, the fibulocalcaneal and posterior talofibular ligaments. The subcutaneous position of these ligaments results in early significant swelling, ecchymosis, and discoloration. The pain is located on the anterolateral fibula, at the insertion site of the anterior talofibular ligament, and often the distal tibiofibular ligament just anterior to the ankle joint is painful. Assessment should include other sites of discomfort, however, to exclude the possibility of associated osseous injuries. Ankle stability is assessed by placing the foot in 20 to 30 degrees of plantar flexion and pulling anteriorly on the posterior aspect of the hindfoot in an attempt to sublux the talar dome from the underlying tibia. Generally, disruption of the anterior talofibular ligament is marked by slight anterior translation of the talus from underneath the tibia in 30 degrees of plantar flexion, but in neutral position it stabilizes. Treatment is directed toward minimizing the edema and swelling; patients should be encouraged to resume ankle motion and to have confidence in weight bearing. Extensive strengthening of the lateral structures of the ankle helps minimize future inversion injuries.

When force applied to the joint surfaces exceeds the resistance of the ligaments and capsule, the joint may subluxate or dislocate. In subluxation, the joint partially separates but spontaneously reduces; in dislocation, the joint surfaces are dislodged. The most common dislocation is that of the shoulder and patellofemoral joint, whereas dislocations of the elbow, hip, and knee are distinctly uncommon. The patient complains of immediate pain, is unable to move the extremity in any effective direction, protects the extremity, and may or may not complain of dysthesias.

Patients with a shoulder dislocation have a squared off appearance, lack the usual deltoid contour, and have a prominence on the anterior aspect of the chest wall, a result of the dislocated humeral head lying anterior and inferior to the glenoid (14). Examination should include an extensive neurologic evaluation of the extremity, as well as assessment of the axillary nerve. Decreased sensation in a small patchy area over the lateral aspect of the upper arm suggests the possibility of concomitant injury. Relocation is accomplished with sedation and traction, but radiographic views should be made first to rule out the possibility of an associated fracture of the tuberosities or upper humeral shaft that could be further displaced by aggressive traction. Neurologic examination should be repeated after reduction.

Considerably less common, but much more devastating, are dislocations of the hip and knee. In an effort to avoid osteonecrosis, a hip dislocation should be considered an emergency and reduction accomplished within the first 6–8 hours after injury. Radiographic studies before and after reduction should be performed to identify associated fractures that could prevent a congruent reduction. If this is suspected, fine-cut computerized tomography scans of the pelvis should be performed to identify intra-articular loose fragments. In knee dislocations, the possibility of neurovascular injury should always be considered. All patients with knee dislocations should have an arteriogram to rule out concomitant vascular injury that may need to be addressed.

OCCUPATIONAL INJURIES

In contrast to the predilection for lower extremity injuries among athletes, the upper extremity, back, and cervical spine are much more commonly affected by injuries sustained in the workforce. In addition, work-related injuries are often based on exposure over time to repetitive tasks. Terms such as repetitive stress injury and cumulative trauma disorder (CTD) are used to describe a wide spectrum of disorders, including many that are similar to chronic overuse syndromes in athletes. With new technology that often mandates repetitive keyboard activity and generous changes in Workers' Compensation benefits, the incidence of CTD has risen dramatically. Currently CTD accounts for more than 50% of all occupational illnesses in the United States with an incidence of 21 cases per 100,000 workers annually (15). This incidence is an exponential increase from the previous decade, possibly a product of the evolving technology in the workplace, improved accuracy of reporting and diagnosis, employees who are more aware of their rights, and with ever-increasing downsizing, employees who are under pressure to perform more tasks, more quickly, in a shorter period of time.

Muscles actively engaged in performing repetitive tasks and distant muscles that must remain contracted for long periods of time to sustain an unsupported extremity are both vulnerable to muscle fatigue and microtears, with associated inflammation, edema, and dysfunction. The following risk factors in the workplace are associated with CTD: 1) repetition, 2) high force, 3) awkward joint posture,

4) direct pressure, 5) vibration, and 6) prolonged constrained posture. The incidence of musculoskeletal complaints and injury rise significantly if two or more risk factors are present (16). Before concluding that an ailment is solely attributable to the work performed, however, it is important to determine whether the patient engages in avocational activities that may also predispose to such injury. In addition, reviewing the nature of the work and possibly even visiting the job site allows the examiner to more accurately determine the causal association between work and physical injury (17).

Treatment of CTD is not limited to active medical intervention to reverse the disorder, but also includes recommendations on alterations at the job site to minimize further injuries to the patient and his or her colleagues. Ergonomics, which is a discipline that devises ways to maximize comfort and productivity while minimizing injury in the workplace, has become a vital adjunct in the management of workplace injuries.

CTDs cover a wide spectrum of disorders, many having a distinctive presentation, predisposing factors, findings on clinical examination, and well-defined and often successful treatment. These injuries include stenosing tenosynovitis of the fingers, de Quervain's tenosynovitis, intersection syndrome, lateral epicondylitis, and rotator cuff tendinitis. Less well-defined are diffuse back and paraspinal complaints, numbness, tingling, perceived weakness, and fatigue. Many of these patients have several, if not all, risk factors. Persistent abnormal posture leads to muscle imbalance and increased tension within the peripheral nerves, which precipitates multi-level nerve compression and symptoms. A more extensive examination of these patients and their work place may have to be conducted, because the inciting factors are likely to be multiple. Evaluation of the patient's posture and position maintained at work often reveals poor support in the seating and arrangement of tools. Additionally, observing the patient at work may help identify both the muscle unit principally involved with the task and remote muscles that support the activity.

Generally the treatment of CTD is to rest the affected part with devices such as night-time splints, neck braces, and lower back supports. Acute management may include the application of ice, nonsteroidal anti-inflammatory drugs, judicious use of local corticosteroid injections, and referral to a physical therapist who can teach appropriate stretching and strengthening exercises and guide the patient through a progressive aerobic program to increase overall physical fitness. To prevent re-injury, assessment of risk factors in the work place should suggest modifications such as using different tools, reducing time on a high-risk task by job rotation, or using protective equipment such as pads and splints (18,19).

Since most of these conditions are compensable under Workers' Compensation, attempts to alleviate the problem expeditiously by surgical intervention should be avoided. Surgery may be considered if all conservative measures have failed after a reasonable trail of at least 3 months. The success of surgery in the Workers' Compensation patient population has consistently been less assured than for non-compensable injuries or maladies.

Injuries to Muscle and Tendon

Sustained muscle contraction and repetitive use often precipitate muscle fatigue, which is associated with decreased strength, coordination, and ability to persist with the activity. This is particularly true in a working situation where arms are held at a distance from the body without support. Such situations are common in automobile assembly workers, mechanics, and electricians who commonly work above their heads while holding heavy equipment. In a similar fashion, workers who are constantly in a static posture and must maintain an arm in abduction or extension for prolonged periods or must sustain a forward thrust of the neck can develop neck torsion syndrome. This syndrome is characterized by pain along the paravertebral segment of the cervical spine extending into the trapezius. On examination these patients have bilateral trapezius spasm, pain on palpation in the area, decreased neck movement, and pain with extreme movement.

Repetitive use of an extremity often precipitates tenosynovitis. The most commonly involved sites are the first dorsal compartment (de Quervain's disease), the area where the mobile wad (abductor pollicis, extensor pollicis longus, extensor pollicis brevis) crosses over the common extensors to the digits in the dorsal distal aspect of the forearm (intersection syndrome), lateral epicondylitis, deltoid tendinitis, and impingement syndrome. Typically, tendinitis is associated with localized discomfort that is increased with passive stretching of the affected muscle tendon unit. There is often pain-induced weakness and crepitation at the site of tendon excursion, and swelling may be apparent in subcutaneous areas.

Injuries of peripheral nerves caused by abnormal posture are common in many job situations and environments. Muscle hypertrophy and atrophy occur simultaneously in muscles challenged and not challenged, respectively. Common entrapments of the upper extremity include the median nerve at the wrist (carpal tunnel syndrome), ulnar nerve at the elbow (cubital tunnel syndrome), and Guyon's canal and radial nerve as it penetrates the supinator in the proximal aspect of the forearm. Direct injury of these nerves can also occur by repeated extrinsic compression.

One of the more common occupational injuries is carpal tunnel syndrome. Patients complain of a tingling sensation along the thumb, index, and middle finger, which may awaken them at night. They also experience weak pinch action and a sensation of spasm in the three digits. Physical examination reveals a positive Tinel's sign at the wrist, decreased muscle bulk in the thenar musculature, decreased sensation along the nerve distribution, and a positive Phalen's test in which wrist flexion reproduces the numbness and tingling. If splints worn at night, NSAIDs, and corticosteroid injections do not alleviate the pain and there ap-

pears to be evidence of electromyographic dysfunction, carpal tunnel release can be performed by either open surgery or endoscopy. However, a quarter of patients experiencing carpal tunnel disease also have symptoms suggestive of other soft tissue injuries such as tendinitis at various sites or even peripheral nerve entrapment (20).

Although consuming literally billions of dollars a year due to loss of productivity and continued compensation, CTD is largely preventable with appropriate assessment of the work environment by well-trained ergonomists.

M.G. ROCK, MD

1. Requa RK: The scope of the problem: the impact of sports-related injuries. Presented at Conference on Sports Injuries in Youth: Surveillance Strategies; April 8-9, 1991; Bethesda, MD

2. Arendt EA, Clohisy DR: The stress injuries of bone. In Nicholas JH, Hershman EB (eds): The Lower Extremity and Spine in Sports Medicine, 2nd ed. St. Louis, Mosby, 1995, 65-81

3. Fullerton LR, Snowdy HA: Femoral neck stress fractures. Am J Sports Med 16:365-377, 1988

4. Sundar M, Carty H: Avulsion fractures of the pelvis in children: a report of 32 fractures and their outcome. Skeletal Rad 23:85-90, 1994

5. Fink RA, Monge JJ: Snowmobiling injuries. Minnesota Med 54:29-32, 1971

6. Paletta GA, Andrish JT: Injuries about the hip and pelvis in a young athlete. Clinics in Sports Med 14:591-628, 1995

7. Abetakis PPM: Muscle soreness in rhabdomyolysis. In Nicholas JA and Hershman EB (eds): The Lower Extremity and Spine in Sports Medicine, 2nd ed. St. Louis, Mosby, 1995, pp 53-63

8. Sim FH, Rock MG, Scott SG: Pelvis and hip injuries in athletes: anatomy and function. In Nicholas JA and Hershman EB (eds): The Lower Extremity and Spine in Sports Medicine, 2nd ed. St. Louis, Mosby, 1995, pp 1025-1065

9. Jackson DW, Feagin JA: Quadriceps contusions in young athletes. J Bone Joint Surg 55A:95-105, 1973

10. Ryan JB, Wheeler JH, Hopkinson WJ, Arclero RA, Kolakowski KR: Quadricep contusion: Westpoint update. Am J Sports Med 19:299-304, 1991

11. Kennedy JC, Roth JH: Major tibial compartment syndromes following minor athletic trauma. Am J Sports Med 7:201-203, 1979

12. Mercier LR: Sports medicine. In Mercier LR (ed): Practical Orthopedics, 4th ed. St. Louis, Mosby, 1995, pp 294-326

13. Noyes F, Basset R: Arthroscopy in acute traumatic hemarthrosis of the knee. J Bone Joint Surg 52A:687-695, 1980

14. Steinberg GG, Akins CM, Baran DT: Shoulder and upper arm. In Steinberg GG, Akins CM (eds): Orthopedics in Primary Care, 2nd ed. Baltimore, Williams & Wilkins, 1992, pp 26-61

15. Bureau of Labor Statistics reports on survey of occupational injuries and illnesses in 1977 through 1989, Washington DC, Bureau of Labor Statitics, U.S. Department of Labor, 1990

16. Armstrong T, Fine L, Goldstein S, Lifshitzid Y, Silverstein B: Ergonomic considerations in hand and wrist tendinitis. Am J Surg Hand 12A:830-837, 1987

17. Rodgers SH: Job evaluation in worker fitness determination. Occupational Health: State of the Art Reviews 3:219-239, 1988

18. Rempel DM, Harrison RJ, Barnhart S: Work-related cumulative trauma disorders of the upper extremity. J Am Med Assoc 267:838-842, 1992

19. Higgs PE, MacKinnon SE: Repetitive motion injuries. Ann Rev Med 46:1-16, 1995

20. Yamaguchi DM, Lipscomb PR, Soule EH: Carpal tunnel syndrome. Minnesota Med 22-33, 1965

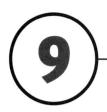

RHEUMATOID ARTHRITIS
A. EPIDEMIOLOGY, PATHOLOGY, AND PATHOGENESIS

Rheumatoid arthritis (RA) is a chronic, inflammatory, systemic disease that produces its most prominent manifestations in the diarthrodial joints. Persistent and progressive synovitis develops in peripheral joints. The initial event inciting the inflammatory response is unknown. An infectious etiology of RA has been vigorously pursued without yielding convincing evidence. Possibly, attempts to identify an etiologic agent have failed because the initial event is not disease-specific and is distinct in different patients. Genetic and environmental factors control the progression, extent, and pattern of the inflammatory response and are thereby responsible for the heterogenous clinical features. RA encompasses a wide spectrum of features, from self-limiting disease to progressively chronic disease with varying degrees of joint destruction to clinically evident extra-articular manifestations. Knowledge of the modulating factors, although still fragmentary, has increased tremendously during the past 10 years and has started to make an impact on the clinical assessment and treatment of patients with RA.

EPIDEMIOLOGY

RA has a worldwide distribution and involves all ethnic groups. Although the disease can occur at any age, the prevalence increases with age and the peak incidence is between the fourth and sixth decade. Data from population-based prevalence and incidence studies have to be interpreted cautiously because there is no unique feature to establish the diagnosis of RA. Therefore, incidence and prevalence studies are based on a set of criteria developed for classification purposes. The most widely used system has been the 1958 American Rheumatism Association criteria and, more recently, the American College of Rheumatology 1987 revised criteria for the classification of RA (1) (see Appendix I). These criteria have a sensitivity and specificity of approximately 90%. Depending on the stringency of the criteria, prevalence estimates vary from 0.3% to 1.5% in the North American population. The prevalence is about 2.5 times higher in females than in males; however, the gender difference is less pronounced among patients who are positive for rheumatoid factor (RF).

Studies of prevalence and incidence have not had a major impact on the understanding of disease pathogenesis. RA appears to be a relatively recent disease. It was first described in the mid-18th century and has not been found in skeletal remains from ancient European or Asian civilizations. However, erosive polyarthritis was documented in the skeletons of prehistoric (3,000–5,000 years ago) Native Americans, which might indicate an infectious agent confined to a small geographic area before the 18th century (2). With this exception, there are no reports of clustering in space or time that would further support an infectious origin. Some Native American populations have a high prevalence rate of 5%–6%, suggesting the alternative explanation

that genetic factors predispose some native Americans to RA. Differences in prevalence rates among other ethnic groups are rather small and are likely explained by variations in disease assessment and age distribution of the study populations. The similar prevalence rates suggest that, rather than one major RA-associated gene, combinations of different genes in different ethnic populations may predispose to disease.

Support for a genetic predisposition comes from studies that RA clusters in families and that there is a high concordance of disease in monozygotic twins (3). It has been estimated that a first-degree relative of an RA patient has about a 16-fold increased risk over the general population. Studies of monozygotic twins have shown a concordance rate between 15% and 30%, which is approximately four times greater than the rate in dizygotic twins, suggesting that more than one gene is important in determining susceptibility. One of these genetic factors is encoded within the major histocompatibility complex (MHC) on chromosome 6. RA is associated with allelic polymorphisms in the HLA-DR region. A second risk factor is linked to gender. Differences in gender and HLA-DR haplotypes account for an estimated 30% of the different concordance rates in dizygotic and monozygotic twins.

PATHOLOGY

The histologic changes in RA are not disease-specific but largely depend on the organ involved. The primary inflammatory joint lesion involves the synovium. In contrast to a hematogenous infectious arthritis, synovial changes are a primary event and do not follow changes of the adjacent bone marrow. The earliest changes are injury to the synovial microvasculature with occlusion of the lumen, swelling of endothelial cells, and gaps between endothelial cells, as documented by electron microscopy. This stage is usually associated with mild proliferation of the superficial lining cell layer. Two cell types constitute the synovial lining: a bone marrow-derived type A synoviocyte, which has macrophage features, and the mesenchymal type B synoviocyte. Both cell types contribute to the synovial hyperplasia, suggesting a paracrine interaction between these two cell types. This stage of inflammation is associated with congestion, edema, and fibrin exudation. Cellular infiltration occurs in early disease and initially consists mainly of T lymphocytes. The T-cell infiltrate is classically described as small nodular aggregates of lymphocytes with a diffuse infiltrate in between. The nodular aggregates consist mainly of CD4 T cells, while CD8 T cells dominate in the diffuse infiltrate. The CD4 T cells mostly express cell-surface antigens characteristic of mature memory cells. Close cell-to-cell contact with dendritic cells and macrophages have been described (4). However, only a minority of T cells express the IL-2 receptor α chain, CD25, and an even smaller percentage express proliferative markers or produce cytokines as a marker of recent cell activation. In later stages, true lymphoid follicles with germinal centers may appear, although rheumatoid synovitis presents with a diffuse lymphocytic infiltrate without follicles or pseudofollicles in many patients. Plasma cells are usually found in more advanced stages of inflammation, and multinucleated giant cells and mast cells are often present. As a consequence of inflammation, the synovium becomes hypertrophic from the proliferation of blood vessels and synovial fibroblasts and from multiplication and enlargement of the synovial lining layers. Granulation tissue extends to the cartilage and is known as *pannus*. The tissue actively invades and destroys the periarticular bone and cartilage at the margin between synovium and bone (Fig. 9A-1).

Clinically evident extra-articular manifestations occur in approximately 20% of RA patients, although subclinical involvement is likely to be more frequent. Rheumatoid nodules have the histologic appearance of a foreign body granuloma with three distinct layers. Multicentric fibrinoid necrosis is surrounded by palisading elongated cells arranged radially and granulation tissue with inflammatory cells. The composition of the necrotic material varies. No conclusions about the necrosis-inducing event can be drawn from histologic examinations, but since nodules frequently occur over pressure points, minor trauma may precipitate the necrosis. The elongated cells in the second layer are modified macrophages that are aligned parallel to collagen fibers.

Tenosynovitis is present in the majority of patients. Involvement of the tendons themselves is common and manifests as a nonspecific inflammatory infiltrate and, less frequently, the formation of characteristic nodules with central necrosis. Similarly, pleurisy and pericarditis are characterized by a diffuse mononuclear cell infiltration and fibrinoid necrosis with occasional nodule formation. Vascular involvement is usually confined to small segments of terminal arteries and lacks distinctive histologic characteristics. Infiltration of mid-size and larger arteries with mononuclear cells can occur, but necrotizing arteritis is infrequent. The

diffuse interstitial pulmonary fibrosis seen in RA cannot be distinguished from the fibrosis in other connective tissue diseases or from primary idiopathic fibrosis. The same is true for the sicca syndrome, frequently seen in RA patients, which cannot be distinguished histologically from primary Sjögren's syndrome. In general, immune complex deposition may contribute to, but does not explain, the spectrum of extracellular manifestations. A common theme appears to be the mononuclear cell infiltrate with varying degrees of fibrinoid necrosis and nodule formations.

PATHOGENESIS

The etiology of the early events in RA remains elusive. The possibility of a bacterial or viral infection has been vigorously pursued. The early pathologic findings of endothelial swelling and synovial hyperplasia are nonspecific, but some investigators have viewed this as evidence for a blood-borne pathogen. Infectious agents induce chronic arthritis in animal models, and deposition of bacterial products in the synovial tissue, as well as chronic infection, have been shown to be responsible for chronic synovial inflammation. This concept received even more attention after several infectious agents were found to induce chronic arthropathy in humans. For example, Lyme disease has been identified as a spirochetal infection. Parvovirus infection in adults frequently results in acute, sometimes protracted, polyarthritis. Rubella virus has been recovered from patients with seronegative chronic polyarthritis. Incorporation of the tax gene into synoviocytes has been postulated as a mechanism to explain the synovial proliferation in HTLV-1-associated arthropathy (5). The search for a putative initiating agent of RA itself has been unrewarding, however. All efforts to associate an infectious agent with RA by isolation, electron microscopy, or molecular biology have failed. It is possible that there is no single primary cause of RA and that different mechanisms may lead to the initial tissue injury and precipitate synovial inflammation. While information on the initiating events is largely missing, substantial progress has been

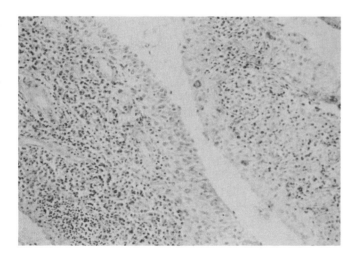

(Figure 9A-1)
Knee synovitis. The multilayerd synovial lining is composed of hyperplastic, hypertrophic synoviocytes with occasional multinucleated giant cells. The enlarged villi are diffusely infiltrated by lymphocytes and plasma cells. Moderate capillary prolifertion is seen. Reprinted from the Revised Clinical Slide Collection on the Rheumatic Diseases with permission of the American College of Rheumatology.

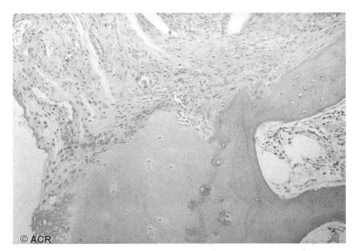

(Figure 9A-2)
Ankle pannus. This microscopic photograph reveals typical pannus formation. Fibrovascular tissue protrudes from the inflamed synovium to the articular cartilage. A portion of the fibrous tissue extends over the surface of the cartilage, which shows death of chondrocytes and loss of basophilia of the matrix. Note the inflammatory exudate in the subchondral bone. Reprinted from the Revised Clinical Slide Collection on the Rheumatic Disease with permission of the American College of Rheumatology.

made in understanding the genetic, molecular, and cellular factors that are involved in perpetuating the primary inflammatory response and the joint destruction process.

GENETIC FACTORS

Family studies and studies in monozygotic and dizygotic twins have shown that RA has several features typical of a complex genetic disease, such as incomplete penetrance, genetic variance, and involvement of multiple genes. The best-studied genes are those of the HLA system. In initial studies, RA was shown to be associated with the HLA-DR4 haplotype (6). Subsequent studies on disease association, genomic organization of the HLA-D region, and molecular characterization of the allelic polymorphisms have provided a more detailed understanding. The actual disease-conferring portion of the D region is confined to a short sequence encompassing amino acid positions 67–74 of the HLA-DRB1 gene (7,8) (see Appendix IV). Studies of different ethnic populations support the concept that a set of HLA-DRB1 alleles is overrepresented among RA patients. Comparison of sequences of HLA-DRB1 showed that all of these alleles share the sequence motif in the third hypervariable region (Table 9A-1). The sequence polymorphism is characterized by a glutamine or an arginine at position 70, a lysine or arginine at position 71, and an alanine at position 74. Negatively charged amino acids at either one of these positions appear not to be associated with RA. The disease-associated alleles include the HLA-DRB1*0401, *0404, and *0408 alleles and HLA-DRB1*0101/2 mainly in the white population, HLA-DRB1*0405 in the Asian population, HLA-DRB1*1402 in some Indian populations, and HLA-DRB1*10 in the Greek population. In the structural model based on the crystalline structure of HLA-DR1, the sequence maps to an α helix that surrounds the antigen-binding cleft of the HLA-DR molecule. The polymorphic residues in the sequence form a pocket that accommodates side chains of the bound peptide. Some of these amino acids also point to the T-cell receptor (TCR) and therefore may be directly involved in HLA–TCR interaction.

(Table 9A-1)
Immumogenetics of rheumatoid arthritis (RA)

- RA is associated with a sequence motif (QR/KRAA) encoded by the HLA-DRB1 gene.

- Different HLA-DRB1 alleles that share the disease-associated sequence motif confer disease susceptibilty in different ethnic populations. The contribution to threshold liability for the disease can be low in some ethnic groups.

- In the crystal structure of the HLA-DR molecule, the RA-associated amino acid stretch maps to a domain that influences T-cell receptor–HLA interaction as well as the binding of antigenic peptides (peptide-binding pocket 4).

- The disease-associated HLA-DRB1 polymorphism determines severity and pattern of disease, suggesting that HLA-DR genes represent progression factors in the disease process.

- The presence of two disease-associated HLA-DRB1*04 alleles is associated with severe articular disease and the presence of extra-articular manifestations.

Based on current knowledge of the biologic function of HLA-DR molecules, three models have been proposed to explain the HLA-DRB1 association with RA (9). In the peptide selection model of RA, the pocket formed by the shared sequences determines whether a putative disease-inducing antigenic peptide would bind to the HLA-DR molecule and would therefore be able to trigger a disease-inducing T-cell response. A second model implies that the disease-associated sequence stretch is directly involved in interacting with contact residues of the TCR. In this model, the disease-associated sequence stretch would influence a large population of the total T-cell compartment, either during T-cell repertoire formation in the thymus or during the peripheral immune response, similar to what has been shown for superantigen-specific T-cell response. In a third model, the disease-associated sequence stretch would not function as part of the whole HLA-DR molecule but as a peptide by itself. HLA-derived peptides are preferentially bound by HLA molecules. These peptides are recognized in the thymus and influence positive and negative selection events of T cells. Molecular mimicry between the disease-associated sequence and several infectious agent-derived proteins have been described. It is therefore possible that the immune response to one of these agents is altered in patients with RA.

Both clinical-association studies and family studies have provided information that may help place the three different models into perspective. These studies have shown that the disease-associated HLA genes modify disease expression. There are currently no convincing data that HLA genes play any other role in disease initiation. Population-based studies have not found any HLA-DR association with RA. Patients with a disease-associated HLA-DR allele who do not have HLA-DR4 develop milder seronegative disease (10). Severity of the disease also appears to be determined by the sequence polymorphism within the disease-associated HLA-DR sequence stretch. Finally, patients with extra-articular manifestations have the strongest HLA-DRB1 association and frequently express two disease-associated HLA-DRB1*04 alleles (11). These data suggest that the disease-associated HLA-DRB1 alleles determine disease progression and severity, and that sequence polymorphisms both inside and outside the disease-associated sequence stretch and a gene-dose effect are important variables influencing the expression of the disease.

The shared epitope hypothesis is based on the assumption that the same sequence stretch functions equally in different ethnic groups. However, recent data suggest that the disease-associated HLA-DRB1 alleles are not completely independent of the genetic background but influence disease pattern in concert with other genes. Family studies have emphasized the importance of the second haplotype in HLA-DRB1*04 positive individuals (11). Concordance rates in siblings sharing both haplotypes are higher than in siblings who shared only one haplotype. Studies of several ethnic groups have found that the disease-associated epitopes, although still associated with RA, are expressed in only a fraction of the patients. These data suggest a more complex model than the peptide selection model. Disease-associated HLA-DRB1 alleles are important in disease progression, rather than in initiating disease, and act in concert with other HLA genes as well as background genes.

Although HLA genes and gender constitute only about 30% of the genetic risk in RA, other genetic factors have not been unequivocally identified. Polymorphism in structural genes or genes that could determine the extent of tissue damage in early stages of disease and thus explain tissue tropism have not been associated with RA. Several candidate genes within the immune system have been explored (including cytokine genes, genes important in the biologic function of HLA molecules, T-cell receptor, and immunoglobulin germline genes) without finding a strong disease association.

T CELLS

The T cell has been described as one of the major infiltrating cells in the synovium. The majority of these cells express the CD4 phenotype. CD4 T cells recognize antigens in restriction to HLA-DR molecules. The finding of CD4 T-cell infiltration together with the HLA-DRB1 association of RA convincingly argues for a central role of the CD4 T cell in the pathogenesis of RA (12). Enormous progress has been made in understanding the mechanism of T-cell migration into the rheumatoid synovium. Several receptor ligand pairs that facilitate adhesion and migration have been described. These receptor ligand pairs are not specific for synovial inflammation but are shared with chronic inflammatory processes in other organs (13). Peripheral blood lymphocytes enter the synovial tissue by binding to the endothelial cells of high endothelial venules. T cells found in synovial tissue have the feature of memory cells and, as such, express a characteristic pattern of cell-surface molecules involved in adhesion and migration. Induction of adhesion molecules on endothelial cells is a primary event in synovial inflammation, and several cytokines have been shown to induce or up-regulate the expression of adhesion molecules on endothelial cells. A number of different families of adhesion molecules, including selectins, intracellular adhesion molecules (β_1 and β_2 integrins, ICAMs), and CD44 have been shown to play a part in the migration. It does not appear that there is a single central interaction in tissue migration, but treatment studies with blocking anti-ICAM antibodies have been based on the hypothesis that up-regulation of ICAM-1 expression on endothelial cells is a critical step in transmigration. Adhesion molecules play important roles in spatial organization within the synovial microenvironment. Many adhesion molecules are able to bind to cell matrix proteins; in particular, integrins bind to collagens, laminin, and fibronectin and are therefore likely involved in the retention of lymphocytes in the tissue.

Cell-to-cell interaction in synovial tissue has been demonstrated for CD4 T cells and macrophages (4), which fits the model that T lymphocytes recognize a locally residing antigen and are activated (Table 9A-2). However, the number of such activated T cells in synovial tissue is small. Approximately 10% of synovial CD4 T cells express the interleukin-2 (IL-2) receptor α chain. It has been difficult to demonstrate T-cell derived lymphokines in synovial inflammation (14). Different models could account for this finding. It is possible that the number of antigen-specific activated T cells within the infiltrate is very small. It is also possible that the T cells are activated but defective in lymphokine production. Optimal lymphocyte activation largely depends on the presence of co-stimulatory receptor ligands. One of the most important co-stimulatory pathways for complete T-cell activation is the interaction between CD28 and CD80/CD86 molecules. The wide expression of CD80 and CD86 in synovial

(Table 9A-2)

Two pathogenetic models of the T-cell response in rheumatoid arthritis (RA)

1. CD4 cells recognize an arthritogenic antigen (exogenous or endogenous) in the synovial tissue and initiate the disease process

   Pro arguments
   - CD4 T cells are the major tissue infiltrating cells.
   - Oligoclonal expansion in the tissue is frequent.
   - The HLA-DRB1 encoded amino acid polymorphism associated with RA contributes to antigen binding.

   Con arguments
   - The synovial T-cell infiltrate is highly heterogeneous.
   - The synovial T-cell receptor repertoire is different among patients.
   - The role of disease-associatied HLA-DRB1 molecules is complex.
   - Evidence for local T-cell activation is scarce.
   - T-cell–depleting therapies are of limited efficacy.

2. CD4 T cells in RA patients have unique functional properties and modulate the inflammatory response.
   - RA patients select a distinct repertoire of naive CD4 T cells.
   - The repertoire of heat-shock–specific T cells is different in RA, possibly secondary to molecular mimicry with the disease-associated HLA-DRB1 motif.
   - Clonal outgrowth of T cells is frequently detected in peripheral blood.
   - Synovial T cells are deficient in IFN-γ production.
   - Rheumatoid factor production shows features of a T-cell–driven response.

tissue does not support the model of defective lymphocyte stimulation involving the CD28 pathway; however, other co-stimulatory molecules may play an important role in the synovial environment and may lead to a distinct repertoire of T-cell effector functions. As a second model, T cells may be down-regulated by inflammatory mediators. Prostaglandins suppress interferon gamma (IFN-γ) and IL-2 secretion, and tumor necrosis factor α (TNF-α) has been implicated as a T-cell suppressive cytokine. Since TNF-α and prostaglandins (PGs) are abundantly produced in synovial inflammation, it is possible that a defective T-cell response, rather than an uncontrolled autoreactive response, is of critical importance in chronic synovial inflammation.

When T cells are activated, they start to proliferate and clonally expand. T-cell activation within a compartment such as synovial tissue should therefore result in a skewing of the TCR repertoire. Consequently, the TCR repertoire has been studied to better understand the nature of T-cell activation. Studies determining the frequencies of TCR Vα and Vβ gene segments in synovial fluid and synovial tissue T cells have yielded conflicting results (9). An expansion of T cells sharing one particular Vβ element would be expected if a superantigen is involved in T-cell activation or if an antigen-specific response results in a major expansion of related T cells. Most of the studies showed some skewing of the synovial TCR repertoire, but these changes were not dramatic and, more importantly, were not consistently found in all studies. Various Vα and Vβ elements have been implicated in individual patients in several studies. Studies analyzing

T cells in the synovial tissue have shown that some T cells undergo clonal expansion; however, based on the TCR structure, the repertoire of these T cells is diverse. The most appropriate interpretation of these observations is that a small subset of synovial T cells proliferate in response to antigens. Proliferating T cells represent a highly diverse population, suggesting that a wide spectrum of antigens is recognized in the lesions. Whether the low concentration of T-cell-derived cytokines is only a reflection of the low number of activated T cells or whether it reflects the functional state of activated T cells is still an issue of debate.

Changes in the T-cell compartment in RA are not restricted to synovial inflammation. Several investigators have concluded that the total T-cell pool is changed in RA, and both progression of synovial inflammation and occurrence of extra-articular manifestations may depend on which type of T cell is available in the repertoire. One attraction of such a model is that it is consistent with the complexity of the HLA-DR association with RA. HLA-DR polymorphisms are controlling the positive and negative selection of CD4 T cells in the thymus. Indeed, it has been shown that the disease-associated HLA-DRB1*04 polymorphism influences the repertoire of peripheral naive T cells (15). Furthermore, the repertoire of CD4 T cells from RA patients could be distinguished from HLA-matched controls, suggesting that additional factors shape the T-cell repertoire in RA. In a second study, a peptide resembling the disease-associated HLA-DRB1 sequence stretch has been implicated in thymic selection. The RA-associated HLA-DR amino acid sequence QKRAA is also present on the heat-shock protein *dnaj* (16). Synovial fluid cells of patients with early disease strongly respond to this bacterial protein and proliferate, suggesting that the disease-associated HLA-DRB1 sequence has a role in positive selection and thereby biases the immune response to bacterial heat-shock proteins. Heat-shock–specific immune responses play an important regulatory role in inflammatory responses, including adjuvant arthritis in animal models and RA. A third line of evidence that the peripheral T-cell repertoire is abnormal in RA comes from studies analyzing oligoclonality in the peripheral T-cell repertoire. Oligoclonal T-cell proliferation was noted in Felty's syndrome several years ago and was subsequently associated with the cytopenia seen in this form of RA. More recent studies have demonstrated clonality within the CD8 and CD4 compartments in RA patients who do not have Felty's syndrome (17,18). Although oligoclonality can also be found in normal healthy individuals, this finding is more pronounced in RA patients. Thus, numerous approaches have demonstrated characteristic features in the repertoire of peripheral T cells in RA patients. It is likely that several distinct mechanisms are responsible for these features. How the T-cell repertoire translates into disease manifestations characteristic of RA is not clear; however, T cells are likely to have a role in fine-tuning the response as well as in disease initiation.

Rheumatoid Factor (RF)

Production of autoantibodies with specificity for the Fc fragment of immunoglobulin G (IgG) is a major immunologic abnormality in RA. RF is not specific for RA. These autoantibodies are also detected in normal individuals and in patients with a variety of conditions including chronic bacterial infection, transplanted organs, and some chronic inflammatory rheumatic diseases. The prevalence in normal individuals increases with age. RF is not present in all patients with RA, and is therefore not a requirement for developing RA. Despite these limitations, RF is the major laboratory hallmark of RA. It is associated with severe disease, and extra-articular manifestations are seen almost exclusively in RF-positive patients. Understanding the mechanisms leading to RF production and its possible effector functions is essential in elucidating the pathogenesis of RA (Table 9A-3).

Many features distinguish RF from other autoantibodies. The autoantigen IgG is soluble and available in high concentrations. It cannot be completely excluded that patients with RA have developed neoantigens on IgG, possibly secondary to a change in the glycolization pattern. However, recent views propose that RF production in RA is closely associated with the biologic function of RFs in normal immune responses (19). B cells, which express RF on their surface, can bind IgG and accumulate the antigen trapped by immunoglobulins (immune complexes). These B cells exist in high frequencies in normal individuals, although they apparently do not secrete large amounts of immunoglobulins. They also are uniquely localized in lymph nodes where they can be found in the mantle zone but not in germinal centers. These findings have provided the basis for a model in which RF-producing B lymphocytes serve as antigen-presenting cells for IgG–antigen complexes but normally do not secrete the cell-surface immunoglobulin.

The mechanisms initiating the secretion of RF are unknown. There is little evidence that immunoglobulin genes are a risk factor for the development of RF. B-cell–derived tumors often secrete RF with very restricted Vκ gene segment usage. In contrast, RFs in RA patients include a heterogeneous set of germline gene elements (20). Many RFs are of the IgM isotype and many immunoglobulin genes sequenced so far are in germline configuration. These data suggest that polyclonal B-cell activation is involved in triggering RF production in early disease. It remains to be determined whether this polyclonal B-cell activation is facilitated by a genetic factor, as exemplified by mutation of the apoptosis gene fas in the lpr mouse, which produces high titers of RF, or whether exogenous factors play a role. Poly-

(Table 9A-3)
Rheumatoid factor (RF)

- RFs are the major autoantibodies in rheumatoid arthritis (RA). They recognize a diverse array of epitopes on the IgG Fc fragment and are associated with more severe and extra-articular disease.

- RF-producing B cells in RA are polyclonal, using a diverse set of immunoglobulin gene segments.

- RF production is a T-cell–dependent phenomenon that is influenced by HLA-DRB1 polymorphism. All immunoglobulin isotypes are represented. Some RFs show evidence of somatic mutation with higher affinity for the IgG Fc fragment.

- RF production and effector functions in RA are likely closely linked to the physiologic function of RF in a normal immune system. B cells expressing RF on the cell surface are important antigen-presenting cells in secondary immune responses. Secreted RF has a role in the stabilization and clearance of immune complexes.

clonal stimulators including lectins and superantigens induce RF production (21). RFs undergo T-cell driven isotype switch and affinity maturation in vivo (20). This differentiation may be under the control of polymorphic HLA-DRB1*04 alleles in which a lysine substitution at position 71 predisposes for RF production (10). Proliferation of RF-positive B cells may occur preferentially in synovial tissue, which is a site of RF production.

The effector functions of RF in the disease process are unclear. It remains an interesting concept that pathologically relevant effector functions correlate with antibody affinity and that the primary defect in RF production in RA patients lies in the deficient T-cell control of affinity maturation. However, most antibodies identified in the clinical setting are of the IgM isotype and may be unmutated. Deposition of immune complexes containing RF occurs in several tissues, and it is likely that activation of the complement cascade by immune complexes contributes to the inflammatory changes in rheumatoid synovium and in rheumatoid vasculitis. However, the evidence for immune complex–mediated tissue injury remains indirect, and the clinical and pathologic features of RA do not suggest an immune complex–mediated disease. Soluble RF may also interfere with the normal regulation of the immune response. Soluble IgM-RF may impair antigen presentation by B cells, whereas soluble IgG-RF facilitates the uptake of antigen by RF-positive B cells by increasing the size of immune complexes.

Effector Mechanisms Leading to Rheumatoid Tissue Destruction

Joint destruction in RA involves articular cartilage, ligaments, tendons, and bone. Several mechanisms contribute to this destructive process. Inflammatory mediators and enzymes are found in synovial fluid, as well as in proliferating synovial membrane. Cartilage and bone are not only the targets of the tissue destructive process, but chondrocytes and osteoclasts actively participate in the loss of extracellular matrix.

Neutrophils are clearly compartmentalized in RA (22). Although very few neutrophils are present in the proliferating synovial tissue, they constitute the major cellular component of synovial fluid. The reasons for this compartmentalization are not entirely clear. Neutrophils adhere to the endothelium of postcapillary venules. This adhesion is activation-dependent. Mediators with neutrophil-activating ability are abundant in synovial fluid. Many of these chemoattractants are cytokines produced by the synovial tissue. The most important mediators for neutrophil adherence and transmigration are transforming growth factor β (TGF-β) and IL-8. Neutrophils can also produce both cytokines and may therefore be responsible for an autocrine loop. Classic chemoattractants such as the complement factor C5a, which is activated as a consequence of immune complex formation, and the leukotriene B4 are present in RA joints. Cytokines and phagocytosis of soluble immune complexes by neutrophils result in prostaglandins and leukotriene production, neutrophil degranulation, and respiratory burst. Immune complex deposition in the upper layers of cartilage may target neutrophils directly to the cartilage and may facilitate a critical concentration of active proteinases and reactive oxygen intermediates.

Tissue destruction in RA is closely related to the production of metalloproteinases and other proteinases, which are able to degrade collagen and proteoglycans (23). The major metalloproteinase-producing cells are synovial fibroblasts and monocytic phagocytes in the synovial lining layer. Production of proteinases is controlled by a number of different cytokines, including IL-1, TNF-α, and TGF-β. Most of these cytokines are secreted by macrophages residing in tissue. Chondrocytes respond to the same cytokines with a decrease in collagen and proteoglycan synthesis while they simultaneously begin synthesizing collagenase and stromolysin and degrading type II collagen and proteoglycans (24). Extracellular matrix in bone is protected from enzyme assault as long as it is mineralized. Activation of osteoclast cells and PGE_2 have been proposed as the major mechanisms facilitating bone resorption.

One of the pathologic hallmarks of RA is the tumor-like expansion of synoviocytes in the synovial lesion. How much of this expansion is due to true proliferation and how much to tissue invasion by monocytic cells is not entirely clear. Both processes most likely contribute to the expansion. Monocyte- and fibroblast-derived cytokines (platelet-derived growth factor, fibroblast growth factor, IL-1, and TNF) are major players in this tissue expansion. In response to these cytokines, the fibroblast-like cells are highly activated. In contrast to the transformation of synoviocytes in HTLV-1-associated arthropathy by the tax gene, there is no clear evidence for a transformation in rheumatoid synovial cells. The expansion of rheumatoid synovium is supported by neovascularization that is controlled by fibroblast- and synovial macrophage-derived cytokines. The resulting picture of the synovial lesion is one of proliferating and expanding mesenchymal and macrophage-derived cells that produce cytokines. Autocrine mechanisms are partially responsible for continuous activation of these cells, production of cytokines, tissue-degrading enzymes, and proliferative activity. This proliferating synovial lesion is not only mainly responsible for tissue destruction but also for attempts at tissue repair. It has been proposed that TNF is a key cytokine controlling this autocrine loop (25). In addition to the autocrine mechanism, activation and proliferation of synoviocytes are likely to be under the control of exogenous mechanisms. The peripheral nervous system produces mediators that modulate the inflammatory response (26). Progression of disease is controlled by T cells and the disease-associated HLA-DRB1 alleles. It is therefore likely that tissue-infiltrating T cells are a major regulator of the activation of cells in the synovial lining layer. The precise nature of this interaction awaits clarification.

JORG J. GORONZY, MD, PhD
CORNELIA M. WEYAND, MD, PhD

1. Arnett FC, Edworthy SM, Bloch DA, et al: The American Rheumatism Association 1987 revised criteria for the classification of rheumatoid arthritis. Arthritis Rheum 31:315-324, 1988

2. Rothschild BM, Turner KR, DeLuca MA: Symmetrical erosive peripheral polyarthritis in the late archaic period of Alabama. Science 241:1498-1502, 1988

3. Winchester R: The molecular basis of susceptibility to rheumatoid arthritis. Adv Immunol 56:389-466, 1994

4. Kurosaka M, Ziff M: Immunoelectron microscopic study of the distribution of T cell subsets in rheumatoid synovium. J Exp Med 158:1191-1210, 1983

5. Nakajima T, Aono H, Hasunuma T, et al: Overgrowth of human synovial cells driven by the human T cell leukemia virus type I tax gene. J Clin Invest 92:186-193, 1993

6. Stastny P: Association of the B-cell alloantigen DRw4 with rheumatoid arthritis. N Engl J Med 298:869-871, 1978

7. Gregersen PK, Silver J, Winchester RJ: The shared epitope hypothesis: an approach to understanding the molecular genetics of susceptibility to rheumatoid arthritis. Arthritis Rheum 30:1205-1213, 1987

8. Nepom GT, Nepom BS: Prediction of susceptibility to rheumatoid arthritis by human leukocyte antigen genotyping. Rheum Dis Clin North Am 18:785-792, 1992

9. Goronzy JJ, Weyand CM: T cells in rheumatoid arthritis: paradigms and facts. Rheum Dis Clin North Am 21:655-674, 1995

10. Weyand CM, McCarthy TG, Goronzy JJ: Correlation between disease phenotype and genetic heterogeneity in rheumatoid arthritis. J Clin Invest 95:2120-2126, 1995

11. Weyand CM, Hicok KC, Conn D, Goronzy JJ: The influence of HLA-DRB1 genes on disease severity in rheumatoid arthritis. Ann Intern Med 117:801-806, 1992

12. Harris ED Jr: Rheumatoid arthritis: pathophysiology and implications for therapy. N Engl J Med 322:1277-1289, 1990

13. Liao H-X, Haynes BF: Role of adhesion molecules in the pathogenesis of rheumatoid arthritis. Rheum Dis Clin N Am 21:715, 1995

14. Firestein GS: The immunopathogenesis of rheumatoid arthritis. Curr Opin Rheumatol 3:398-406, 1991

15. Walser-Kuntz DR, Weyand CM, Weaver AJ, O'Fallon WM, Goronzy JJ: Mechanisms underlying the formation of the T cell receptor repertoire in rheumatoid arthritis. Immunity 2:597-605, 1995

16. Albani S, Keystone E, Nelson JL, et al: Positive selection in autoimmunity: abnormal immune responses to a bacterial dnaj antigenic determinant in patients with early rheumatoid arthritis. Nature Med 1:448-452, 1995

17. DerSimonian H, Sugita M, Glass DN, Maier AL, Weinblatt ME, Reme T, Brenner MB: Clonal V α 12.1+ T cell expansions in the peripheral blood of rheumatoid arthritis patients. J Exp Med 177:1623-1631, 1993

18. Goronzy JJ, Bartz-Bazzanella P, Hu W, Jendro MC, Walser-Kuntz DR, Weyand CM: Dominant clonotypes in the repertoire of peripheral CD4+ T cells in rheumatoid arthritis. J Clin Invest 94:2068-2076, 1994

19. Carson DA, Chen PP, Kipps TJ: New roles for rheumatoid factor. J Clin Invest 87:379-383, 1991

20. Randen I, Thompson KM, Pascual V, et al: Rheumatoid factor V genes from patients with rheumatoid arthritis are diverse and show evidence of an antigen-driven response. Immunol Rev 128:49-71, 1992

21. He X, Goronzy JJ, Zhong W, Xie C, Weyand CM: VH3-21 B cells escape from a state of tolerance in rheumatoid arthritis and secrete rheumatoid factor. Molecular Med 1:768-780, 1995

22. Pillinger MH, Abramson SB: The neutrophil in rheumatoid arthritis. Rheum Dis Clin North Am 21:691-714, 1995

23. Krane SM: Mechanisms of tissue destruction in rheumatoid arthritis. In McCarty DJ, Koopman WJ (eds): Arthritis and Allied Conditions, 12th ed. Malvern, Lea & Febiger, 1993, pp 763-779

24. Lotz M, Blanco FJ, von Kempis J, Dudler J, Maier R, Villiger PM, Geng Y: Cytokine regulation of chondrocyte functions. J Rheumatol 43:104-108, 1995

25. Elliott MJ, Maini RN, Feldmann M, et al: Randomised double-blind comparison of chimeric monoclonal antibody to tumor necrosis factor alpha (cA2) versus placebo in rheumatoid arthritis. Lancet 344:1105-1110, 1994

26. Lotz M, Vaughan JH, Carson DA: Effect of neuropeptides on production of inflammatory cytokines by human monocytes. Science 241:1218-1221, 1988

B. CLINICAL AND LABORATORY FEATURES

Clinical features of rheumatoid arthritis (RA) vary not only from one patient to another but also in an individual patient over the disease course. The most common mode of onset is the insidious development of symptoms over a period of several weeks (1,2). Explosive acute polyarticular onset evolving over several days also occurs, but acute monarticular arthritis as the initial manifestation is decidedly rare. The initial presentation often lacks the characteristic symmetry seen as the disease progresses to a more chronic state.

DIAGNOSIS

Diagnosis during the early weeks of the disease is essentially one of exclusion, although characteristic features such as symmetric sterile synovitis with typical serologic features strongly suggest RA. Radiographic evidence of erosions becomes apparent only after the disease has been present for several months or more than a year.

The American College of Rheumatology has established criteria for the diagnosis of RA, the classification of severity by roentgenography, functional class, and the definition of remission (see Appendix I). Although not designed for managing individual patients, the criteria are useful both as a frame of reference and in describing clinical phenomena.

By definition, the diagnosis of RA cannot be made until the disease has been present for at least several weeks. Moreover, many extra-articular features of RA, the characteristic symmetry of inflammation, and the typical serologic findings may not be evident in the first month or two of the disease. Therefore the diagnosis of RA is usually presumptive early in its course.

Although extra-articular manifestations may dominate in some patients, documentation of an inflammatory synovitis is essential for a diagnosis. Inflammatory synovitis can be documented by demonstrating synovial fluid leukocytosis, defined as white blood cell (WBC) count greater than 2000/mm³, histologic evidence of synovitis, or radiographic evidence of characteristic erosions.

Other causes of synovitis must be excluded. Although this can often be done upon initial evaluation, conditions such as systemic lupus erythematosus (SLE), psoriatic arthritis, and the seronegative spondyloarthropathies may initially be indistinguishable from RA. Usually it is the development of extra-articular features of these disorders, rather than characteristics of the synovitis, that allows a differential diagnosis.

Synovial biopsies are seldom performed or required for diagnosis, and radiographic changes are not apparent in early disease when the diagnosis is in doubt. If a palpable effusion is detected, the joint should be aspirated to document synovial fluid leukocytosis and to exclude the presence of crystals.

Effusions and synovial thickening are difficult to detect in joint spaces deep below the surface, such as the hip, often the shoulder, and occasionally the metatarsophalangeal (MTP) joints. For this reason, the examiner must depend on demonstrating limited motion of the joint. The presence of a joint deformity is not specific evidence of inflammatory synovitis because deformities can also occur in other inflammatory conditions such as SLE, and even in noninflammatory disorders such as osteoarthritis. However, in a nonweight-bearing joint such as the elbow or wrist, the examiner can usually assume that, unless a patient has a history of unique joint trauma, a deformity results from synovitis.

LABORATORY FEATURES

No laboratory test, histologic finding, or radiographic feature confirms a diagnosis of RA. Rather, the diagnosis is established by a constellation of findings observed over a period of time.

Rheumatoid factor (RF) is found in the serum of about 85% of patients with RA. Studies indicate that RF titers tend to correlate with severe and unremitting disease, nodules, and extra-articular lesions. In the individual patient, however, the RF titer is of little prognostic value; moreover, serial titers are of no value in following the disease process. Therefore, when a patient is known to be RF-positive, repeating the test at a later date serves no purpose. However, a small percentage of patients who are initially RF-negative become positive as the disease progresses, and their clinical features and prognosis parallel those of patients who were RF-positive in early disease. Rheumatoid factors can also be found in other diseases, including several inflammatory disorders also associated with synovitis (Table 9B-1).

The erythrocyte sedimentation rate (ESR) is a measurement of the rate at which red blood cells settle and is related to several factors in the serum (see Chapter 7B). Typically, the ESR correlates with the degree of synovial inflammation, but it varies greatly from patient to patient; and a rare patient with active inflammatory RA may even have a normal ESR. However, it is generally a useful objective measure to follow the course of inflammatory activity in an individual patient. C-reactive protein, an acute-phase reactant, may also be used to monitor the level of inflammation.

Other laboratory abnormalities observed in RA include hypergammaglobulinemia, hypocomplementemia, thrombocytosis, and eosinophilia. These states occur more often in patients with severe disease, high RF titer, rheumatoid nodules, and extra-articular manifestations.

ARTICULAR MANIFESTATIONS

The articular manifestations of RA can be placed in two categories: reversible signs and symptoms related to inflammatory synovitis and irreversible structural damage caused by synovitis. This concept is useful not only for staging disease and determining prognosis but also for selecting medical or surgical treatment. Structural damage in the typical patient usually begins sometime between the first and second year of the disease (3). Although synovitis tends to follow a fluctuating pattern, structural damage progresses as a linear function of the amount of prior synovitis (Fig. 9B-1).

Morning Stiffness

Morning stiffness is an almost universal feature of synovial inflammation, both in RA and other systemic rheumatic disorders. In contrast to the brief (5–10 minutes) period of gelling seen in osteoarthritis, morning stiffness is prolonged, usually lasting more than 2 hours. This phenomenon depends on extended immobilization during sleep and is not related to hours of the day or periods of sunlight. The duration tends to correlate with the degree of synovial inflammation and disappears when a remission occurs. For this reason, documenting the presence and length of morning stiffness is part of the patient's database and is useful in following the disease course. Patients should be asked, "After you have gotten up, how long does it take until you're feeling as good as you'll ever feel?"

Synovial Inflammation

Clinical signs of synovitis may be subtle and are often subjective. Warm, swollen, obviously inflamed joints are usually seen only in the most active phases of inflammatory synovitis. Moreover, these observations are usually restricted to superficial joints with an easily distensible capsule, such as the knee and, occasionally, the wrist and proximal interphalangeal (PIP) joints. Deeply buried joints such as the hip rarely present with a tense effusion that is apparent on physical examination. Ankle effusion is also difficult to detect because the joint capsule is restricted by numerous tendons and retinacula. Even when swelling is present, it is often difficult to distinguish ankle effusion from edema or cellulitis.

The pathologic and clinical picture of chronic rheumatoid synovitis differs considerably from synovitis in early disease. As the inflammation continues, vascularity of the synovium decreases as granulation tissue and fibrosis develop. The resultant joint immobility brought on by the disease process further reduces synovial vascularity, and the degree of obvious inflammation apparent on examination is significantly reduced. This phenomenon has been called "burned-out" RA, a faulty concept describing patients with long-

(Table 9B-1)
Selected diseases associated with elevated serum rheumatoid factors

Chronic bacterial infections
  Subacute bacterial endocarditis
  Leprosy
  Tuberculosis
  Syphilis
  Lyme disease
Viral diseases
  Rubella
  Cytomegalovirus
  Infectious mononucleosis
  Influenza
Parasitic diseases
Chronic inflammatory disease of uncertain etiology
  Sarcoidosis
  Periodontal disease
  Pulmonary interstitial disease
  Liver disease
Mixed cryoglobulinemia
Hypergammaglobulinemic purpura

Modified from Koopman WJ, Schrohenber RE: Rheumatoid factor. In Utsinger PD, Zvaifler NJ, Ehrlich GE (eds): Rheumatoid Arthritis: Etiology, Diagnosis and Therapy. Philadelphia, JB Lippincott, 1985, pp 217-241.

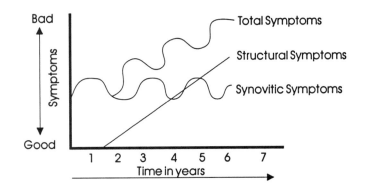

(Figure 9B-1)
Symptomatic course of rheumatoid arthritis.

standing RA whose joints are not warm or noticeably swollen. Further observation of these patients reveals that they continue to experience prolonged morning stiffness, generalized malaise, and chronic fatigue; have anemia and elevated ESR; and, most important, demonstrate progressive joint destruction on serial radiographs. Therefore, clinical assessments based on joint swelling and tenderness in the later stages of RA may be overly optimistic (4). In fact, RA rarely spontaneously remits after the first year (5).

Structural Damage

Cartilage loss and erosion of periarticular bone are the characteristic features of structural damage. The clinical features related to structural damage are marked by progressive deterioration functionally and anatomically. Structural damage to the joint is irreversible and additive. Objective evidence of cartilage destruction can be obtained either by radiographs showing total loss of joint space or by demonstrating "bone-on-bone crepitus," which produces a high-pitched screech detectable on palpation or auscultation. Nothing else makes this sound.

Symptoms that fail to respond to aggressive anti-inflammatory therapy also indicate that irreversible structural damage exists. When such damage is suspected, corticosteroids may be injected into the joint. The failure to benefit from this treatment provides good evidence that other anti-inflammatory therapies are unlikely to be beneficial in the future.

MANIFESTATIONS IN SPECIFIC JOINTS

Principles of the role of synovitis in creating joint destruction are applicable to all joints. However, certain unique aspects are pertinent to specific joints.

Cervical Spine

Although RA of the thoracic and lumbar spine is exceptionally rare, cervical spine involvement is common. The inflammatory process involves diarthrodial joints and is neither palpable nor visible to the examiner. Clinical manifestations of early disease consist primarily of neck stiffness that is perceived through the entire arc of motion; generalized loss of motion may also develop. Tenosynovitis of the transverse ligament of C1, which stabilizes the odontoid process of C2, may produce significant C1–C2 instability. Cervical myelopathy may develop as a result of erosion of the odontoid process, ligament laxity, or ligament rupture. Disease of the apophyseal joints may also contribute to cervical instability. Clinical evaluation of patients with RA should always include a careful neurologic examination. Neck pain without neurologic features tends to be self-limited and usually improves, even when radiographic evidence of joint destruction is present. This may be related to the fact that the neck is a nonweight-bearing structure. Conversely, pain does not always accompany cervical instability, even when myelopathy is significant. Frequently, the course of neck pain and neurologic symptoms are not synchronous.

Shoulders

Because the shoulder capsule lies beneath the muscular rotator cuff, an effusion is difficult to detect on physical examination. Typically, the only objective finding is loss of motion. The patient responds to shoulder pain by unconsciously restricting shoulder motion. Because basic activities of daily living do not require extremes of shoulder movement, frozen shoulder syndrome can develop rapidly. An aggressive program of range of motion exercises may prevent this. Symptoms related to frozen shoulder are usually much more severe at night when movements during sleep stretch the tightened joint capsule. If irreversible joint damage occurs the shoulder symptoms do not necessarily parallel cartilage destruction, possibly because the shoulder is a relatively unconstrained and nonweight-bearing joint that is not as dependent as other joints on the cartilage surface for useful function (6).

Elbow

The elbow is one of the easiest of all joints in which to detect inflammation. Because this joint is superficial, synovitis is evident by palpating fullness and thickening in the radial-humeral joint. Flexion deformities of the elbow may develop in early RA. The ulnar nerve passes posteromedially to the elbow, and compressive neuropathies may develop at this site related to the synovitis. Symptoms include paresthesia over the fourth and fifth fingers and weakness in the flexor muscle of the little finger. When structural symptoms begin to develop, the physician should distinguish symptoms of radiohumeral disease (which is accentuated by pronation–supination) from those related to ulnohumeral disease (which is brought on by flexion–extension).

Hand

The wrists are affected in virtually all patients with RA. The metacarpophalangeal (MCP) and PIP joints are often involved, whereas the distal interphalangeal (DIP) joints are usually (although not always) spared. Ulnar deviation at the MCP joints is often associated with radial deviation at the wrists. Swan-neck deformities (Fig. 9B-2) can develop, as can the boutonnière deformity in which flexion at the PIP and hyperextension at the DIP joints occurs.

In addition to symptoms related to synovitis, pain or dysfunction may be caused by compression of a peripheral nerve entrapped in a confined area by synovitis. The most common site is the carpal tunnel of the wrist. Patients with early wrist disease may develop carpal tunnel syndrome

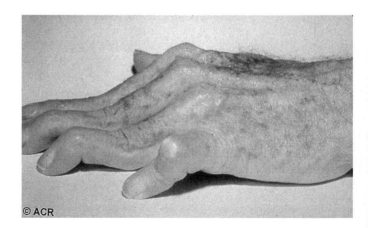

(Figure 9B-2)
Rheumatoid arthritis: hand, swan-neck and boutonnière deformity. Swan-neck deformities are seen in the second, third, and fourth digits of a patient with chronic rheumatoid arthritis. A boutonnière deformity of the fifth digit is present. Reprinted from the Revised Clinical Slide Collection on the Rheumatic Diseases, with permission of the American College of Rheumatology.

from compression of the median nerve. As the disease progresses, the retinaculum distends and symptoms may improve. A similar neuropathy involves the ulnar nerve, which passes through Guyon's canal within the wrist. Guyon's canal syndrome may be distinguished from entrapment neuropathy at the elbow by the absence of weakness of the fifth finger when flexed against resistance.

Tenosynovitis and the formation of rheumatoid nodules within tendon sheaths can interfere with finger flexion. Nodular thickening, which may be palpated along the flexor tendons of the palm, may cause symptoms that patients describe as "locking and catching" as the nodule slides along its sheath. Tendon rupture may occur if inflammatory tenosynovitis erodes through the tendon, an event that is most common in the extensor muscle of the DIP joint of the thumb. Another cause of tendon rupture at the wrist is the so-called attrition rupture of extensor tendons in the third, fourth, and fifth fingers. This rupture occurs because these tendons, which cross the dorsal surface of the ulnar styloid process, are subjected to abrasion if the ulnar styloid erodes to jagged bone. Tendon ruptures present with a history of an abrupt, usually painless, loss of a highly specific function (eg, inability to flex or extend) on active motion, although passive range of motion is unaffected.

Hip

Although hip involvement is common in RA, early manifestations of hip disease are typically not apparent, even to a skilled examiner. Because the joint is located deep within the pelvis, evidence of palpable distention or synovial thickening is absent. Furthermore, early hip disease is often asymptomatic, although a subtle reduction in range of motion may be observed. Typically, the initial dysfunction is first noticed when the patient has difficulty putting on shoes or socks on the affected side. When pain develops, it usually appears in the groin or thigh but may also be felt in the buttock, low back, or medial aspect of the knee. If cartilage destruction does occur, the symptoms may accelerate more rapidly than in other joints.

Knee

Effusions and synovial thickening of the knee are usually easily detected on examination. Posterior herniation of the capsule creating a popliteal (Baker's) cyst may be associated with dissection or rupture into the calf, producing symptoms suggestive of thrombophlebitis. However, the characteristic history, absence of engorged collateral veins, and a distinct border of edema below the knee distinguish this syndrome from thrombophlebitis. Ultrasonography can readily define a Baker's cyst but may show little after rupture or dissection has occurred. Arthrography, with a film of the calf musculature taken after a brief period of exercise, may be required to demonstrate a herniation of the calf musculature (Fig. 9B-3).

Foot and Ankle

Because lower extremity joints are weight-bearing structures, involvement of the foot and ankle causes greater dysfunction and pain than occur in upper extremity joints. In descending order of frequency, RA characteristically affects the MTP, talonavicular, and ankle joints. MTP arthritis causes "cock-up" deformities of the toes and subluxations of the MTP heads on the sole. As a result, the normally smooth, flowing transmission of forces across the metatarsal heads is

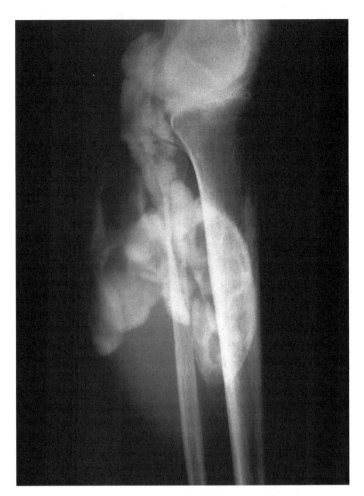

(Figure 9B-3)
Rheumatoid arthritis: popliteal cyst (arthrogram). This is the lateral projection of the arthrogram of the left knee of a patient with a popliteal cyst. Good filling is noted of the suprapatellar bursa and knee joint proper. The contrast medium extends posteriorly into the distended gastrocnemio-semimembranosus bursa with extension and/or rupture distally into the calf.

interrupted, causing gait problems. Inflammation of the talonavicular joint causes pronation and eversion of the foot. Flexion and extension of the ankle is usually preserved in early RA. The tarsal tunnel, which is posteroinferior to the medial malleolus and contains the posterior tibial nerve, is often compressed by synovitis. Entrapment of this nerve causes burning paresthesias on the sole of the foot, which are made worse by standing or walking (7).

JOINT DEFORMITIES

Joint deformities in RA occur from several different mechanisms, all related to synovitis and the patient's attempt to avoid pain by keeping the joint in the least painful position. These mechanisms are joint immobilization, destruction of cartilage and bone, and alterations in muscles, tendons, and ligaments.

Any joint — normal or abnormal — that is subjected to prolonged immobilization loses motion because of tendon shortening and contraction of the articular capsule. By maintaining motion, the development of deformities may be avoided. The value of continued movement is illustrated by such joints as the knee and ankle, which seldom lose motion in early RA because walking, the act of sitting, and climbing stairs put these joints through their full range of motion. In contrast, joints whose full range of motion is less critical to basic function, such as the shoulder, wrist, and elbow, often develop deformities in early disease because patients are able to function with reduced range of motion. By holding these joints in a position that maximizes the volume within the joint cavity, patients reduce pain by decreasing intra-articular pressure.

Muscles and tendons around an inflamed joint may spasm and shorten in response to inflammation. This phenomenon is easiest to observe in abnormalities of intrinsic muscles of the hand and anterior peroneal muscle tendons over the arch of the foot. Spasms and shortening in these areas contribute to deformities of MCP flexion and tarsal pronation.

Ligaments that stabilize the joint may be weakened or severed by the erosive properties of inflamed synovium or pannus, which release enzymes that lyse collagen. Damaged ligaments destabilize the joint, altering the lines of force and the axis of rotation. MCP subluxations and ulnar deviation are related to this mechanism.

The tenosynovium lining the tendon sheath is commonly inflamed in RA leading to joint deformities related to thickening of the tendon sheath, the formation of obstructing tendon nodules, or tendon ruptures. Characteristically, tendon ruptures are abrupt and painless. On physical examination, tendon dysfunction is detected by a discrepancy between active and passive motion.

Synovitis and pannus denude the surface of cartilage and erode juxta-articular bone, creating incongruous articular surfaces. Once cartilage is completely gone the opposing bone surfaces may fuse when immobilized, much as a bone fracture fuses during splinting.

EXTRA-ARTICULAR MANIFESTATIONS

Rheumatoid arthritis is a systemic disease, and most patients experience generalized malaise or fatigue. Significant inflammation of other organ systems also occurs predominantly in patients who are RF positive. Other risk factors that generally correlate with the development of extra-articular manifestations include rheumatoid nodules, severe articular disease, and probably, the MHC class II HLA-DRB1*0401 allele (8).

Skin Manifestations

Rheumatoid nodules develop at some time in up to 50% of RA patients. Virtually all patients with nodules are RF-positive. The nodules tend to develop in crops during active phases of the disease and form subcutaneously, in bursae, and along tendon sheaths. Although they have been described in almost every region and may occur in the viscera, nodules are typically located over pressure points, such as the extensor surface of the forearm (Fig. 9B-4), Achilles tendon, ischial area, over the MTP joint, and the flexor surface of the fingers. These lesions may develop gradually or abruptly and are generally associated with some signs of inflammation. Nodules and gouty tophi both have a predilection for the olecranon, but tophi tend to develop insidiously and grow slowly, often without apparent inflammation. Biopsy of the nodule may be necessary if the diagnosis is uncertain. Over time, rheumatoid nodules often either disappear or involute. Methotrexate may enhance or accelerate the development of rheumatoid nodules (9).

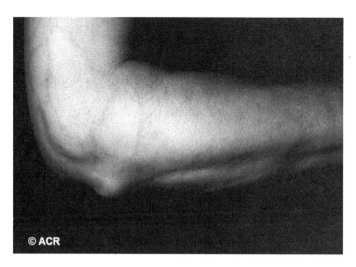

(Figure 9B-4)
A large subcutaneous nodule is located on the extensor surface of the forearm near the elbow. Reprinted from the Revised Clinical Slide Collection on the Rheumatic Diseases, with permission of the American College of Rheumatology.

Vasculitic lesions are often seen in RA, particularly various forms of dermal vasculitis. The most common are leukocytoclastic vasculitis and palpable purpura. Although dermal vasculitis does not generally indicate a coexistent systemic vasculitis, patients should be examined for evidence of involvement of other organ systems, especially renal and neurologic dysfunction. Ischemic ulcers, however, often occur with systemic involvement.

Drugs used to treat RA can also create skin abnormalities. Ecchymoses may occur as a consequence of either platelet dysfunction related to nonsteroidal anti-inflammatory drugs (NSAIDs) or capillary fragility from corticosteroids. Petechiae may be a sign of thrombocytopenia from disease-modifying drugs such as gold, penicillamine, or sulfasalazine. Chrysiasis, a cyanotic hue most apparent on the forehead, is a manifestation of long-term gold therapy.

Ocular Manifestations

Keratoconjunctivitis sicca as a manifestation of associated Sjögren's syndrome is common in RA, but because patients are not always aware of the symptoms the clinician should ask questions about eye dryness and should institute prophylactic measures. Episodes of episcleritis are common and usually run a benign self-limited course. Scleritis has a more morbid prognosis, however. This inflammation, which histologically resembles that of rheumatoid nodules, may erode through the sclera into the choroid causing scleromalacia perforans.

Respiratory Manifestations

Inflammation of the cricoarytenoid joint is a common finding in RA. The symptoms are usually episodic and consist of laryngeal pain, dysphonia, and occasionally pain on swallowing, all of which may be accentuated in the morning (10). Laryngeal obstruction is rare but may occur after extubation for endotracheal anesthesia.

Autopsy studies have found histologic evidence of interstitial lung disease in most people who had RA. The prevalence of clinical symptoms is significantly lower. Because RA imposes limitations that make physical exertion difficult

(11), respiratory involvement may be asymptomatic. However, the mortality from pulmonary disease in RA is twice that of the general population (12). Radiographic features of respiratory involvement include interstitial fibrosis, which has a predilection for basal involvement, and solitary or multiple nodules in the lung parenchyma. Cavitation of these nodules can be identified on computed tomography. On rare occasions, a subpleural nodule may rupture, creating a bronchopleural fistula, which may progress to a pneumothorax or empyema.

Pulmonary involvement identical to that seen in RA alone has also been described in association with penicillamine and with gold therapy, but the significance of this observation is uncertain. A similar process has been reported with methotrexate therapy; respiratory symptoms tend to improve when the drug is stopped. Bronchiolitis obliterans may also be associated with RA or a complication of drug therapy.

Inflammation of the pleura occasionally causes typical symptoms of pleurisy, which is usually a self-limited, episodic event. Inflammatory pleural disease may also be asymptomatic, and the small pleural effusions are discovered incidentally on chest radiographs. Laboratory evaluation of the pleural fluid demonstrates markedly low glucose level compared with serum levels and a WBC count usually less than 5000/mm^3.

Cardiac Manifestations

Echocardiographic evidence of a pericardial effusion or other pericardial abnormality is seen in almost 50% of RA patients who have no clinical symptoms of heart involvement (13). Symptomatic pericarditis, manifested either by pain or altered cardiovascular physiology, is rare. Although pericarditis may occur at any time, these episodes usually develop during a generalized disease flare. An occasional patient may progress to chronic constrictive pericarditis, manifested by peripheral edema and signs of right-sided heart failure. Inflammatory lesions similar to rheumatoid nodules may develop on the myocardium and valve leaflets. Clinical manifestations include valvular dysfunction, embolic phenomena, conduction defects, and perhaps myocardiopathy. Aortitis involving segments or the entire aorta has been described and is associated both with aortic insufficiency related to dilation of the aortic root and with aneurysmal rupture (14).

Gastrointestinal Manifestations

No gastrointestinal abnormalities are related specifically to RA, with the exception of xerostomia seen in patients with associated Sjögren's syndrome and ischemic bowel complications of rheumatoid vasculitis. However, gastritis and peptic ulcer disease are major complications of NSAID therapy and a significant cause of morbidity and mortality in RA.

Renal Manifestations

In contrast to SLE, glomerular disease is exceedingly rare in RA. Proteinuria, if it develops, is usually either related to drug toxicity (gold or penicillamine) or secondary to amyloidosis. Interstitial renal disease may occur in Sjögren's syndrome, but in RA patients, it is more often related to the use of NSAIDs, acetaminophen, or other analgesics. Papillary necrosis may occur as a result of chronic exposure to these agents.

Neurologic Complications

Nervous system involvement is common in RA but is usually subtle in presentation, which can make it difficult to distinguish between articular and neuropathic lesions (15). The pathogenesis of neurologic disorders is fundamentally related to one of three mechanisms: cervical spine instability, peripheral nerve entrapment, and vasculitis resulting in mononeuritis multiplex.

Cervical spine instability most commonly occurring at C1–C2, is related to destruction of the transverse ligament of C1 or the odontoid process itself. A "step-off" subluxation related to apophyseal joint destruction may also occur, most commonly at C4–C5 or C5–C6. Lateral radiographs taken in flexion and extension are required to demonstrate the instability. Magnetic resonance imaging or computed tomography is then performed to further evaluate the precise anatomy and to document spinal cord compression.

Symptoms of cervical myelopathy typically are gradual in onset and often unrelated to either the development of or accentuation in neck pain. When neck pain does occur, it frequently radiates over the occiput in the distribution of the C1–C3 nerve roots. *L'hermitte's sign*, the sudden development of tingling paresthesias that descend the thoracolumbar spine as the cervical spine is flexed, may occur. In patients with long-standing destructive RA, the most common symptom of cervical myelopathy is the development over weeks to months of bilateral sensory paresthesias of the hands and motor weakness. Physical examination may demonstrate pathologic reflexes, such as Babinski's sign, Hoffmann's sign, and hyperactive deep-tendon reflexes.

When a peripheral nerve passes through a compartment that is also occupied by synovium or tendon sheaths, the potential exists for nerve compression by synovitis or tenosynovitis. Symptoms are related to fluctuations in synovial inflammation and the joint posture. In addition to compression of the median nerve in the carpal tunnel or the ulnar nerve in Guyon's canal, neuropathies may involve the posterior interosseous nerve in the antecubital fossa, the femoral nerve anterior to the hip joint, the peroneal nerve adjacent to the fibular head, and the interdigital nerve at the MTP joint. Compression syndromes of these nerves may be confirmed by neurophysiologic studies.

The syndrome of *mononeuritis multiplex* is marked by abrupt onset of a persistent peripheral neuropathy that is unaltered by either change in the joint position or reduction in synovial inflammation, thus distinguishing it from a compression neuropathy. Concurrent evidence of rheumatoid vasculitis is often seen. Neurophysiologic studies reveal an axonal lesion and frequently demonstrate several clinically inapparent mononeuropathies. A sural nerve biopsy may confirm the diagnosis.

Hematologic Manifestations

A hypochromic-microcytic anemia with low serum ferritin and low or normal iron-binding capacity is an almost universal finding in patients with active RA. Because most patients are taking ulcerogenic NSAIDs and therefore often test positive for occult blood on stool tests, distinguishing this anemia from an iron-deficiency anemia is difficult. To compound the problem, patients with iron deficiency may fail to respond vigorously to iron therapy with a brisk reticulocytosis. Serum ferritin levels also fail to distinguish the two. Only an examination of the bone marrow for iron stores provides a definitive answer. More aggressive evaluation should generally be restricted to patients whose pattern of gastrointestinal symptoms, degree of anemia, or documented loss of blood via the gastrointestinal tract seems to require gastrointestinal or hematologic studies.

Felty's syndrome was originally described as the combination of RA, splenomegaly, leukopenia, and leg ulcers. Subsequent observations have shown an association with lymphadenopathy, thrombocytopenia, and the HLA-DR4 haplotype (16). Felty's syndrome is most common in patients with severe, nodule-forming RA. The precise pathogenesis of the leukopenia, which selectively involves neutrophils, is poorly understood. The large granular lymphocyte (LGL) syndrome shares many of the same features of Felty's syndrome (17), but it is not exclusive to RA. LGL syndrome may represent a process that permits RA to develop, rather than being a result of the disease itself. An increased incidence of non-Hodgkin's lymphoma has been reported in patients with Felty's syndrome (18).

Thrombocytopenia may also occur in RA as a result of marrow suppression due to immunosuppressive or cytotoxic therapy, or it may be related to an autoimmune process in gold, penicillamine, or sulfasalazine therapy.

COURSE AND PROGNOSIS

Studies of prognosis in RA patients are difficult because of the chronic nature of the disease, its inherent variability, and the difficulty of identifying milder or subclinical forms. Many patients never seek medical care. In addition, the diagnosis of RA is often not included on the death certificate.

Criteria for remission have been established (see Appendix I), but the prevalence of remission is unknown. A population study on the prevalence of RA was unable to substantiate the diagnosis in well over one-half of patients who had originally been diagnosed with the disease several years earlier (19). Although some of these patients may have experienced spontaneous remission, interpreting such studies is difficult because both therapy and patient selection can influence epidemiologic findings. In a classic monograph on the clinical picture of RA patients treated only with salicylates and simple orthopedic measures, Short and Bauer found that only 10% of patients experienced clinical remission during more than a decade of follow-up (20). This observation is similar to that of Ragan, who also found a low rate of spontaneous remission and also noted that when remissions did occur, they did so in the first 2 years of disease onset (5). Both studies, which focused on patients seeking medical care from rheumatologists, seem to closely parallel current clinical observations. Factors that predict a more severe, persistent disease course are the presence of rheumatoid factor, nodules, and the HLA-DR4 haplotype (21). In patients who do not undergo spontaneous remission, the prognosis in regard to joint destruction seems to depend on the severity of synovial inflammation.

Almost 90% of the joints ultimately affected in a given patient are involved during the first year of disease (6). There-

fore, a patient who has had RA for several years may be assured, given the worst-case scenario, which joints will or will not be involved in the future.

Several studies over the past decade have demonstrated increased mortality rates in RA patients and have shown that patients with severe forms of the disease die 10–15 years earlier than expected. The causes of death that were disproportionately high compared with the US population were infections, pulmonary and renal disease, and gastrointestinal bleeding (12).

RONALD J. ANDERSON, MD

1. Fleming A, Benn RT, Corbett M, Wood PHN: Early rheumatoid disease. Patterns of joint involvement. Ann Rheum Dis 35:361-364, 1976
2. Schumacher HR: Palindromic onset of rheumatoid arthritis. Arthritis Rheum 25:361-365, 1982
3. van der Heijde DM, van Riel PL, van Leeuwen MA, van't Hof MA, van Rijswijk MH, van de Putte LB: Prognostic factors for radiographic damage and physical disability in early rheumatoid arthritis. A prospective study of 147 patients. Br J Rheumatol 31:519-525, 1992
4. Pincus T, Brooks RH, Callahan LF: Measurements of inflammatory activity in rheumatoid arthritis may indicate no change or improvement over 5 years while measures of damage indicate disease progression: implications for assessment of long-term outcomes [Abstract]. Arthritis Rheum 38:S630, 1995
5. Ragan C, Farrington E: The clinical features of rheumatoid arthritis. Prognostic indices. JAMA 2:16, 1959
6. Roberts WN, Daltroy LH, Anderson RJ: Stability of normal joint findings in persistent classical rheumatoid arthritis. Arthritis Rheum 31:267-271, 1988
7. McGuigan L, Burke D, Fleming A: Tarsal tunnel syndrome and peripheral neuropathy in rheumatoid disease. Ann Rheum Dis 42:128-131, 1983
8. Weyand CM, Hicok KC, Conn DL, Goronzy JJ: The influence of HLA-DR B1 genes on disease severity in rheumatoid arthritis. Ann Intern Med 117:801-806, 1992
9. Kerstens PJ, Boerbooms AM, Jeurissen ME, Fast JH, Assman KJ, van de Putte LB: Accelerated nodulosis during long term methotrexate therapy for rheumatoid arthritis: an analysis of 10 cases. J Rheumatol 19:867-871,1992
10. Bienenstock H, Ehrlich GE, Freyberg RH: Rheumatoid arthritis of the cricoarytenoid joint: a clinicopathological study. Arthritis Rheum 6:48-63, 1963
11. Walker WC, Wright V: Pulmonary lesions and rheumatoid arthritis. Ann Rheum Dis 28:252-258, 1969
12. Pincus T, Callahan LF: Early mortality in RA predicted by poor clinical status. Bull Rheum Dis 41(4):1-4, 1992
13. John JT Jr, Hough A, Sergent JS: Pericardial disease in rheumatoid arthritis. Am J Med 66:385-390, 1979
14. Gravallese EM, Corson JM, Coblyn JS, Pinkusas, Weinblatt ME: Rheumatoid aortitis: a rarely recognized but clinically significant entity. Medicine: 68:95-106, 1989
15. Nakano KK, Schoene WC, Baker RA, Dawson DM: The cervical myelopathy associated with rheumatoid arthritis. Am Neuro Assoc 3:144, 1978
16. Dinant HJ, Muller WH, van den Berg-Loonen EM, Nijenhuis LE, Engelfriet CP: HLA Drw4 in Felty's syndrome. Arthritis Rheum 23:1336, 1980
17. Barton JC, Prasthofer EF, Egan ML, Heck LW, Koopman WJ, Grossic E: Rheumatoid arthritis associated with expanded populations of granular lymphocytes. Ann Intern Med 104:314-323, 1986
18. Gridley G, Klippel JH, Hoover RN, Fraumeni JF: Incidence of cancer among men with Felty's syndrome. Ann Intern Med 120:35-39, 1994
19. O'Sullivan JB, Cathcart ES: The prevalence of rheumatoid arthritis. Follow-up evaluation of the effect of criteria on rates in Sudbury, Mass. Ann Intern Med 76:573-577, 1972
20. Short CL, Bauer W, Reynolds WE: Rheumatoid Arthritis. Cambridge, Harvard University Press, 1957
21. Van Zeben D, Hazes JM, Zwinderman AH, Cats A, Schrender GM, D'Amaro J, Breedveld FL: Association of HLA-DR4 with a more progressive disease course in patients with rheumatoid arthritis. Results of a follow-up study. Arthritis Rheum 34:822-830, 1991

C. TREATMENT

Although knowledge of the immunologic and inflammatory processes involved in rheumatoid arthritis (RA) has expanded greatly, progress in developing treatments that alter the natural history of the disease has lagged far behind. Most of the current drug therapies continue to be based on empiric observations, with little understanding of the drugs' mechanisms of action (1).

In most patients, RA is a severe, chronic disorder that predictably leads to joint erosions with progressive joint damage, functional limitations, and work disability during the initial 5 years of the disease. At least 50% of RA patients are refractory to current treatment, have variable degrees of systemic disease, and eventually need surgical intervention. Increased mortality is apparent, not only from the disease process itself, but also as a result of treatments and co-morbid disease. Encouragingly, recent studies have demonstrated that the severity of RA appears to be decreasing, due either to early aggressive treatment or to societal trends (2).

The prognosis of individual RA patients can best be estimated from long-term observational studies that use quantitative data derived from serial health assessment questionnaires. Information gleaned from these sources emphasize how patients function in their environment and workplace. Such functional scales also guide the physician with regard to the effectiveness of a treatment regimen (3). Although the results of laboratory tests and radiographs will continue to be factored into the therapeutic equation, their lack of sensitivity to change or correlation with function has diminished their use. Individual prognostic profiles derived from clinical, laboratory, and socioeconomic data can guide physicians in tailoring treatment decisions. Lower economic and educational status are associated with a higher prevalence, morbidity, and mortality of many chronic disorders, including RA (4).

TREATMENT GUIDELINES

Data from longitudinal clinical and epidemiologic studies provide guidelines for treatment. These studies emphasize 1) the need for early diagnosis, 2) identification of prognostic factors, and 3) early aggressive treatment. Recent studies have shown that the median lag time between the onset of RA symptoms and diagnosis is 36 weeks, with a range from 4 weeks to more than 10 years (5). Earlier diagnosis and treatment, preferably within the first several months after the onset of symptoms, may help prevent irreversible joint damage. The identification of prognostic factors and co-morbidities should include using sensitive tools to define disease activity, functional state, and response to treatment (6). Poor prognostic features include the early onset of severe synovitis with functional limitation, joint erosions, extra-articular manifestations, rheumatoid factor positivity, and a family history of severe RA. Finally, because joint destruction is most pronounced in the first years after disease onset, early and aggressive institution of disease-modifying treatments may prevent severe disability.

Mild Disease, No Poor Prognostic Features

The following treatment is recommended for patients with mild disease in the absence of poor prognostic features.

1. Initiate a program of education and physical and occupational therapy.
2. Institute a nonsteroidal anti-inflammatory drug (NSAID). The choice of drug should be based on the patient's medication history, co-morbidities, and age. The drug requiring the fewest daily doses, costing the least, and having the most acceptable toxicity profile should be chosen. Prophylactic measures against gastric toxicity should be included, if indicated.
3. Administer a disease-modifying antirheumatic drug (DMARD). Medications with a low toxicity potential such as hydroxychloroquine, sulfasalazine, or auranofin (oral gold) should be considered and should include appropriate surveillance for toxicity.

Moderately Severe Disease, Poor Prognostic Indicators

In RA patients with moderately severe disease and poor prognostic features, the following regimen is recommended.

1. Emphasize the importance of education, compliance, and physical and occupational therapy.
2. Institute an NSAID.
3. Institute a DMARD such as parenteral gold, auranofin, or weekly methotrexate.
4. Institute a short course (3 to 5 days) of corticosteroids (eg, oral prednisone 10 mg twice a day initially, followed by a rapid taper to zero).

Severe Disease, Poor Prognostic Features

For RA patients with severe disease and the presence of poor prognostic features, the following therapy is recommended.

1. Institute an extensive, ongoing program of education and physical and occupational therapy. Although a multidisciplinary approach to the RA patient is always desirable, it is mandatory for patients in this category.
2. Start an NSAID.
3. Start a DMARD. The drug(s) chosen in this situation should have the greatest likelihood of controlling severe disease for the longest period of time. Such agents include parenteral gold and weekly oral or parenteral methotrexate. Azathioprine and penicillamine are alternative considerations. Although not supported by short-term studies, the addition of a second DMARD such as hydroxychloroquine is appropriate for these patients.
4. Start corticosteroids. A slightly longer course may be considered, or intermittent short courses may be appropriate, depending on the patient's clinical status.

LONGITUDINAL ASSESSMENT

Longitudinal assessments are critical for gathering objective measurements to evaluate response to treatment. These must include assessments of both clinical disease activity and functional status. Quantitative clinical assessments of disease activity traditionally include tender and swollen joint count, range of motion, walking time, duration of morning stiffness, severity of fatigue, and grip strength. Certain laboratory tests are good measures of the state of inflammation. The presence of anemia, thrombocytosis, an elevated Westergren erythrocyte sedimentation rate or C-reactive protein, especially in the setting of clinically apparent disease activity, clearly represent poorly controlled disease. Persistent joint swelling and laboratory manifestations of active inflammation are forerunners of erosive disease and demand the physician's attention and response. The finding of joint erosions on radiographs and their association with progressive joint deformities further supports disease activity and progression.

Quantitative assessment of functional, social, pain, and emotional status can be easily determined with a health assessment questionnaire. Comparison of assessments is very helpful in monitoring the disease course and in defining improvement, lack of change, or worsening in reference to therapeutic interventions. Physician and patient global assessments that use visual analog scales may be applied to assessments of pain, stiffness, and fatigue, and limitations of function.

The treatment regimen should be altered if there is clear lack of improvement or worsening of clinical, functional, and laboratory response parameters, despite an adequate therapeutic trial. The definition of *adequate* differs from drug to drug, but generally it means several weeks for an NSAID and several months for a DMARD.

SPECIFIC TREATMENT MODALITIES
Education and Physical and Occupational Therapy

The importance of initial and ongoing education in the overall treatment plan for all RA patients needs to be stressed. In some patients, the type, extent, and manner in which educational material is presented may be more important than drug therapy. Physical and occupational therapy, underused and underappreciated, have an important impact on a) joint protection, optimal joint use and range of motion, and the performance of activities of daily living; b) exercise leading to maintenance or improvement in joint range of motion and function; c) splinting of inflamed or painful joints leading to reduction of inflammation, decreased joint trauma, and improved alignment of joint components; and d) postoperative range of motion, joint protection, and muscle strengthening.

Drugs Used to Treat RA
Nonsteroidal Anti-inflammatory Drugs

NSAIDs are regarded as one of the foundation medications used in the long-term treatment of RA. By inhibiting the synthesis of pro-inflammatory prostaglandins, they control inflammation and pain. There is no evidence that these agents alter the natural history of the disease, however. Each NSAID appears to be effective in certain patients and toxic in others. Although NSAIDs have major differences in overall toxicity index scores, all NSAIDs tend to have similar rates of discontinuation for toxicities. NSAID-associated gastropathy is one of the most prevalent serious drug toxicities in the United States; the chance of hospitalization or death due to a gastrointestinal event is 1.3% to 1.6% over the course of 12 months, or 1 in 3 RA patients over the entire

course of disease. The major risk factors are increased age, concomitant use of corticosteroids, prior NSAID-related side effects, level of disability, and NSAID dose. In these high-risk groups, the prophylactic use of misoprostol, a prostaglandin analog, appears to deliver cost-effective protection against gastric toxicity.

As a general rule, NSAIDs are prescribed for all RA patients at the onset of joint pain and inflammation. A practical approach is to begin an NSAID that has the optimal profile of toxicity, cost, simplicity of dosing, and high likelihood for compliance (see Chapter 52 and Appendix V). A common practice is to try several different NSAIDs over a 3–4 week course to determine which drug provides the best balance between effectiveness and toxicity for the individual patient. Monitoring for toxicity should include complete blood cell counts and biochemical profiles every 3–4 months with close observation for abnormalities in liver function tests, hemoglobin, and renal function, as well as stool guaiac assessment for occult blood every 4 months.

Corticosteroids

A recent placebo-controlled trial using accepted radiographic scoring systems showed a statistically significant difference between prednisone-treated and placebo-treated RA patients in the development of new erosions over 2 years (7). These findings are somewhat at odds with extensive clinical experience with patients who developed severe and progressive deformities despite taking corticosteroids for decades. Although some studies have demonstrated the relative safety of long-term, low-dose corticosteroids (5 mg/day prednisone or less), many others highlight the cumulative toxicity that leads to osteoporosis, infections, peptic ulcer disease, and shortened lifespan (8).

Short courses of corticosteroids (20 mg/day prednisone initially, with a rapid taper over 5 days) may be effective for controlling disease flares and for bridging treatment periods in which DMARDs have not yet controlled disease. Every attempt should be made to avoid long-term corticosteroid use. If necessary, severely limited function may improve with low-dose (5 mg or less) prednisone daily or every other day. Intravenous pulse methylprednisolone (ie, 250 mg over 1 hour for 1 to 3 consecutive days) is sometimes helpful in controlling refractory disease. Intra-articular corticosteroid injections are highly effective for treating monarticular synovitis.

Disease-modifying Antirheumatic Drugs

The members of this class of drugs (Table 9C-1) differ greatly in their chemical structure and pharmacokinetics, presumed modes of action, clinical indications and position in the treatment algorithm, and toxicity profiles (1). Debate continues over whether these drugs have the capacity to heal active erosions and prevent the development of new ones, reverse or prevent deformities, aid normal function, and prolong life (9). To be designated a DMARD, a drug must change the course of RA for at least 1 year as evidenced by sustained improvement in physical function, decreased inflammatory synovitis, and slowing or prevention of structural joint damage.

All of the DMARDs currently in clinical use have been shown by short-term (36–48 weeks) randomized controlled trials to be more effective than placebo or equally effective to

(Table 9C-1)

Disease-modifying antirheumatic drugs used to treat rheumatoid arthritis

Type of Drug	Recommended Dosage
Gold compounds	
Gold sodium thiomalate (Solganal)	One intramuscular dose of 10 mg, followed by 25 mg 1 week later to test for sensitivity; maintenance therapy, 50 mg/week for 20 weeks, then taper to every 4 weeks
Aurothioglucose (Myochrysine)	Same as above
Auranofin (Ridaura)	3–9 mg daily; available in 3-mg tablets
Antimalarial drugs	
Hydroxychloroquine (Plaquenil)	6 mg/kg/day, taken in two divided doses with meals; available in 200-mg tablets
Penicillamine (D-Pen, Cuprimine)	125–250 mg/day, increased to a maximum of 750–1000 mg/day; available in 250-mg tablets
Methotrexate (Rheumatrex)	7.5–15 mg/week; may increase to 17.5–25 mg; available in 2.5-mg tablets. In unresponsive patients or patients with gastric toxicity, switch to subcutaneous, intramuscular, or intravenous route
Azathioprine (Imuran)	50–100 mg/day; maximum dose 2.5 mg/kg/day; available in 50-mg tablets
Sulfasalazine (Azulfidine entabs)	500 mg/day, then increase dose to a maximum of 3000 mg/day in two divided doses with meals; available in 500-mg enteric-coated tablets
Alkylating agents	
Cyclophosphamide (Cytoxan)	50–100 mg/day; maximum dose 2.5 mg/kg/day; available in 50-mg tablets
Cyclosporine (Sandimmune)	2.5–5 mg/kg/day; available in 25 mg, 50 mg, 100 mg capsules; oral solution 2 mg/ml

Adapted from Cash and Klippel (1), with permission.

another DMARD with regard to controlling inflammatory parameters (ie, joint counts, acute-phase reactants, and global patient and physician scores) and functional assessment scales. Many studies now define improvement in quantitative terms using specific criteria, with a significant change being greater than 20%–50% improvement in the outcome compared with baseline data (10,11). Few studies have consistently shown true DMARD capacity on the basis of strict radiographic criteria. However, it is generally accepted that erosions and joint deformities are less likely to develop when a patient's systemic inflammatory state is controlled and joint synovitis is absent.

The physician must make balanced decisions in prescribing DMARDs, weighing potential drug toxicity profiles with disease severity (12-14) (Table 9C-2, Chapter 54, Appendix V). Toxicity index scores, which are derived from symptoms, laboratory abnormalities, and hospitalizations attributable to DMARDs and adjusted for disease severity and comorbidities, have demonstrated substantial differences in toxicity among specific DMARDs (Tables 9C-2 and 9C-3). Hydroxychloroquine appears to be the least toxic, followed by intramuscular gold. More toxic are penicillamine, methotrexate, and azathioprine. But perhaps surprisingly, the toxicity of methotrexate and azathioprine is similar to that of the most toxic NSAID, indomethacin, whereas hydroxychloroquine is substantially less toxic than most NSAIDs. Although hematologic toxicities due to intramuscular gold, methotrexate, and azathioprine are uncommon, they have the largest impact on cost.

The optimal DMARD combines a high degree of disease-modifying capacity, minimal toxicity, and a high probability that a patient will be able to continue the drug for 2–5 years, the time period in which deformities and disability develop most rapidly. Long-term studies from practice databases have demonstrated that, whereas 50% or more of RA patients are still taking methotrexate at 5 years, fewer than 20% are on other DMARDs (14). The reasons for discontinuation vary from one drug to another, but most are due to drug toxicities.

Determining the cost of DMARD therapy in RA includes not only the direct cost of the drug itself but also the cost of monitoring for and treating toxicities (15). If all these factors are included, oral gold is the least expensive DMARD ($927/patient/6 months of therapy) and parenteral gold the most expensive ($1,768/patient/6 months of therapy). The cost of monitoring comprises more than 50% of the total cost for all DMARDs except azathioprine and injectable gold. Monitoring and treating toxicity account for more than 60% of the total cost with the exception of injectable gold.

Hydroxychloroquine

The antimalarial drug hydroxychloroquine is widely used in treating RA patients. It has a very acceptable toxicity profile and can be safely combined with other DMARDs. Maculopathy occurs almost exclusively at higher than recommended doses (6 mg/kg/day), although eye examinations are recommended every 6 months during therapy. Hydroxychloroquine is particularly effective in the early treatment of patients with mild to moderate and/or seronegative RA. Its true disease-modifying capacity is probably weak, however.

Sulfasalazine

This DMARD shares many attributes with hydroxychloroquine. Sulfasalazine has an acceptable toxicity profile, and its clinical effectiveness has led to its use in early mild disease at doses of 2–3 grams/day, taken with meals to limit gastric intolerance. The potential for developing leukopenia demands close hematologic monitoring for the first 2

(Table 9C-2)
Effectiveness and toxicity profiles of drugs used in rheumatoid arthritis

Level of Potential Toxicity	Disease Severity			
	Mild	Moderate	Severe	Refractory
Low	Hydroxychloroquine Sulfasalazine Auranofin	Hydroxychloroquine Sulfasalazine Steroids (short course)	Steroids (short course)	Steroids (short course)
Moderate	NSAIDs	Parenteral gold Methotrexate Azathioprine NSAIDs	Parenteral gold Methotrexate (7.5–15 mg) Combination DMARD Azathioprine NSAIDs	Parenteral gold Methotrexate (15–25 mg) Azathioprine Combination DMARD NSAIDs
Moderate to high			Daily steroids	Daily steroids
High			Penicillamine Cyclosporine	Penicillamine Cyclosporine Cyclophosphamide

months with laboratory surveillance every 6 weeks thereafter.

Gold Salts

Parenteral gold preparations (gold sodium aurothioglucose and thiomalate) are effective, generally safe, and one of the few drugs shown to result in short-term or intermediate disease remissions. Long-term studies demonstrate clinical effectiveness, but erosions continue to develop. Blood and urine monitoring is mandatory. Thrombocytopenia is responsive to corticosteroids and leukopenia to granulocyte colony-stimulating factors.

Although the incidence of severe toxicity from oral gold is low, the clinical effectiveness of this drug is disappointing. The role of auranofin should be limited to early mild RA, or it should be used in combination with other medications.

Methotrexate

Long-term clinical studies have clearly demonstrated the efficacy and safety of methotrexate in managing RA. Its true disease-modifying capacity, however, continues to be questioned.

The use of folinic acid (expensive) or folic acid (inexpensive and may also protect against atherosclerosis) reduces the incidence of common side effects, especially gastrointestinal toxicities, without decreasing the effectiveness of methotrexate. Early fears about hepatic fibrosis and cirrhosis have been allayed by the absence of severe liver toxicity in follow-up liver biopsies of methotrexate-treated RA patients. A position paper from the American College of Rheumatology recommends not performing a liver biopsy during therapy unless the clinician notes persistently abnormal alanine aminotransferase or albumin levels (16) (see Appendix II). Increasing the dosage to as high a dose as 15–20 mg/week or switching to a parenteral route may markedly improve the clinical response. Although the majority of RA patients take methotrexate and physicians prescribe it earlier in the disease course because of its rapid onset of action and long-term acceptability, some concerns still exist. Its use as a first-line DMARD in early RA is still somewhat controversial (17,18).

Several common practical problems with methotrexate therapy should be considered. Once started, it is very difficult to stop the drug because a disease flare occurs in more

(Table 9C-3)
Toxic effects common to disease-modifying antirheumatic drugs*

Drug	Gastrointestinal	Mucocutaneous	Hematologic
Parenteral gold	+	+++	++
Oral gold	+++	+	+
Hydroxychloroquine	++	+	+
Penicillamine	++	+++	++
Methotrexate	+++	+++	+
Azathioprine	+++	+	++
Sulfasalazine	+++	++	++
Cyclophosphamide	+++	+	+++
Cyclosporine	++	+	+

* The relative importance of the toxic effect is indicated as follows: + = rare and an infrequent cause of discontinuing the drug, ++ = common but infrequent cause of discontinuing the drug, and +++ = common and frequent cause of discontinuing the drug.
Adapted from Cash and Klippel (1), with permission.

(Table 9C-4)

*Toxic effects of individual disease-modifying antirheumatic drugs**

Drug	Liver	Lung	Renal Function	Infection	Terato-genicity	Cancer Degree of Association	Miscellaneous Disorders
Parenteral gold	+	+	++	None	None	None	—
Oral gold	–	–	+	None	None	None	—
Hydroxychloro-quine	–	–	–	None	Weak	None	Uncommon association with retinopathy, neuromyopathy
Penicillamine	+	++	++	None	Moderate	None	Uncommon association with myasthenic syndrome, lupus, myositis
Methotrexate	++	++	–	Moderate	Strong	Weak to moderate[†]	Association with nodulosis, osteoporosis (?)
Azathioprine	++	–	–	Moderate	Weak	Moderate	Early leukopenia
Sulfasalazine	+	+	–	None	None	None	Weak association with oligospermia
Cyclophosphamide	–	–	–	Strong	Strong	Strong	Strong association with hemorrhagic cystitis, ovarian and testicular failure
Cyclosporine	+	–	+++	Weak	?	Weak	Strong association with hypertension, neuro-pathy, osteoporosis (?)

* The relative importance of the toxic effect is indicated as follows: – = not reported or extremely rare, + = rare and infrequent cause of discontinuing the drug, ++ = common but infrequent cause of discontinuing the drug, and +++ = common and frequent cause of discontinuing the drug.

[†]ref 27

Adapted from Cash and Klippel (1), with permission.

than 75% of patients within 6–8 weeks. Often, it is difficult to regain disease control with an alternative DMARD. This common withdrawal problem may be one reason why the drug is continued longer than other DMARDs. Hypersensitivity pneumonitis occurs in 3%–5% of patients and can be life-threatening, especially on reexposure to the drug. This complication is usually responsive to corticosteroid treatment. Preexisting pulmonary disease may predispose to this adverse reaction (19). Opportunistic infections may occur, including *Pneumocystis carinii* pneumonitis. Patients may develop progressive and painful nodules, particularly on the fingers; colchicine may help prevent or treat methotrexate-induced nodules. Finally, more than 50 cases worldwide have described the development of B cell, non-Hodgkin's lymphoma in methotrexate-treated patients. A cause-and-effect relationship between the drug and the tumor is supported by some cases that resolved spontaneously after patients stopped methotrexate therapy. Close surveillance for such tumors is indicated, and patients should be told of the potential oncogenicity of the drug (20).

Azathioprine

Azathioprine is used to treat moderate to severe RA. Long-term studies have demonstrated that it is well tolerated without an obvious increased risk of tumor development. This drug is used primarily in patients who have disease refractory to other DMARDs or have severe extra-articular manifestations.

Penicillamine

Although numerous studies have shown penicillamine to be safe and effective in low doses (250 mg/day), it is not routinely used to treat RA, except for patients with marked, refractory extra-articular disease manifestations. Penicillamine has a slow onset of action and a high frequency of side effects such as leukopenia and autoimmune disorders.

Cyclosporine

Despite many studies demonstrating the clinical effectiveness of cyclosporine, its cost and potential for irreversible renal toxicity, even at low doses (2.5–5.0 mg/kg/day), have limited its use to severe, progressive RA refractory to all other DMARDs. A recent multicenter short-term study comparing RA patients treated with methotrexate alone to those receiving both cyclosporine and methotrexate demonstrated a clinically important (20%) improvement in disease activity, without substantial differences in side effects (21).

Cyclophosphamide

The alkylating agent cyclophosphamide is highly effective for treating RA. However, this drug has been abandoned for routine use because of its high toxicity profile (ie, oncogenicity, bladder hemorrhage, bone marrow toxicity, infertility). Cyclophosphamide is the drug of choice in RA vasculitis unresponsive to corticosteroids.

Combination Protocols

Traditional drug combinations for RA commonly include an NSAID, a DMARD, and short intermittent courses of oral corticosteroids. Medications are changed after either an appropriate course has failed to control disease or an initial improvement fades. Increasingly, two (or more) DMARDs are being used to treat RA patients. This approach is based on the reasoning that drug resistance, which develops with single agents, may be overcome by the use of multiple drugs. There are reports of all types of DMARD combinations, but many include hydroxychloroquine because of its benign safety profile. Most studies have failed to demonstrate a significant additive effect of combining DMARDs, however, and some have shown an increased frequency of side effects. Most of these have been short-term studies and may not adequately reflect the efficacy that may occur in long-term analysis (22). A variation of DMARD combination therapy is the "step-down, bridge approach" in which multiple drugs are initiated simultaneously to effect a rapid control of the disease (23). Once the disease is brought under control, drugs are discontinued one at a time until the patient remains on the least toxic medication. Randomized controlled long-term trials evaluating this approach are lacking, and the cost and potential side effects are of concern.

Antibiotics

Minocycline, a tetracycline drug, has both antibacterial and metalloproteinase-inhibitory capacity. Several clinical trials recently demonstrated mild-to-moderate clinical improvement in RA patients (24–26).

TREATMENT OF SPECIFIC RA-RELATED PROBLEMS

Rheumatoid nodules are treated as a component of the overall inflammatory state. Rarely is there a need for surgical removal because of severe pain or infection. Visceral nodules causing organ dysfunction are treated as part of the active systemic process.

In Felty's syndrome, the response of granulocytopenia to corticosteroid treatment is usually disappointing and may be associated with an increased risk of infection. DMARDs such as gold and methotrexate or lithium carbonate have been helpful in isolated cases. The use of granulocyte colony-stimulating factor has been quite effective in cases of treatment resistant or severe Felty's syndrome. Recurrent infections and pancytopenia may be indications for splenectomy, a procedure that is effective in only 50% of patients.

Pleuritis and pericarditis may occur during episodes of active disease. These complications usually respond to NSAIDs or a course of oral corticosteroids. Rarely, pericardial tamponade may occur, necessitating pericardiocentesis, local corticosteroid injection, or a pericardial window. In rare instances, constrictive pericarditis may demand pericardial stripping. Interstitial inflammatory fibrotic disease, which seldom dominates the clinical picture, may result from infection or drug reactions to intramuscular gold, methotrexate, or penicillamine.

Rheumatoid vasculitis is a potentially life-threatening disorder necessitating high-dose oral or intravenous corticosteroids (equivalent to 60 mg/day prednisone in divided doses) and, commonly, a cytotoxic drug (oral cyclophosphamide is the most effective). When the disease is controlled, a switch to oral methotrexate (15–25 mg/week) is appropriate.

The orthopedic surgeon plays a major role in treating patients who develop severe, progressive disease with permanent joint damage and dysfunction. The spectrum of surgical intervention varies from carpal tunnel release and tendon rupture repair to total joint replacement and treatment of cervical myelopathy. When surgery is planned, the internist and rheumatologist are responsible for coordinating the patient's overall medical care, guiding drug therapy, and maintaining surveillance for infection and thromboembolic disease.

STEPHEN A. PAGET, MD

1. Cash JM, Klippel JH: Second-line drug therapy for rheumatoid arthritis. N Engl J Med 330:1368-1375, 1994
2. Ward MM, Leigh JP, Fries, JF: Progression of functional disability in patients with rheumatoid arthritis. Associations with rheumatology subspecialty care. Arch Int Med 153:2229-2237, 1993
3. Pincus T: Why should rheumatologists collect patient self-report questionnaires in routine rheumatologic practice? Rheum Dis Clin North Am 21:271-319, 1995
4. Combe B, Eliaou JF, Daures JP, Meyer O, Clot J, Sany J: Prognostic factors in rheumatoid arthritis: comparative study of two subsets of patients according to severity of articular damage. Br J Rheumatol 34:529-534, 1995
5. Chan KW, Felson DT, Yood RA, Walker AM: The lag time between onset of symptoms and diagnosis of rheumatoid arthritis. Arthritis Rheum 37:814-820, 1994
6. van Leewen MA, van der Heijde DM, van Rikswijk, Houtman PM, van Riel PL, vande Putte, Limburg PC: Interrelationships of outcome measures and process variables in early rheumatoid arthritis: a comparison of radiologic damage, physical disability, joint counts, and acute phase reactants. J Rheumatol 21:425-429, 1994
7. Kirwan JR: The effect of glucocorticoids on joint destruction in rheumatoid with regard to early and aggressive treatment of people with RA: The Arthritis and Rheumatism Council Low-dose Glucocorticoid Study Group. N Engl J Med 333:142-146, 1995
8. Saag KG, Koehnke R, Caldwell JR, Brashington R, Burmeister LF, Zimmerman B, Kohler JA, Furst DE: Low-dose, long-term corticosteroid therapy in rheumatoid arthritis: an analysis of serious adverse events. Am J Med 96:115-123, 1994
9. Epstein WV: Efficacy of standard slow-acting anti-rheumatic drugs. Semin Arthritis Rheum 23:32-38, 1994
10. Conaghan PG, Brooks P: Disease-modifying antirheumatic drugs, including methotrexate, gold, antimalarials, and D-penicillamine. Curr Opin Rheumatol 7:167-173, 1995
11. Ward MM: Clinical measures in rheumatoid arthritis: which are the most useful in assessing patients? J Rheumatol 21:17-27, 1994
12. Felson DT, Anderson JJ, Meenan RF: Use of short-term efficacy/toxicity tradeoffs to select second-line drugs in rheumatoid arthritis: a meta-analysis of published clinical trials. Arthritis Rheum 35: 1117-1125, 1992
13. Fries JF, Williams CA, Ramey DR, Bloch DA: The relative toxicities of disease-modifying antirheumatic drugs. Arthritis Rheum 36:297-306, 1993
14. Pincus T, Marcum S, Callahan LF: Long-term drug therapy for rheumatoid arthritis in seven rheumatology private practices: II. Second line drugs and prednisone. J Rheumatol 19:1885-1894, 1992
15. Prashker MJ, Meenan RF: The total costs of drug therapy for rheumatoid arthritis. Arthritis Rheum 38:318-325, 1995
16. Kremer JM, Alarcon GS, Lightfoot RW, Willkens RF, Furst DE, William HJ, Dent PB, Weinblatt ME: Methotrexate for rheumatoid arthritis: suggested guidelines for monitoring liver toxicity. Arthritis Rheum 37:316-328, 1994
17. Weinblatt ME, Kaplan H, Germain BF, et al: Methotrexate in rheumatoid arthritis: a five-year prospective multicenter study. Arthritis Rheum 37:1492-1498, 1994
18. Furst DE: Should methotrexate be used to treat early rheumatoid arthritis? Semin Arthritis Rheum 23:39-43, 1994
19. Carroll GJ, Thomas R, Phatouros CC: Incidence, prevalence, and possible risk factors for pneumonitis in patients with rheumatoid arthritis receiving methotrexate. J Rheumatol 21:51-54, 1994
20. Kamel OW, van deRijn M, Weiss GJ, Del Zappo AJ, Hench PIC, Robbins BA, Montgomery PG, Warnke RA: Reversible lymphomas associated with Epstein-Barr virus occurring during methotrexate therapy for rheumatoid arthritis and dermatomyositis. N Engl J Med 328:1317-1321, 1993
21. Tugwell P, Pincus T, Yocum D, et al: Combination therapy with cyclosporine and methotrexate in severe rheumatoid arthritis: The Methotrexate-Cyclosporine Combination Study Group. N Engl J Med 333:137-141, 1995

22. Pincus T: Limitations of randomized clinical trials to recognize possible advantages of combination therapies in rheumatoid arthritis. Semin Arthritis Rheum 23:11-18, 1993

23. Wilske KR: Inverting the therapeutic pyramid: observations and recommendations on new directions in rheumatoid arthritis therapy based upon the author's experience. Semin Arthritis Rheum 23:11-18, 1993

24. Kloppenberg M, Breedveld FC, Terweil JP, Malleec, Dijikmacs BAC: Minocycline in active rheumatoid arthritis: a double-blind, placebo-controlled trial. Arthritis Rheum 37:629-636, 1994

25. Tilley BC, Alarcón GS, Heyse SP, et al: Minocycline in rheumatoid arthritis: a 48 week, placebo-controlled trial. Ann Intern Med 122:81-89, 1995

26. O'Dell JR, Haire CE, Palmer W, et al: Treatment of early rheumatoid arthritis with minocycline or placebo: results of a randomized, double-blind, placebo-controlled trial. Arthritis Rheum 40:842-848, 1997

PSORIATIC ARTHRITIS

The arthropathy associated with psoriasis combines features of both rheumatoid arthritis (RA) and the seronegative spondyloarthropathies. The disease may present with a variety of forms including monarthritis, asymmetric oligoarthritis or polyarthritis, or symmetric polyarthritis resembling RA. Spinal and sacroiliac disease may also occur alone or in combination with peripheral arthritis. Rheumatoid factor is usually absent (Fig. 10-1). Although there is no uniform agreement on classification, clinical, epidemiologic, genetic, and radiographic studies suggest that psoriatic arthritis is a separate disease entity distinct from other inflammatory arthritides (1,2).

EPIDEMIOLOGY

The overall prevalence of psoriatic arthritis is approximately 0.1% in the United States. Arthritis occurs in approximately 5%–7% of patients with psoriasis, but it may affect up to 40% of hospitalized patients with extensive skin involvement (3). Psoriasis is common in whites (overall prevalence is about 2%), but it is relatively uncommon in Asians. Psoriatic arthritis has been described in African blacks, but adequate prevalence data are not available for this population. The male-to-female ratio is equal, but this ratio varies in different subsets of the disease. Females predominate in the group with symmetric polyarthritis and males predominate in the group with spinal involvement. In contrast to psoriasis where the peak age of onset is between 5 and 15 years, the peak age of onset for psoriatic arthritis is between 30 and 55 years, which is similar to that of RA.

PATHOGENESIS

The etiology of both psoriasis and psoriatic arthritis are not known. Genetic, environmental, and immunologic factors appear to influence the susceptibility of the disease and its expression. In fact, the marked heterogeneity of the disease may not only reflect differences in genetic background but also the involvement of multiple etiologic factors in the pathogenesis. Given the similarities of the disease with both RA and the spondyloarthropathies, etiopathogenetic mechanisms involved in these diseases are likely operative in different subgroups of patients.

Genetic Factors

Convincing evidence of a genetic basis for psoriasis comes from population surveys, twins studies, and analysis of individual pedigrees (4). The pattern of inheritance does not follow single-gene Mendelian inheritance patterns, but it is suggestive of a polygenic influence. A gene involved in conferring susceptibility to psoriasis has been mapped to the distal region of human chromosome 17 (5) (see Appendix IV). Although the concordance between monozygotic twins with psoriasis is high (about 70%) compared with RA (about 30%), the lack of complete concordance suggests an additional role for environmental factors. Formal twin studies have not been undertaken in patients with psoriatic arthritis, and thus the relative importance of genetic and environmental factors is not known. Family studies suggest an approximately 50-fold increased risk of psoriatic arthritis in first degree relatives of patients with the disease. Within a family, there may be some members who develop only psoriasis or arthritis and some who develop both conditions.

Psoriatic arthritis is associated with HLA-Cw6, but the association is weaker than that between HLA-Cw6 and psoriasis alone (5). There is an association between HLA-B27 and both the peripheral arthropathy and the spinal disease in which radiologic sacroiliitis is present. The associations between HLA-B16 (or its splits HLA-B38 and HLA-B39) and peripheral arthritis, and between HLA-DR4 and symmetric polyarthritis are not conclusive. An important role for class I HLA antigens in the pathogenesis of psoriatic arthritis is supported by data derived from the HLA-B27 transgenic rat model where psoriasiform skin and nail lesions have been observed (6). Of interest, these lesions develop in animals

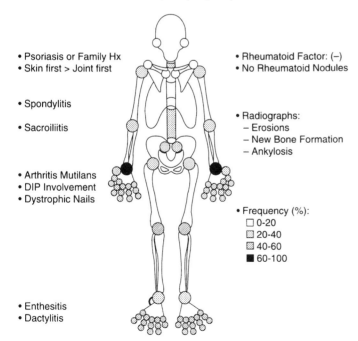

PSORIATIC ARTHRITIS

- Peripheral and/or Axial Disease
- Prevalence: 0.1%
- Male/Female: 1/1
- Caucasians > Non-Caucasians
- Peak Age: 20-40
- HLA: Cw6, B27 (B16, DR4)

- Psoriasis or Family Hx
- Skin first > Joint first

- Spondylitis

- Sacroiliitis

- Arthritis Mutilans
- DIP Involvement
- Dystrophic Nails

- Enthesitis
- Dactylitis

- Rheumatoid Factor: (–)
- No Rheumatoid Nodules

- Radiographs:
  – Erosions
  – New Bone Formation
  – Ankylosis

- Frequency (%):
  □ 0-20
  ▨ 20-40
  ▩ 40-60
  ■ 60-100

(Figure 10-1)
Epidemiology and clinical manifestations of psoriatic arthritis. The disease combines features of both rheumatoid arthritis and the spondyloarthropathies. DIP = distal interphalangeal.

grown in germ-free environments in which gut or joint involvement does not occur.

Environmental Factors

Environmental factors including infectious agents and physical trauma are likely to be important in the pathogenesis of the disease. The clinical similarities of reactive arthritis with psoriatic arthritis and the precipitation of psoriasis by streptococcal infections in children are some of the evidence supporting a role for infectious agents in the pathogenesis of the disease. The notion that psoriatic arthritis may be a reactive arthritis to psoriatic plaque flora (*Streptococci* and *Staphylococci*) has been widely discussed. Microbial antigens could act as superantigens or result in generating T-cell cross-reactivity with autoantigens (such as keratin, laminin, type II collagen, and heat-shock proteins). In this model, activated keratinocytes of the involved skin, which are known to express HLA class II antigens, may be presenting these antigens to T cells infiltrating the dermis (7). The possibility that trauma may precipitate psoriatic arthritis (the deep Koebner effect) has been suggested by several case series. Trauma could result either in the release of putative autoantigens or the expression of heat-shock proteins resembling bacterial antigen.

Immunologic Factors

The histopathologic changes in psoriatic skin are remarkably similar to those observed in the synovium and entheses with hyperproliferation of epithelial cells (keratinocytes and synoviocytes), accumulation of inflammatory cells (T cells, macrophages, B cells, and neutrophils), and elongation and increased tortuosity of blood vessels (8). There is considerable debate as to whether the initiating event is due to a defect in keratinocytes (leading to their abnormal activation and attraction of inflammatory cells) or to specific T-cell clones that may be activated at distant sites but preferentially accumulate in the skin or the joints in an antigen-driven process. There is uniform agreement that T cells are essential for initiating and perpetuating the disease (8,9). An important role for CD8 T cells is favored by: 1) the linkage of psoriasis to certain MHC alleles (especially HLA-Cw6); 2) the skewing of the CD8 (but not the CD4) T-cell receptor to specific V β subtypes, suggesting an antigen-driven process (10,11); and 3) the observed association of HIV-1 infection with an explosive onset of psoriasis and psoriatic arthritis (12). Similar to RA, perpetuation of the disease most likely results from a complex interplay between T cells, keratinocytes, fibroblasts, and type A (macrophage-like) and type B (fibroblast-like) synoviocytes with the relative contribution of each cell differing with the duration of the disease and the individual patient.

CLINICAL FEATURES

Given the wide spectrum of clinical manifestations, it is helpful to classify patients with psoriatic arthritis into different clinical subgroups. From a diagnostic and therapeutic point of view, patients may be classified into the following three groups: 1) asymmetric oligoarthritis or monarthritis (observed in about 30%–50% of patients); 2) polyarthritis often symmetric resembling RA (about 30%–50%); and 3) predominantly axial disease (spondylitis, sacroiliitis, and/or arthritis of hip and shoulder joints resembling ankylosing spondylitis) with or without peripheral joint disease (about 5%).

Distal interphalangeal (DIP) joint involvement (overall prevalence about 25%), arthritis mutilans (about 5%), sacroiliitis (about 35%), and spondylitis (about 30%) may occur with any of these subgroups. Transition of one pattern into another is not uncommon and may result in heterogenous combinations of joint disease.

Clinical Presentation

In about 70% of patients psoriasis is present many years before or appears concomitantly (in about 15%) with the onset of arthritis. Although the arthritis is usually insidious in onset, approximately one-third of patients have an acute onset. Constitutional symptoms are uncommon. In a small percentage of adults (about 15%), and more often in children, the arthritis appears before the skin or nail changes (arthritis sine psoriasis). Most patients have a family history of psoriasis as well as certain clinical features that may provide important clues for its diagnosis.

Joint Disease

Oligoarticular Arthritis or Monarthritis

The most common initial manifestation, observed in up to two-thirds of patients, is a mono- or oligoarticular arthritis similar to the peripheral arthritis that complicates the other spondyloarthropathies; in approximately one-third to one-half of these patients, this will evolve into a more symmetric polyarthritis indistinguishable from RA. A classic presentation includes oligoarticular arthritis involving a large joint, such as a knee, with one or two interphalangeal joints and dactylitis of a digit or toe, the latter resulting from a combination of tenosynovitis and arthritis of the DIP or proximal interphalangeal (PIP) joints. In some cases, the arthritis may follow an episode of trauma, leading to the erroneous diagnosis of "post-traumatic" or "mechanical" arthritis. If a careful history reveals either a family history of psoriasis or guttate psoriasis in childhood, a search for hidden areas of psoriasis (scalp, umbilicus, and perianal area) and characteristic radiologic findings (see below) will provide important clues to the correct diagnosis. Psoriatic lesions may be limited to one or two small psoriatic patches, with or without nail involvement. Involvement of the DIP joints is characteristic of the disease; DIP joint involvement is almost always associated with psoriatic changes in the nails.

Polyarthritis

Symmetric polyarthritis involving the small joints of the hands and feet, wrists, ankles, knees, and elbows is the most common pattern of psoriatic arthritis. The arthritis may be indistinguishable from RA, but there is a higher frequency of DIP joint involvement and a tendency for bony ankylosis of the DIP and PIP joints, which may lead to "claw" or "paddle" deformities of the hands. Patients who have symmetric polyarthritis and psoriasis but without the characteristic clinical (dactylitis, enthesitis, DIP or sacroiliac joint involvement) or radiologic features and who are positive for rheumatoid factor probably have coincident RA.

Arthritis mutilans

Arthritis mutilans due to osteolysis of the phalanges and metacarpals of the hand (or in rare cases of the phalanges and metatarsals of the feet) is a rare but highly characteristic feature of the disease that results in "telescoping" of the involved finger. It occurs in about 5% of patients with psoriatic arthritis.

Axial disease

Axial disease may occur in rheumatoid factor-negative patients with peripheral arthritis and is often asymptomatic. Both genders are affected equally. Although axial disease may occur independently of peripheral arthritis, usually it manifests after several years of peripheral arthritis. Spine symptoms are rarely a presenting feature. Symptoms of inflammatory low-back pain or chest wall pain may be absent or minimal, despite advanced radiographic changes. Sacroiliitis has been observed in up to one-third of patients, frequently is asymptomatic and asymmetric, and may occur independently of spondylitis. Spondylitis may also occur without sacroiliitis, may affect any portion of the spine in a random fashion, and may result in fusion of the spine. In rare cases, involvement of the cervical spine results in atlantoaxial and subaxial subluxations. Another pattern of spondylitis develops in HLA–B27-positive patients with late-onset psoriasis, iritis, sacroiliitis, rarely peripheral arthritis, and progressive spinal involvement from the sacroiliac joints toward the cervical spine (cephalad). Such patients most likely have coincident ankylosing spondylitis.

Other Manifestations

Inflammation at the attachment of tendons and ligaments to bones (enthesitis), a characteristic feature of the spondyloarthropathies, is common especially at the insertions of the Achilles tendon and plantar fascia into the calcaneus. Enthesopathies tend to occur more frequently in the oligoarthritis form of disease. Ocular involvement, predominantly conjunctivitis, is not uncommon and may be observed in up to one-third of patients. As with ankylosing spondylitis, complications such as aortic insufficiency, uveitis, pulmonary fibrosis involving the upper lobes, and amyloidosis may occur but are rare.

Dermatologic Features

The typical psoriatic skin lesion is a sharply demarcated erythematous plaque with a well-marked, silvery scale. The lesions typically appear on the extensor surfaces of the elbow, knees, in the scalp, ears, and the presacral areas, but they are also found anywhere on the body including palms and soles, flexor sites, lower back, hair line, the perineum, and the genitalia. Their size is variable, ranging from 1 mm or less in early acute psoriasis to several centimeters in well-established disease. Gentle scraping usually produces pinpoint bleeding (Auspitz's sign).

Nail involvement is the only clinical feature that identifies patients with psoriasis who are likely to develop arthritis. Clinical signs of psoriatic involvement of the nails include pitting, onycholysis (separation of the nail from the underlying nail bed), transverse depression (ridging) and cracking, subungual keratosis, brown-yellow discoloration (oil-drop sign), and leukonychia with rough surface. None of these dystrophic nail abnormalities are specific for psoriatic arthritis. Although nail pitting is not uncommon in healthy individuals, multiple pits (usually more than 20) in a single nail of a digit affected by dactylitis or an inflamed DIP joint is characteristic of psoriatic arthritis.

Radiographic Features

Several radiographic features are characteristic of the disease (Fig. 10-2). The bone changes in psoriatic arthritis are a unique combination of erosion, which helps in differentiat-

ing it from ankylosing spondylitis, and bone production in a specific distribution, which distinguishes it from RA (13). The distinguishing features are: fusiform soft tissue swelling in a bilateral asymmetric distribution with maintenance of normal mineralization; dramatic joint space loss with or without ankylosis of the interphalangeal (IP) joints of the hands and feet; destruction of IP joints with widening of the joint spaces; bone proliferation of the base of the distal phalanx and resorption of the tufts of the involved distal phalanges; joint erosion with tapering of the proximal phalanx and bone proliferation of the distal phalanx (pencil-in-cup deformity); and "fluffy" periostitis. In decreasing order of frequency, the radiographic abnormalities are distributed in the hands, feet, sacroiliac joints, and spine. Sacroiliitis may

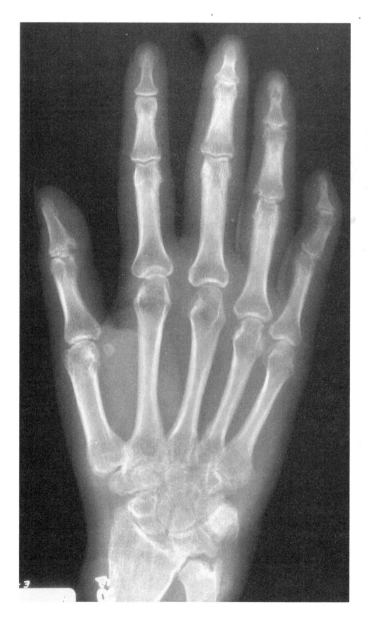

(Figure 10-2)
Radiographic findings in psoriatic arthritis. This hand radiograph demonstrates classic changes of psoriatic arthritis with involvement of the first, third, fourth, and fifth rays and wrists. Marginal erosions are seen at the distal and proximal interphalangeal joints with new bone formation. Involvement of the carpus with joint space narrowing and new bone formation around the ulnar styloid are also present. Courtesy of Dr. Mark D. Murphy-Armed Forces Institute of Pathology, Washington, DC.

be unilateral or symmetric in early stages but may progress to bilateral fusion. Spondylitis may occur with or without involvement of the sacroiliac joints. Isolated, sometimes unusually bulky and irregular marginal or nonmarginal syndesmophytes may appear at any portion of the spine.

Differential Diagnosis

Differential diagnosis must include other causes of spondyloarthropathy and RA. Spine disease is less severe than in ankylosing spondylitis and appears at a later age (30 years or older); other differences are psoriatic skin or nail disease, a family history of psoriasis, and less-symmetric radiologic features, which help distinguish between these two diseases. The presence of dactylitis and enthesitis, signs of psoriatic skin or nail disease, family history of psoriasis, involvement of the DIP joints, lack of rheumatoid factor, presence of spinal disease or sacroiliitis, and radiographic evidence of new bone formation or bone ankylosis help distinguish the disease from RA.

More problematic is the distinction between psoriatic arthritis and other seronegative spondyloarthropathies. Reactive arthritis, the arthritis associated with inflammatory bowel disease, and psoriatic arthritis share many common features. The lack of a preceding infectious episode, the predilection for joints of the upper extremities, and the absence of balanitis and urethritis may help distinguish psoriatic arthritis from reactive arthritis. Although hyperkeratotic skin and nail changes may occur in reactive arthritis, in most cases these lesions involve only the soles and palms. Keratoderma blennorrhagica and palmoplantar postural psoriasis are clinically and histologically identical. Since both psoriasis and psoriatic arthritis may be presenting features of undiagnosed HIV infection, this should be ruled out especially in patients with unusually severe disease.

TREATMENT
Skin Disease

The initial treatment for stable plaque psoriasis is topical. However, topical therapy may be impractical for patients with extensive psoriasis (more than 20% involvement) and systemic therapy may be indicated at the onset (14). Topical treatment includes emollients and keratolytic agents alone or in combination with anthralin, corticosteroids, and vitamin D derivatives such as calcipotriene. Stress and certain drugs (β-adrenergic blockers, angiotensin-converting enzyme inhibitors, lithium, and antimalarial drugs) may exacerbate psoriasis and should be used with caution.

Joint Disease

The general principles of managing patients with RA or spondylitis also apply to patients with psoriatic arthritis. The treatment depends on the type of the joint disease (axial versus peripheral) and the severity of joint and skin involvement. Simultaneous joint and skin disease activity has been observed in up to one-third of patients, particularly those with nonspondylitic disease (15).

Nonsteroidal anti-inflammatory drugs (NSAIDs) are effective in most patients and should be tried first. For patients whose response to NSAIDs is inadequate and patients with progressive, erosive, polyarticular disease, disease-modifying antirheumatic drugs (DMARDs) should be initiated as early as possible (2). Methotrexate is effective for both the skin disease and peripheral arthritis in patients with

oligo- or polyarticular disease (16). Dosage and monitoring are the same as for patients with RA. Sulfasalazine (2–3 gm/day) is helpful for both axial and peripheral arthritis (17,18); some data suggest the drug is of greater benefit for patients with symmetric polyarthritis (18). Sulfasalazine does not have any significant effect on the skin disease. Photochemotherapy (PUVA therapy) is effective for both skin and joint disease, but only in nonspondylitic disease (15), and may be especially helpful for patients with extensive skin involvement. Antimalarials, gold, azathioprine, cyclosporine, etretinate, and calcitriol are also effective according to small, open-label, uncontrolled trials. Azathioprine, cyclosporine, etretinate, and calcitriol are likely to improve both skin and joint disease. Etretinate should probably be avoided in patients with axial disease because spinal ligamentous calcification is associated with long-term use. Corticosteroids may be used in low doses, either in combination with DMARDs or as bridge therapy while waiting for onset of action of DMARDs (19). Combination therapy may be considered in patients with aggressive, destructive disease who have an inadequate response to single agent therapy.

As in RA, flares that affect only one or two joints can be effectively treated with local corticosteroid injections. Intra-articular injections through psoriatic lesions should be avoided because the skin may be colonized with *Staphylococci* and *Streptococci*. If such injections are unavoidable, careful preparation of the skin is essential. For patients with intractable pain or loss of joint function, surgery is indicated. Although several reports have raised concerns about a higher risk of infections, recurrent contracture or stiffness, or excessive bone formation after surgery, most of these fears seem ill-founded and surgery should not be withheld.

PROGNOSIS

In general, patients with psoriatic arthritis are less likely to complain about pain than patients with RA. Although it is widely accepted that patients with psoriatic arthritis may have a more benign course than patients with RA, earlier studies may have underestimated the actual disease morbidity (20). Clearly defined prognostic factors are not available; a family history of psoriatic arthritis, disease onset before age 20, the presence of HLA-DR3 or -DR4, erosive or polyarticular disease, and extensive skin involvement have been associated with a worse prognosis, and these patients may require more aggressive treatment.

DIMITRIOS T. BOUMPAS, MD
IOANNIS O. TASSIULAS, MD

1. O'Neil T, Silman AJ: Historical background and epidemiology. Bailliere's Clin Rheumatol 8:245-261, 1994

2. Gerber LH, Espinoza LR: Psoriatic Arthritis, New York, Grune and Stratton, 1985

3. Cuellar ML, Silveira LH, Espinoza LR: Recent development in psoriatic arthritis. Curr Opin Rheumatol 6:378-384, 1994

4. Eastmont CJ: Genetics and HLA antigens. Bailliere's Clin Rheumatol 8:263-276, 1994

5. Tomfrhde J, Silverman A, Barnes R, et al: Gene for familial psoriasis susceptibility mapped to the distal end of human chromosome 17q. Science 264:1141-1145, 1994

6. Hammer RE, Maika SD, Richardson JA, Tang JP, Taurog JD: Spontaneous inflammatory disease in transgenic rats expressing HLA-B27 and human β2m: an animal model of HLA-B27-associated human disorders. Cell 63:1099-1112, 1990

7. Nickoloff BJ, Turka LA: Immunological functions of non-professional antigen-presenting cells: new insights from studies of T-cell interactions with keratinocytes. Immunol Today 15:464-469, 1994

8. Panayi GS: Immunology of psoriasis and psoriatic arthritis. Bailliere's Clin Rheumatol 8:419-427, 1994

9. Gottlieb SL, Gilleaudeau P, Johnson R, Estes L, Woodworth TG, Gottlieb AB, Krueger JG: Response of psoriasis to a lymphocyte selective toxin (DAB389 IL-2) suggests a primary immune but not keratinocyte, pathogenic basis. Nature Medicine 1:442-447, 1995

10. Leung DYM, Travers JB, Giorno R, et al: Evidence for a streptococcal superantigen-driven process in acute guttate psoriasis. J Clin Invest 96:2106-2112, 1995

11. Chang JCC, Smith LR, Froning KJ, et al: CD8+ T cells in psoriatic lesions preferentially use T-cell receptor Vβ3 and Vβ13.1 genes. Proc Natl Acad Sci (USA) 91:9282-9286, 1994

12. Calabrese LH: Human immunodeficiency virus (HIV) infection and arthritis. Rheum Dis Clin N Am 19:477-488, 1993

13. Brower AC: Psoriatic Arthritis. In Brower AC (ed): Arthritis in Black and White, W.B. Saunders, 1988

14. Greaves MW, Weinstein GD: Treatment of psoriasis. N Engl J Med 332:581-588, 1995

15. Perlman SG, Gerber L, Roberts M, Nigra TP, Barth WF: Photo-chemotherapy and psoriatic arthritis. A prospective study. Ann Intern Med 91:717-722, 1979

16. Espinoza LR, Oui LZ, Espinoza CG, et al: Psoriatic arthritis: clinical response and side effects to methotrexate. J Rheumatol 16:872-877, 1992

17. Dougados M, Van Der Linden S, Leirisalo-Repo M, et al: Sulfasalazine in the treatment of spondyloarthropathy. A randomized, multicenter, double-blind, placebo-controlled study. Arthritis Rheum 38:618-627, 1995

18. Farr M, Kittas GD, Waterhouse L, Jubb R, Felix-Davis D, Bacon AP: Sulfasalazine in psoriatic arthritis: a double-blind placebo-controlled study. Br J Rheumatol 29:46-49, 1990

19. Pioro MH, Cash JM: Treatment of refractory psoriatic arthritis. Rheum Dis Clin N Am 21:129-149, 1995

20. Gladman DD, Stafford-Brady F, Chang HC, Levandowski K, Russel LM: Longitudinal study of clinical and radiological progression in psoriatic arthritis. J Rheumatol 17:809-812, 1990

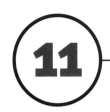

SERONEGATIVE SPONDYLOARTHROPATHIES

A. EPIDEMIOLOGY, PATHOLOGY, AND PATHOGENESIS

The seronegative spondyloarthropathies are an interrelated group of multisystem inflammatory disorders. As rheumatic disorders, they affect the spine, peripheral joints, periarticular structures, or all three. They are also variably associated with characteristic extra-articular manifestations, which include acute or chronic gastrointestinal or genitourinary inflammation, sometimes due to bacterial infection; anterior ocular inflammation; psoriasiform skin and nail lesions; and, uncommonly, lesions of the aortic root, cardiac conduction system, and pulmonary apices (1). Most but not all of these disorders show an increased prevalence among individuals who have inherited the HLA-B27 gene.

Recognized diagnostic entities within the spondyloarthropathies include ankylosing spondylitis (AS), reactive arthritis, spondylitis and peripheral arthritis associated with psoriasis or inflammatory bowel disease, juvenile onset spondyloarthropathy, and a variety of less easily classifiable disorders often termed *undifferentiated spondyloarthropathy* or, simply, *spondyloarthropathy* (Table 11A-1). Sets of diagnostic criteria for the various spondyloarthropathies have been put forth during the past three decades. The most recent additions are criteria for the undifferentiated disorders, proposed by the European Spondyloarthropathy Study Group (2) (see Appendix I). In none of these diseases is the etiology or pathogenesis well understood. Any concept of their pathogenesis must explain, on the one hand, the striking association that most of the disorders share with HLA-B27, and, on the other hand, the observation that B27 by itself seems neither universally necessary nor sufficient for the development of any of the individual diseases. The association of the various disorders with B27 is summarized in Table 11A-2.

EPIDEMIOLOGY

Among the spondyloarthropathies, AS has been the most extensively studied disorder in epidemiologic surveys. It is estimated that the prevalence of AS in white North Americans is 0.1%–0.2%. In large population surveys in Holland and Australia, 1%–2% of adults inheriting HLA-B27 were found to have AS. In contrast, in families of patients with AS, 10%–20% of adult first-degree relatives inheriting HLA-B27 have been found to have the disease. The concordance rate of AS in identical twins is estimated to be 60% or less (3). These epidemiologic findings indicate that both genetic and environmental factors play a role in the pathogenesis of the disease, and that the genetic factors may include allelic genes in addition to HLA-B27. Recent evidence that certain clinical subsets of the spondyloarthropathies show some association with HLA-encoded alleles other than B27 seems to support this latter concept (4,5).

Epidemiology of HLA-B27

HLA-B27 is a serologically defined allele of the HLA-B locus, one of the three classical HLA loci encoding class I major histocompatibility complex (MHC) gene products (HLA-A, B, and C), which are 44-kD molecules expressed on cell surfaces in noncovalent association with β_2-microglobulin (β_2m). Eleven allelic subtypes of B27 have been identified, designated B*2701 through B*2711 (1, 5–7). B*2705 is the predominant subtype in most non-Asian populations, whereas B*2704 is the most prevalent subtype in Chinese and several other Asian populations (5) (see Appendix IV). The prevalence of B27 in different racial groups is indicated in Table 11A-3.

It is generally accepted that the B27 molecule itself is involved in disease pathogenesis. This supposition is based on a large body of indirect evidence from clinical epidemiology and on the direct demonstration that transgenic rats expressing HLA-B*2705 spontaneously develop a broad spectrum of disease manifestations resembling human B27-associated disease. The propensity of the B27 molecule to induce disease thus presumably derives from one or more unique features of its structure. It might therefore be expected that analysis of the structure–function relationships of the B27 molecule and a detailed dissection of its unique features should provide insight into its role in the pathogenesis of the spondyloarthropathies. Such investigations are the focus of many researchers. It is striking that strong associations have been found between the spondyloarthropathies and several of the B27 subtypes, and yet there is no persuasive evidence thus far that any B27-related disease is associated preferentially with one or more of the B27 subtypes. A firm association with both AS and reactive arthritis, based on large population surveys, has been shown for B*2702, -04, and -05, and there is anecdotal association with B*2701, -03, -06, and -07. B*2708, -09, -10, and -11 have only recently been described, and no decisive data regarding disease association are yet available for these subtypes.

Structure and Function of HLA-B27

The surface-expressed class I molecule consists of a complex of HLA-encoded heavy chain, β_2m, and endogenously synthesized peptide, usually a nonamer (7). The complex is assembled during biosynthesis in the endoplasmic reticulum so that the heavy chain α_1 and α_2 domains are folded to form a cleft in which the peptide is bound. The polymorphic residues along the antigen binding cleft form six pockets, A through F, that accommodate side chains of the bound peptide. In this way, a distinct spectrum of peptides binds each different class I allele. The peptides can be derived from either normal cellular constituents or intracellular infectious agents or tumors. The bound peptides are displayed along with the class I molecule itself on cell surfaces, where they can be recognized as either self or foreign by T lymphocytes. The same molecular structure is also thought to participate in thymic selection.

The consensus B27 sequence shared by the different B27 subtypes contains a cluster of amino acids within the pep-

(Table 11A-1)

Comparison of ankylosing spondylitis and related disorders

	Disorder				
Characteristic	Ankylosing Spondylitis	Reactive Arthritis (Reiter's Syndrome)	Juvenile Spondyl-oarthropathy	Psoriatic Arthropathy*	Enteropathic Arthropathy†
Usual age at onset	Young adult <40	Young to middle-age adult	Childhood onset, ages 8 to 18	Young to middle-age adult	Young to middle-age adult
Sex ratio	3 times more common in males	Predominantly males	Predominantly males	Equally distributed	Equally distributed
Usual pattern of onset	Gradual	Acute	Variable	Variable	Gradual
Sacroiliitis or spondylitis	Virtually 100%	<50%	<50%	≈20%	<20%
Symmetry of sacroiliitis	Symmetric	Asymmetric	Variable	Asymmetric	Symmetric
Peripheral joint involvement	≈25%	≈90%	≈90%	≈95%	Frequent
Eye involvement‡	25–30%	Common	20%	Occasional	Occasional
Cardiac involvement	1–4%	5–10%	Rare	Rare	Rare
Skin or nail involvement	None	Common	Uncommon	Virtually 100%	Uncommon
Role of infectious agents as triggers	Unknown	Yes	Unknown	Unknown	Unknown

* About 5–7% of patients with psoriasis develop arthritis, and psoriatic spondylitis accounts for about 5% of all patients with psoriatic arthritis.
† Associated with chronic inflammatory bowel disease.
‡ Predominantly conjunctivitis in reactive arthritis and acute anterior uveitis in the other disorders listed.
Adapted from Arnett Jr. FC, Khan MA, Willkens RF: A new look at ankylosing spondylitis. Patient Care, Nov. 30, 1989, pp 82-101.

tide-binding cleft, including two B27-unique residues Lys70 and Asn97 (except B*2707, which lacks Asn97), as well as His9, Thr24, Glu45, Cys67, Ala69, and Ala71 (6-8). These residues either form or lie contiguous to the B pocket, which is formed by residues 9, 24, 45, and 67, and this pocket constitutes the most distinctive feature of B27 structure. For peptides that bind to B27, arginine at position 2 appears to be a dominant anchor residue, the side chain of which fits snugly into the B pocket, forming hydrogen bonds with the surrounding B27 side chains. However, B27-bound antigenic peptides lacking Arg at position 2 have also been found.

Recently, an unusual allele, HLA-B73, has been identified that has a B pocket very similar to HLA-B27, although differing from B*2705 by 16 amino acids elsewhere in the α_1 and β_2 domains (9). Nothing is yet known regarding poten-

(Table 11A-2)

HLA-B27 associations among the spondyloarthropathies

Disorder	B27 Frequency
Ankylosing spondylitis	90%
With uveitis or aortitis	Nearly 100%
Reactive arthritis	50-80%
With sacroiliitis or uveitis	90%
Juvenile spondyloarthropathy	80%
Inflammatory bowel disease	Not increased
With peripheral arthritis	Not increased
With spondylitis	50%
Psoriasis vulgaris	Not increased
With peripheral arthritis	Not increased
With spondylitis	50%
Unaffected whites	6-8%

Modified from Kahn MA: Ankylosing spondylitis and related spondyl-oarthropathies. In: Spine: State of the Art Review. Philadelphia, Hanley and Belfus, 1990.

(Table 11A-3)

Racial distribution of HLA-B27 subtypes

Subtype	Racial Group	Occurrence of B27 within Group
B*2701	Whites, ? others	Rare
B*2702	Whites (especially Jews)	10%–15%
B*2703	West Africans	60%–70%
B*2704	Asians	50%–90%
B*2705	Whites	85%–90%
	Asians	10%–50%
	West Africans	30%–40%
	African Americans	>90%
	Native Americans, Eskimos	100%
B*2706	Asians	≤10%
B*2707	Asian Indians, Asians	≤10%
B*2708	Not known	Rare
B*2709	Whites, ? others	Rare
B*2710	Whites, ? others	Rare
B*2711	Asians, ? others	Rare

Modified from Kanga et al (5), with permission.

(Table 11A-4)
Evidence linking B27-associated disease with gastrointestinal (GI) inflammation

---

Triggering of reactive arthritis by GI pathogens

Increased prevalence of AS in patients with inflammatory bowel disease

Increased prevalence of inflammatory bowel disease in family members of patients with AS

Acute GI inflammation occurring in the setting of venereally acquired reactive arthritis

Persistent elevation of IgA levels in AS

Presence of microscopic bowel inflammation in the majority of patients with B27-associated spondyloarthropathies, even in the absence of arthropathy

Antigenic cross-reactivity between the HLA-B27 molecule and components of enteric bacteria

Triggering of inflammatory arthritis in rats by injection of peptidoglycan from normal bowel flora

High prevalence of early GI inflammation in transgenic rats expressing HLA-B27

Absence of arthritis and GI inflammation in germ-free B27 transgenic rats

---

tial disease associations with this allele. A central unanswered question regarding the role of B27 in disease pathogenesis is whether B27-associated disease derives from a particular peptide or family of peptides binding to B27, or whether another mechanism is involved that is independent of peptide specificity.

PATHOLOGY

Sacroiliitis is the pathologic hallmark and usually one of the earliest manifestations of AS. The early lesion consists of subchondral granulation tissue that ultimately erodes the joint, which is gradually replaced by fibrocartilage regeneration and then by ossification. The initial lesion in the spine is thought to consist of inflammatory granulation tissue at the junction of the annulus fibrosus of the intervertebral disc and the margin of vertebral bone. The outer annular fibers may eventually be replaced by bone, forming a syndesmophyte. Ascending progression of this process leads to the *bamboo spine* observed radiographically. Other lesions in the spine include diffuse osteoporosis, erosion of vertebral bodies at the disc margin (Romanus lesion), "squaring" of vertebrae, and inflammation and destruction of the disc-bone border. Inflammatory arthritis of the apophyseal joints is common, with erosion progressing to bony ankylosis. Similar axial pathology can occur in the other spondyloarthropathies as well, although with some differences, which will be discussed under the individual syndromes.

The pathology of peripheral joint arthritis in AS shows synovial hyperplasia, lymphoid infiltration, and pannus formation, but the process lacks a number of features commonly seen in rheumatoid arthritis, including proliferation of synovial villi, fibrin deposits, and ulceration. Central cartilaginous erosions due to proliferation of subchondral granulation tissue is a common finding in AS. Similar synovial pathology is seen in the other spondyloarthropathies.

Enthesitis, ie, inflammation at sites of tendinous or ligamentous attachment to bone, is another pathologic hallmark of the spondyloarthropathies. In AS, it is especially common at sites localized around the spine and pelvis, where it may eventually undergo ossification. In the other spondyloarthropathies, enthesitis is more common at peripheral sites, such as the calcaneal attachment of the Achilles tendon.

PATHOGENESIS
Microbes and Reactive Arthritis

Reactive arthritis has traditionally been considered a sterile inflammatory response to an infection remote from the site of inflammation. This concept was based on the consistent failure to culture the inciting organisms from inflamed joints. Recent studies have indicated that, although intact organisms appear to be absent from the inflamed joints, antigens derived from these organisms can indeed be detected, largely within intrasynovial cells, by immunofluorescence or electron microscopy (10, 11). This phenomenon has been demonstrated for *Chlamydia trachomatis*, *Yersinia enterocolitica*, and *Salmonella typhimurium Shigella flexneri*. In cases of disease induced by *Yersinia* and by *Chlamydia*, antigen has been detected within synovial cells or tissue years after the acute attack. Thus, persistence of microbial antigens is likely to play an important role in the pathogenesis of the acute and chronic inflammation characteristic of reactive arthritis. How these antigens reach the joints, and possibly other sites of inflammation such as periarticular structures and the anterior ocular chamber, is not known. The persistence of *C. trachomatis* within joints appears to be qualitatively different from that of the other known triggering organisms, because it is only in *C. trachomatis* infection that synovium-associated microbial nucleic acid has been detected, along with evidence of bacterial replication (11).

In addition to persistence of the triggering agents, the pathogenesis of reactive arthritis is also associated with the presence of T cells within synovial fluid with antigenic specificity for the specific microbial triggers (12). Most such T cells that have been analyzed are CD4+ CD8- and MHC class II-restricted. However, B27-restricted CD4- CD8+ and MHC-unrestricted γδ T cells have also been identified. The antigenic targets of the CD4+ T cells include, in the case of *C. trachomatis*, an 18-kD histone protein, a 61-kD heat shock protein, and an as yet unidentified 30-kD protein; in *Y. enterocolitica* infection, the antigenic targets are the β subunit of urease and the 50S subunit of the ribosomal L23 protein.

Despite the evidence for bacterial persistence in reactive arthritis, trials of long-term antibiotic therapy for these patients have been disappointing (13).

Spondyloarthropathies and the Gut

A large body of evidence, summarized in Table 11A-4, suggests an intimate association between the pathogenesis of the B27-associated diseases and intestinal bacteria or intestinal inflammation. Several important questions will need to be answered before the basis for this connection can be understood. Perhaps most fundamental is the question of whether some gut-related process is a necessary precursor to the development of some or all of the spondyloarthropathies. Furthermore, it is not yet known whether the usually mild and often asymptomatic inflammation seen in patients with B27-associated arthropathy (14) represents one end of the spectrum of Crohn's disease or ulcerative colitis, or whether it represents an altogether different process. Progress in understanding the link with the gut will undoubtedly help unravel the mystery of the pathogenesis of the spondyloarthropathies.

HLA-B27 and Molecular Mimicry

A few years after the association of B27 with the spondyloarthropathies was established, it was hypothesized that the association might be explained by antigenic mimicry (often termed "molecular mimicry") between the B27 molecule and a triggering microorganism, most likely a Gram-negative bacillus. Although it has never been explained how mimicry of a class I MHC molecule would lead to the anatomically localized disease seen in the spondyloarthropathies, several investigators have sought and obtained evidence that antigenic determinants were shared between HLA-B27 and different bacterial products. Some early reports of mimicry and B27 were questionable, but in recent years this phenomenon has been more convincingly demonstrated (15). Another finding that has remained controversial for almost 20 years is the reported presence of elevated serum antibodies levels, primarily IgA, to *Klebsiella pneumoniae* in patients with AS. There continues to be little clinical or experimental evidence supporting the hypothesis that molecular mimicry plays a role in the pathogenesis of B27-associated disease, and thus the significance of these findings remains unclear.

Transgenic Animals Expressing HLA-B27

Both rats and mice transgenic for HLA-B27 have been extensively investigated. Rats expressing high levels of B27 and human β_2m show striking, spontaneously arising inflammatory abnormalities. These include peripheral and axial arthritis, gastrointestinal inflammation and diarrhea, psoriatic-like skin changes, cardiac inflammation, and genital inflammation in males. Histologically, the joint, gut, skin, and heart lesions resemble the lesions seen in B27-associated disease in humans. These findings provide direct evidence that the HLA-B27 molecule participates in disease pathogenesis (16, 17). The gut and joint abnormalities in these rats are prevented by raising the rats in a germ-free environment (18). This finding suggests that normal gut bacteria, in addition to the pathogens described above, may also participate in the pathogenesis of the spondyloarthropathies.

Early studies with B27 transgenic mice failed to identify any B27-specific disease phenotype. However, it has recently been observed that the presence of the B27 gene increases the incidence of spontaneous ankylosis of the tarsal joints in certain strains of mice (19). Moreover, B27 transgenic mice lacking mouse β_2-microglobulin have been reported to show a male-predominant peripheral arthritis (20, 21). Continued investigation of these animal models should provide useful insight into the pathogenesis, therapy, and prevention of the spondyloarthropathies.

SUMMARY

A large collection of observations has accumulated regarding the pathogenesis of the spondyloarthropathies, concurrent with advances in the diagnosis and management of these disorders. Nonetheless, an experimentally validated model of pathogenesis that integrates the available data has so far proved elusive (22). The role of the B27 molecule remains to be clarified. Perhaps an even greater enigma of the

spondyloarthropathies is their pathologic diversity. Any complete answer to the role of B27 must explain how the same molecule can predispose to the acute, microbially triggered, asymmetric peripheral arthritis and extra-articular phenomena of reactive arthritis, on the one hand, and to the insidious, progressive axial phenomena of AS, on the other. Such an answer also must explain how virtually the same clinical manifestations can occur in the absence of B27. To investigators in this area, these questions loom as the challenge for the future.

JOEL D. TAUROG, MD

1. Calin A , Taurog JD, (eds): The Spondarthritides. Oxford University Press: Oxford, UK, 1997

2. Dougados M, van der Linden S, Juhlin R, et al: The European Spondyloarthropathy Study Group preliminary criteria for the classification of spondyloarthropathy. Arthritis Rheum 34:1218-1227, 1991

3. Jarvinen P: Occurrence of ankylosing spondylitis in a nationwide series of twins. Arthritis Rheum 38:381-383, 1995

4. Rubin LA, Amos CI, Wade JA, et al: Investigating the genetic basis for ankylosing spondylitis: linkage studies with the major histocompatibility complex region. Arthritis Rheum 37:1212-1220, 1994

5. Kanga U, Mehra NK, Larrea CL, Lardy NM, Kumar A, Feltkamp TEW: Seronegative spondyloarthropathies and HLA-B27 subtypes: a study in Asian Indians. Clinical Rheumatol 15(Suppl 1):13-18, 1996

6. Hildebrand WH, Domena JD, Shen SY, et al: The HLA-B7Qui antigen is encoded by a new subtype of HLA-B27 (B*2708). Tissue Antigens 44:47-51, 1994

7. Lopez de Castro JA: Structural polymorphism and function of HLA-B27. Curr Opin Rheumatol 7:270-278, 1995

8. Madden DR, Gorga JC, Strominger JL, Wiley DC: The three-dimensional structure of HLA-B27 at 2.1Å resolution suggests a general mechanism for tight peptide binding to MHC. Cell 70:1035-1048, 1992

9. Parham P, Arnett KL, Adams EJ, et al: The HLA-B73 antigen has a most unusual structure that defines a second lineage of HLA-B alleles. Tissue Antigens 43:302-313, 1994

10. Granfors K, Jalkanen S, Von Essen R, et al: Yersinia antigens in synovial-fluid cells from patients with reactive arthritis. N Engl J Med 320:216-221, 1989

11. Nanagara R, Li F, Beutler A, Hudson A, Schumacher HR, Jr: Alteration of *Chlamydia trachomatis* biologic behavior in synovial membranes: suppression of surface antigen production in reactive arthritis and Reiter's syndrome. Arthritis Rheum 38:1410-7, 1995

12. Burmester GR, Daser A, Kamradt T, Krause A, Mitchison NA, Sieper J, Wolf N: Immunology of reactive arthritides. Annu Rev Immunol 13:229-250, 1995

13. Leirisalo-Repo M: Are antibiotics of any use in reactive arthritis? APMIS 101:575-581, 1993

14. Mielants H, Veys EM, Cuvelier C, et al: The evolution of spondyloarthropathies in relation to gut histology #3. Relation between gut and joint. J Rheumatol 22:2279-2284, 1995

15. Scofield RH, Kurien B, Gross T, Warren WL, Harley JB: HLA-B27 binding of peptide from its own sequence and similar peptides from bacteria: implications for spondyloarthropathies. Lancet 345:1542-1544, 1995

16. Hammer RE, Maika SD, Richardson JA, Tang J-P, Taurog JD: Spontaneous inflammatory disease in transgenic rats expressing HLA-B27 and human β_2-m: an animal model of HLA-B27-associated human disorders. Cell 63:1099-1112, 1990

17. Taurog JD, Hammer RE: Experimental spondyloarthropathy in HLA-B27 transgenic rats. Clinical Rheumatol 15(Suppl 1):22-27, 1996

18. Taurog JD, Richardson JA, Croft JT, et al: The germfree state prevents development of gut and joint inflammatory disease in *HLA-B27* transgenic rats. J Exp Med 180:2359-2364, 1994

19. Weinreich S, Eulderink F, Capkova J, et al: HLA-B27 as a relative risk factor in ankylosing enthesopathy in transgenic mice. Human Immunol 42:103-115, 1995

20. Khare SD, Luthra HS, David CS: Spontaneous inflammatory arthritis in HLA-B27 transgenic mice lacking β_2-microglobulin: a model of human spondyloarthropathies. J Exp Med 182:1153-1158, 1995

21. Khare SD, Hansen J, Luthra HS, David CS: HLA-B27 heavy chains contribute to spontaneous inflammatory disease in B27/human β_2-microglobulin double transgenic mice transgenic mice with disrupted mouse β_2m. J Clin Invest 98:2746-2763, 1996

22. Sieper J, Braun J: Pathogenesis of spondyloarthropathies: persistent bacterial antigen, autoimmunity, or both? Arthritis Rheum 38:1547-1554, 1995

B. REACTIVE ARTHRITIS (REITER'S SYNDROME) AND ENTEROPATHIC ARTHRITIS

REACTIVE ARTHRITIS (REITER'S SYNDROME)

Reactive arthritis and Reiter's syndrome are both designations for a form of peripheral arthritis, often accompanied by one or more extra-articular manifestations, which appear shortly after certain infections of the genitourinary or gastrointestinal tracts. The majority of affected individuals, usually young men, have inherited the human leukocyte antigen (HLA) B27. Reiter's syndrome originally referred to the clinical triad of nongonococcal urethritis, conjunctivitis, and arthritis that occurred in a young German officer after a bout of bloody dysentery and reported by Hans Reiter in 1916 (1). Subsequently, more cases were observed following epidemics or sporadic outbreaks of diarrheal illnesses caused by *Shigella, Salmonella,* and *Campylobacter* microorganisms, as well as by venereally acquired genitourinary infections, usually *Chlamydia trachomatis* (2). The term *reactive arthritis* was first used in 1967 to describe similar cases following *Yersinia* gastroenteritis (3).

A high frequency of HLA-B27 was discovered in patients with Reiter's syndrome or reactive arthritis in 1973–1974 (2). HLA-B27 typing was utilized to confirm the concept that Reiter's syndrome occurred frequently in the absence of clinically apparent urethritis or conjunctivitis (incomplete Reiter's syndrome) (4). Increasingly, the term "reactive arthritis" is supplanting the use of the designation Reiter's syndrome, although the terms should be considered synonymous. Because of many overlapping clinical, epidemiologic, and genetic features, reactive arthritis is classified as a seronegative spondyloarthropathy that is distinct from rheumatoid arthritis (Table 11B-1) (5).

Clinical Presentation

Reactive arthritis typically begins acutely 2–4 weeks after venereal infections or bouts of gastroenteritis (2). A history of either in the month preceding onset is useful diagnostically, but frequently venereal infection is asymptomatic. Most endemic cases occur in young men (9:1) and are believed to result from venereally acquired infections (2,6), whereas cases following food-borne enteric infections affect both genders equally. Whites are affected more commonly than African Americans or other racial groups who have a lower frequency of HLA-B27. Recent preliminary evidence suggests that preceding respiratory infections with *Chlamydia pneumoniae* also may trigger the disease (7).

Nongonococcal urethritis, when present, is usually the first manifestation and occurs in both postvenereal or postenteric forms of the disease. Mild dysuria and a mucopurulent urethral discharge are most typical in men, but occasionally prostatitis and/or epididymitis are present. Women may have dysuria, vaginal discharge, and purulent cervicitis and/or vaginitis. Patients who are asymptomatic for genital inflammation are often found to have sterile pyuria, especially when a first-voided morning urine sample is examined. *C. trachomatis* is frequently the cause of the urethritis or cervicitis and is the triggering agent of the reactive arthritis. *Neisseria gonorrhoeae* also may be found in the genital tract, as it frequently coexists with chlamydia infections, but does not cause reactive arthritis. *Ureaplasma urealyticum* may be a cause of reactive arthritis, but a definite etiologic role has not been established (8). Sterile genital inflammation may occur in postenteric reactive arthritis as an inherent disease feature and is unrelated to any sexually acquired infection.

Conjunctivitis, when present, usually accompanies or follows urethritis by several days. Since symptoms and signs are often mild and transient, patients should be questioned about recent crusting of the eyelids, especially in the morning, which suggests subtle ocular inflammation. Some patients develop obvious conjunctival redness, usually bilateral, with a burning sensation and exudation. Acute anterior uveitis (iritis), typically affecting one eye, may occur contemporaneously with, later than, or instead of conjunctivitis and is characterized by severe ocular erythema, pain, and photophobia.

The articular manifestations typically appear last, often after symptoms of urethral and ocular inflammation have subsided. In cases following gastroenteritis, the bowel symptoms usually have resolved 1–3 weeks earlier, and the inciting enteric pathogen cannot be cultured from the stool.

Articular Manifestations

Reactive arthritis is characteristically additive, asymmetric, and oligoarticular, affecting an average of four joints. Lower limb joints, especially knees, ankles, and small joints of the feet, are affected more commonly than those of the upper extremities (wrists, elbows, and hand joints). In fact, at least one third of patients have an exclusively lower limb arthritis; only rarely does a patient have upper extremity involvement alone (4). Hip disease is uncommon, but sternoclavicular, shoulder, and temporomandibular joints are occasionally affected.

Joints affected with reactive arthritis are typically swollen, warm, tender, and painful on active and passive movement. They often display a dusky blue discoloration or frank erythema accompanied by exquisite tenderness suggestive of a septic joint. When toes or fingers are affected, the entire digit is usually diffusely swollen, a phenomenon referred to as sausage digits or *dactylitis.*

In addition to arthritis, inflammation also typically occurs at bony sites where tendons, ligaments, or fascia have their attachments or insertions (entheses). Enthesitis (or enthesopathy) most commonly occurs at the insertions of the plantar aponeurosis and Achilles tendon on the calcaneus, thus leading to one of the most frequent, distinctive, and disabling manifestations of the disease—heel pain. Other common sites for enthesitis include ischial tuberosities, iliac crests, tibial tuberosities, and ribs, thus causing musculoskeletal pain at sites other than joints.

Low-back and buttock pain are also common in reactive arthritis, occurring in approximately 50% of cases. Low-back symptoms are probably caused primarily by sacroiliac or other spinal joint involvement; however, radiographically

Frequencies of demographic, clinical, laboratory and radiographic features in 69 consecutive patients with Reiter's syndrome (reactive arthritis) evaluated at a referral medical center

	Reiter's Syndrome
Demographic features	
Age at onset	
Range	13–60 years
Mean	26 years
Median	24 years
Male	87%
Race	
White	80%
African American	20%
Preceding diarrhea	6%
Clinical features	
Nongonococcal urethritis	46%
Conjunctivitis	31%
Peripheral arthritis	
Upper limbs only	0
Lower limbs only	39%
Both upper and lower limbs	61%
Knees	68%
Ankles	49%
Small joints of feet	64%
Small joints of hands	42%
Wrists	25%
Elbows	22%
Shoulders	19%
Temporomandibular joints	6%
Sternoclavicular joints	6%
Hips	<1%
Mean no. of affected joints	4.5
Sausage digits	52%
Heel pain	61%
x-ray changes of calcaneus	16%
Spinal arthritis	
Low-back pain	61%
Sacroiliitis (on x-ray)	17%
Spondylitis (on x-ray)	7%
Mucocutaneous lesions (any)	43%
Keratoderma blennorrhagicum	23%
Circinate balanitis	26%
Oral ulcers	14%
Nail changes	13%
Other clinical features	
Fever ≥101°F	32%
Weight loss (≥4.5 kg)	19%
Uveitis	12%
Aortitis	6%
Amyloidosis	<1%
Laboratory findings	
Anemia	39%
Leukocytosis (>10,000/mm³)	34%
Thrombocytosis (>400,000/mm³)	27%
Elevated erythrocyte sedimentation rate	72%
Rheumatoid factor	0
HLA-B27	81%

Adapted from Arnett (4), with permission.

demonstrable sacroiliitis eventually develops in only 20% of patients. Other potential causes of back pain are enthesitis or prostatitis. With time, approximately 10% of patients progress to clinically evident ankylosing spondylitis, but it is unclear whether this represents the continuation of reactive arthritis or the independent development of ankylosing spondylitis, which also is genetically linked to HLA-B27 (4,9).

Extra-Articular Manifestations

Several other mucocutaneous and visceral manifestations are highly distinctive of reactive arthritis. *Keratoderma blennorrhagicum* is a papulosquamous skin rash that appears most commonly on the soles or palms but may affect any cutaneous area (Fig. 11B-1). Raised, waxy, papular lesions that resemble mollusk shells or pustules are the usual earliest findings. Later, these lesions become hyperkeratotic and scaly, often coalescing into large patches indistinguishable from psoriasis. In fact, keratoderma blennorrhagicum is a form of pustular psoriasis, which may occur in the absence of reactive arthritis, but is also associated with HLA-B27. In a few patients with reactive arthritis, the rash affects large areas of the skin and/or evolves into a generalized exfoliative dermatitis.

The toe and/or finger nails also may become thickened, opacified and crumble, thus resembling mycotic infection or psoriatic onychodystrophy. Unlike in psoriasis, however, "Reiter's nails" do not demonstrate pitting. *Circinate balanitis* is the characteristic lesion involving the glans or shaft of the penis. In uncircumcised men, the lesions appear as moist, shallow ulcers that are often serpiginous and surround the meatus. In circumcised men, the rash is dry, plaque-like, hyperkeratotic, and resembles keratoderma or psoriasis (Fig. 11-2). Oral ulcers, which are shallow and usually painless, may appear on the tongue or hard palate. The patient may be unaware of their presence. All of these mucocutaneous manifestations are similar histopathologically, showing spongiosiform changes similar to psoriasis and differing only in the degree of hyperkeratosis. Profound weight loss and even cachexia occurs in some patients, and its cause is unknown.

Acute anterior uveitis occurs episodically in 20% of patients at any time during the course of reactive arthritis. A

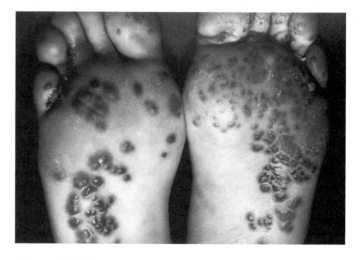

(Figure 11B-1)
Typical cutaneous lesions of keratoderma blennorrhagicum on feet of a patient with Reiter's syndrome.

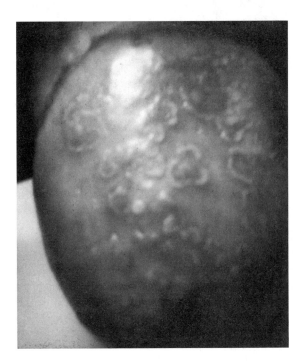

(Figure 11B-2)
Circinate balanitis in a patient with Reiter's syndrome.

few patients develop chronic uveitis that ultimately results in visual impairment or loss.

Aortitis occurs in 1%–2% of patients, typically after long-standing active arthritis, but occasionally earlier during the acute phase. Aortic valve regurgitation and heart block are the clinical consequences of inflammatory thickening of the proximal aortic root and valves which may extend to the atrioventricular node or adjacent conducting system (10). Less commonly, the interventricular septum is also involved, leading to mitral valve regurgitation. The majority of patients with aortic regurgitation have relentless progression of valvular incompetence leading to left-sided heart failure and ultimately require aortic valve replacement. Those who develop complete heart block need immediate cardiac pacemaker placement.

Amyloidosis of the *serum amyloid* A variety has been reported in a few cases and usually presents as proteinuria or the nephrotic syndrome. An IgA nephropathy occurs occasionally.

Some patients with Reiter's syndrome have been reported to have neurologic complications, including peripheral neuropathies, encephalopathy, and transverse myelitis. However, it is unclear whether these nervous system syndromes were truly related to the reactive arthritis process.

Clinical Course and Prognosis

Reactive arthritis runs a self-limited course of from 3 to 12 months in the majority of patients; however, some studies suggest that many patients continue to be plagued by minor residual musculoskeletal symptoms (9,11). Relapses may occur in up to 15% of cases, but it is unclear whether this is the result of reinfection. Approximately 15% of patients continue to have chronic, often destructive and disabling arthritis or enthesitis. Long-term disability is most often related to chronic foot pain or deformities from arthritis, heel pain (enthesitis), or vision loss. Ankylosing spondylitis develops in approximately 10% of cases. Mortality from reactive arthri-

tis is infrequent and results most often from the cardiac complications or amyloidosis (2).

Relation to HIV Infection

Reiter's syndrome has been reported frequently in patients with human immunodeficiency virus (HIV) infection (12). Recent epidemiologic surveys suggest that HIV itself does not cause the disease, but rather, the association is an indirect one due to sexually acquired diseases, either *C. trachomatis* or enteric pathogens, which are common to both diseases (13).

Observations that Reiter's syndrome is likely to be more severe in HIV-positive individuals, especially those with AIDS, are probably correct. In such patients, severe polyarticular arthritis and disabling enthesitis, as well as extensive cutaneous manifestations, have been described. HLA-B27 occurs in the same frequency (approximately 75%) in HIV-positive patients with Reiter's syndrome as in HIV-negative cases (12).

Laboratory Features

A mild normocytic, normochromic anemia due to chronic inflammation is not uncommon. Leukocytosis with total white blood cell counts ranging from 10,000 to 15,000/mm³ is typical during the acute phase, and thrombocytosis with platelet counts of 400,000-600,000/mm³ range is not unusual. Acute phase reactants, including C-reactive protein and erythrocyte sedimentation rate, are typically abnormal. Serum globulins, especially IgA, are frequently elevated. A recent study has shown that the IgA antibodies are directed against the specific bacterium triggering the disease (14). When clinically available, testing for specific bacterial IgA antibodies may be useful in diagnosis. Tests for rheumatoid factor and antinuclear antibodies are negative. Typing for HLA-B27 is positive in two-thirds to three-quarters of white patients with reactive arthritis, but is less common (30%–50%) in African Americans (15). HLA-B27 is more likely to be found in patients with a chronic or relapsing course, as well as those with complicating sacroiliitis, spondylitis, iritis, or aortitis (9). Among B27-negative patients with reactive arthritis, HLA-B7 cross-reactive antigens are often reported, including HLA-B7, B22 (now B54, B55, or B56), B40 (now B60), or B42 (15).

Synovial fluid typically shows highly inflammatory changes including turbidity, poor viscosity or poor mucin clot tests, white blood cell counts ranging from 5,000 to 50,000/mm³ with a polymorphonuclear cell predominance, and high total protein and complement levels. The synovial fluid glucose level, in contrast to a true septic arthritis, is not significantly reduced compared with serum levels. Gram stains show no microorganisms, and bacterial cultures are sterile. Occasionally, large mononuclear cells containing several ingested polymorphonuclear leukocytes containing inclusion bodies are seen and have been called "Reiter's cells." Recent data now suggest that the intracellular inclusions represent bacterial antigens (16). In fact, bacterial antigens and perhaps viable microorganisms have been detected in synovial fluid, but more often in synovial tissue, in patients with reactive arthritis, even after years of disease (16,17). Research techniques such as polymerase chain reaction to detect bacterial RNA or DNA in joint fluid and tissue can identify the specific bacteria causing reactive arthritis. These technologies are likely to be adapted for clinical testing in the near future.

Radiographic Manifestations

Abnormalities on joint X-ray should not be expected early in disease, but only after symptoms have been present for at least several months. The most distinctive radiographic findings are a fluffy periosteal reaction and, at times, bony erosions of the calcaneus at the insertions of the plantar and/or Achilles tendons in patients who have symptoms of heel pain (Fig. 11B-3). Similar radiographic findings occasionally may be found in patients with ankylosing spondylitis or psoriatic arthritis. Periostitis and new bone formation also may be seen at other symptomatic sites of enthesitis or around affected joints or adjacent bony shafts. Such changes are most commonly seen in the feet, involving metatarsophalangeal bones and joints where there may be joint destruction with or without bony fusion across former joints. "Pencil-in-cup" deformities of small joints in feet or hands occasionally are found resembling deformities more typically seen in psoriatic arthritis.

Spinal radiographic abnormalities include sacroiliitis, which is often unilateral, and atypical ossified ligaments (syndesmophytes), which tend to be more asymmetrical and spotty than those seen in ankylosing spondylitis.

Diagnosis

The diagnosis of reactive arthritis or Reiter's syndrome is made on clinical grounds, based on the disease manifestations and laboratory findings. Preliminary criteria for Reiter's syndrome were developed by the American College of Rheumatology (ACR), which defined the disease as the combination of nongonococcal urethritis or cervicitis and a sterile peripheral arthritis occurring within 1 month of one another. As about 40% of patients have no symptoms or signs of genital inflammation, these criteria are not very sensitive (4). The presence of a seronegative, asymmetrical oligoarthritis, especially in a young person, should alert the physician to the possibility of this syndrome. The presence of an antecedent diarrheal illness or venereal exposure adds additional weight to the diagnosis, but is often absent. The presence of heel pain or other symptoms of enthesitis, dactylitis, or any of the mucocutaneous lesions increase the likelihood of reactive arthritis. Testing for HLA-B27 may be a useful adjunct in diagnosis and shows a reasonable predictive value only if the clinical data support a strong likelihood of the disease. However, only two-thirds of white patients with reactive arthritis are B27-positive (15).

Care must be taken to exclude gonococcal and other forms of septic arthritis. All patients with symptoms or signs of genital tract inflammation should have urethral or cervical smears tested for both N. gonorrhoeae and C. trachomatis using Gram's stain, culture, or molecular probe. When possible, synovial fluid should also be cultured for N. gonorrhoeae and other pathogens, since gonococcal or other septic arthritides may mimic reactive arthritis. Psoriatic arthritis may be difficult or impossible to discriminate from reactive arthritis, although it is usually a more indolent process. The presence of distal interphalangeal joint involvement, pitting of the nails, and plaque-like psoriatic lesions over elbows or knees are strongly supportive of psoriatic arthritis. Atypical presentations of ankylosing spondylitis beginning with peripheral joint symptoms or so-called undifferentiated spondyloarthropathies, which have overlapping clinical features of several of these diseases, may be impossible to distinguish from reactive arthritis unless a specific bacterium can be identified (18).

IDIOPATHIC INFLAMMATORY BOWEL DISEASE
Clinical Features

Peripheral arthritis occurs in approximately 10%–20% of patients with Crohn's disease or ulcerative colitis. Not infrequently, arthritis with or without other extraintestinal manifestations is the first clinical symptom of inflammatory bowel disease (IBD), especially Crohn's disease. However, in retrospect, the patient may recall subtle symptoms of abdominal cramping, occasional diarrhea, and weight loss (19). IBD most often affects young adults and children, both males and females.

The typical pattern of joint inflammation is migratory arthralgias or arthritis. Less often, the arthritis is additive, oligoarticular, usually asymmetric, and affects predominantly the lower extremity joints. Knees, ankles, and feet are most commonly affected, but any peripheral joint may be involved, including the hip. Large-joint effusions, especially of the knee, are common. Deformities are rare. Peripheral arthritis always reflects active IBD and typically subsides with treatment of the bowel inflammation. In fact, surgical colectomy in ulcerative colitis results in permanent remission of the arthritis; however this is not the case in Crohn's disease, in which other bowel areas may be affected. Rare instances of a chronic granulomatous synovitis, which may be destructive, have been described in Crohn's disease. HLA-B27 is not associated with the peripheral arthritis of IBD or with Crohn's disease or ulcerative colitis (15).

Spinal arthritis, including sacroiliitis or frank spondylitis, occurs in approximately 10% of IBD patients and is frequently asymptomatic (19). Males develop this complication more often than females (3:1). Unlike the peripheral arthritis, spondylitis does not necessarily reflect active bowel inflammation, and it tends to run an independent course. Even colectomy does not halt its progression. The clinical symptoms, signs, and radiographic features of IBD-associated spondylitis are indistinguishable from those of idiopathic ankylosing spondylitis, except that HLA-B27 is found much less frequently in the former (approximately 50%).

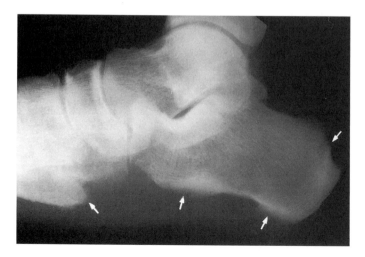

(Figure 11B-3)
Radiograph of the lateral foot in a patient with Reiter's syndrome and heel pain. Arrows indicate enthesitis with periosteal reaction (arrows) at sites of tendon insertions.

Extra-articular manifestations of IBD also typically reflect active bowel disease and tend to occur at the same time as the peripheral arthritis. The most common cutaneous complication of Crohn's disease is erythema nodosum, while that of ulcerative colitis is pyoderma gangrenosa. Painful, deep oral ulcers may occur in both disorders, as may attacks of acute anterior uveitis. Fever and weight loss also are common during active disease periods.

Laboratory Features

Anemia is common in IBD and reflects both chronic inflammation and chronic gastrointestinal blood loss. Leukocytosis is also common, and an extreme thrombocytosis (platelet counts of 700,000/mm³ to more than 1 million/mm³) sometimes occurs. Acute-phase reactants, such as C-reactive protein and erythrocyte sedimentation rate, are typically elevated. Serum rheumatoid factor and antinuclear antibodies are not found; however, positive tests for antineutrophil cytoplasmic antibodies (ANCA), usually pANCA, have been reported in approximately 60% of patients with ulcerative colitis and less commonly in Crohn's disease (20). pANCA is directed against lactoferrin autoantigens rather than proteinase-3 (cANCA) or myeloperoxidase (the usual ANCA). The frequency of HLA-B27 is no greater in patients with IBD or with IBD-associated arthritis than in the general population. However, approximately half of the patients with complicating spondylitis are B27 positive (15). Synovial fluid findings have been reported infrequently, but show nonspecific inflammatory changes and are sterile on culture.

INTESTINAL BYPASS ARTHRITIS

A form of peripheral arthritis was recognized earlier to occur frequently in patients undergoing intestinal bypass surgery (jejunocolostomy or jejunoileostomy)—formerly a popular treatment for morbid obesity (21). The arthritis was described as migratory or additive, nondeforming, polyarticular, and symmetrical, becoming chronic in approximately one-third of these patients. Cutaneous vasculitis often accompanied the arthritis, and more serious hepatic, renal, and hematologic complications eventually led to the discontinuation of these procedures.

WHIPPLE'S DISEASE

Whipple's disease is a rare multisystem disease, usually affecting men, that is characterized by fever, diarrhea, steatorrhea, and profound weight loss. A variety of extra-intestinal manifestations may occur, especially joint disease, which can appear as migratory arthralgias or transient episodes of an additive, symmetrical polyarthritis. Rarely, the arthritis is chronic but is typically nondeforming. There are some reports of sacroiliitis and HLA-B27 positivity, but it is unclear whether these are true associations. Other features may include serositis (pleural effusions), lymphadenopathy, cutaneous hyperpigmentation, anterior and/or posterior uveitis, nervous system disease (ocular palsies or encephalopathy), leukocytosis, and thrombocytosis.

Diagnosis traditionally has been based on finding characteristic periodic acid-Schiff staining deposits in macrophages of the small intestine and less commonly in lymph node or joint synovial biopsies. On electron microscopy, rod-shaped bacillary organisms have been seen in the same cells. Although all attempts to culture these organisms have failed, a unique bacterial RNA sequence has been found, which has led to its classification as a Gram-positive actinomycete now named *Tropheryma whippelii*. Thus, Whipple's disease appears to be a systemic infection. Diagnosis is now possible using polymerase chain reaction of affected tissues or even blood samples (22), and remission can be achieved using long-term antibiotic treatment with tetracyclines.

FRANK C. ARNETT, MD

1. Reiter H: Ueber eine bisher unbekannte spirochaeten-infektion (spirochaetosis arthritica). Dtsche Med Wschr 42:1535-1536, 1916
2. Keat A: Reiter's syndrome and reactive arthritis in perspective. N Engl J Med 309:1606-1615, 1983
3. Ahvonen P, Sievers K, Aho K: Arthritis associated with *Yersinia enterocolitica* infection. Acta Rheum Scand 15:232-253, 1967
4. Arnett FC: Incomplete Reiter's syndrome: clinical comparisons with classical triad. Ann Rheum Dis 38(Suppl 1):73-78, 1979
5. Moll JMH, Haslock I, MacRae I, Wright V: Associations between ankylosing spondylitis, psoriatic arthritis, Reiter's disease, the intestinal arthropathies, and Behcet's syndrome. Medicine 53:343-364, 1974
6. Iliopoulos A, Karras D, Ioakimidis D, et al: Change in the epidemiology of Reiter's syndrome (reactive arthritis) in the post-AIDS era? An analysis of cases appearing in the Greek army. J Rheumatol 22:252-254, 1995
7. Braun J, Laitko S, Treharne J, Eggens U, Wu P, Distler A, Sieper J: Chlamydia pneumoniae: a new causative agent of reactive arthritis and undifferentiated oligoarthritis. Ann Rheum Dis 53:100-105, 1994
8. Horowitz S, Horowitz J, Taylor-Robinson D, et al: Ureaplasma urealyticum in Reiter's syndrome. J Rheumatol 21:877-882, 1994
9. Leirsalo M, Skylv G, Kousa M, et al: Followup study on patients with Reiter's disease and reactive arthritis, with special reference to HLA-B27. Arthr Rheum 25:249-258, 1982
10. Bulkley BH, Roberts WC: Ankylosing spondylitis and aortic regurgitation. Circulation 48:1014-1027, 1973
11. Thomson GTD, DeRubeis DA, Hodge MA, Rajanayagam C, Inman RD: Post-salmonella reactive arthritis: late clinical sequelae in a point source cohort. Am J Med 98:13-21, 1995
12. Winchester R, Bernstein DH, Fischer HD, Enlow R, Solomon G: The co-occurrence of Reiter's syndrome and acquired immunodeficiency. Ann Intern Med 106:19-26, 1987
13. Clark MR, Solinger AM, Hochberg MC: Human immunodeficiency virus infection is not associated with Reiter's syndrome: data from three large cohort studies. Rheum Dis Clin North Am 18:267-276, 1992
14. Kingsley G, Panayi G: Antigenic responses in reactive arthritis. Rheum Dis Clin North Am 18:49-66, 1992
15. Arnett FC: Histocompatibility testing in the rheumatic diseases: diagnostic and prognostic implications. Rheum Dis Clin North Am 18:187-202, 1992
16. Granfors K: Do bacterial antigens cause reactive arthritis? Rheum Dis Clin North Am 18:37-48, 1992
17. Nanagara R, Feng LI, Beutler A, Hudson A, Schumacher HR: Alteration of chlamydia trachomatis biologic behavior in synovial membranes. Arthritis Rheum 38:1410-1416, 1995
18. Zeidler H, Mau W, Khan MA: Undifferentiated spondyloarthropathies. Rheum Dis Clin North Am 18:187-202, 1992
19. Gravallese EM, Kantrowitz FG: Arthritic manifestations of inflammatory bowel disease: clinical review. Am J Gastroenterol 83:703-709, 1988
20. Duerr RH, Targan SR, Landers CJ, LaRusso NF, Lindsay KL, Wiesner RH, Shanahan F: Neutrophil cytoplasmic antibodies: a link between primary sclerosing cholangitis and ulcerative colitis. Gastroenterol 100:1385-1391, 1991
21. Stein HB, Schlappner OLA, Boyko W, Gourlay RH, Reeve CE: The intestinal bypass arthritis-dermatitis syndrome. Arthritis Rheum 24:684-689, 1981
22. Lowsky R, Archer GL, Fyles G, et al: Diagnosis of Whipple's disease by molecular analysis of peripheral blood. N Engl J Med 331:1343-1346, 1994

C. ANKYLOSING SPONDYLITIS

Ankylosing spondylitis (AS) is a chronic, systemic inflammatory disorder of the axial skeleton, affecting sacroiliac (SI) joints and the spine. The presence of sacroiliitis is its hallmark. Hip and shoulder joints, and less commonly, peripheral joints or extra-articular structures may also be involved (1). The term is derived from the Greek words *angkylos,* meaning "bent" (the word ankylosis now means joint stiffening or fusion) and *spondylous,* meaning spine. However, spinal ankylosis appears only in very late stages of the disease and may not occur in patients with mild disease. The etiology of AS is as yet not fully understood, but there is a strong genetic predisposition associated with the histocompatibility antigen, HLA-B27 (2). The disease sometimes occurs in association with reactive arthritis (Reiter's syndrome), psoriasis, ulcerative colitis, or Crohn's disease—the so called secondary forms of AS. Most patients, however, show no evidence of these diseases and are characterized as having primary or uncomplicated AS.

The earliest, most typical, consistent findings are seen in the SI joints; other axial sites characteristically affected include discovertebral, apophyseal, costovertebral, and costotransverse joints and the paravertebral ligamentous structures. The inflammation appears to originate in ligamentous and capsular sites of attachment to bones (*enthesitis*), juxta-articular ligamentous structures, and the synovium, articular cartilage, and subchondral bones of involved joints (3). The inflammatory process frequently results in gradual fibrous and bony ankylosis.

CLINICAL FEATURES

The symptoms usually begin in late adolescence or early adulthood; onset after age 45 is uncommon. The disease is three times more common in men than women, and the clinical and radiographic features of the disease probably evolve more slowly in women (4). A small subset of patients have juvenile-onset spondylitis (before age 16), which is relatively more common among Native Americans, Mexican Mestizos, and in many developing countries (5).

The major clinical features of AS can be divided into skeletal and extraskeletal manifestations (Table 11C-1).

Skeletal Manifestations

Back complaints are the first clinical manifestations in approximately 75% of patients with adult-onset AS. The back pain is usually of insidious onset, dull in character, difficult to localize, and felt deep in the gluteal area or the sacroiliac region. Pain at this early stage can be quite severe and accentuated on coughing, sneezing, or sudden twisting of the back. It can be unilateral or intermittent at first, but within a few months it becomes persistent and bilateral. The lower lumbar area becomes stiff and painful and may even be tender. For some patients, pain and stiffness in the lumbar area, rather than the more typical buttock-ache, is the initial symptom. Backache and stiffness tend to worsen after prolonged periods of inactivity, at night or early morning. Patients may experience considerable difficulty in getting out

of bed, rolling sideways to avoid flexing or rotating the spine. Pain may at times interfere with sleep, and some patients have difficulty sleeping well or find it necessary to exercise at night or move about for a few minutes before returning to bed. The back stiffness tends to be eased by moving about, a hot shower, or exercise. Some patients may complain of easy fatigability, perhaps resulting in part from disturbed sleep pattern. The presence of AS should be suspected when the following features in the clinical history are present: insidious onset of back pain and stiffness; onset before age 40 years; persistence of symptoms for more than 3 months; accentuation of back symptoms in the morning or after periods of inactivity; and improvement of back symptoms with exercise.

Occasionally, back pain is absent or too mild to impel the patient to seek medical care. Some patients may complain only of back stiffness, fleeting muscle aches, or musculotendinous tender spots that become worse on exposure to cold or dampness. Such patients are often diagnosed as having "rheumatism" or "fibrositis." Pain in the buttocks or down the back of the thigh can be misdiagnosed as "lumbago" or "sciatica," although neurologic examination is within normal limits. Some patients in the early stages of their disease may have mild constitutional symptoms (eg, anorexia, malaise, weight loss, and even mild fever), especially those with juvenile-onset AS in developing countries.

Enthesitis can result in extra-articular or juxta-articular bony tenderness, a major and often a presenting complaint in some patients, affecting costosternal junctions, spinous processes, iliac crests, greater trochanters, ischial tuberosities, tibial tubercles, Achilles tendon insertion, or the site of plantar fascial attachment to the calcaneus. Recent data indicate that juvenile-onset spondyloarthropathies are much more prevalent than previously realized, and that persistent or recurrent bouts of enthesitis or peripheral arthritis may precede the onset of definite axial disease by many years (5).

The first symptoms may result from involvement of the hips and shoulders. These joints are affected at some stage of disease in one-third of patients, but this is relatively more common among patients with juvenile-onset AS. The in-

(Table 11C-1)
Clinical features of ankylosing spondylitis

Skeletal	Extraskeletal
Axial arthritis, such as sacroiliitis and spondylitis	Eyes (acute iritis)
Arthritis of hip and shoulder joints	Heart and ascending aorta
Peripheral arthritis	Lung (apical fibrosis) Cauda equina syndrome
Others: enthesitis, osteoporosis, spinal fracture, spondylodiscitis, pseudoarthrosis	Amyloidosis

volvement is usually bilateral. If the hips have not been affected in the first 10 years of disease, they are unlikely to be involved later (6). Some degree of flexion contractures at the hip joints is common in most AS patients at later stages of disease, giving rise to a characteristic rigid gait with flexion at the knees to maintain an erect posture.

Involvement of the shoulder girdle (glenohumeral, acromioclavicular, or sternoclavicular joints) is less common and often leads to only minor disability, mostly resulting from some loss of thoracoscapular movement. Inflammation of the thoracic spine (including the costovertebral joints), costosternal areas, and manubriosternal or sternoclavicular joints may cause chest pain that may be accentuated on coughing or sneezing. Some patients notice an inability to expand the chest fully. Stiffness and pain in the cervical spine generally tend to develop after some years, but they occasionally occur in the early stages of disease. Involvement of peripheral joints, other than hips and shoulders, is infrequent. When present it is usually asymmetric, mild and transient, rarely persistent or erosive, and tends to resolve without any residual joint deformity. Occasionally, peripheral joint involvement occurs after the axial disease has become inactive (7). Temporomandibular joint pain and tenderness may occur in about 10% of patients, sometimes resulting in decreased range of motion of the joint. Late-onset undifferentiated spondyloarthropathy has recently been described in which there is little or no clinical involvement of the axial skeleton early, but eventually bilateral sacroiliitis develops (8).

The diagnosis of AS is based on clinical (including radiographic) findings, which can sometimes be minimal in the early stages of the disease. Tenderness of SI joints or soreness of spinal processes or paraspinal muscles may be present, and some limitation of spinal motion is common. Sometimes sacroiliac pain may be elicited by pressure over the anterior superior iliac spines and by compressing the two iliac bones of the pelvis toward or away from each other while the patient is supine. The pain can also be elicited by maximal flexion of one hip joint and hyperextension of the other. The loss of mobility of the lumbar spine is best assessed by checking lateral flexion, hyperextension, axial rotation, and forward flexion. Early loss of spinal mobility is usually due to pain and muscle spasm rather than bony ankylosis, and therefore marked improvement in spinal mobility can occur after treatment with nonsteroidal anti-inflammatory drugs (NSAIDs) and proper physical therapy. Some additional early, but often overlooked, physical findings resulting from enthesitis include tenderness over ischial tuberosities, greater trochanters, costochondral or manubriosternal junctions, anteriosuperior iliac spines or the iliac crest, and sometimes even over calcanei, tibial tubercles, or pubic symphysis.

Involvement of costovertebral and costotransverse joints results in restriction of respiratory excursion, and therefore most patients with AS breathe primarily by using their diaphragms. Limited chest expansion in an individual with insidious onset of chronic low-back pain and without chest disease such as emphysema or scoliosis should strongly raise the possibility of AS. The entire spine becomes increasingly stiff after many years of disease progression, and the patient loses normal posture because of flattening of the lumbar spine and development of thoracic kyphosis. The anterior chest becomes flattened, the abdomen protuberant, and the breathing increasingly diaphragmatic. Involvement of the cervical spine results in progressive limitation of neck motion, and a forward stoop of the neck gradually develops. Spinal ankylosis develops at a variable rate and pattern; occasionally the disease may remain confined to one part of the spine. With fusion, the pain from spinal involvement diminishes and morning stiffness lessens. In extreme cases, the entire spine may be fused in a flexed position, making it difficult for some patients to look ahead as they walk.

Extraskeletal Manifestations

Acute anterior uveitis (also called acute iritis or iridocyclitis) is the most common extraskeletal involvement in patients with AS. It occurs in 25%–30% of patients at some time in the course of disease. Uveitis is virtually always unilateral and has a strong tendency to recur, sometimes in the contralateral eye. The symptoms are usually acute and include pain, increased lacrimation, photophobia, and blurred vision. There is circumcorneal congestion, the iris is edematous and appears discolored, and the pupil is small but may become irregular if posterior synechiae form. Copious exudate in the anterior chamber of the eye can be seen on slit-lamp examination. Individual attacks of uveitis usually subside within 2–3 months. Residual visual impairment is rare but may occur if treatment is inadequate or delayed. Occasionally acute iritis may be the presenting symptom, which draws attention to the diagnosis of AS.

Cardiovascular involvement can occur in some patients, usually those with severe long-standing AS with peripheral joint involvement (9,10). Aortitis of the ascending aorta and resulting fibrosis can cause dilation of the aortic ring and aortic valve incompetence. On rare occasions, acute aortic insufficiency with rapid deterioration of cardiac function in relatively young patients with minimal spondylitis has been noted. Fibrosis can affect the subaortic area and cause cardiac conduction abnormalities from involvement of the bundle of His or the atrioventricular node; very rarely, fibrosis involves the anterior leaflet of the mitral valve and results in mitral valve incompetence. Complete heart block causing Stokes-Adam's attacks may occur in some patients, necessitating implantation of a cardiac pacemaker.

Rigidity of the chest wall in patients with AS results in an inability to expand the chest fully on inspiration. However, this inability does not usually cause ventilatory insufficiency because diaphragmatic breathing contributes to maintaining respiratory competence. A rare pleuropulmonary complication is a slowly progressive, usually asymptomatic and bilateral, apical pulmonary fibrosis, which is diagnosed as an incidental radiographic finding (11). These lesions can cavitate and may subsequently become colonized by fungi or bacteria, resulting in cough, increasing dyspnea, and occasionally hemoptysis.

Neurologic involvement may occur in patients with AS, most often related to spinal fracture, atlantoaxial subluxation, or cauda equina syndrome. Fracture is most common in the cervical spine, and the resulting quadriplegia is the most dreaded complication of AS because mortality is high. The clinician should exclude the possibility of spinal fracture in any patient with advanced AS who experiences neck or back pain after even a mild trauma. Sometimes the undiagnosed or improperly treated fracture causes spondylodiscitis and pseudoarthrosis. Other well-recognized but uncommon complications of long-standing AS include spontaneous anterior atlantoaxial subluxation, presenting as occipital pain with or without signs of spinal cord compression, and a slowly progressive cauda equina syndrome.

Amyloidosis (secondary type) is a very rare complication of AS, especially in the United States. It should be considered in the differential diagnosis in AS patients with proteinuria, with or without progressive azotemia. A few cases of IgA nephropathy have been reported in AS patients (12).

LABORATORY AND IMAGING STUDIES

An elevated erythrocyte sedimentation rate (ESR) or serum C-reactive protein (CRP) is noted in up to 75% of patients with AS, which typically correlates with clinical disease activity; CRP may be a better marker of disease activity than ESR. Mild-to-moderate elevations of serum IgA are frequently observed, and the level generally correlates with acute phase reactants. There is no association with rheumatoid factor or antinuclear antibodies. A mild, normocytic, normochromic anemia is present in 15% of patients. Mild elevations of serum alkaline phosphatase (primarily derived from bone) or creatine phosphokinase (with normal levels of serum aldolase) may be seen in some patients, but neither correlates with disease activity or treatment. The synovial fluid does not show markedly distinctive features compared with other inflammatory arthropathies.

The radiographic changes of AS evolve over many years, and the earliest, most consistent and most characteristic findings are seen in the SI joints. Sacroiliitis is bilateral and usually symmetric, consisting of blurring of the subchondral bone plate, followed by bony erosions and sclerosis resembling postage-stamp serrations (Fig. 11C-1). They are typically seen first and tend to be more prominent on the iliac side because the cartilage covering that side of the joint is much thinner than that covering the sacral side. Progression of subchondral bone erosions can lead to "pseudo-widening" of the joint space, and with time there is gradual fibrosis, calcification, interosseous bridging, and ossification. After several years there may be complete bony ankylosis of the SI joints, and even resolution of the juxta-articular bony sclerosis.

Bony erosions and osteitis (whiskering) at sites of osseous attachment of tendons and ligaments are frequently observed (3). They result from enthesitis and are seen particularly at the ischial tuberosities, iliac crest, calcanei, femoral trochanters, and spinous processes of the vertebrae. The inflammatory lesions in the vertebral column affect the superficial layers of the annulus fibrosus, at their attachment to corners of vertebral bodies, the apophyseal joints, and intervertebral ligaments. Reactive bone sclerosis can be seen on radiographs as highlighting of the corners of vertebral bodies, and subsequent bone resorption can lead to squaring of the vertebral bodies. This can be followed by a gradual ossification of the superficial layers of the annulus fibrosus and eventual bridging between vertebrae; these vertical bony bridges are called syndesmophytes (Fig. 11C-2). Concomitant inflammatory changes often occur, causing ankylosis in the apophyseal joints and ossification of some of the spinal ligaments. These processes can ultimately result in virtually complete fusion of the vertebral column ("bamboo spine") and spinal osteoporosis.

Hip joint involvement leads to symmetric concentric joint-space narrowing, irregularity of the subchondral bone plate with subchondral sclerosis, osteophyte formation at the outer margins of the articular surfaces (both the acetabulum and the femoral head), and ultimate bony ankylosis. Shoulder girdle involvement can result in concentric narrowing of the glenohumeral joint space (rarely osseous ankylosis), erosions on the superolateral aspect of the humeral head, erosive abnormalities or osseous ankylosis of the acromioclavicular joint, and osseous proliferation at the acromial attachment of the acromioclavicular ligament ("bearded acromion"). Absent are periarticular or widespread osteopenia in the involved hip or shoulder girdles.

The evaluation of SI joints and the spine by radionuclide scintigraphy, computed tomography, and magnetic resonance imaging (MRI) has been attempted in patients with early disease in whom standard radiography of the SI joints may show normal or equivocal changes (13). Quantitative scintigraphy has generally been found to be too sensitive and too nonspecific to be of much clinical value. Computed tomography is more sensitive and as specific as conventional radiography in identifying sacroiliitis, but this technology should be reserved for those few patients

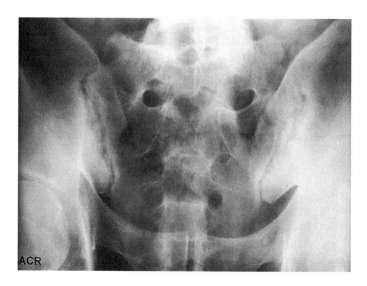

(Figure 11C-1)
Early sacroiliitis in ankylosing spondylitis. Note subchondral bone resorption and irregularity of sacroiliac joints. Reprinted from Berens DL: Roentgen features of ankylosing spondylitis. Clin Orthop 74:20-33, 1971, with permission.

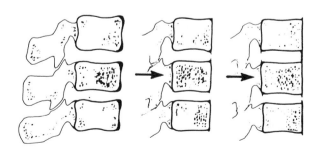

(Figure 11C-2)
Schematic representation of the lateral view of lumbar spine showing progressive squaring and fusion of vertebral bodies anteriorly (syndesmophytes) and gradual fusion of the apophyseal (facet) joints posteriorly.

whose conventional radiographs show normal or equivocal results when AS is strongly suspected on clinical grounds. Magnetic resonance imaging in such a clinical situation also produces excellent, although costly, computer-generated imaging and has the added advantages of lack of ionizing radiation, and is able to detect early lesions in articular cartilage and edema of adjacent bone marrow. MRI is also useful in diagnosing spinal fractures in AS and for demonstrating arachnoid diverticula in cauda equina syndrome.

The overwhelming majority of patients with AS can be readily diagnosed clinically and do not need to be tested for HLA-B27. However, the SI joints on routine pelvic radiographs may not always be easy to interpret in the early phase of disease, especially in adolescent patients. In such relatively uncommon situations, HLA-B27 determination can be used to further minimize the degree of uncertainty of the diagnosis by Bayesian analysis. It should be noted, however, that the prevalence of HLA-B27 in the general population, and the strength of its association with AS, differ appreciably among ethnic and racial groups (1,14). In addition, the test also does not help distinguish AS from other spondyloarthropathies, because all these diseases are associated with HLA-B27, although the strength of the association varies. Differentiation between these diseases is based primarily on clinical grounds.

Clinical assessment of disease activity in patients with AS is difficult, especially in uncomplicated disease confined to the SI joints and spine (15). Functional indices have been proposed that correlate reasonably well with the overall (global) assessment by the patient and the physician.

DISEASE COURSE

The course of AS is highly variable and can be characterized by spontaneous remissions and exacerbations, particularly in early disease. The outcome is generally favorable because the disease is often relatively mild or self-limited, and the majority of the patients remain fully employed. Only rarely does AS show persistent disease activity that results in early and severe disability. Patients with hip joint involvement or completely ankylosed cervical spine with kyphosis are more likely to be disabled. In recent years, the results of total hip arthroplasty are gratifying in preventing partial or total disability in many such patients.

There is an excess mortality among patients, but only more than 20 years after the diagnosis of AS (16,17). A population-based study, which included milder cases not seen at referral centers, did not show premature mortality (18). It is quite likely that the survival of patients with mild disease, who make up the majority of patients with AS, is comparable to the general population. However, spinal fracture, surgery, cardiovascular involvement, associated medical conditions including ulcerative colitis and Crohn's disease, as well as complications of treatment with NSAIDs, may contribute to premature death in some patients.

MANAGEMENT

Currently, no preventive cure or measures for AS are available, but most patients can be managed well (Table 11C-2), and prognosis has improved in recent years. An early diagnosis, a compliant patient, and a competent physician can substantially influence the outcome of the disease (19). NSAIDs should be used regularly in full therapeutic anti-in-

(Table 11C-2)
Principles of management of ankylosing spondylitis

1. There is no cure, but most patients can be well managed.
2. Educating patients about the disease helps increase compliance.
3. Early diagnosis is very important, as is the early recognition and treatment of extraskeletal manifestations, such as acute iritis, and of the associated diseases or complications.
4. Nonsteroidal antiinflammatory drugs may be used to control pain and suppress inflammation.
5. Daily exercises preserve good posture, minimize deformity, and maintain good chest expansion. Swimming is the best overall exercise.
6. Surgical measures such as hip arthroplasty or correction of spinal deformity can be helpful.
7. Psychosocial and vocational supportive measures and counseling, family and genetic counseling, and patient support groups are sources of help and information for patients.
8. Thorough family history and, if possible, physical examination of the patient's relatives may sometimes disclose remarkable disease aggregation and many undiagnosed or misdiagnosed affected relatives.

flammatory doses, during active phases of the disease (see Chapter 52, Appendix V). Patients differ in their responses, as do side effects, and it is worthwhile to search out the best NSAID for each individual. Aspirin seldom provides an adequate therapeutic response. Oral corticosteroids have no therapeutic value in the long-term management of the musculoskeletal aspects of AS because of their serious side effects, and they do not halt disease progression. Acute anterior uveitis can usually be managed by dilation of the pupil and instilling corticosteroid eye drops; on rare occasions, systemic steroids are required. Recalcitrant enthesitis and persistent synovitis often respond well to a local corticosteroid injection.

Sulfasalazine may be effective in some AS patients, particularly those with peripheral arthritis. This drug may be tried when the disease is not adequately controlled by NSAIDs, and for patients unable to tolerate NSAIDs. Because of its efficacy in inflammatory bowel disease and psoriasis, sulfasalazine appears to be especially useful for AS associated with these diseases. A small number of patients with severe AS and peripheral joint involvement who are unresponsive to NSAIDs and sulfasalazine have sometimes responded to oral methotrexate therapy (20).

Regular exercises are of fundamental importance to prevent or minimize deformity. Patients with AS should keep the spine as straight as possible, walk erect, avoid prolonged stooped posture, and sleep on a firm mattress with as thin a pillow as possible. They should do spinal extension exercises and deep breathing exercises once or twice daily and not smoke. Physiotherapy is valuable for teaching patients the proper exercises and making sure that the exercise program is maintained. Group exercise sessions that include hydrotherapy and swimming are very helpful. Many patients with impaired neck mobility have difficulty driving and find special wide-view mirrors very helpful. Radiotherapy has no role in the modern management of patients with AS because of the high risk of leukemia and aplastic anemia. Splints, braces, and corsets are generally not helpful and are not advised. There is no special diet and there is no evidence that any specific food contributes to the initiation or exacerbation of AS. Pregnancy does not usually affect the symptoms of AS, and fertility, course of pregnancy, and childbirth have been reported to be normal.

Total hip arthroplasty prevents partial or total disability from severe hip disease. Vertebral wedge osteotomy may be needed to correct severe kyphosis in some patients, although it carries a relatively high risk of paraplegia.

MUHAMMAD ASIM KHAN, MD

1. Khan MA. Ankylosing spondylitis: Clinical features. In Klippel JH, Dieppe PA (eds): Rheumatology, lst edition. London: Mosby-Wolfe, 1994, 3.25.1-3.25.10

2. Feltkamp TEW, Khan MA, de Castro JAL: The pathogenetic role of HLA-B27. Immunol Today, 1996, 7:5-7

3. Resnick D, Niwayama G: Ankylosing spondylitis. In Resnick D (ed): Diagnosis of Bone and Joint Disorders, 3rd edition. Philadelphia, WB Saunders, 1995, 1008-1074

4. Kidd B, Mullee M, Frank A, Cawley M: Disease expression of ankylosing spondylitis in males and females. J Rheumatol 15:1407-1409, 1988

5. Burgos-Vargos R, Vasquez-Mellado J: The early clinical recognition of juvenile-onset ankylosing spondylitis and its differentiation from juvenile rheumatoid arthritis. Arthritis Rheum 38:835-844, 1995

6. Carette S, Graham DC, Little H, et al: The natural disease course of ankylosing spondylitis. Arthritis Rheum 26:186-190, 1983

7. Cohen MD, Ginsburg WW: Late-onset peripheral joint disease in ankylosing spondylitis. Ann Rheum Dis 41:574-578, 1982

8. Olivieri I, Padula A, Pierro A, et al: Late onset undifferentiated spondyloarthropathy. J Rheumatol 22:899-903, 1995

9. O'Neil TW, Bresnihan B: The heart in ankylosing spondylitis. Ann Rheum Dis 51:705-706, 1992

10. Arnason JA, Patel AK, Rahko PS, Sundstrom WR: Transthoracic and transesophageal echocardiographic evaluation of the aortic root and subvalvular structures in ankylosing spondylitis. J Rheumatol 23:120-123, 1996

11. Rosenow EC III, Strimlan CV, Muhm JR, et al: Pleuropulmonary manifestations of ankylosing spondylitis. Mayo Clin Proc 52:641-649, 1977

12. Bruneau C, Villiaumeocy J, Avouac B, et al: Seronegative spondyloarthropathies and IgA glomerulonephritis: A report of four cases and a review of the literature. Semin Arthritis Rheum 15:179-184, 1986

13. Blum U, Buitargo-Tellcz C, Mundinger A, et al: Magnetic resonance imaging for detection of active sacroiliitis. A prospective study comparing conventional radiography, scintigraphy, and contrast enhanced MRI. J Rheumatol 23:2107-2115, 1996.

14. Khan MA: HLA-B27 and its subtypes in world populations. Curr Opinion Rheumatol 7:263-269, 1995

15. Calin A: The individual with ankylosing spondylitis: Defining disease status and the impact of the illness. Br J Rheumatol 34:663-672, 1995

16. Callahan LF, Pincus T: Mortality in the rheumatic diseases. Arthritis Care Res 8:229-241, 1995

17. Khan MA, Khan MK, Kushner I: Survival among patients with ankylosing spondylitis: a life-table analysis. J Rheumatol 8:86-90, 1981

18. Carter ET, McKenna CH, Brian DD, Kurland LT: Epidemiology of ankylosing spondylitis in Rochester, Minnesota, 1935-1973. Arthritis Rheum 22:365-370, 1979

19. Toivanen A, Khan MA: Therapeutic dilemma in ankylosing spondylitis and related spondylarthropathies. Rheumatol Rev 3:21-27, 1994

20. Creemers MCW, Franssen MJAM, van de Putte LBA, et al: Methotrexate in severe ankylosing spondylitis: an open study. J Rheumatol 22:1104-1107, 1995

D. TREATMENT

Patient education is the cornerstone of treatment for patients with seronegative spondyloarthropathy. Patients with ankylosing spondylitis (AS) should be informed of the chronic nature of the disease and the possible clinical outcomes. The patient who is engaged in physically demanding work may need career counseling. Functional assessments by questionnaire (1) and a functional index (2) provide useful measures for quantitating functional impact of the disease. Exercise to maintain spinal mobility and optimum posture helps prevent deformity. Swimming is the ideal exercise for patients with AS. An experienced physiotherapist can assist greatly in achieving the goal of preventing deformity. Group physical therapy is superior to individualized therapy in improving thoracolumbar mobility and enhancing overall health (3). Patients should be instructed to sleep with a straight back (prone or supine) and avoid sleeping curled up on one side. Deep breathing exercises and not smoking will help maintain chest expansion.

Education also is a key element in the comprehensive care of patients with reactive arthritis. If the disorder was initiated by a sexually transmitted infection, the clinician may also need to address emotional elements. For example, a particularly stressful circumstance with potential for marital discord can arise with the onset of urethritis or balanitis following a gastrointestinal infection acquired during foreign travel. The clinician should initiate a frank discussion of the current concepts of infection. A second area of concern is prognosis, since reactive arthritis often occurs in young, active individuals for whom athletic activity is a priority. There is a general recognition that reactive arthritis has a

greater propensity for chronicity than previously appreciated, which should temper an overly optimistic prognosis. One study reported that at one year, 40% of patients with post-genitourinary-acquired reactive arthritis and 20% of post-gastrointestinal-acquired reactive arthritis still had active disease, but almost all had recovered at 2-year follow-up (4). In a 5-year follow-up a group of patients with reactive arthritis caused by *Salmonella*, two-thirds continued to have subjective complaints and 37% demonstrated objective joint changes (5). This variability in clinical course should be included in discussions with the patient.

ANTI-INFLAMMATORY AGENTS

Most patients experience significant improvement in joint inflammation with the use of nonsteroidal anti-inflammatory drugs (NSAIDs). In general, newer NSAIDs are more effective than salicylate. Indomethacin or diclofenac, up to 200 mg daily in divided doses, are usually well tolerated and do not necessitate cytoprotective therapy in the absence of specific risk factors. In the patients with AS, the goal of NSAID therapy is to achieve sufficient control of pain and stiffness to allow an active, sustained program of exercise and physical therapy.

In the treatment of seronegative spondyloarthropathy, corticosteroids may be given as intra-articular injections into acutely inflamed joints. The response to local steroid injection is often neither as dramatic nor as sustained as in patients with rheumatoid arthritis, however, so this therapy constitutes only one part of a comprehensive treatment program. Corticosteroid injection of the sacroiliac joint is usually performed under fluoroscopic guidance. Maugars and colleagues reported that in 24 such injections, 79% of patients achieved a good response and improvement could persist over many months (6). This procedure can on occasion obviate the need for initiating second-line agents. Systemic corticosteroids (either orally or as an intravenous bolus protocol) have been used with some success in severe symptomatic flares of ankylosing spondylitis, but no controlled trials have been conducted. The goal should be to promptly taper the dose when symptomatic control is achieved.

SECOND-LINE AGENTS
Sulfasalazine

This drug has been used with moderate success in each clinical subset of the seronegative spondyloarthropathy family of diseases. In AS, sulfasalazine has been reported to improve symptoms and reduce the frequency of peripheral arthritis in placebo-controlled trials (7,8). There is no evidence, however, that sulfasalazine maintains spinal mobility or retards radiologic progression of disease. It is of interest that sulfasalazine is associated with a decrease in IgA antibodies to certain intestinal organisms, but this did not correlate with laboratory or clinical parameters (9). Published experience of this agent in reactive arthritis is more limited. Sulfasalazine has been associated with an improvement in CD4 lymphocyte count in a small number of patients with reactive arthritis and human immunodeficiency virus (HIV) infection (10).

A comprehensive double-blind, placebo-controlled trial with 251 spondyloarthropathy patients recently evaluated the efficiency of sulfasalazine (11). Patients' overall assessment of disease activity showed a significant difference, with 60% of the group receiving the drug showing improvement versus 44% in the placebo group. Laboratory markers of inflammation were also significantly changed in favor of sulfasalazine. In subgroup analysis, patients with psoriatic arthritis demonstrated more impressive benefits than either those with reactive arthritis or with AS for the four primary efficacy variables of pain, morning stiffness, patient overall assessment, and physician overall assessment. Adverse effects were more frequent in the sulfasalazine group, but all were transient or reversible after cessation of treatment. In general, the response to therapy was more demonstrable in polyarticular disease than oligoarticular disease, and in peripheral joints than in axial disease. Although this was a 6-month trial, efficacy seemed to plateau at 16 weeks after initiation of treatment.

More recently a 36-week trial of sulfasalazine (2000 mg/day) versus placebo in the spondyloarthropathies was published in three sequential articles. In patients with ankylosing spondylitis (12), there was no difference between sulfasalazine and placebo at the end of the trial. In the subgroup of these patients with peripheral arthritis, improvement favored sulfasalazine. In psoriatic arthritis (13), response rate at the end of 36 weeks was 57.8% for sulfasalazine compared with 44.6% for placebo (P = 0.05). In reactive arthritis (14), response rate was 62.3% for sulfasalazine compared with 47.7% for placebo (P = 0.09). In all three areas of the study, the erythrocyte sedimentation rate declined more with sulfasalazine than placebo (P < 0.0001), and the adverse reactions were fewer than expected and were mainly due to nonspecific gastrointestinal complaints (dyspepsia, nausea, vomiting, diarrhea).

Methotrexate

Coincident with the increasing use of methotrexate in rheumatoid arthritis, there has been wider use of the drug in patients with seronegative spondyloarthropathy. Generally responses have been good, but there are few studies to substantiate these impressions. The onset of action appears to be rapid in most cases, with mucocutaneous lesions more responsive than arthritis in general. In patients with reactive arthritis, in which young males predominate, coincident alcohol habits are common and a serious discussion of the hazards of methotrexate and alcohol must precede initiating drug therapy in each patient.

Methotrexate for the treatment of AS has recently been reported in a 24-week open study of 11 patients (15). Clinical improvement was noted at 24 weeks compared with baseline. Of five patients who discontinued treatment, three had disease flares and restarted methotrexate therapy. Side effects were mild and reversible. These early beneficial results warrant a placebo-controlled study. Efficacy is most likely to be perceived early in the disease course

Other Disease-Modifying Agents

There have been several reports of alternative agents as options for second-line therapy in reactive arthritis. A placebo-controlled crossover study of azathioprine in eight patients was reported (16). Patients were randomized to receive azathioprine or placebo. Of six patients completing the crossover, five reported subjective improvement on active drug, and joint scores fell during azathioprine treatment but rose during placebo. Bromocriptine has been used in postdysenteric reactive arthritis (17). The rationale for using this drug was based on the recognized immunoregulatory properties of prolactin and a report of hyperprolactinemia in some patients with reactive arthritis. Of the four patients treated, two demonstrated dramatic improvement after 24 hours of treatment, and two did so after 4 days of treatment. All patients had a prolonged beneficial effect lasting at least 4 months following the short course of treatment. One patient with chronic reactive arthritis was reported to have a beneficial response to meselamine (18), which is bioavailable in the small bowel and used in the treatment of inflammatory bowel disease. This implicates the anti-inflammatory effect of salicylate, rather than the antimicrobial effect of the sulfa moiety, in accounting for the efficacy of sulfasalazine. A larger study is needed to define the role of 5'-ASA in treating seronegative spondyloarthropathy.

Antibiotic Therapy

The current concept of the pathogenesis of reactive arthritis postulates that a bacterial infection, usually genitourinary or gastrointestinal, is the triggering event in an immunogenetically susceptible host. For the other spondyloarthropathies, there is less compelling evidence to implicate infection in a causal role. It would appear logical that eradication of the source of microbial antigens would have a salutory effect on reactive arthritis, but there are few studies to definitely support the role of antibiotics. It is sound clinical practice to treat a culture-proven Chlamydia urethritis, in conjunction with treating the patient's sexual partners. A recent randomized control study of 166 adults with Chlamydia-induced urethritis or cervicitis found that azithromycin, 1 gm as a single dose, was equivalent to doxycycline 100 mg twice daily for 7 days in achieving bacteriological eradication (19). While some infectious disease consultants argue that antibiotic treatment based on stool cultures positive for *Salmonella* or *Yersinia* may prolong the carrier state, the patient's general degree of illness often dictates the need for antibiotic therapy. A double-blind study described 36 patients with chronic reactive arthritis, most caused by *Yersinia*, who were treated with ciprofloxacin for 3 months. There was a variable effect on joint symptoms but no clear effect on erythrocyte sedimentation rate or Ritchie index (20). In *Chlamydia*-induced reactive arthritis the evidence is more supportive. A retrospective review of 109 patients in Greenland concluded that 37% of episodes of urethritis not treated with anti-Chlamydial agents were associated with reactive arthritis, whereas only 10% of such episodes treated with tetracycline progressed to the disease (21). Lymecycline (a form of tetracycline) was evaluated in a double-blind, placebo-controlled study of 40 patients with chronic reactive arthritis, for a 3-month treatment period (22). The antibiotic therapy significantly decreased the duration of illness in patients with *Chlamydia*-induced disease but not in patients with reactive arthritis triggered by enteric infection. These observations support the notion that *Chlamydia* plays a role in the arthritis, although nonantimicrobial effects of tetracycline could well contribute to the effect. It would seem prudent to treat patients with *Chlamydia*-induced reactive arthritis with doxycycline or tetracycline, as well as their sexual partners, on the basis of these reports. However, the role of antibiotics in postdysenteric reactive arthritis is unresolved.

EXTRA-ARTICULAR FEATURES

The ocular inflammation of seronegative spondyloarthropathy most often is acute anterior uveitis. This inflammation may be the first occasion for a medical assessment, and only at a later time does the associated spondyloarthropathy become apparent (23). Such complications should be managed jointly by the rheumatologist and the ophthalmologist. Topical steroid drops are first-line treatment, but occasionally systemic corticosteroids are needed. The goal is to resolve the inflammation promptly and to prevent synechiae formation and subsequent glaucoma. Steroid-sparing agents for refractory ocular disease include methotrexate, azathioprine, and cyclosporin A. The oral mucosa and genital lesions are best managed with topical corticosteroid preparations. This is also true for keratoderma blennorrhagica. Although second-line agents have been used for extra-articular features, the reported experience is small and treatment is often empirical (24).

ROBERT D. INMAN, MD

1. Abbott CA, Helliwell PS, Chamberlain MA: Functional assessment in ankylosing spondylitis: evaluation of a new self-administered questionnaire and correlation with anthropomorphic variables. Br J Rheum 33:1060-1066, 1994

2. Calin A, Garrett S, Whitelock H, et al: A new approach to defining functional ability in ankylosing spondylitis: the development of the Bath ankylosing spondylitis functional index. J Rheumatol 21:2281-2285, 1994

3. Hidding A, van der Linden S, Boers M, et al: Is group physical therapy superior to individual therapy in ankylosing spondylitis? A randomized controlled trial. Arthritis Care and Research 6:17-1123, 1993

4. Glennas A, Kvien T, Melby K, et al: Reactive arthritis: a favorable 2 year course of outcome, independent of triggering agent and HLA-B27. J Rheumatol 21:2274-2280, 1994

5. Thomson GTD, DeRubeis DA, Hodge MA, et al: Post-Salmonella reactive arthritis: late clinical sequelae in a point source cohort. Am J Med 98:13-21, 1995

6. Maugars Y, Mathis C, Vilon P, et al: Corticosteroid injection of the sacroiliac joint in patients with seronegative spondyloarthropathy. Arthritis Rheum 35:564-568, 1992

7. Kirwan J, Edwards A, Huitfeldt B, et al: The course of established ankylosing spondylitis and the effects of sulfasalazine over 3 years. Br J Rheumatol 32:729-733, 1993

8. Bosi Ferraz M, Tugwell P, Goldsmith C, et al: Meta-analysis of sulfasalazine in ankylosing spondylitis. J Rheumatol 17:1482, 1990

9. Nissila M, Lahesmaa R, Leirisalo-Repo M, et al: Antibodies to *Klebsiella pneumoniae, Esherichia coli,* and *Proteus mirabilis* in ankylosing spondylitis: effect of sulfasalazine treatment. J Rheumatol 21:2082-2087, 1994

10. Disla E, Rhim HR, Reddy A, et al: Improvement in CD4 lymphocyte count in HIV-Reiter's syndrome after treatment with sulfasalazine. J Rheumatol 21:662-664, 1994

11. Dougados M, van der Linden S, Leirisalo-Repo M, et al: Sulfasalazine in the treatment of spondyloarthropathy. A randomized, multicenter, double-blind, placebo controlled study. Arthritis Rheum 38:618-627, 1995

12. Clegg DO, Reda DJ, Weisman MH, et al: Comparison of sulfasalazine and placebo in the treatment of ankylosing spondylitis. Arthritis Rheum 39:2004-2012, 1996

13. Clegg DO, Reda DJ, Mejias E, et al: Comparison of sulfasalazine and placebo in the treatment of psoriatic arthritis. Arthritis Rheum 39:2013-2020, 1996

14. Clegg DO, Reda DJ, Weisman MH, et al: Comparison of sulfasalazine and placebo in the treatment of reactive arthritis (Reiter's syndrome). Arthritis Rheum 39:2021-2027, 1996

15. Creemers MC, Franssen MJ, van de Putte LB, et al: Methotrexate in severe ankylosing spondylitis: an open study. J Rheumatol 22:1104-1107, 1995

16. Calin A: A placebo-controlled crossover study of azathioprine in Reiter's syndrome. Ann Rheum Dis 45:653-655, 1986

17. Bravo G, Zazueta B, Lavalle C: An acute remission of Reiter's syndrome in male patients treated with bromocriptine. J Rheumatol 19:747-750, 1992

18. Thomson GT, McKibbon C, Inman RD: Meselamine therapy in Reiter's syndrome. J Rheumatol 21:570-572, 1995

19. Martin DH, Mroczkowski TF, Dalu AZ, et al: A controlled trial of a single dose of azithromycin for the treatment of chlamydial urethritis and cervicitis. New Engl J Med 327:921-925, 1992

20. Toivanen A, Kli-Kerttula T, Luukainen R, et al: Effect of antimicrobial treatment on chronic reactive arthritis. Clin Exp Rheum 11:301-307, 1993

21. Bardin T, Enel C, Cornelis F, et al: Antibiotic treatment of venereal disease and Reiter's syndrome a Greenland population. Arth Rheum 35: 190-194, 1992

22. Lauhio A, Leirisalo-Repo M. Lahdevirta J, et al: Double-blind, placebo-controlled study of three-month treatment with lymecycline in reactive arthritis, with special reference to *Chlamydia trachomatis.* Arth Rheum 34:6-14, 1991

23. Careless DJ, Inman RD: Acute anterior uveitis: clinical and experimental aspects. Semin Arth Rheum 24:432-441, 1995

24. Creemers MCW, van Riel PLCM, Franssen MJ, et al: Second-line treatment in seronegative spondyloarthropathies. Semin Arth Rheum 24:71-81, 1994

INFECTIOUS DISORDERS
A. SEPTIC ARTHRITIS

The clinical picture of acute bacterial arthritis includes the rapid onset (from a few hours to a few days) of moderate to severe joint pain, warmth, tenderness, and restricted motion in a patient who may or may not have other symptoms of a serious infection. Delay in diagnosing these vulnerable patients reduces the likelihood of a successful treatment outcome. Despite the availability of new effective antibiotics and joint drainage techniques, septic arthritis continues to be a serious cause of morbidity, mortality, joint damage, and functional disability.

PATHOGENIC MECHANISMS IN ARTICULAR INFECTION

Bacteria reach joints by direct inoculation as a result of trauma, surgery, or arthrocentesis; by migration into the joints from a contiguous focus of osteomyelitis, soft tissue abscess, infected prosthesis, or wound infection; or via subsynovial blood vessels during bacteremia from a remote focus of infection.

After they are directly inoculated into the joint cavity, bacteria rapidly multiply in the liquid culture medium of the synovial fluid and are phagocytosed by synovial lining cells. Bacteria are either killed by the synovial cells or form microabscesses within the synovial membrane. Organisms that reach the synovium via the bloodstream multiply in enlarging subsynovial microabscesses until they break into the articular cavity.

Some bacteria can produce bone tissue and collagen adhesions, permitting certain bacterial strains to localize in bone and joints (1). Bacterial products such as endotoxin (lipopolysaccharide) from gram-negative organisms, cell wall fragments, exotoxins from gram-positive organisms, and immune complexes stimulate synovial cells to release tumor necrosis factor α (TNF-α) and interleukin (IL) 1 β. These cytokines up-regulate expression of adhesion ligands (ICAM-1) in synovial membrane vessel endothelial cells, resulting in leukocyte attachment and migration into articular tissues and synovial fluid. In synovial fluid and synovial tissues, the bacteria are phagocytosed and killed by polymorphonuclear leukocytes. Bacterial fragments may form antigen–antibody complexes that activate the classic pathway of complement, and bacterial toxins activate the alternative complement pathway to produce the pro-inflammatory split products C3a and C5a. The phagocytic killing of bacteria also results in autolysis of neutrophils with release of lysosomal enzymes into the joint which causes synovial, ligament, and cartilage damage. In the process, arachidonic acid metabolism is stimulated, collagenase and proteolytic enzymes are released, and more IL-1 is generated to amplify the inflammatory response (2). Cellular immune mechanisms also appear to play a role in acute joint infection. After 48 hours of synovial infection, T lymphocytes infiltrate the synovium, IL-6 levels are in-

creased, and polyclonal B-cell activation results in IgG antibody production (3).

Bacterial products damage articular cartilage via direct effects on chondrocytes inhibiting proteoglycan synthesis and increasing protease activity. Chondrocytes are stimulated by IL-1 and *Staphylococcus aureus* polysaccharides to increase proteinase activity. *Haemophilus influenza* type B (HiB) lipo-oligosaccharide induces production of TNF-α and IL-1, which regulate secretion of the metalloproteases, stromelysin and collagenases, from chondrocytes and synovial tissue. These metalloproteases participate in degradation of proteoglycan in the cartilage matrix. TNF-α and IL-1 also reduce chondrocyte synthesis of proteoglycan. The chondrocyte proteases persist in the cartilage and continue proteolytic degradation of cartilage with release of collagen and proteoglycan from the matrix, even after the infection is eradicated by antibiotics (4).

Bacterial toxins also activate the coagulation system, causing intravascular thrombosis in the subsynovial vessels and fibrin deposition on the surface of the synovium and articular cartilage. The layer of fibrin provides an acellular gelatinous nidus for bacterial replication. Subsynovial microvascular obstruction causes ischemia and necrosis, permitting further abscess formation. Activation of the coagulation system and fibrin deposition activates the fibrinolytic mechanism with formation of plasmin, which destroys the protein core and polysaccharides in cartilage matrix.

After the initial acute necrotic inflammatory synovitis, the synovial membrane proliferates (pannus) and erodes articular cartilage and subchondral bone. A chronic inflammatory synovitis may persist even after the infection has been eradicated by antibiotics. It has been theorized that cartilage is altered by infection to become antigenic, and, together with the adjuvant effects of bacterial components, causes a persistent, immune-mediated, sterile inflammatory synovitis.

CLINICAL PRESENTATION

Most articular infections involve a single joint but 15%–20% of cases are polyarticular (5). With monarticular septic arthritis, most common sites are the knee (40%–50%), hip (13%–20%), shoulder (10%–15%), wrist (5%–8%), ankle (6%–8%), elbow (3%–7%), and the small joints of the hand or foot (5%). In patients with polyarticular septic arthritis, the knees are most commonly involved. Twenty percent of patients are afebrile, and shaking chills are reported by only 20% of patients. With acute bacterial arthritis, joint pain is moderate to severe and is markedly worsened by movement or palpation unless the patient is profoundly immunosuppressed. Most infected joints are visibly swollen, warm to the touch, and often red. Comorbidity factors not only modify the risk and frequency of septic arthritis, but also may alter the severity of presenting symptoms. Potential risk factors associated with septic arthritis include advanced age, coexistent diseases, prosthetic joints, joint surgery, arthrocentesis, and intravenous drug abuse. Comorbid conditions associated with septic arthritis include rheumatoid arthritis (RA), diabetes mellitus, malignancy, sickle cell disease, anemia, systemic lupus erythematosus, chronic liver disease, skin infections, and hemophilia (6). In patients with polyarticular joint infection, 84% have a pre-existing rheumatic disease or are immunosuppressed by drug treatment or systemic illness. *S. aureus* is the causative organism in 80%. Mortality rate is 30%–40% compared with 4%–8% for monarticular septic arthritis.

SEPTIC ARTHRITIS IN CHILDREN

Septic arthritis in an infant may present with limited spontaneous movement of a limb (pseudoparalysis), irritability, and low-grade or no fever. Joint infections tend to involve the large joints of the lower extremities, such as the knee, hip, and ankle. In the vast majority of children, joint infection is monarticular. Septic arthritis may occur with otitis media, infected umbilical catheters or central lines, femoral venipunctures, meningitis, or adjacent osteomyelitis. Septic arthritis often occurs with osteomyelitis because metaphyseal vessels communicate with epiphyseal vessels. *S. aureus* and group B streptococci are the most common organisms in neonates and in children older than 2 years. From 6 months to 2 years, *H. influenzae* and *Kingella kingae* are the most common organisms (7). Immunization has reduced *H. influenzae* infections by 95% but may still be causative in incompletely immunized children. *Neisseria gonorrhoeae* causes less than 10% of septic arthritis in children, but it is the most common cause if the infection is polyarticular.

Synovial fluid gram stain is positive in one-third of patients and culture is positive in two-thirds. Blood cultures are positive in one-half of patients and may be the only method for identifying the causative organism. In one-third of children with septic arthritis, the causative organism is not identified.

SEPTIC ARTHRITIS IN THE ELDERLY

Forty to fifty percent of adults with septic arthritis are over age 60 (8). In this older age group, 75% of the infections occur in joints with prior arthritis, most of which involve the hip, knee, or shoulder. Many of the elderly also have significant comorbidity from diabetes, malignancy, renal failure, chronic lung disease, alcoholism, or other rheumatic disease. Only 10% of the elderly patients are febrile, and only one-third have marked leukocytosis. The erythrocyte sedimentation rate is usually significantly elevated. Joint culture and/or blood culture is positive in most cases. The source of joint infection is from another focus of infection in approximately three-fourths of the patients (urinary tract infection, pneumonia, osteomyelitis) or from direct inoculation from trauma or wound infections. Permanent joint damage is substantial, with 30% progressing to osteomyelitis, and half the survivors have a poor functional outcome.

JOINT INFECTION IN RHEUMATOID ARTHRITIS

Patients with RA are at increased risk of joint infections, with an annual incidence of 0.5%. Infection is polyarticular (5) in nearly one-half the patients and periarticular signs such as infected adjacent bursae, spontaneous drainage, and sinus tract formation are common presenting manifestations. Fever and leukocytosis are not prominent, but the sedimentation rate is usually elevated and declines with appropriate therapy. Blood cultures are positive in 50%–80% of patients. The most common organism is *S. aureus*, which is seen in 93% of those with polyarticular infection and 72% with monarticular infection. The primary sources of infection in RA patients are infected rheumatoid nodules, calluses of the foot, lung infections, or urinary tract infection. Recurrence of infection in the same joint occurs in up to one-third of patients. The mortality rate is higher in polyarticular (49%) than in monarticular (16%) involvement.

JOINT INFECTION IN DRUG ABUSERS

Intravenous drug abuse is increasingly associated with infection of joints. In a recent report, approximately one-third of septic arthritis cases occurred in drug users, and many of these patients were HIV-positive (9). Joint infection occurs predominantly in the joints and bones of the axial skeleton (sternoclavicular, costochondral, hip, shoulder, vertebrae, symphysis pubis, and sacroiliac joints), but can also occur in the peripheral joints. Most infections are due to *S. aureus* or gram-negative organisms such as *Enterobacter, P. aeruginosa,* and *Serratia marcescens.* Gram-negative joint infections tend to be more indolent and difficult to diagnose. Outbreaks of acute systemic candidiasis in addicts using contaminated brown heroin produce a clinical syndrome of ocular, cutaneous, and costochondral junction or sternoclavicular joint infection. An elevated sedimentation rate and leukocytosis are present in more than 60% of patients, but radiographic abnormalities are present in only 30%. 99m-Technetium bone scans are usually abnormal and especially helpful in evaluating the axial skeleton joints.

JOINT INFECTION AFTER ARTHROSCOPY AND INTRA-ARTICULAR INJECTIONS

Joint infection rates following arthroscopy range from 0.04% to 4.0% with increased risk if intra-articular steroids are used, time of arthroscopy is prolonged, multiple excisional procedures are performed, or equipment disinfectant times are shortened. Organisms causing postarthroscopy infections are *S. aureus, S. epidermidis,* and gram-negative organisms. Onset of joint pain, with or without erythema and fever, within 2 weeks of arthroscopy should prompt evaluation for possible joint infection (10).

The risk of joint infection following intra-articular corticosteroid injection is well-recognized, but is uncommon (probably less than 0.01%). Early acute septic arthritis, within 1 week after arthrocentesis, occurs from direct bacterial inoculation during the arthrocentesis or from bacteremia contamination of the injection tract. The acute infection is usually associated with suggestive clinical signs of fever, abrupt increase in pain, and swelling of the joint. Systemic symptoms may be absent and local joint symptoms may not be severe or may be disregarded, especially in patients with underlying arthritis and/or those on immunosuppressive drugs.

INFECTIONS IN PROSTHETIC JOINTS

Infection of a prosthetic joint causes loosening of the prosthesis and sepsis with significant morbidity and mortality.

The rate of early prosthetic joint infections (less than 12 months) is 2% or less, and the annual rate of late infection (more than 12 months) is 0.60% (11). Two-thirds of prosthetic joint infections occur within 1 year of surgery and are due to intra-operative inoculations of bacteria into the operated joint or postoperative bacteremias. There is a substantially increased risk of prosthetic joint infection in patients with RA, psoriasis, and prior joint infection. Infection risk also increases with concurrent infection at a distant site, corticosteroid therapy, prolonged operative duration, use of large bone grafts, and delayed wound healing (11). The presence of infection anywhere in the body is a contraindication to elective prosthesis implantation. Joint replacement should be delayed until infection is eradicated.

The early infection rates have been substantially reduced by the administration of perioperative antibiotics so that bactericidal levels of antibiotics are present in the tissues during surgery; the use of clean air systems in operating rooms; and improved surgical technique or experience (ie, reduced time for the surgery) (12,13). The most common organisms causing early prosthetic infections are S. aureus (50%), mixed infections (33%), gram-negative bacteria (10%), and anaerobes (5%) (12).

With prosthesis infection, patients often require removal of hardware. Reimplantation of a new prosthesis is often complicated by reinfection (60% recurrence in RA patients). Organisms isolated in late infection are predominantly gram-positive, mostly staphylococcal and streptococcal species. Escherichia coli and anaerobes account for the remainder (11).

Treatment options for joint prosthesis infection are arduous and prolonged. They include: 1) long-term suppression of infection with antibiotics in patients who are not fit for surgery; 2) excision arthroplasty, with or without fusion (for those with uncontrolled infection or insufficient bone stock remaining); 3) arthrotomy for prosthesis removal with meticulous debridement of all cement, abscesses, and devitalized tissues, followed by prolonged antibiotics; 4) immediate or delayed (1–3 months) reimplantation of a new prosthesis using antibiotic impregnated cement. There is a high rate of reinfection (38%) in new implants, whether they are replaced immediately or after 2–3 months of antibiotic therapy (14).

DISSEMINATED GONOCOCCAL INFECTIONS

N. gonorrhoeae, a gram-negative intracellular and extracellular diplococcus, produces septic arthritis in the small joints of the hands, wrists, elbows, knees, ankles, and, rarely, the axial skeletal joints. There are 1–3 million cases of gonococcal infection per year in the United States, and approximately 1% of patients develop bacteremia and arthritis (disseminated gonococcal infection, or DGI). DGI is generally discussed as a separate entity from other forms of suppurative bacterial arthritis because it is the most common form of acute bacterial arthritis, has a distinctive clinical picture, and responds well to appropriate therapy.

Understanding of the pathogenesis of DGI is based on experimental animal studies in which nonviable bacteria and N. gonorrhoeae lipopolysaccharide produce arthritis in rabbits. The early phase of DGI is likely an immune complex disease that resolves spontaneously. Affected individuals presumably have foci of infection within mucosal surfaces that can cause intermittent bacteremia and the clinical manifestations of DGI. In some cases the bacteremia is sufficient

to establish a synovial infection and cause true septic arthritis. N. gonorrhoeae may also cause gonococcal osteomyelitis with a subacute pattern of pain or swelling without fever or rash, often in the small joints of the hands or feet.

A common presentation of gonococcal arthritis occurs in a sexually active individual with a 5–7 day history of fever, shaking chills, multiple skin lesions (petechiae, papules, pustules, hemorrhagic bullae, or necrotic lesions), fleeting migratory polyarthralgias, and tenosynovitis in the fingers, wrists, toes, and ankles that typically evolves into a persistent monarthritis or oligoarthritis. Up to half the patients have skin lesions that begin as an erythematous macule that progresses to a papule, then a pustule with necrosis or ulceration. These lesions appear on the trunk and extremities, including the palms and soles, but spare the oral mucosa. Lesions at different stages are usually present at the same time (Fig. 12A-1). Symptoms of genitourinary tract infection are frequently absent; 80% of men and women have asymptomatic local infection. Urethritis is asymptomatic in about 50% of patients, cervicitis is usually asymptomatic, proctitis is asymptomatic in 90%, and pharyngitis is usually asymptomatic. Women are often menstruating or pregnant. Other risk factors for disseminated gonococcal infection include inherited deficiencies of the late complement components C5, C6, C7, and C8.

Isolation of the organism can be difficult because it is very sensitive to drying. Blood cultures are often positive during the first week, but cultures from joints with early tenosynovitis are often negative. Cultures of synovial fluid from joints with frank purulent arthritis are usually positive, as is fluid from skin lesions. The operational rule for diagnosis is to culture synovial fluid, blood, and smears from the cervix, urethra, rectum, pharynx, and skin lesions on chocolate or Thayer–Martin medium. Culture requires 24 hours, but treatment should be initiated on the basis of characteristic clinical features. Antibiotics should be administered to eradicate all foci of infection and prevent further recurrences of bacteremia. Treatment is the same for both the early febrile tenosynovitis phase or the later frank arthritis. The strains that cause DGI have pili on their surface and are resistant to phagocytosis, but they are generally sensitive to penicillin.

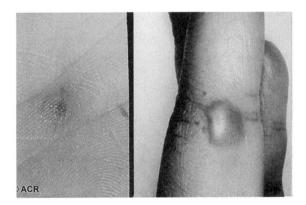

(Figure 12A-1)
Vesicopustular and hemorrhagic skin lesions in disseminated gonococcal infection. **Left,** *a pustule with a necrotic center surrounded by inflammation.* **Right,** *large hemorrhagic blister (bulla) with fluid that may be positive for the inciting organism. Reprinted from Clinical Slide Collection on the Rheumatic Diseases, with permission of the American College of Rheumatology.*

Strains that carry a plasmid for production of beta-lactamase (penicillinase) are resistant to penicillin but sensitive to spectinomycin. The strains of penicillinase-producing *N. gonorrhoeae* are found predominantly in patients in the Far East and West Africa, but these strains are rapidly increasing in the United States and Europe, especially among prostitutes and the urban poor.

Current treatment recommendations are initial ceftriaxone 1 gram/day for 7 days; if the strain is found to be sensitive, penicillin 10–20 million units/day or ampicillin 4 grams/day for 7 days (15). If synovial fluid continues to accumulate, daily needle aspiration may be required. Gonococcal infections usually do not require surgical debridement or drainage and usually do not produce any permanent joint damage.

A similar arthritis–dermatitis syndrome may be caused by *N. meningitidis,* which may be increasing in frequency in urban areas. This gram-negative diplococcus may cause septic arthritis in patients with relatively mild upper respiratory tract infection or in those with severe clinical illness, shock, and meningoencephalitis. Petechial lesions on mucosal surfaces, trunk, and lower extremities should suggest this as a diagnostic possibility.

ANAEROBIC INFECTIONS

Anaerobic joint infections are uncommon, accounting for only 1% of septic arthritis cases. Often, several organisms are involved. Anaerobic infections can occur after trauma or penetrating injury to the limbs, in prosthetic joints, in immunocompromised patients, or after gastrointestinal surgery for malignancy (16). The most common anaerobes in postoperative or trauma-induced joint infection are *Peptococcus* and *Peptostreptococcus* species. *Bacteroides fragilis* is the most common pathogen found in anaerobic infections in patients with debilitating illnesses. Other anaerobic organisms include *Fusobacterium* species, anaerobic diphtheroids or corynebacteria, and clostridium species. One-half of the anaerobic infections are mixed.

Most cases of anaerobic joint infection are monarticular and involve the hip or knee. Foul smelling synovial fluid and air within the joint or surrounding soft tissue on radiographs suggest anaerobic infection. Infection of the hip may occur by direct extension of a retroperitoneal or pelvic abscess, often in the setting of malignancy or chemotherapy. Extra-articular sites of anaerobic infection include the abdomen, genital tract, periodontal abscesses, sinusitis, and decubiti.

DIAGNOSTIC APPROACH

Clinical suspicion and an extra-articular focus of infection should prompt a search for septic arthritis. A positive Gram stain and culture of the synovial fluid are the fundamental criteria for diagnosing bacterial arthritis, but they are revealing in only 50%–75% of patients. Delay in diagnosis occurs when the anticipated clinical picture is altered. Fever may be absent or only low-grade in half the patients, and results of blood tests are usually nonspecific. Peripheral white blood cell (WBC) count is elevated in about 50% of the patients. ESR and C-reactive protein are usually elevated. Blood cultures are positive in approximately half of the patients and are sometimes the only way to identify the causative organism.

Synovial fluid analysis is the most important test in acute septic arthritis. The fluid is intensely inflammatory (more than 50,000 WBC/mm^3) in 50%–70% of patients and moderately inflammatory (2000–50,000/mm^3) in the remainder. The percent of polymorphonuclear leukocytes is usually higher than 85%. Synovial fluid WBC count may be low within the first 72 hours, but is higher 12–48 hours later. Synovial fluid glucose is often less than 50% of the serum glucose in joint infection, but may also be low in RA and reactive arthritis. Lactic acid is usually elevated because of increased glucose utilization and anaerobic conversion to lactic acid (17). Lactic acid levels usually correlate with a fall in synovial fluid pH, but they may be normal in gram-negative infections or if antibiotics have been administered. Urate and calcium pyrophosphate crystals may be seen in infected synovial fluids, presumably because intra-articular deposits "leach out" during infection. The finding of crystals should not dissuade the clinician from the diagnosis of joint sepsis.

Gram stain of synovial fluid reveals organisms in 50%–70% of infected joints and distinguishes gram-positive from gram-negative organisms, although not staphylococci from streptococci. Fluid should be cultured aerobically and anaerobically. If gonococcal infection is likely, chocolate agar or Thayer–Martin media should be plated as soon as the specimen is obtained, taking care to avoid drying. The use of blood culture bottles for synovial fluid may improve the frequency of bacteria isolation. The operational rule should be to culture all orifices, body fluids, and foci of infection.

Early in acute bacterial arthritis, the only radiographic abnormality evident is soft tissue swelling and signs of synovial effusions. A plain radiograph should be obtained at the time of diagnosis to search for a contiguous focus of osteomyelitis and to provide a baseline for monitoring treatment. After 10 to 14 days, destructive changes become evident, including joint space narrowing (reflecting cartilage destruction) and erosions or foci of subchondral osteomyelitis (Fig. 12A-2). Gas formation within the joints suggests infection with *E. coli* or anaerobes.

^{99m}Technetium methylene diphosphonate bone scans demonstrate increased uptake with increased blood flow in the septic synovial membrane and at metabolically active bone (Fig. 12A-3). ^{67}Gallium citrate or ^{111}indium-labeled WBC scans may demonstrate enhanced activity in septic

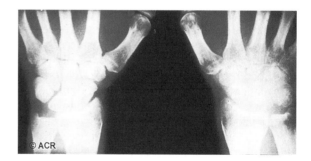

(Figure 12A-2)
Staphylococcus arthritis of the right wrist. The carpus and adjacent bones reveal soft tissue swelling and localized osteopenia. There is narrowing of multiple joints and irregularity of adjacent bony margins. The left wrist is normal. Reprinted from Clinical Slide Collection on the Rheumatic Diseases, with permission of the American College of Rheumatology.

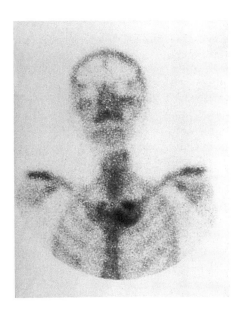

(Figure 12A-3)
Technetium radioisotope scan of septic left sternoclavicular joint shows increased uptake in medial clavicle and first rib. Reprinted from Clinical Slide Collection on the Rheumatic Diseases, with permission of the American College of Rheumatology.

joints. Gallium concentrates at sites of increased protein concentration and leukocytes, whereas technetium uptake results from increased blood flow. Fluoroscopy can be helpful during aspiration of the axial joints. Bone scans show abnormal uptake for 1 year after a prosthesis has been inserted, but thereafter, increased uptake occurs with septic or aseptic loosening of the prosthesis. Gallium scans have a low sensitivity for prosthesis infection, and the utility of indium-labeled WBC scans has not been established.

THERAPEUTIC APPROACH

The initial selection of antibiotics for bacterial arthritis is directed by the clinical setting, including age, history, extra-articular foci of infection, comorbidity factors, and synovial fluid Gram stain findings. The initial antibiotic regimen should be adjusted when culture identifies the causative organism (usually available in 24–48 hours) and adjusted again when sensitivities of the causative organism are known (usually available by day 3 or 4). Parenteral administration should be continued for 2 weeks, followed by oral antibiotics for 2–6 weeks given at two or three times the usual dose. The duration of antibiotic therapy is determined by the clinical response (18). Infections caused by streptococci and *Haemophilus* can be eradicated usually in 2 weeks. Staphylococcal infections require 3 weeks or longer, especially in patients with arthritis. Parenteral antibiotics produce synovial fluid antibiotic concentrations adequate to eradicate bacteria, and therefore intra-articular injections of antibiotics are unnecessary. Synovial fluid bactericidal levels should be measured if response to therapy is not prompt.

Acute nongonococcal septic arthritis cannot be treated successfully by antibiotics alone. The joint must be aspirated to drain intra-articular pus. Adequate drainage is accomplished by large-bore needle aspiration one or more times per day, lavage of peripheral joints, or arthroscopic lavage and debridement of axial and larger peripheral joints (19). Surgical arthrotomy is usually required for drainage and debride-

ment of septic hips and shoulders, septic joints with co-existent osteomyelitis, and joint infections that are not controlled within 5–7 days by needle or arthroscopic drainage. Arthroscopy permits disruption of abscesses, removal of necrotic synovium, lysis of intra-articular adhesions, and irrigation with visualization. The outcome of needle drainage is comparable to arthrotomy and arthroscopy in accessible joints (19). In children, arthroscopy has been shown to be as good as arthrotomy, and it allows for earlier recovery and avoids the need for repeated aspirations.

Patients with painful joint infections hold the joint in flexion, which can lead to contractures. It has been standard therapy to splint infected joints to reduce pain. However, recent studies advocate continued passive and active range of motion with muscle-strengthening exercises when the effusion is reduced.

The clinical outcome depends on several factors, including the duration of symptoms before treatment. Only one-fourth of patients have complete recovery if treatment is delayed more than 7 days. Other factors include the number of infected joints, the patient's age, the patient's immunocompetence, normalcy of the joint architecture before infection, the sensitivity of the infecting organism to minimally toxic antibiotics, the duration of positive synovial fluid cultures, the extent of surgical debridement or drainage required to control infection, and the treatability of the extra-articular site of infection.

MAREN LAWSON MAHOWALD, MD

1. Patti JM, Bremmel T, Krajewska-Poetrasik D, et al: The Staphylococcus aureus collagen adhesin is a virulence determinant in experimental septic arthritis. Infec Imm 62:152-161, 1994
2. Saez-Lorens X, Jafari H, Olsen K, et al: Induction of suppurative arthritis in rabbits by Haemophilus endotoxin, tumor necrosis factor-alpha, and interleukin-1 beta. J Inf Dis 163:1267-1272, 1991
3. Bremell T, Abdelnour A, Tarkowski A: Histopathological and serological progression of experimental S. aureus arthritis. Infect Imm 60:2976-2985, 1992
4. Williams RI, Smith R, Schurman D: Septic arthritis: staphylococcal induction of chondrocyte proteolytic activity. Arthritis Rheum 33:533-541, 1990
5. Dubost J, Fis I, Denis P, et al: Polyarticular septic arthritis. Medicine (Baltimore) 72: 296-310, 1993
6. Goldenberg DL: Infectious arthritis complicating rheumatoid arthritis and other chronic rheumatic disorders. Arthritis Rheum 32:496-502, 1989
7. Yagupsky P, Dagan R, Howard C, et al: Epidemiology, etiology and clinical features of septic arthritis in children younger than 24 months. Arch Pediat Adol Med 149:537-40.5, 1995
8. Youssef P, York J: Septic arthritis: a second decade of experience. Aust NZ J Med 24:307-311, 1994
9. Brancos MA, Peris P, Miro JM, et al: Septic arthritis in heroin addicts. Semin Arthritis Rheum 21:81-87, 1991
10. Armstrong RW, Bolding F, Joseph R: Septic arthritis following arthroscopy: clinical syndromes and analysis of risk factors. J Arthro Related Surg 8:213-223, 1992
11. Maderazo EG, Judson S, Pasternak H: Late infections of total joint prostheses: a review and recommendations for prevention. Clin Orthop 229:131-142, 1988
12. Maguire JH: Advances in the control of perioperative sepsis in total joint replacement. Rheum Dis Clin North Am 14:519-535, 1988
13. Medical Letter: Antimicrobial prophylaxis in surgery. Medical Letter 37:79-82, 1995
14. Ross AC: Salvage of the infected arthroplasty. Annals Rheum Dis 51:910-913, 1992
15. Handsfield H, Sparling P (eds): Neisseria gonorrhoeae. In Mandell G, Bennett J, DR: Principles and Practice of Infectious Iiseases, 4th ed. New York, Churchill Livingstone, 1995
16. Brook I, Frazier EH: Anaerobic osteomyelitis and arthritis in a military hospital: a 10-year experience. Am J Med 94:21-28, 1993
17. Gratacos J, Vila J, Maya F, et al: d-Lactic acid in synovial fluid: a rapid diagnostic test for bacterial synovitis. J Rheumatol 22:1504-1508, 1995
18. Smith J: Infectious arthritis. Infec Dis Clin North Amer 4:523-538, 1990
19. Broy SB, Schmid FR: A comparison of medical drainage (needle aspiration) and surgical drainage (arthrotomy or arthroscopy) in the initial treatment of infected joints. Rheum Dis Clin North Am 12:501-522, 1986

The occurrence of acute arthritis as a feature of some viral infections has long been recognized. The development in some patients of chronic arthralgia or arthritis following a viral infection has spurred investigators to search for virally induced alterations in the immune system or persistent viral infection to explain the chronic sequelae of acute viral infections. The number of patients in the rheumatic disease population with postviral arthralgia or arthritis may be significant, but diagnosis of the acute infection is rarely confirmed by acute-phase serology or viral isolation because patients often present late in the disease course. As advances in biotechnology provide simpler, more sensitive tests for viruses and options for specific antiviral treatment become available, it will become necessary to consider specific viruses in the differential diagnosis of arthritis.

PARVOVIRUS B19

Infection with human parvovirus, designated B19, may be responsible for as many as 12% of patients presenting with recent onset polyarthralgia or polyarthritis (1). Parvovirus B19 is common and widespread, causing the childhood febrile *exanthem erythema infectiosum,* or fifth disease, characterized by "slapped cheeks" face rash (Fig. 12B-1) and a lacy or blotchy rash of the torso and extremities. Up to 60% of adults have serologic evidence of past infection. Up to 10% of children with fifth disease have arthralgias, and 5% have arthritis, usually short-lived. However, up to 78% of infected symptomatic adults develop joint symptoms. Outbreaks of erythema infectiosum occur in late winter and spring, but summer and fall outbreaks have also been observed. Sporadic cases may occur throughout the year (2).

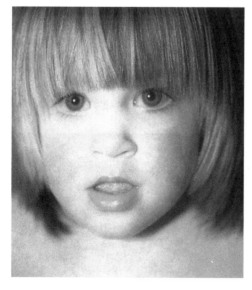

(Figure 12B-1)
Erythema infectiosum rash showing bright red "slapped cheeks." Note that the rash spares the nasolabial folds. Circumoral pallor may be present. Reproduced from Feder HM, Jr: Fifth disease. N Engl J Med 331:1062, 1994, with permission.

Whereas parvovirus B19 infection is usually asymptomatic or mild in children, adults tend to have a more severe flu-like illness. Adults usually lack the facial rash, and the reticular rash on the torso and extremities may be subtle or absent. Arthralgia is more prominent than frank arthritis. The distribution of involved joints is rheumatoid-like. Symmetric involvement of metacarpophalangeal (MCP), proximal interphalangeal (PIP), knee, wrist, and ankle joints are prominent. Patients usually experience sudden onset polyarthralgia or polyarthritis followed in 2 weeks by improvement. Joint symptoms in infected adults are usually self-limited, but up to 10% may have prolonged symptoms. Chronic arthropathy may last up to 10 years, the longest follow-up to date. The disease course in patients with chronic symptoms is characterized by intermittent flares. Only one-third are completely symptom-free between flares (1). Morning stiffness is prominent. About half of patients meet American College of Rheumatology diagnostic criteria for rheumatoid arthritis (RA) (see Appendix I). Rheumatoid factor is usually absent in parvovirus B19 arthropathy, but transiently low- to moderate-titer rheumatoid factor as well as antinuclear, anti-DNA, antilymphocyte, or anticardiolipin antibodies may be found in some patients. Joint erosions and rheumatoid nodules have not been described. Specific serologic diagnosis is possible; however, there is a brief window of opportunity to make the diagnosis based on the presence of anti-B19 IgM antibodies, which may be elevated for only 2 months following an acute infection. Joint symptoms appear 1–3 weeks following initial infection; anti-B19 IgM antibodies are usually present at the time of onset of rash or joint symptoms. The high prevalence of anti-B19 IgG antibodies in the adult population limits the diagnostic usefulness of serologic testing. Treatment is limited to nonsteroidal anti-inflammatory drugs (NSAIDs). Parvovirus B19 has also been shown to cause most cases of transient aplastic crisis in patients with chronic hemolytic anemias, some cases of hydrops fetalis with fetal loss, and, in immunocompromised patients, chronic bone marrow suppression (3). Parvovirus B19 infection has also been associated with cases of Henöch–Schönlein purpura, thrombotic thrombocytopenic purpura, vasculitis, and acute non-A, non-B, non-C fulminant liver failure.

HEPATITIS VIRUSES

Hepatitis B virus (HBV) infection may cause an immune complex–mediated arthritis. Significant viremia occurs early in infection; soluble immune complexes with circulating antihepatitis B surface antigen are formed as antihepatitis B surface antigen antibodies are produced. The onset of arthritis is usually sudden and often severe. Joint involvement is usually symmetric and migratory or additive, but simultaneous involvement of several joints at onset does occur. The joints of the hands and the knees are most often affected, but wrists, ankles, elbows, shoulders, and other large joints may be involved as well. Arthritis and urticaria may precede jaundice by days to weeks and may persist several weeks after jaundice. While arthritis is usually limited to the pre-icteric prodrome, patients who develop chronic active hepatitis or chronic HBV viremia may have recurrent arthralgias or arthritis. Polyarteritis nodosa may be associated with chronic hepatitis B viremia (4). Hepatitis A infection is rarely associated with arthralgia or rash during acute infection or cryoglobulinemia in chronic infection (5). Hepatitis C virus is often associated with type II cryoglobulinemia. It may present as essential mixed cryoglobulinemia, a triad of arthritis, palpable purpura, and cryoglobulinemia.

RUBELLA VIRUS

Rubella virus is the sole member of the genus rubivirus in the *Togaviridae* family of RNA viruses. Rubella infection leads to a high incidence of joint complaints in adults, especially in women. Joint symptoms may occur 1 week before or after onset of the characteristic rash. Joint involvement is usually symmetric and may be migratory, resolving over a few days to 2 weeks. Arthralgias are more common than frank arthritis. Stiffness is prominent. The PIP and MCP joints of the hands, the knees, wrists, ankles, and elbows are most frequently involved. Periarthritis, tenosynovitis, and carpal tunnel syndrome are known complications. In some patients, the symptoms may persist for several months or years (6).

Live attenuated vaccines have been used in rubella vaccines. A high frequency of postvaccination arthralgia, myalgia, arthritis, and paraesthesias have been associated with all vaccine preparations. The HPV77/DK12 strain was the most arthritogenic of the vaccines that have been available in the United States. The currently used vaccine RA 27/33 may cause postvaccination joint symptoms in 15% or more of recipients (7). The pattern of joint involvement is similar to natural infection. Arthritis usually appears 2 weeks after inoculation and lasts less than a week. However, symptoms may persist in some patients for more than a year.

In children, two rheumatologic syndromes may occur. In the "arm syndrome," a brachial radiculoneuritis causes arm and hand pain and dysthesias that are worse at night. The "catcher's crouch syndrome" is a lumbar radiculoneuropathy characterized by popliteal fossa pain on arising in the morning. Those affected assume a catcher's crouch position with flexed knees. The pain gradually decreases through the day. Both syndromes occur 1–2 months postvaccination. The initial episode may last up to 2 months, but recurrences are usually shorter in duration. Episodes of catcher crouch syndrome may recur for up to 1 year, but there is no permanent damage (7,8).

HUMAN IMMUNODEFICIENCY VIRUS

Several musculoskeletal syndromes have been described in patients infected with human immunodeficiency virus (HIV) (9). Whether reactive arthritis, Reiter's syndrome, and psoriatic arthritis are more prevalent in HIV-infected populations remains somewhat controversial. The incidence and prevalence of these rheumatic diseases may vary among populations studied and may depend on geography, mode of HIV transmission, exposure to different infectious agents, other risk factors, and how HIV-infected patients are identified (10). Reiter's syndrome may have a prevalence as high as 11% in some HIV-infected populations. These patients differ from other patients with Reiter's syndrome in that they do not have sacroiliitis or anterior uveitis, nor do they present with the classic triad of arthritis, urethritis, and

uveitis. The prevalence of HLA-B27 positivity appears to be lower in the HIV-infected patients than in non-HIV–associated Reiter's syndrome (11). In Africa, the route of HIV transmission is predominantly heterosexual; approximately 40% of HIV patients with joint symptoms in Zimbabwe have Reiter's syndrome, and another 40% have a pauciarticular presentation without the extra-articular features characteristic of Reiter's syndrome (12,13). In the United States, psoriatic arthritis limited to a pattern of asymmetric oligoarthritis may be seen in as many as one-third of HIV-infected patients with psoriasis, but the overall incidence of psoriasis does not appear to be significantly increased. Whether the different patterns of rheumatic disease expression are attributable to HIV infection itself or to co-infection with other agents remains controversial. The caprine arthritis–encephalitis virus, a goat retrovirus, causes an inflammatory destructive arthritis and lends support to the notion that HIV infection alone may have musculoskeletal manifestations.

Initial HIV infection may be associated with a transient flu-like illness with arthralgias. Several more chronic rheumatic syndromes also occur. The concurrence of RA and HIV is thought to be very rare. An acute symmetric polyarthritis involving small joints of the hands and wrists has been described in a very small number of patients, but many have periosteal new bone formation around the involved joints, a feature not seen in RA. A subacute oligoarticular arthritis primarily of the knees and ankles may cause severe arthralgia and disability, but it is transient, peaks in intensity within 1–6 weeks, and responds to NSAIDs. The synovial fluid is noninflammatory. Mononuclear cell infiltrates may be seen in the synovium of involved joints. As many as 10% of HIV-infected patients may experience "painful articular syndrome," which lasts less than a day and is characterized by intermittent severe joint pain predominantly of the shoulders, elbows, and knees. The pain may be incapacitating and require short-term narcotic analgesics. Fibromyalgia has been reported in HIV-infected patients, with a prevalence as high as 29% in one series. The role of HIV and other infectious agents in these syndromes remains to be clarified (10).

Human T cell leukemia virus (HTLV) is endemic in Japan, where it is associated with oligoarthritis and a nodular rash. These patients have positive serologies for anti-HTLV antibodies, and type C viral particles may be seen in skin lesions. The presence of atypical synovial cells with lobulated nuclei and T-cell synovial infiltrates suggests direct involvement of the synovial tissue by the leukemic process (14).

ALPHAVIRUSES

The alphavirus genus of the *Togaviridae* family includes a number of arthritogenic viruses responsible for major epidemics of febrile polyarthritis in Africa, Australia, Europe, and Latin America. All are mosquito-borne, the specific species depending on the virus and the locale. The known viral pathogens in this genus include Sindbis virus, Chikungunya fever virus, O'nyong-nyong virus, Ross River virus, Barmah Forest virus, and Mayaro virus (15,16).

Sindbis virus was first discovered in a *Culex univittatus* mosquito in Egypt, 1952. Sindbis virus was associated with vesicular rash in Uganda in 1961 and subsequently with epidemic arthralgia and rash in South Africa and Australia. There is a high seroprevalence of anti-Sindbis virus antibody in Africa and Asia where sporadic cases and small outbreaks occur. In Europe, disease occurs in northern European forests, where it is known as Okelbo disease in Sweden, Pogosta disease in Finland, and Karelian fever in the Karelian isthmus of Russia. Sindbis virus infection is characterized by low-grade fever, malaise, joint and tendon pain, myalgia, and rash. The rash is maculopapular, involving the torso and extremities but sparing the face. The rash may evolve to vesicles and pustules, which may be hemorrhagic, especially on the hands and feet. Recovery is full but sometimes prolonged. The rash may recur during convalescence.

Chikungunya fever virus causes febrile arthritis in sporadic cases and in large-scale outbreaks. It is transmitted from its reservoir hosts (baboons, monkeys, and in Senegal, *scotophilus* bat species) to humans by *Aedes* mosquitoes in south and west-central Africa, Thailand, Vietnam, and India. Following a 3–12 day incubation period after a bite by an infected mosquito, Chikungunya fever virus causes abrupt onset of fever to 104°F lasting 2–4 days, flushing for 1–2 days, headache, myalgia, nausea, vomiting, coryza, lymphadenopathy, conjunctivitis, photophobia, retrobulbar pain, and sudden severe pain in one or more joints. Chikungunya is Swahili for "that which bends up." The wrists and ankles are most commonly affected followed by MCP, PIP, and knee joints, and then distal interphalangeal joints, shoulders, elbows, and neck. Synovial fluid shows decreased viscosity with poor mucin clot, and 2000–5000 white cells/mm³. Joint erosions do not occur. A maculopapular skin eruption occurs 2–4 days after onset of illness, and petechiae may occur. A tourniquet sign may be positive. A diagnosis is confirmed by serology showing high titer Chikungunya antibody. Acute disease resolves within 10 days, but joint pain and swelling may last weeks to months. About 10% of patients have chronic or recurrent joint symptoms.

O'nyong-nyong virus first appeared in an outbreak in northwest Uganda in 1959 and quickly spread by *Anopheles* mosquitoes to Kenya, Tanzania, Sudan, Nyasaland, Zaire, and the Central African Republic at a rate of 1.7 km/day, ultimately affecting 2 million people before the outbreak ended in 1962. The infection rate was 90% with more than 70% of infections being symptomatic. Following an incubation period of up to 28 days, the individual develops sudden onset headache, retro-orbital pain, chills, and symmetric severe polyarthralgia. The polyarthralgia is disabling, hence the term O'nyong-nyong, meaning "joint breaker" in Acholi. A majority of patients develop a morbilliform rash by day 4 of their illness. The rash is often pruritic; 60–70% of patients have facial involvement with conjunctivitis. Postcervical lymphadenitis is often prominent. Mild fever may last up to 5 days; one-third have fever greater than 101°F. Residual joint pain often persists.

Ross River virus is responsible for epidemics of acute febrile polyarthritis in the islands of the South Pacific, including Australia and New Zealand, where it is endemic. The virus is transmitted by the *Aedes vigilex* mosquito. Outbreaks occur most frequently in the late summer and fall. Patients experience sudden onset of chills, arthralgias, myalgias, mild fever, and joint pain. Wrists, ankles, MCP, interphalangeal joints, knees, and elbows are most commonly effected. The majority of patients develop a macular, papular, or maculopapular rash, although vesicular or petechial lesions may also be seen. Most patients improve within 2–3 days, but some have numerous recurrences of arthralgias,

joint swelling, and weakness steadily decreasing in severity for up to 1 year. Barmah Forest virus is another alphavirus originally isolated from mosquitoes in Australia and recently shown to cause febrile polyarthritis (16).

Mayaro virus has a monkey reservoir and is transmitted to humans by *Haemagogus* mosquitoes feeding in the South American tropical rain forest. It was first recognized in Trinidad in 1954 and has caused epidemics in Bolivia and Brazil. Mayaro virus was responsible for an outbreak among 800 of 4000 exposed latex gatherers in Belterra, Brazil, in 1988, with 80% of infections being symptomatic. Patients had sudden onset of fever, headache, dizziness, chills, and arthralgias in the wrists, fingers, ankles, and toes. About 20% had joint swelling. Unilateral inguinal lymphadenopathy was seen in some patients. Leukopenia was common. During the first 1–2 days of illness, viremia was present. After 2–5 days, resolution of fever was associated with onset of a maculopapular rash on the trunk and extremities, which lasted about 3 days. Recovery was complete, although some had persistent arthralgias at 2 months. Of interest, Mayaro virus has been isolated from a bird in Louisiana.

OTHER VIRUSES

A host of commonly encountered viral syndromes can occasionally cause joint involvement. In rare instances, children with varicella have been reported to develop brief monarticular or pauciarticular arthritis that is thought to be viral in origin. This is to be differentiated from the occasional bacterial arthritis due to contiguous bacterial spread from an infected vesicle. Adults who develop mumps occasionally develop small- or large-joint synovitis lasting up to several weeks. Arthritis may precede or follow parotitis by up to 4 weeks.

Infection with adenovirus and coxsackieviruses A9, B2, B3, B4, and B6 have been associated with recurrent episodes of polyarthritis, pleuritis, myalgia, rash, pharyngitis, myocarditis, and leukocytosis. Epstein–Barr virus–associated mononucleosis is frequently accompanied by polyarthralgia, but frank arthritis is rare. Polyarthritis, fever, and myalgias due to echovirus infection has been reported in only a few cases. Arthritis associated with herpes simplex virus or cytomegalovirus infections are likewise rare. Vaccinia virus has been associated with postvaccination knee arthritis in only two reported cases.

STANLEY J. NAIDES, MD

1. White DG, Woolf AD, Mortimer PP, et al: Human parvovirus arthropathy. Lancet 1:419-421, 1985

2. Naides SJ: Erythema infectiosum (fifth disease) occurrence in Iowa. Am J Public Health 78:1230-1231, 1988

3. Naides SJ, Scharosch LL, Foto F, et al: Rheumatologic manifestations of human parvovirus B19 infection in adults. Initial two-year clinical experience. Arthritis Rheum 33:1297-1309, 1990

4. Inman RD: Rheumatic manifestations of hepatitis B virus infection. Sem Arthritis Rheum 11:406-420, 1982

5. Inman RD, Hodge M, Johnston ME, et al: Arthritis, vasculitis, and cryoglobulinemia associated with relapsing hepatitis A virus infection. Ann Intern Med 105:700-703, 1986

6. Smith CA, Petty RE, Tingle AJ: Rubella virus and arthritis. Rheum Dis Clin N Am 13:265-274, 1987

7. Howson CP, Howe CJ, Fineberg HV, eds: Adverse Effects of Pertussis and Rubella Vaccines. A Report of the Committee to Review the Adverse Consequences of Pertussis and Rubella Vaccines. National Academy Press, Washington, DC, 1991, pp 187-205

8. Schaffner W, Fleet WF, Kilroy AW, et al: Polyneuropathy following rubella immunization: a follow-up study and review of the problem. Am J Dis Child 127:684-688, 1974

9. Winchester R, ed: AIDS and Rheumatic Disease. Rheum Dis Clin N Am, 17:1-195, 1991

10. Calabrese LH: Human immunodeficiency virus (HIV) infection and arthritis. Rheum Dis Clin N Am 19:477-488, 1993

11. Berman A, Reboredo G, Spindler A, et al: Rheumatic manifestations in populations at risk for HIV infection: the added effect of HIV. J Rheumatol 18:1564-1567, 1991

12. Adebajo A, Davis P: Rheumatic diseases in African blacks. Semin Arthritis Rheum 24:139-153, 1994

13. Davis P, Stein M: Human immunodeficiency virus related connective tissue diseases: a Zimbabwean perspective. Rheum Dis Clin N Am 17:89-97, 1991

14. Nishioka K, Nakajima T, Hasunuma T, et al: Rheumatic manifestation of human leukemic virus infection. Rheum Dis Clin N Am 17:489-503, 1993

15. Peters CJ, Dalrymple JM: Alphaviruses. In Fields BN, Knipe DM, Chanock RM, et al (eds): Virology, 2nd ed. Raven Press, New York, 1990, pp 713-761

16. Nash P, Harrington T: Acute Barmah Forest polyarthritis. Aust N Zealand J Med 21:737-738, 1991

C. LYME DISEASE

Lyme disease is a potentially multisystem inflammatory disease caused by the tick-borne spirochete *Borrelia burgdorferi* (1). The disease was originally described in 1975 from the evaluation of an outbreak of presumed juvenile rheumatoid arthritis that occurred in and around Lyme, Connecticut (2). Lyme disease may develop in a variety of ways. The classic pattern begins with *erythema migrans,* the characteristic rash, which develops within a month of a tick bite. This can be followed by neurologic, cardiac, and articular manifestations (3).

EPIDEMIOLOGY

Lyme disease has been reported in North America, Europe, and Asia. More than 90% of all Lyme disease in the United States is reported from the eight states of New York, New Jersey, Connecticut, Rhode Island, Massachusetts, Pennsylvania, Wisconsin, and Minnesota, although within these states the distribution is not uniform; there are endemic areas, but in other areas the risk of Lyme disease is negligible (Fig. 12C-1). However, someone can visit an endemic area, acquire infection, and return home to a nonendemic area for clinical presentation and diagnosis.

Three etiologic agents for Lyme disease are included within *Borrelia burgdorferi sensu lato.* These are *B. burgdorferi sensu stricto, B. afzelii* (formerly known as VS461), and *B. garinii.* All are present in Europe and Asia, but only *sensu stricto* has been identified in North America. Differences in the organism (4) and in the immunogenetics of the affected human populations have been implicated as causes for the differences between European and North American Lyme disease.

When Lyme disease was first described, the vector in the Northeast was identified as *Ixodes dammini,* thought to be different from *I. scapularis* in the Southeast and Midwest. Recent studies suggest that these vectors are identical. The vector in the Pacific states is *I. pacificus* (the black legged tick); *I. ricinus* and *I. persulcatus* are the vectors in Europe and Asia, respectively.

CLINICAL FEATURES

The clinical manifestations of Lyme disease can be divided into three overlapping phases: early localized, early disseminated, and late disease. There are many examples of patients presenting with later features as the first manifestations of Lyme disease.

Early Localized Disease

Early localized disease includes erythema migrans (EM) and associated findings (5). Erythema migrans occurs in 50% to 80% of patients (although recent studies suggest that EM may be much more common) within one month after the tick bite (mean delay, 7 days). Only about 30% of patients recall the tick bite at the site of EM. The lesion is generally found in or near the axilla, or belt line, as ticks take their meals in warm, moist regions of the body. It is usually asymptomatic, although it may burn, itch, or hurt, and it typically expands over the course of a few days. There may be central clearing or the EM may be uniformly red. Only a minority of patients have the so-called "classic" bull's eye lesion. Lesions that mimic EM include fixed drug eruption, ringworm, tick- or arthropod-bite reaction, granuloma annulare, and cellulitis. Early studies suggested that approximately one-half of patients with EM have multiple skin lesions, due to spirochetemia, although more recent experience suggests this occurs less often. Patients with early localized disease may describe nonspecific complaints resembling a viral syndrome, such as fatigue, malaise, headache, myalgias, and arthralgias. Physical examination occasionally reveals regional or generalized lymphadenopathy or organomegaly. Prompt treatment of EM with appropriate antibiotics prevents progression to later features of disease in the vast majority of patients.

Early Disseminated Disease

Early disseminated disease occurs days to months after the tick bite and may occur without preceding EM. The two

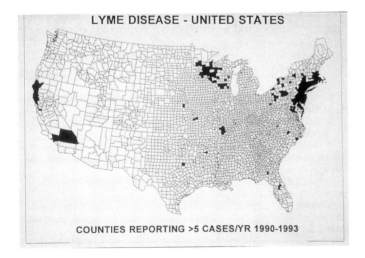

(Figure 12C-1)
Endemic areas for Lyme disease: US counties averaging more than 5 cases of Lyme disease per year during the period 1990–1993. Data courtesy of CDC-DVBID. Reprinted from Fish D: Environmental risk and prevention of Lyme disease. Am J Med 1995;98 (Suppl 4A): 2S-9S, with permission

most common manifestations are cardiac and neurologic features. In the absence of prior treatment, approximately 8% of patients with EM develop cardiac manifestations, including heart block of any degree (or combination of degrees) and/or mild myopericarditis. In the majority of cases, cardiac disease begins to resolve during or even before antibiotic therapy, although there is evidence suggesting that *B. burgdorferi* can very rarely cause chronic cardiomyopathy, or persisting heart block.

Neurologic damage occurs in about 10% of untreated EM patients. Findings include lymphocytic meningitis, cranial nerve palsies—especially of the facial nerve (occasionally bilateral)—and radiculoneuritis. Meningitis typically resolves spontaneously. Treatment of early, disseminated neurologic disease can speed resolution and prevent progression to later features of Lyme disease. Mononeuritis multiplex, plexitis, and myelitis have also been described. Even in endemic areas, the majority of facial nerve palsy is not due to *B. burgdorferi*.

Late Disease

Late disease occurs months to years after onset of the infection and may not be preceded by other features of Lyme disease. Musculoskeletal complaints are reported by the majority of patients with EM who are not treated with antibiotic therapy (6). Intermittent, migratory episodes of polyarthritis occur in 50%—a pattern which mimics juvenile rheumatoid arthritis as described in the original cluster of cases of "Lyme arthritis." Many patients with true arthritis have prior arthralgias. Chronic arthritis, usually monarticular disease affecting the knee, occurs in approximately 10% and can cause erosion of bone and cartilage. Joint fluid analysis reveals a white blood cell count of 25,000 cells/mm³ (range 500–100,000), most of which are polymorphonuclear cells. Chronic inflammatory joint disease due to *B. burgdorferi* typically lasts 5–8 years, although brief episodes of arthralgia may persist thereafter. The incidence of arthritis in patients appropriately treated with antibiotics for earlier features of Lyme disease is not known, but is certainly quite low. In many cases of Lyme arthritis, there may have been no prior clinical problems to suggest Lyme disease.

Late neurologic features of *B. burgdorferi* infection, called "tertiary neuroborreliosis" (drawing on possible analogies with tertiary neurosyphilis), include encephalopathy, neurocognitive dysfunction, and peripheral neuropathy (8). The encephalopathy may be subtle, causing cognitive, mood, and sleep disturbances. Neuropsychological testing can demonstrate changes suggestive (but not diagnostic) of Lyme disease. Such testing can also provide the basis for cognitive rehabilitation should it prove necessary. Patients may complain of distal paresthesias and/or radicular pain; somatosensory evoked potentials may be useful in identifying changes in the former, whereas nerve conduction velocity/electromyography studies help with the latter. Spinal fluid changes include elevated levels of protein and specific antibodies; lymphocytic pleocytosis is usually not present. These patients are typically strongly seropositive.

Other Clinical Features

Fibromyalgia is common in patients with preceding Lyme disease and in many who never had Lyme disease but who carry that diagnosis. Fibromyalgia following Lyme disease is not a manifestation of ongoing infection and does not respond to antibiotic therapy (7). The achiness of fibromyalgia has been mistaken for Lyme arthritis, and fatigue and forgetfulness has been misinterpreted as neurologic Lyme disease.

Nonspecific complaints (such as headache, fatigue, and arthralgia) may persist after treatment of Lyme disease, often lingering for months with slow spontaneous resolution. Such complaints do not require further antibiotic treatment.

Other problems linked to Lyme disease, often on the basis of a positive enzyme-linked immunoadsorbent assay (ELISA) not corroborated by Western blot, include panniculitis resembling erythema nodosa, acrodermatitis, atrophicans, lymphocytoma, myositis, bursitis and tendinitis, hepatitis, inflammation of various structures of the eye, and splenitis.

PREGNANCY AND LYME DISEASE

Pregnancy complicated by Lyme disease remains a major concern. Initial case reports suggested that maternal–fetal transmission might cause congenital anomalies or fetal demise (9,10). However, where Borrelial forms were found in tissue, there was no inflammation, in marked contrast to the histologic findings of inflammation in congenital lues. Large-scale prospective studies have suggested that there is little, if any, risk to the fetus and that there is no definable "congenital Lyme disease syndrome" (11).

PATHOGENESIS

How *B. burgdorferi* causes Lyme disease is unclear. The organism does not make toxins or cause local tissue damage. It may, in fact, bind and activate host proteolytic enzymes to escape the inoculation site and allow dissemination by spirochetemia (12), which may occur within days of the local infection. *B. burgdorferi* has been identified in EM lesions, myocardium, and spinal and synovial fluids, by culture, polymerase chain reaction, or histologic examination (13). Local inflammation is presumably due to the host response. It is likely that poorly degraded antigens on dead or effete organisms can be the focus of inflammation, analogous with the antigen-induced model of rheumatoid arthritis. Local cytokine production may cause preseveration of local immune reaction and may modify local cells' immune and other functions (14). There is an immunogenetic linkage of chronic Lyme arthritis with HLA-DR4 and secondarily with HLA-DR2, although how this is involved in the pathogenesis and persistence of the synovitis is not clear.

Vasculitis has been implicated in some cases of peripheral neuropathy, and a vascular lesion resembling endarteritis obliterans has been identified in meninges and synovium. Early in Lyme disease there is polyclonal B cell activation, with immune complex and cryoglobulin production, although no serum sickness-like illness occurs. Finally, there is in vitro evidence implicating molecular mimicry as a mechanism in neurologic Lyme disease. The organism's flagellin contains an epitope that cross-reacts with a human axonal protein, and a monoclonal antibody to this epitope modifies neural cell lines in vitro (14).

LABORATORY FINDINGS

The diagnosis of Lyme disease is made on clinical grounds; serologic testing should be used for confirmation only. Current practice is to confirm all positive or equivocal ELISA results with Western blot analysis. Individuals with positive ELISA not corroborated by Western blot are considered to have false-positive results, which occur in up to 5% of the normal population. Thus, the costs to society of testing and treating patients with poorly defined symptoms and no objective findings would be substantial and ill-advised. False-positive ELISA results have been reported in patients with other spirochetal infections (such as relapsing fever, syphilis, pinta, yaws, bejel, leptospirosis), Epstein–Barr virus infection, non-spirochetal endocarditis, rheumatoid arthritis, and systemic lupus erythematosus. Even if a positive ELISA is corroborated by a positive Western blot, the significance of true seropositivity in a healthy person, that is, an asymptomatic seropositive, is not established. Furthermore, serologic testing has not been standardized, so comparison between different laboratories is problematic.

Antibody responses may be undetectable in infection of less than 6 weeks duration. Moreover, early or even incomplete antibiotic therapy may abrogate the humoral response, rendering that person permanently seronegative, despite having active infection. Serologic reactivity may persist long after the infection has been adequately treated with antibiotics. Most patients with late manifestations are strongly seropositive, and seronegativity in patients with possible late features of Lyme disease should raise doubts about the diagnosis. Testing of the synovial or spinal fluid for concentration, relative to the serum, of specific antibodies is the only way to be assured that the local inflammation is due to B. burgdorferi.

MANAGEMENT

Antibiotic treatment of B. burgdorferi infection is usually curative (1). Prompt therapy in early disease usually prevents progression to later features. Suggested drug regimens for each stage of Lyme disease are given in Table 12C-1. There is no evidence to suggest that oral therapy in follow-up of intravenous therapy or, more prolonged, higher dose, or combination therapies are needed. Of note, 5% to 10% of patients with early disease experience a Jarisch–Herxheimer reaction within the first several days of treatment. This reaction is usually mild, lasting for less than a day. Therapy during pregnancy should be as appropriate for the features of Lyme disease, although some clinicians treat all such women parenterally. Current studies suggest that the risk of contracting Lyme disease from a known tick bite is very small, so prophylactic therapy is not recommended. As noted, some patients with arthritis are refractory to antibiotic therapy and some of these patients benefit from intra-articular corticosteroid injections, hydroxychloroquine, or synovectomy (15).

Nonspecific complaints may persist for many months following successful therapy. Recovery from neurologic damage may be very slow, as peripheral neurons regenerate at a rate of 1 to 2 mm/day. There is no example of B. burgdorferi resistant to the standard agents, nor is there evidence that the organism can hide in vivo or become dormant, thereby avoiding antibiotics. Lack of response to appropriate antibiotic therapy should prompt a re-examination of the diagnosis, initial and current (13).

PREVENTION STRATEGIES

The best technique for avoiding Lyme disease is to take personal precautions to avoid the risk of tick bite, including

(Table 12C-1)

Current recommendations for therapy in Lyme disease

Oral Therapy of Early Lyme Disease		
Adults		
Doxycycline*	100 mg b.i.d.	3 to 4 weeks§
Tetracycline*†	250 to 500 mg q.i.d.	3 to 4 weeks
Amoxicillin†‡	250 to 500 mg q.i.d.	3 to 4 weeks
Children		
Amoxicillin	40 mg/kg/day, divided dose	3 to 4 weeks
Erythromycin	30 mg/kg/day, divided dose	3 to 4 weeks
Penicillin G	25 to 50 mg/kg/day, divided dose	3 to 4 weeks

Intravenous Therapy of Early Disseminated and Late Lyme Disease¶		
Adults		
Third generation cephalosporins		
Ceftriaxone	2 g q.d. or 1 g b.i.d.	2 to 4 weeks
Cefotaxime	3 g b.i.d.	2 to 4 weeks
Penicillin		
Penicillin G	20 million units in 6 divided doses	2 to 4 weeks
Chloramphenicol	50 mg/kg/day in 4 divided doses	2 to 4 weeks
Children		
Third generation cephalosporins		
Ceftriaxone	75 to 100 mg/kg/day	2 to 4 weeks
Cefotaxime	90 to 180 mg/kg/day	2 to 4 weeks
Penicillin		
Penicillin G	300,000 U/kg/day in 6 divided doses	2 to 4 weeks

* No studies comparing doxycycline with tetracycline have been done.

† Dosage determined by size of patient

‡ No studies comparing amoxicillin with amoxicillin plus probenecid have been done; cefuroxime axetil and azithromycin have also been studied in Lyme disease.

§ There is no proof that isolated facial nerve palsy or carditis must be treated with intravenous therapy. Oral doxycycline for early Lyme neuroborreliosis has been shown to be effective in European studies. Especially in children, oral treatment for Lyme arthritis may suffice.

¶ There is no proof that this the optimal duration of therapy or that more than 10 to 14 days of treatment is necessary.

Modified from Sigal LH: Current drug therapy recommendations for the treatment of Lyme disease. Drugs 43:683-699, 1992.

detailed tick checks at the end of the day (to remove the tick before it can bite), wearing light clothes (so ticks will be visible) with cuffs tucked into the socks (so ticks cannot gain access to the skin), and proper use of repellents such as DEET (N,N-diethyl-m-toluamide).

In animal studies inoculation with recombinant outer-surface protein A (ospA) has been shown to successfully prevent subsequent B. burgdorferi infection (16). In preliminary clinical trials recombinant ospA inoculation appears to be safe and immunogenic (17). Even if effective, however, the vaccine should not represent the primary prevention strategy in endemic or non-endemic areas.

LEONARD H. SIGAL, MD

1. Steere AC: Lyme disease. N Engl J Med 321:586-596, 1989
2. Steere AC, Malawista SE, Snydman DR, Shope RE, Andiman WA, Ross MR, Steele FM: Lyme arthritis: an epidemic of oligoarticular arthritis in children and adults in three Connecticut communities. Arthritis Rheum 20:7-17, 1977
3. Sigal LH: Summary of the first one hundred patients seen at a Lyme disease referral center. Am J Med 88:577-81, 1990
4. van Dam AP, Kuiper H, Vos K, et al: Different genospecies of Borrelia burgdorferi are associated with distinct clinical manifestations of Lyme Borreliosis. Clin Infect Dis 17:708-717, 1993
5. Steere AC, Bartenhagen NH, Craft JE, et al: The early clinical manifestations of Lyme disease. Ann Intern Med 99:76-82, 1983
6. Steere AC, Schoen RT, Taylor, E: The clinical evolution of Lyme arthritis. Ann Intern Med 107:725-731, 1987
7. Hsu V, Patella SJ, Sigal LH: "Chronic Lyme disease" as the incorrect diagnosis in patients with fibromyalgia. Arthritis Rheum 36:1493-1500, 1993
8. Logigian EL, Kaplan RF, Steere AC: Chronic neurological manifestations of Lyme disease. N Engl J Med 323:1438-1444, 1990
9. Markowitz LE, Steere AC, Benach JL, Slade JD, Broome CV: Lyme disease during pregnancy. JAMA 255:3394-3396, 1986
10. Weber K, Bratzke H, Neubert U, Wilske B, Duray PH: Borrelia burgdorferi in a newborn despite oral penicillin for Lyme borreliosis during pregnancy. Pediatr Infect Dis J 7:286-289, 1988
11. Gerber MA, Zalneraitis EL: Childhood neurologic disorders and Lyme disease during pregnancy. Pediatr Neurol 11:41-43, 1994
12. Coleman JL, Sellati TJ, Testa JE, Kew RR, Furie MB, Benach JL: Borrelia burgdorferi binds plasminogen, resulting in enhanced penetration of endothelial monolayers. Infect Immunol 63:2478-2484, 1995
13. Sigal LH: Persisting complaints attributed to Lyme disease: possible mechanisms and implications for management. Am J Med 96:365-374, 1994
14. Sigal LH: The immunology and potential mechanisms of immunopathogenesis of Lyme disease. Annu Rev Immunol 15:63-92, 1997
15. Schoen RT, Aversa JM, Rahn DW, Steere AC: Treatment of refractory chronic Lyme arthritis with arthroscopic synovectomy. Arthritis Rheum 34:1056-1060, 1991
16. Fikrig E, Barthold SW, Kantor FS, et al:. Long-term protection of mice from Lyme disease by vaccination with ospA. Infect Immunol 60:773-777, 1992
17. Keller D, Koster FT, Marks DH, Hosbach P, Erdile LF, Mays JP: Safety and immunogenicity of a recombinant outer surface protein A Lyme vaccine. JAMA 271:1764-1768, 1994

D. MYCOBACTERIAL, FUNGAL, AND PARASITIC ARTHRITIS

Mycobacteria, fungi, and parasites are infrequent causes of musculoskeletal infections (1). However, because of increasing numbers of persons immunosuppressed as a result of human immunodeficiency virus (HIV) infection, aging, or debilitating diseases, and greater immigration from developing countries endemic for these infections, musculoskeletal infections from these organisms are increasing. These agents should be considered in patients with chronic monarticular arthritis, but they may present with other manifestations, including spondylitis, osteomyelitis, tendinitis, and erythema nodosum (Table 12D-1). Definitive diagnosis usually depends on identification of the responsible organism in pus, synovial fluid, or tissue.

MYCOBACTERIA
Mycobacterium tuberculosis

Infection with *M. tuberculosis* is usually acquired by inhalation and begins with an initial nonspecific pneumonitis, followed by lymphatic and hematogenous spread to upper lobes and other organs. In immunocompetent hosts, infection is limited by cellular immunity. Reactivation may occur during a period of diminished host immunity, with multiplication of bacilli in dormant foci and may spread via lymphatics or blood. Osteoarticular involvement occurs in 1% to 5% of patients with tuberculosis (2). Of these, up to 30% have infection in other organs. Men are at slightly greater risk that women. Bone infection typically occurs via hematogenous seeding, during primary pulmonary infection (in children) or from a quiescent pulmonary focus or an extrapulmonary site (in adults). Tuberculin skin tests are positive in most patients with osteoarticular tuberculosis, but chest radiographs are often normal. The definitive diagnosis is made by the demonstration of *M. tuberculosis* in tissue of synovial fluid.

The classic presentation of osteoarticular infection is spinal tuberculosis, or Pott's disease. Infection of peripheral joints, especially weight-bearing joints, tendons, or bursae, may also occur, and reactive arthritis (Poncet's disease) has been reported. Tuberculosis must also be considered in cases of chronic arthritis in patients with underlying connective tissue disease (3).

Spinal Tuberculosis

Tuberculous spondylitis, or Pott's disease, is the most common form of osteoarticular infection with *M. tuberculosis*. Thoracic vertebrae are involved most frequently, followed by lumbar, and less commonly, cervical and sacral vertebrae. In endemic areas, spinal tuberculosis is primarily a disease of children and young adults. In the United States and Europe, most cases are seen in adults (4), occurring by reactivation of dormant foci.

Infection usually begins in the anterior portion of the vertebral bodies, with subsequent disc involvement, disc space narrowing, destruction of vertebral end-plates, and collapse of the anterior portion of the vertebral body, causing the characteristic gibbus deformity (Fig. 12-1) (5). Infection often extends to adjoining discs or vertebrae, or to distant sites. Localized soft tissue inflammation or abscesses involving local structures may occur, such as paravertebral or psoas abscesses, and sinus tracts may be formed. Neurologic injury may be caused by pressure on the spinal cord from a paraspinal abscess, inflammatory vasculitis with thrombosis of spinal vessels, cord transection from vertebral collapse, or spinal root compression from arachnoiditis or abscess (5).

(Table 12D-1)

Typical presentations of osteoarticular infections caused by mycobacteria and fungi.

Mycobacteria

Tuberculosis	Spondylitis (Pott's disease)
	Monarticular arthritis of large weight-bearing joints
	Osteomyelitis
	Bursitis, tenosynovitis
	Reactive arthritis (Poncet's disease)
Bacillus Calmette–Guérin	Migratory arthritis or arthralgias
Atypical mycobacteria	Arthritis or tendinitis of hand or wrist
	Multifocal bone, joint, or tendon infection
Leprosy	Polyarthritis with erythema nodosum leprosum
	Destruction of small bones and joints of hands and feet
	Neuropathic arthritis of wrist or ankles

Fungi

Candidiasis	Polyarthritis with osteomyelitis in seriously ill infants
	Monarthritis of knee in seriously ill patients past infancy
Coccidioidomycosis	Polyarthritis with erythema nodosum
	Monarthritis of knee
	Osteomyelitis
Sporotrichosis	Monarthritis of knee, wrist, or hand
	Polyarthritis with disseminated skin lesions
Blastomycosis	Monarthritis of large weight-bearing joints associated with pulmonary involvement and skin abscesses
	Osteomyelitis
	Spondylitis
Cryptococcosis	Monarthritis secondary to osseous infection
	Spondylitis
Histoplasmosis	Polyarthritis with erythema nodosum

Modified from Perrone et al (6), with permission.

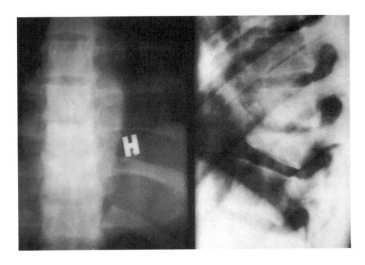

(Figure 12D-1)

Tuberculous spondylitis (Pott's disease). **Left,** *An antero-posterior projection of the thoracic spine shows a paravertebral soft-tissue mass due to a tuberculous cold abscess. The ribs extend out radially, indicating a gibbus deformity.* **Right,** *A lateral radiograph of the thoracic spine showing bone destruction of adjacent vertebral end-plates. Narrowing of the disc space and vertebral collapse have caused a gibbus deformity. Reproduced from the Clinical Slide Collection on the Rheumatic Diseases, with permission of the American College of Rheumatology.*

Back pain is present in most patients. Neurologic manifestations from compression of spinal cord or roots occur in 12% to 50% (5). Fever may be present. Active pulmonary tuberculosis may be absent, but there is often evidence of past disease.

Radiographs typically show disc space narrowing with vertebral collapse and paraspinous abscess (6). Computerized tomography (CT) can define the bony anatomy and paraspinal masses, and magnetic resonance imaging can show impingement of neural structures. The differential diagnosis is broad, including other infections such as brucellosis or pyogenic bacterial infection, neoplasm, and sarcoidosis; bacteriologic confirmation is recommended. Diagnosis is best made by examination of biopsy material, obtained by CT-guided or open biopsy.

Therapy is complicated by the increase in drug-resistant tuberculosis. Nine to twelve months of combination chemotherapy is recommended (7), although there are no definitive studies to support this. Indications for surgery include the presence of motor deficits, spinal deformity, a nondiagnostic needle biopsy, and noncompliance with or lack of response to medical therapy (4).

Tuberculous Arthritis

Tuberculous arthritis occurs mainly in the hips and knees, but may involve other joints (8). Most patients are middle-aged or older, often with underlying medical disorders or previous intra-articular corticosteroid injections. Arthritis is typically monarticular and insidious. Joint pain and swelling are usually present, but signs of inflammation may be limited. A delay in diagnosis of 3–4 years is not unknown. Articular tuberculosis is usually due to reactivation of a hematogenously seeded focus and need not be associated with active disease elsewhere.

Articular tuberculosis is often secondary to adjacent osteomyelitis. Tuberculous osteomyelitis can occur without joint involvement. In adults, a single lesion is most common, usually involving the metaphysis of a long bone. In children, the hands and feet may be involved, causing tuberculous dactylitis.

Characteristic radiographic findings of tuberculous arthritis are juxta-articular osteoporosis, marginal erosions, and gradual joint space narrowing (Phemister's triad). Similar changes can occur in other forms of infection or rheumatoid arthritis. Additional radiographic findings include soft tissue swelling, subchondral cysts, bony sclerosis, periostitis, and calcifications.

Synovial fluid is usually turbid, but may be bloody. The white blood cell count is generally elevated, with a predominance of polymorphonuclear cells and a low glucose. Synovial fluid acid-fast smears are positive in about 20% of cases, and culture is positive in up to 80% (1). The diagnosis of tuberculous arthritis is best made by histologic and microbiologic examination of synovium. Histology may demonstrate caseating or noncaseating granulomas.

Tuberculous arthritis usually responds to combination chemotherapy (8). Surgery may be needed for synovectomy, debridement, joint stabilization, or removal of infected prostheses.

Poncet's Disease

Poncet's disease is a form of reactive arthritis occurring during active tuberculosis (9). *M. tuberculosis* cannot be isolated from joints. Polyarticular arthritis typically involves the hand and feet. Joint symptoms abate with antituberculous treatment.

Mycobacterium bovis and Bacillus Calmette—Guérin

M. bovis infection is now rare, but musculoskeletal symptoms have been related to attenuated *M. bovis* as a component of Bacillus Calmette–Guérin (BCG) (10). Intravesicular BCG instillation for bladder cancer has been associated with fever, malaise, and migratory polyarticular arthralgias or arthritis in up to 6% of patients. Symptoms worsen with repeated treatments and can be prevented by isoniazid. Other syndromes include systemic BCG infection, including monarticular arthritis with *M. bovis* isolated from joints, and reactive arthritis. *M. bovis* infection of a prosthetic joint has been described.

Atypical Mycobacteria

Musculoskeletal involvement with atypical (non-tuberculous) mycobacteria can mimic tuberculosis and include bone, joint, tendon, and bursal infection. Infections are indolent, with insidious onset. The peak age incidence is 40–69 years, with a male-to-female ratio of 3:1 (11). Photochromogens account for the majority of infections, with 32% caused by *Mycobacterium marinum* and 24% due to *M. kansasii. M. avium* complex accounts for an additional 11%. Various other mycobacterial species are identified in the remaining cases, including *M. gordonae, M. scrofulaceum, M. szulgai, M. xenopi, M. terrae, M. foruitum, M. chelonei*, and unclassified mycobacterial. A history of prior trauma, operation, or intra-articular injection is usual, but occasionally hematogenous seeding occurs. Corticosteroid use and underlying arthritis are additional risk factors. *M. marinum* infections are often associated with aquatic exposure.

Any joint, bursa, or tendon sheath may be infected, but the hands are most frequently involved, followed by the wrists and knees. Polyarticular involvement occurs in less than one-fourth of patients, most often with *M. kansasii, M. avium* complex, and *M. marinum*. Delayed diagnosis is typical; delays of up to 10 years have been reported. The most common presenting complaint is joint swelling, followed by joint pain and limited motion. A slow healing wound may be present. Constitutional symptoms, including fever, chills, weight loss, and malaise, are infrequent. Carpal tunnel syndrome may arise from synovitis involving the flexor tendons of the wrist.

Radiographs of affected joints are often normal. If abnormalities are identified, they are usually soft tissue swelling, joint destruction, effusion, bony erosion, or destruction. A pattern of preservation of the central joint space with marginal erosion with sclerotic borders of adjacent bone has been described.

Synovial fluid may be noninflammatory or markedly inflammatory. Pathology typically demonstrates noncaseating granulomatous inflammation, but the absence of granulomas does not exclude the diagnosis. Diagnosis is made by demonstration of the responsible mycobacterium in synovial fluid or tissue. Negative cultures do not rule out infection, as these organisms can be difficult to cultivate.

Treatment of atypical mycobacterial joint infections involves a combination of chemotherapy and surgery. Most strains of notuberculous mycobacteria are resistant to antituberculous drugs to some degree; combination chemotherapy is required for most (1).

Mycobacterium leprae

Leprosy can cause several forms of arthritis (12). Erythema nodosum leprosum occurs in patients with lepromatous leprosy. Manifestations include crops of subcutaneous nodules, fever, and polyarticular arthralgias or arthritis; joint symptoms are immunologically mediated. Septic arthritis, with *M. leprae* found in synovial fluid, occurs infrequently. Chronic erosive arthritis of large and small joints resembling rheumatoid arthritis, which improves with treatment of the leprosy, is also described. In late stages of leprosy, development of Charcot joint due to sensory neuropathy and repeated trauma is a classic finding.

FUNGI

Most fungal musculoskeletal infections have an insidious onset, indolent course, and generally mild inflammation. Other than positive cultures, most laboratory findings are nonspecific.

Candidae

Candida species rarely cause septic arthritis. Arthritis can arise from direct inoculation or hematogenous dissemination of organisms (13,14). Intra-articular inoculation may occur during arthrocentesis or joint surgery. When related to injection, arthritis is typically chronic, monarticular, and caused by species other than *Candida albicans*. The knee is most frequently involved. Intra-articular inoculation can also occur during joint surgery. Fungi cause only 1% of infected prosthetic joints (14). *C. albicans* is the most frequent organism. Infection is usually indolent, monarticular, and chronic. Symptoms may not develop until two years after surgery. Radiographs demonstrate loosening of prosthetic components.

Hematogenous spread of *C. albicans* to joints can occur with disseminated candidiasis. Disseminated candidiasis is associated with drug abuse; among non-drug abusers, it is seen in seriously ill patients receiving intensive medical care, notably hospitalized infants (14). In infants, *Candida* arthritis is usually polyarticular and associated with local osteomyelitis. Past infancy, patients with disseminated candidiasis typically have a serious illness treated with antibiotics, chemotherapy, and/or immunosuppressive agents. The clinical course may be acute with marked synovitis, or more indolent and milder. Arthritis is monarticular in about

75% of cases; most often involving a knee. Bursitis also has been associated with disseminated candidiasis.

The diagnosis is made by culture of *Candida* from synovial fluid or tissue. Treatment with systemic or intra-articular amphotericin B has been successful. 5-fluorocytosine may be helpful as an adjunct to amphotericin B, but should not be used alone because of resistance. Ketoconazole and fluconazole have been successful in treating candidal infection, but the *Candida* species causing infection must by identified because some non-albicans species are resistant. Treatment of infected prosthetic joints usually requires removal of the prosthesis and debridement.

Coccidioidomycosis

Coccidioidomycosis is caused by *Coccidioides immitis*, a soil fungus found in semi-arid areas of the southwestern US, Central America, and South America. Osteoarticular involvement can occur during primary or disseminated infection.

Primary infection is often asymptomatic; about 40% develop self-limited symptoms ranging from flu-like complaints to pneumonia. "Valley fever" or "desert rheumatism" are terms used for erythema nodosum, erythema multiforme, and arthralgias or arthritis caused by coccidioidomycosis. Arthritis is usually polyarticular and migratory, lasting less than four weeks (15).

Chronic pulmonary infection occurs in about 2% of patients, and disseminated disease is seen in about 0.2%. Arthritis and osteomyelitis can occur during disseminated infection. Chronic arthritis of one knee is the most frequent articular manifestation, most often occurring in men. Pathologic features include villous hypertrophy, pannus formation, and bony erosions. Delay in diagnosis averages 4.5 years. Osteomyelitis occurs in 10% to 20% of patients with disseminated disease, most often involving ends of long bones, the skull, vertebrae, and ribs.

Synovial fluid samples rarely yield *C. immitis*. The diagnosis is best made by demonstration of organisms in tissue. Amphotericin B followed by ketoconazole, or long-term ketoconazole can treat osteoarticular coccidioidomycosis, but infection may recur after stopping therapy. Intra-articular amphotericin B has been reported to be useful. Surgical drainage of pus, debridement, or synovectomy may be necessary.

Sporotrichosis

Sporotrichosis, caused by *Sporothrix schenckii*, is usually limited to cutaneous disease, presenting as a painful erythematous nodule at the site of a thorn scratch or puncture. Infection is spread by lymphatic drainage or local extension.

Most localized extracutaneous disease affects musculoskeletal structures, causing arthritis, tenosynovitis, osteitis, or granulomatous myositis (15). Cutaneous findings are present in most patients with musculoskeletal involvement. Arthritis is usually chronic; it may be mon- or polyarticular, and may involve knees, wrists, small joints of the hands, ankles, and elbows. (16). Disseminated sporotrichosis usually occurs in immunouppressed or systemically ill patients. Most patients with disseminated sporotrichosis have bone or joint involvement or both. Radiographs show single or multiple lytic lesions with minimal periostitis.

Synovial pathology demonstrates chronic noncaseating granulomatous inflammation. Diagnosis is based on culture of organisms from joint fluid or tissue. Amphotericin B, with or without surgical debridement, is often curative, but prolonged treatment may be necessary. Intra-articular amphotericin B, itraconazole, and ketoconazole have been reported to be effective.

Blastomycosis

Blastomyces dermatitidis is endemic in the Ohio and Mississippi River valleys and in mid-Atlantic states of the US. Primary pulmonary infection occurs after inhalation of infectious spores; other sites are seeded by hematogenous or lymphatic spread. Osteomyelitis occurs in one-half of patients and arthritis in about 10% (17). Arthritis is typically monarticular, usually associated with pulmonary disease and cutaneous abscesses. In contrast to other fungal causes of arthritis, patients with blastomycosis usually have constitutional symptoms, and arthritis is more often acute, leading to quicker diagnosis. A knee is most frequently involved, followed by an ankle or elbow. In most cases articular disease arises from hematogenous spread, but about one-third are due to nearby osteomyelitis. Osteomyelitis frequently involves vertebrae, ribs, tibia, and skull. Vertebral infection involves the thoracic and/or lumbar spine, and mimics tuberculosis.

Synovial fluid smears and stains may reveal organisms, but definitive diagnosis requires culture. Blastomycosis can be treated with amphotericin B, ketoconazole, or itraconazole. Surgery may be required for patients who fail treatment with these drugs.

Cryptococcosis

Inhalation of *Cryptococcus neoformans* can cause clinically silent or overt pulmonary infection. Hematogenous spread may seed other organs, notably the central nervous system. Most clinically apparent disseminated cases occur in immunosuppressed patients. Osseous infection occurs in 5% to 10% with dissemination, involving the long bones, vertebrae, ribs, tarsals, and carpals with a subacute or chronic course (15). Vertebral infection may mimic tuberculosis. Radiographs show lytic lesions with little periosteal reaction. Cryptococcal arthritis is infrequent, usually due to direct extension of adjacent osteomyelitis (18). The diagnosis is made by demonstration of organisms in synovial fluid or tissue. Treatment is usually with amphotericin B, with or without 5-flourocytosine. Fluconazole may be sufficient for immunocompetent hosts.

Histoplasmosis

Histoplasmosis, caused by *Histoplasma capsulatum*, is endemic in the Mississippi and Ohio River valleys. Most infections are subclinical and self-limited. Dissemination occurs in less that 0.1%, usually in the elderly or immunosuppressed populations (15). During primary infection, acute self-limited migratory polyarticular arthralgia or arthritis may occur, with or without erythema nodosum or erythema multiforme. Arthritis in these cases is immunologically mediated. Arthritis, osteomyelitis, tenosynovitis, and carpal tunnel syndrome occur infrequently in disseminated histoplasmosis. Diagnosis is based on the culture of *H. capsulatum* from tissue or histologic demonstration of organisms. Successful treatment has been accomplished with amphotericin B, itraconazole, and fluconazole, but surgical debridement may be required.

Other Fungal and Related Organisms

Maduromycosis, or mycetoma, is a chronic infection of skin, subcutaneous tissue, and bone. The foot is most often involved. Maduromycosis is caused by a variety of organisms, including actinomyces or true fungi. Infection begins with subcutaneous inoculation of organisms and local extension, with eventual development of granule-draining sinus tracts.

Invasive *Aspergillus* infection can involve a variety of organs, most often the lungs and sinuses. Direct extension of infection can result in osteomyelitis of vertebrae, ribs, or skull. Vertebral involvement can mimic Pott's disease. Articular involvement is rare.

A variety of other fungi have been reported rarely as causes of infectious arthritis, including *Petriellidium boydii* (*Allesheria boydii*), *Fusarium solani*, *Saccharomyces cerevisiae*, and *Torulopsis glabrata* (15).

The actinomycetes are strictly anaerobic bacilli, but they have properties similar to fungi. Actinomycosis, caused most often by *Actinomyces israelii*, is manifest as abscess formation in the abdomen, lung, or soft tissues of the neck. Skeletal infection occurs by local extension, involving the mandible or spine. Usually several vertebrae are involved, with sparing of discs. Diagnosis is made by demonstration of characteristic sulfur granules on Gram's stain, and culture of organisms. The actinomycetes are sensitive to penicillin and tetracycline.

PARASITES

Parasites are organisms that live on or in another and derive their nourishment from the host. They can be grouped as protozoa, helminths, and arthropods (19). Protozoa are unicellular organisms lacking a cell wall. They can replicate within the host. Helminths are multicellular organisms that vary in size from a few millimeters to several meters. Most do not replicate within the host. Arthropods can infest human skin; manifestations are usually limited to the skin but they can also serve as vectors for transmission of other infections.

Some parasites may persist in the host for extended periods. Immune responses induced by parasitic infections can cause tissue injury and musculoskeletal manifestations, including hypersensitivity reactions and immune complex deposition. Such manifestations are usually benign and often resolve with treatment of the underlying infection. Arthralgia is more common than arthritis, but the frequency of joint involvement is not known.

Among protozoa, *Giardia lamblia* has been reported as a cause of acute-onset, mild, recurrent seronegative arthritis, similar to reactive arthritis at times. Other protozoa associated with arthralgias and arthritis include *Entamoeba histolytica*, *Trichomona vaginalis*, and *Toxoplasma gondii*.

Several helminths have been associated with joint symptoms. *Strongyloides stercoralis* can cause reactive arthritis. *Taenia saginata* (beef tapeworm) has been associated with oligo- and polyarticular findings, with evidence of an immune-mediated mechanism and response to antiparasitic therapy. Cysticercosis has been associated with localized myalgias and arthralgias. *Echinoccus granulosus*, which causes hydatid cysts, can involve the spine or long bones. Schistosomiasis has been associated with arthritis and sacroiliitis (20). Articular involvement occurs in about 10% of patients with filariasis, usually monarticular arthritis of the knee or ankle (19). Nonsteroidal anti-inflammatory drugs are not helpful, but symptoms improve with anti-infective agents. Dracunculosis can produce a variety of musculoskeletal symptoms, including myalgias, arthralgia, and acute or chronic monarticular arthritis.

STEVEN R. YTTERBERG, MD

1. Meier JL, Hoffman GS: Mycobacterial and fungal infections. In Sledge CB, Ruddy S, Harris ED, Jr., Kelley WN (eds): Arthritis Surgery. Philadelphia, WB Saunders, 1994, 513-529
2. Grosskopf I, Ben David A, Charach G, Hochman I, Pitlik S: Bone and joint tuberculosis: a 10-year review. Isr J Med Sci 30:278-283, 1994
3. Stecher DR, Gusis SE, Maldonado Cocco JA: Tuberculous arthritis in the course of connective tissue disease: report of 4 cases. J Rheumatol 19:1418-1420, 1992
4. Rezai AR, Lee M, Cooper PR, Errico TJ, Koslow M: Modern management of spinal tuberculosis. Neurosurgery 36:87-97, 1995
5. Mahowald ML, Messner RP: Arthritis due to mycobacteria, fungi and parasites. In Koopman WJ (ed): Arthritis and Allied Conditions, 13th ed. Baltimore, Williams & Wilkins, 1997, pp 2305-2320
6. Perronne C, Saba J, Behloul Z, Salmon-Ceron D, Leport C, Vilde JL, Kahn MF: Pyogenic and tuberculous spondylodiskitis (vertebral osteomyelitis) in 80 adult patients. Clin Infect Dis 19:746-750, 1994
7. American Thoracic Society: Treatment of tuberculosis and tuberculosis infection in adults and children. Am J Respir Crit Care Med 149:1359-1374, 1994
8. Garrido G, Gomez-Reino JJ, Fernandez-Dapica P, Palenque E, Prieto S: A review of peripheral tuberculous arthritis. Semin Arthritis Rheum 18:142-149, 1988
9. Dall L, Long L, Stanford J: Poncet's disease: Tuberculous rheumatism. Rev Infect Dis 11:105-107, 1989
10. Torisu M, Miyahara T, Shinohara N, Ohsato K, Sonozaki H: A new side effect of BCG immunotherapy - BCG-induced arthritis in man. Cancer Immunol Immunother 5:77-83, 1978
11. Yangco BC, Espinoza CG, Germain BF: Nontuberculous mycobacterial joint infections. In Espinoza L (ed): Infections in the Rheumatic Disease. Orlando, Grune & Stratton, 1988, 139-157
12. Chavez-Legasip M, Gomez-Vasquez A, Garcia-De La Torre I: Study of rheumatic manifestations and serologic abnormalities in patients with lepromatous leprosy. J Rheumatol 12:738-741, 1985
13. Cuende E, Barbadillo C, E-Mazzucchelli R, Isasi C, Trujillo A, Andreu JL: Candida arthritis in adult patients who are not intravenous drug addicts: report of these cases and review of the literature. Semin Arthritis Rheum 22:224-241, 1993
14. Silveira LH, Cuellar ML, Citera G, Cabrera GE, Scopelitis E, Espinoza LR: Candida arthritis. Rheum Dis Clin North Am 19:427-437, 1993
15. Cueliar ML, Silveira LH, Citera G, Cabrera GE, Valle R: Other fungal arthritides. Rheum Dis Clin North Am 19:439-455, 1993
16. Bayer AS, Scot VJ, Guz LB: Fungal arthritis. III. Sporotrichal arthritis. Semin Arthritis Rheum 9:66-74, 1979
17. Bayer AS, Scot VJ, Guze LB: Fungal arthritis. IV. Blastomycotic arthritis. Semin Arthritis Rheum 9:145-151, 1979
18. Ricciardi DD, Sepkowitz DV, Berkowitz LB, Bienenstock H, Maslow M: Cryptoccal arthritis in a patient with acquired immune deficiency syndrome. Case report and review of the literature. J Rheumatol 13:455-458, 1986
19. Bocanegra TS: Rheumatic manifestations of parasitic diseases. In Espinoza L (ed): Infections in the Rheumatic Diseases. Orlando, Grune & Stratton, 1988, 243-261
20. Bassiouni M, Kamel M: Bilharzial arthropathy. Ann Rheum Dis 43:806-809, 1984

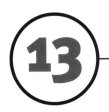

RHEUMATIC FEVER

Acute rheumatic fever is a delayed, non-suppurative sequela of a pharyngeal infection with the group A streptococcus. Onset is usually characterized by an acute febrile illness that may manifest itself in several ways: 1) migratory arthritis predominantly involving the large joints; 2) clinical and laboratory signs of carditis and valvulitis; 3) involvement of the central nervous system (eg, Sydenham's chorea); or 4) a combination of the above. The clinical episodes are self limiting, but damage to the valves may be chronic and progressive, resulting in cardiac dysfunction.

Although there has been a dramatic decline in both the severity and mortality of acute rheumatic fever since the turn of the century, there have been recent reports of its resurgence in this country (1), reminding us that the disease remains a public health problem even in developed countries. In addition, the disease continues essentially unabated in many of the developing countries, and current estimates suggest there will be 10–20 million new cases per year in those countries where two-thirds of the world population lives.

EPIDEMIOLOGY

The incidence of rheumatic fever began to decline before the introduction of antibiotics into clinical practice, decreasing from 250 to 100 patients per 100,000 population from 1862–1962 in Denmark (2). The introduction of antibiotics in 1950 rapidly accelerated this decline; in 1980, the incidence ranged from 0.23 to 1.88 patients per 100,000, primarily in children and teenagers. A notable exception to this has been in the Hawaii, New Zealand, and Maori populations, which are predominantly of Polynesian ancestry, where the rate continues to be 13.4/100,000 hospitalized children/year (3).

While there is little evidence for the direct involvement of group A streptococci in the affected tissues of patients with acute rheumatic fever, there is significant epidemiologic evidence indirectly implicating the group A streptococcus in the initiation of disease. It is well known that outbreaks of acute rheumatic fever closely follow epidemics of either streptococcal sore throats or scarlet fever. In patients with documented streptococcal pharyngitis, adequate antibiotic treatment markedly reduces the incidence of subsequent rheumatic fever. Moreover, appropriate antimicrobial prophylaxis prevents the recurrence of disease (4). If one tests the sera of the majority of acute rheumatic fever patients for three antistreptococcal antibodies (streptolysin O, hyaluronidase, and streptokinase), the majority of acute rheumatic fever patients (whether or not they recall an antecedent streptococcal sore throat) will have elevated antibody titers to these antigens.

Caution is necessary when documenting (either clinically or microbiologically) an antecedent streptococcal infection. The rate of isolation of group A streptococci from the oropharynx is extremely low even in populations that generally do not have access to microbial antibiotics. Further, there appears to be an age-related discrepancy in the clinical documentation of an antecedent pharyngitis. In older children and young adults, the recollection of pharyngitis approaches 70%; in younger children, this rate approaches only 20% (5). Thus, it is important to have a high index of suspicion of rheumatic fever in children or young adults presenting with signs of arthritis and/or carditis even in the absence of a documented pharyngitis.

Another intriguing, and as yet unexplained, observation has been the association of rheumatic fever only with streptococcal *pharyngitis*. Group A streptococci are grouped into two main classes based on differences in the C repeat regions of the M protein (6). One class is clearly associated with streptococcal pharyngeal infection, the other (with some exceptions) belongs to strains commonly associated with impetigo. While there have been many outbreaks of impetigo, rheumatic fever almost never occurs following infection with these streptococcal strains. Thus, the particular strain of the streptococcus may be crucial in initiating the disease process.

The pharyngeal site of infection, with its large repository of lymphoid tissue, may also be important in the initiation of the abnormal humoral response by the host to those antigens cross-reactive with target organs. While impetigo strains do colonize the pharynx, they do not appear to elicit as strong an immunologic response to the M protein moiety as do the pharyngeal strains (7). Streptococcal strains capable of causing pharyngitis are almost always potentially capable of causing rheumatic fever. Whether or not certain strains are more "rheumatogenic" than others remains unresolved.

Only a few M serotypes (types 5, 14, 18, 24) have been implicated in outbreaks of rheumatic fever. Several different M types were isolated from patients seen during an outbreak in Utah, the strains were both mucoid and non-mucoid in character (8). In Trinidad, types 41 and 11 have been the most common strains associated with rheumatic fever.

Increased frequencies of the MHC class II alleles HLA-DR4 and DR2 have been noted in Caucasian and black patients with rheumatic heart disease (9). Other studies have implicated DR1 and DRw6 as susceptibility factors in South African black patients with rheumatic heart disease (10). Most recently, associations of HLA-DR7 and Dw53 have been noted in rheumatic fever patients in Brazil (11). These apparently different results concerning HLA antigens and rheumatic fever susceptibility prompts speculation that these reported asociations might be for genes close to but not identical to the rheumatic fever susceptibility gene.

Monoclonal antibodies have been prepared by immunizing mice with B cells from rheumatic fever patients. One of these antibodies, D8/17, was found to identify a marker expressed on increased numbers (>20%) of B cells in 100% of rheumatic fever patients of diverse ethnic origins (12). While approximately 90% to 95% of non-affected normals had a range of 4% to 6% D8/17 B cells, there was a distinct population (4% to 7%) of non-affected normals in which the number of D8/17 B cells was one standard deviation above normal (10% to 12% positive cells) and thus could be considered rheumatic fever-susceptible individuals. The antigen defined by this monoclonal antibody showed no association with or linkage to any known MHC allele, nor did it appear to be related to B cell activation antigens.

CLINICAL FEATURES
Arthritis

In the classic, untreated case, the arthritis of rheumatic fever affects several joints in quick succession, each for a short time. The legs are usually affected first and later the arms. The terms "migrating" or "migratory" are often used to describe the polyarthritis of rheumatic fever, as the various localizations usually overlap and the onset, as opposed to the full course of the arthritis, "migrates" from joint to joint.

Joint involvement is more common and more severe in adolescents and young adults than in children. This involvement occurs early in the rheumatic illness, and is usually the earliest symptomatic manifestation of the disease, although asymptomatic carditis may precede it. Rheumatic polyarthritis may be painful, but is almost always transient. The pain is usually more prominent that the objective signs of inflammation. Classically, each joint is inflamed for a week at the most, and inflammation may be present in multiple joints. The inflammation decreases and then disappears. Radiographs taken at this point may show a slight effusion, but most likely will be unremarkable.

In routine practice, however, many patients with arthritis and/or arthralgias are treated empirically with salicylates or other nonsteroidal anti-inflammatory drugs. Accordingly, arthritis subsides quickly in the joint(s) already affected and does not "migrate" to new joints. Thus, therapy may deprive the diagnostician of a useful sign.

Carditis

Cardiac valvular and muscle damage can be manifested in a variety of signs or symptoms. These include heart murmurs, cardiomegaly, congestive heart failure, and pericarditis. Mild to moderate chest discomfort, pleuritic chest pain, or a pericardial friction rub are indications of pericarditis. On examination, the patient may have new or changing murmurs. If valvular damage is severe and occurs concurrently with cardiac dysfunction, congestive heart failure can occur. This is the most life-threatening clinical syndrome of acute rheumatic fever. Electrocardiographic abnormalities encompass all degrees of heart block, including atrioventricular dissociation. The most common radiologic manifestation of carditis is cardiomegaly. Studies of patients using echocardiographic techniques suggest that when these more sensitive measurements of cardiac dysfunction are used, nearly all patients with acute rheumatic fever have signs of acute carditis.

Rheumatic Heart Disease

Rheumatic heart disease is the most severe sequela of acute rheumatic fever. Occurring 10 to 20 years after the original attack, it is the major cause of acquired valvular disease in the world (13). The mitral valve is mainly involved and aortic valve involvement occurs less often. Mitral stenosis, due to severe calcification of the mitral valve, is a classic finding and needs to be treated surgically, especially when symptoms of left atrial enlargement are seen. However, younger patients with mitral stenosis but no valvular calcification may be spared valve replacement for some time by the use of percutaneous (balloon) mitral valvuloplasty. This may have great potential in countries where cardiac surgery is less likely to be available.

The incidence of rheumatic heart disease in patients with a history of acute rheumatic fever has varied. In our experience, valvular damage manifesting as organic murmur later in life is still likely to occur in almost one-half of patients if they had evidence of carditis at initial diagnosis.

Chorea

Sydenham's chorea, chorea minor, or "St. Vitus dance" is a neurologic disorder consisting of abrupt, purposeless, non-rhythmic involuntary movements, muscular weakness, and emotional disturbances. The movements are usually more marked on one side and are occasionally completely unilateral (hemichorea).

The muscular weakness is best revealed by asking the patient to squeeze the examiner's hands: the pressure of the patient's grip increases and decreases continuously and capriciously, a phenomenon known as relapsing grip, or "milking sign." Emotional changes manifest themselves in outbursts of inappropriate behavior, including crying and restlessness. In rare cases, the psychological manifestations may be severe and may result in transient psychosis.

The neurologic examination fails to reveal sensory losses or involvement of the pyramidal tract. Diffuse hypotonia may be present. Chorea may follow streptococcal infections after a latent period that is longer, on average, than the latent period of other rheumatic manifestations. Some patients with chorea have no other symptoms; however, careful examination of the heart may reveal murmurs.

Subcutaneous Nodules

The subcutaneous nodules of rheumatic fever are firm and painless. They range from a few millimeters to 1 or even 2 cm in diameter. The overlying skin is not inflamed and can usually be moved over the nodules. They are most commonly located over bony surfaces or prominences, or near tendons, and their number varies from a single nodule to a few dozen. When numerous, they are usually symmetric. These nodules are present for one or more weeks, rarely for more that a month. They are smaller and more short-lived than the nodules of rheumatoid arthritis. Although in both diseases the elbows are most frequently involved, the rheumatic nodules are more common on the olecranon, and the rheumatoid nodules are usually found 3 or 4 cm distal to it. Rheumatic subcutaneous nodules generally appear only after the first weeks of illness, usually in patients with carditis.

Erythema Marginatum

Erythema marginatum is an evanescent, nonpruritic skin rash, pink or faintly red, affecting usually the trunk, sometimes the proximal parts or the limbs, but not the face (Fig. 13-1). This lesion extends centrifugally while the skin in the center returns to normal; hence, the name. The outer edge of

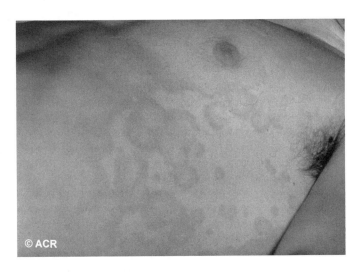

(Figure 13-1)
Rheumatic fever: erythema marginatum. This circinate eruption extends centrifugally, sometimes leaving residual hyperpigmentation. Individual lesions appear principally as open or closed rings with sharp outer edges, but macular rings with pale centers also occur. Fusion of adjacent rings produces a polycyclic configuration. Although a major criterion for the diagnosis of acute rheumatic fever, erythema marginatum is not often seen. Reprinted from the Clinical Slide Collection on the Rheumatic Diseases, with permission from the American College of Rheumatology.

the lesion is sharp, whereas the inner edge is diffuse. Because the margin of the lesion is usually continuous, making a ring, it is also known as *erythema annulare*.

The individual lesions may appear and disappear in a matter of hours, usually to return. A hot bath or shower may make them more evident or may even reveal them for the first time.

Erythema marginatum usually occurs early in the disease. It often persists or recurs, even when all other manifestations of disease have disappeared. Occasionally, the lesions appear for the first time or, more likely, are noticed for the first time, late in the course of the illness or even during convalescence. This disorder usually occurs only in patients with carditis.

LABORATORY FINDINGS

The diagnosis of rheumatic fever cannot be established readily by laboratory tests. Serial chest radiographs may be helpful in following the course of carditis, and electrocardiograms may reflect the inflammatory process on the conduction system.

Throat cultures are usually negative by the time rheumatic fever appears, but an attempt should be made to isolate the organism. Streptococcal antibodies are more useful for several reasons: 1) they reach a peak titer at about the time of onset of rheumatic fever; 2) they indicate true infection rather than transient carriage; and 3) any significant recent streptococcal infection can be detected by making several tests of different antibodies. It is useful to take one serum specimen on admission and a second two weeks later for comparison. The antibody usually tested for is the antistreptolysin O titer. If negative, one should also test for anti-DNAse B, anti-DNAse, and antihyaluronidase antibodies.

Titers of antistreptolysin vary with age, season, and geography. Titers of 200 to 300 Todd units/ml are common in

healthy children of elementary school age. After a streptococcal pharyngitis, the antibody response peaks at about 4 to 5 weeks, which is usually during the second or third week of rheumatic fever (depending on how early it is detected). Thereafter, antibody titers decline rapidly in the next several months and, after 6 months, they decline more slowly. Because only 80% of patients with rheumatic fever show a rise in the titer of antistreptolysin, it is recommended that other antistreptococcal antibody tests be made in the absence of a positive titer for antistreptolysin. Streptococcal antibodies, when increased, support but do not prove the diagnosis of acute rheumatic fever.

Acute-Phase Reactants

Acute-phase reactants are increased during acute rheumatic fever, just as they are during other inflammatory conditions. Both the C-reactive protein and the erythrocyte sedimentation rate (ESR) are invariably abnormal during the active rheumatic process, if not suppressed by antirheumatic drugs. When treatment has been discontinued or is being tapered, the C-reactive protein or ESR are useful in monitoring inflammation. If either the C-reactive protein or ESR remain normal a few weeks after discontinuing antirheumatic therapy, the attack may be considered ended unless chorea appears.

Anemia

A mild normochromic, normocytic anemia of chronic inflammation may be seen during acute rheumatic fever. Suppressing the inflammation usually improves the anemia; thus, iron therapy is usually not indicated.

TREATMENT

The mainstay of treatment for acute rheumatic fever has always been anti-inflammatory agents, most commonly aspirin. Dramatic improvement in symptoms is usually seen after the start of therapy. Usually 80 to 100 mg/day in children and 4 to 8 g/day in adults are required to achieve a serum salicylate concentration of 20 to 30 mg/dl. Anti-inflammatory therapy should be maintained until all symptoms are absent and ESR or C-reactive protein is normal. If severe carditis is also present, as indicated by significant cardiomegaly, congestive heart failure, or third-degree heart block, corticosteroid therapy can be instituted. The usual dosage is 2 mg/kg/day of oral prednisone during the first one to two weeks. Depending on clinical and laboratory improvement, the dosage of prednisone is then tapered over the next several weeks. As the dose of prednisone is being tapered, aspirin may be added in the dosage recommended above.

Whether or not signs of pharyngitis are present at the time of diagnosis, antibiotic therapy with penicillin should be started and maintained for at least 10 days, given in doses recommended for the eradication of a streptococcal pharyngitis. In addition, all family contacts should be cultured, and individuals positive for beta-hemolytic streptococci should also be treated. If compliance is an issue, depot penicillins, eg, benzathine penicillin G (600,000 units in children, 1.2 million units in adults) should be given. Recurrences of acute rheumatic fever are most common within 2 years of the original attack but can happen at any time; the risk of recurrence decreases with age. Recurrence rates have been decreasing, from 20% to between 2% and 4% in recent outbreaks. This may be due to better surveillance and treatment.

Prophylaxis

Antibiotic prophylaxis with penicillin should be started immediately after the resolution of the acute episode. The optimal regimen consists of oral penicillin VK, 250,000 units twice daily, or injection of depot penicillin (1.2 million units of penicillin G) intramuscularly every four weeks. If the patient is allergic to penicillin, erythromycin (250 mg/day) can be substituted.

Guidelines for long-term prophylaxis are unclear; most believe it should continue at least until the patient is a young adult (18–20 years), which is usually 10 years from an acute attack with no recurrence. In our opinion, individuals with documented evidence of rheumatic heart disease should be continued on prophylaxis indefinitely; as rheumatic fever can recur even in the fifth or sixth decade of life.

An attractive alternative to long-term prophylaxis in an individual with rheumatic fever would be a streptococcal vaccine designed not only to prevent recurrent infections in rheumatic-susceptible individuals but also to prevent streptococcal disease in general.

POST-STREPTOCOCCAL REACTIVE ARTHRITIS

Recently, several investigators have speculated whether post-streptococcal reactive arthritis, both in adults and children, is really acute rheumatic fever (14,15). Arguments in favor of regarding post-streptococcal reactive arthritis as a distinct clinical entity include the following. First, the latent period between the antecedent streptococcal infection and the onset of migratory arthritis is shorter (1–2 weeks) than

the 2–3 weeks usually seen in the classic acute rheumatic fever. Second, the response of the arthritis to aspirin and other nonsteroidal drugs is poor in comparison to the dramatic response seen in acute rheumatic fever. Third, evidence of carditis is not usually seen in patients with post-streptococcal reactive arthritis, and the severity of the arthritis is quite marked. Finally, extra-articular manifestations such as tenosynovitis and renal abnormalities are often seen in these patients.

While these cases (admittedly rare) do exist, migratory arthritis without evidence of other major Jones Criteria (Table 13-1), if supported by two minor manifestations, must still be considered acute rheumatic fever especially in children. Variations in the response to aspirin in these children often are not documented with serum salicylate levels and an unusual clinical course is not sufficient to exclude the diagnosis of acute rheumatic fever. In our opinion, appropriate antibiotic prophylaxis should be prescribed (16).

ALLAN GIBOFSKY, MD
JOHN B. ZABRISKIE, MD

1. Veasy IG, Tani LY, Hill HR: Persistence of acute rheumatic fever in the intermountain area of the United States. J Pediatr 124:9-16, 1994

2. Gordis L: The virtual disappearance of rheumatic fever in the United States: lessons in the rise and fall of disease. Circulation 72:1155-1162, 1985

3. Pope RM: Rheumatic fever in the 1980s: Bull Rheum Dis 38:1-8, 1989

4. Shulman ST, Gerber MA, Tanz, RR, Markowitz M: Streptococcal pharyngitis: the case for penicillin therapy. Pediatr Infect Dis 13:1-7, 1994

5. Veasy LG, Wiedmeier SE, Orsmond GS, Ruttenberg HD, Boucek MM, Roth SJ, Tait VF, Thompson JA, Daly JA, Kaplan EL, Hill HR: Resurgence of acute rheumatic fever in the intermountain region of the United States. N Engl J Med 316:421-427, 1987

6. Bessen D, Jones KF, Fischetti VA: Evidence for the distinct classes of streptococcal m protein and their relationship to rheumatic fever. J Exp Med 169:269-283, 1989

7. Kaplan EL, Anthony BF, Chapman SS, Ayoub MM, Wannamaker LW: The influence of the site of infection on the immune response to group A streptococci. J Clin Invest 49:1405-1414, 1970

8. Kaplan EL, Anthony BF, Chapman SS, Ayoub EM, Wannamaker LW: Group A streptococcal serotypes isolated from patients and sibling contacts during the resurgence of rheumatic fever in the United States in the mid-1980s. J Infect Dis 159:101-103, 1989

9. Ayoub EA, Barrett DJ, Maclaren NK, Krischer JP: Association of class II human histocompatibility leucocyte antigens with rheumatic fever. J Clin Invest 77:2019-2026, 1986

10. Maharaj B, Hammond MG, Appadoo B, Leary WP, Pudifin DJ: HLA-A, B, DR and DQ antigens in black patients with severe chronic rheumatic heart disease. Circulation 765:259-261, 1987

11. Guilherme L, Weidenbach W, Kiss M II, Snitcowsky R, Kalil J: Association of human leucocyte class II antigens with rheumatic fever or rheumatic heart disease in a Brazilian population. Circulation 83:1995-1998, 1991

12. Khanna AK, Buskirk DR, Williams RC Jr, Gibofsky A, Crow MK, Mennon A: Presence of a non-HLA B cell antigen in rheumatic fever patients and their families as defined by a monoclonal antibody. J Clin Invest 83:1710-1716, 1989

13. United Kingdom and United States joint report on rheumatic heart disease: The natural history of rheumatic fever and rheumatic heart disease. Circulation 32:457-476, 1965

14. Schaffer FM, Agarwal R, Helm J, Gingell RL, Roland JMA, O'Neil KM. Post-streptococcal-reactive arthritis and silent carditis: a case report and review of the literature. Pediatrics 93:837-839, 1994

15. Arnold MH, Tyndall A: Post-streptococcal-reactive arthritis. Ann Rheum Dis 48:681-688, 1989

16. Gibofsky A, Zabriskie JB: Rheumatic fever: new insights into an old disease. Bull Rheum Dis 42:5-7, 1994

(Table 13-1)
Revised Jones criteria (1992) for diagnosis of acute rheumatic fever*

Major Manifestations	Minor Manifestations
Carditis	Clinical findings
Polyarthritis	Arthralgia
Chorea	Fever
Erythema marginatum	Laboratory findings
Subcutaneous nodules	Elevated acute phase reactants
	Erythrocyte sedimentation rate
	C-reactive protein
	Prolonged PR interval

Plus:

Supporting evidence of antecedent group A streptococcal infection
    Positive throat culture or rapid streptococcal antigen test
    Elevated or rising streptococcal antibody titer

*If supported by evidence of preceding group A streptococcal infection, the presence of two major manifestations or of one major and two minor manifestations indicates a high probability of acute rheumatic fever.

14

OSTEOARTHRITIS
A. EPIDEMIOLOGY, PATHOLOGY, AND PATHOGENESIS

EPIDEMIOLOGY

Osteoarthritis (OA) is the most common form of arthritis and the second most common cause of long-term disability among adults in the United States (1,2). The prevalence varies among different populations (Table 14A-1), but it is a universal problem of humans. Both prevalence and severity parallel age in most individuals. Over one-half of all people older than age 65 have radiographic changes of OA in the knees (3), and virtually everyone has these changes in at least one joint after age 75. Most individuals have no symptoms. However, OA should not be considered a "normal" feature of aging; and changes found in cartilage from asymptomatic older subjects are quite different from those seen in osteoarthritic cartilage.

Other epidemiologic factors besides age are involved in OA. Occupations that subject particular joints to repetitive trauma predispose individuals to OA in those joints. Continuous overuse of a particular joint can be related to the subsequent development of OA (4). For example, baseball pitchers tend to develop OA of shoulders and elbows, football players have more problems with hips and knees, and ditch diggers experience arthritis of the wrists. In addition, isolated trauma such as fracture at the joint space or surgery to remove a torn meniscus is commonly followed by OA in the joint later in life.

Gender and race play roles in the prevalence and severity of OA. The frequency of OA is about equal in the genders between age 45 and 55, but after age 55 OA is much more common in women (5). The prevalence of knee osteoarthritis is more common in African-American women than in whites. Additionally, women are more prone to the inflammatory form of OA of the hands, involving the distal interphalangeal (DIP) and proximal interphalangeal (PIP) joints, producing Heberden's and Bouchard's nodes, respectively (6). Studies in mice have suggested that estrogens might play a protective role against OA (7,8). However, studies in rabbits (9) and in postmenopausal women (10) have failed to document any beneficial effects of estrogen replacement on disease progression.

Obesity appears to correlate best with OA of the knee (11,12). Interestingly, OA seems to be inversely related to osteoporosis, perhaps as a result of alterations in the transmission of stresses across joints in the presence of abnormal bone density (13). Weight-bearing joints including the lumbosacral spine, hips, knees, and feet are most commonly involved in OA. The cervical spine, PIP, and DIP joints are also frequently affected. Joints such as the elbows and shoulders are involved only when predisposed by trauma, inflammation, or overuse.

Other factors associated with OA include a history of trauma, other bone and joint disorders, rare inherited genetic mutations of collagen, a history of inflammatory arthritis, and some metabolic disorders. Congenital hip dysplasias or slipped capital femoral epiphyses alter the mechanics of joint function. Similar changes occur in Paget's disease of bone and in osteonecrosis. Polymorphisms of the type II collagen gene (Col2A1), as well as for types IX and XI collagen, lead to the formation of cartilage that cannot withstand the various forces transmitted across the joint (14,15). Additional support for the role of heredity in some individuals is found in the tendency of inflammatory OA of the hands to run in families. Cartilage damaged by inflammation in rheumatoid arthritis or by urate or calcium pyrophosphate crystals is further altered by OA. Certain metabolic and endocrine disorders such as hemochromatosis, ochronosis, acromegaly, and chondrocalcinosis are associated with OA.

PATHOLOGY

At the gross level, OA is manifested first by cartilage irregularity, followed by eburnation or ulceration of the cartilage surface, and eventually by frank cartilage loss. The latter results in "bone-on-bone" contact in the joint, with even more rapid deterioration in movement and function. At the microscopic level, early changes include fibrillation, or irregularity, of the cartilage surface; later loss of Safranin O staining represents depletion of glycosaminoglycans. Clefts in the cartilage surface then develop, and eventually loss of cartilage can be seen, paralleling the gross findings (Fig. 14A-1). Very early in the osteoarthritic process, inflammatory cells may be seen, but this finding is transient and inflammation is not a significant component of OA (with the exception of the inflammatory variant in the hands, especially in women).

Biochemically, OA is associated with decreased glycosaminoglycan content (including chondroitin sulfate, keratan sulfate, and hyaluronic acid) (16), increased water content (resulting from the increased ability of water to diffuse into the cartilage as glycosaminoglycans are lost) (17), and increased matrix metalloproteinase (MMP) activity. The MMP enzymes, in particular, appear to play a significant role in the degradation of the extracellular matrix of cartilage that occurs in OA and participate in the breakdown of both proteoglycan and collagen (18,19).

PATHOGENESIS

Osteoarthritis is primarily a disease of cartilage. The major constituents of cartilage are water, proteoglycans, and collagens. The proteoglycans contain a protein core with glycosaminoglycan side chains, predominantly chondroitin sulfate and keratan sulfate. The proteoglycans form aggregates with hyaluronic acid, another glycosaminoglycan, and link proteins (MW 40,000–45,000), which contribute to the stability and strength of cartilage. The collagens also are important in the structural integrity and functional capabilities

(Table 14A-1)
Prevalence of osteoarthritis in different populations.

	Age (Years)	Female (%)	Male (%)
English population	35 and over	70	69
US whites	40 and over	44	43
Alaskan Eskimos	40 and over	24	22
Jamaican rural population	35–64	62	54
Pima Indians	30 and over	74	56
Blackfoot Indians	30 and over	74	61
South African blacks	35 and over	53	60
Mean of 17 populations	35 and over	60	60

Reprinted from Peyron et al (2), with permission.

of cartilage. The major collagen found in hyaline cartilage, the cartilage of the joints, is type II collagen. Lesser amounts of types I, IX, and XI collagen also are present.

Many theories have been proposed to explain the degradation of cartilage in OA. The initiating event is usually attributed to mechanical stress that leads to altered chondrocyte metabolism, the production of proteolytic enzymes such as MMPs, and disruption of matrix properties. The first pathologic event may be the development of multiple microfractures, which leads to degradation and gradual loss of the articular cartilage, alteration of joint architecture, and osteophyte formation (20).

In early OA the chondrocytes exhibit a transient proliferative response, undergoing clonal growth forming brood clusters. Chondrocytes also produce increased quantities of cytokines such as interleukin-1 (IL-1), tumor necrosis factor α (TNF-α), and other growth factors; matrix-degrading enzymes such as the metalloproteinase family of collagenases, gelatinases, and stromolysins, and other enzymes including lysozyme and cathepsins. IL-1 and TNF-α promote cartilage degradation by inducing enzymes that degrade collagen and proteoglycans and block the synthesis of cartilage matrix proteins. The MMP enzymes are normally inhibited by naturally occurring small proteins, called tissue inhibitors of metalloproteinases (TIMPS).

In theory, an imbalance between production of MMPs and TIMPs, that tips the scales in favor of increased proteolysis of the extracellular matrix could promote osteoarthritic changes. Similar imbalances between other regulatory molecules and the factors they modulate may likewise be invoked.

As OA progresses, crystals of basic calcium phosphate (primarily hydroxyapatite) are shed into the joint fluid. These crystals are commonly found in joint fluids of very severe osteoarthritic joints (for example, in Milwaukee shoulder syndrome) and have been implicated in the pathogenesis of the disease. One hypothesis proports the basic calcium phosphate crystals are endocytosed by synovial lining cells, resulting in the release of prostaglandin E_2, collagenases, stromelysin, and other proteases into the joint space and amplifying the cartilage degeneration.

Once initiated, the osteoarthritic process continues unchecked. As cartilage architecture changes, the mechanics of joint use are further altered, leading to more stress, further joint damage, and release of damaging degradative enzymes. As a consequence, the process of OA becomes self-perpetuating.

ROSE S. FIFE, MD

1. Bland JH, Cooper SM: Osteoarthritis: A review of the cell biology involved and evidence for reversibility. Semin Arthritis Rheum 14:106-133, 1984

2. Peyron JG, Altman RD: The epidemiology of osteoarthritis. In Moskowitz RW, Howell DS, Goldberg VM, Mankin HJ (eds): Osteoarthritis: Diagnosis and Medical/Surgical Management, 2nd ed. Philadelphia: WB Saunders Inc, 1992, pp 15-37

3. Peyron JG: Epidemiologic and etiologic approach to osteoarthritis. Semin Arthritis Rheum 8:288-306, 1979

4. Fife RS: Osteoarthritis. In Hazzard WR, Bierman EL, Blass JP, Ettinger WH Jr, Halter JB (eds): Principles of Geriatric Medicine and Gerontology, 3rd ed. New York, McGraw-Hill, 1994, pp 981-986

5. Acheson RM, Collart AB: New Haven survey of joint diseases. Ann Rheum Dis 34:379-387, 1975

6. Stecher RM: Heberden's nodes: A clinical description of osteoarthritis of the finger joints. Ann Rheum Dis 14:1-10, 1955

7. Silberberg R, Thomasson R, Silberberg M: Degenerative joint disease in castrate mice. Arch Pathol 65:442-444, 1958

8. Silberberg M, Silberberg R: Role of sex hormones in the pathogenesis of osteoarthrosis of mice. Lab Invest 12:285-289, 1963

9. Sokoloff L, Varney DA, Scott JF: Sex hormones, bone changes and osteoarthritis in DBA/2JN mice. Arthritis Rheum 8:1027-1038, 1965

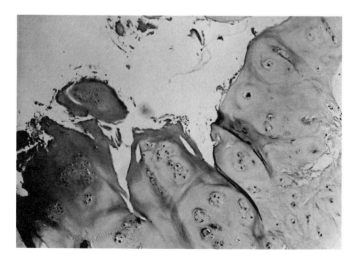

(Figure 14A-1)
Osteoarthritic human cartilage. Pathologic changes include surface fibrillation, vertical fissures, and clusters of proliferating cells. Cartilage components are being released into the synovial cavity.

10. Hannan MT, Felson DT, Anderson JJ, Naimark A, Kannel WB: Estrogen use and radiographic osteoarthritis of the knee in women: The Framingham Osteoarthritis Study. Arthritis Rheum 33:525-532, 1990

11. Davis MA, Ettinger WH, Neuhaus JM: Obesity and osteoarthritis of the knee: Evidence from the National Health and Nutrition Examination Survey (NHANES I). Semin Arthritis Rheum 20 (suppl):34-41, 1990

12. Felson DT, Anderson JJ, Naimark A, Walker AM, Meenan RF: Obesity and knee osteoarthritis: The Framingham Study. Ann Int Med 109:18-24, 1988

13. Cooper C, Cook PL, Osmond C, Fisher L, Cawley MI: Osteoarthritis of the hip and osteoporosis of the proximal femur. Ann Rheum Dis 50:540-542, 1991

14. Knowlton RG, Katzenstein PL, Moskowitz RW, Weaver EJ, Malemud CJ, Pathria MN, Jimenez SA, Prockop DJ: Genetic linkage of a polymorphism in the type II procollagen gene (COL2A1) to primary osteoarthritis associated with mild chondrodysplasia. N Engl J Med 322:526-530, 1990

15. Eyre DR, Weis MA, Moskowitz RW: Cartilage expression of a type II col-lagen mutation in an inherited form of osteoarthritis associated with a mild chondrodysplasia. J Clin Invest 87:357-361, 1991

16. Brandt KD: Osteoarthritis. Clin Geriatric Med 4:279-293, 1988

17. Venn M, Maroudas A: Chemical composition and swelling of normal and osteoarthrotic femoral head cartilage. Ann Rheum Dis 36:121-129, 1977

18. Sapolsky AI, Keiser H, Howell DS, Woessner JF Jr: Metalloproteases of human articular cartilage that digest cartilage proteoglycans at neutral and acid pH. J Clin Invest 58:1030-1041, 1976

19. Pelletier J-P, Martel-Pelletier J, Howell DS, Ghandur-Mnaymneh L, Enis JE, Woessner JF Jr: Collagenase and collagenolytic activity in human osteoarthritic cartilage. Arthritis Rheum 26:63-68, 1983

20. Woo SL-Y, Kwan MK, Cutts RD, Akeson WH: Biochamical considera-tions. In Moskowitz RW, Howell DS, Goldberg VM, Mankin HJ (eds): Osteoarthritis: Diagnosis and Medical/Surgical Management, 2nd ed. Philadelphia, WB Saunders, 1992, pp 191-211

B. CLINICAL FEATURES AND TREATMENT

The definition of osteoarthritis, published in the proceedings of a 1994 conference sponsored by the American Academy of Orthopaedic Surgeons and National Institutes of Health, highlights the clinical features of the disease (1):

Osteoarthritis (OA) is the result of both mechanical and biologic events that destabilize the normal coupling of degradation and synthesis of articular cartilage and subchondral bone. Although it may be initiated by multiple factors including genetic, developmental, metabolic and traumatic, OA involves all of the tissues of the diarthrodial joint. Ultimately, OA is manifested by morphologic, biochemical, molecular and biomechanical changes of both cells and matrix which lead to a softening, fibrillation, ulceration and loss of articular cartilage, sclerosis and eburnation of subchondral bone, osteophytes and subchondral cysts. When clinically evident, OA is characterized by joint pain, tenderness, limitation of movement, crepitus, occasional effusion, and variable degrees of local inflammation.

SYMPTOMS AND SIGNS

The typical patient with OA is middle-aged or elderly with pain and stiffness in and around a joint accompanied by limitation of function. The pain is gradual or insidious in onset, is usually mild in intensity, worsens by using the involved joint(s), and improves or is relieved with rest. Initially, the pain may be intermittent and self-limited; pain at rest or during the night is a feature of severe disease. The mechanisms of pain in OA are multifactorial; pain may originate from periostitis at sites of bony remodeling, subchondral microfractures, irritation of sensory nerve endings in the synovium from osteophytes, periarticular muscle spasm, bone angina due to decreased blood flow and elevated intraosseus pressure, and synovial inflammation accompanied by the release of prostaglandins, leukotrienes, and various cytokines (2).

Although morning stiffness is common in OA patients, the duration is shorter, often less than 30 minutes, than in patients with active rheumatoid arthritis (RA). Gel phenomenon (stiffness after periods of rest and inactivity) is also common in OA and resolves within several minutes. Most patients note that both pain and stiffness are modified by changes in the weather; characteristically, symptoms worsen in damp, cool, and rainy weather. This feature has been attributed to changes in intra-articular pressure associated with changes in atmospheric barometric pressure.

Patients with OA of the knees often complain of instability or buckling, especially when descending stairs or stepping off curbs. Osteoarthritis of the hip usually causes problems with gait and pain that is usually localized to the groin and may radiate down the anterior thigh to the knee. Patients with OA of the hands may have problems with manual dexterity, especially if the joints at the thumb base—ie, first carpometacarpal (CMC) and trapezioscaphoid—are involved. Involvement of the apophyseal or facet joints of the lower cervical and lumbar spine may cause symptoms of neck and low-back pain, respectively. In addition, osteophytes can narrow the foramens and compress nerve roots, producing radicular symptoms including pain, weakness, and numbness.

On physical examination, findings are usually localized to symptomatic joints and vary with the severity of disease. Bony enlargement is common, causing tenderness at the joint margins and the attachments of the joint capsule and periarticular tendons. Limitation of motion is usually related to osteophyte formation, severe cartilage loss leading to joint surface incongruity, or periarticular muscle spasm or contracture. Joint instability can be detected by excess motion. Locking of a joint during range of motion is likely due to loose bodies or floating cartilage fragments within the joint.

Crepitus, which is felt on passive range of motion, is due to irregularity of the opposing cartilage surfaces. This sign is present in more than 90% of patients with OA of the knee. Almost 50% of patients with knee OA have a malalignment of the joint, most commonly a varus deformity due to loss of articular cartilage in the medial compartment. Pain on motion may be due to joint capsule irritation, periarticular muscle spasm, or periostitis.

Signs of local inflammation include warmth and soft-tissue swelling due to joint effusion. Patients with erosive OA may have signs of inflammation in the interphalangeal joints of the hands. However, the presence of a hot, erythematous, markedly swollen joint suggests either septic arthritis or a superimposed microcrystalline process, such as gout, pseudogout, or basic calcium phosphate (hydroxyapatite) arthritis.

RADIOGRAPHIC FEATURES

The clinical diagnosis of OA is usually confirmed with radiographs of the affected joint (Fig. 14B-1). The classic radi-

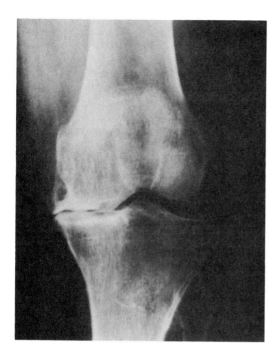

(Figure 14B-1)
Radiograph of the knee showing moderate-to-severe osteoarthritis. Note the marked joint-space narrowing in the medial compartment, osteophyte formation, and sclerosis of subchondral bone.

ographic finding is bony proliferation (ie, osteophyte formation or spurs) at the joint margin. Asymmetric joint space narrowing and subchondral bone sclerosis develop as the disease progresses. Joint space narrowing may result from loss of articular cartilage or progression of the tidemark region of calcified cartilage bone remodeling. Later changes include the formation of subchondral cysts with sclerotic walls and bone remodeling with alteration in the shape of bone ends. Because bone demineralization (periarticular osteoporosis) and marginal erosions are not radiographic features of OA, their presence strongly suggests a diagnosis of RA or other inflammatory arthritis. Central erosions and cortical collapse in the distal and, less commonly, proximal interphalangeal (PIP) joints of the hands can be seen on radiographs in some patients with erosive OA.

LABORATORY FINDINGS

The diagnosis of OA can almost always be made by history and physical examination. Results of routine laboratory tests are normal and are therefore useful in screening for associated conditions and for establishing baseline for monitoring therapy. For example, patients with radiographic evidence of chondrocalcinosis should have levels of serum calcium, phosphorous, magnesium, and thyroid-stimulating hormone measured. Measurements of serum hemoglobin, creatinine, potassium, and aspartate aminotransferase levels may be obtained before initiating therapy with nonsteroidal anti-inflammatory drugs (NSAIDs).

Clinicians often routinely order tests for rheumatoid factor (RF) and erythrocyte sedimentation rate (ESR) for all patients with joint complaints. However, neither the presence of RF nor mildly elevated ESR excludes a diagnosis of OA in the older patient. About 20% of healthy elderly individuals are RF-positive in low titer, and ESR tends to rise with age. Patients with a markedly elevated ESR, however, should be

evaluated for polymyalgia rheumatica, underlying malignancy such as multiple myeloma, and chronic infection.

Synovial fluid analysis usually reveals a white blood cell (WBC) count below 2000 cells/mm^3. Occasionally, patients with OA have a mildly inflammatory effusion with elevated protein and higher WBC levels. The finding of inflammatory fluid with an elevated WBC count suggests either a superimposed microcrystalline process or septic arthritis.

DIFFERENTIAL DIAGNOSIS

The major challenges to the physician in the diagnosis of OA are two-fold: 1) to distinguish patients with OA from those with inflammatory disorders such as RA and polymyalgia rheumatica, and 2) to identify those few patients who have a secondary form of OA (3).

Osteoarthritis involves a characteristic pattern of axial and peripheral joints in which one or more of the following joint groups are affected: distal interphalangeal (DIP), PIP, and first CMC joints of the hands; cervical and lumbar spine; and first metatarsophalangeal (MTP) joints of the feet, knees, and hips. The number of involved joints varies; patients who have three or more joint groups affected are considered to have generalized OA.

Generalized OA is frequently associated with bony enlargement of the DIP and PIP joints called Heberden's nodes and Bouchard's nodes, respectively (nodal osteoarthritis). Generalized OA most often affects middle-aged to elderly women and is inherited in an autosomal dominant fashion. Patients with non-nodal generalized OA often have a history of mild inflammatory joint disease. Generalized OA can be distinguished from RA by the pattern of joint involvement in the hands; RA typically involves the metacarpophalangeal (MCP) and PIP joints but spares the thumb base and DIP joints.

The American College of Rheumatology (ACR) has developed algorithms for the classification of patients with OA of the hands, hips, and knees (4-6). Although not designed for diagnosis of the individual patient, the classifications highlight major differences between groups of OA patients and patients with other causes of pain at these sites.

Patients with OA of the axial skeleton who have symptoms of muscle aching in the neck and shoulder girdle and the low back and pelvic girdle should be evaluated for polymyalgia rheumatica. This diagnosis is based on history and laboratory tests; patients with polymyalgia rheumatica usually have prolonged morning stiffness, a markedly elevated ESR, and mild normochromic, normocytic anemia.

Patients with OA involving atypical joints (eg, MCP joints, wrists, elbows, shoulders, or ankles) should be evaluated for an underlying disorder such as calcium pyrophosphate deposition disease or hemochromatosis.

TREATMENT

The underlying principles of managing OA patients are: 1) relieving symptoms, 2) maintaining or improving function, 3) limiting physical disability, and 4) avoiding drug toxicity. Numerous treatment options exist (Table 14B-1), and treatment should be based on the distribution and severity of joint involvement, as well as the presence of comorbid conditions. Recently, the ACR published guidelines for the medical management of patients with OA of the hip and knee (7,8) (see Appendix II).

Nonpharmacologic therapy
    Patient education and self-management programs
    Social support via telephone contact
    Physical and occupational therapy
    Range-of-motion and strengthening exercises
    Aerobic conditioning
    Weight loss
    Assistive devices for ambulation and activities of daily
      living
Pharmacologic therapy
    Oral non-opioid analgesics (eg, acetaminophen)
    Topical analgesics (eg, capsaicin cream)
    Nonsteroidal anti-inflammatory drugs
    Intra-articular steroid injections
    Opioid analgesics
Surgical therapy
    Closed tidal joint lavage
    Arthroscopic debridement and joint lavage
    Osteotomy
    Total joint arthroplasty

Nonpharmacologic Modalities

Patient education materials, including pamphlets published by the Arthritis Foundation, provide basic information to help patients understand and cope with OA. Patients should be encouraged to participate in self-management programs, such as the Arthritis Self-Help Course, which is administered by local chapters of the Arthritis Foundation. Studies have shown that patients who participate in this program have better outcomes and lower health care costs than patients who receive traditional care.

Patients with physical disabilities and difficulties in performing activities of daily living may benefit from consultation with an occupational and physical therapist. The occupational therapist evaluates the patient's ability to perform activities of daily living, provides assistive devices as needed, and teaches joint protection techniques and energy conservation skills. In addition, splints can be designed to either stabilize or reduce inflammation in finger joints, especially the thumb base. The physical therapist teaches the patient how to use therapeutic heat and massage and provides an individualized exercise program. A recent meta-analysis supported a central role for exercise in managing patients with lower-limb OA, especially of the knee (9). Exercise programs stress range of motion and muscle strengthening (eg, quadriceps strengthening exercises for patients with OA of the knees to improve stability). Braces, canes, walkers, and other ambulation aids and devices are provided if needed. Physical therapy also plays a crucial role in the pre- and postoperative management of patients undergoing reconstructive orthopedic surgery.

Overweight patients should be encouraged to lose weight, because increased weight is associated with progression of knee and hip OA. Referral for dietary instruction and enrollment in an aerobic exercise program, either fitness walking or swimming, may be helpful. Local chapters of the Arthritis Foundation sponsor aquatic exercise programs in heated pools under the direction of a trained therapist.

Pharmacologic Therapy

The main indication for drug therapy in OA patients is relief of pain. Simple analgesics, such as acetaminophen, are currently the drug of choice. Two studies demonstrated that the short-term efficacy of acetaminophen is comparable with that of ibuprofen and naproxen in patients with OA of the knee (10,11). Patients who fail to respond to acetaminophen should be considered candidates for treatment with an NSAID, unless contraindicated. Since the different NSAIDs are about equally effective in relieving pain, the choice of a specific NSAID is largely influenced by differences in toxicity profiles, frequency of drug dosing, and cost (12,13). The major concern about the routine use of NSAIDs in OA patients is the increased risk of upper gastrointestinal toxicity (eg, gastric and duodenal ulcers, gastrointestinal bleeding) and renal toxicity (eg, reversible renal insufficiency, fluid retention, hyperkalemia) (14).

Intra-articular corticosteroid injections are useful in treating a joint effusion or local inflammation that is limited to a few joints. Local injections are beneficial as an adjunct to NSAID therapy and may be used for patients who are unable to take NSAIDs. Injections should be performed using aseptic technique, and aspirated fluid should be sent for appropriate bacteriologic culture, if infection is suspected. Repeated intra-articular injections at a frequency of more than two or three times a year have been discouraged because of concern about the potential for progressive cartilage damage and pseudo-Charcot arthropathy. In reality, very few such complications have been reported.

Other medical modalities available for treating OA include topical analgesic creams (eg, 0.025% capsaicin cream). Patients with OA of the knee who have failed to respond to other therapies may benefit from closed tidal joint lavage with saline.

Surgery

Patients whose symptoms are not adequately controlled with medical therapy and who have moderate-to-severe pain and functional impairment are candidates for orthopedic surgery. OA of the knee that is complicated by internal derangement may be treated with arthroscopic debridement and, if indicated, lavage with meniscectomy. High tibial osteotomy is indicated for young patients with knee OA complicated by significant angular deformity and malalignment; femoral osteotomy is indicated for young patients with unilateral OA of the hip.

Total joint arthroplasty has markedly improved the quality of life of patients with knee and hip OA and is one of the major advances in the management of OA over the past 30 years (15). These operations almost always provide significant, if not excellent, pain relief. Function is less consistently restored to normal, however. Therefore, the most satisfying results are obtained when the operation is performed for the primary purpose of pain relief. Perioperative mortality is generally below 1%, and short-term complications, including thromboembolic disease and infection, occur in fewer than 5% of patients. A major concern is the long-term complication of loosening due to deterioration of the bone–cement interface. The recent developments of porous coated prostheses, which allow fixation by bone ingrowth, and newer techniques for cementing noncoated prostheses may eventually reduce the need for revision surgery due to loosening.

Experimental Agents

Presently, no drugs that reverse the structural or biochemical abnormalities of OA have been approved by the Food and Drug Administration. Such disease-modifying drugs have been studied in several animal models of OA, however (16), and may be available in the future for use in humans (17). Examples include oral doxycycline, intra-articular injection of hyaluronate, intramuscular injection of pentosan polysulfate and polysulfated glycosaminoglycans, and cartilage transplants.

MARC C. HOCHBERG, MD, MPH

1. Keuttner KE, Goldberg V (eds): Osteoarthritic Disorders. Rosemont, IL, American Academy of Orthoaedic Surgeons, 1995, pp xxi-xxv

2. Altman RD (ed): Pain in osteoarthritis. Semin Arthritis Rheum 18(suppl 2):1-104, 1989

3. Schumacher HR Jr: Secondary osteoarthritis. In Moskowitz RW, Howell DS, Goldberg VM, Mankin HJ (eds): Osteoarthritis: Diagnosis and Surgical Management. Philadelphia, WB Saunders, 1993, pp 367-398

4. Altman RD, Asch E, Bloch D, et al: Development of criteria for the classification and reporting of osteoarthritis: classification of osteoarthritis of the knee. Arthritis Rheum 29:1039-1049, 1986

5. Altman R, Alarcon G, Appelrough D, et al: The American College of Rheumatology criteria for the classification and reporting of osteoarthritis of the hand. Arthritis Rheum 33:1601-1610, 1990

6. Altman R, Alarcon G, Appelrough D, et al: The American College of Rheumatology criteria for the classification and reporting of osteoarthritis of the hip. Arthritis Rheum 34:505-514, 1991

7. Hochberg MC, Altman RD, Brandt KD, et al: Guidelines for the medical management of osteoarthritis: Part I. Osteoarthritis of the hip. Arthritis Rheum 38:1535-1540, 1995

8. Hochberg MC, Altman RD, Brandt KD, et al: Guidelines for the medical management of osteoarthritis: Part II. Osteoarthritis of the knee. Arthritis Rheum 38:1541-1546, 1995

9. Puett DW, Griffin MR: Published trials of nonmedicinal and noninvasive therapies for hip and knee osteoarthritis. Ann Intern Med 121:133-140, 1994

10. Bradley JD, Brandt KD, Katz BP, Kalasinski LA, Ryan SL: Comparison of an inflammatory dose of ibuprofen, an analgesic dose of ibuprofen and acetaminophen in the treatment of patients with osteoarthritis of the knee. N Engl J Med 325:87-91, 1991

11. Williams HJ, Ward JR, Egger MJ, et al: Comparison of naproxen and acetaminophen in a two-year study of treatment of osteoarthritis of the knee. Arthritis Rheum 36:1196-1206, 1993

12. Brooks P, Day R: Nonsteroidal antiinflammatory drugs: differences and similarities. N Engl J Med 324:1716-1725, 1991

13. Furst DE: Are there differences among nonsteroidal antiinflammatory drugs? Comparing acetylated salicylates, nonacetylated salicylates, and nonacetylated nonsteroidal antiinflammatory drugs. Arthritis Rheum 37:1-9, 1994

14. Griffin MR, Brandt KD, Liang MH, Pincus T, Ray WA: Practical management of osteoarthritis: integration of pharmacologic and nonpharmacologic measures. Arch Family Med 4:1049-1055, 1995

15. Buckwalter JA, Lohmander S: Operative treatment of osteoarthritis: current practice and future development. J Bone Joint Surg 76A:1405-1418, 1994

16. Howell DS, Altman RD, Pelletier JP, et al: Disease modifying antirheumatic drugs: current state of their application in animal models of osteoarthritis. In Keuttner K, Goldberg V (eds): Osteoarthritic Disorders. Rosemont, IL, American Academy of Orthopaedic Surgeons, 1995, pp 365-377

17. Brandt KD: Toward pharmacologic modification of joint damage in osteoarthritis. Ann Intern Med 122:874-875, 1995

APATITES AND MISCELLANEOUS CRYSTALS

15

A wide variety of crystalline particles other than monosodium urate monohydrate (MSUM, the gout crystal) and calcium pyrophosphate dihydrate (CPPD) can be found in joint tissues and fluids under certain conditions (1) (Table 15-1). Of those listed, the basic calcium phosphates, particularly carbonated apatites (hydroxyapatite, $Ca_{10}(PO_4)_6.OH$, with CO_3 substituting for OH groups) are encountered most frequently. Lipid deposits and cholesterol crystals are also a relatively common finding in diseased joints.

The relationships between the deposition of these crystals and other miscellaneous crystals in articular and periarticular tissues and the etiopathogenesis of rheumatic diseases is complex, controversial, and poorly understood (2). Crystal deposition can be secondary to local tissue damage, as well as contributing to it. Furthermore, mixtures of different types of basic calcium phosphates and other crystals, including CPPD, are frequently seen in the same tissue, making it difficult to correlate the presence of a particular crystal species with a disease state.

BASIC CALCIUM PHOSPHATES
Sites of Deposition and Epidemiology

Basic calcium phosphates are frequently deposited in periarticular tendons, intervertebral discs, and intra-articular

(Table 15-1)
Some crystals and other particles identified in joint tissues and synovial fluids*

Monosodium urate monohydrate crystals

Spherulites of urates

Calcium pyrophosphate dihydrate crystals

Basic calcium phosphates

    Apatites

    Tricalcium phosphate

    Octacalcium phosphate

Dicalcium phosphate dihydrate (Brushite)

Calcium magnesium phosphate (Whitlokite)

Calcium carbonates (Calcite and Aragonite)

Calcium oxalates (monohydrate and dihydrate)

Lipids

    Cholesterol crystals

    "Liquid lipid crystals"

    Lipid spherulites

Protein crystals such as cryoglobulins, hematoidin crystals, and Charcot–Leyden crystals

Steroid crystals

Plant thorns, sea urchin spines, and other extrinsic particles

Metal, plastic, and cement fragments from implants

Cartilage fragments

* Combinations or mixtures of two or more types of particle in the same joint are seen more commonly than would be expected by chance

tissues including the cartilage (3). Periarticular calcification can occur at almost any joint site, is sometimes seen at multiple sites, and is rarely familial. The most common form of periarticular calcification occurs around one or both shoulder joints in adults (4). The true incidence or prevalence of this phenomenon is unknown. Intra-articular deposition has been associated with chronic joint damage, but recent studies indicate that some forms of basic calcium phosphates, particularly whitlokite crystals, are also found in most normal articular cartilage (5).

Identification of Basic Calcium Phosphates Deposits and Crystals

Compensated polarized light microscopy, which is the standard technique used to identify MSUM and CPPD crystals in synovial fluid and tissue, is of no value in the identification of basic calcium phosphates. Most apatite and other basic calcium phosphates crystals are small rod-shaped particles, varying in length from 50–500 nm, and they are below the size of resolution of the light microscope. However, they do tend to clump together to form aggregates that appear as shiny, coin-like objects of around 1–5 µm. Special stains have been used in an attempt to screen fluids and tissues for the presence of these aggregates. The most popular has been Alizarin red S (6), a calcium stain that can produce a characteristic appearance from basic calcium phosphates crystal aggregates, with a pale center and an "onion skin" surrounding. However, both false-positive and false-negative results can occur using this technique, and the stain is not crystal specific.

Other techniques that have been used to recognize these crystals include electron microscopy, infra-red spectroscopy with Fourier transformation, a binding assay using (14C) ethane-1-hydroxy-1, 1-diphosphonate (EHDP), Raman microscopy, and atomic force microscopy. However, the only techniques that can give precise crystal identification require powder or individual crystal diffraction patterns to be obtained. This can be achieved by first extracting the crystals from the tissues or fluids and examining the deposits by x-ray powder diffraction (7).

Etiology and Pathogenesis of Basic Calcium Phosphate-Related Disorders

Crystal formation requires a sufficient local concentration of solutes (supersaturation), nucleation of crystals, and their subsequent growth. Body fluids are normally close to or at the point of supersaturation with respect to a number of basic calcium phosphates. Despite this crystal formation is uncommon, due to the presence of natural inhibitors of crystal formation in connective tissues and body fluids. Formation of crystal deposits can occur as a result of metabolic disturbances that raise solute concentrations, from loss of the natural inhibitors, or from the appearance of nucleation or growth promoters.

The mechanisms behind periarticular and subcutaneous basic calcium phosphate crystal formation are largely unknown. In most patients there is no obvious local, genetic, or metabolic cause. Crystal deposition may be related to local tissue damage and tends to occur in relatively avascular areas. Calcifying tendinitis may be an active, cell-mediated process. In articular cartilage, it is likely that basic calcium phosphates arise from chondrocyte-derived matrix vesicles with nucleation on collagen fibers, similar to the mechanisms thought to be involved in normal matrix calcification in bones and teeth. Other mechanisms are likely to be involved in the formation of the tiny whitlokite and other particles seen near the surface of normal articular cartilage.

Crystal-related tissue damage could be induced by basic calcium phosphate crystals in several ways. Showers of crystals can initiate an acute inflammatory response through the interaction of the crystal surfaces with inflammatory mediators and cells, as in the case of MSUM and CPPD. In addition, there is in vitro evidence that basic calcium phosphate particles can be phagocytosed by a number of cell types, resulting in mitogenesis as well as increased formation of proteases (8). Finally, the presence of excess mineral in the cartilage or synovial fluid of a joint might result in mechanical damage through surface wear or a loss of the normal mechanical resistance of the tissues (9).

Clinical Associations

Acute Calcific Periarthritis

The majority of periarticular deposits of basic calcium phosphate aggregates found on routine radiographs are not associated with articular symptoms. In a minority, crystal shedding leads to the release of a shower of particles into surrounding tissue spaces, leading to an acute inflammatory response, and the clinical syndrome of acute calcific periarthritis. This is most common at the shoulder, where the basic calcium phosphate aggregates found in the supraspinatus or other periarticular tendons rupture into the subacromial bursa or surrounding tissues (Fig. 15-1) (4).

Patients present with the sudden onset of severe pain. The affected area may become red, hot, and swollen; severe local tenderness and loss of function may also occur. Untreated, the symptoms gradually resolve over a period of a few days or weeks. The differential diagnosis includes other forms of crystal-related disease, trauma, and sepsis. Radiographs will generally show the presence of calcific deposits, although their nature changes as the attack evolves. They can even disappear, causing diagnostic confusion. Inert deposits appear as sharp, well defined nummular deposits on the radiograph. As the attack begins the edges of these deposits become fluffy and ill-defined. Subsequently they appear smaller, presumably due to the crystals shedding into the surrounding tissues. If the diagnosis is uncertain, it may be appropriate to try to aspirate fluid from the affected area. The specimens obtained may look like toothpaste or chalk. Polarized light microscopy will help rule out the presence of other types of crystal such as MSUM, CPPD, or cholesterol.

A special form of acute calcific periarthritis affecting the base of the big toe can mimic gout, and is sometimes known as "pseudo-pseudo-podagra" (10). This is most common in premenopausal females, and is the likely diagnosis in any case of suspected gout in this gender and age-group. Attacks can also occur around other small joints of the hands (11) or feet, and occasionally around the spine. These attacks

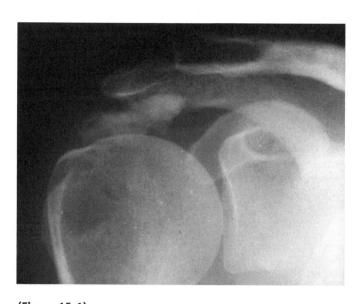

(Figure 15-1)
Shoulder radiograph showing a large periarticular deposit of calcific material in the area of the supraspinatus tendon and subacromial bursa. Note that the deposit has no trabeculae (indicating that it is not bony) and that it has clear edges—when an acute attack of calcific periarthritis occurs, the edges become blurred and the deposit smaller as crystals are shed into the surrounding soft tissues.

may recur, and multiple sites are occasionally involved. Acute calcific periarthritis has also been associated with the development of erosive changes in the adjacent bone in rare cases (12).

Treatment with nonsteroidal anti-inflammatory drugs and rest is usually sufficient. If attempted, aspiration may also help to alleviate symptoms. The use of local corticosteroids is controversial. They help in the resolution of the acute attack, but may contribute to further local calcification subsequently. In severe or prolonged cases, surgical removal of the deposit is sometimes indicated.

Chronic Calcific Periarthritis

Acute calcific periarthritis is sometimes followed by the development of a chronic "frozen" shoulder, or chronic periarthritis. It has been estimated that up to 7% of chronic shoulder disorders might be related to periarticular calcific deposits, but in the absence of good data on the frequency of deposition in normal individuals, it is difficult to know what contribution basic calcium phosphate deposits make to chronic periarticular syndromes.

Acute Articular Inflammation

Basic calcium phosphate crystals can cause acute synovitis of small or large joints. This is rarely recognized in clinical practice, however, because the diagnosis is difficult to substantiate due to the problem of identifying the crystals, and the low of volume synovial fluid in small joints. In the finger joints in particular, basic calcium phosphate crystals have been associated with a more chronic inflammatory monarthritis, resulting in erosive changes (13).

Osteoarthritis

Basic calcium phosphates crystals have been most closely associated with osteoarthritis (OA). Using Alizarin red S staining or analytical electron microscopy, these particles can be found in 30%–60% of synovial fluid samples from patients with OA. Furthermore, there is an association between the severity of radiographic joint damage and the presence of the particles (14). However, there is controversy about the relationship between the disease process and crystal deposition, and the possible contribution of crystals to the joint damage; they may simply be shed from the bone or other joint tissues as part of the OA disease process. Recent work, with more sensitive methods for detecting the crystals, indicates that nearly all OA tissue samples and fluids contain basic calcium phosphates (15), and that some degree of crystal deposition may also be common in normal joints (5). The apparent presence or absence of these crystals does not influence the therapy of OA.

Large Joint Destructive Arthropathies

A distinctive form of large joint destructive arthropathy has been described in older people, predominantly females, and most commonly affects the shoulder. This condition has been described under a variety of names, including "les caries seniles hemorrhagique" and "L'arthropathie destructice rapide de l'epaule" in French literature and "apatite-associated destructive arthritis," "idiopathic destructive arthritis," or "Milwaukee shoulder" in the English literature (16–18).

Patients present with a history of pain, swelling, and loss of function of the affected joint, most commonly the dominant shoulder. Examination reveals extensive damage to both the joint and soft tissues and large, cool effusions. Aspiration yields large volumes of synovial fluid, which is often blood-stained, contains large quantities of basic calcium phosphate crystals, and has a low, predominantly mononuclear cell content. Radiographs show extensive damage to both sides of the joint, with resorption of bone across the joint surfaces (Fig 15-2). The condition may stabilize after a few years, with resolution of the effusion, but the patient is left with a completely destroyed joint. Management is difficult; analgesic and anti-inflammatory therapy may provide some help, but aspiration and local injection is usually of transient benefit. A more prolonged improvement has recently been reported following joint lavage (19).

Calcinosis Cutis

Many of the connective tissue disorders are associated with the formation of calcific deposits of basic calcium phosphate crystals in the subcutaneous tissues, particularly in the hands. Raynaud's phenomenon is usually a concomitant feature. The most frequent associations are with limited scleroderma or CREST (calcinosis, Raynaud's phenomenon, esophageal disease, sclerodactyly, and telangiectasia) and childhood dermatomyositis. The deposits may be associated with intermittent mild inflammation, and can rupture through the skin, leading to extrusion of "chalk." Occasionally, the calcification is very severe, leading to much pain and major disruption of hand function.

MISCELLANEOUS CRYSTALS AND OTHER PARTICLES

A variety of different minerals can be deposited in joints. Other particles, such as plant thorns, may enter joints through the skin, and particulate matter from joint prostheses and other implants may be shed into joint spaces. In each case the crystal or particle may then induce an inflammatory response or contribute to tissue damage in other ways.

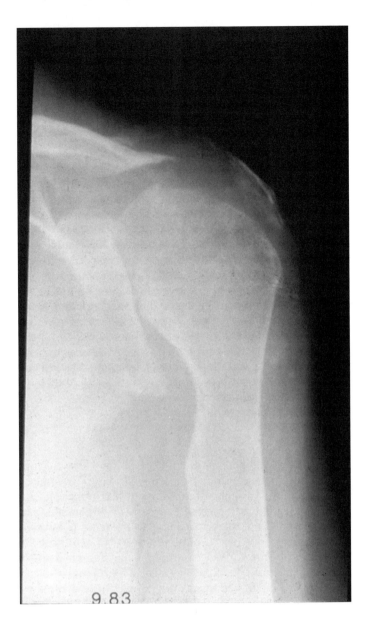

(Figure 15-2)
Shoulder radiograph showing upward subluxation of the humerus and extensive bony destruction of the acromium and of both sides of the glenohumeral joint, with soft tissue evidence of an effusion and calcific deposits. These are the characteristic features of advanced "apatite associated destructive arthritis" or "Milwaukee shoulder."

However, caution must be used in the interpretation of particles identified by light microscopy in synovial fluids or joint tissues. Inexperienced observers may have difficulty differentiating cartilage fragments, steroid crystals, contaminants from syringes and containers, and dust contamination from genuine pathogenic crystals and particles.

Cholesterol and Other Lipids

Cholesterol crystals form relatively large pleiotropic plate-shaped crystals that are easily identified by polarized light microscopy. They are most often seen in chronic cysts or effusions in patients with rheumatoid arthritis or another chronic arthropathy, and there is probably relatively little clinical significance to their presence. Various other forms of lipid spherules can also be found in synovial fluids, particularly following joint trauma; they may give rise to the striking "Maltese Cross" appearance on microscopy, and can contribute to synovitis (20).

Calcium Oxalate

Calcium oxalate crystals can be deposited in musculoskeletal tissues in both primary and secondary hyperoxaluria (21). Primary hyperoxaluria is a rare syndrome associated with premature death and widespread organ involvement. The secondary form is associated with chronic renal failure, especially in patients on hemodialysis and those given ascorbic acid supplements (ascorbic acid metabolizes to oxalate). The crystals can be deposited in joints and tendon sheaths as well as bones and other periarticular tissues, causing arthritis and tenosynovitis. The condition has a predilection for the hands. The deposits may be seen as soft nummular shadows on radiographs, and the crystals can be identified by polarized light microscopy.

PAUL DIEPPE, MD

1. Dieppe PA, Calvert P: Crystals and joint disease. London, Chapman and Hall, 1983
2. Dieppe PA, Watt I: Crystal deposition in osteoarthritis: an opportunistic event ? Clin Rheum Dis, 11:367-392, 1985
3. McCarty DJ, Hogan JM, Gatter RA, Grossman M: Studies on pathological calcifications in human cartilage. J Bone Joint Surg 48(A):309-325, 1966
4. Faure G and Dalcusi G: Calcific tendonitis: a review. Ann Rheum Dis 42 (suppl):49-53, 1983
5. Scotchford CA, Ali SY: Magnesium whitlokite deposition in articular cartilage: a study of 80 specimens from 70 patients. Ann Rheum Dis 54:339-344, 1995
6. Paul H, Reginato AJ, Schumacher HR: Alizarin red S staining as a screening test to detect calcium compounds in synovial fluid. Arthritis Rheum 26:191-200, 1983
7. Swan AJ, Heywood BR, Dieppe PA: Extraction of calcium containing crystals from synovial fluids and articular cartilage. J Rheumatol 19:1763-1773, 1992
8. Caporali R, Rossi S, Montecucco C: Tidal irrigation in Milwaukee shoulder syndrome. J Rheumatol 21:1781-1782, 1994
9. McCarthy GM, Mitchell PG, Struve JS, Cheung HS: Basic calcium phosphate crystals cause co-ordinated induction and secretion of collagenase and stromelysin. J. Cell Physiol 153:140-146, 1992
10. Fam AG, Rubenstein J: Hydroxyapatite pseudopodagra. A syndrome of young women. Arthritis Rheum 32:741-747, 1989
11. McCarthy GM, Carrera GF, Ryan LM: Acute calcific periarthritis of the finger joints: a syndrome of women. J Rheumatol 20:1077-1080, 1993
12. Fritz P, Bardin T, Laredo J-D et al: Paradiaphyseal calcific tendonitis with cortical bone erosion. Arthritis Rheum 37:718-723, 1994
13. Schumacher HR, Miller JL, Ludivico C, Jessar RA: Erosive arthritis associated with apatite crystal deposition. Arthritis Rheum 24:31-37, 1981
14. Halverson PB, McCarty DJ: Patterns of radiographic abnormalities associated with basic caclium phosphate and caclium pyrophosphate crystal deposition in the knee. Ann Rheum Dis 45:603-605, 1986
15. Swan AJ, Chapman B, Heap P et al: Submicroscopic crystals in osteoarthritic synovial fluids. Ann Rheum Dis 53:467-470, 1994
16. Lequesne M, Fallut M, Couloumb R et al: L'arthropathie destructrice rapide de L'epaule. Rev Rheum 49:427-437, 1982
17. Campion GV, McCrae F, Alwan W et al: Idiopathic destructive arthritis of the shoulder. Semin Arthritis Rheum 17:232-245, 1988
18. Halverson PB, Carrera GF, McCarty DJ: Milwaukee shoulder syndrome: fifteen additional cases and a description of contributing factors. Arch Intern Med 150:677-682, 1990
19. Hayes A, Harris B, Dieppe PA. Clift SE: Wear of articular cartilage: the effect of crystals. J Eng Med 207:41-58, 1993
20. Reginato AJ. Lipid microspherule associated acute monoarticular arthritis. Arthritis Rheum 26:1166, 1986
21. Hoffman G, Schumacher HR, Paul H et al: Calcium oxalate micro-crystalline associated arthrits in end stage renal disease. Ann Intern Med 97:36-42, 1982

CALCIUM PYROPHOSPHATE DIHYDRATE CRYSTAL DEPOSITION

16

Specific identification of calcium pyrophosphate dihydrate (CPPD) crystals ($Ca_2P_2O_7 \bullet H_2O$) in synovial fluid or articular tissue allows the clinician to differentiate between CPPD deposition disease and other inflammatory and degenerative arthritides (1). The term *chondrocalcinosis* refers to the presence of calcium-containing crystals detected as radiodensities in articular cartilage. Calcium-containing crystals other than CPPD may also deposit in articular cartilages, producing both radiographically detectable densities in cartilage and joint inflammation or degeneration. Deposition of CPPD crystals is not limited to articular cartilage; less frequently CPPD crystals are deposited in synovial lining, ligaments, tendons, and on rare occasions, periarticular soft tissue much like gouty tophi.

CPPD deposition disease may be asymptomatic or may manifest in a variety of ways. The term *pseudogout* refers to the acute gout-like attacks of inflammation that occur in some patients with CPPD deposition disease. CPPD deposition may also cause symptoms similar to septic arthritis, polyarticular inflammatory arthritis, or osteoarthritis.

Pathologic surveys indicate that about 4% of the adult population have articular CPPD deposits at the time of death (1). Radiologic surveys show a steadily increasing prevalence with age, and by their ninth decade, nearly 50% of individuals have chondrocalcinosis.

CLASSIFICATION

Arthritis associated with CPPD crystal deposition can be classified as hereditary, sporadic (idiopathic), or associated with various metabolic diseases or trauma. Most patients with familial disease show an autosomal dominant pattern of inheritance. A thorough study of patients with sporadic disease would likely result in reclassifying many people as having heritable or disease-associated deposition. Because of the high prevalence of CPPD crystal deposition, the condition has often been reported as associated with other conditions. The most likely "true" associations include hyperparathyroidism, hemochromatosis, hypothyroidism, amyloidosis, hypomagnesemia, and hypophosphatasia. However, none of these associations has been proved in rigorously controlled studies. An association with aging is best documented.

The routine study of a patient newly diagnosed with CPPD crystal deposition should include evaluation of serum calcium, ferritin, magnesium, phosphorous, alkaline phosphatase, and thyroid-stimulating hormone. Further studies should be obtained if abnormal values are found. Hypomagnesemia and hypophosphatasia need not be considered in patients over age 60 years at the time of first clinical symptoms.

CLINICAL FEATURES

Acute pseudogout is marked by inflammation in one or more joints lasting for several days to 2 weeks. These self-limited attacks can be as abrupt in onset and as severe as acute gout. Almost one-half of all attacks involve the knees, although attacks have been documented in nearly all other joints, including the first metatarsophalangeal (the most common site for gout). As with gout, pseudogout attacks can occur spontaneously or be provoked by trauma, surgery, or severe illness such as stroke or myocardial infarction. Patients are usually asymptomatic between episodes. Differentiation from gout or joint infection may be difficult and requires arthrocentesis, examination of the synovial fluid for crystals, and culture. About 25% of patients with CPPD deposition disease exhibit the pseudogout pattern of disease.

About 5% of patients with CPPD deposition manifest a "pseudo-rheumatoid" presentation with multiple joint involvement with symmetric distribution and low-grade inflammation. Accompanying morning stiffness, fatigue, synovial thickening, flexion contractures, and elevated erythrocyte sedimentation rate often lead to a misdiagnosis of rheumatoid arthritis. In addition, 10% of patients with CPPD deposits have low titers of rheumatoid factor, which provide further diagnostic confusion. The presence of high titer rheumatoid factor and radiographic evidence of typical rheumatoid bony erosions favor the diagnosis of rheumatoid arthritis.

Nearly one-half of patients with CPPD deposits have progressive degeneration of numerous joints. The knees are most commonly affected, followed by the wrists, metacarpophalangeal joints, hips, shoulders, elbows, and ankles. Although there is some overlap with the pattern of joint involvement in primary osteoarthritis (eg, hip and knee), the distribution of joint degeneration with CPPD deposition is distinctive. Involvement of distal interphalangeal and proximal interphalangeal joints manifested by Heberden's and Bouchard's nodes and first carpometacarpal joint—all characteristic of primary osteoarthritis—are no more common in patients with CPPD deposition disease than would be expected by chance alone in an elderly population. Symmetric involvement is the rule, although degeneration may be more advanced on one side. Flexion contractures of the affected joints and deformities of the knees are common. Valgus knee deformities are especially suggestive of underlying CPPD crystal deposits. Patients with chronic symptoms of this pseudo-osteoarthritis pattern may have superimposed episodes of joint inflammation.

Neurologic manifestations of CPPD crystal deposition in the axial skeleton can occur. A syndrome of acute neck pain ascribed to CPPD (or to basic calcium phosphate) deposits associated with a tomographic appearance of calcification surrounding the odontoid process has been termed the *crowned dens* syndrome (2). At times, neck pain may be accompanied by stiffness and fever that mimic meningitis. This may occur in the postoperative period after parathyroidectomy. Other patients have developed long tract signs and symptoms related to deposits of CPPD crystals and adjacent tissue hypertrophy in the cervical spine (3). The ligamentum flavum has been the most regularly reported cervical site of CPPD crystal deposition (4). Crystal deposits, ligament hypertrophy, and chondroid metaplastic growths all contribute to encroachment on the cord. Infrequently, lumbar spine involvement manifests as acute radiculopathy or neurogenic claudication from spinal stenosis.

Systemic findings during an acute attack of pseudogout are frequent but not invariable. These include a fever of 99–103°F, leukocytosis of 12,000–15,000/mm^3, and elevated erythrocyte sedimentation rate and serum acute-phase reactants. Interleukin-6 may mediate some of these systemic effects (5).

Many patients with CPPD crystal deposits have no joint symptoms. Even patients who have symptoms in some joints have other joints with CPPD deposits that are completely asymptomatic and clinically normal.

RADIOLOGIC FEATURES

The typical appearance of punctate and linear densities in articular hyaline or fibrocartilaginous tissues is diagnostically helpful. The most characteristic sites of crystal deposition are illustrated in Fig. 16-1. When the deposits are typical and unequivocal, the radiologic appearance is nearly specific, but interpretation of atypical or faint deposits is

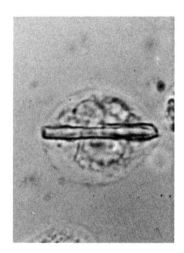

(Figure 16-2)
Neutrophilic leukocyte in fresh preparation of synovial fluid from an 84-year-old woman with acute inflammation of the knee (pseudogout). Note rod-shaped crystal of calcium pyrophosphate dihydrate.

often difficult. Calcific deposits may also appear in the articular capsule, ligaments, and tendons. Although the earliest calcific deposits occur in radiographically normal cartilage, degenerative changes often supervene. A patient can be screened for CPPD crystal deposits with four roentgenograms: an anteroposterior (AP) view of both knees, an AP view of the pelvis for visualization of the symphysis pubis and hips, and a posteroanterior view of both hands to include the wrists. If these views show no evidence of crystal deposits, it is most unlikely that further study will prove fruitful.

Changes in the metacarpophalangeal joints, such as squaring of the bone ends, subchondral cysts, and hook-like osteophytes, are characteristic features of the arthritis associated with hemochromatosis but are also found in patients with CPPD crystal deposition alone. These changes occur more frequently in patients with CPPD crystal deposits and hemochromatosis than in those with only crystal deposits. In addition to the difference in the pattern of affected joints, CPPD may be differentiated from osteoarthritis by the finding of isolated patellofemoral joint space narrowing or isolated wrist degeneration. Such differences may provide helpful clinical clues and are incorporated into the diagnostic criteria given in Table 16-1.

PATHOGENESIS OF INFLAMMATION AND CARTILAGE DEGENERATION

Acute pseudogout is thought to represent a dose-related inflammatory host response to CPPD crystals shed from cartilaginous tissues contiguous with the synovial cavity (Fig. 16-2) (6). Phagocytosis of crystals by neutrophils results in release of lysosomal enzymes and cell-derived chemotactic factors. Phagocytosis by synovial lining cells leads to cell proliferation and release of prostaglandins, cytokines, and proteases such as collagenase and stromelysin.

Colchicine in therapeutic concentrations is remarkably effective in blocking the release of chemotactic factors for neutrophils and mononuclear cells and inhibits neutrophil–endothelial cell binding, a step in the ingress of neutrophils into the synovial space.

The frequency of association of CPPD crystal deposits and degenerative joint disease may result from the biologic properties of cell interaction with calcium-containing crystals (7). Ingestion of such crystals by fibroblasts or mononuclear synovial lining cells is followed by intracellular dissolution, raising intracellular free-calcium levels. This

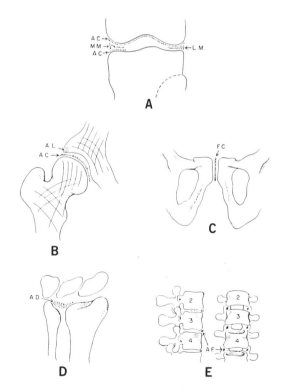

(Figure 16-1)
Diagrammatic representation of characteristic sites of CPPD crystal deposition. A, A.C. = articular cartilage; L.M. and M.M. = lateral and medial meniscus in knee joint shown in anteroposterior projection. B, A.L. = acetabular labrum in anteroposterior projection of hip joint. C, F.C. = fibrocartilaginous symphysis pubis in anteroposterior projection of pelvis. D, A.D. = articular disc of the wrist in anteroposterior projection. E, A.F. = anulus fibrosus of intervertebral discs in anteroposterior and lateral views. Reprinted from Bulletin on the Rheumatic Diseases with permission.

Criteria

I. Demonstration of CPPD crystals in tissue or synovial fluid by definitive means (eg, characteristic X-ray diffraction or chemical analysis)

II. (a) Identification of monoclinic or triclinic crystals showing no or weakly positive birefringence by compensated polarized light microscopy

   (b) Presence of typical radiographic calcifications

III. (a) Acute arthritis, especially of knees or other large joints

   (b) Chronic arthritis, especially of knee, hip, wrist, carpus, elbow, shoulder, or metacarpophalangeal joint, especially if accompanied by acute exacerbations. The chronic arthritis shows the following features helpful in differentiating it from osteoarthritis:

     1. Uncommon site—wrist, metacarpophalangeal, elbow, shoulder

     2. Radiographic appearance—radiocarpal or patellofemoral joint space narrowing, especially if isolated (patella "wrapped around" the femur)

     3. Subchondral cyst formation

     4. Severity of degeneration—progressive, with subchondral bony collapse and fragmentation with formation of intra-articular radiodense bodies

     5. Osteophyte formation—variable and inconstant

     6. Tendon calcifications, especially triceps, Achilles, obturators

Categories

A. Definite disease: Criteria I or II(a) plus (b) must be fulfilled.

B. Probable disease: Criteria II(a) or II(b) must be fulfilled

C. Possible disease: Criteria III(a) or III(b) should alert the clinician to the possibility of underlying CPPD deposition

sequence predictably engenders a mitogenic response, resulting in tissue hypertrophy. Moreover, stimulated lining cells secrete proteolytic enzymes (collagenase, stromelysin, and gelatinase), which may damage cartilage and other articular structures. Cytokine release can lead to further protease release by lining cells or chondrocytes. Such effects have been demonstrated for CPPD crystals in vitro. That these events occur in vivo is suggested by synovial fluid studies indicating that fluids containing CPPD crystals have on average the highest concentration of proteoglycan breakdown products and the highest ratio of protease-to-protease inhibitor of all forms of arthritis tested.

PATHOGENESIS OF CRYSTAL DEPOSITION

Plasma levels and urinary excretion of inorganic pyrophosphate (PPi) are not elevated in patients with CPPD crystal deposition disease. Synovial fluid PPi concentration, however, is elevated in most joints with CPPD crystal deposition. Articular chondrocytes likely contribute to the PPi, which accumulates in joint fluids, since cartilage slices and chondrocyte cell cultures liberate PPi into the ambient media, while nonarticular tissues do not. The liberation of

PPi is stimulated by ascorbate and transforming growth factor β (8) and inhibited by probenecid (9), insulin-like growth factor (10), inhibitors of protein synthesis, and interleukin-1 (11). Kinetic studies indicate that much of the extracellular PPi may be generated by an ectoenzyme, NTPPase (12). This enzyme is found in elevated amounts in cartilage extracts (13), synovial fluids (14), and cell cultures (15) from patients with CPPD deposits. It generates PPi from nucleoside triphosphate substrates such as adenosine triphosphate (ATP), which is also present in elevated concentrations in CPPD-containing joint fluids (16). Vesicles derived from chondrocytes are particularly enriched in NTPPase activity and are able to nucleate and grow monoclinic CPPD crystals in vitro in the presence of ATP (17). ATP added to cartilage explants likewise induces formation of perichondral CPPD-like crystals, many of which appeared to form within membranous structures (18). The vesicle-associated form of NTPPase is distinct from two other forms found on many cells including chondrocytes (19,20).

Unlike gout, a disease generally associated with a systemic abnormality of excess anion (hyperuricemia), CPPD crystal deposition is driven by a local abnormality of excess articular anion production. In either condition, local factors determine the foci of crystal deposition. Local factors favoring CPPD crystal deposition could include bursts of increased PPi generation by selected chondrocytes, leading to a pericellular increase in anion; synthesis of molecules or particulates capable of heterologous CPPD crystal nucleation; or absence of physiologic crystal inhibitors.

TREATMENT

Unlike gout, there is no practical way to remove CPPD crystals from joints. Treatment of putative associated diseases such as hyperparathyroidism, hemochromatosis, or myxedema does not result in resorption of CPPD crystal deposits. Acute attacks in large joints can be treated through aspiration alone or aspiration combined with injection of microcrystalline corticosteroid esters. Intravenous colchicine is effective in the treatment of pseudogout, but nonsteroidal anti-inflammatory drugs are recommended for most patients. The effectiveness of oral colchicine is less predictable in pseudogout than in gout, but both the number and duration of acute attacks are significantly reduced by colchicine taken on a daily basis for prophylaxis. ACTH or corticosteroid treatment has been used successfully in patients with both gout and pseudogout (21). Whether removing crystals may prevent or slow the degenerative cartilaginous and bony changes is an important but unanswered question.

LAWRENCE M. RYAN, MD

1. Ryan LM, McCarty DJ: Calcium pyrophosphate crystal deposition disease: pseudogout: articular chondrocalcinosis. In McCarty DJ, Koopman WJ (eds): Arthritis and Allied Conditions. Philadelphia, Lea and Febiger, 1992, p 1711

2. Bouvet J, le Parc J, Michalski B, Benlahrache C, Auquier L: Acute neck pain due to calcifications surrounding the odontoid process: the crowned dens syndrome. Arthritis Rheum 28:1417-1420, 1985

3. Kawano N, Matsuno T, Miyazawa S, Iida H, Yada K, Kobayashi N, Iwasaki Y: Calcium pyropophate dihydrate crystal deposition disease in the cervical ligamentum flavum. J Neurosurg 68:613-620, 1988

4. Baba H, Maezawa Y, Kawahara N, Tomita K, Furusawa N, Imura: Calcium crystal deposition in the ligamentum flavum of the cervical spine. Spine 18:2174-2181, 1993

5. Guerne P, Terkeltaub R, Zuraw B, Lotz M: Inflammatory microcrystals stimulate interleukin-6 production and secretion by human monocytes and synoviocytes. Arthritis Rheum 32:1443-1452, 1989

6. Terkeltaub RA: Pathogenesis and treatment of crystal-induced inflammation. In McCarty DJ, Koopman WJ (eds): Arthritis and Allied Conditions. Philadelphia, Lea and Febiger, 1993, p 1819

7. Cheung HS, Ryan LM: Role of crystal deposition in matrix degradation. In Woessner FJ, Howell DS (eds): Joint Cartilage Degradation: Basic and Clinical Aspects. New York, Marcel Dekker, Inc. 1995, p209

8. Rosenthal AK, Cheung HS, Ryan LM: Transforming growth factor B1 stimulates inorganic pyrophosphate elaboration by porcine cartilage. Arthritis Rheum 34:904-911, 1991

9. Rosenthal AK, Ryan LM: Probenecid inhibits transforming growth factor B1 induced pyrophosphate elaboration by chondrocytes. J Rheumatol 21:896-900, 1990

10. Olmez U, Ryan LM, Kurup IV, Rosenthal AK: Insulin-like growth factor-1 suppresses pyrophosphate elaboration by transforming growth factor B1 stimulated chondrocytes and cartilage. Osteoarthritis and Cartilage 2:149-154, 1994

11. Lotz M, Rosen F, McCabe G et al: Interleukin 1 beta suppresses transforming growth factor-induced inorganic pyrophosphate (PPi) production and expression of the PPi-generating enzyme PC-1 in human chondrocytes. Proc Natl Acad Sci USA 92:10364-10368, 1995

12. Ryan LM, McCarty DJ: Understanding inorganic pyrophosphate metabolism - toward prevention of calcium pyrophosphate dihydrate crystal deposition. Ann Rheum Dis 54:939-941, 1995

13. Tenenbaum J, Muniz O, Schumacher HR, Good AE, Howell DS: Comparison of pyrophosphohydrolase activities from articular cartilage in calcium pyrophosphate deposition disease and primary osteoarthritis. Arthritis Rheum 24:492-500, 1981

14. Rachow JW, Ryan LM, McCarty DJ, Halverson PB: Synovial fluid inorganic pyrophosphate concentration and nucleotide pyrophosphohydrolase activity in basic calcium phosphate deposition arthropathy and Milwaukee shoulder syndrome. Arthritis Rheum 31:408-413, 1988

15. Ryan LM, Wortmann RL, Karas B, Lynch MP, McCarty DJ: Pyrophosphohydrolase activity and inorganic pyrophosphate content of cultured human skin fibroblasts. Elevated levels in some patients with calcium pyrophosphate dihydrate deposition disease. J Clin Invest 77:1689-1693, 1986

16. Ryan LM, Rachow JW, McCarty DJ: Synovial fluid ATP: a potential substrate for the production of inorganic pyrophosphate. J Rheumatol 18:716-720, 1991

17. Derfus BA, Rachow JW, Mandel NS, Boskey AL, Buday M, Kushnaryov VM, Ryan LM: Articular cartilage vesicles generate calcium pyrophosphate dihydrate-like crystals in vitro. Arthritis Rheum 35:231-240, 1992

18. Ryan LM, Kurup IV, Derfus BA, Kushnaryov VM: ATP-induced chondrocalcinosis. Arthritis Rheum 35:1520-1525, 1992

19. Masuda I, Hamada J, Haas AL, Ryan LM, McCarty DJ: A unique ectonucleotide pyrophosphohydrolase associated with porcine chondrocyte-derived vesicles. J Clin Invest 95:699-704, 1995

20. Huang R, Rosenbach M, Vaughn R, Provvedini D, Rebbe N, Hickman S, Goding J, Terkeltaub R: Expression of the murine plasma cell nucleotide pyrophosphohydrolase PC-1 is shared by human liver, bone and cartilage cells. J Clin Invest 94:560-567, 1994

21. Ritter J, Kerr LD, Valeriano-Marcet J, Spiera H: ACTH revisited: effective treatment for acute crystal induced synovitis in patients with multiple medical problems. J Rheumatol 21:696-699, 1994

17 | GOUT

A. EPIDEMIOLOGY, PATHOLOGY, AND PATHOGENESIS

Gout is a heterogeneous group of diseases resulting from tissue deposition of crystals of monosodium urate (MSU) or of uric acid in supersaturated extracellular fluids. Clinical manifestations include: 1) recurrent attacks of articular and periarticular inflammation, also called gouty arthritis; 2) accumulation of articular, osseous, soft tissue, and cartilaginous crystalline deposits, called tophi; 3) uric acid calculi in the urinary tract; and 4) interstitial nephropathy with renal function impairment, called gouty nephropathy (1). The metabolic disorder underlying gout is hyperuricemia, which is defined as serum urate concentration more than two standard deviations (SD) above the mean, as established by individual laboratories according to gender (generally more than 7.0 mg/dl for men and 6.0 mg/dl for women). By itself, hyperuricemia is not sufficient for the expression of gout, however, and asymptomatic hyperuricemia in the absence of gout is not a disease.

EPIDEMIOLOGY

Gout is predominantly a disease of adult men, with a peak incidence in the fifth decade. The disease rarely occurs in men before adolescence or in women before menopause. It is a common disorder that frequently results in significant short-term disability, occupational limitations, and utilization of medical services. In 1986, the prevalence of self-reported gout in the United States was estimated to be 13.6 per 1000 men and 6.4 per 1000 women. The prevalence has increased over the past few decades in the United States, as well as in other countries that have a high standard of living. Prevalence among black men may be higher than among white men, possibly reflecting the relative prevalence of hypertension (2).

Beginning in puberty, serum urate concentration in males rises from childhood mean values of 3.5 mg/dl and reach adult levels of 4.0 mg/dl. In contrast, urate levels remain rather constant in females until menopause, at which time concentrations begin to rise. This discrepancy during the reproductive years appears to stem from the action of estrogen, which promotes renal excretion of uric acid (1). Because of increased longevity and the frequent long-term use of thiazide diuretics, the prevalence of gout is believed to be rising among elderly women in Western countries (3).

Hyperuricemia is present in at least 5% of asymptomatic Americans on at least one occasion during adulthood. However, it appears that fewer than one in four hyperuricemic individuals will, at any point, develop clinically apparent urate crystal deposition. The most likely reasons, at least in part, are that increases in urate levels are relatively mild in most individuals (serum urate less than 9.0 mg/dl) and are often transient in response to dietary alterations or to ingestion of certain drugs.

The duration and magnitude of hyperuricemia directly correlate not only with the likelihood of subsequent development of gouty arthritis and uric acid urolithiasis but also with age of onset of initial clinical gouty manifestations (1,4). Nevertheless, recent data on the long-term effects of hyperuricemia and gout indicate that, in the absence of uric acid overproduction, severe hyperuricemia (at least up to 13 mg/dl in men and 10 mg/dl in women) is tolerated with little apparent jeopardy to renal function (4).

PATHOGENESIS OF HYPERURICEMIA

Uric acid is the normal end-product of the degradation of purine compounds (1). The limit of solubility of monosodium urate in plasma is approximately 6.7 mg/dl at 37°C. Thus, the normal adult mean (± SD) serum urate concentrations (5.1 ± 1.0 mg/dl in men and 4.0 ± 1.0 mg/dl in women) provide a narrow margin of safety for urate deposition. In humans gout is a consequence of the species-wide lack of the enzyme uric acid oxidase, or uricase. Uricase oxidizes uric acid, which is only sparingly soluble in body fluids, to the highly soluble compound allantoin. Knockout mice that are homozygous for absence of the uricase gene exhibit a marked increase in serum urate—from approximately 1.0 mg/dl to about 11.0 mg/dl—and develop severe uric acid nephrolithiasis and renal dysfunction during the first month of life (5). Multiple genetic and environmental influences prompt the chain of events that governs uric acid formation, transport, and disposal. Single or combined derangements in these delicately balanced processes can lead to hyperuricemia and gout. Among environmental factors modifying serum urate concentration are body weight, diet, lifestyle, social class, and hemoglobin level. An example of the interplay of genetic and environmental factors in determining hyperuricemia is provided by the higher mean serum urate levels encountered among Filipinos living in the United States versus individuals of identical racial background living in the Philippines. The limited ability of members of this population group to excrete uric acid supports the hypothesis that a tendency toward hyperuricemia is inherited and is manifested when a diet with a relatively high purine content, such as the usual American diet, is ingested. The familial occurrence of gout, known for nearly 2000 years, is reported by about 20% of affected patients, and hyperuricemia has been demonstrated in one-fourth of first-degree relatives of gout patients (1).

Purine Metabolism and Biochemistry

In humans, uric acid is derived both from the ingestion of foods containing purines and from the endogenous synthesis of purine nucleotides, which are building blocks in the synthesis of nucleic acids. The synthesis of purine nucleotides involves biochemical pathways that are closely regulated (Fig. 17A-1). In the pathway of purine synthesis de novo, a purine ring is synthesized from small molecule precursors, sequentially added to a ribose–phosphate backbone donated by 5-phosphoribosyl-1-pyrophosphate (PRPP). The first reaction of this pathway is catalyzed by

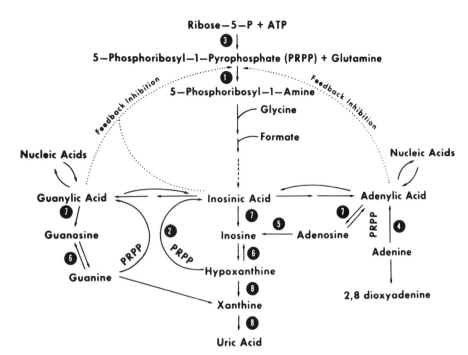

Ribose—5—P + ATP
3|
5—Phosphoribosyl—1—Pyrophosphate (PRPP) + Glutamine
1|
5—Phosphoribosyl—1—Amine

Feedback Inhibition   Feedback Inhibition

— Glycine

— Formate

Nucleic Acids   Nucleic Acids

Guanylic Acid   ←→   Inosinic Acid   →   Adenylic Acid
7   **7**   **7**
Guanosine   **2**   **5**   Adenosine   **4**
6   PRPP   PRPP   Inosine   ←   Adenosine   PRPP   Adenine
Guanine   **6**
Hypoxanthine   2,8 dioxyadenine
8
Xanthine
|**8**
Uric Acid

(Figure 17A-1)
Schematic outline of purine metabolism: 1) amidophosphoribosyltransferase; 2) hypoxanthine–guanine phosphoribosyltransferase; 3) PRPP synthetase; 4) adenine phosphoribosyltransferase; 5) adenosine deaminase; 6) purine nucleoside phosphorylase; 7) 5'-nucleotidase; 8) xanthine oxidase. Adapted from Seegmiller, Rosenbloom, and Kelley: Science 155:1682-1684, 1967, with permission.

amidophosphoribosyltransferase (reaction 1 in Fig. 17A-1). This reaction is the major site of the regulation of the pathway by means of an antagonistic interaction between inhibition by purine nucleotide products and activation by PRPP, a substrate usually present in limited concentrations in the cell. Other sites of control of purine nucleotide production have been identified at the level of PRPP synthesis (reaction 3 in Fig.17A-1) and at the distal branch point governing distribution of newly formed nucleotides into adenylate and guanylate derivatives (1).

Purine nucleotide synthesis can also occur through the activities of adenine phosphoribosyltransferase (reaction 4 in Fig. 17A-1) and hypoxanthine–guanine phosphoribosyltransferase (HGPRT) (reaction 2 in Fig. 17A-1). Each enzyme catalyzes the reaction between PRPP and the respective purine base substrate in the single-step synthesis of purine nucleotides. Among the factors governing the relationship between rates of purine base salvage and purine synthesis are the availability of PRPP and the concentrations of the nucleotide products common to both pathways (1).

The catabolic steps that generate uric acid from nucleic acids and free purine nucleotides involve degradation through purine nucleoside intermediates to hypoxanthine and xanthine. The latter are ultimately oxidized to uric acid in sequential reactions catalyzed by the enzyme xanthine oxidase (reaction 8 in Fig. 17A-1).

Urate circulates in the plasma mainly in unbound form. The total miscible urate pool averages about 1200 mg (range 800–1600 mg) in normal men and about one-half this value in normal women. Since uric acid synthesis averages about 750 mg/day in men, an estimated two-thirds of the urate pool is turned over daily (1). Chronic hyperuricemia in gout is invariably characterized by substantial expansion of the total body urate and uric acid pool and urate supersaturation of the extracellular space.

The major route of uric acid disposal is renal excretion, which accounts for about two-thirds of urate loss. Normal adult men receiving a purine-free diet excrete about 425 ± 80 mg/day in the urine. Substantial increases in urinary uric acid excretion are normally possible in response to increased filtered urate load. Bacterial oxidation of urate secreted into the gut is the principal mechanism of extrarenal urate disposal. This pathway has a relatively limited ability to compensate for changes in urate pool size until serum urate values rise above 14.0 mg/dl.

Causes and Classification of Hyperuricemia

Increased uric acid production and diminished uric acid excretion by the kidney, operating alone or in combination, contribute substantially to the hyperuricemia of patients with gout. Thus, patients with hyperuricemia and gout can be subclassified according to the mechanism responsible for hyperuricemia—that is, overproduction or underexcretion of uric acid, or both mechanisms (Table 17A-1). In this scheme, primary hyperuricemia refers to inherently disordered uric acid metabolism not associated with another acquired disorder. Such classification is particularly useful in directing diagnostic attention and may be used to guide therapy.

Urate Overproduction

Approximately 10% of patients with hyperuricemia or gout excrete excessive quantities of uric acid in a 24-hour urine collection, commonly defined as more than 800 mg of uric acid excreted while on a normal diet. Isotopic labeling studies generally demonstrate increased rates of uric acid synthesis (overproduction) in such individuals. Overproduction of urate occurs with some frequency in a variety of acquired and genetic disorders that are characterized by excessive rates of cell and, therefore, nucleic acid turnover, such as myeloproliferative and lymphoproliferative diseases, hemolytic anemias, and anemias associated with ineffective erythropoiesis, Paget's disease of bone, and psoriasis. These disorders constitute examples of secondary hyperuricemia and gout with uric acid overproduction.

Inherited derangements in mechanisms regulating purine nucleotide synthesis account for a very small minority of patients with urate overproduction. Early adult-onset gout and a high incidence of uric acid urinary tract stones constitute the usual clinical phenotype in both partial deficiency of

HGPRT and milder forms of superactivity of PRPP synthetase (1,6,7). Severe HGPRT deficiency is associated with spasticity, choreoathetosis, mental retardation, and compulsive self-mutilation (Lesch–Nyhan syndrome) (1,6). In some individuals, regulatory defects in PRPP synthetase are accompanied by sensorineural deafness and neurodevelopmental defects (1,7). Intracellular accumulation of PRPP is a result of diminished utilization of this regulatory substrate in purine base salvage. This drives purine synthesis at an increased rate in HGPRT deficiency (Fig. 17A-1). In the case of variant forms of PRPP synthetase with excessive activity, increased PRPP availability for purine synthesis results from increased rates of PRPP generation (1). Thus, aberrations of both of these enzymes result in increased uric acid synthesis by increasing PRPP availability and altering the balance of control of purine synthesis toward increased production. Both of these enzymes are produced from X-linked genes, and thus homozygous males are affected. In addition, postmenopausal gout and urinary tract stones can occur as the phenotype of carrier females. Hyperuricemia in prepubertal boys always suggests that one of these enzymatic defects could be the cause.

Uric Acid Underexcretion

Most patients with primary hyperuricemia or gout (more than 90%) have a relative deficit in the renal excretion of uric acid. Excretion of normal amounts of uric acid is accomplished in these individuals only when serum urate concentrations are inappropriately high (1).

Virtually all plasma urate is filtered at the glomerulus, with more than 95% of the filtered load undergoing proximal tubular (presecretory) reabsorption (1). Subsequent proximal tubular secretion (of about 50% of the filtered urate load) contributes the major share of excreted uric acid. Postsecretory tubular reabsorption (of about 40% of the filtered urate load) is another primary mechanism of renal uric acid handling.

Renal urate excretion can be influenced by heredity (8), and a number of kindreds with relatively early-onset gout and a reduced fractional excretion of urate have been described (9). However, there is no evidence to suggest that most primary uric acid underexcreters with gout constitute a population with a single genetic or acquired renal defect. A diminished tubular secretory rate may contribute to hyperuricemia in some of these patients, and the possibilities of increased tubular reabsorption or diminished uric acid filtration in other patients with renal urate retention have not been dismissed.

Pharmacologic agents that alter renal tubular function also contribute to the occurrence of gout with uric acid underexcretion. Among the offending agents (Table 17A-1) are diuretics (3), cyclosporine (10), and low-dose salicylates (1). Cryptic forms of acquired renal impairment can also be manifested initially by gouty arthritis, as exemplified by the high incidence of this disorder in patients with chronic lead intoxication. Decreased excretion of uric acid also occurs in diabetic ketoacidosis, starvation, ketosis, ethanol intoxication, and lactic acidosis. The organic acids that accumulate in these conditions compete with urate tubular secretion. Finally, patients with gout tend to have a relatively high incidence of other diseases that predispose to renal insufficiency, such as hypertension and diabetes mellitus (1).

Combined Overproduction and Underexcretion

Alcohol consumption promotes hyperuricemia by increasing urate production and decreasing uric acid excretion. The higher purine content in some alcoholic beverages is a factor and, in addition, excessive alcohol consumption causes accelerated hepatic breakdown of adenosine triphosphate (ATP) and increased urate production (11). High alcohol intake may lead to hyperlactic acidemia, which blocks uric acid secretion.

Two inborn errors of metabolism can also produce hyperuricemia by a combined mechanism. These include glucose-6-phosphatase deficiency and fructose-1-phosphate aldolase deficiency. The defect in the former causes accelerated purine biosynthesis, and in the latter, accelerated purine nucleotide degradation. Lactic acidemia is a consequence of each.

PATHOGENESIS OF GOUT

In most instances, urate crystallizes as a monosodium salt in oversaturated joint tissues (1). As mentioned above, only a minority of individuals with sustained hyperuricemia develop tophi and gouty arthropathy. Furthermore, gout has been observed in a few individuals who have not previously had evidence of hyperuricemia (12). The reasons for these exceptions are poorly understood at present. The decreased solubility of sodium urate at the lower temperatures of peripheral structures such as the toes and ears may help explain why urate crystals deposit in these areas (1,13). However, the predilection for marked urate crystal deposition in the first metatarsophalangeal (MTP) joint may also relate to repetitive minor trauma.

The observations that hemiplegia appears to have a sparing effect on the development of tophi and acute gout on the paretic side, and that tophi and acute gout occur in interphalangeal joints at the location of Heberden's nodes (14), suggest the potential importance of connective tissue structure and turnover in urate crystal deposition. Provocative findings have raised the possibility that immunoglobulin plays a role in urate crystal deposition in vivo (14).

Urate tophi can usually be found in the synovial membrane at the time of the first gouty attack (13). Urate crystals in joint fluid at the time of the acute attack may derive from rupture of preformed synovial deposits, or they may have precipitated de novo (15). Declines in serum urate levels, as effected by antihyperuricemic drugs, may promote the release of urate crystals from tophi via a decrease in the size of crystals; the packed crystals may consequently loosen, forming gaps at the periphery of deposits.

In some individuals with gout, urate crystals can be found in asymptomatic MTP and knee joints that have never been involved in an acute attack (13). Furthermore, asymptomatic patients with hyperuricemia may have urate crystals in MTP joint fluid. These findings confirm that gout can exist in an asymptomatic state.

PATHOLOGY OF GOUT

The histopathology of the tophi (Fig. 17A-2) shows a chronic foreign body granuloma surrounding a core of monosodium urate crystals. The inflammatory reaction around the crystals consists mostly of mononuclear cells and giant cells. A fibrous capsule is usually prominent. Crystals within the tophi are needle-shaped and are often arranged radially in small clusters. These crystals can be dissolved by formalin-based fixatives (16), so caution must be

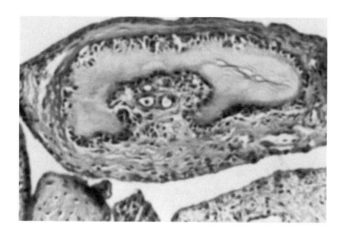

(Figure 17A-2)
Photomicrograph of synovium (knee) of a 46-year-old man who sustained repeated attacks of gouty arthritis for 15 years. Note large tophaceous deposit in the synovial villus with surrounding histiocytic reaction. Crystals are dissolved from tophi unless tissue is processed with absolute alcohol.

exercised in handling these specimens. The DeGolantha stain can be used to stain urates black; crystals can also be identified by compensated polarized light microscopy in frozen or alcohol-fixed specimens. Other potentially important components in tophi include lipids, glycosaminoglycans, and plasma proteins.

In the parenchymal renal disease of gout, the kidneys are usually small and equally affected. The cortical area is reduced in width, and scars can been seen through the capsule. Many of these changes can be related to associated hypertension and infection (1). Even before the availability of effective urate-depleting drugs, renal parenchymal urate deposits were only occasionally present. The renal pelvis may contain uric acid stones.

Histologic examination of kidneys from patients with gouty nephropathy reveals urate crystals located primarily in the medullary interstitium, papillae, and pyramids. Like other tophi, they may be surrounded by a chronic inflammatory reaction with foreign-body giant cells. Nephrosclerosis and other evidence of hypertensive disease are also common.

PATHOGENESIS OF GOUTY INFLAMMATION

Gout was the first disease in which crystals were identified in joint effusions and subsequently incriminated in the pathogenesis of the arthritis. Intra-articular injection of urate crystals was shown to induce gout-like attacks, even in normal subjects. However, the finding of crystals in synovial fluids of asymptomatic joints (13) illustrates that factors other than simply the presence of crystals may be important in modulating the inflammatory reaction.

Urate crystals are directly able to initiate and sustain intense attacks of acute inflammation because of their capacity to stimulate the release of numerous inflammatory mediators (13). These include mediators from phagocytes, synovial cells, and other constituents such as cyclooxygenase and lipoxygenase metabolites of arachidonic acid, phospholipase A_2-activating protein, lysosomal proteases, interleukin (IL)-1, IL-6, IL-8, and tumor necrosis factor α (TNF-α). In addition, urate crystals generate soluble mediators (including C5a, bradykinin, and kallikrein) via proteolysis of serum proteins (13).

The ability of urate crystals to activate cells is likely due to nonspecific activation of certain signal transduction pathways (including membrane G protein activation, cytosolic calcium mobilization, and tyrosine kinase signaling) that are used in a more specific manner by receptor-mediated signals such as growth factors (13,17).

In acute gout, neutrophil influx is believed to be promoted both by endothelial–neutrophil adhesion triggered by IL-1 and TNF-α and by inducting expression of chemotactic factors including IL-8, the activated fifth component of complement (C5a), and crystal-induced chemotactic factor. The ingress of neutrophils appears to be the most important event for developing acute urate crystal-induced synovitis; indeed, effects at the level of neutrophil–endothelial interaction likely represent a major locus for the prophylactic and therapeutic effects of colchicine (18). Intra-articular neutrophils can be activated both by direct contact with crystals and by exposure to the rich soup of soluble mediators. These events support continuing ingress of neutrophils, which is probably vital for perpetuating acute gouty inflammation because of the limited functional lifespan (days) of normal neutrophils. In this regard, the rate at which neutrophils undergo apoptosis in the acute gouty joint is likely to be accelerated by TNF-α and certain other mediators.

The systemic release from the gouty joint into the venous circulation of IL-1, TNF-α, IL-6, and IL-8 appears to be responsible for systemic manifestations (eg, fever, leukocytosis, hepatic acute-phase protein response) and may help explain the capacity of the acute gouty attack to affect joints in more than one region.

The acute gouty attack may be self-limited by certain changes in not only the physical properties and proteins coating intra-articular urate crystals, but also in the balance between pro- and anti-inflammatory factors (eg, release of IL-1 receptor antagonist and transforming growth factor β) (13,19). However, the precise mechanisms that spontaneously limit acute gouty inflammation remain to be defined.

ROBERT A. TERKELTAUB, MD

1. Becker MA, Levinson D: Clinical gout and pathogenesis of hyperuricemia. In Koopman WJ (ed): Arthritis and Allied Conditions, 13th ed. Baltimore, Williams & Wilkins, 1996, pp 2041-2072

2. Hochberg MC, Thomas JT, Thomas DJ, Mead L, Levine DM, Klag MJ: Racial differences in the incidence of gout: the role of hypertension. Arthritis Rheum 38:628-632, 1995

3. Langford HG, Blaufox MD, Borhani NO, Curb JD, Molteri A, Schneider KA, Pressel S: Is thiazide-produced uric acid elevation harmful? Arch Intern Med 147:645-649, 1987

4. Campion EW, Glynn RJ, DeLabry LO: Asymptomatic hyperuricemia. Risks and consequences in the normative aging study. Am J Med 82:421-426, 1987

5. Wu X, Wakamiya M, Vaishnav S, et al: Hyperuricemia and urate nephropathy in urate oxidase-deficient mice. Proc Nat Acad Sci USA 91:742-746, 1994

6. Wilson JM, Stout JT, Palella TD, Davidson BL, Kelley WN, Caskey CT: A molecular survey of hypoxanthine-guanine phosphoribosyltransferase deficiency in man. J Clin Invest 77:188-195, 1986

7. Becker MA, Puig JG, Mateos FA, Jimenez ML, Kim M, Simmonds HA: Inherited superactivity of phosphoribosylpyrophosphate synthetase: association of uric acid overproduction and sensorineural deafness. Am J Med 85:383-390, 1988

8. Emmerson BT, Nagel SL, Duffy DL, Martin NG: Genetic control of the renal clearance of urate: a study of twins. Ann Rheum Dis 51:375-377, 1992

9. Calabrese G, Simmonds HA, Cameron JS, Davies PM: Precocious familial gout with reduced fractional urate clearance and normal purine enzymes. Q J Med 75:441-450, 1990

10. Lin H, Rocher LL, McQuillan MA, Schmaltz S, Palella TD, Fox IH: Cyclosporine-induced hyperuricemia and gout. N Engl J Med 321:287-292, 1989

11. Faller J, Fox I: Ethanol induced hyperuricemia: evidence for increased urate production by activation of adenine nucleotide turnover. N Engl J Med 307:1598-1602, 1982

12. McCarty DJ: Gout without hyperuricemia. JAMA 271:302-303, 1994

13. Terkeltaub R: Pathogenesis and treatment of crystal-induced inflammation. In McCarthy DJ, Koopman WJ (eds): Arthritis and Allied Conditions, 13th ed. Baltimore, Williams & Wilkins, 1996, pp 2085-2102

14. Kam M, Perl-Treves D, Caspi D, Addadi L: Antibodies against crystals. FASEB J 6:2608-2613, 1992

15. Fiechtner JJ, Simkin PA: Urate spherulites in gouty synovia. JAMA 245:1533-1536, 1981

16. Simkin PA, Bassett JE, Lee QP: Not water, but formalin, dissolves urate crystals in tophaceous tissue samples. J Rheumatol 21:2320-1, 1994

17. Roberge C, Gaudry M, Medicis R, Lussier A, Poubelle P, Naccache P: Crystal-induced neutrophil activation. IV. Specific inhibition of tyrosine phosphorylation by colchicine. J Clin Invest 92:1722-1729, 1993

18. Cronstein BN, Molad Y, Reibman J, Balakhane E, Levin RI, Weissmann G: Colchicine alters the quantitative and qualitative display of selectins on endothelial cells and neutrophils. J Clin Invest 96:994-1002, 1995

19. Liote F, Prudhommeaux F, Schiltz C, Champy R, Herbelin A, Oritz-Bravo E, Bardin T: Inhibition and prevention of monosodium urate monohydrate crystal-induced acute inflammation in vivo by transforming growth factor beta-1. Arthritis Rheum 36:1192-1198, 1996

B. CLINICAL AND LABORATORY FEATURES

Gout is a disease caused by the deposition of monosodium urate crystals in the tissues of and around joints. The natural course of classic gout passes through three distinct stages: asymptomatic hyperuricemia, acute intermittent gout, and chronic tophaceous gout (Fig. 17B-1). The rate of progression from asymptomatic hyperuricemia to chronic tophaceous gout varies considerably from one patient to another and is dependent on numerous endogenous and exogenous factors.

STAGES OF CLASSIC GOUT
Asymptomatic Hyperuricemia

Hyperuricemia is a very common biochemical abnormality and can be defined in either physiologic or epidemiologic terms. In extracellular fluids, 98% of uric acid is in the form of monosodium urate (MSU) at pH 7.4. The solubility of MSU in human serum (or plasma) reaches saturation at concentrations of 7 mg/dl; serum concentrations greater than this are considered supersaturated. However, it is common for clinical laboratories to define hyperuricemia as a serum urate level that is greater than two standard deviations above the mean value in a gender- and age-matched healthy population (above 8.1 mg/dl in adult men or 7.2 mg/dl in adult women). In males, adult levels are reached during puberty. Serum urate levels for women run approx-imately 1 mg/dl lower than those for men but rise to a similar level after menopause.

In the Normative Aging Study, subjects with urate levels between 7.0 and 8.0 mg/dl had a cumulative incidence of gouty arthritis of 3%, while those with urate levels of 9.0 mg/dl or more had a 5-year cumulative incidence of 22% (1). Thus, the incidence of gout increases with age as well as with the degree of hyperuricemia. It should be remembered, however, that the vast majority of subjects with hyperuricemia never develop symptoms associated with uric acid excess, including gouty arthritis, tophi, or kidney stones.

Acute Intermittent Gout

The initial episode of acute gout usually follows decades of asymptomatic hyperuricemia (Fig. 17B-1). Thomas Sydenham, the famous 17th century physician writing of his personal experiences with gout (2), eloquently described the initial hours of an acute attack in the following way:

> He goes to bed and sleeps well, but about Two a Clock in the Morning, is waked by the Pain, seizing either his great Toe, the Heel, the Calf of the Leg, or the Ankle; this Pain is like that of dislocated Bones, with the Sense as it were of Water almost cold, poured upon the Membranes of the part affected, presently shivering and shaking follow with a feverish Disposition; the Pain is first gentle, but increased by degrees— till dash towards Night it comes to its height, accompanying

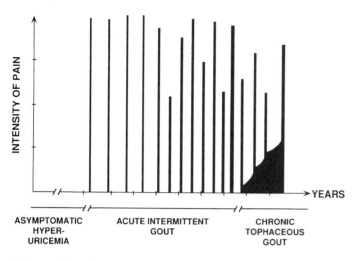

(Figure 17B-1)
The three stages of disease progression in classic gout. The period of asymptomatic hyperuricemia lasts decades, followed by acute intermittent gout with painless intercritical segments finally leading to chronic tophaceous gout with progressive background pain and joint destruction.

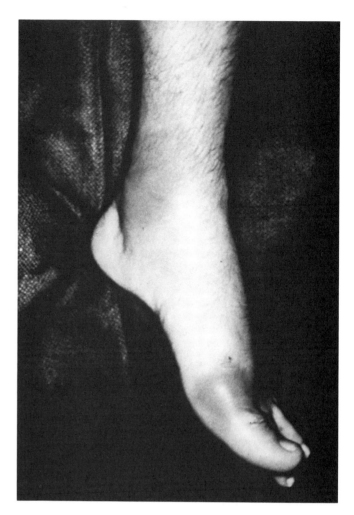

(Figure 17B-2)
Acute gouty arthritis involving the first metatarsophalangeal joint and ankle joint.

itself neatly according to the Variety of the bones of the Tarsus and Metatarsus, whose Ligaments it seizes, sometimes resembling a violent stretching or tearing of those ligaments, sometimes gnawing of a dog, and sometimes a weight; more over, the Part affected has such a quick and exquisite Pain, that it is not able to bear the weight of the cloths upon it, nor hard walking in the Chamber (1).

This classic description captures the exquisite pain frequently associated with acute gouty arthritis, and it is this clinical picture most commonly evoked by the term *gout*.

In men, the first attacks usually occur between the fourth and sixth decades of life. In women, age at onset is older and varies with several factors, the most important of which is age at menopause. The onset of a gouty attack is usually heralded by the rapid development of warmth, swelling, erythema, and exquisite pain in the affected joint. Pain escalates from its faintest twinges to its most intense level over an 8- to 12-hour period. The initial attack is usually monarticular and in one-half of patients involves the first metatarsophalangeal (MTP) joint. Eventually this joint is affected in 90% of individuals with gout. Other joints that are frequently involved in this early stage are the midfoot, ankles, heels, and knees and less commonly the wrists, fingers, and elbows. The intensity of pain is characteristically very severe, but may vary among subjects. Classically, patients cannot stand even the weight of a bed sheet, and most find walking difficult or impossible when lower extremity joints are involved.

Systemic symptoms such as fever, chills, and malaise may accompany acute gout. The cutaneous erythema associated with the gouty attack may extend beyond the involved joint and resemble bacterial cellulitis (Fig. 17B-2). The natural course of untreated acute gout varies from episodes of mild pain that resolve in several hours ("petit attacks") to severe attacks lasting 1–2 weeks. Early in the acute intermittent stage, episodes of acute arthritis are infrequent and intervals between attacks sometimes last for years. The mean time interval is 11 months between the initial attacks and the subsequent acute episode. Over time, the attacks typically become more frequent, longer in duration, and involve more joints.

The intercritical periods of acute intermittent gout are just as characteristic of this stage as are the acute attacks. The previously involved joints are virtually free of symptoms. Despite this, monosodium urate crystals can often be identified in the synovial fluid. In one study, these crystals were found in the synovial fluids of 36 of 37 knees that had previously been inflamed. Synovial fluids containing crystals also had a higher mean cell count than those with no crystals, 449 cells/mm³ versus 64 cells/mm³ (3). These subtle differences may reflect ongoing subclinical inflammation.

Chronic Tophaceous Gout

This stage of gouty arthritis usually develops after 10 or more years of acute intermittent gout, although patients have been reported with tophi as their initial clinical manifestation (4). The transition from acute intermittent gout to chronic tophaceous gout occurs when the intercritical periods are no longer free of pain. The involved joints are now persistently uncomfortable and swollen, although the intensity of these symptoms is much less than during acute flares. Gouty attacks continue to occur against this painful background, and without therapy they may recur as often as every few weeks. The amount of background pain also steadily increases with time if appropriate intervention is not started (Fig 17B-3). Clinically evident tophi may or may not be detected on physical examination during the first few

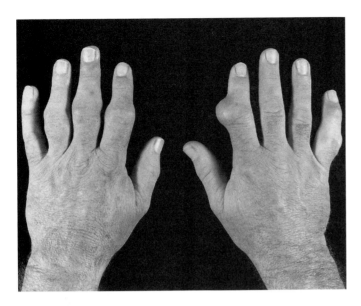

(Figure 17B-3)
The hands of a patient with chronic tophaceous gout reveal large tophi over the right second and fifth proximal interphalangeal (PIP) joints and the left second through fourth PIPs.

years of this stage of gout. However, periarticular tophi detected by magnetic resonance imaging (5) and synovial "microtophi" discovered through the arthroscope are certainly present early in this stage of gout. Polyarticular involvement becomes much more frequent during this time. With diffuse and symmetric involvement of small joints in the hands and feet, chronic tophaceous gout can occasionally be confused with the symmetric polyarthritis of rheumatoid arthritis.

The development of tophaceous deposits of monosodium urate is a function of the duration and severity of hyperuricemia (6). Hench found that untreated patients developed tophi an average of 11.7 years after the onset of acute gout (7). In another study of 1165 patients with primary gout, patients without tophi had serum uric acid levels of 10.3 ± 1.3 mg/dl and those with extensive deposits had levels of 11.0 ± 2.0 mg/dl. Other factors associated with the development of tophi include early age of gout onset, long periods of active but untreated gout, an average of four attacks per year, and a greater tendency toward upper extremity and polyarticular episodes (8).

Subcutaneous gouty tophi may be found anywhere over the body but occur most commonly in the fingers, wrists, ears, knees, olecranon bursa, and pressure points such as the ulnar aspect of the forearm and the Achilles' tendon. In patients with nodal osteoarthritis, tophi have a propensity for forming in Heberden's nodes. Tophi may also occur in connective tissues at other sites, such as renal pyramids, heart valves, and sclerae. Before antihyperuricemic agents were available, as many as 50% of patients with gout eventually developed clinical or radiographic evidence of tophi. Since the introduction of allopurinol and the uricosuric agents, the incidence of tophaceous gout has declined.

UNUSUAL PRESENTATIONS
Early-Onset Gout

Between 3% and 6% of patients with gout have symptom onset before age 25. Early-onset gout represents a special subset of patients who generally have a genetic component,

a more accelerated clinical course, and require more aggressive antihyperuricemic therapy. In large epidemiologic studies of classic gout, a family history of gout and/or nephrolithiasis is present in 25%–30% of cases. In early-onset gout, the incidence of family history is about 80%. In this younger group, detailed questioning about the kindred over several generations may yield enough information to suggest a mode of inheritance (X-linked or autosomal dominant or recessive).

Like classic gout, early-onset gout may be due to either overproduction of urate or reduced renal clearance of uric acid. Diseases associated with overproduction of urate in children and young adults include enzymatic defects in the purine pathway, glycogen storage diseases, and hematologic disorders such as hemoglobinopathies and leukemias. The complete deficiency of hypoxanthine-guanine phosphoribosyl transferase (HGPRT) is an X-linked inherited inborn error of purine metabolism with a characteristic clinical presentation known as the Lesch–Nyhan syndrome. In addition to severe neurologic abnormalities, these boys develop gout and kidney stones in their first decade of life if they are not treated early with allopurinol. The partial deficiency of HGPRT (the Kelley–Seegmiller syndrome) results in early-onset gout or uric acid nephrolithiasis and is also X-linked in its inheritance. Patients with this syndrome have minor or no neurologic problems.

Glycogen storage disease types I, III, V, and VII are associated with early-onset gout and are inherited as autosomal recessive diseases. Sickle cell disease, beta-thalassemia, and nonlymphocytic leukemias may all be complicated by gouty arthritis in the young adult years.

Conditions associated with uric acid underexcretion in young patients include a specific renal tubular disorder known as familial urate nephropathy (9). This autosomal dominant disorder causes hyperuricemia from a very young age, before any evidence of renal insufficiency. The condition may lead to progressive renal failure and end-stage kidney disease by age 40. Other nephropathies associated with early-onset gout include polycystic kidney disease, chronic lead intoxication, medullary cystic disease, and focal tubulointerstitial disease.

Transplantation Gout

Hyperuricemia reportedly develops in 75%–80% of heart transplant recipients who routinely take cyclosporine for preventing allograft rejection (10). A slightly lower frequency (approximately 50%) of kidney and liver transplant recipients develop hyperuricemia, presumably because lower doses of cyclosporine are used in these individuals. Whereas in the general population asymptomatic hyperuricemia progresses to clinical gout in 1 out of 30 subjects, cyclosporine-induced hyperuricemia leads to gout in 1 of 6 patients (11). Other differences between primary and cyclosporine-induced gout include the marked shortening of the asymptomatic hyperuricemia and acute intermittent gout stages with the rapid appearance of tophi. The stage of asymptomatic hyperuricemia lasts for 2–3 decades in classic gout but is present for only 6 months to 4 years in cyclosporine-induced disease. Similarly, the duration of the acute intermittent stage is only 1–4 years in transplant recipients, whereas it may last 8–15 years in classic gout. Because other medications are being used by organ transplant patients such as systemic corticosteroids and azathioprine, their gouty symptoms are frequently less dramatic than those of classic gouty subjects.

Gout in Women

Unlike most other rheumatic conditions, gout is less common in women. In most large reviews, women account for no more than 5% of all gouty subjects (12). Ninety percent of women are postmenopausal at the time of their initial attack. Postmenopausal gout is clinically similar in presentation and course of classic gout except that the age of onset is later in women than in men (mean age 60 years in women versus 49 years in men). Several associated conditions are much more common in postmenopausal women with gout than in men. Diuretic use (95%), hypertension (73%), and renal insufficiency (50%) have strong associations with postmenopausal gout, as does preexisting joint disease such as osteoarthritis (13).

Premenopausal gout has a strong hereditary component, as does early-onset gout in men. Most women who develop gout before menopause have hypertension and renal insufficiency but are not using diuretic therapy. The rare woman with premenopausal gout and normal renal function should be evaluated for the autosomally inherited familial hyperuricemia nephropathy (9) or the even more rare non-X-linked inborn errors of purine metabolism (13).

"Normouricemic" Gout

The two most frequent explanations for gout with normal levels of uric acid are: 1) the patient doesn't have gout, or 2) the serum urate is normal at the time measured, but the patient is actually chronically hyperuricemic.

Several articular conditions can closely mimic gout, including other crystalline arthropathies of calcium pyrophosphate dihydrate, basic calcium (apatite), and liquid lipid (14). Other causes of acute monarthropathies such as infection, sarcoidosis, and trauma should also be considered (15). The clinical suspicions of gout should be confirmed by crystal analysis of synovial fluid. Without this confirmation, the diagnosis remains in question.

A misunderstanding of the definition of hyperuricemia also contributes to the misdiagnosis of normouricemic gout. A sustained serum urate level above 7.0 mg/dl is a permissive environment for MSU crystal formation. For various reasons, patients with acute and chronic gout occasionally have urate values below this biochemical definition of hyperuricemia. It is, in fact, rather common for a patient presenting with acute gout to have a normal serum urate during the episode of severe pain. This finding probably results from the uricosuric effect of adrenocorticotropic hormone release and adrenal stimulation caused by the stress of the painful process. Normalization of serum urate values during acute gouty flares may be more common in alcoholics than in nondrinkers. Aside from the standard urate lowering agents (allopurinol, probenecid, and sulfinpyrazone), other drugs such as high-dose salicylates, corticosteroids, dicumarol, glycerol guaiacholate, and x-ray contrast agents may also lower serum urate values in patients with gout and lead to the false impression of normouricemic gout.

Yü reported that 1.6% of 2145 gouty patients had sustained normouricemia even after not taking allopurinol or uricosuric agents for months (16). In most of these cases, hyperuricemia eventually returned, although several patients with very mild gouty symptoms remained normouricemic over a prolonged period.

PROVOCATIVE FACTORS OF ACUTE ATTACKS

Why crystals form in some hyperuricemic fluids and not in others is still unclear. When synovial fluids are balanced for urate concentrations, the fluids from gouty patients have a far greater propensity for promoting crystal formation than similar fluids from patients with either osteoarthritis or rheumatoid arthritis (RA). A number of synovial fluid proteins have been reported to function as promoters or inhibitors of crystal nucleation. The current list of physiologically important nucleators is short, with the leading contenders being type I collagen and a gamma globulin subfraction (17).

The degree of hyperuricemia is positively correlated with the overall risk of acquiring gout. However, rapid increases or decreases in the concentration of synovial fluid urate are more closely related to the actual precipitation of the acute gouty attack. A rapid flux in urate level is a triggering mechanism in gout induced by trauma, alcohol ingestion, and drugs.

Trauma is frequently reported to be an inciting event for acute gouty episodes. The trauma may be as minor as a long walk and may not have caused pain during the activity, but it caused intra-articular swelling. When the joint is allowed to rest, there is a relatively rapid efflux of free water from the joint fluid. This results in a sudden increase in synovial fluid urate concentration that may allow precipitation of urate crystals and a gout attack to develop. This mechanism may also explain why gouty attacks commonly occur at night.

Alcohol ingestion may predispose to gout through several mechanisms. The consumption of lead-tainted moonshine results in chronic renal tubular damage that leads to secondary hyperuricemia and "saturnine" gout. The ingestion of any form of ethanol can acutely raise uric acid production by accelerating the breakdown of intracellular adenosine triphosphate (8). Beer consumption has an added impact on gout because it contains large quantities of guanosine, which is catabolized to uric acid.

Drugs may precipitate gout by rapidly raising or lowering urate levels. Thiazide diuretics are frequent offenders by selectively interfering with urate excretion at the proximal convoluted tubule. Low-dose aspirin (less than 2 gm/day) can also raise serum urate levels, whereas higher doses have a uricosuric effect and may lower the serum urate concentration. Either a rapid increase or reduction in the serum urate level can provoke gouty attacks; allopurinol is the drug most often responsible for this effect. The mechanism for this paradoxic response appears to be the destabilizing of microtophi in the gouty synovium when the urate concentration of the synovial fluid is rapidly changed. As the microtophi break apart, crystals are shed into the synovial fluid and the gouty episode is initiated (19).

CLINICAL ASSOCIATIONS
Renal Disease

The only consistent visceral damage caused by hyperuricemia is its effect on the kidneys. Several distinct forms of hyperuricemia-induced renal disease are recognized, including chronic urate nephropathy, acute uric acid nephropathy, and uric acid nephrolithiasis.

Progressive renal failure is common in the gouty population and accounts for up to 10% of deaths. Hypertension, chronic lead exposure, and ischemic heart disease are the most important contributing factors to this complication; the role of hyperuricemia as a single factor in chronic parenchymal disease of the kidney remains controversial. Chronic urate nephropathy is a distinct entity that is caused by the deposition of monosodium urate crystals in the renal medulla and pyramids and is associated with mild albuminuria. Although chronic hyperuricemia is thought to be the cause of urate nephropathy, this form of kidney involvement is essentially never seen in the absence of gouty arthritis.

Acute renal failure can be caused by hyperuricemia in the acute tumor lysis syndrome, which occurs in patients given chemotherapy for rapidly proliferating lymphomas and leukemias. With massive liberation of purines during cell lysis, uric acid precipitates in the distal tubules and collecting ducts of the kidney. Acute uric acid nephropathy can result in oliguria or anuria. This form of acute renal failure can be distinguished from other forms by a ratio of uric acid to creatinine greater than 1.0 in a random or 24-hour urine collection.

Uric acid renal stones occur in 10%–25% percent of all patients with gout. The incidence correlates strongly with the serum urate level; the likelihood of developing stones reaches 50% when the serum urate is above 13 mg/dl. Symptoms of renal stones precede the development of gout in 40% of patients. Calcium-containing renal stones occur 10 times more frequently in gouty subjects than in the general population.

Hypertension

Hypertension is present in 25%–50% of gouty patients, and 2%–14% of hypertensive subjects have gout. Since serum urate concentration correlates directly with peripheral and renal vascular resistance, reduced renal blood flow may account for the association between hypertension and hyperuricemia. Factors such as obesity and male gender also link hypertension and hyperuricemia.

Obesity

Hyperuricemia and gout are highly correlated with body weight for both men and women, and individuals with gout are commonly overweight compared to the general population. Obesity may be a common factor linking hyperuricemia, hypertension, hyperlipidemia, and atherosclerosis.

Hyperlipidemia

Serum triglycerides are elevated in 80% of patients with gout. The association between hyperuricemia and serum cholesterol is controversial, although serum levels of high-density lipoprotein (HDL) are generally decreased in patients with gout. These abnormalities of serum lipids likely reflect overindulgence rather than a genetic link.

RADIOLOGIC FEATURES

The radiographic findings of gout are often unremarkable early in the disease course. In acute gouty arthritis, the only finding may be soft tissue swelling around the affected joint. In most instances, bone and joint abnormalities develop only after many years of disease and are indicative of the deposition of urate crystals. The abnormalities are most frequently asymmetric and seen in the feet, hands, wrists, elbows, and knees.

The bony erosions of gout are radiographically distinct from the erosive changes of other inflammatory arthritides such as RA. Gouty erosions are usually slightly removed

from the joint whereas rheumatoid erosions are typically in the immediate proximity of the articular surface (Fig. 17B-4). The characteristic gouty erosion has features that are both atrophic and hypertrophic leading to erosions with an "overhanging edge." The joint space is preserved in gout until very late in the disease process. Juxta-articular osteopenia, a common and early finding in RA, is absent or minimal in gout.

LABORATORY FEATURES AND DIAGNOSIS

Elevated serum urate level has long been considered a cornerstone in the diagnosis of gout. In reality, the actual utility of this laboratory finding in establishing the diagnosis is limited. The vast majority of hyperuricemic subjects will not develop gout, and the serum urate may be normal during gouty attacks. Far too many patients are diagnosed with gout based on the clinical triad of an acute monarthritis, hyperuricemia, and a dramatic improvement of articular symptoms in response to colchicine. A "diagnosis" by these parameters is only presumptive, and the physician should remain alert to other possibilities. A clinical response to colchicine, which was once considered to be strong evidence of gout, is frequently observed with other types of arthritis including calcium pyrophosphate pseudogout and basic calcium phosphate (hydroxyapatite) tendinitis. Serum urate determinations are helpful and necessary in following the effects of antihyperuricemic therapy.

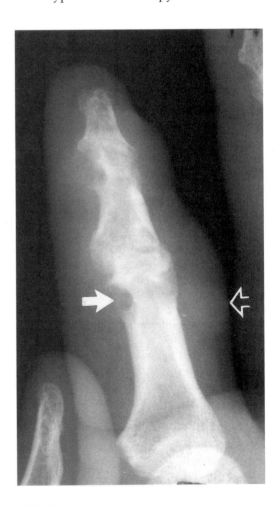

(Figure 17B-4)
Radiographic changes of chronic gout include a typical gouty erosion with overhanging edge (solid arrow) and a soft tissue tophus (open arrow).

The definitive diagnosis of gout is possible only by aspiration and inspection of either synovial fluid or tophaceous material and the demonstration of characteristic monosodium urate crystals (Fig. 17B-5). The crystals are usually needle or rod-shaped. On compensated polarized microscopy, they appear as bright, birefringent crystals that are yellow when parallel to the axis of slow vibration on the first order color compensator. The crystals are usually intracellular during acute attacks, but small, truncated extracellular crystals commonly appear as the attack subsides and during the intercritical periods.

The synovial fluid findings are consistent with moderate to severe inflammation. The leukocyte count usually falls between 5000 and 80,000 cells/mm^3 with an average between 15,000 to 20,000. The cells are predominantly neutrophils. Synovial aspirates should be sent for culture if there is any hint of a septic process. Bacterial infection can coexist with gouty crystals.

A 24-hour urine uric acid measurement is not required of all patients presenting with gout. This measurement is useful for patients being considered for uricosuric therapy (benemid or sulfinpyrazone) or when the cause of marked hyperuricemia (>11 mg/dl) is being investigated. On a regular diet, urinary uric acid excretion of more than 800 mg/24

hours suggests a problem of urate overproduction. In children and young adults, this overproduction may be caused by enzymatic defects. In older patients, this level of urinary uric acid suggests one of the diseases associated with rapid cellular turnover such as the myelo- or lymphoproliferative disorders. Certain drugs, contrast dyes, and alcohol interfere with urinary uric acid measurements and should be avoided for several days before the study.

N. LAWRENCE EDWARDS, MD

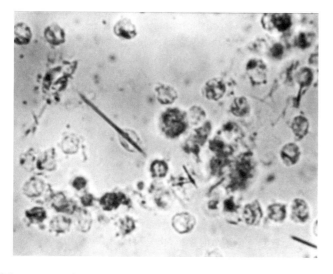

(Figure 17B-5)
Photomicrograph of fresh preparation of synovial fluid obtained from the inflamed knee of a 45-year-old man with acute gouty arthritis. Note numerous small and large needle-shaped crystals of monosodium urate monohydrate that have been engulfed by neutrophilic leukocytes.

1. Campion EW, Glynn RV, DeLabry LO: Asymptomatic hyperuricemia: risks and consequences in the Normative Aging Study. Am J Med 82:421-426,1987

2. Sydenham T: The whole works of that excellent practical physician, Dr. Thomas Sydenham. 7th ed translated by John Pechey. London, Feals, 1717

3. Pascual E: Persistence of monosodium urate crystals and low-grade inflammation in the synovial fluid of patients with untreated gout. Arthritis Rheum 34:141-145,1991

4. Wernick R, Winkler C, Campbell S: Tophi as the initial manifestation of gout: report of six cases and review of the literature. Arch Intern Med 152:873-876 ,1992

5. Popp JD, Bidgood WD, Edwards NL: Magnetic resonance imaging of tophaceous gout in the hands and wrists. Seminars Arthritis Rheum 25:282-289,1996

6. Popp JD, Bidgood WD, Edwards NL: The gouty tophus. Rheumatology Rev 2,163-168, 1993

7. Hench PS: The diagnosis of gout and gout arthritis. J Lab Clin Med 22:48-55, 1936

8. Nakayama DA, Barthelemy C, Carrera G, Lightfoot RW, Wortmann RL: Tophaceous gout: a clinical and radiographic assessment. Arthritis Rheum 27:468-471, 1984

9. Moro F, Ogg CS, Simmonds HA, et al: Familal juvenile gouty nephropathy with renal urate hypoexcretion preceding renal disease. Clin Nephrol 35:263-269, 1991

10. Burack DA, Griffith BP, Thompson ME, et al: Hyperuricemia and gout among heart transplant recipients receiving cyclosporine. Am J Med 92:141-146, 1992

11. Howe S, Edwards NL: Controlling hyperuricemia and gout in cardiac transplant recipients. J Musculoskel Med 12(4):15-24, 1995

12. Lally EV, Ho G, Kaplan SR: The clinical spectrum of gouty arthritis in women. Arch Intern Med 146:2221-2225, 1986

13. Puig JG, Michán AD, Jiménez ML, et al: Female gout: clinical spectrum and uric acid metabolism. Arch Intern Med 151:726-732, 1991

14. Reginato AJ, Schumacher HR, Allan DA, Rabinowitz JL: Acute monarthritis associated with lipid liquid crystals. Ann Rheum Dis 44:537-543, 1985

15. Baker DG, Schumacher HR: Acute monarthritis. N Engl J Med 329:1013-1020, 1993

16. Yü T-F: Diversity of clinical features in gouty arthritis. Semin Arthritis Rheum 13:360-368, 1984

17. McGill NW, Dieppe PA: The role of serum and synovial fluid components in the promotion of urate crystal formation. J Rheumatol 18:1042-1045, 1991

18. Puig JG, Fox IH: Ethanol induced activations of adenine nucleotide turnover. Evidence for a role of acetate. J Clin Invest 74:936-941, 1984

19. Popp JD, Edwards NL: New insights into gouty arthritis. Contemp Intern Med 7:55-64, 1995

C. TREATMENT

Gout progresses naturally through three stages: asymptomatic hyperuricemia, acute intermittent gout, and chronic tophaceous gout. Effective medical management exists for each stage (1). Goals of treatment include providing rapid and safe pain relief, preventing further attacks, and preventing formation of tophi, kidney stones, and destructive arthropathy. Optimal management requires a well-informed patient. Unless clear explanations are provided, patients may misuse their medications or confuse drugs used for acute gouty flares with those used for treatment of hyperuricemia. In most situations treatment is highly successful and without complications.

ACUTE GOUT

The goal of treating the acute gout attack is to eliminate the pain and other symptoms caused by the intense inflammation. Many agents can be used effectively, including colchicine, nonsteroidal anti-inflammatory drugs (NSAIDs), and corticosteroids. The sooner after onset of an attack that any of these agents are given, the more rapidly the signs of inflammation will resolve.

Colchicine

Colchicine is an effective agent for the treatment of acute gout, and pain subsides within 48 hours in the majority of patients treated with this drug (1,2). Colchicine inhibits the polymerization of microtubules by binding their protein subunits and preventing their aggregation. Membrane-dependent functions such as chemotaxis and phagocytosis may, therefore, be disrupted. Colchicine also inhibits the production of crystal-induced chemotactic factor and interleukin-6. After an intravenous dose, plasma levels decay rapidly as colchicine is concentrated intracellularly, with only 10% excreted during the first 24 hours. With sensitive assays, colchicine can be detected in granulocytes and in urine 10 days after administration. Thus, an important determinant of toxicity is the cumulative dose over 7–10 days relative to renal function (3). Colchicine enters enterohepatic circulation, and liver disease or extrahepatic biliary obstruction may potentiate its toxic effects.

In the typical patient, colchicine is administered as 0.5- or 0.6-mg tablets taken hourly until one of three endpoints is reached: 1) significant improvement of pain and inflammation, 2) gastrointestinal toxicity, or 3) a maximum total dose of 6.0 mg, assuming normal renal and hepatic function. Oral colchicine may cause gastrointestinal toxicity in up to 80% of patients. Nausea, vomiting, diarrhea, and cramping abdominal pain may be severe, leading to hypovolemia, electrolyte disturbances, and metabolic alkalosis. The gradual use of small, repeated doses is intended only to minimize gastrointestinal toxicity, but affords no therapeutic advantage.

Intravenous colchicine may be useful, particularly in the postoperative patient in whom oral intake is restricted. Intravenous use has the dual advantages of rapid onset of action and no gastrointestinal toxicity, provided oral colchicine is not being used concomitantly. The drug should be diluted for intravenous use in 20 ml of normal saline (not D5W) and administered over 10 to 20 minutes through a secured intra-venous line to avoid thrombophlebitis or extravasation. Thrombophlebitis may develop if the intravenous colchicine is not diluted properly, and skin sloughing may occur if it extravasates.

The improper use of colchicine, particularly the intravenous form, has led to serious toxicities and even fatalities. Excessive dosage may produce bone marrow suppression, renal failure, disseminated intravascular coagulation, hypocalcemia, cardiopulmonary failure, seizures, and death (3-5). In these patients, colchicine-induced granulocytopenia is a major contributor to a fatal outcome. All reported cases of death, severe toxicity, or neuromuscular disease have involved unusually high doses of colchicine, renal insufficiency, advanced age, or the use of both oral and intravenous preparations during a short period of time.

Intravenous colchicine should be administered with care, following these basic guidelines (6). A single intravenous dose should not exceed 3 mg, and the total cumulative dose for an attack should not exceed 4 mg in a 24-hour period. Patients should not receive additional colchicine by any route for 7 days after a full intravenous dose. The drug dosage should be reduced in the presence of renal or hepatic disease and in the older patient with apparently normal renal function. Finally, absolute contraindications to intravenous colchicine include combined renal and hepatic disease, a glomerular filtration rate of <10 ml/min, and extrahepatic biliary obstruction.

Relative contraindications include significant intercurrent infection, pre-existing bone marrow suppression, and immediate prior use of oral colchicine. In patients with estimated glomerular filtration rates <50–60 ml/min, doses should be halved (5). In general, it is better not to mix oral and intravenous colchicine during any attack or in a 7–10 day time period. In none of the reported cases of extreme toxicity were these requirements fulfilled. Their application should greatly increase the safety of intravenous colchicine administration.

Nonsteroidal Anti-inflammatory Drugs

Nonsteroidal anti-inflammatory drugs are probably used more often than colchicine for acute gout. Many physicians prefer to use indomethacin for acute gout, but other NSAIDs may be just as effective. In general, NSAIDs are started in their recommended maximal doses at the first sign of an attack. The dose may be lowered as symptoms resolve, but medication should be continued until the arthritis has resolved totally for at least 48 hours. When used in this way, the response rate of NSAIDs approaches that of oral colchicine. NSAIDs may cause significant side effects, most commonly gastrointestinal symptoms. These appear to be less common when NSAIDs are used to treat acute gout compared to their use in other conditions.

Nonsteroidal anti-inflammatory drugs should be avoided in patients with active or recent peptic ulcer disease and in patients requiring anticoagulation therapy. Caution should be used in prescribing NSAIDs in patients with renal insufficiency or conditions associated with impaired renal blood flow. These drugs may exacerbate renal insufficiency and cause hyperkalemia by inducing hyporeninemic hypoaldosteronism through inhibition of intrarenal prostaglandin formation. They may worsen hypertension, induce sodium retention, and exacerbate edematous states. Rarely, NSAIDs may cause interstitial nephritis or papillary necrosis. See Chapter 52 for more information on NSAIDs.

Corticosteroids and Adrenocorticotropic Hormone

Corticosteroids and adrenocorticotropic hormone (ACTH) are usually reserved for patients in whom colchicine or NSAIDs are contraindicated or ineffective. There are reports of relapse or early recurrence complicating their use; however, a recent study of corticosteroids in acute gout noted relapse infrequently (7). Response time was comparable to that of NSAIDs. A single unblinded trial compared ACTH with indomethacin in monarticular gout and reported similar efficacy (8).

For acute gout, 20–40-mg doses of prednisone or its equivalent are administered daily for three to four days and then gradually tapered over 1–2 weeks. If oral administration is problematic, the hospitalized patient can be treated with equivalent doses of intravenous methylprednisolone. Adrenocorticotropic hormone is given as an intramuscular injection of 40–80 IU; some have recommended following the initial dose with 40 IU every 6–12 hours for several days if necessary.

Aspiration and intra-articular corticosteroid injection with 10–40 mg of triamcinolone or 2–10 mg dexamethasone is a useful alternative in the patient who has gout in one or two large joints. Full drainage of the joint alone may be helpful. If septic arthritis is suspected after aspiration, injection should be deferred until synovial fluid has been cultured, because septic and gouty arthritis can occur simultaneously. Joint aspiration and injection may be a nontoxic therapeutic option in the elderly patient with renal insufficiency, peptic ulcer disease, or other intercurrent illness. It is also an appropriate option for recalcitrant gout.

Most often, gout will respond to colchicine, NSAIDs, or corticosteroids alone. In some situations, however, one agent may not be sufficient because of delay in therapy or severity of the attack. When this occurs, these agents may be used in combination, and pain medications including narcotics may be added to the regimen.

PROPHYLACTIC TREATMENT OF INTERMITTENT GOUT

Modification of diet, drug regimen, and lifestyle may reduce the frequency of acute attacks and render daily drug therapy unnecessary. Weight loss may yield beneficial reduction in serum urate, and dietary purine restriction may be an important adjunct to therapy, although plasma urate reduction is usually modest. Alcohol should be avoided because it may both increase production and impair excretion of uric acid. Dehydration and repetitive trauma (as encountered in certain exercises or occupations) may be avoidable causes of gouty attacks. Furthermore, diuretics and other drugs known to contribute to hyperuricemia should be eliminated if possible.

The decision to employ prophylactic therapy in individual patients depends on issues such as toxicity, cost, adherence, and patient tolerance of acute attacks. Prophylactic therapy ought not be considered until one has decided to add an antihyperuricemic agent to the regimen. The use of prophylactic colchicine without controlling the hyperuricemia allows tophi to develop without the usual warning signs of acute gouty attacks.

A single double-blind, placebo-controlled study supports the prophylactic efficacy of one 0.5 mg colchicine tablet twice daily (9). Prophylactic therapy reduces the frequency of attacks by 75% to 85% and moderates the severity of attacks that do occur. The smallest daily dose providing acceptable control of attacks should be used to minimize the risk of toxicity.

The protracted use of small daily doses of colchicine appears to be relatively safe, although prophylactic use of colchicine has been associated with a neuromuscular syndrome. Colchicine-induced myopathy resembles polymyositis with proximal muscle weakness, elevated creatine kinase levels, and abnormalities on electromyogram. The myopathy may resolve spontaneously over several weeks, but more subtle polyneuropathy caused by colchicine resolves more slowly (5). When used long-term for familial Mediterranean fever, few serious problems have been reported with doses of 1.0–1.5 mg daily, although diarrhea occurs commonly and steatorrhea rarely. There have been rare reports of colchicine-associated azoospermia, but the literature does not document any clear effect on fertility.

HYPERURICEMIA AND URATE-LOWERING AGENTS

The treatment of hyperuricemia in patients with recurrent or chronic gout implies a long-term commitment to daily therapy and behavioral change. The antihyperuricemic agents available are sufficiently potent that dietary restriction of purines is not necessary, nor is the automatic avoidance of medications that have hyperuricemic properties.

The goal of treatment is consistent maintenance of serum urate <5.0 mg/dl to allow solubilization of crystalline urate. One recent study examined radiographic changes occurring over 10 years of urate-lowering therapy (10). As achieving "normouricemia" did not appear to translate into radiographic improvement of intraosseous tophi as often as expected, the authors expressed concern that greater reductions of serum urate may be necessary even when symptoms are controlled.

Appropriate antihyperuricemic agents include uricosuric drugs and xanthine oxidase inhibitors. In either instance, the lowest dose that maintains the serum urate in acceptable ranges should be employed. Because fewer than 10% of patients are overproducers of uric acid, uricosuric therapy is rarely inappropriate. However, because allopurinol is effective in both overproducers and underexcretors and is given in a single daily dose, it is generally recommended. Both allopurinol and uricosuric drugs are available in generic form with roughly comparable prices for average effective doses.

Allopurinol is the agent of choice for patients who have urate overproduction, tophus formation, nephrolithiasis, or other contraindications to uricosuric therapy. It is the preferred drug in cases of renal insufficiency, but its toxicity occurs most frequently when the glomerular filtration rate is reduced. Toxicity can almost always be avoided if dosages are restricted appropriately. Typically, a dosage of 300 mg/day can be started as initial therapy; however, doses of 100 mg or less are appropriate in the elderly, in those with frequent attacks, or in patients with glomerular filtration rate <50 ml/minute (1).

In addition to dyspepsia, headache, and diarrhea, a pruritic papular rash occurs in 3% to 10% of those receiving allopurinol. Additional toxicities include fever, urticaria, leukocytosis, eosinophilia, interstitial nephritis, acute renal failure, granulomatous hepatitis, and toxic epidermal necrolysis.

The syndrome of allopurinol hypersensitivity is a rare but serious toxicity with a mortality rate of 20% to 30% (1). In situations where the need to reduce hyperuricemia is great, allopurinol hypersensitivity may be overcome through cautious desensitization. In an oral regimen, slow daily escalations of dose from 8 μg to 300 mg over 30 days may be successful. A rapid intravenous regimen for desensitization has been used successfully in a patient who failed oral desensitization (11). After a 0.1 μg intradermal skin test, intravenous allopurinol was infused in five increments from 0.1 μg to 500 μg at 15-minute intervals. Doses were advanced at 30-minute intervals from 1.0 mg to 50 mg in five further increments. One hour later, 100 mg was given intravenously; the following morning, 300 mg was given orally. Thereafter, daily 300 mg doses of allopurinol were tolerated without incident. Symptoms of hypersensitivity can recur after full desensitization and resumption of the drug at full dosage (12). Oxypurinol, the active metabolite of allopurinol, will be tolerated by some patients sensitive to allopurinol.

Uricosuric agents are effective for patients who 1) have a glomerular filtration rate exceeding 50–60 ml/min; 2) are willing to drink at least 2 liters of fluids daily and maintain good urine flow even at night; 3) have no history of nephrolithiasis or excessive urine acidity; and 4) can avoid all salicylate ingestion, because even low doses can inhibit the drug's effect. With advancing age, glomerular filtration rate falls and few patients over 65 years of age can adequately respond to most uricosuric drugs.

Probenecid is the uricosuric agent used most often. It is started at 0.5 g/day and is advanced slowly to not more than 1 g twice daily or until target urate level is reached. The most common side effects of probenecid therapy are rash and gastrointestinal upset. The adverse effect of most concern, however, is urate nephrolithiasis. Despite patient efforts to maintain high urine volume, stones may form, indicating that uricosuric therapy may be inappropriate. Allopurinol is preferred in such patients. If a uricosuric is absolutely necessary, urinary alkylinization to pH 6.0–6.5 may be effective in increasing urate solubility. Potassium citrate in doses of 30–80 mEq/day may help prevent nephrolithiasis. Sulfinpyrazone, a potent uricosuric agent, promotes urate nephrolithiasis and should be used with similar precautions. Gastrointestinal side effects are seen in approximately 5% of patients (1). A congener of phenylbutazone, sulfinpyrazone may be ulcerogenic, and in rare cases, bone marrow suppression may occur. The drug is slowly advanced from 100 mg to approximately 800 mg daily in divided doses until the desired level of serum urate is reached. Available in Europe, benzbromarone is a more potent uricosuric that may be effective even in the face of moderate renal insufficiency or salicylate use. Several drug interactions involving urate-lowering agents should be noted. For unknown reasons, the concomitant administration of allopurinol and ampicillin is associated with increased frequency of rash. Probenecid inhibits the excretion of the penicillins as well as of indomethacin, dapsone, and acetazolamide. Probenecid may also affect the metabolism of rifampin and heparin. If probenecid is used to enhance urate excretion in the tophaceous gout patient on allopurinol, dosage adjustment is necessary to avoid the interaction of these two drugs. Allopurinol may increase the half life of probenecid, and probenecid accelerates the excretion of allopurinol. Thus, higher allopurinol doses may be needed, and probenecid may be effective in relatively low doses. It is reasonable to question whether the initiation of urate-lowering therapy implies the need for lifelong treatment. Gast (13) reported his experience with 10 patients of whom five had experienced no recurrence 33 months after the discontinuation of urate-lowering therapy. The other five patients had recurrent attacks first occurring at 15.8 months on average. Such data suggest that discontinuation of urate-lowering therapy may be well tolerated after years of normouricemia and presumed depletion of total body urate.

ASYMPTOMATIC HYPERURICEMIA

Hyperuricemia alone is seldom a reason for treatment. However, over a period of years moderate hyperuricemia may lead to gouty arthritis, tophus formation, and less commonly, nephrolithiasis. Although there is little long-term risk of tophus formation in the patient with a plasma urate level of 7–8 mg/dl, there is increasing risk with higher levels. Up to 50% of nonselected gout patients develop tophi by examination or radiography if left untreated. In as much as individuals almost always experience attacks of acute gout before tophi develop, the finding of asymptomatic hyperuricemia is not an indication for treatment with urate-lowering drugs. The cause for hyperuricemia should be determined (hematologic disorder or renal disease, for example) and associated problems such as hypertension, alcoholism, hyperlipedemia, or obesity should be addressed.

GOUT IN THE TRANSPLANT HOST

The prevalence of gout in recipients of organ transplants has greatly increased with the use of cyclosporine. Treatment of the acute attack and reduction of hyperuricemia may be difficult in the transplant host. Without regard to the organ transplanted, renal function is often impaired. Like NSAIDs, cyclosporine may interfere with renal prostaglandin formation, thus decreasing renal blood flow; when used together they may have an additive effect on renal function (14). Colchicine use may be hazardous in the patient on azathioprine whose granulocyte count is decreased. Corticosteroids and ACTH may be ineffective, because most transplant patients are on long-term corticosteroid therapy at the time of their attack. In the patient with marginal renal function or white blood cell count, the safest alternative to colchicine and NSAIDs may be articular injection. Synovial fluid culture should be performed routinely in such patients.

The management of hyperuricemia in the transplant host is similarly complex. The patient with glomerular filtration rate below 50 ml/min will not respond to uricosuric agents. Tophi may be present, dictating the use of allopurinol even in the patient with an adequate glomerular filtration rate. Yet allopurinol causes potentiation of azathioprine, which as a purine analogue is metabolized by xanthine oxidase. The use of allopurinol requires a 50% to 75% reduction of azathioprine dose (14), and even with frequent monitoring of white cell count, the therapeutic margin between leukopenia and inadequate immunosuppression is dangerously narrow.

PARKS W. PRATT, MD
GENE V. BALL, MD

1. Emmerson BT: The management of gout. N Engl J Med 344:445-451, 1996.

2. Gutman AB: Treatment of primary gout: the present status. Arthritis Rheum 8:911-20, 1965

3. Moreland LM, Ball GV: Colchicine and gout. Arthritis Rheum 34:782-786, 1991

4. Roberts WN, Liang MH, Stein SH: Colchicine in acute gout: reassessment of risks and benefits. JAMA 257:1920-1922, 1987

5. Putterman C, Ben-Chetrit E, Caraco Y, et al: Colchicine intoxication: clinical pharmacology, risk factors, features, and management. Semin Arthritis Rheum 21:143-55, 1991

6. Wallace SL, Singer JZ: Review: systemic toxicity associated with the intravenous administration of colchicine-guidelines for use. J Rheumatol 15:495-499, 1988

7. Groff GD, Franch WA, Raddaty DA: Systemic steroid therapy for acute gout: a clinical trial and review of the literature. Semin Arthritis Rheum 19:329-336, 1990

8. Axelrod D, Preston S: Comparison of parenteral adreno-corticotropic hormone with oral indomethacin in the treatment of acute gout. Arthritis Rheum 31:803-5, 1988

9. Paulus HE, Schlosstein LH, Godfrey RC, et al: Prophylactic colchicine therapy of intercritical gout. A placebo-controlled study of probenecid-treated patients. Arthritis Rheum 17:609-614, 1987

10. McCarthy GM, Barthelemy CR, Veum JA, et al: Influence of antihyperuricemic therapy and the clinical and radiographic progression of gout. Arthritis Rheum 34:1489-1494, 1991

11. Halz-LeBlanc BAE, Reynolds WJ, MacFadden DK: Allopurinol hypersensitivity in a patient with chronic tophaceous gout: Success of intravenous desensitization after failure of oral desensitization. Arthritis Rheum 34:1329-1331, 1991

12. Unsworth J, Blake DR: Desensitization to allopurinol: a cautionary tale. Ann Rheum Dis 46:646, 1987

13. Gast LF: Withdrawal of longterm antihyperuricemic therapy in tophaceous gout. Clin Rheumatol 6:70-73, 1987

14. West C, Carpenter BJ, Hakala TR: The incidence of gout in renal transplant recipients. Am J Kidney Dis 10:369-372, 1987

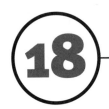

UNDIFFERENTIATED CONNECTIVE TISSUE SYNDROMES

18

The concept of undifferentiated connective tissue syndromes has grown from the recognition that systemic rheumatic diseases have several properties which make a specific diagnosis difficult (1,2).

Of most importance is the occurrence of several clinical features that are shared to a variable extent by rheumatoid arthritis (RA), systemic lupus erythematosus (SLE), systemic sclerosis (scleroderma), polymyositis and dermatomyositis (PM and DM), and Sjögren's syndrome. These include Raynaud's phenomenon, polyarthritis, interstitial lung disease, pleuritis or pericarditis, and vasculitis. Patients who present with one or more of these features often do not satisfy criteria for any of the recognized systemic rheumatic diseases. In addition, evolution to a recognizable connective tissue disease may require years or may never occur. Alternatively, the signs and symptoms may disappear, removing the necessity for any disease designation.

In addition to the shared clinical features, serologic features are also shared to a variable extent by all of these diseases. Chief among these are the presence of antinuclear antibodies (ANA), measured by indirect immunofluorescence, and rheumatoid factors, autoantibodies directed to the Fc fragment of immunoglobulin G (IgG). This frequent sharing of clinical features and serologic findings makes early diagnosis difficult in a group of diseases for which no etiology has been established. Moreover, no definitive diagnostic tests exist in the absence of a cluster of clinical features that lead to the diagnosis of the differentiated form of each of these diseases. In addition to these complexities, each of the systemic rheumatic diseases is extremely heterogeneous. It is very clear that, especially for SLE, systemic sclerosis, PM, and DM, numerous subsets can be classified on the basis of a combination of clinical characteristics and the recognition of specific autoantibodies directed to well-defined molecular target antigens.

Finally, there are numerous instances of overlap, with the presence of two or more diseases, that are more or less fully expressed. An example that has generated much controversy is the concept of mixed connective tissue disease in which there may be the presence of SLE, PM, DM, and systemic sclerosis in various combinations, in association with high titers of autoantibodies to the nRNP or U_1RNP antigen (3,4). There are, however, many known instances of overlap among and between these diseases unaccompanied by antibodies to U_1RNP. Conversely, these specific antibodies occur to a variable extent with each of these diseases when they occur alone. Reports that antibodies to the 70 kD polypeptide of the U_1RNP antigen are characteristic of mixed connective tissue disease have been confirmed, but these also occur in at least one-half of SLE patients with anti-U_1RNP precipitins who do not have overlap features (5).

RECOGNITION OF DIFFERENTIATED CONNECTIVE TISSUE DISEASES

A reasonable approach to clinical investigation in the systemic rheumatic diseases requires that criteria be established to classify patients for the purposes of clinical research (see Appendix I). Patients with undifferentiated connective tissue syndromes generally are not entered into such studies, because they do not satisfy criteria for a specific disease.

In the investigation of individual patients for clinical diagnosis, characteristic differentiated features are sought that comprise the disease picture for each of the systemic connective tissue diseases. While these are discussed in detail in other chapters, a brief review is presented so that the specific clinical and serologic features of these diseases can be contrasted with the nonspecific clinical and serologic findings that lead to the designation of undifferentiated connective tissue syndrome, a waystation for the numerous incomplete connective tissue syndromes that cannot be classified.

Systemic Lupus Erythematosus

In SLE, the "differentiated" features rarely seen in the other connective tissue diseases are glomerulonephritis, photosensitivity, characteristic skin rashes, central nervous system disease, and various cytopenias such as Coombs' positive hemolytic anemia, leukopenia, and thrombocytopenia. These are all very unusual in systemic sclerosis, RA, and PM/DM. Pleuropericarditis and peritonitis are most common in SLE, but they are seen to a variable extent in the other systemic rheumatic diseases. Serologically, antibodies to double-stranded DNA, Sm, and ribosomal P proteins are seen almost exclusively in SLE, while precipitating antibodies to U_1RNP, Ro(SS-A) and La(SS-B), which are present in aggregate in 85% of SLE patients, are present in other rheumatic diseases. Precipitating antibodies to Ro(SS-A) and La(SS-B) are seen more commonly in primary Sjögren's syndrome than in SLE. There are numerous combinations of these clinical findings in association with several defined autoantibodies that would definitively make the diagnosis of SLE.

Systemic Sclerosis

There is less heterogeneity in systemic sclerosis than in SLE, but the diagnosis depends strongly on the presence of thickened skin due to dermal collagen accumulation in a diffuse pattern, in which the thickening extends proximal to the wrists and also involves the trunk and face. Patients with diffuse skin involvement have an increased risk of sclerosis of the internal organs such as the heart, lungs, and bowel, as well as renal nephrosclerosis with malignant hypertension. Virtually all patients with systemic sclerosis have Raynaud's phenomenon, and a subset called limited cutaneous scleroderma exists, which has limited skin involvement restricted to the hands (sclerodactyly) and face, calcinosis, esophageal motility disturbances, and telangiectasia (CREST syndrome). Patients with limited skin disease may have various combinations of these findings (such as REST and RST), constituting limited forms of the syndrome.

There is also a family of antinuclear antibodies highly specific for systemic sclerosis, which include antibodies to various nucleolar antigens, Scl_{70} or topoisomerase I, and the centromere antigens. Antibodies to the centromere antigens correlate highly with the presence of the CREST or limited cutaneous variants. There is no serologic marker that occurs in the majority of patients with diffuse skin disease, although antibodies to topoisomerase I occur more frequently in diffuse disease than in limited skin disease or CREST (6).

Polymyositis/Dermatomyositis

In the differentiated forms of polymyositis and dermatomyositis, there is a family of disease specific autoantibodies, many of which are disease specific and are associated with clinical subsets (see Chapter 21, Inflammatory and Metabolic Myopathies). Patients with PM and interstitial lung disease produce antibodies to a set of translation-related proteins that include Jo-1, PL-7, and PL-12, which are histidyl, threonyl, and alanyl tRNA synthetases respectively, as well as the translation component KJ. Antibodies to signal recognition particle occur in patients with PM without interstitial lung disease, and antibodies to Mi2, a nuclear protein complex, occur specifically in patients with DM. These antibodies have not been reported in the other connective tissue diseases to any significant extent even when sensitive tests are employed in their detection (7).

THE DIAGNOSTIC PROBLEM

Patients who do not clearly express the clinical features of any disease or who have partial overlap of features of two or more diseases probably account for 15% to 25% of tertiary referrals in patients with suspected systemic rheumatic diseases. An example of this conundrum is illustrated by the patients who present with Raynaud's phenomenon and no other clinical findings, a common clinical problem for rheumatologists. The first issue is whether the Raynaud's phenomenon is an isolated phenomenon or is the harbinger of a systemic rheumatic disease. Should a thorough laboratory and physical exam fail to reveal evidence of a systemic rheumatic disease, a positive ANA indicates high risk (and absence of ANA indicates low risk) for the development of a systemic rheumatic disease. If the positive ANA is anti-centromere antibody, it is likely that systemic sclerosis will develop in those patients. Prospective studies are in

progress and, in the coming years, physicians will be able to tell patients with isolated Raynaud's phenomenon and anti-centromere antibody what their risk and time frame are for the development of systemic sclerosis. Similarly, patients with Raynaud's phenomenon and any of the disease-specific autoantibodies are likely to develop the differentiated connective tissue disease associated with that particular autoantibody. Another common conundrum is the patient with an inflammatory polyarthritis without bone erosions and with or without a positive ANA, but no rheumatoid factor and no disease-specific autoantibodies or other clinical findings that define the clinical syndrome.

Patients with any of the incompletely expressed rheumatic diseases accompanied by autoantibodies that are not diagnostic are best designated as having undifferentiated connective tissue syndrome. Such patients are not well served by making a definitive diagnosis before the clinical data indicate the nature of the disease, because in many instances the disease remits permanently, or the undifferentiated nature of the malady may be long lasting or evolve slowly, requiring only that symptomatic therapy be given as the prognosis and course are unknown.

As our knowledge expands, etiologies, and disease specific autoantibodies that antedate clinical disease with certain disease specificity may be discovered. This type of knowledge should reduce the numbers of patients diagnosed with undifferentiated connective tissue syndrome, but for the reasons cited, such a category serves as a constant reminder of our incomplete knowledge of the systemic rheumatic diseases. For the present, it is important to help the patient deal with uncertainty. Treatment can be directed at manifestations present, even without a firm diagnosis.

MORRIS REICHLIN, MD

1. LeRoy EC, Maricq HR, Kahaleh MB: Undifferentiated connective tissue syndromes. Arthritis Rheum 23:341-343, 1980
2. Christian CL: Connective tissue disease: overlap syndromes. In Cohen A, Bennett JC (eds): Rheumatology and Immunology, 2nd ed. New York, Grune & Stratton, 1986, pp 175-179
3. Sharp GC, Irwin WS, May CH, et al: Association of antibodies to ribonucleoprotein and Sm antigens with connective tissue disease, systemic lupus erythematosus, and other rheumatic diseases. N Engl J Med 295:1149-1154, 1976
4. Sharp GC, Irvin WS, Tan EM, et al: Mixed connective tissue disease—an apparently distinct rheumatic disease syndrome associated with a specific antibody to extractable nuclear antigen (ENA). Am J Med 52:148-159, 1972
5. Reichlin M, van Venrooij WJ: Autoantibodies to the URNP particles: relationship to clinical diagnosis and nephritis. Clin Exp Immunol 83:286-290, 1991
6. Reichlin M: Progressive Systemic Sclerosis in Systemic Autoimmunity. In Bigazzi PL, Reichlin M(eds): Systemic Autoimmunity. New York, Marcel Dekker, 1991, pp 275-287
7. Targoff IN: Polymyositis in Systemic Autoimmunity. In Bigazzi PL, Reichlin M (eds): Systemic Autoimmunity. New York, Marcel Dekker, 1991, pp 201-246

19

SYSTEMIC LUPUS ERYTHEMATOSUS
A. EPIDEMIOLOGY, PATHOLOGY, AND PATHOGENESIS

EPIDEMIOLOGY

Systemic lupus erythematosus (SLE) is a prototypic autoimmune disease characterized by the production of antibodies to components of the cell nucleus in association with a diverse array of clinical manifestations. SLE is primarily a disease of young women. Peak incidence occurs between the ages of 15 and 40 during the childbearing years, with a female-to-male ratio of approximately 5:1. However, the onset can range from infancy to advanced age; in both pediatric and older onset patients, the female-to-male ratio approximates 2:1. In a general outpatient population, SLE affects approximately 1 in 2000 individuals, although the prevalence varies with race, ethnicity, and socioeconomic status (1).

SLE shows a strong familial aggregation with a much higher frequency among first-degree relatives of patients. Moreover, in extended families SLE may coexist with other autoimmune conditions such as hemolytic anemia, thyroiditis, and idiopathic thrombocytopenia purpura. SLE occurs concordantly in approximately 25%–50% of monozygotic twins and 5% of dizygotic twins. Despite the influence of heredity, most cases appear sporadic.

IMMUNOPATHOLOGY

The pathologic findings of SLE occur throughout the body and are manifested by inflammation, blood vessel abnormalities that encompass both bland vasculopathy and vasculitis, and immune complex deposition. The best-characterized organ pathology is the kidney. By light, electron, and immunofluorescence microscopy, the kidney in SLE displays increases in mesangial cells and mesangial matrix, inflammation, cellular proliferation, basement membrane abnormalities, and immune complex deposition. These deposits are comprised of immunoglobulins M, G, and A (IgM, IgG, and IgA) as well as complement components. On electron microscopy, the deposits can be visualized in the mesangium as well as subendothelial and subepithelial sides of the glomerular basement membrane (Fig. 19A-1).

Pathologic findings in the kidney are classified according to two grading schemes, which together provide information for clinical staging. The World Health Organization (WHO) system is based on the extent and location of proliferative changes within glomeruli as well as alterations in the basement membrane. These patterns are not static, and transitions between categories can be observed. A second classification system is based on signs of activity and chronicity (2). This system is useful in predicting outcome, although it is based on nonspecific indicators (Table 19A-1). With either scheme, lupus nephritis exhibits marked variability, differing in severity and pattern among patients, as illustrated in Fig. 19A-2.

Skin lesions in SLE demonstrate inflammation and degeneration at the dermal–epidermal junction with the basal or germinal layer as the primary site of injury. In these lesions, granular deposits of IgG, as well as complement components, can be demonstrated in a band-like pattern by immunofluorescence microscopy. Necrotizing vasculitis involving small- and medium-sized vessels may also cause skin lesions.

Other organ systems affected by SLE usually display nonspecific inflammation or vessel abnormalities, although pathologic findings are sometimes minimal. For example, despite the varied and dramatic clinical manifestations of central nervous system involvement, typically the only findings are cortical microinfarcts and a bland vasculopathy with degenerative or proliferative changes; inflammation and necrosis indicative of vasculitis are only rarely found.

The heart may also show nonspecific foci of inflammation in the pericardium, myocardium, and endocardium, even in the absence of clinically significant manifestations. Verrucous endocarditis, known as Libman–Sacks endocarditis, is a classic pathologic finding of SLE and is manifested by vegetations, most frequently at the mitral valve. These vegetations consist of accumulations of immune complexes, inflammatory cells, fibrin, and necrotic debris.

Occlusive vasculopathy causes both venous and arterial thrombosis in SLE and is a common pathologic finding. Although coagulation can be a sequel of inflammation, autoantibodies to clotting system components may also directly trigger thrombotic events. The most notable of these are designated antiphospholipid antibodies. These antibodies are part of the spectrum of lupus anticoagulants and bind complexes of phospholipids in association with the serum protein β_2-glycoprotein 1 (3). Vessel abnormalities in SLE may also result from increases in endothelial cell adhe-

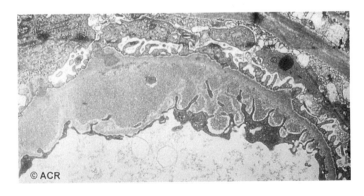

(Figure 19A-1)
Immune deposits in lupus nephritis. This electron micrograph illustrates large granular subendothelial immune deposits as well as smaller subepithelial and intramembranous deposits. Broadening and fusion of the foot processes are also present. Reprinted from the Revised Clinical Slide Collection on the Rheumatic Diseases, with permission of American College of Rheumatology.

Activity Index	Chronicity Index
Proliferative change	Sclerotic glomeruli
Necrosis/karyorrhexis	Fibrous crescents
Cellular crescents	Tubular atrophy
Leukocyte infiltration	Interstitial fibrosis
Hyaline thrombi	
Interstitial inflammation	

siveness by a mechanism analogous to the Schwartzman reaction (4).

Several other pathologic findings that are prominent in SLE have an uncertain relationship to inflammation. Patients with longstanding disease, including women without the usual risk factors for cardiovascular disease, frequently develop atherosclerosis. It is unclear whether these lesions result from steroid-induced metabolic abnormalities, hypertension, or vascular changes caused by a chronic burden of immune complexes. Similarly, osteonecrosis, as well as neurodegeneration in patients with chronic severe disease, may arise from vasculopathy, drug side effects, or persistent immunologic insults.

Immunopathogenesis of Antinuclear Antibodies

The central immunologic disturbance in SLE patients is autoantibody production. These antibodies are directed to a host of self molecules found in the nucleus and cytoplasm of cells, as well as on their surface. In addition, SLE sera contain antibodies to soluble molecules such as IgG and coagulation factors. Because of the wide range of its antigenic targets, SLE is classified as a disease of generalized autoimmunity.

Among autoantibodies expressed in patient sera, those directed against components of the cell nucleus (antinuclear antibodies or ANA) are the most characteristic of SLE and are found in more than 95% of patients (5). These antibodies bind DNA, RNA, nuclear proteins, and protein–nucleic acid complexes. Many of these autoantigenic molecules are highly conserved among mammalian species because of their key roles in cell metabolism (Table 19A-2).

Among ANA specificities in SLE, two appear unique to this disease. Antibodies to double-stranded (ds) DNA and an RNA–protein complex termed Sm are found essentially only in SLE patients and are included as serologic criteria in the classification of SLE (see Appendix I). Although both anti-DNA and anti-Sm are serologic markers, they differ significantly in their pattern of expression and clinical associations. These antibodies are produced independently by patients and, although anti-DNA levels frequently fluctuate over time and may even disappear, anti-Sm levels remain more constant.

The anti-Sm and anti-DNA responses also differ in the nature of their target antigens. The Sm antigen, which is designated an snRNP (small nuclear ribonucleoprotein), is composed of a unique set of uridine-rich RNA molecules (U1, U2, U4, U5, U6) bound to a common group of core proteins as well as unique proteins specifically associated with the RNA molecules. Whereas anti-DNA antibodies react to a conserved nucleic acid determinant widely present on DNA, anti-Sm antibodies specifically target snRNP core proteins (B, B′, D, and E) and not RNA.

Perhaps the most remarkable feature of the anti-DNA response is its association with immunopathologic events in SLE—in particular, glomerulonephritis. This role has been established by the correlation of serum levels of anti-DNA with periods of disease activity, the isolation of anti-DNA in enriched form from glomerular eluates of patients with active nephritis, and the induction of nephritis by administering anti-DNA antibodies to normal animals. The relationship between levels of anti-DNA and active renal disease is not invariable, however; some patients with active nephritis may lack serum anti-DNA, whereas others with high levels of anti-DNA are clinically discordant and escape nephritis (6).

The occurrence of nephritis without anti-DNA may be explained by the pathogenicity of other autoantibody specificities (eg, anti-Ro or anti-Sm). The converse situation of clinical quiescence despite serologic activity has suggested that only some anti-DNA provoke glomerulonephritis. Studies to delineate the basis of renal pathogenicity initially focused on the respective roles of antibodies to single-stranded (ss) DNA and dsDNA. Whereas anti-dsDNA antibodies are essentially exclusive to SLE, anti-ssDNA antibodies have wider expression among inflammatory and infectious diseases. Both specificities frequently coexist in SLE, however, because many anti-DNA antibodies bind a common antigenic determinant present on both ssDNA and dsDNA. Since renal eluates show antibody activity to both DNA forms, it appears likely that, although the diagnostically important anti-dsDNA are pathogenic, antibodies to ssDNA may also have a similar pathogenic role.

Studies correlating immunochemical properties of anti-DNA antibodies with nephritis suggest that several features, including isotype, ability to fix complement, and capacity to bind glomerular preparations, promote pathogenicity (7).

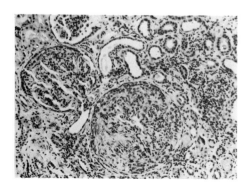 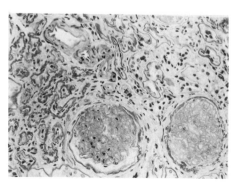

(Figure 19A-2)
Left: Signs of "active" lupus nephritis showing glomerular proliferation, crescents, abundant inflammatory cell infiltration, and interstitial cell infiltrates (hematoxylin-eosin). Right: Signs of "chronic" lupus nephritis showing glomerular sclerosis, vascular thickening, tubular atrophy, and interstitial fibrosis (periodic acid–Schiff).

(Table 19A-2)

Principle antinuclear antibodies in systemic lupus erythematosus (SLE)*

Specificity	Target Antigen	Function	Frequency in SLE (%)
Native DNA	dsDNA	Genetic information	40
Denatured DNA	ssDNA	Genetic information	70
Histones	H1, H2A, H2B, H3, H4	Nucleosome structure	70
Sm	snRNP proteins B, B', D, E	Splicesome component, RNA processing	30
U1RNP	snRNP proteins A, C, 70K	Splicesome component, RNA processing	32
SS-A/Ro	60 and 52 kD proteins, complexed with Y1-Y5 RNA	Unknown	35
SS-B/La	48 kD protein complexed with various small RNA	Regulation of RNA polymerase 3 transcription	15
Ku	86 and 66 kD proteins	DNA binding	3
PCNA/cyclin	36 kD protein	Auxillary protein of DNA polymerase d	10
Ribosomal RNP	38, 16, and 15 kD phosphoproteins, associated with ribosomes	Protein synthesis	10

* Modified from Tan (5), with permission.

Although assays to detect these properties have been developed, they are not used routinely for clinical monitoring. Indeed, most assays for anti-DNA are designed for their utility in diagnosis rather than for assessing disease activity. In contrast to their role in nephritis, anti-DNA antibodies have not been clearly associated with other clinical events.

Although many ANA have never been adequately evaluated for pathogenicity, there is nevertheless evidence that certain autoantibodies other than anti-DNA have a clinical impact. Associations of other autoantibodies with disease events include antibodies to ribosomal P proteins (anti-P) with neuropsychiatric disease and hepatitis; antibodies to Ro with neonatal lupus and subacute cutaneous lupus; antibodies to phospholipids with vascular thrombosis, thrombocytopenia, and recurrent abortion; and antibodies to blood cells with specific cytopenias.

The contribution of ANA to clinical events in SLE has been difficult to understand as the intracellular location of the target antigens should protect them from antibody interactions. The location of these antigens may not be fixed, however, and some may be translocated to the membrane and be accessible to antibody attack; damage to cells by ultraviolet radiation, for example, may lead to such movement. There is some evidence to suggest, however, that ANA may enter cells, bind nuclear antigens, and perturb cell function (8).

Of clinical events in SLE, nephritis has been most intensively studied mechanistically because of the impact of kidney disease on morbidity and mortality. Clinical observations strongly suggest that SLE renal disease results from the deposition of immune complexes containing anti-DNA, since active nephritis is marked by elevated anti-DNA levels with a corresponding depression of total hemolytic complement. Furthermore, since anti-DNA shows preferential renal deposition, these findings suggest that DNA–anti-DNA immune complexes are a major pathogenic species (9).

Although renal injury in SLE may result from immune complexes that contain anti-DNA, the constituents of circulating complexes have been difficult to characterize because of their low concentration in serum. The formation of immune complexes in situ, rather than within the circulation, could explain the paucity of DNA–anti-DNA complexes in serum. According to this mechanism, immune complexes would be assembled in the kidney on pieces of DNA adherent to the glomerular basement membrane. These DNA pieces may be attached to histones, which also bind strongly to glomerular sites.

Another mechanism by which anti-DNA antibodies may mediate nephritis is direct interaction with glomerular antigens. Many anti-DNA antibodies are polyspecific and interact with molecules other than DNA. Among its interactions, anti-DNA can bind heparan sulfate and laminin, two glomerular constituents. The binding of anti-DNA to these molecules could directly activate complement to incite local inflammatory damage; this binding could also anchor immune complexes to kidney sites, whether they are formed in the circulation or in situ.

The pathogenesis of other SLE manifestations is less well understood, although immune complex deposition at relevant tissue sites has generally been considered a likely mechanism. Indeed, the frequent association of depressed complement levels and signs of vasculitis with active SLE suggests that immune complexes are important agents for initiating or exacerbating organ damage. These considerations do not exclude the possibility that tissue injury results from either cell-mediated cytotoxicity or direct antibody attack on target tissues.

Determinants of Disease Susceptibility

Studies on patients suggest that SLE is caused by genetically determined immune abnormalities that can be triggered by both exogenous and endogenous factors. While the predisposition to disease is hereditary, it is likely to be multigenic in origin and involve different sets of genes in different individuals. Analysis of genetic susceptibility has been based primarily on the search for gene polymorphisms occurring with greater frequency in patients than in control populations. Most of the markers tested have involved genes for known immune response phenomena.

Of these genetic elements, the major histocompatibility complex (MHC) has been most intensively scrutinized for its contribution to human SLE. Using a variety of MHC gene markers, population-based studies indicate that the susceptibility to SLE, like many other autoimmune diseases in humans, involves class II gene polymorphisms. An association of HLA DR2 and DR3 (and recently defined subspecificities) with SLE has been commonly observed, with these alleles producing a relative risk of disease of approximately 2 to 5.

This analysis of MHC gene associations is complicated, however, by the existence of extended HLA haplotypes in which class II genes are in linkage disequilibrium with other potential susceptibility genes. Since the MHC is rich in genes for immune system elements, the association of disease with a class II marker does not denote a specific functional abnormality promoting pathogenesis. Indeed, a contribution of class II genes to susceptibility to SLE has been difficult to conceptualize because these genes regulate responses in an antigen-specific manner, whereas SLE is characterized by responses to a host of self antigens of unrelated sequence and structure.

In contrast to their uncertain role in disease susceptibility, class II genes appear to exert a more decisive influence on the production of particular ANA. The response to several SLE autoantigens has been associated with particular class II alleles, as well as short amino acid sequences found in different class II specificities. These sequences, which are denoted shared epitopes, may influence antigen-specific responses by virtue of their location at contact points of class II molecules with processed peptides (10).

Among other MHC gene systems, inherited complement deficiencies also influence disease susceptibility. Like class I and II molecules, complement components, in particular C4a and C4b, show striking genetic polymorphism, with a deficiency of C4a molecules (null alleles) a common occurrence in the population. As many as 80% of SLE patients have null alleles irrespective of ethnic background, with homozygous C4a deficiency conferring a high risk for SLE. Since C4a null alleles are part of an extended HLA haplotype with the markers HLA-B8 and DR3, the influence of these class I and class II alleles of disease susceptibility may reflect linkage disequilibrium with complement deficiency. SLE is also associated with inherited deficiency of C1q, C1r/s, and C2 (11).

An association of SLE with inherited complement deficiency may seem surprising because of the prominence of immune complex deposition and complement consumption in this disease. However, a decrease in complement activity could promote disease susceptibility by impairing the neutralization and clearance of foreign antigen. With a burden of persistent antigen, the immune system would be excessively stimulated, allowing the emergence of autoreactivity. Since C4a and C4b differ in their interaction with antigens based on chemical composition, absence of either molecule would create only a selective deficiency state without jeopardizing overall host defenses.

Immunoglobulin (Ig) and T-cell receptor (TCR) gene systems have also been investigated as possible susceptibility factors in SLE, although given the enormous diversity inherent in the Ig and TCR systems, it would seem unlikely that structural gene polymorphisms could promote autoimmunity. Nevertheless, an association of SLE with a polymorphism in the genes for the T-cell α receptor chain has been demonstrated in population studies. Furthermore, the production of certain autoantibodies, including anti-Ro, appears linked to the β chain locus of the T-cell receptor (12). These observations suggest that the array of TCR expressed by an individual may be genetically constrained and could affect the generation of T cells that recognize self. The contribution of Ig genes to an SLE diathesis is less clear, although studies of heavy-chain allotypes suggest that patients may preferentially express certain Gm markers.

Genetics of Murine SLE

Several strains of inbred mice with inherited lupus-like disease have been described and studied as models to elucidate the human disease. These mice all display features that mimic human SLE such as ANA production, immune complex glomerulonephritis, lymphadenopathy, and abnormal B- and T-cell function. These strains differ in the expression of certain serologic and clinical findings (eg, anti-Sm, hemolytic anemia, and arthritis), as well as the occurrence of disease among males and females. Among various lupus strains described (NZB, NZB/NZW, MRL-lpr/lpr, BXSB, and C3H-gld/gld), the development of a full-blown lupus syndrome requires multiple unlinked genes (13).

In mice, single mutant genes (lpr, gld, and Yaa) can promote anti-DNA production as well as alter the number and functional properties of both B and T cells. In lpr and gld mice, these abnormalities result from mutations in proteins involved in apoptosis. This process, also known as programmed cell death, plays a critical role in the development of the immune system, as well as the establishment and maintenance of tolerance. The lpr mutation leads to the absence of Fas, a cell-surface molecule that triggers apoptosis in lymphocytes, while gld affects a molecule termed the Fas ligand that interacts with Fas. These gene defects appear to operate in peripheral, in contrast to central, tolerance and allow the persistence of autoreactive cells (14).

In contrast to human SLE, the lupus strains lack a common MHC class I or II marker that can be identified as a susceptibility factor. MHC molecules may nevertheless contribute to pathogenesis as shown by formal genetic analysis of disease in New Zealand mice (NZB, NZB/NZW) as well as the pattern of disease expression in congenic NZB mice with mutations in their class II genes. Such mice have dramatically enhanced anti-DNA production as well as nephritis, suggesting that self antigen presentation may be influenced by the structure of the class II molecules (15). Among lupus mice, New Zealand strains have an MHC-linked deficiency in the expression of the proinflammatory cytokine tumor necrosis factor α (TNF-α). This deficiency state, which has a counterpart in humans, may be pathogenic because administration of TNF-α to mice with low endogenous production ameliorates disease (16).

Immune Cell Disturbances

Autoantibody production in SLE occurs in the setting of generalized immune cell abnormalities that involve the B cell, T cell, and monocyte lineages. Together, these immune cell disturbances appear to promote B-cell hyperactivity, leading to hyperglobulinemia, increased numbers of antibody-producing cells, and heightened responses to many antigens, both self and foreign. Generalized or polyclonal B-cell activation appears sufficient to induce certain autoantibodies since the magnitude of these responses is proportional to the degree of hyperglobulinemia. The induction of anti-DNA by polyclonal activation also occurs in normal mice treated with the B-cell mitogen lipopolysaccharide and reflects the presence in the normal B-cell repertoire of a large precursor population for so-called natural autoantibodies. These IgM antibodies bind polyspecifically to both foreign and self antigens and are generally considered to be non-pathogenic.

Although nonspecific immune activation can provoke certain ANA responses, it does not appear to be the major mechanism for inducing pathogenic autoantibodies, especially anti-DNA. Levels of these antibodies far exceed the extent of hyperglobulinemia. In addition, anti-DNA antibodies have features indicative of in vivo antigen selection by a receptor-driven mechanism—most significantly, variable region somatic mutations of the replacement type. These mutations can produce sequence changes in the complementarity determining regions of an antibody that increase DNA binding activity and specificity for dsDNA (17).

The ability of DNA to drive autoantibody production in SLE contrasts with the poor immunogenicity of mammalian DNA when administered to normal animals. This discrepancy suggests that SLE patients either have a unique capacity to respond to DNA or are exposed to DNA in a form that is much more immunogenic than the preparations used for experimental immunization. This DNA may be in the form of nucleosomes, which have enhanced immunologic activity and appear to stimulate at least some ANA during the course of disease (18). Alternatively, bacterial or viral DNA may stimulate this response because they contain base sequences that are absent from the host and are therefore immunogenic (19).

The specificity of ANA directed to nuclear proteins supports the hypothesis that these responses are antigen-driven, as these antibodies bind multiple independent determinants found in different regions of these proteins. In this respect, ANA responses resemble those arising during experimental immunization. Spontaneous ANA responses may differ from responses induced in normal animals, however, in their specificity for antigenic determinants of functional significance (eg, catalytic sites of enzymes) as well as their ability to bind to very short linear peptides.

The pattern of ANA binding minimizes the possibility that molecular mimicry is the exclusive etiology for autoimmunity in SLE. According to this mechanism, autoantibody production might be stimulated by a foreign antigen bearing an amino acid sequence or antigenic structure resembling a self molecule. This type of cross-reactivity has been hypothesized for many different autoimmune diseases and has been suggested for SLE because of the sequence similarity between certain nuclear antigens and viral and bacterial proteins (eg, Ro protein and the nucleocapsid protein of vesicular stomatitis virus).

If SLE autoantibodies resulted from molecular mimicry, however, they would be expected to bind self antigen only at sites of homology with foreign antigen rather than the entire molecule, as has been observed. These arguments suggest that self antigen, rather than a mimic, sustains autoantibody production, but they do not eliminate the possibility that a cross-reactive response to a foreign antigen initiates an ANA response. Thus, the foreign antigen may induce a population of B cells that bind both foreign and self antigen. These B cells could process self antigen and present determinants that are not subject to tolerance and therefore are able to stimulate autoreactive T-cell responses (20).

Studies analyzing the genetics of SLE and the pattern of ANA production both strongly suggest that T cells are critical to disease pathogenesis. In the murine models of lupus, the depletion of helper T cells by monoclonal antibody treatment abrogates autoantibody production and clinical disease manifestations. The nature of the T cells helping ANA responses, the mechanisms by which they escape tolerance, and the process of self-antigen presentation have not yet been elucidated, however. Indeed, it is unclear whether self antigen is presented from endogenous sources or whether it is first released from damaged or dying cells and then processed and presented by conventional antigen-presenting cells.

The basis of T-cell help in autoantibody responses may differ from conventional responses because of the physical chemical nature of the antigens. Most SLE antigens exist as complexes or particles, such as nucleosomes, containing multiple protein and nucleic acid species. Because these antigens may effectively trigger B-cell activation by multivalent binding, T-cell help for autoimmune responses could be delivered by nonspecifically activated T cells. Alternatively, T-cell reactivity to these antigens could be elicited to only one protein on a complex, allowing a single helper T cell to collaborate with B cells for multiple protein and nucleic acid determinants.

Triggering Events

Although inheritance and the hormonal milieu may create a predisposition toward SLE, the initiation of disease and its temporal variation in intensity likely result from environmental and other exogenous factors. Among these potential influences are infectious agents, which could both induce specific responses by molecular mimicry and perturb overall immunoregulation; stress, which can provoke neuroendocrine changes affecting immune cell function; diet, which can affect production of inflammatory mediators; toxins including drugs, which could modify cellular responsiveness and the immunogenicity of self antigens; and physical agents such as sunlight, which can cause inflammation and tissue damage. The impingement of these factors on the predisposed individual is likely to be highly variable and could be a further explanation for disease heterogeneity, as well as its alternating periods of flare and remission.

DAVID S. PISETSKY, MD, PhD

1. Ward MM, Pyun E, Studenski S: Long-term survival in systemic lupus erythematosus. Patient characteristics associated with poorer outcomes. Arthritis Rheum 38:274-283, 1995

2. Austin III HA, Boumpas DT, Vaughan EM, Balow JE: Predicting renal outcomes in severe lupus nephritis: contributions of clinical and histologic data. Kidney Int 45:544-550, 1994

3. Boumpas DT, Fessler BJ, Austin III HA, Balow JE, Klippel JH, Lockshin MD: Systemic lupus erythematosus: emerging concepts. Part 2: Dermatologic and joint disease, the antiphospholipid antibody syndrome, pregnancy and hormonal therapy, morbidity and mortality, and pathogenesis. Ann Intern Med 123:42-53, 1995

4. Belmont HM, Buyon J, Giorno R, Abramson S: Up-regulation of endothelial cell adhesion molecules characterizes disease activity in systemic lupus erythematosus. The Schwartzman phenomenon revisited. Arthritis Rheum 37:376-383, 1994

5. Tan EM: Antinuclear antibodies: diagnostic markers for autoimmune diseases and probes for cell biology. Adv Immunol 44:93-151, 1989

6. Pisetsky DS: Anti-DNA antibodies in systemic lupus erythematosus. Rheum Dis Clin NA 18:437-454, 1992

7. Bernstein KA, Kahl LE, Balow JE, Lefkowith JB: Serologic markers of lupus nephritis in patients: use of a tissue-based ELISA and evidence for immunopathogenic heterogeneity. Clin Exp Immunol 98:60-65, 1994

8. Vlahakos D, Foster MH, Ucci AA, Barrett KJ, Datta SK, Madaio MP: Murine monoclonal anti-DNA antibodies penetrate cells, bind to nuclei, and induce glomerular proliferation and proteinuria in vivo. J Amer Soc Nephrol 2:1345-1354, 1992

9. Foster MH, Cizman B, Madaio MP: Biology of Disease. Nephritogenic autoantibodies in systemic lupus erythematosus: immunochemical properties, mechanisms of immune deposition, and genetic origins. Lab Invest 69:494-507, 1993

10. Reveille JD, Macleod MJ, Whittington K, Arnett FC: Specific amino acid residues in the second hypervariable region of HLA-DQA1 and DQB1 chain genes promote the Ro (SS-A)/LA (SS-B) autoantibody responses. J Immunol 146:3871-3876, 1991

11. Atkinson JP: Complement activation and complement receptors in systemic lupus erythematosus. Springer Semin Immunopathol 9:179-194, 1986

12. Scofield RH, Frank MB, Neas BR, Horowitz RM, Hardgrave KL, Fujisaku A, McArthur R, Harley JB: Cooperative association of T cell β receptor and HLA-DQ alleles in the production of anti-Ro in systemic lupus erythematosus. Clin Immunol Immunopath 72:335-341, 1994

13. Theofilopoulos, AN, Kofler, R, Singer PA, Dixon FJ: Molecular genetics of murine lupus model. Adv Immunol 46:61-109, 1989

14. Nagata S, Suda T: Fas and Fas ligand: lpr and gld mutations. Immunol Today 16:39-43, 1995

15. Chiang G-L, Bearer E, Ansari A, Dorshkind K, Gershwin ME: The bm12 mutation and autoantibodies to dsDNA in NZB. H-2bm12 mice. J Immunol 145:94-101, 1990

16. Jacob CO: Tumor necrosis factor and interferon gamma: relevance for immune regulation and genetic predisposition to autoimmune disease. Sem Immunol 4:147-154, 1992

17. Radic MZ, Weigert M: Genetic and structural evidence for antigen selection of anti-DNA antibodies. Annu Rev Immunol 12:487-520, 1994

18. Mohan C, Adams S, Stanik V, Datta, SK: Nucleosome: a major immunogen for pathogenic autoantibody-inducing T cells of lupus. J Exp Med 177:1367-1381, 1993

19. Gilkeson GS, Pippen AMM, Pisetsky DS: Induction of cross-reactive anti-dsDNA antibodies in preautoimmune NZB/NZW mice by immunization with bacterial DNA. J Clin Invest 95:1398-1402, 1995

20. Mamula MJ, Fatenejad S, Craft J: B cells process and present lupus autoantigens that initiate autoimmune T-cell responses. J Immunol 152:1453-1461, 1994

B. CLINICAL AND LABORATORY FEATURES

The frequencies of various clinical manifestations at presentation or at any time during the course of systemic lupus erythematosus (SLE) are shown in Table 19B-1. Malaise, overwhelming fatigue, fever, and weight loss are nonspecific manifestations that affect most patients at some time during the course of the disease. Despite their frequency, these features alone are not helpful in diagnosing SLE or identifying a flare, bacause they may just as likely indicate the development of infection or fibromyalgia.

SKIN MANIFESTATIONS

The most recognized skin manifestation of SLE is the butterfly rash (Fig. 19B-1), which usually presents as an erythematous, elevated, pruritic, and painful lesion in a malar distribution. Histologically the lesions may show only nonspecific inflammation, although immune deposits at the dermal–epidermal junction may be seen by immunoflourescence. Other acute lesions include generalized erythema, which may or may not be photosensitive, and bullous lesions (1). The majority of patients are photosensitive, with skin and other systemic manifestations exacerbated by sun exposure.

Subacute cutaneous lupus erythematosus (SCLE) is a relatively distinct cutaneous lesion that is nonfixed, nonscarrieing, and exacerbating and remitting (1). Lesions commonly occur in sun-exposed areas either as the papulosquamous variant, which mimics psoriasis or lichen planus, or as polycyclic or annular lesions, which may mimic erythema annulare centrifugum (Fig. 19B-2). Patients with SCLE commonly have antibody to Ro (SS-A), which also has been demonstrated in the lesion.

Discoid lesions may occur in the absence of any systemic manifestations (called discoid lupus) or may be a manifestation of SLE. The lesions often begin as erythematous papules or plaques, with thick, adherent scaling and a hypopigmented central area. Scarring with central atrophy is common (Fig. 19B-3).

Alopecia may be diffuse or patchy. If associated with disease flares, hair tends to regrow once the disease is under control. If it results from the extensive scarring of discoid lesions, hair loss may be permanent.

Mucous membrane lesions include mouth ulcers, vaginal ulcers, and nasal septal erosions. Panniculitis, urticarial lesions, and vasculitis may also be seen. Vasculitic lesions manifest as palpable purpura, nail-fold or digital ulcerations, splinter hemorrhages; lesions of the digital pulp and palm simulate Osler's nodes and Janeway spots.

(Table 19B-1)
Frequency of systemic lupus erythematosus manifestations*

Manifestations	Onset (376)*	Anytime (750)*
Constitutional	53%	77%
Arthritis	44%	63%
Arthralgia	77%	85%
Skin	53%	78%
Mucous membranes	21%	52%
Pleurisy	16%	30%
Lung	7%	14%
Pericarditis	13%	23%
Myocarditis	1%	3%
Raynaud's	33%	60%
Thrombophlebitis	2%	6%
Vasculitis	23%	56%
Renal	38%	74%
Nephrotic syndrome	5%	11%
Azotemia	3%	8%
Central nervous system	24%	54%
Cytoid bodies	2%	3%
Gastrointestinal	18%	45%
Pancreatitis	1%	2%
Lymphadenopathy	16%	32%
Myositis	3%	3%

*University of Toronto data. Frequency at onset based on 376 patients diagnosed at Lupus Clinic, and frequency at anytime during the course of the disease for 750 patients registered prior to July, 1995.

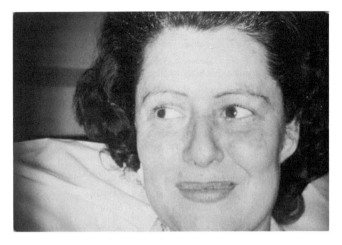

(Figure 19B-1)
Malar rash in a patient with systemic lupus erythematosus.

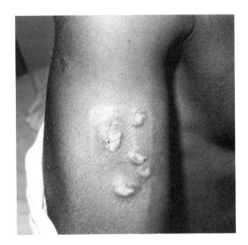

(Figure 19B-3)
Discoid lupus lesions.

MUSCULOSKELETAL MANIFESTATIONS

Arthralgias and arthritis are the most common presenting manifestations of SLE. Acute arthritis may involve any joint, but typically the small joints of the hands, wrists, and knees are symmetrically involved. It may be migratory or persistent and chronic (2). Soft-tissue swelling is common, but effusions tend to be minimal. There may occasionally be subcutaneous nodules similar to those seen in rheumatoid arthritis (RA). Synovial analysis reveals a mildly inflammatory fluid with a positive antinuclear antibody test and diminished complement levels. Unlike that seen in RA, the arthritis of SLE typically is not erosive or destructive of bone or cartilage. However, deforming arthritis may occur with ulnar deviation of the fingers, subluxations, and contractures (Fig. 19B-4). Initially, subluxations in the small joints of the hands are reversible, but can become fixed. This pattern of nonerosive but deforming disease is called *Jaccoud's arthritis*. Radiographic findings in such patients reveal no erosions even when subluxations are present.

Patients with SLE may complain of muscle pain and weakness. True muscle inflammation may be seen; however, the histologic features of myositis in SLE is not as striking as those found in idiopathic polymyositis/dermatomyositis. Patients with SLE may develop a drug-related myopathy secondary to corticosteroid use or as a complication of anti-

malarial therapy. Fibromyalgia is often seen in people with SLE and must be considered in patients presenting with musculoskeletal complaints.

RENAL MANIFESTATIONS

Patients seldom report specific symptoms related to the kidney until there is advanced nephrotic syndrome or renal failure. Clinical renal disease is marked by any or all of the following: the presence of proteinuria (more than 500 mg/24 hours, or more than 3+ on a dipstick if quantitation is not done); the presence of casts (including red blood cells, hemoglobin, granular, tubular, or mixed); the presence of hematuria (more than 5 red blood cells per high power field) or pyuria (more than 5 white blood cells/high power field) in the absence of infection; and an elevated serum creatinine.

Most SLE patients manifest some abnormality on renal biopsy, although in some cases it is only possible to document it with special techniques such as immunofluorescence or electron microscopy (3–5). In a study of clinical and morphologic features in 148 patients with SLE, only three patients with truly normal biopsies were found (3) (Table 19B-2). Specific morphologic features seen on kidney biopsies have prognostic implications (6). The presence of chronic le-

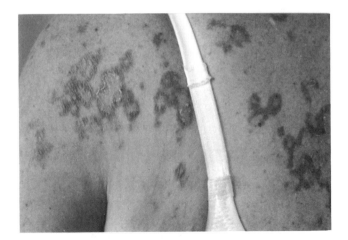

(Figure 19B-2)
Subacute cutaneous lupus lesions.

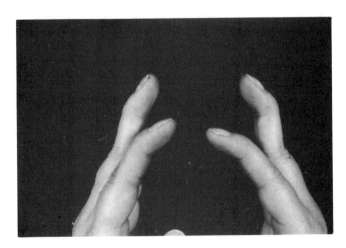

(Figure 19B-4)
Correctable swan neck deformities of Jaccoud's arthropathy in a patient with systemic lupus erythematosus.

(Table 19B-2)

World Health Organization classification of lupus nephritis in 148 biopsies

Classification	Number
I. Normal glomeruli	12
a) Nil (by all techniques)	3
b) Normal by light but deposits on electron microscopy or immunofluorescence	9
II. Pure mesangial alterations (mesangiopathy)	62
a) Mesangial widening and/or mild hypercellularity	51
b) Moderate hypercellularity	11
III. A. Focal segmental glomerulonephritis	19
a) "Active" necrotizing lesions	14
b) "Active" and sclerosing lesions	5
III. B. Focal proliferative glomerulonephritis	3
a) "Active" necrotizing lesions	1
b) "Active" and sclerosing lesions	2
IV. Diffuse glomerulonephritis	37
a) Without segmental lesions	9
b) With "active" necrotizing lesions	13
c) With "active" and sclerosing lesions	14
d) With sclerosing lesions	1
V. Diffuse membranous glomerulonephropathy	11
a) Pure membranous glomerulonephropathy	2
b) Associated with lesions of category II	7
c) Associated with lesions of category III	0
d) Associated with lesions of category IV	2
VI. Advanced sclerosing glomerulonephritis	4

sions is associated with reduced survival, both for the patient and for the kidney.

NEUROPSYCHIATRIC MANIFESTATIONS

Neuropschiatric manifestations are common in SLE, and may present in the context of active SLE or as an isolated event (4,7). There is a wide spectrum of clinical manifestations (Table 19B-3) that may be grouped into neurologic (including the central nervous system [CNS], cranial, and peripheral nerves) and psychiatric (including psychosis and severe depression). Many patients present with mixed neurologic and psychiatric manifestations, making classification difficult.

(Table 19B-3)

Neuropsychiatric manifestations*

Manifestation	At Presentation (376)	Anytime (750)
Headache	12%	36%
Seizures	4%	10%
Cerebral vascular accidents	2%	4%
Cranial neuropathy	2%	4%
Peripheral neuropathy	2%	14%
Organic brain syndrome	7%	15%
Psychosis	2%	5%

* University of Toronto data. Frequency at onset based on 376 patients diagnosed at Lupus Clinic, and frequency at anytime during the course of the disease for 750 patients registered prior to December, 1995.

Intractable headaches, often unresponsive to narcotic analgesics, are common features both at presentation and at follow-up. The headaches may be migrainous and may accompany other neuropsychiatric features. Seizures may be either focal or generalized. Chorea, resembling Sydenham's chorea, may occur early in the disease, particularly in patients with anticardiolipin antibody. Cerebrovascular accidents, including paresis or subarachnoid hemorrhage, have also been related to anticardiolipin antibody syndrome. Visual defects, blindness, papilledema, nystagmus or ptosis, tinnitus and vertigo, or facial palsy may be presenting symptoms of cranial neuropathies.

Peripheral neuropathy may be motor, sensory (stocking glove distribution), or mixed motor and sensory polyneuropathy or mononeuritis multiplex. An acute ascending motor paralysis indistinguishable from Guillain-Barré has been reported. Rare instances of transverse myelitis, presenting with lower extremity paralysis, sensory deficits, and loss of sphincter control have been reported.

Organic brain syndrome in SLE is defined as a state of disturbed mental function with delirium, emotional inadequacy, and impaired memory or concentration in the absence of a drug, infectious, or metabolic cause. Systematic studies of neurocognitive function in SLE found that more than 80% of patients with either active or inactive neuropsychiatric involvement, and 42% of patients who had never had neuropsychiatric manifestations, demonstrated significant cognitive impairment. This compares with 17% of patients with RA and 14% of controls (8).

The diagnosis of neuropsychiatric lupus is primarily clinical. Exclusion of other possible etiologies such as sepsis, uremia, and severe hypertension is mandatory. Evidence of disease activity in other organs is helpful but not always present. Nonspecific cerebrospinal fluid (CSF) abnormalities such as elevated white blood cell count, elevated protein, or reduced glucose may be present in one-third of the patients (9). Electroencephalogram (EEG) abnormalities are common, but are nonspecific; evoked potentials have been proposed as a sensitive measure of CNS involvement in SLE. Radionuclide scans have not been uniformly helpful. Positron emission tomography (PET) showing areas of low attenuation that may represent areas of disturbed cerebral circulation and metabolism appear promising (10). Computed tomography (CT) findings such as evidence of cerebral infarction and hemorrhage may reflect specific pathologic processes. Cortical atrophy may be found in SLE, but does not necessarily reflect CNS disease. Magnetic resonance imaging (MRI) is particularly useful in patients with diffuse presentations. The small focal areas of increased signal intensity in both the cerebral white matter and the cortical gray matter tend to disappear after therapy with corticosteroids. These lesions may therefore represent areas of local edema, or inflammatory infiltrates, that resolve with treatment. A more advanced technique, ^{31}P nuclear magnetic resonance spectroscopy, may provide better demonstration of brain lesions in neuropsychiatric lupus (11).

SEROUS MEMBRANE MANIFESTATIONS (SEROSITIS)

Serositis in SLE is common and may present as pleurisy, pericarditis, or peritonitis. Pleural rubs are less common than either clinical pleurisy or radiographic abnormalities. Pleural effusions are frequently bilateral and usually small, but occasionally can be massive. Pleural effusions are seen more often in older patients and in drug-induced lupus. When fluid is available for examination, it is usually an exudate with a normal glucose level. When pleural effusions are significant, other causes of effusion (such as infection) must be ruled out by thoracentesis before therapy is begun.

Pericarditis is the most common presentation of heart involvement in SLE, but is less frequent than pleurisy as a feature of serositis. Clinical pericarditis has an incidence of 20%–30% in most large series, but may be found in more than 60% of SLE patients at autopsy. The clinical diagnosis is frequently difficult and depends on a constellation of clinical findings including typical percordial chest pain and a pericardial rub. However, pericarditis may also be painless and clinically silent. Constrictive pericarditis can occasionally develop in patients with pericardial involvement, although this is rare.

GASTROINTESTINAL MANIFESTATIONS

Gastrointestinal problems are common and symptoms include abdominal pain, anorexia, nausea, and occasionally vomiting. Etiologies for such symptoms include diffuse peritonitis, bowel vasculitis, pancreatitis, and inflammatory bowel disease. In the majority of patients, peritoneal inflammation causes the symptoms. When ascites presents in conjunction with abdominal pain and active lupus elsewhere, it generally follows the course of and responds to treatment for the other features of SLE. However, in a small number of patients, ascites may become chronic. When infection or malignancy is suspected, aspiration of ascitic fluid may be necessary.

Patients with mesenteric vasculitis generally present with insidious lower abdominal pain that may come and go over a period of weeks or months. Arteriography may reveal the presence of vasculitis. Rectal bleeding can occur, and colonoscopy may reveal both small bowel and colonic ulcerations. Intestinal perforations from mesenteric vasculitis have been described. If mesenteric vasculitis is suspected, perforation must be avoided through intensive investigation and treatment. However, if perforation is suspected or does occur, surgical intervention is necessary.

Hepatomegaly occurs commonly in SLE, but overt clinical liver disease is uncommon. Liver enzyme elevations have been associated with active SLE and nonsteroidal anti-inflammatory drug (NSAID) use, especially salicylates. Liver enzyme levels return to normal when the SLE is under control and the NSAIDs are stopped. Symptoms typical of acute pancreatitis are abdominal pain, nausea, vomiting, and an elevated serum amylase. Elevated serum amylase levels have also been detected in patients without clinical signs of pancreatitis.

PULMONARY MANIFESTATIONS

Pulmonary involvement in SLE may consist of pneumonitis, pulmonary hemorrhage, pulmonary embolism, pulmonary hypertension, and shrinking lung syndrome. Lupus pneumonitis may present as either an acute or a chronic illness. The acute illness simulates pneumonia and may present with classic symptoms of fever, dyspnea, cough, and occasionally hemoptysis. Acute pneumonitis must be differentiated from infection. Invasive investigation including bronchoalveolar lavage is indicated when doubt persists. The chronic form of lupus pneumonitis presents as a diffuse interstitial lung disease and is characterized by dyspnea on exertion, nonproductive cough, and basilar rales.

Pulmonary hemorrhage presenting with cough and hemoptysis or as a pulmonary infiltrate is an uncommon but very serious feature of SLE. It is presumed to be due to pulmonary vasculitis. Other causes of hemorrhagic pneumonia, particularly viral pneumonia, must be considered in the differential diagnosis.

Lupus pulmonary involvement may also give rise to a syndrome of pulmonary hypertension similar to idiopathic pulmonary hypertension (12). Patients present with dyspnea, a normal chest radiograph, and a restrictive pattern on pulmonary function testing. Raynaud's phenomenon is frequently present. Doppler studies and cardiac catheterization confirm pulmonary hypertension. Secondary causes of pulmonary hypertension must be ruled out. Searching for multiple pulmonary emboli and sites of deep venous thrombosis is particularly important. When there is any doubt, pulmonary angiography should be performed. One must also rule out the antiphospholipid antibody syndrome with intrapulmonary clotting.

CARDIAC MANIFESTATIONS

Cardiac involvement in SLE may consist of pericarditis, myocarditis, endocarditis, or coronary artery disease. Myocarditis may be suspected in patients who present with arrhythmias or conduction defects, unexplained cardiomegaly with or without congestive heart failure, or an unexplained tachycardia. Most patients have associated pericarditis. Congestive heart failure is a less common feature and is usually secondary to a combination of factors that may include myocarditis. However, associated hypertension and the use of corticosteroid medication are usually more important contributing factors. Myocardial involvement may be subtle; noninvasive investigations may reveal reversible defects suggesting ischemia and persistent defects suggesting scarring (13). If myocarditis is suspected, endomyocardial biopsy may help confirm the diagnosis. The true incidence of endocarditis is very difficult to discern in SLE because the majority of murmurs heard clinically are not associated with any organic valvular disease. Endocarditis diagnosed on the basis of a murmur plus abnormal echocardiographic studies is infrequent. The nonbacterial verrucous vegetations described by Libman and Sacks are much less common than they were in the presteroid era. Vegetations may vary from mere valvular thickening detected by two-dimensional echocardiography to very large lesions causing significant valvular dysfunction. Valve replacement has been required on occasion. Acute and subacute bacterial endocarditis may occur on previously damaged valves. For this reason, prophylactic antibiotics for surgical and dental procedures is advisable in patients with lupus endocarditis.

Coronary vasculitis is not common in SLE. When it occurs, it is usually associated with other features of active disease. Conversely, atherosclerotic coronary artery disease is usually associated with inactive lupus.

RETICULOENDOTHELIAL SYSTEM MANIFESTATIONS

Splenomegaly is a common finding in patients with SLE. In addition, splenic atrophy, presumably secondary to infarction, and splenic lymphoma have also been recognized.

Lymphadenopathy may occur in single or multiple sites. The nodes are usually soft, nontender, and variable in size. In some patients, there may be fluctuation of the lymphadenopathy with disease exacerbations. The lymph nodes demonstrate reactive hyperplasia on pathologic examination.

LABORATORY FEATURES
Hematologic Abnormalities

Cytopenias including anemia, leukopenia, lymphopenia, and thrombocytopenia are frequent manifestations of SLE. Anemia may have many different etiologies, including those secondary to chronic inflammatory disease, renal insufficiency, blood loss, or drug use. Acute autoimmune hemolytic anemia resulting from autoantibodies directed against red blood cell antigens is frequently associated with a positive Coombs' test, but occasionally Coombs' will be negative. Conversely, one may find a positive Coombs' test in the absence of any evidence of hemolysis.

Leukopenia with white blood cell counts ranging between $2500/mm^3$ and $4000/mm^3$ are often associated with active disease. Other causes for leukopenia such as drug use and infection must be considered. The white blood cell count rarely falls below $1500/mm^3$ in active SLE unless there is an additional cause. Lymphocytopenia is usually associated with antibodies to lymphocytes and often correlates with disease activity.

Thrombocytopenia, as with anemia, requires that other etiologies such as infection or drug use be ruled out before ascribing the finding to SLE. Although anti-platelet antibodies are a frequent finding, they are not always associated with thrombocytopenia. There are two distinct subsets of patients with lupus thrombocytopenia (14). In one subset, the thrombocytopenia follows the course of acute SLE and responds to treatment. The second subset of patients usually presents with a platelet count of around $50,000/mm^3$ and has no serious bleeding or active lupus elsewhere in the body.

A variety of clotting abnormalities have been reported in SLE. The most common is the lupus anticoagulant with a prolonged partial thromboplastin time (which is not corrected by mixing patient plasma with normal plasma), anticardiolipin antibody, and a false-positive VDRL test for syphilis. The false-positive VDRL test may precede onset of the other symptoms of SLE by many years. Anticardiolipin antibodies have been associated with specific manifestations such as thromboembolic phenomena and recurrent fetal loss (see Chapter 27).

The erythrocyte sedimentation rate (ESR) is frequently elevated in active SLE, but it does not mirror lupus activity and may remain elevated in patients with prolonged clinical remissions. A positive C-reactive protein (CRP), at one time purported to measure infection in lupus, has not proved a reliable indicator of a superimposed infection.

Serologic Abnormalities

Complement levels measured as either total hemolytic complement or complement components C3 and C4 are depressed in patients with active SLE. Complement levels are often used as a surrogate for disease activity and are particularly useful when followed serially to detect early, preclinical changes in disease.

Some autoantibodies seen in SLE are useful in diagnosis (15). These include antibodies to double-stranded DNA; anti-Sm, which is seen primarily in SLE; anti-histone antibody, which is seen primarily in drug-induced lupus; and anti-Ro and anti-La antibodies, which are seen in Sjögren's syndrome as well as in SLE.

Antibodies such as those to DNA were initially thought to reflect disease activity in SLE, and therefore were considered monitors of therapy. There are indeed a large number of patients who are clinically and serologically concordant. In these patients, worsening of serology predicts an impending flare in clinical disease. However, in many patients DNA antibodies are an imperfect predictor of clinical disease activity, and elevated levels do not consistently correlate with any clinical feature except renal disease (16). Elevated DNA antibody levels and low complement levels may persist for long periods before the flare is recognized clinically. Thus, in any patient being seen for the first time, it is most appropriate to treat the clinical state and not the serologic abnormalities. If observations confirm that these patients are clinically and serologically concordant, one might then consider treating serologic changes.

A small minority of patients with SLE do not have antinuclear antibody or lupus erythematosus (LE) cells (ANA-negative lupus). These patients tend to have increased prevalence of skin rash, photosensitivity, Raynaud's phenomenon, and serositis (17). Some of these patients subsequently have been shown to have the anti-Ro (SS-A) antibody.

EVOLVING SPECTRUM OF SLE
Latent Lupus

Latent lupus describes a group of patients who present with a constellation of symptoms suggestive of SLE, but who do not qualify by classification or a rheumatologist's intuition as having classic SLE (18). These patients usually present with either one or two of the American College of Rheumatology classification criteria for SLE and disease features not included among the criteria. These may include lymphadenopathy; fever; headache; nodules; Sjögren's syndrome; fatigue; neuropathy; fewer than two active joints; an elevation in partial thromboplastin time, gammaglobulin, and ESR; depressed complement; positive rheumatoid factor; or aspirin-induced hepatotoxicity. Many of these patients will persist with their constellation of signs and symptoms over many years without the disease evolving into classic SLE. These patients generally do not respond well to therapy for SLE and are best treated symptomatically. It is not clear that any of the presenting features of the illness can predict which patients will eventually develop classic SLE. Patients with latent lupus tend to have a milder form of disease, and typically do not present with CNS or renal disease.

Drug-Induced Lupus

Drug-induced lupus may be diagnosed in a patient with no history suggesting SLE, whose clinical and serologic manifestations of SLE appear while taking the drug, and whose clinical symptoms improve quickly on discontinuing the drug. Serologic abnormalities resolve more slowly. Drugs associated with drug-induced lupus have been classified into three categories: drugs for which proof of the association is definite (chlorpromazine, methyldopa, hydralazine, procainamide, and isoniazid); drugs that are only possibly associated (dilantin, penicillamine, and quinidine);

and drugs where the association is still questionable (represented by a wide variety of drugs including gold salts, a number of antibiotics, and griseofulvin).

The clinical features of drug-related lupus are usually less severe than those of idiopathic SLE (19). The most commonly reported clinical features are constitutional symptoms, fever, arthritis, and serositis. Central nervous system and renal involvement are distinctly uncommon. Laboratory examinations reveal the presence of cytopenias, a positive LE prep, and positive antinuclear antibody and rheumatoid factor tests. Antibodies to single-stranded DNA are commonly found, but antibodies to double-stranded DNA are not typically present. In addition, complement levels are generally not depressed. Antihistone antibodies occur in more than 90% of cases. However, antihistone antibodies are not specific—they are also found in 20%–30% of patients with idiopathic SLE.

Antiphospholipid Antibody Syndrome

The antiphospholipid antibody syndrome describes the association of arterial and venous thrombosis, recurrent fetal loss, and immune thrombocytopenia with a variety of antibodies directed against cellular phospholipid components (see Chapter 27). This syndrome may be part of the clinical spectrum of SLE, or may occur as a primary form without other clinical features of SLE.

Late-Stage Lupus

Although short-term prognosis in SLE has improved dramatically over the past three decades, the mortality rates in patients surviving more than 5 years and especially more than 10 years have not shown similar dramatic improvement. Patients with disease duration of greater than 5 years tend to die of causes other than active SLE. Mortality and morbidity are affected by long-term complications of SLE that result either from the disease itself or as a consequence of its therapy. These changing patterns in morbidity and mortality are illustrated in Table 19B-4.

The nephropathy of late-stage lupus involves the development of end-stage renal disease after many months of stable renal function. These patients have no signs of multisystem SLE, and serologic abnormalities have generally converted to normal. Renal biopsies in these patients reveal glomerular hyalinization, vascular pathology, fibrinoid necrosis, and interstitial inflammation. Clinical problems usually relate to severe hypertension and recurrent congestive heart failure.

Deaths occurring late in the course of SLE are often related to myocardial infarction and atherosclerosis in the absence of other evidence of active SLE. These complications generally occur in premenopausal women and also have been reported in adolescents. Thus far cardiovascular complications have been reported primarily as atherosclerotic coronary artery disease with either angina or myocardial infarction, as peripheral vascular atherosclerotic disease with intermittent claudication, or as vascular insufficiency and gangrene. The atherosclerotic process may be severe enough to require angioplasty or bypass surgery.

Acute joint pain presenting in the later stages of SLE, especially localized to a very few areas, may indicate the development of osteonecrosis. In most large series, osteonecrosis is recognized as an important cause of musculoskeletal disability in late SLE. Patients with osteonecrosis are generally in the younger age group and have an interval between diagnosis of SLE and osteonecrosis of about 4 years. The hip is the most commonly involved joint, although reports have noted involvement of most joints in the body. One-half to two-thirds of patients with osteonecrosis will have multiple sites. Corticosteroid use, particularly in high doses, is a risk factor for osteonecrosis. Because osteonecrosis is not related to active SLE, the systemic disease may be active or inactive at the time of osteonecrosis presentation. There is no general agreement as to the predictive role of any specific manifestation of SLE (such as Raynaud's phenomenon or vasculitis) in the subsequent development of osteonecrosis.

In late-stage lupus, when there is no longer any evidence of active disease and the patient is taking low-dose or no corticosteroids, neurocognitive disabilities remain a frequent complaint. Patients often present with decreased memory, difficulty doing simple mathematic calculations, and increased speech disabilities. They often have significant impairments on formal neurocognitive testing. Cortical atrophy may be seen on CT scans, both in patients with previous CNS disease and in those without.

In the late stages of lupus, patients may present with increasing dyspnea although a chest examination is normal. Chest radiographs may reveal an elevated diaphragm but normal lung fields. Pulmonary function tests will usually reveal small lung volumes and a restrictive pattern. This syndrome, called shrinking lung syndrome, is a result of altered respiratory mechanics either on the basis of impaired respiratory muscle or diaphragm function or problems in the respiratory skeletal apparatus.

PREGNANCY AND SLE

Fertility rates in patients with SLE are reportedly the same as in the general population. Although a lupus patient may conceive normally, her chances of carrying a pregnancy through to term are reduced, due to greater incidence of spontaneous abortion, prematurity, and intrauterine death. In all large series of SLE patients, there are large numbers of therapeutic abortions, most for psychosocial reasons, but some out of concern for the effects of pregnancy on the disease.

Early studies of SLE and pregnancy in the steroid era perpetuated the idea that pregnancy had an adverse effect on the clinical course of the disease. However, recent studies have shown that the frequency of flares in pregnant SLE patients is the same as the frequency in nonpregnant patients (20). Disease activity should be controlled before conception.

Another issue that arises in pregnant SLE patients is the differentiation between lupus flares, particularly renal dis-

(Table 19B-4)
Late complications of systemic lupus erythematosus

Glomerulonephritis	End-stage renal disease, dialysis, transplantation
Vasculitis	Atherosclerosis, venous syndromes, pulmonary emboli
Arthritis	Osteonecrosis
Cerebritis	Neuropsychological dysfunction
Pneumonitis and myopathy	Shrinking lung syndrome

ease, and pre-eclampsia and eclampsia. The presence of other features of SLE, as well as laboratory abnormalities such as anti-DNA antibody or depressed complement levels, may favor the diagnosis of a flare.

CRITERIA

Criteria for the Classification of SLE

For a disease with such protean manifestations and variable course as SLE, the need for classification criteria that would allow comparison of patients from different centers is obvious (21) (Appendix I).

Criteria for Disease Activity in SLE

Although the criteria for the classification of SLE help distinguish patients with SLE from patients with other connective tissue diseases, and thus allow for comparison of patients from different centers, these criteria have not been helpful in assessing disease activity or disease exacerbations. Multiple systems to assess clinical disease activity in SLE have been devised, but there have been only a handful of validated instruments. Three indices, the SLEDAI (SLE disease activity index), SLAM (systemic lupus activity measure), and BILAG (British Isles lupus assessment group), have been validated against each other during a series of conferences (6). Although these disease activity instruments were arrived at independently by the participating groups, they were found to be comparable.

Health Status Criteria in SLE

Measurements of health status include quality of life assessments, psychological and social impact of the disease, and physical disability. To date, the Arthritis Impact Measurement Scales (AIMS), and the Health Assessment Questionnaire (HAQ), among other questionnaires, have been used. It has recently been suggested that the Medical Outcome Survey Short-Form 36 be adopted to assess health status in patients with SLE. A damage index, reflecting the accumulated damage occurring in patients with SLE as a result of previous inflammation or its treatment, has been developed and validated (22).

DAFNA D. GLADMAN, MD
MURRAY B. UROWITZ, MD

1. Sontheimer RD, Gilliam JN: Systemic lupus erthematosus and the skin. In Lahita RG (ed): Systemic Lupus Erythematosus, 2nd ed. New York, Churchill Livingstone, 1992, pp 657-681

2. Boumpas DR, Fessler BJ, Austin HA, Balow JE, Klippel JH, Lockshin MD: Systemic lupus erythematosus: emerging concepts. Part 2: dermatologic and joint disease, the antiphospholipid antibody syndrome, pregnancy and hormonal therapy, morbidity and mortality, and pathogenesis. Ann Intern Med 123:42-53, 1995

3. Gladman DD, Urowitz MB, Cole E, Ritchie S, Chang CH, Churg J: Kidney biopsy in SLE. I. A clinical-morphologic evaluation. Quart J Med 73:1125-1153, 1989

4. Boumpas DT, Austin HA, Fessler BJ, Balow JE, Klippel JH, Lockshin MD: Systemic lupus erythematosus: emerging concepts. Part 1: Renal, neuropsychiatric, cardiovascular, pulmonary and hematologic disease. Ann Intern Med 122:940-950, 1995

5. McLaughlin JR, Bombardier CB, Farewell VT, Gladman DD, Urowitz MB: Kidney biopsy in systemic lupus erythematosus. III. Survival analysis controlling for clinical and laboratory variables. Arthritis Rheum 37:559-567, 1994

6. Gladman DD: Prognosis and treatment of systemic lupus erythematosus. Curr Opin Rheumatol 7:402-408, 1995

7. Kovacs JAJ, Urowitz MB, Gladman DD: Dilemmas in neuropsychiatric lupus. Rheum Dis Clin North Am 19:795-814, 1993

8. Denburg SD, Denburg JA, Carbotte RM, Fisk JD, Hanly JG: Cognitive deficits in systemic lupus erythematosus. Rheum Dis Clin North Am 19:815-831, 1993

9. West SG, Emelen W, Wener MH, Kotzin BL: Neuropsychiatric lupus erythematosus: 10-year prospective study on the value of diagnostic tests. Am J Med 99:153-163, 1995

10. Kovacs JAJ, Urowitz MB, Gladman DD, Zeman R: The use of SPECT in neuropsychiatric SLE: a pilot study. J Rheumatol 22:1247-1253, 1995

11. Griffey RH, Brown MS, Bankhurst AD, Sibbitt RR, Siggitt WL Jr: Depletion of high-energy phosphates in the central nervous system of patient with systemic lupus erythematosus, as determined by phosphorus-31 nuclear magnetic resonance spectroscopy. Arthritis Rheum 33:827-833, 1990

12. Winslow TM, Ossipov MO, Fazio GP, Simonson JS, Redberg RF, Schiller NB: Five-year follow-up study of the prevalence and progression of pulmonary hypertension in systemic lupus erythematosus. Am Heart J 129:510-515, 1995

13. Sasson Z, Rasooly Y, Chow CW, Marshall S, Urowitz MB: Impairment of left ventricular diastolic function in systemic lupus erythematosus. Am J Cardiol 69:1629-1634, 1992

14. Miller MH, Urowitz MB, Gladman DD: The significance of thrombocytopenia in systemic lupus erythematosus. Arthritis Rheum 26:1181-1186, 1983

15. Reeves WH, Satoh M, Wang J, Chou CH, Ajmani AK: Antibodies to DNA, DNA-binding proteins, and histones. Rheum Dis Clin North Am 20:1-28, 1994

16. Walz-Leblanc B, Gladman DD, Urowitz MB, Goodman PJ: Serologically active clinically quiescent SLE. J Rheumatol 21:2239-2241, 1994

17. Urowitz MB, Gladman DD: Anti-nuclear antibody negative lupus. Systemic lupus erythematosus. In Lahita RG (ed): Systemic Lupus Erythematosus. New York, Churchill Livingstone, 1992, pp 561-567

18. Ganczarczyk L, Urowitz MB, Gladman DD: Latent lupus. J Rheumatol 16:475-478, 1989

19. Yung RL, Richardson BC: Drug-related lupus. Rheumatic Dis Clin North Am 20:61-86, 1994

20. Gladman DD, Urowitz MB: Rheumatic disease in pregnancy. In Burrow JN, Ferris TF (eds): Medical Complications During Pregnancy, 4th ed. Philadelphia, WB Saunders 1995, pp 501-529

21. Tan EM, Cohen AS, Fries JF, et al: The 1982 revised criteria for the classification of systemic lupus erythematosus. Arthritis Rheum 25:1271-1277, 1982

22. Gladman D, Ginzler E, Goldsmith C, et al: The development and initial validation of the SLICC/ACR damage index for SLE. Arthritis Rheum 39:363-369, 1996

C. TREATMENT

Advances in the treatment of systemic lupus erythematosus (SLE) have been a major factor in improvements in patient survival and reductions in disease morbidity over the past several decades (1).

GENERAL PRINCIPLES OF MANAGEMENT

Patient education and psychosocial interventions are an important aspect of managing SLE, particularly in newly diagnosed patients. Books and pamphlets specifically written for patients are helpful for providing basic information about the disease (2). In many hospitals and communities, lupus support groups have been organized. Besides the educational function offered by these groups, many patients benefit enormously simply by having the opportunity to interact with others who have the disease.

Many lupus patients are photosensitive and should be reminded of the need to avoid intense sun exposure. They should be instructed in the liberal use of sun screens and given practical advice such as wearing long-sleeved clothing and large-brimmed hats and going outdoors mainly during early morning or evening hours. Office workers may need to avoid sunlight from windows or even exposure to overhead fluorescent lights. Care also must be taken in the use of photosensitizing drugs, particularly antibiotics.

Because infections are common in SLE, patients should be reminded of the importance of prompt evaluation of unexplained fever. This is especially necessary for patients treated with high-dose corticosteroids or cytotoxic drugs and patients with renal failure, cardiac valvular vegetations, or ulcerative skin or mucous membrane lesions. Patients should be immunized with influenza vaccine yearly, and pneumococcal vaccine should be given after splenectomy. Antibiotic prophylaxis should be instituted for all dental, genitourinary, and other invasive procedures.

Birth control is important in women with active SLE, particularly with nephritis, and in patients treated with drugs contraindicated during pregnancy such as antimalarial agents and cyclophosphamide. Pregnancy poses concerns of potential disease exacerbations in the mother and separate risks to the fetus. This requires more careful monitoring of disease activity than usual in the pregnant patient, including the provision of obstetrical care by a specialist trained in the management of high-risk pregnancies.

DRUG THERAPIES

Primary drug management of SLE involves the use of drugs that suppress end-organ inflammation or interfere with immune function. Very few drug therapies have been subjected to testing by randomized controlled trials, however. The type and severity of clinical manifestations serve to guide treatment. In addition, it is important to recognize the critical role of aggressive management of comorbid conditions that commonly occur in SLE patients, such as hypertension, infections, seizures, hyperlipidemia, and osteoporosis.

Nonsteroidal Anti-inflammatory Drugs

Nonsteroidal anti-inflammatory drugs (NSAIDs) are used for musculoskeletal symptoms, mild serositis, and constitutional signs such as fever. In addition, low-dose aspirin (80 to 325 mg/day) is used for prophylaxis in patients with the antiphospholipid syndrome. The onset of action of NSAIDs is prompt, with clinical improvement typically evident within days of beginning drug treatment. As with other rheumatic diseases, response to individual NSAIDs varies markedly. There is no reason to believe that one NSAID is better than another, and factors such as cost, convenience, and how well the patient tolerates the drug are important practical considerations.

Several adverse effects of NSAIDs may be easily confused with active SLE. Nonsteroidal drugs inhibit prostaglandin synthesis within the kidney and impair renal blood flow. Patients with lupus nephritis are particularly susceptible because of a heightened dependency on prostaglandins to maintain renal function compromised by glomerular inflammation. In rare instances, NSAIDs may cause membranous nephropathy, acute interstitial nephritis, or acute tubular necrosis. Thus, when SLE patients present with loss of renal function or proteinuria, the possibility of NSAID-induced nephropathies should be considered before ascribing the changes to active lupus nephritis. These patients also should be questioned about their use of nonprescription NSAIDs. Renal abnormalities produced by NSAIDs, particularly impaired renal function, are generally promptly and completely reversible.

Nonsteroidal drugs may cause various neuropsychiatric signs and symptoms such as headache, dizziness, and depression that may be confused with central nervous system (CNS) lupus. An aseptic meningitis syndrome has been reported with several NSAIDs, particularly ibuprofen, which presents with headache, meningismus, and fever. Pruritus, facial edema, and conjunctivitis may occur on occasion. Lymphocytosis, elevated protein, and a sterile culture are findings in the cerebrospinal fluid. The syndrome promptly resolves when the NSAID is discontinued.

Nonsteroidal drugs, particularly aspirin, can cause a reversible hepatitis characterized by elevated hepatic transaminase levels. Other uncommon side effects of NSAIDs include skin rashes, pancytopenia, and pancreatitis.

Corticosteroids

There are many uses for corticosteroids in SLE patients, including topical or intralesional preparations for rashes, intra-articular injections for acute arthritis, and oral or parenteral therapy for systemic disease manifestations (Table 19C-1). Improvement is noted in most instances within the first several days, and corticosteroids may indeed be lifesaving in severely ill patients. The actual type of corticosteroid used is less important than the dose; however, long-acting corticosteroids such as dexamethasone are generally avoided. Most physicians prefer prednisone since it is available in multiple strengths that facilitate dose changes. Oral corticosteroid therapy is usually started as a single daily dose taken in the morning. As a general rule, minor manifestations of lupus such as arthritis, serositis, and constitutional signs readily respond to prednisone doses of 0.5 mg/kg daily or less, whereas more serious major organ in-

(Table 19C-1)

The multiple uses of corticosteroids in systemic lupus erythematosus

Indication	Corticosteroid Regimen
Cutaneous manifestations	Topical or intralesional corticosteroids
Minor disease activity	Prednisone (or equivalent) at a dose of <0.5 mg/kg in a single or divided daily dosage
Major disease activity	Oral: Prednisone (or equivalent) at a dose of 1 mg/kg in single or divided daily dosage; duration should not exceed 4 weeks
	IV bolus: Methylprednisolone (1 g or 15 mg/kg) over 30 minutes; dose often repeated for 3 consecutive days

volvement such as nephritis or CNS disease are indications for high-dose prednisone in the range of 1.0 mg/kg daily. Intravenous methylprednisolone (bolus therapy) is a commonly used alternative to high-dose oral therapy. In patients who fail to show improvement, the dose of corticosteroids may be either increased or given in divided doses two or three times daily. Patients who fail to show substantial improvement after a 4-week course of high-dose corticosteroids are candidates for immunosuppressive drugs or other aggressive forms of management.

Corticosteroid toxicities are a major problem in SLE, and once disease activity is judged to be under control, gradual reduction of the dosage (tapering) is essential. Patients on a multiple daily dose regimen should first be converted to a single morning dose before attempting to reduce the actual drug dose. Patients need to be carefully monitored during tapering for signs of increasing disease activity, which may necessitate temporary increases in the dose. Some patients appear to have a corticosteroid threshold below which disease activity predictably develops. In patients with prolonged periods of disease remission, eventual discontinuation of the corticosteroid should be a goal of patient management.

Antimalarial Drugs

Hydroxychloroquine, chloroquine, and quinacrine are especially useful in managing cutaneous manifestations of lupus, but these antimalarial compounds are also helpful for treating musculoskeletal and constitutional symptoms. Additional reported benefits of hydroxychloroquine in SLE include lowering serum cholesterol and reducing the risks of venous thrombosis and coronary artery disease. Antimalarials should be used with caution in SLE patients with glucose-6-phosphate dehydrogenase (G6PD) deficiency and in patients with liver disease. Quinacrine (100 mg daily) and hydroxychloroquine (200–400 mg daily) are the best studied and most widely used antimalarial agents. Although there are some differences in onset of action and toxicities, the choice between these two agents is largely a matter of physician preference. Improvements in cutaneous manifestations, including discoid, subacute cutaneous, and erythematous

inflammatory lesions, can be remarkably rapid, often evident within days of starting therapy. Patients who fail to respond to a particular antimalarial may benefit from either substituting or adding an alternative antimalarial drug. Discontinuation of antimalarials is associated with an increased risk of lupus flares, including major exacerbations such as vasculitis, transverse myelitis, and nephropathy (3). As a consequence, there is a general reluctance to ever completely discontinue antimalarials in stable patients who have clearly benefited from the drug.

The low doses of antimalarials used in SLE are well tolerated and rarely associated with adverse reactions. Minor gastrointestinal complaints and skin rashes are infrequent, although quinacrine has a propensity to turn the skin yellow. Because rare instances of CNS toxicities have been reported, including headache, emotional lability, psychoses, ataxia, and seizures, antimalarials should be discontinued in patients with suspected neuropsychiatric involvement. Long-term antimalarial therapy may cause a mitochondrial neuromyopathy with progressive proximal and distal muscle weakness. Although hematologic toxicities with antimalarials are distinctly uncommon, complete blood counts should be obtained occasionally.

Much of the concern about the use of antimalarials in SLE has focused on potential ocular toxicities. As a precaution, ophthalmologic examination is recommended prior to therapy and every 6 to 12 months thereafter. Evaluation should include visual acuity, slit-lamp, fundoscopic, and visual field testing. However, the risk of retinal toxicity in patients taking the low doses of antimalarials used in SLE is extremely small (4).

Antimalarials cross the placenta, and rare instances of congenital defects such as cleft palate, sensorineural hearing loss, and posterior column defects have been reported. In general, antimalarials are contraindicated during pregnancy. However, the SLE patient treated with antimalarials who wishes to become pregnant faces the risk of disease flare from discontinuing the drug. The safety of antimalarials during pregnancy has been noted in a small series of SLE patients (5).

Methotrexate

Weekly low-dose oral methotrexate (7.5–15 mg) appears to be useful in managing arthritis, skin rashes, serositis, and constitutional signs and symptoms (6,7). Because methotrexate is eliminated by both glomerular filtration and tubular secretion, it must be used with caution in patients with evidence of lupus nephritis. Although recent studies have indicated a more primary role for weekly methotrexate in various types of systemic vasculitis such as polyarteritis, Wegener's granulomatosis, and Takayasu's arteritis, the efficacy of methotrexate in lupus nephritis and other forms of lupus vasculitis has not been established.

Cyclophosphamide

High-dose intravenous bolus cyclophosphamide regimens (0.5–1.0 g/m²) are widely used in the treatment of major SLE organ involvement; low-dose oral therapy (1–4 mg/kg daily) is much less commonly prescribed. The alkylating metabolites of cyclophosphamide are excreted by the kidneys, and dosages must be reduced in patients with impaired renal function. In addition, the drug must be given with caution to patients with leukopenia, and regular monitoring of white blood cell counts, hematocrit, and platelet counts are essential. Cyclophosphamide is a potent teratogen, and a pregnancy test before starting therapy and birth control measures during therapy are essential.

In randomized controlled trials of patients with diffuse proliferative lupus nephritis, monthly infusion of intravenous cyclophosphamide has been shown to retard progressive scarring within the kidney, prevent loss of renal function, and reduce the risk of end-stage renal failure (1) (Fig. 19C-1). The rate of relapse following a 6-month course of cyclophosphamide is high, however, and most patients need extended therapy or substitution of maintenance oral immunosuppressive therapy. Intravenous cyclophosphamide has reportedly been effective in managing most other serious forms of the disease, including hematologic, CNS, and vascular manifestations (1,8,9).

The toxicities of cyclophosphamide are substantial. Nausea and vomiting, particularly following intravenous therapy, are common, and most patients require antiemetic drugs. Alopecia may occasionally be severe and require the use of a wig; however, patients should be reassured that the hair will regrow even with continued therapy. Patients treated with cyclophosphamide are at heightened risk for infections, especially herpes zoster, and require careful evaluation for unexplained fever. Long-term cyclophosphamide therapy may damage gonadal tissue and lead to ovarian failure or azoospermia. The risk of ovarian failure increases with a woman's age and is a nearly universal complication in patients older than age 30 who are treated with cyclophosphamide (10). The recovery of ovarian function or spermatogenesis is unpredictable. Estrogen supplements or gonadotropin releasing hormone (GnRH) analogs theoretically should protect the ovary from the effects of cyclophosphamide. However, neither of these has been carefully studied. Recent evidence suggests thast testosterone may prevent cyclophosphamide-induced azoospermia (11). Before begin-

ning cyclophosphamide therapy in very young patients, some consideration should be given to ova or sperm storage.

Acrolein, which is a metabolite of cyclophosphamide, damages bladder mucosa and may cause acute hemorrhagic cystitis, bladder fibrosis, and transitional and squamous cell carcinoma. Bladder complications are mainly seen with long-term oral drug administration, but the risks are substantially reduced with intermittent intravenous regimens. Generous fluid intake will reduce concentrations of acrolein in the bladder and minimize these complications. The sulfhydryl compound mesna binds acrolein and is increasingly being used as a uroprotective agent with intravenous therapy, particularly in patients with known cyclophosphamide-induced bladder damage who require drug administration. Patients treated with prolonged courses of cyclophosphamide, especially oral drug therapy, should be screened indefinitely for malignant changes in the bladder (12). Hematuria, particularly of new onset after prolonged drug administration, should be assessed by urine cytology and cystoscopy. Patients treated with cyclophosphamide who develop evidence of reduced bladder capacity, such as increased frequency and small urinary volumes, should undergo complete cystometric evaluation.

The major established malignancy risk with cyclophosphamide is bladder and skin cancer, although it is generally believed that malignancies of hematopoietic or lymphoreticular origin are also increased. The actual risks of these malignancies have not been established, however (13).

Azathioprine

The purine analog azathioprine (1–3 mg/kg daily) is generally considered to be a less effective but far less toxic drug than cyclophosphamide. In SLE the drug is used primarily as an alternative to cyclophosphamide for the treatment of nephritis and as a steroid-sparing agent in nonrenal manifestations.

The most common side effects of azathioprine are gastrointestinal intolerance and bone marrow toxicity. The onset of anemia or leukopenia may be abrupt, and blood counts must be monitored regularly during therapy. Bone marrow toxicity is generally reversible by reducing the dose or discontinuing the drug. Azathioprine can produce elevated liver enzymes, particularly the pyruvic and glutamic oxaloacetic transaminases, that are occasionally accompanied by a syndrome of fever, diffuse abdominal pain, diarrhea, and maculopapular skin rash. The hepatotoxicity is thought to result from drug hypersensitivity, and hepatocellular necrosis and mild biliary stasis may be seen on liver biopsy. Hepatic abnormalities are typically reversible on discontinuing the drug.

Azathioprine is associated with an increased risk of hematopoietic and lymphoreticular malignancies. Case reports of non-Hodgkin's lymphoma and leukemia and a fourfold increase in uterine cervical atypia have been documented in SLE patients following treatment with azathioprine.

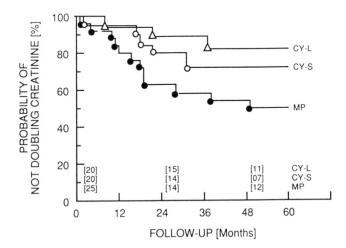

(Figure 19C–1)
Cumulative probability of not doubling serum creatinine in patients with lupus nephritis treated with methylprednisolone (MP), monthly intravenous cyclophosphamide for 6 months (CY-S), or cyclophosphamide given for a total of 30 months (CY-L). CY-L is significantly different from MP, p = 0.037. Reproduced from Boumpas DT, Austin HA, Vaughn EM, et al: Severe lupus nephritis: controlled trial of pulse methylprednisolone versus two different regimens of pulse cyclophosphamide. Lancet 340:741-744, 1992, with permission.

Cyclosporin A

Although several different macrolides have been shown to modify murine models of autoimmunity, studies in SLE patients are currently limited only to cyclosporin A. Experiences with low-dose cyclosporin A (3–6 mg daily) in both nonrenal manifestations (14) and membranous nephropathy are encouraging (15). Toxicities of the drug were minimal; no nephrotoxicity was observed in either study.

Hormonal Therapies

Danazol, the attenuated androgen, has been shown to be useful in managing lupus thrombocytopenia (16). The mechanism of action of the drug has not been defined, but it is thought to involve endocrine influences such as suppression of pituitary follicle-stimulating hormone and luteinizing hormone on immune or reticuloendothelial functions. Pregnancy, breast feeding, or unexplained vaginal bleeding are absolute contraindications to danazol therapy, and the drug must be used with caution in patients with liver or renal involvement. The major adverse reactions relate to hormonal changes induced by the drug, such as vaginitis, irregular menses including amenorrhea, virilization, and emotional lability. Drug effects on the liver require monitoring of liver chemistries. Hepatic tumors have been reported with long-term therapy.

Prolactin levels are increased in some patients with SLE and reportedly parallel lupus activity. The ergot derivative bromocriptine inhibits prolactin secretion from the anterior pituitary through antagonism of dopamine receptors. Bromocriptine has been shown to be immunosuppressive in several murine models of autoimmunity and may have a role in the treatment of nonlife-threatening lupus manifestations (17).

Low levels of dehydroepiandrosterone (DHEA), an adrenal steroid with limited androgenic activity, have been reported in patients with SLE. In a murine model of lupus, DHEA ameliorated nephritis through a mechanism thought to involve influences on cytokine secretion (18). A placebo-controlled trial of DHEA has reported benefits in patients with mild to moderate lupus activity (19).

Immunoglobulins

Intravenous immunoglobulin has been shown to be useful for managing severe lupus thrombocytopenia (20). The platelet count rises rapidly within hours of administration, occasionally peaking with extraordinarily high counts in which thrombotic events become a clinical concern. The rate of relapse of thrombocytopenia following treatment is high, however. The primary role for immunoglobulin therapy is to control acute bleeding associated with lupus thrombocytopenia or to rapidly increase the platelet count to allow for splenectomy or other surgery. The role of immunoglobulin for treating other lupus manifestations has not been studied.

A typical dose schedule for lupus thrombocytopenia is 300–400 mg/kg/day given for 5 consecutive days, often followed by monthly maintenance therapy in an attempt to prevent relapse. The major contraindication is IgA deficiency, an occasional finding in SLE patients. Adverse reactions include fever, chills, myalgias, fluid retention, and abdominal and chest pain; true anaphylactic reactions are rare. The mechanism of action of immunoglobulin in reversing lupus thrombocytopenia is uncertain, but it may involve interference with Fc receptor-mediated functions or the interaction of anti-idiotype antibodies contained within the gamma globulin fractions with antibody-producing cells or secreted antiplatelet antibodies. Other effects of immunoglobulin on immune function that have been described include suppression of T-lymphocyte proliferation and reduction of natural killer cell activity.

Dapsone

Dapsone has been used to manage cutaneous manifestations of lupus, including discoid, subacute cutaneous lupus, bullous, and lupus profundus lesions. Therapy is typically started at 50 mg daily with gradual increases of the dose to a maximum of 150 mg daily. Hematologic side effects, in particular a dose-related hemolysis, are common and require careful monitoring. Because patients with G6PD deficiency are at heightened risk for hematologic toxicities, routine screening for this condition prior to therapy is recommended. Methemoglobinemia with weakness, tachycardia, nausea, headache, and abdominal pain is a rare complication of therapy.

PLASMA EXCHANGE

The role of plasma exchange in SLE is limited to rare, acute conditions associated with a high mortality such as thrombotic thrombocytopenic purpura and pulmonary hemorrhage (21). There is no evidence that plasma exchange is beneficial in the long-term management of lupus, particularly lupus nephritis. One of the problems with plasma exchange is that concentrations of autoantibodies and immune complexes are typically only transiently reduced; once plasma exchange is stopped, abnormal levels resume rapidly. A strategy to stimulate pathologic immune clones is to follow plasma exchange with intravenous cyclophosphamide ("stimulation-depletion"). This experimental therapy is reportedly associated with long-term lupus remissions (22).

DIALYSIS AND TRANSPLANTATION

Patients with end-stage lupus nephropathy are managed with dialysis or kidney transplantation. There is a tendency for decreased clinical and serologic lupus activity following the onset of end-stage renal disease. Survival of lupus patients and other end-stage renal patients is comparable. Most studies note an increased incidence of infections among SLE patient on dialysis. Kidney transplantation during an acute exacerbation of SLE is controversial and may increase the risk of a poor outcome. Recurrence of lupus nephritis in transplanted allografts, often with the same histopathology as in the native kidney, develops in 2%–4% of transplanted kidneys (23).

JOHN H. KLIPPEL, MD

1. Boumpas DT, Austin HA, Fessler BJ, Balow JE, Klippel JH, Lockshiu MD: Systemic lupus erythematosus: renal, neuropsychiatric, cardiovascular, pulmonary, and hematologic disease. Ann Intern Med 122:940-950, 1995

2. Wallace DJ: The Lupus Book: A Guide for Patients and Their Families. New York, Oxford University Press, 1995.

3. The Canadian Hydroxychloroquine Study Group: A randomized study of the effect of withdrawing hydroxychloroquine sulfate in systemic lupus erythematosus. N Engl J Med 324:150-154, 1991

4. Spalton DJ, Verdon Roe GM, Hughes GRV: Hydroxychloroquine, dosage parameters and retinopathy. Lupus 2:355-358, 1993

5. Levy M, Buskila D, Gladman DD, Urowitz MB, Koren G: Pregnancy outcome following first trimester exposure to chloroquine. Am J Perinatol 8:174-178, 1991

6. Wilson K, Abeles M: A 2-year, open-ended trial of methotrexate in systemic lupus erythematosus. J Rheumatol 21:1674-1677, 1994

7. Waltz-LeBlanc BA, Dagenais P, Urowitz MB, Gladman DD: Methotrexate in systemic lupus erythematosus. J Rheumatol 21:836-838, 1994

8. Klippel JH: Is aggressive therapy effective for lupus? Rheum Dis Clin N Amer 19:249-261, 1993

9. Neuwelt CM, Lacks S, Kaye BR, Ellman JB, Borenstein DG: Role of intravenous cyclophosphamide in the treatment of severe neuropsychiatric systemic lupus erythematosus. Am J Med 98:32-41, 1995

10. Wang CL, Wang F, Bosco JJ: Ovarian failure in oral cyclophosphamide treatment for systemic lupus erythematosus. Lupus 4:11-14, 1995

11. Masala A, Faedda R, Alagna S, et al: Use of testosterone to prevent cyclophosphamide-induced azoospermia. Ann Intern Med 126:292-295, 1997

12. Talar-Williams C, Hijazi Y, Walther M, et al: Cyclophosphamide-induced

bladder toxicity in patients with Wegener's granulomatosis. Ann Intern Med 124:477-484, 1996

13. Sweeney DM, Manzi S, Janosky J, Selvaggi KJ, Ferri W, Medsger TA, Jr., Ramsey-Goldman R: Risk of malignancy in women with systemic lupus erythematosus. J Rheumatol 22:1478-1482, 1995

14. Tokuda M, Kurata N, Mizoguchi A, Inoh M, Seto K, Kinashi M, Takahara J: Effect of low-dose cyclosporin A on systemic lupus erythematosus. Arthritis Rheum 37:551-558, 1994

15. Radhakrishnan J, Kunis CL, D'Agati V, Appel GB: Cyclosporine treatment of lupus membranous nephropathy. Clin Nephrol 42:147-154, 1994

16. West SG, Johnson SC: Danazol for the treatment of refractory autoimmune thrombocytopenia in systemic lupus erythematosus. Ann Intern Med 108:703-706, 1988

17. McMurray RW, Weidensaul D, Allen SH, Walker SE: Efficacy of bromocriptine in an open-label therapeutic trial for systemic lupus erythematosus. J Rheumatol 22:2084-2091, 1995

18. Suzuki T, Suzuki N, Engleman EG, Mizushima Y, Saleane T: Low serum levels of dehydro-epiandrosterone may cause deficient IL-2 production by lymphocytes in patients with systemic lupus erythematosus. Clin Exp Immunol 99:251-255, 1995

19. van Vollenhoven RF, Engleman EG, McGuire JL: Dehydroepiandrosterone in systemic lupus erythematosus: results of a double-blinded, placebo-controlled, randomized clinical trial. Arthritis Rheum 38:1826-1831, 1995

20. Maier WP, Gordon DS, Howard YP, Saleh MN, Miller SB, Lieberman JD, Woodlee PM: Intravenous immunoglobulin therapy in systemic lupus erythematosus-associated thrombocytopenia. Arthritis Rheum 33:1233-1239, 1990

21. Stricker RB, Davis JA, Gershow J, Yamamoto KS, Kiprov DD: Thrombotic thrombocytopenic purpura complicating systemic lupus erythematosus: case report and literature review from the plasmapheresis era. J Rheumatol 19:1469-1473, 1992

22. Euler HH, Schroeder JO, Harten P, Zeuner RA, Gutschmidt HJ: Treatment-free remission in severe lupus erythematosus following synchronization of plasmapheresis with subsequent pulse cyclophosphamide. Arthritis Rheum 37:1784-1794, 1994

23. Mojcik CF, Klippel JH: End-stage renal disease and systemic lupus erythematosus. Am J Med 101:100-107, 1996

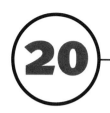

SYSTEMIC SCLEROSIS AND RELATED SYNDROMES
A. EPIDEMIOLOGY, PATHOLOGY, AND PATHOGENESIS

Scleroderma—literally hard (*skleros*) skin (*derma*)—encompasses both disease restricted to the skin (localized scleroderma) and disease with internal organ involvement (diffuse scleroderma). Diffuse scleroderma is also called systemic sclerosis. Subcategories of disease are defined by the extent of skin involvement, which predicts clinical course (1). Patients with limited cutaneous sclerosis have skin thickening below the elbows and knees, sometimes with face and neck involvement as well. Patients with diffuse cutaneous systemic sclerosis have more extensive skin thickening that involves the upper extremities or trunk.

EPIDEMIOLOGY

Although the etiology of systemic sclerosis is unknown, epidemiologic studies have provided insight into factors that regulate disease susceptibility and clinical course. Susceptibility appears to be controlled by a complex interaction between environmental encounters and genetic and nongenetic host factors. The clinical course is influenced by genetic factors.

Systemic sclerosis is an acquired, noncontagious, rare disease that occurs worldwide in sporadic cases. The incidence of definite systemic sclerosis in the United States is estimated at 19 cases per million people per year (2). Disease incidence may have increased during the last half of the 20th century. The prevalence is 19–75 cases per 100,000 people (2). Thus, 40,000 to 165,000 people in the United States have definite systemic sclerosis. Prevalence figures rise three- to fourfold when patients are included who have mild systemic sclerosis-like illnesses (2) but do not meet classification criteria (3) (see Appendix I).

Inhaled or ingested chemicals and viruses are environmental factors that may be involved in disease susceptibility (4). Occupational exposure to silica dust is associated with a relative risk of 25 and frank silicosis with a relative risk of 110. Cases have been reported in individuals exposed to organic solvents, biogenic amines including appetite suppressants, and urea formaldehyde. Fibrosing illnesses with scleroderma-like features occur after exposure to vinyl chloride, bleomycin, tainted rape seed oil, and L-tryptophan. Limited studies suggest lifestyle factors of smoking, moderate alcohol consumption, and ownership of more than one pet are associated with increased risk of developing systemic sclerosis. Several retrospective studies have not found an increased incidence of silicone implants in women with systemic sclerosis.

Homology between viruses and autoantigens in systemic sclerosis suggests a potential role of viruses in disease susceptibility (5). There are homologies between DNA topoisomerase 1 and the p30^{gag} protein from feline sarcoma virus and cytomegalovirus. Regions of the PM-Scl antigen are homologous to SV-40 large T antigen and human immunodeficiency virus tat protein. U1 RNP shares an amino acid segment with herpes simplex virus type I ICP4 protein. There are also homologies between fibrillarin and a capsid protein encoded by herpes simplex virus type 1 and Epstein–Barr virus nuclear antigen 1.

Host factors that modify disease susceptibility are age and female gender (4). Systemic sclerosis is very rare in the first two decades of life, with peak occurrence in individuals in their 40s and 50s. Excess involvement of women is most pronounced during the mid- and late-childbearing years, between age 30 and 55, where ratios of females to males may reach 7–12:1. This characteristic suggests female sex hormones influence disease susceptibility. The ratio is less dramatic at other ages, although women predominate in all groups.

There is no evidence of a strong genetic contribution, other than gender, to disease susceptibility. Weak associations of systemic sclerosis with HLA-DQA2, the C4A null allele, an allele of the Cγ 2 T-cell antigen receptor gene, and low activity of P-450 enzymes have been noted. Unlike rheumatoid arthritis and systemic lupus erythematosus, families with more than one case of systemic sclerosis are rare; only about 20 cases with affected first-degree relatives have been documented. The incidence of systemic sclerosis appears higher in African Americans than in Nigerian blacks and higher in Oklahoma Choctaw Indians than in Missouri Choctaw Indians. These disparities could arise from genetic differences between ethnically related populations or from different environmental exposures. The importance of environmental factors in disease susceptibility is further suggested by equal concordance rates for systemic sclerosis in monozygotic and dizygotic twins and the occurrence of disease in conjugal pairs.

Genetic factors influence the clinical course of systemic sclerosis. Studies in different populations show that autoantibody specificities are associated with particular HLA alleles. For example, in white Americans, the production of anticentromere antibodies is associated with HLA-DQB1 molecules with a polar glycine or tyrosine at position 26 (6). The production of antitopoisomerase I antibodies is associated with a tyrosine residue at position 30 (7). HLA genes influence other disease manifestations such as pulmonary fibrosis, which is associated with the B8, DR3, DR52, DQB2 haplotype.

PATHOLOGY

Widespread small-vessel vasculopathy and fibrosis set systemic sclerosis apart from other connective tissue diseases. Both processes occur in the skin and internal organs, causing symptoms and organ dysfunction. The vasculopathy and fibrosis of systemic sclerosis arise in the setting of autoimmunity.

The small-vessel vasculopathy is a proliferative, obliterative process that preferentially affects small arteries, arterioles, and capillaries (Fig. 20A-1). The process starts in the endothelium, with evidence of both activation and damage (8).

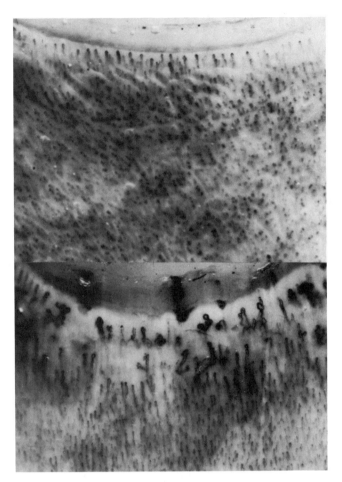

(Figure 20A-1)
*Nailfold capillary bed in a normal subject (**top**) and in a patient with systemic sclerosis (**bottom**). Note the bottom photograph shows both enlarged capillaries and avascular areas, as well as capillary hemorrhages and staining of the cuticle. Reprinted from Dermatologica 168:73-77; 1984, with permission.*

Nonspecific collapse of vimentin intermediate filaments of the cytoskeleton is followed by vacuolization of the cytoplasm and blebbing of the endothelial cell membrane. Tight junctions disappear, and endothelium sloughs into the lumen. Some endothelial cells show an active biosynthetic state, suggesting attempts at repair, but the net outcome is endothelial cell loss. Increased cell-surface expression of HLA class II molecules, β_1 integrins, intercellular adhesion molecule-1 (ICAM-1), endothelial cell adhesion molecule-1 (ELAM-1), and P-selectin indicates activation of the endothelial cells. Even in clinically normal skin, cytoskeletal and cell-membrane abnormalities of endothelial cells are undeniable (8,9). Elevated serum or plasma levels of ICAM-1, ELAM-1, P-selectin, endothelin-1, tissue plasminogen activator, and factor VIII/von Willebrand factor antigen all reflect endothelial cell activation or injury.

Smooth-muscle–like myointimal cells proliferate within the intima of small vessels, in a bed of ground substance and loose fibrils (8). Luminal narrowing develops and is exacerbated when the damaged endothelium induces platelet activation and thrombosis. Platelet activation is responsible for release of mediators, such as platelet-derived growth factor (PDGF) and thromboxane A_2, which can induce vasoconstriction and stimulate growth of endothelial cells and fibroblasts. Basement membranes thicken and reduplicate,

and proteinaceous perivascular edema seeps through the vessels. Fibrin is deposited within and around the vessels. These events are likely to reduce transfusion of nutrients through the vessels.

Fibrosis in systemic sclerosis is caused by increased deposition of collagen, fibronectin, and glycosaminoglycans by activated fibroblasts (10). In the skin, fibrosis is more marked in the lower dermis and the subcutaneous tissue (Fig. 20B-2). Synthesis of collagen types I, III, V, and VI mRNAs and proteins is increased (11). In contrast, collagenase activity appears normal. Other evidence of fibroblast activation in systemic sclerosis is increased cell-surface expression of HLA-DR molecules and ICAM-1. Evidence of fibroblast activation is seen even in clinically normal skin (9). Here, increased expression of procollagen type 1 mRNA occurs without fibrosis. Fibrosis may represent the final, but not inevitable, consequence of fibroblast activation in patients.

An activated immune system is an early, universal event in systemic sclerosis. Antinuclear antibodies are present at clinical presentation in 95% of patients. Some autoantibody systems are quite specific for systemic sclerosis, including the topoisomerase 1, centromere, RNA polymerase I, RNA polymerase III, and U3 RNP systems (Table 20A-1) (5). Many other nonspecific targets of autoantibodies in patients have been identified.

T cells, B cells, macrophages, mast cells, eosinophils, basophils, and platelets are present in increased numbers or in an activated state in the blood or tissues of patients (12). A perivascular mononuclear cell infiltrate is present at all stages of skin involvement in systemic sclerosis, except in clinically normal skin (8). The infiltrate consists predominately of T cells, with some pericytes, Langerhan cells, plasma cells, and macrophages, and, in rare cases, B cells. Invasion of the vessel wall by mononuclear cells is uncommon, and the vascular disease is not considered a vasculitis.

Underappreciated pathologic processes in systemic sclerosis are acquired DNA damage and increased susceptibility to cell damage by free radicals. Increased chromosomal breaks, deletions, and acentric fragments occur in both lymphocytes and fibroblasts from patients and family members (13). Increased mutations in variable number tandem repeats are seen in patients, their siblings, and offspring. Cir-

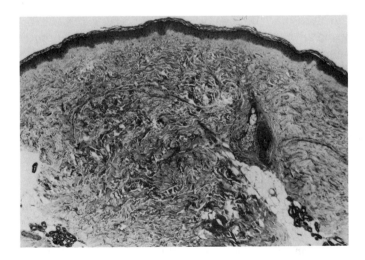

(Figure 20A-2)
Thinning of the epidermis with loss of rete pegs and marked increase in dermal thickness due to increased extracellular matrix.

Anticentromere antibodies
Antinuclear antibodies (speckled, nucleolar, other)
Antinucleolar antibodies
   RNA polymerases I, II, III
   Fibrillarin (U3 RNA protein complex)
   Nucleolar 4-65 RNA
   U2 RNA protein complex
Polymyositis/SSc overlay (Pm/Scl)
Antitopoisomerase I (formerly Scl-70)
Anticollagen type I (interstitial collagen, ubiquitous)
Anticollagen type IV (basement membrane structure)
Antilaminin (basement membrane attachment protein)
Antiribonucleoprotein (RNP)
Jo-1 (Anti-histidyl-transfer RNA [tRNA] synthetase)
SS-A(Ro), SS-B(La)
Ku
Anti Th (nucleolar)

culating clastogenic factors and increased susceptibility to clastogens that generate free radicals occur in systemic sclerosis. Low-density lipoproteins from patients are also more susceptible to oxidation by free radicals.

PATHOGENESIS

Any model of the pathogenesis of systemic sclerosis must account for small-vessel vasculopathy, fibrosis, and autoimmunity. Interactions among cells in small blood vessels, fibroblasts, and the immune system are undoubtedly complex in patients. One of many possible models of the pathogenesis of systemic sclerosis is presented in Fig. 20A-3.

Role of the Immune System

Activation of the immune system in systemic sclerosis may be facilitated by an increased expression of adhesion molecules and integrins on lymphocytes, vascular endothelium, and fibroblasts. Dermal endothelial cells from patients have increased expression of ELAM-1, which is involved in the homing of T cells to the skin. Perivascular lymphocytes in systemic sclerosis skin show increased expression of β_1 and β_2 integrins, including lymphocyte function antigen-1 (LFA-1). Interactions between LFA-1 and ICAM-1 mediate

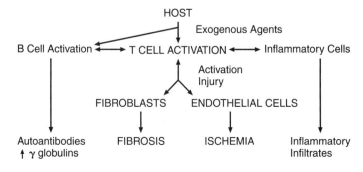

(Figure 20A-3)
Model of the immunopathogenesis of systemic sclerosis.

T-cell binding to fibroblasts, and fibroblasts of patients have increased expression of ICAM-1.

Activated T cells appear pivotal in the pathogenesis of systemic sclerosis. They provide specificity to the immune response and regulate functions of other immune cells. Moreover, they are the predominant infiltrating cell in the perivascular areas. Different T-cell subsets may contribute to the disease process in different organs and at different stages. CD4 T cells are more common than CD8 T cells in the skin of patients with systemic sclerosis at all stages of disease (8). Patients with active interstitial lung disease have increased numbers and percentages of CD8 T cells in their bronchoalveolar lavage (BAL) fluid, with oligoclonal expansion of some CD8 T cells. The γδ T-cell repertoire is skewed in both the peripheral blood and BAL of patients with systemic sclerosis, with evidence of an oligoclonal expansion of the Vδ1+ subset (14). CD8 and γδ T cells are particularly adherent to fibroblasts.

It is likely that the activated T cells in the tissues of patients with systemic sclerosis are responding specifically to initiating antigens or antigens exposed by the disease process. T cells from patients can be activated by skin extracts and purified type I and type IV collagen. Cellular antigens on fibroblasts, epithelial cells, and muscle cells are reported to stimulate cytotoxic T-cell responses, although this is not consistently observed.

There is limited evidence that activated B cells cause tissue damage in systemic sclerosis. Patient sera contain antibodies that bind to both endothelial cells and fibroblasts and promote antibody-dependent cellular cytotoxicity in vivo. Many autoantibodies in systemic sclerosis sera do not activate the complement cascade, and serum complement levels are normal. Immune complexes may be present in the sera, but there is scant evidence of tissue deposition.

Inflammatory cells besides T cells contribute to tissue damage in systemic sclerosis. Mast cell degranulation occurs in the skin of systemic sclerosis patients. Neutrophils infiltrate the lungs during alveolitis. Activated eosinophils and basophils are found in increased numbers in the lungs of patients with alveolitis.

Cytokines

It is likely that multiple cytokines contribute to the sclerodermatous process and that key cytokines may vary with the stage of disease. Tumor necrosis factor α (TNF-α) and several interleukins (IL), notably IL-1α, IL-1β, IL-2, IL-4, IL-6, and IL-10, have all been proposed as contributors to the pathogenesis of systemic sclerosis. They are often present in patients' sera or their production by peripheral blood mononuclear cells is increased. IL-8 mRNA and protein are increased in BAL from systemic sclerosis patients with pulmonary fibrosis, where IL-8 may be responsible for influx of neutrophils. Increased levels of transforming growth factor β (TGF-β) mRNA and pro α1(I) collagen mRNA co- localize within inflammatory skin infiltrates from patients in the early phase of disease. This finding is important because TGF-β stimulates fibrosis and angiogenesis. However, increased production of TGF-β in involved skin and lung tissue is not a consistent finding. Platelet-derived growth factor (PDGF) is an attractive candidate for mediating tissue damage in systemic sclerosis. It stimulates the proliferation of both endothelial cells and fibroblasts and enhances chemotaxis. Increased amounts of PDGF are found in the skin of patients with systemic sclerosis, along with increased PDGF type β receptors (15).

Endothelial Cell Damage

Endothelial cell activation and damage may result from both the effects of soluble mediators or cellular cytotoxicity (10). Many cytokines capable of altering endothelial cell function are found in increased amounts in sera or tissues of systemic sclerosis patients. These include IL-1, IL-2, IL-4, IL-6, IL-8, lymphotoxin, TNF-α, TGF-β, and PDGF. Sera from some patients may contain nonspecific substances cytotoxic to endothelial cells. Granzyme 1 (a lysosomal protein released by cytotoxic T cells), leukotriene B$_4$, and endothelin-1 are circulating factors that may damage or alter function of small vessels in systemic sclerosis. Antibodies against endothelial cells have the potential to cause damage through antibody-dependent cellular cytotoxicity.

The endothelial cell itself is likely to contribute to activating cells of the immune system and fibroblasts. Endothelial cells can present antigen to T cells and stimulate T-cell production of cytokines. Factors produced by the endothelium, such as endothelin-1 and TGF-β, can stimulate extracellular matrix production by fibroblasts.

Fibroblast Abnormalities

Fibrosis in fibroblasts from patients with systemic sclerosis results from at least two events: stimulation of extracellular matrix production by cytokines, and outgrowth of fibroblasts that produce higher basal amounts of extracellular matrix. Fibroblast explant cultures from clinically thickened skin produce higher amounts of extracellular matrix on a per cell basis than normal fibroblasts when initially placed in culture (11). They revert to production of normal levels of extracellular matrix production with passage. Fibroblasts that are making procollagen mRNA are next to infiltrating T cells (16) and TGF-β mRNA (17). Other cytokines that stimulate extracellular matrix production, such as IL-1 and IL-4, may contribute to fibrosis in systemic sclerosis patients. Fibroblasts from patients with systemic sclerosis have increased IL-1 receptors. Decreased production of interferon-γ, which reduces collagen synthesis, may contribute to the profibrotic milieu. It remains possible that these fibroblasts are inherently abnormal in their responsiveness to cytokine stimulation. Only a subset of fibroblasts may contribute to fibrosis in systemic sclerosis. In situ hybridization studies of patients' skin show that only some fibroblasts are actively producing procollagen mRNA (16). This is supported by electron microscopic findings that only some fibroblasts appear metabolically active, with dilated endoplasmic reticulum and increased numbers of cytoplasmic microvesicles (18). Fibroblasts with a similar morphology can be identified in cultured dermal fibroblast lines from systemic sclerosis patients. They produce more collagen on a per cell basis than do other fibroblasts within the same line. A higher percentage of fibroblasts cloned from patients produce greater amounts of collagen than do fibroblasts cloned from controls (19).

BARBARA WHITE, MD

1. LeRoy EC, Black C, Fleishmajer R, Jablonska S, Krieg T, Medsger TA Jr, Rowell N, Wollheim F: Scleroderma (systemic sclerosis): classification, subsets, and pathogenesis. J Rheumatol 15:202-205, 1988

2. Maricq HR, Weinrich MC, Keil JE, Smith EA, Harper FE, Nussbaun AL, LeRoy EC, McGreger AR, Diat F, Rosal EJ: Prevalence of scleroderma spectrum disorders in the general population of South Carolina. Arthritis Rheum 32:998-1006, 1989

3. Subcommittee for Scleroderma Criteria of the American Rheumatism Association Diagnostic and Therapeutic Criteria Committee: Preliminary criteria for classification of systemic sclerosis (scleroderma). Arthritis Rheum 23:581-590, 1980

4. Silman AJ: Scleroderma: Disease definition and criteria. In Silman AJ, Hochberg MC (eds): Epidemiology of the Rheumatic Diseases. Oxford, Oxford University Press, 1993, pp 192-219

5. Douvas A: Pathogenesis: serologic correlates. In Clements PJ, Furst DE (eds): Systemic Sclerosis. Baltimore, Williams & Wilkins, 1996, pp 175-202

6. Reveille JD, Owerbach D, Goldstein R, Moreda R, Isern RA, Arnett FA: Association of polar amino acids at position 26 of the HLA-DQB1 first domain with the anticentromere autoantibody response in systemic sclerosis (scleroderma). J Clin Invest 89:1209-12, 1992

7. Reveille JD, Durban E, MacLeod-St. Clair MJ, Goldstein R, Moreda R, Altman RD, Arnett FA: Association of amino acid sequences in the HLA-DQB1 first domain with the antitopoisomerase I autoantibody response in scleroderma (progressive systemic sclerosis). J Clin Invest 90:973-80, 1992

8. Prescott RJ, Freemont AJ, Jones CJP, Hoyland J, Fielding P: Sequential dermal microvascular and perivascular changes in the development of scleroderma. J Pathol 166:255-263, 1992

9. Claman HN, Giorno RC, Seibold JR: Endothelial and fibroblast activation in scleroderma: the myth of the "uninvolved skin." Arthritis Rheum 34:1495-501, 1991

10. Rodnan GP, Lipinski E, Luksick J. Skin thickness and collagen content on progressive systemic sclerosis (scleroderma) and localized scleroderma. Arthritis Rheum 22:130-140, 1979

11. LeRoy EC, McGuire M, Chen N: Increased collagen synthesis by scleroderma fibroblasts in vitro. A possible defect in the regulation or activation of the scleroderma fibroblast. J Clin Invest 54:880-9, 1974

12. White B: Pathogenesis: immune aspects. In Clements PJ, Furst DE (eds): Systemic Sclerosis. Baltimore, Williams & Wilkins, 1996, pp 229-250

13. Emerit I: Chromosomal breakage in systemic sclerosis and related disorders. Dermatologica 153:145-56, 1976

14. Yurovsky VV, Sutton PA, Schulze DH, Wigely FM, Wise RA, White B: Expansion of selected Vδ1+ γ/δ T cells in systemic sclerosis patients. J Immunol 153:881-91, 1994

15. Klareskog L, Gustafsson R, Schneyius A, Hallgren R: Increased expression of platelet derived growth factor type ß receptors in the skin of patients with systemic sclerosis. Arthritis Rheum 33:1534-41, 1990

16. Kahari V-M, Sandberg M, Kalimo H, Vuorio T, Vuorio E: Identification of fibroblasts responsible for increased collagen production in localized scleroderma by in situ hybridization. J Invest Dermatol 90:664-70, 1988

17. Higley H, Persichitte K, Chu S, Waegell W, Vancheeswaran R, Black C: Immunocytochemical localization and serologic detection of transforming growth factor β1. Association with type I procollagen and inflammatory cell markers in diffuse and limited systemic sclerosis, morphea, and Raynaud's phenomenon. Arthritis Rheum 37:278-88, 1994

18. Fleishmajer R, Perlish JS, West JP: Ultrastructure of cutaneous cellular infiltrates in scleroderma. Arch Dermatol 113:1161-6, 1977

19. Whiteside TL, Ferrarini M, Hebda P, Buchingham RB: Heterogeneous synthetic phenotype of cloned scleroderma fibroblasts may be due to aberrant regulation in the synthesis of connective tissue. Arthritis Rheum 31:1221-9, 1988

B. CLINICAL FEATURES

Systemic sclerosis (scleroderma) is a chronic multisystem disease (1). The initial symptoms are typically nonspecific and include Raynaud's phenomenon, lack of energy or fatigue, and musculoskeletal complaints. These symptoms may persist for weeks or months before other signs emerge. The first specific clinical clue to suggest a diagnosis of scleroderma is skin thickening that begins as swelling or "puffiness" of the fingers and hands. The subsequent course of clinical events is highly variable, but significant skin, pulmonary, cardiac, gastrointestinal, or renal disease can occur.

Scleroderma is classified into subsets of disease defined by the degree of clinically involved skin (Table 20B-1). Patients with "limited" scleroderma have cutaneous thickening of the distal limbs without truncal involvement. The CREST syndrome of Calcinosis, Raynaud's phenomenon, Esophageal dysmotility, Sclerodactyly, and Telangiectasia falls within the limited subset of scleroderma. Patients with "diffuse" disease have skin thickening over distal and proximal limb sites and/or the trunk. Criteria have been established for a diagnosis of systemic sclerosis that require skin thickening proximal to the metacarpophalangeal joints or signs of digital ischemia and pulmonary fibrosis (See Appendix I). The criteria capture most patients with scleroderma, but exclude some patients with limited scleroderma or the CREST syndrome.

Patients with limited scleroderma usually have Raynaud's phenomenon for years (often 5 to 10 years) before other signs of scleroderma are seen. They are less likely than patients with diffuse disease to develop severe lung, heart, or kidney disease, although all can occur. Most patients with limited scleroderma gradually develop features of the CREST syndrome. Subcutaneous calcinosis presents as small, localized, hard masses on fingers, forearms, or other pressure points (Fig. 20B-1). Telangiectasia frequently become numerous, particularly on the face, mucous membranes, and hands. Pulmonary hypertension, sometimes in the absence of severe pulmonary fibrosis, and large-artery occlusive disease manifested by digital ischemia and amputation are serious manifestations of limited scleroderma (2).

In contrast to limited scleroderma, patients with diffuse scleroderma have a short interval between the onset of Raynaud's phenomenon and significant other organ involvement. Inflammatory signs that appear in the early stages include edematous skin, painful joints and muscles, and, in some cases, tendon friction rubs. Relatively rapid progressive skin changes occur during the first months of disease and continue for approximately 2 to 3 years, after which the skin tends to soften and either thin or return toward normal texture. Severe fibrosis of the skin causes irreversible atrophic changes and tethering to deeper tissue. This is particularly a problem in the fingers and hands and causes significant disability (Fig. 20B-2).

The overall course of scleroderma is highly variable, and disease activity is difficult to measure. However, once a remission occurs, relapse is uncommon. The diffuse form of the disease generally has a worse prognosis with a 10-year survival rate of approximately 40%–60%, compared with a ≥70% 10-year survival rate in the limited form (3). Car-diopulmonary disease is the leading cause of death. Factors suggesting a poor prognosis include diffuse skin involvement, late age of onset at disease, African or Native American race, the presence of tendon rubs, pulmonary function demonstrating a diffusing capacity <40% predicted, or significant renal disease.

Serologic studies can help predict clinical features and survival. Scleroderma patients with anticentromere antibody associated with CREST syndrome have a relatively good prognosis, but they may develop pulmonary hypertension, digital amputation, or biliary cirrhosis. Anti-RNA polymerase increases the risk of cardiac or renal disease, and antifibrillarin is associated with heart and lung involvement; the presence of either of these antibodies predicts a poor prognosis. Patients with antitopoisomerase and anti-

(Table 20B-1)
Subsets of systemic sclerosis

Diffuse Cutaneous Scleroderma
- Proximal skin thickening involving face/neck, trunk, and symmetrically the fingers, hands, arms and legs
- Rapid onset of disease following appearance of Raynaud's phenomenon
- Significant visceral disease: lung, heart, gastrointestinal, or kidney
- Associated with antinucleolar antibodies and absence of anticentromere antibody
- Variable disease course but overall poor prognosis: survival 40%–60% at 10 years

Limited Cutaneous Scleroderma
- Skin thickness limited to symmetrical change of fingers, distal arms, legs, and face/neck.
- Progression of disease after onset of Raynaud's phenomenon
- Late visceral disease with prominent hypertension and digital amputation
- CREST syndrome
- Association with anticentromere antibody
- Relatively good prognosis: survival ≥70% at 10 years

Overlap Syndromes
- Diffuse or limited scleroderma with typical features of one or more of the other connective tissues diseases
- Mixed connective tissue disease: features of systemic lupus erythematosus, scleroderma, polymyositis, rheumatoid arthritis, and presence of anti-U$_1$ RNP

Undefined Connective Tissue Disease
- Patients with features of systemic sclerosis (scleroderma) who do not have definite clinical or laboratory findings to make a diagnosis

Localized Scleroderma
- Morphea: plaques of fibrotic skin and subcutaneous tissue without systemic disease
- Linear scleroderma: longitudinal fibrotic bands that occur predominantly on extremities and involve skin and deeper tissues

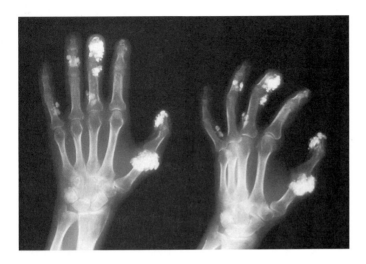

(Figure 20B-1)
Radiograph demonstrating subcutaneous calcinosis on the fingers of a patient with CREST syndrome.

U1-RNP have intermediate survival and a high risk of pulmonary disease.

RAYNAUD'S PHENOMENON

Patients with Raynaud's phenomenon experience of cold hands and feet associated with color changes of the skin of the digits (4). These symptoms appear suddenly as attacks that are triggered by cold temperature or emotional stress. Closure of the muscular digital arteries, precapillary arterioles, and arteriovenous shunts of the skin in response to temperature and neural signals cause skin pallor, followed by cyanosis. Reversal of the vasospastic period generally occurs 10 to 15 minutes after the stimulus has ended (rewarming); the digits then return to normal color, have a blushed appearance, or appear mottled.

Surveys have found that 4%–15% of the general population have symptoms of Raynaud's phenomenon (5). However, in most instances it is mild and not associated with either structural vascular changes or ischemic tissue damage. When the attacks are intense or have an onset after the age

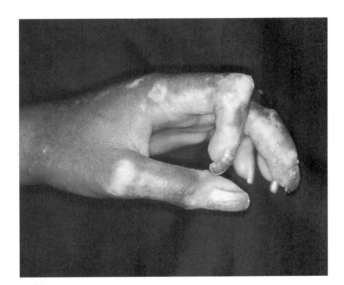

(Figure 20B-2)
Severe scleroderma of the hand with fibrosis of the skin causing finger contractures, depigmentation, and ulceration.

of 20, there is a greater likelihood that Raynaud's phenomenon is secondary to an underlying medical problem (Table 20B-2). Enlarged capillary loops and loss of normal capillaries in the nailfold of the digits are helpful physical signs to distinguish scleroderma from primary Raynaud's phenomenon. Other features of primary Raynaud's phenomenon include normal findings on physical examination and laboratory testing.

More than 90% of scleroderma patients have Raynaud's phenomenon that is associated with tissue fibrosis of the fingers and loss of digital pad (sclerodactyly), digital ulceration, and, on occasion, ischemic demarcation and digital amputation. In addition to the vasospasm of Raynaud's phenomenon, vascular occlusion occurs because of fibrosis of the intimal layer of the vessel, platelet activation, perturbation of the clotting cascade, and fibrin deposition. In scleroderma, there is good evidence of "systemic" Raynaud's phenomenon, a generalized vasospastic disorder involving vasculopathy of the terminal arterial circulation of the lungs, kidneys, and heart.

SKIN

In the earliest stage (the edematous stage) the skin appears mildly inflamed with nonpitting edema and, in some cases, erythema. Pruritus and swelling are associated with

(Table 20B-2)
Causes of secondary Raynaud's phenomenon

Connective Tissue Diseases
    Polymyositis and dermatomyositis
    Scleroderma
    Sjögren's syndrome
    Systemic lupus erythematosus
    Systemic vasculitis
    Undifferentiated connective tissue disease
Drugs and Toxins
    Amphetamines
    Clonidine
    Ergotamines
    Vinblastine and bleomycin
    Vinyl chloride exposure
Structural Arterial Disease
    Athero-emboli
    Atherosclerosis
    Thoracic outlet syndrome
    Thromboangiitis obliterans (Buerger's disease)
Occupational Disorders
    Hand-arm vibration syndrome
    Hypothenar hammer syndrome
Hematologic Diseases
    Cold agglutinin disease
    Cryoglobulinemia
    Paraproteinemia
Other
    Hypothyroidism
    Paraneoplastic
    Post-frostbite
    Reflex sympathetic dystrophy

skin lymphocyte infiltration, fibroblast and mast cell activation, and local release of a variety of cytokines into the skin. Collagen deposition from activated fibroblasts thickens the dermis, and normal skin and its appendages gradually become damaged. The patient feels progressive tightening of the skin and decreased flexibility. In the diffuse form of disease, the skin changes are widespread, and varying degrees of hypo- and hyperpigmentary changes may occur, giving the skin a "salt and pepper" appearance.

As scleroderma progresses into the fibrotic stage, the skin becomes more thickened, and severe surface drying provokes pruritus. This stage may persist and progress over a 1- to 3-year period or longer. Finally, inflammation and further fibrosis seem to cease as the atrophic stage begins. The skin then becomes atrophic and thinned with tethering secondary to fibrotic tissue binding to underlying structures. Painful ulcerations can occur at sites of flexion contractures (eg, the proximal interphalangeal joints) (Fig. 20B-2). In this late stage, other areas of the skin gradually remodel and may appear clinically normal, especially the trunk and proximal limbs.

Subcutaneous calcinosis composed of amphorous calcium hydroxyapatite is more prominent in limited scleroderma (Fig. 20B-1). This crystalline material can ulcerate the skin or cause recurrent episodes of local inflammation that mimic infection. Often, digital lesions seen in scleroderma include fissures, paronychia, and both traumatic and ischemic ulceration.

MUSCULOSKELETAL

Nonspecific musculoskeletal complaints such as arthralgias and myalgias are one of the earliest symptoms of scleroderma. Frank arthritis can also occur, but pain and stiffness over joints are generally greater than objective inflammatory signs would predict. Discomfort can extend along tendons and into muscles of the arms and legs. Pain on motion of the ankle, wrist, knee, or elbow may be accompanied by a coarse friction rub caused by inflammation and fibrosis of the tendon sheath or adjacent tissues. These rubs are almost always seen in diffuse skin disease and may predict a worse overall clinical outcome.

The dominant musculoskeletal problem in late scleroderma is muscle atrophy and muscle weakness (6). Disuse and deconditioning caused by contractures from fibrotic skin and malnutrition are the major causes, but muscle fibrosis associated with a mild elevation in serum creatine kinase may also occur. An "overlap" syndrome with an inflammatory myopathy typical of dermatomyositis or polymyositis is frequently overlooked because of the severity of the other more obvious causes of weakness. Myopathy secondary to drugs (e.g., corticosteroids, D-penicillamine) used in the treatment of scleroderma can mimic inflammatory or scleroderma muscle disease.

PULMONARY

Some impairment of lung function is almost universal in scleroderma (7). However, it is often clinically silent until later stages of the disease when it may become a major cause of morbidity and mortality. The most common initial symptom is shortness of breath on exertion, and later a nonproductive cough can develop. Chest pain is generally not caused by scleroderma lung disease, but may occur because of another process such as musculoskeletal pain, reflux esophagitis, pleurisy, or pericarditis.

Impaired gas exchange in the lung is caused by fibrosing alveolitis proceeding to interstitial fibrosis or a vasculopathy of pulmonary vessels characterized by intimal layer fibrosis and smooth muscle hypertrophy. Although most patients have both pathologic processes, pulmonary interstitial fibrosis is more likely to be severe in patients with diffuse skin disease, while isolated pulmonary hypertension is associated with the CREST syndrome.

Pulmonary disease is best detected by pulmonary function testing or high resolution computed tomography. Chest radiographs are relatively insensitive, but may show bilateral lower lobe fibrosis of the lung parenchyma. Pulmonary function testing usually demonstrates low lung volumes, causing a restrictive ventilatory defect. Frequently, an isolated low diffusing capacity is seen either as a manifestation of early restrictive disease or as the first signs of pulmonary vascular disease. Pulmonary hypertension can also be detected by echocardiographic studies before physical findings become obvious. The presence of clinical signs of pulmonary hypertension and/or a low diffusing capacity (less than 40% predicted) is associated with high mortality.

The course of lung disease in scleroderma is highly variable; the majority of patients have an early but modest decline in lung function and then follow a stable course or improve (8). Approximately one-third have a more severe progressive decline in lung function that continues for 4 to 5 years and then appears to stabilize. Less common problems of the lung include aspiration pneumonia secondary to severe esophageal dysfunction, respiratory failure from muscle weakness, pulmonary hemorrhage, and pneumothorax. Scleroderma patients also have an increased risk of lung cancer.

GASTROINTESTINAL

Difficulties with the gastrointestinal tract are some of the most common problems encountered in scleroderma and are present in both diffuse and limited disease (9). A small oral aperture (Fig. 20B-3), dry mucosal membranes, and periodontal disease can lead to problems with chewing foods, loss of teeth, and poor nutrition. Dysphagia with heartburn are the most common gastrointestinal symptoms found in scleroderma, but severe esophageal reflux and esophagitis can also occur with few symptoms. Studies with esophageal

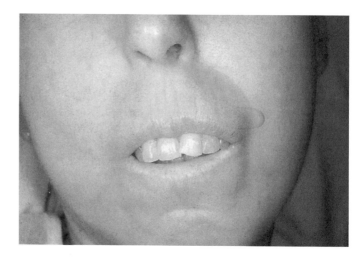

(Figure 20B-3)
Scleroderma has caused perioral fibrosis and a tight pursed-lip appearance with small oral aperture. Facial telangiectasia are also present.

manometry have correlated loss of secondary peristalsis in the distal esophagus with loss of normal esophageal clearance and serious reflux. Untreated or persistent esophagitis can lead to erosions and bleeding, stricture, Barrett's metaplasia, or possibly adenocarcinoma. Other uncommonly recognized complications of esophageal disease include aspiration, unexplained coughing, hoarseness, and atypical chest pain.

In the early stages of scleroderma, abnormal function of the smooth muscle in the distal two-thirds of the esophagus is likely secondary to neuromuscular dysfunction; later, there is smooth muscle atrophy and fibrosis, as well as excess collagen deposition in the lamina propria and submucosa. Esophageal disease is associated with a low pressure in the lower esophageal sphincter and poor gastric emptying. Delayed emptying of the stomach associated with retention of solid foods aggravates reflux and is also a frequent cause of bloating, nausea, vomiting, and early satiety.

Dysmotility of the small intestine may be asymptomatic or it can cause serious chronic pseudo-obstruction of the intestine, presenting with severe distension, abdominal pain, and vomiting. Mild abdominal distension, crampy abdominal pain, diarrhea, weight loss, and malnutrition can also be consequences of malabsorption caused by bacterial overgrowth in stagnant intestinal fluids. Occasionally patients with advanced bowel disease have pneumatosis cystoides intestinalis caused by intestinal gas dissecting into the bowel wall or, on occasion, into the peritoneal cavity mimicking a ruptured bowel. Although the presence of pneumatosis cystoides intestinalis is a poor prognostic sign, medical (not surgical) management is indicated.

The large intestine and rectum are also affected by scleroderma. As a consequence of muscular atrophy of the large bowel wall, asymptomatic wide mouth diverticula unique to scleroderma are commonly found in the transverse and descending colon (Fig. 20B-4). Fecal incontinence that is difficult to manage can be a consequence of fibrosis of the rectal sphincters.

CARDIAC

The clinical manifestations of scleroderma heart disease are quite variable, usually subtle in expression, and often not seen until late in the course of the disease (10). Symptoms include dyspnea on exertion, palpitations, and, less frequently, chest discomfort. Pathologic studies of the scleroderma heart and sensitive diagnostic testing have documented that the myocardium, myocardial blood vessels, and the pericardium are commonly involved—particularly in patients with diffuse disease. Overt clinical signs of any cardiac disease are a poor prognostic sign.

Patchy fibrosis throughout the entire myocardium that is unrelated to extramural coronary artery disease is characteristic of scleroderma. Areas of contraction band necrosis are thought to occur as a consequence of hypoxia/reperfusion injury due to vasospasm of distal coronary vessels. Supporting this theory of vascular heart disease is the finding, during thallium scintigraphy, of perfusion defects that increase in number during cold provocation of a Raynaud's attack. Despite these findings, a decline in left ventricular ejection fraction is a late clinical manifestation.

Small and large pericardial effusions can be demonstrated by echocardiography in 30%–40% of primarily asymptomatic scleroderma patients. Clinically overt pericarditis is uncommon. Although a large pericardial effusion is considered a

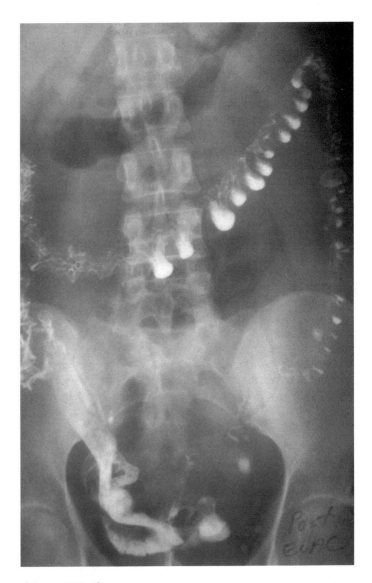

(Figure 20B-4)
Wide-mouth diverticuli of the colon is seen on this barium study of a patient with scleroderma.

poor prognostic sign, cardiac tamponade is a rare event. Electrocardiograms often demonstrate conduction system disease and arrhythmias that are usually clinically silent.

RENAL

Although pathologic disease of the kidney is almost always present in scleroderma, the most important clinical manifestation is accelerated hypertension and/or rapidly progressive renal failure: the scleroderma renal crisis (11). Approximately 80% of cases of renal crisis occur within the first 4 to 5 years of disease, usually in patients with diffuse disease. Blood pressure is usually abnormal (>150/90), but occasionally a normotensive crisis can occur. Laboratory data demonstrate normal or high creatinine levels, proteinuria, or microscopic hematuria. Poorer outcomes are more likely in men, patients with an older age of onset, and those who present with creatinine greater than 3 mg/dl. Risk factors for renal crisis include diffuse skin disease, new unexplained anemia, and the presence of anti-RNA polymerase III antibody. Scleroderma patients may have reduced creatinine clearance, proteinuria, microscopic hematuria, and nonmalignant hypertension, but often, another cause for these abnormalities is discovered.

OTHER SIGNS

A recent survey has found that nearly 50% of patients with scleroderma have symptoms of depression, often major depression that is responsive to treatment (12). Sexual dysfunction is also common in scleroderma. Impotence among male patients is usually secondary to organic neurovascular disease. The sicca complex is a frequent problem, with associated Sjögren's syndrome accounting for the majority of cases. Aggressive dental care and frequent use of topical natural tears to protect the cornea are important. Neuropathy from carpal tunnel syndrome is seen and may require surgical release. Trigeminal neuralgia has been reported and may respond to tricyclic antidepressants or a neuroleptic drug. Hypothyroidism secondary to thyroid fibrosis or autoimmune thyroiditis is a common problem. Liver disease is infrequent, but primary biliary cirrhosis has been associated with the CREST syndrome.

SCLERODERMA-LIKE DISORDERS
Localized Scleroderma

Localized scleroderma is an uncommon fibrotic reaction limited to the skin and adjacent structures that does not involve other organ systems (13). It is seen more frequently among children and young women (14). Localized scleroderma has been classified into two major groups: morphea and linear scleroderma. Morphea presents in different ways, including an isolated 1–15 cm plaque lesion and generalized morphea (multiple lesions). Some patients have both linear scleroderma and morphea lesions.

Localized scleroderma usually presents as a nonspecific area of erythema and pain that then expands with an ivory-like fibrotic center surrounded by a margin of hyperpigmentation with a lilac appearance. The lesion is characterized by infiltration of lymphocytes, mast cells, plasma cells, and eosinophils with excess collagen deposition extending into the dermis, the subcutaneous fat, and, in some forms, deeper structures. Lesions are distributed asymmetrically, or they can become confluent in generalized morphea. Morphea lesions remain active for weeks to several years, but spontaneous softening leaving a pigmented area is the rule.

Linear scleroderma is more common on the lower extremities. It appears as a nondermatomal fibrotic band that infiltrates skin, subcutaneous fat, fascia, and muscle. The fibrotic band disrupts normal bone growth and can cause disabling joint contractures. Midline facial involvement has been termed "en coup de sabre" to describe a deformity similar to the wound of a sword. This lesion may progress over years, causing severe facial hemiatrophy and linear hair loss.

The cause of localized scleroderma is unknown, but genetic, infectious, and autoimmune mechanisms have been suggested. Autoantibodies are seen frequently in localized scleroderma, usually antinuclear antibody and antibody to single-stranded DNA and histone. No treatment has been proved to alter the natural course of localized scleroderma, but moderate doses of systemic or locally injected corticosteroids, D-penicillamine, and, recently, photochemotherapy with 8-methoxypsoralen have been reported helpful.

Environmentally Associated Disorders

An association between silica (silicon dioxide) exposure and diffuse scleroderma has been reported in stone masons, gold miners, and coal miners. The clinical features of these individuals are the same as idiopathic scleroderma with typical skin changes, Raynaud's phenomenon, and pulmonary fibrosis. Antitopoisomerase has been reported in approximately 50% of these cases.

The association of silicone (a synthetic polymer containing silicon) and scleroderma or another connective tissue disease has been suggested by anecdotal case reports of autoimmune disease in women who were exposed to silicone following breast augmentation. However, recent case-control studies of large populations of women and patients with scleroderma have not found any association between breast implants and scleroderma or other connective tissue disease (15).

Occupational acro-osteolysis is a scleroderma-like illness that is associated with industrial exposure to vinyl chloride. Association of typical scleroderma has also been reported following exposure to organic solvents (eg, trichlorethylene, perchlorethylene) that have a similar structure to vinyl chloride. Exposure to amines in epoxy resins have also been implicated in causing a scleroderma-like illness.

Diffuse Fasciitis with Eosinophilia

Diffuse fasciitis with eosinophilia (DFE; also called eosinophilic fasciitis or Shulman's syndrome) occurs sporadically and mimics scleroderma with swelling, stiffness, and decreased flexibility of the limbs associated with thickening of the subcutaneous tissue (16). Although the process can be widespread and involves the trunk and limbs, the fingers, hands, and face are usually spared. Raynaud's phenomenon, visceral involvement, and microvascular disease are absent, thus distinguishing DFE from scleroderma. Fibrosis puckers the overlying tissues ("peau d' orange" skin) and entraps subcutaneous veins, but the overlying skin still wrinkles. A diagnosis of DFE is dependent on histologic findings from a deep biopsy that includes skin, subcutaneous tissue, and muscle. Inflammation in the subcutaneous tissue is characterized by mononuclear cell infiltration and, in some cases, striking tissue eosinophilia. Autoantibodies are usually absent, but a striking peripheral eosinophilia and hypergammaglobulinemia is typical.

The cause of DFE is unknown, although approximately 30% of case series have reported the onset of DFE following vigorous exercise. There has also been a temporal association with various hematologic conditions including aplastic anemia, myelomonocytic and chronic lymphocytic leukemia, thrombocytopenia, monoclonal gammopathy, myeloproliferative syndrome, and lymphomas. DFE has been seen in late graft-versus-host disease and in association with some solid tumors. Toxin(s) and drug exposure have also been suggested as triggers for DFE.

The natural course of DFE is not well defined, but patients seem to spontaneously regress or remain unchanged for years. Responses have been seen with corticosteroid treatment, hydroxycholoquine, methotrexate, D-penicillamine, and cimetidine. Physical therapy and careful vigilance for an associated hematologic problem are highly recommended.

Epidemic Scleroderma-like Disorders

Eosinophilia-myalgia syndrome (EMS) and toxic oil syndrome (TOS) are toxin-induced disorders that mimic scleroderma (17,18). Both syndromes are associated with subcutaneous tissue fibrosis, which provides indirect evidence that environmental toxins could cause idiopathic scleroderma. EMS was first reported in 1989 in association with the use of the amino acid L-tryptophan for conditions such as insomnia and depression. It is now known that certain batches of the L-tryptophan were contaminated with several potential toxins including 1,1'-ethylidenebis (L-tryptophan) (EBT) and 3-(phenyl-amino)alanine. EMS presented as a multisystem disease with intense myalgias, arthralgias, fever, and a papular rash associated with eosinophilia. Subcutaneous edema with woody induration occurred that is similar to DFE and mimics scleroderma. A chronic phase of EMS is now recognized and is characterized by scleroderma-like skin changes, recurrent myalgias, paresthesias with peripheral neuropathy, neurocognitive dysfunction, and chronic fatigue. Treatment with corticosteroids appears to have helped in the acute inflammatory phase, but it is not clear that any agent alters the course or the chronic phase of EMS. A variety of agents have been used including nonsteroidal antiinflammatory drugs, D-penicillamine, methotrexate, cyclophosphamide, azathioprine, and cyclosprin A.

An epidemic of toxic oil syndrome (TOS) occurred in 1981 following individuals' ingestion of rapeseed oil denatured with aniline. TOS causes widespread vasculopathy in almost every organ, which is characterized by inflammatory cells in the vessel wall and subintimal fibrosis. After an acute illness characterized by pulmonary infiltrates and myalgias, patients developed a chronic disease with Raynaud's phenomenon, muscle atrophy, fatigue, and musculoskeletal pain. Biopsy material from both EMS and TOS patients has demonstrated the presence of the profibrotic cytokines transforming growth factor β and platelet-derived growth factor AA, which suggests that toxins can induce the production of these mediators of fibrosis. While corticosteroids appear to help the acute phase of TOS, no therapy has been proven to alter the course of the disease.

Other Scleroderma-Like Disorders

Scleredema can be a transient illness of unknown cause or a fibrotic condition of the skin in association with insulin-dependent diabetes. The distribution of scleredema is typically the neck, shoulder girdle, and upper back, with relative sparing of the hands and the absence of Raynaud's phenomenon. Sclerodactyly and fibrosis of the palmar fascia can also occur in insulin-dependent diabetes, particularly the juvenile onset type. Scleroderma-like skin changes have been reported in a variety of other disorders including the carcinoid syndrome, myeloma or paraproteinemia, scleromyxedema (papular mucinosis), chronic graft-versus-host disease, porphyria cutanea tarda, Werner's syndrome, progeria, phenylketonuria, bleomycin exposure, local lipodystrophies, and POEMS syndrome (*P*lasma cell dyscrasia, *P*olyneuropathy, *O*rganomegaly, *E*ndocrinopathy, *M*onoclonal spikes, and *S*cleroderma-like skin changes) (19).

FREDRICK M. WIGLEY, MD

1. Clements PJ, Furst DE: Systemic Sclerosis, Baltimore, Williams and Wilkins, 1996

2. Wigley FM, Wise RA, Miller R, Needleman BW, Spence RJ: Anticentromere antibody as a predictor of digital ischemic loss in patients with systemic sclerosis. Arth Rheum 35:688-693, 1992

3. Medsger TA Jr.: Epidemiology of systemic sclerosis. Clin Dermatol 12:207-216, 1994

4. Wigley FM: Is Raynaud's an isolated phenomenon? Contemporary Intern Med 7:43-56, 1995

5. Maricq HR, Carpentier PH, Weinrich MC, Keil JE, Franco A, Dronet P, Proncot OCM, Maines MU: Geographic variation in the prevalence of Raynaud's phenomenon: Charleston, SC, USA vs. Tarentaise, Savoie France. J Rheumatol 20:70-76, 1993

6. Clements PJ, Furst DE, Carapion DS, Bohan A, Harris R, Levy J, Paulus HE: Muscle disease in systemic sclerosis. Diagnostic and therapeutic considerations. Arth Rheum 21:62-71, 1978

7. Black CM, DuBois RM: Organ involvement: pulmonary. In Clements PJ, Furst DE (eds): Systemic Sclerosis. Baltimore, Williams and Wilkins, 1996, pp 299-331

8. Schneider PD, Wise, RA, Hochberg MC, Wigley FM: Serial pulmonary function test in systemic sclerosis. Am J Med 73:385-394, 1982

9. Sjögren RW: Gastrointestinal motility in scleroderma. Arth Rheum 37:1265-1282, 1994

10. Clements PJ, Furst DE: Heart involvement in systemic sclerosis. Clin Dermatol 12:267-275, 1994

11. Steen VD: Renal involvement in systemic sclerosis. Clin Dermatol 12:253-258, 1994

12. Roca RP, Wigley FM: Psychosocial aspects in systemic sclerosis. In Clements PJ, Furst DE (eds): Systemic Sclerosis. Baltimore, Williams and Wilkins, 1996, pp 501-511

13. Dehen L, Roujeau JC, Cosnes A, Revuz J: Internal involvement in localized scleroderma. Medicine 73:241-245, 1994

14. Vziel Y, Kvafchik B, Silverman ED, Thorner PS, Laxer RM: Localized scleroderma in childhood: a report of 30 cases. Semin Arth Rheum 23:328-240, 1994

15. Gabriel SE, O'Fallon WM, Kurland LT, Beard CM, Woods JE, Melton LJ III: Risk of connective tissue diseases and other diseases after breast implantation. N Engl J Med 330:1697-1702, 1994

16. Lakhanpal S, Ginsburg WW, Michet CJ, Doyle JA, Moore SB: Eosinophilia fasciitis: clinical spectrum and therapeutic response in 52 cases. Semin Arth Rheum 17:221-231, 1988

17. Silver RM: The eosinophilia-myalgia syndrome. Clin Dermatol 12:457-465, 1994

18. Kaufman LD, Krupp LB: Eosinophilia-myalgia syndrome, toxic-oil syndrome and diffuse fasciitis and eosinophilia. Curr Opin Rheumatol 7:560-567, 1995

19. Jablonska S, Blaszczyk: Differential diagnosis of scleroderma-like disorders. In Clements PJ, Furst DE (eds): Systemic Sclerosis. Baltimore, Williams and Wilkins, 1996, pp 99-120

C. TREATMENT

Therapy in systemic sclerosis has been a major challenge. The relative rarity of the disease makes performing double-blind, controlled trials difficult. Moreover, systemic sclerosis has a wide spectrum of clinical manifestations and severity as well as a variable course. Spontaneous improvement occurs frequently, rendering interpretation of therapeutic interventions difficult without untreated comparison groups. Only recently have objective measures been used to quantify changes in the disease. These techniques include methods of measuring changes in skin thickening (1), pulmonary function, cardiac contractility, and renal function.

DISEASE-MODIFYING DRUGS

Many drugs are used in systemic sclerosis, but no single agent has been proved convincingly effective. Potential sites of drug actions are shown in Fig. 20C-1. Although vascular abnormalities are believed to be important in the pathogenesis, aspirin and dipyridamole, which alter platelet function, are ineffective. Ketanserin, an experimental serotonin antagonist, reduces the frequency and severity of Raynaud's phenomenon and promotes the healing of digital ulcers, but the drug has no effect on skin thickening or internal organ damage. Iloprost, a prostacyclin analog, is a promising new agent for Raynaud's phenomenon and digital ulcers (2).

Immune mechanisms (lymphocytic infiltration, lymphokine stimulation of fibroblasts, and production of au-

toantibodies) have all been considered potential sites for intervention in systemic sclerosis. The immunosuppressive agents chlorambucil and 5-fluorouracil have been evaluated in double-blind controlled trials and found to be ineffective (3,4). Methotrexate and cyclosporin A (5) have been studied in several small series with promising results, but nephrotoxicity of the latter may be a limiting factor.

Penicillamine, an immunomodulating agent that also interferes with cross-linking of collagen, is the most widely used drug in treating systemic sclerosis. A large retrospective study showed significant improvement in skin thickening after 2 years of therapy and improved 5-year survival compared with untreated patients (6). A reevaluation several years later confirmed these results (Fig. 20C-2). Clinical studies of interferon gamma (7), which down-regulates fibroblast proliferation and collagen production in vitro, and colchicine, which affects procollagen transport and secretion by fibroblasts, have shown variable but not exciting results. Ketotifen, a mast cell stabilizing agent, prevents skin fibrosis in the tight skin mouse, but a double-blind study of patients with systemic sclerosis failed to show any significant changes (8).

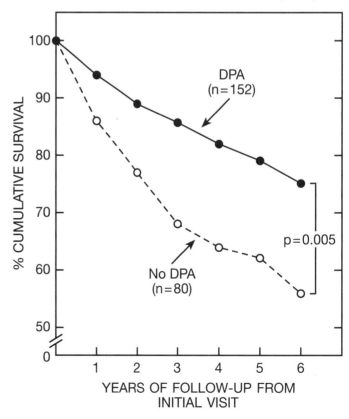

(Figure 20C-1)
Pathogenesis of systemic sclerosis and potential sites of drug use.

(Figure 20C-2)
Comparison of patients treated with D-penicillamine versus untreated patients; shows improved 5-year survival rate of treated patients.

MANAGEMENT OF AFFECTED ORGAN SYSTEMS

Raynaud's Phenomenon

The most common symptom in patients with systemic sclerosis is Raynaud's phenomenon. Total abstinence from smoking, avoiding cold exposure, keeping the entire body (not just hands) warm, and biofeedback training (9) are common sense measures that are usually effective for mild to moderate symptoms. When Raynaud's phenomenon becomes complicated by the occurrence of digital tip ulcers or when it interferes with daily activities, the use of vasodilators, particularly the calcium channel blockers, is recommended. These drugs, especially nifedipine, which relaxes vascular smooth muscle, are very effective in decreasing the frequency and severity of Raynaud's phenomenon in double-blind studies (10). Slow-release preparations of calcium channel blockers are better tolerated and less likely to cause hypotensive episodes. Other agents including amlodipine, prazosin, and topical nitroglycerin have also been useful in some patients.

Treatment of digital tip ulcers includes soaking the fingers in antiseptic fluid such as half-strength hydrogen peroxide, air drying, covering only the ulcer with antibiotic ointment, and applying a bandage. This occlusive type of dressing is particularly helpful with large uninfected ulcers. Oral anti-staphylococcal antibiotics should be given for an infected ulcer. For deeper infections, surgical debridement of devitalized tissue and intravenous antibiotics may be necessary; amputation is the last resort.

Skin Involvement

Local skin care includes avoiding excessive bathing, which dries skin, and using moisturizing creams containing lanolin. Pruritus is often a serious problem, particularly early in the course of diffuse disease. There is no effective treatment, but fortunately this complaint almost always disappears with time. Calcinosis cannot be prevented and the deposits cannot be dissolved despite encouraging reports using probenecid, warfarin, or cardizen. However, the inflammatory reaction often associated with hydroxyapatite crystal deposition may be reduced by a brief course of colchicine.

Musculoskeletal Involvement

Joint and tendon sheath involvement is common. Treatment with nonsteroidal anti-inflammatory drugs (NSAIDs) is generally helpful, but relief is often more difficult to achieve than in other connective tissue diseases. In early diffuse disease, tenosynovitis causing tendon rubs can be very painful, and limit joint movement. When NSAIDs are inadequate in controlling pain, low-dose corticosteroids (prednisone less than 10 mg/day) or narcotic analgesics may be necessary. In patients with tenosynovitis, early aggressive physical therapy with emphasis on stretching exercises is very important. However, it is often quite painful, and analgesics are frequently required to maximize a patient's participation in such an exercise program. Dynamic splinting is not effective. Carpal tunnel symptoms, which often appear before systemic sclerosis is diagnosed, can be successfully treated with resting wrist splints and, if necessary, local steroid injections without surgery. Myositis is treated with corticosteroids and, in resistant patients, the addition of methotrexate. The bland fibrotic myopathy of systemic sclerosis is best managed with strengthening and range of motion exercises alone.

Gastrointestinal Symptoms

Esophageal dysmotility most commonly causes heartburn and lower esophageal dysphagia. Adequate relief may be obtained by elevating the head of the bed on 4–8 inch blocks, eating small frequent meals in an upright position, abstaining from nocturnal eating, and using antacids frequently. However, the mainstay of therapy is proton pump blockade with agents such as omeprazole, which completely eliminates heartburn in most patients (11). Calcium channel blockers, which decrease lower esophageal sphincter pressure, and NSAIDs often aggravate reflux symptoms. Prokinetic drugs such as cisapride are used to stimulate esophageal muscle contraction, but these agents have limited effectiveness. Distal esophageal stricture is managed with periodic dilatations. Surgical procedures for reflux have not achieved general acceptance, but new laparoscopic reflux procedures hold some promise.

Primary small-bowel involvement with delayed transit and bacterial overgrowth may cause abdominal distention or bloating, diarrhea, weight loss, and malabsorption. Broad spectrum antibiotics such as ampicillin, tetracycline, trimethoprim–sulfamethoxazole (Bactrim), metronidazole, or ciprofloxacin, given in tandem in 2-week courses or continuously in low doses may produce a dramatic effect on these symptoms. Cisapride may be helpful in this circumstance. Supplemental fat-soluble vitamins and calcium are often required, and patients with serious malnutrition may need hyperalimentation. In patients with clinical signs of bowel obstruction, the initial management should be conservative non-surgical decompression with nasogastric suction.

Cardiopulmonary Involvement

Most patients with pulmonary interstitial disease have a mild, nonprogressive process that does not require treatment. Attempts to reverse advanced, fixed fibrosis have been uniformly unsuccessful. In contrast, inflammatory alveolitis identified by bronchoalveolar lavage or high resolution computed tomography scan may be reversible. The use of corticosteroids and more recently cyclophosphamide (12) has had variable success in altering the progression of lung disease in such patients. Controlled studies are in progress to determine the best therapy. Another option with severe, advanced pulmonary interstitial fibrosis is single- or double-lung transplantation.

Isolated pulmonary arterial hypertension without significant interstitial fibrosis has the worst prognosis of all visceral problems in systemic sclerosis. No therapy, including potent vasodilators, anti-inflammatory, or immunosuppressive agents, has been shown to alter the mortality of this complication, which is uniformly fatal within 6 months to 5 years after onset. Intravenous prostacyclin, which improves survival and reduces morbidity in patients with primary pulmonary hypertension (13), is being studied in patients with pulmonary hypertension secondary to systemic sclerosis. Most patients die from arrhythmias due to hypoxia, in situ pulmonary arterial thrombosis, or cor pulmonale due to

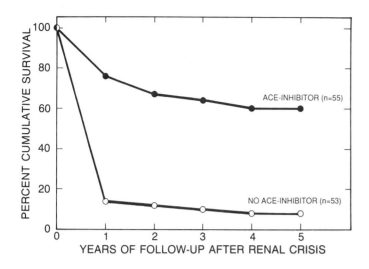

(Figure 20C-3)
Improved survival of scleroderma renal crisis as a result of ACE inhibitors.

tients now have an 80% 1-year and 60% 5-year survival, in contrast to a 15% 1-year survival without the use of ACE inhibitors (14). The key to successful treatment is early detection and rapid normalization of blood pressure. ACE inhibitors are the most reliably effective agents, but other new and potent antihypertensives can be added if needed. In some patients, renal failure ensues despite early and vigorous intervention; however, approximately 50% of patients treated with ACE inhibitors who progress to dialysis have enough improvement in renal function to discontinue dialysis after 6–18 months.

VIRGINIA D. STEEN, MD

1. Clements PJ, Lauchenbruch P, Seibold JR, et al: Inter and intraobserver variability of total skin score thickness score (Modified Rodnan TSS) in systemic sclerosis. J Rheumatol 22:1281-1285,1995
2. Wigley FM, Seibold JR, Wise RA, et al: Intravenous iloprost treatment of Raynaud's phenomenon and ischemic ulcers secondary to systemic sclerosis. J Rheumatol 19:1407-1414, 1992
3. Furst DE, Clements PJ, Hillis S, et al: Immunosuppression with chlorambucil, versus placebo, for scleroderma. Results of a three-year parallel, randomized, double-blind study. Arthritis Rheum 32:584-593, 1989
4. Torres MA, Furst DE: Treatment of generalized systemic sclerosis. Rheum Dis Clin N Am 16:217-241, 1990
5. Zachariae H, Halkier-Sorensen L, Heickendorff L, et al: Cyclosporin A treatment of systemic sclerosis. Br J Dermatol 122:677-681, 1990
6. Steen VD, Medsger TA Jr, Rodan GP: D-penicillamine therapy in progressive systemic sclerosis (scleroderma). Ann Intern Med 97:652-659, 1984
7. Kahan A, Amor B, Menkes CJ, et al: Recombinant interferon-gamma in the treatment of systemic sclerosis. Am J Med 87:273-277, 1989
8. Gruber BL, Kaufman LD: A double-blind randomized controlled trial of ketotifen versus placebo in early diffuse scleroderma. Arthritis Rheum 34:362-366, 1991
9. Yocum DE, Hodes R, Sundstrom WR, et al: Use of biofeedback training in treatment of Raynaud's disease and phenomenon. J Rheumatol 12:90-93, 1985
10. Finch MB, Dawson J, Johnston GD: The peripheral vascular effects of nifedipine in Raynaud's syndrome associated with scleroderma: a double-blind crossover study. Clin Rheumatol 5:493-498, 1986
11. Olive A, Maddison PJ, Davis M: Treatment of oesophagitis in scleroderma with omeprazole. Br J Rheumatol 28:553, 1989
12. Silver RM, Warrick JH, Kinsella MB, et al: Cyclophosphmide and low-dose prednisone therapy in patients with systemic sclerosis (scleroderma) with interstitial lung disease. J Rheumatol 20:838-844,1993
13. Barst RJ, Rubin LJ, McGoon MD, et al: Survival in primary pulmonary hypertension with long term continuous intravenous prostacyclin. Ann Intern Med 121: 463-4, 1994.
14. Steen VD, Constantino, JP, Shapiro AP, Medsger TA Jr: Outcome of renal crisis in systemic sclerosis: relation to availability of converting enzyme (ACE) inhibitors. Ann Intern Med 113:352-357, 1990

respiratory insufficiency. Supplemental oxygen, anticoagulation (to prevent pulmonary thromboembolism), and control of right-sided heart failure are supportive measures. Combined heart–lung or single lung transplantation is the only other therapeutic option.

Pericarditis, congestive heart failure, and serious arrhythmias are the major cardiac complications in systemic sclerosis. All are treated as they would be in any patient. Mild to moderate pericardial effusions and other asymptomatic cardiac abnormalities are generally not progressive and often require no treatment.

Renal Crisis

In previous decades, renal crisis was the most feared visceral complication of systemic sclerosis. Renal failure was the usual outcome, since there was no effective pharmacologic method of managing the malignant hypertension. With the introduction of angiotensin-converting enzyme (ACE) inhibitors, which are capable of reversing underlying hyperreninemia and controlling hypertension, the outcome of renal crisis has dramatically changed (Fig. 20C-3). Pa-

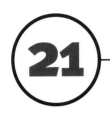

INFLAMMATORY AND METABOLIC DISEASES OF MUSCLE

21

Inflammatory diseases of muscle are a heterogeneous group of disorders characterized by proximal muscle weakness and nonsuppurative inflammation of skeletal muscle. Traditionally, the terms *polymyositis* and *dermatomyositis* have been used to represent these diseases. Today, it is more appropriate to use the term *idiopathic inflammatory myopathy* to describe the entire group and reserve the terms polymyositis and dermatomyositis for more specific conditions or subsets.

CLASSIFICATIONS

The generally accepted criteria for the diagnosis of idiopathic inflammatory myopathies include 1) proximal muscle weakness, 2) elevated serum levels of enzymes derived from skeletal muscle, 3) myopathic changes demonstrated by electromyography, and 4) muscle biopsy evidence of inflammation. The addition of a skin rash (criterion 5) allows the diagnosis of dermatomyositis (1) (see Appendix I). Patients are assigned to categories based on their age or the coexistence of another disease. Today the idiopathic inflammatory myopathies are classified clinically among seven groups based upon clinical criteria (2) (Table 21-1). More recently, circulating myositis-specific autoantibodies have been identified in some patients with idiopathic inflammatory myopathy (3) (Table 21-2). It appears that the presence of these antibodies may define relatively homogeneous groups of patients with regard to disease manifestations and prognosis (4). Although promising, the clinical usefulness of a classification scheme based on these antibodies must be determined by future study.

EPIDEMIOLOGY

The idiopathic inflammatory myopathies are relatively rare diseases. Accurate estimates of their prevalence are difficult to obtain because the diseases are uncommon and lack universally accepted specific diagnostic criteria. Estimates of incidence range from 0.5 to 8.4 cases per million. The incidence appears to be increasing, although this may simply reflect increased awareness and more accurate diagnosis.

Overall, the age at onset for the idiopathic inflammatory myopathies has a bimodal distribution, with peaks between ages 10 and 15 years in children and between 45 and 60 years in adults. However, the mean ages for specific groups differ. The age at onset for myositis associated with another collagen vascular disease is similar to that for the associated condition. Both myositis associated with malignancy and inclusion body myositis are more common after age 50. Women are twice as commonly affected as men, with the exception of inclusion body myositis, which affects men twice as often. Racial differences are apparent. In adults the lowest rates are reported in the Japanese and the highest in blacks. Although no direct relationships have been established between an inflammatory myopathy and a specific genetic marker, several associations have been recognized. The strongest associations are for HLA-B8, HLA-DR3, and DRW52 phenotypes with polymyositis and dermatomyositis in all age groups.

CLINICAL FEATURES

The dominant clinical feature of the idiopathic inflammatory myopathies is symmetric proximal muscle weakness. The weakness can be accompanied by systemic symptoms of fatigue, morning stiffness, and anorexia. Laboratory investigation reveals elevated levels of serum enzymes derived from skeletal muscle, especially creatine kinase (CPK). Electromyography (EMG) demonstrates myopathic changes consistent with inflammation, and muscle

(Table 21-1)

Clinical classification of the idiopathic inflammatory myopathies

Polymyositis
Dermatomyositis
Amyopathic dermatomyositis
Juvenile dermatomyositis
Myositis associated with neoplasia
Myositis associated with collagen vascular disease
Inclusion body myositis

(Table 21-2)

Syndromes associated with myositis-specific autoantibodies

Autoantibody	Clinical Features	Treatment Response
Antisynthetase*	Polymyositis or dermatomyositis with Relatively acute onset Interstitial lung disease Fever Arthritis Raynaud's phenomenon	Moderate with disease persistence
Anti-SRP†	Polymyositis with Very acute onset Often in fall Severe weakness Palpitations	Poor
Anti-Mi2	Dermatomyositis with V sign and shawl sign Cuticular overgrowth	Good

* Anti-Jo1 is the most common myositis-specific autoantibody. Other antisynthetase antibodies are anti-PL-7, anti-PL-12, anti-EJ, and anti-OJ.
† SRP = signal recognition particle.

histology shows inflammatory changes. These manifestations can occur in a variety of combinations or patterns, and no single feature is specific or diagnostic.

Polymyositis in Adults

The clinical features of polymyositis in the adult are representative of all the inflammatory myopathies (5). Adult-onset polymyositis begins insidiously over 3–6 months with no identifiable precipitating event. Shoulder and pelvic girdle muscles are most affected. Weakness of neck muscles, particularly the flexors, occurs in about half the patients, but ocular and facial muscles are virtually never involved. Dysphagia may develop secondary to esophageal dysfunction or cricopharyngeal obstruction. Pharyngeal muscle weakness may cause dysphonia and difficulty swallowing. Myalgias and arthralgias are not uncommon, but severe tenderness and frank synovitis are unusual. Raynaud's phenomenon is sometimes present, and periorbital edema may occur.

Pulmonary and cardiac manifestations may develop at any time during the course of disease. Velcro-like crackles may be heard on chest auscultation with interstitial fibrosis or interstitial pneumonitis. Aspiration pneumonia may complicate the disease course in patients with swallowing difficulties. Cardiac involvement is usually restricted to asymptomatic electrocardiographic abnormalities, although supraventricular arrhythmia, cardiomyopathy, and congestive heart failure may develop.

The CK level is elevated at some time during the course of disease. Normal levels of CK may be found very early in the course of disease, in advanced cases with significant muscle atrophy, or as a result of circulating inhibitors of its activity. Elevation of serum CK level is a reasonable indicator of disease severity. Other muscle enzymes are also elevated in most cases including aldolase, serum glutamic-oxaloacetic transaminase (SGOT), serum glutamic-pyruvic transaminase (SGPT), and lactate dehydrogenase (LDH). The erythrocyte sedimentation rate is normal in 50% of patients with polymyositis and is elevated above 50 mm/hour (Westergren's method) in only 20%.

Electromyography classically reveals the following triad: 1) increased insertional activity, fibrillations, and sharp positive waves; 2) spontaneous, bizarre high-frequency discharges; and 3) polyphasic motor unit potentials of low amplitude and short duration. This triad is characteristic but not diagnostic. The complete triad is seen in approximately 40% of patients. In contrast, 10%–15% of patients may have completely normal EMGs. In a small number of patients, abnormalities are limited to the paraspinal muscles.

In classical polymyositis, muscle fibers are found to be in varying stages of necrosis and regeneration (6). The inflammatory cell infiltrate is predominantly focal and endomysial. T lymphocytes, especially CD8 cytotoxic cells accompanied by a smaller number of macrophages, are found surrounding the invading initially non-necrotic fibers. In other cases, degeneration is seen in the absence of inflammatory cells in the immediate area. Intact fibers may vary in size. Destroyed fibers are replaced by fibrous connective tissue and fat. However, in some cases no fiber necrosis is observed, and the only recognized change is type 2 fiber atrophy.

Dermatomyositis in Adults

The clinical features of dermatomyositis include all those described for polymyositis plus a variety of cutaneous manifestations (7). Rashes may antedate the onset of muscle weakness by more than a year. Skin involvement varies widely from patient to patient. Gottron's papules or sign—symmetric lacy pink or violaceous raised or macular areas typically found on the dorsal aspect of interphalangeal joints, elbows, patellae, and medial malleoli—are considered pathognomonic. Characteristic changes include heliotrope (violaceous) discoloration of the eyelids often with associated periorbital edema; macular erythema of the posterior shoulders and neck (shawl sign), anterior neck and upper chest (V-sign), face, and forehead; dystrophic cuticles; and "mechanic's hands," darkened or dirty-appearing horizontal lines seen across the lateral and palmar aspects of the fingers. Periungual telangiectasias and nailfold capillary changes similar to those observed in patients with scleroderma or systemic lupus erythematosus and Raynaud's phenomenon can be seen.

The muscle biopsy histopathology of classic adult dermatomyositis shows a perivascular infiltration of inflammatory cells, composed of higher percentages of B lymphocytes and CD4 T helper lymphocytes. Occasionally, biopsies reveal perifascicular atrophy (6).

Amyopathic Dermatomyositis

Some patients with biopsy-confirmed classic cutaneous findings of dermatomyositis have no clinical evidence of muscle disease. The terms *amyotrophic dermatomyositis* and *dermatomyositis sine myositis* have been used to describe these patients. Such patients may constitute 10% of all patients with dermatomyositis. Although overt muscle weakness is not demonstrable, fatigue may be a dominant complaint, and analysis of energy-containing compounds (such as ATP) by magnetic resonance spectroscopy reveals abnormal muscle energy metabolism and altered exercise capacities (8).

Juvenile Dermatomyositis

The usual inflammatory myopathic process observed in children has a highly characteristic pattern, although a disease similar to adult polymyositis occasionally occurs (9). This process differs from the adult form because of the coexistence of vasculitis, ectopic calcification, lipodystrophy, and muscle weakness. In juvenile dermatomyositis, the skin lesions and weakness are almost always coincidental, but the severity and progression of each can vary greatly from patient to patient. In some, remission is complete with little or no therapy. However, in dermatomyositis accompanied by vasculitis, progression may be devastating despite therapy. Gastrointestinal ulcerations resulting from vasculitis may cause hemorrhage or perforation of a viscus. Ectopic calcifications may occur in the subcutaneous tissues or in the muscles.

The histologic changes in muscle of patients with juvenile dermatomyositis are essentially the same as those for the adult form, although perifascicular atrophy is much more prevalent (6). Endothelial hyperplasia and deposition of IgG, IgM, and complement (C3) within the vessel wall are also prominent.

Myositis and Other Collagen Vascular Diseases

Muscle weakness is a common finding in patients with collagen vascular diseases. The features of idiopathic inflammatory myopathy may dominate the clinical picture in some patients with scleroderma, systemic lupus erythematosus, mixed connective tissue disease, and Sjögren's syndrome. In other cases, weakness may be accompanied by normal enzyme levels and an absence of EMG abnormalities. The full picture of polymyositis is less common but can occur in rheumatoid arthritis, adult Still's disease, Wegener's granulomatosis, and polyarteritis nodosa. In vasculitic syndromes, muscle weakness is more commonly related to arteritis and nerve involvement than to non-suppurative inflammatory changes of muscles.

Myositis and Malignancy

A subset of patients with inflammatory myopathies develop muscle weakness with an underlying malignancy. The true incidence of this relationship is not clear (10). Malignancy may precede or follow the onset of muscle weakness. The association is rare in childhood but has occurred in patients of all ages in all subsets of disease, although associated malignancy may be more common with dermatomyositis. It appears that the sites or types of malignancy that occur in association with myositis are those expected for age and gender of the individual. Ovarian cancer may prove the exception because it is over-represented in women with dermatomyositis.

Inclusion Body Myositis

Inclusion body myositis mainly affects older individuals (11). The symptoms begin insidiously and progress slowly. Symptoms may have been present for 5–6 years before diagnosis. The clinical picture in some patients differs from that of typical polymyositis in that it may include focal, distal, or asymmetric weakness and neurogenic or mixed neurogenic and myopathic changes on EMG. Dysphagia is noted in over 20% of patients. As the muscle weakness becomes severe, it is accompanied by atrophy and diminished deep-tendon reflexes. In some patients, the disease continues a slow, steady progression, while it seems to plateau in others, leaving the individual with fixed weakness and atrophy of the involved musculature.

The characteristic change in inclusion body myositis is the presence of intracellular vacuoles (6). On paraffin sections, the vacuoles appear lined with eosinophilic material, but on frozen preparations they appear lined with basophilic granules. Lined vacuoles are not specific for inclusion body myositis. Electron microscopy reveals either intracytoplasmic or intranuclear tubular or filamentous inclusions. These structures are straight and rigid-appearing with periodic transverse and longitudinal striations. Myelin figures (also called myeloid bodies) and membranous whorls are also common.

PATHOGENESIS

The idiopathic inflammatory myopathies are believed to be immune-mediated processes that are triggered by environmental factors in genetically susceptible individuals. Two observations have provided strong support for the hypothesis that the idiopathic inflammatory myopathies are disorders of autoimmunity. First is the recognized association with other autoimmune diseases, including Hashimoto's thyroiditis, Graves' disease, myasthenia gravis, type I diabetes mellitus, primary biliary cirrhosis, and connective tissue diseases. Second is the high prevalence of circulating autoantibodies (3,4). The autoantibodies

associated with polymyositis and dermatomyositis include the myositis-specific autoantibodies (MSAs) found almost exclusively in these diseases (Table 21-2), autoantibodies that occur more commonly in myositis but are not specific for these disorders, and those found in patients with overlap syndrome.

The MSAs can be categorized as those directed at aminoacyl-tRNA synthetases, nonsynthetase cytoplasmic antigens, and nuclear antigens. The antisynthetases are the most commonly recognized MSAs; antihistidyl-tRNA synthetase, termed anti-Jo-1, is the most common of these. The antisynthetases show immunochemical properties characteristic of autoantibodies. They immunoprecipitate tRNA, inhibit enzyme function, and react with conformational epitopes. The antisynthetases do not cross-react or occur together. An individual patient will have only one MSA.

The cause or triggering event of the idiopathic inflammatory myopathies is unknown, but viruses have been strongly implicated. The seasonal variation in the onset of disease among different MSA subsets (first half of the year for antisynthetase syndrome and latter half for anti-SRP) is indirect evidence that infectious agents may play a role. The most striking evidence of a viral cause for the idiopathic inflammatory myopathies is found in animal models. Chronic myositis develops following infection with a picornavirus and persists long after the virus can no longer be detected in the tissue. The best described model is produced by injecting coxsackievirus B1 into neonatal Swiss mice. Infection of adult BALB/C mice with encephalomyocarditis virus-221A produces a virus dose–dependent model of polymyositis as well.

The importance of genetic factors is evident in mouse models of disease and in studies of class II immunohistocompatibility antigens. Individuals with HLA-DR3 are at increased risk for developing inflammatory muscle disease, including polymyositis and juvenile dermatomyositis. All patients with anti-Jo-1 antibodies have the HLA antigen DR52, and white patients also have a high prevalence of HLA-B8, HLA-DR3, and DR6. Inclusion body myositis is more likely associated with HLA-DR1, DR6, and DQ1.

The pathologic changes in muscle provide the strongest evidence that these diseases have an immune-mediated pathogenesis (6,12). The changes in polymyositis and inclusion body myositis appear to result from cell-mediated antigen-specific cytotoxicity. Non-necrotic muscle fibers are seen surrounded by and invaded by CD8 mononuclear cells, with cytotoxic cells outnumbering suppressor cells by a ratio of 3 to 1 in the CD8 cell population. B cells and natural killer cells do not appear to play a significant role in polymyositis or inclusion body myositis. The fibers invaded by T cells show increased major histocompatibility complex class I expression, a necessary condition for T-cell-mediated cytotoxicity. These findings suggest that the pathology of polymyositis and inclusion body myositis involves recognition of an antigen on the surface of muscle fibers by antigen-specific T cells.

In contrast to polymyositis, humoral immune mechanisms appear to play a greater role in dermatomyositis. Invasion of nonnecrotic fibers is quite universal, and the cellular infiltrates are predominantly perivascular in location. B cells outnumber T cells. Among T lymphocytes, CD4 cells are common, whereas CD8 cells and activated T cells are rare. The vasculopathy that is so prominent in juvenile dermatomyositis and occasionally present in the adult form of the disease also appears to be immune-mediated through humoral mechanisms. Immunoglobulins and complement components including the C5-9 membrane attack complex are deposited in the capillaries and small arterioles in this disease, but not in polymyositis.

The rimmed vacuoles and cytoplasmic and intranuclear filamentous inclusions that characterize inclusion body myositis indicate unique pathogenetic mechanisms for this group. Amyloid deposits have been identified in the vacuolated muscle fibers in inclusion body myositis. In addition, abnormal accumulation of ubiquitin, β-amyloid protein, β-amyloid precursor protein, and prion protein have been found in the rimmed vacuoles.

TREATMENT OF IDIOPATHIC INFLAMMATORY MYOPATHIES

The treatment of the inflammatory myopathies is largely empirical (13,14). Before initiating treatment, the patient's clinical status should be evaluated as objectively as possible. Pretreatment testing of the strength of individual muscle groups provides valuable information, and these baseline measures can be compared with those obtained after therapy is initiated. Chest radiography, pulmonary function studies, and fluoroscopic swallowing studies may be indicated. Muscle enzymes, including CK, aldolase, SGOT, SGPT, and LDH, should be measured in addition to other laboratory values that might be affected by therapy. Cancer screening tests indicated by the patient's age and gender should not be overlooked.

Physical therapy may play an important role in therapy. Bed rest may be required during intervals of severe inflammation. Passive range of motion exercise is encouraged during these intervals to maintain movement and prevent contractures. With improvement, therapy should include active-assisted, and then active exercises.

Glucocorticoids are the standard first-line medication for any idiopathic inflammatory myopathy. Initially prednisone is usually given in a single dose of 1 mg/kg/day, but in severe cases the daily dose can be divided or intravenous methylprednisolone used. Clinical improvement may be noted in the first weeks or gradually over 3–6 months. Generally, the earlier in the disease course prednisone is started, the faster and more effectively it works. As many as 90% of patients improve, at least partially, with glucocorticoid therapy, with 50%–75% of those achieving complete remission.

If a patient fails to respond to glucocorticoid therapy, another agent is added, usually either azathioprine or methotrexate. Methotrexate is generally given on a weekly schedule at doses of 5–15 mg orally or 15–50 mg intravenously. The typical dose of azathioprine is 2–3 mg/kg/day (maximum of 150 mg/day). Other immunosuppressive agents have been used in steroid-resistant patients. Cyclophosphamide, 6-mercaptopurine, chlorambucil, cyclospor- ine, plasmapheresis, lymphapheresis, total-body (or total-nodal) irradiation, and intravenous immunoglobulin have also been used. Hydroxychloroquine can be used to treat the cutaneous lesions of dermatomyositis, although it has no recognized effect on the myositis.

METABOLIC MYOPATHIES

Metabolic myopathies are a heterogenous group of conditions that have in common abnormalities in muscle energy metabolism that result in skeletal muscle dysfunction (15). Some metabolic myopathies should be considered primary, since they are associated with known or postulated biochemical defects that affect the ability of the muscle fibers to maintain adequate levels of ATP. The prevalence of these disorders appears to be greater than previously appreciated. Secondary metabolic myopathies may be caused by various endocrine disorders such as thyroid or adrenal diseases or electrolyte abnormalities.

Primary Metabolic Myopathies
Disorders of Glycogen Metabolism

Myophosphorylase deficiency (McArdle's disease) is one of nine diseases that share an underlying defect in glycogen synthesis, glycogenolysis, or glycolysis. These disorders are often referred to as the glycogen storage diseases, because each defect results in abnormal deposition and accumulation of glycogen in skeletal muscle (16). The classic clinical manifestation of a glycogen storage disease is exercise intolerance, which may be attributed to pain, fatigue, stiffness, weakness, or intense cramping. Most affected persons are well at rest and can function without difficulty at low levels of exercise. Symptoms tend to develop when the majority of energy for muscular work is derived from carbohydrate—that is, following activities of high intensity and short duration or activities of less intensity for longer intervals. Some patients experience a "second wind" phenomenon; although they must stop an activity because of symptoms, they are often able to resume the exercise after resting.

Symptoms develop during childhood in some patients, but significant problems including severe cramping or exercise-induced rhabdomyolysis and myoglobinuria with renal failure may not develop until adolescence. A subset of patients develops progressive proximal muscle weakness in adulthood that may be difficult to differentiate from polymyositis, because patients with glycogen storage disease have elevated CK levels and myopathic changes on EMG. The diagnosis of glycogen storage diseases may be suggested by finding the classic changes of glycogen deposition on muscle biopsy. The forearm ischemic exercise test is a useful method of screening for glycogen storage disease (Table 21-3). The putative diagnosis should always be confirmed by specific enzyme analysis of muscle tissue whenever it is suspected, either by histology or ischemic exercise

(Table 21-3)
*Forearm ischemic exercise test**

1. Venous blood is drawn without a tourniquet for baseline levels of lactate and ammonia.
2. A sphygmomanometer is placed around the upper arm and inflated to 20–30 mm Hg above systolic pressure.
3. The subject vigorously exercises the hand by squeezing until reaching complete fatigue or for a minimum of 2 minutes with the cuff inflated.
4. At the completion of exercise, the cuff is deflated and venous blood samples for lactate and ammonia are collected 2 minutes later.

* In normal subjects, both lactate and ammonia levels increase at least threefold above baseline. The major reason for a false-positive result is insufficient exercise effort. A positive result should always be confirmed by analysis of the putative enzyme activity in skeletal muscle.

testing. Inherited deficiency of acid maltase presents in infantile, childhood, and adult forms. Acid maltase activity is localized to lysosomes and does not affect cytosolic glycogen metabolism. Therefore, the results of ischemic exercise testing are normal in this deficiency. The diagnosis of adult acid maltase deficiency should usually be suspected because of characteristic electromyographic changes.

Disorders of Lipid Metabolism

The recognized disorders of lipid metabolism that cause myopathic problems are due to abnormalities in the transport and processing of fatty acids for energy. Carnitine palmityltransferase (CPT) is necessary for the transport of long-chain fatty acids into mitochondria. CPT deficiency is an autosomal recessive disorder that causes attacks of myalgia and myoglobinuria. These attacks are typically associated with vigorous physical activity but may occur with fasting, infection, or cold exposure. Serum CK levels, electromyograms, and muscle histology are normal except during episodes of rhabdomyolysis. The diagnosis is made by assaying muscle tissue for enzyme activity.

Carnitine is an essential intermediate that acts as a carrier of long-chain fatty acids into mitochondria where they undergo β-oxidation. Carnitine deficiency causes abnormal lipid deposition in skeletal muscle and can result from inherited or acquired causes. Primary carnitine deficiencies can be divided into systemic and muscle types. Patients with muscle carnitine deficiency present with chronic muscle weakness in late childhood, adolescence, or early adulthood. The process affects mainly proximal muscles but may also involve facial and pharyngeal musculature. Muscle carnitine deficiency may be confused with polymyositis because serum CK levels are elevated in more than half the patients, and electromyography often reveals myopathic changes. Acquired carnitine deficiencies have been reported with pregnancy, renal failure requiring long-term hemodialysis, end-stage cirrhosis, myxedema, adrenal insufficiency, and therapy with valproate or pivampicillin.

Mitochondrial Myopathies

These clinically heterogeneous disorders cause morphologic abnormalities in the number, size, or structure of mitochondria (17). The metabolic abnormalities described in these conditions are numerous and can be attributed to defects in pyruvate and acyl-CoA processing, β-oxidation, the respiratory chain, or energy conservation. Many mitochondrial myopathies are inherited through maternal transmission and are caused by defects in mitochondrial DNA. The clinical spectrum of these conditions is quite diverse and includes progressive muscular weakness, external ophthalmoplegia with or without proximal myopathy, progressive exercise intolerance, and multisystem disease. More than 25 specific enzyme abnormalities have been described, of which at least six may present with exercise intolerance or progressive muscle weakness in adults. Ragged-red fibers are the histologic hallmark of these diseases.

Myoadenylate Deaminase Deficiency

This disorder may be primary or secondary. The primary form is inherited in an autosomal recessive pattern. Patients report symptoms of exercise intolerance with post-exercise myalgia and cramping. When rested, patients are asymptomatic. Symptoms are usually mildly restrictive. Patients with primary myoadenylate deaminase deficiency will usually have normal serum CK levels, EMGs, and muscle histology. Results of the forearm ischemic exercise test are, however, abnormal. The primary deficiency is due to a nonsense mutation at codon 12 of the adenosine monophosphate (AMP) deaminase 1 gene, which has been identified in 22% of normal individuals (18). Thus, at least three-fourths of patients with myoadenylate deaminase deficiency are asymptomatic. The secondary form appears to be acquired in the course of a variety of neuromuscular diseases and collagen vascular diseases, including polymyositis, dermatomyositis, systemic sclerosis, and systemic lupus erythematosus.

OTHER CAUSES OF MUSCLE WEAKNESS

Although the inflammatory and metabolic myopathies are relatively rare, the list of diseases that cause myopathic symptoms for which patients seek medical attention is long (Table 21-4).

Neurologic diseases can generally be differentiated because they cause asymmetric weakness, distal extremity involvement, altered sensorium, or abnormal cranial nerve function. In contrast, myopathies cause only proximal and symmetric weakness. Exceptions include some mitochondrial myopathies, which may be accompanied by ocular problems, and inclusion body myositis, which may have neuropathic features.

Cancer must be considered in the evaluation of patients with myopathic symptoms. Although weakness and fatigue can occur in neoplastic disease from the systemic effects of cytokines released by tumor cells or as a result of immune response to the malignancy, prominent neuromuscular changes can also develop as features of paraneoplastic syndromes.

Numerous drugs can cause myopathic changes by a variety of mechanisms. Some, such as D-penicillamine and procainamide, are immune-mediated. Some, such as alcohol, may have direct toxic effects. Still others may cause metabolic or electrolyte abnormalities. Clofibrate, lovastatin, gemfibrozil, and other lipid-lowering agents probably alter muscle fiber energetics. Thiazide diuretics induce hypokalemia, which can cause weakness, myalgias, and cramps. Zidovudine (AZT) can induce a mitochondrial myopathy.

Numerous infections can cause a myopathy, with viruses being the most common. Children with influenza A and B viral infections can experience severe myalgias associated with very high CK levels. Weakness is a common finding in patients suffering from AIDS and may be due to cachexia, central or peripheral nervous system diseases, polymyositis emerging as a consequence of altered immune function, AZT toxicity, or opportunistic infections (eg, cytomegalovirus, *Mycobacterium avium-intracellulare*, *Cryptococcus*, *Trichinella*, *Toxoplasma*, pyomyositis).

TESTING FOR MUSCLE DISEASE
Chemistries

Elevated serum enzymes derived from skeletal muscle including CK, aldolase, AST, ALT, and LDH help confirm the presence of a myopathic process (19). High levels of these enzymes are found in the inflammatory diseases of muscle but are not specific for those diagnoses. CK is generally the most useful enzyme to follow, since elevated serum levels result from muscle necrosis or leaking membranes. Trauma is a well-recognized cause of high CK levels, as are isometric and aerobic exercise (especially in poorly conditioned individuals). Occasionally, elevated CK levels are observed in

(Table 21-4)
*Differential diagnosis of muscle weakness**

Neuropathic diseases
  Muscular dystrophies
  Denervating conditions
  Neuromuscular junction disorders
  Proximal neuropathies
  Myotonic diseases
Neoplasm
  Paraneoplastic syndromes
  Eaton–Lambert syndrome
Drug-related conditions
  Alcohol
  Amiodarone
  Clofibrate
  Cocaine
  Colchicine
  Cyclosporine
  Enalapril
  Fenofibrate
  Gemfibrozil
  Glucocorticoids
  Heroin
  Hydroxychloroquine
  Ketoconazole
  Levodopa
  Lovastatin
  Nicotine acid
  D-Penicillamine
  Phenytoin
  Valproic acid
  Zidovudine (AZT)
Infections
  Viral
    Advenovirus
    Coxsackievirus
    Cytomegalovirus
    Echovirus
    Epstein–Barr virus
    Human immunodeficiency virus (HIV)
    Influenza viruses
    Rubella virus
  Bacterial
    Clostridium welchii
    Mycobacterium tuberculosis
  Spirochetal
    Borrelia burgdorferi (Lyme spirochete)
  Fungal
    Cryptococcus
  Parasitic
    Toxoplasma gondii
  Helminthic
    Trichinella
Inborn errors of metabolism
  Nutritional-toxic
  Endocrine disorders
Miscellaneous causes
  Sarcoidosis
  Atherosclerotic emboli
  Behçet's disease
  Fibromyalgia
  Psychosomatic

* Does not include inflammatory or metabolic causes described in the text.

asymptomatic individuals. Racial differences in normal CK levels must be considered in this context because healthy black males have higher CK levels than whites or Hispanics, with the majority of values appearing abnormal by usual laboratory values.

Electromyography

Electromyography is a valuable technique for determining the classification, distribution, and severity of diseases affecting skeletal muscle (20). Although the changes identified are not specific, EMG can allow differentiation between myopathic and neuropathic conditions and can localize the site of the neurologic abnormality to the central nervous system, spinal cord anterior horn cell, peripheral nerves, or neuromuscular junction. In addition, knowledge of the distribution and severity of abnormalities can guide selection of the most appropriate site to biopsy.

Muscle Biopsy

Four types of evaluation can be performed on skeletal muscle: histology, histochemistry, electron microscopy, and assays of enzyme activities or other constituents. Hematoxylin and eosin and modified Gomori's trichrome stains are used for most histology. The latter stain is useful in identifying ragged-red fibers, typical findings in many mitochondrial myopathies. A wide variety of stains is used for histochemistry. ATPase stains determine fiber type. NADH and succinic dehydrogenases reflect the mitochondria. Periodic acid–Schiff stains are used for glycogen, and oil red O for lipid.

This combination of histologic and histochemical analysis is generally useful in differentiating myopathic from neuropathic processes. Myopathic changes include rounding and variation of fiber size, internal nuclei, fiber atrophy, degeneration and regeneration, fibrosis, and fatty replacement. Neuropathic conditions that cause denervation produce small, atrophic, angular fibers and target fibers. Reinnervation causes fiber-type grouping—that is, aggregation of fibers all of the same type.

Enzyme deficiency states may be identified with appropriate histochemical stains but are best diagnosed by subjecting the tissue protein to assays for the specific enzyme activity. Ultrastructural analysis shows characteristic changes in cases of inclusion body myositis, increased numbers of altered morphology of mitochondria in mitochondrial myopathies, and abnormal glycogen or lipid deposition.

Forearm Ischemic Exercise Testing

During vigorous ischemic exercise, skeletal muscle functions anaerobically, generating lactate and ammonia. Lactate is the product of glycolysis and ammonia is a co-product of myoadenylate deaminase activity. The forearm ischemic exercise test takes advantage of this physiology and has been standardized for use in screening glycogen storage diseases (except acid maltase deficiency) and myoadenylate deaminase deficiency (Table 21-3). In individuals with a glycogen storage disease, the ammonia level increases normally, but lactate levels remain at baseline. In contrast, in myoadenylate deaminase deficiency, lactate levels increase but ammonia levels do not.

Imaging Techniques

Neither conventional radiography nor radionuclide imaging have proved particularly useful in patients with muscle

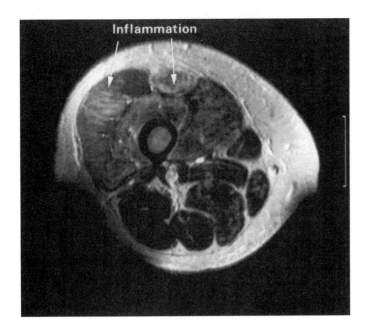

Inflammation

(Figure 21-1)
T2-weighted image of upper leg muscle from patient with dermatomyositis revealing inflammatory changes (8).

diseases. However, computer-based image analysis using ultrasonography, computed tomography, and magnetic resonance imaging (MRI) provide useful images. Of these, MRI offers the best imaging of soft tissue and muscle. Since MRI can detect early or subtle disease changes and show patchy muscle involvement, it may prove superior to EMG in determining the site for muscle biopsy. MRI can be used to semi-quantitatively grade muscle involvement, and therefore can be used to follow the response to therapy of several muscle diseases (Fig. 21-1) (8).

NANCY J. OLSEN, MD
ROBERT L. WORTMANN, MD

1. Bohan A, Peter JB: Polymyositis and dermatomyositis: first of two parts. N Engl J Med 292:344-347, 1975

2. Wortmann RL: Inflammatory diseases of muscle and other myopathies. In Kelley WN, Harris ED Jr., Ruddy S, Sledge CB (eds): Textbook of Rheumatology, 5th ed. Philadelphia, WB Saunders, 1996

3. Targoff IN: Immune manifestations of inflammatory muscle disease. Rheum Dis Clin North Am 20:857-880, 1994

4. Love LA, Leff RL, Fraser DD, et al: A new approach to the classification of idiopathic inflammatory myopathy: myositis-specific autoantibodies define useful homogeneous patient groups. Medicine 70:360-374, 1991

5. Bohan A, Peter JB, Bowman BS, Pearson CM: A computer-assisted analysis of 153 patients with polymyositis and dermatomyositis. Medicine 56:255-286, 1977

6. Engel AG, Hohfeld R, Banker BQ: The polymyositis and dermatomyositis syndromes. In Engel AG, Franzini-Armstrong C (eds): Myology, 2nd ed. New York, McGraw-Hill, 1994, pp 1335-1383

7. Euwer RL, Sontheimer RD, Braverman IM: Dermatomyositis and polymyositis. In Demis DJ (ed): Clinical Dermatology, 1st ed. Philadelphia, JB Lippincott, 1994, pp 1-14

8. Park JH, Vital TZ, Ryder NM, et al: Magnetic resonance imaging and P-31 magnetic resonance spectroscopy provide unique quantitative data useful in the longitudinal management of patients with dermatomyositis. Arthritis Rheum 37:736-746, 1994

9. Pachman LM: Inflammatory myopathy in childhood. Rheum Dis Clin North Am 20:919-942, 1994

10. Airio A, Puklaala E, Isomaki A: Elevated cancer incidence in patients with dermatomyositis: a population based study. J Rheumatol 22:1300-1303, 1995

11. Leff RL, Miller FW, Hicks J, et al: The treatment of inclusion body myositis: a retrospective review and a randomized, prospective trial of immunosuppressive therapy. Medicine 72:225-235, 1993

12. Kalovidouris AP: Mechanisms of inflammation and histopathology in inflammatory myopathy. Rheum Dis Clin North Am 20:881-897, 1994

13. Oddis CV: Therapy of inflammatory myopathy. Rheum Dis Clin North Am 20:899-918, 1994

14. Wortmann RL: Idiopathic inflammatory diseases of muscles. In Weisman MH, Weinblatt ME (eds): Treatment of the Rheumatic Diseases, 1st ed. Philadelphia, WB Saunders, 1995, pp 201-216

15. Wortmann RL: Metabolic diseases of muscle. In Koopman W (ed): Arthritis and Allied Conditions, 13th ed. Baltimore, Williams & Wilkins, 1996

16. DiMauro S, Tsujino, S: Nonlysosomal glycogenoses. In Engel AE, Franzini-Armstrong C (eds): Myology, 2nd ed. New York, McGraw-Hill, 1994, pp 1554-1576

17. Johns JR: Mitochondrial DNA and disease. N Engl J Med 333:638-644, 1995

18. Morisake T, Gross M, Morisaki H, et al: Molecular basis of AMP deaminase deficiency in skeletal muscle. Proc Natl Acad Sci USA 89:6457-6461, 1992

19. Bohlmeyer TJ, Wu AH, Perryman MB: Evaluation of laboratory tests as a guide to diagnosis and therapy of myositis. Rheum Dis Clin North Am 22:845-856, 1994

20. Daube JR: Electrodiagnosis of muscle disorders. In Engel AG, Franzini-Armstrong C (eds): Myology, 2nd ed. New York, McGraw-Hill, 1994, pp 764-794

22 SJÖGREN'S SYNDROME

Sjögren's syndrome (SS) is an immune-mediated disorder of exocrine glands. The most common clinical presentation is the combination of dry eyes (keratoconjunctivitis sicca) and dry mouth (xerostomia). It is divided into primary and secondary forms. The latter form affects patients with sicca symptoms in association with other autoimmune diseases, most commonly rheumatoid arthritis, systemic lupus erythematosus (SLE), or systemic sclerosis (1).

CLASSIFICATION CRITERIA

Several different sets of criteria for SS have been developed (2-4) see Appendix I. The San Diego criteria (Table 22-1) consist of a combination of clinical and laboratory features that include objective evidence of keratoconjuctivitis (KCS) and evidence of a systemic autoimmune disorder, as manifest by characteristic autoantibodies and minor salivary gland biopsy. Exclusions to the diagnosis of SS in the

(Table 22-1)
San Diego criteria for Sjögren's syndrome (SS)*

I. Primary Sjögren's syndrome
  A. Symptoms and objective signs of ocular dryness
    1. Schirmer's test less than 8 mm wetting per 5 minutes, and
    2. Positive Rose Bengal staining of cornea or conjunctiva to demonstrate keratoconjunctivitis sicca.
  B. Symptoms and objective signs of dry mouth
    1. Decreased parotid flow rate using Lashley cups or other methods, and
    2. Abnormal findings from biopsy of minor salivary gland (focus score of ≥2 based on average of four evaluable lobules).
  C. Serologic evidence of a systemic autoimmunity
    1. Elevated rheumatoid factor >1:320 or
    2. Elevated antinuclear antibody >1:320 or
    3. Presence of anti-SS-A(Ro) or anti-SS-B(La) antibodies.
II. Secondary Sjögren's syndrome
  Characteristic signs and symptoms of SS (described above) plus clinical features sufficient to allow a diagnosis of rheumatoid arthritis, systemic lupus erythematosus, polymyositis, scleroderma, or biliary cirrhosis.
III. Exclusions
  Sarcoidosis, preexistent lymphoma, human immunodeficiency virus, hepatitis virus B or C, primary fibromyalgia, and other known causes of autonomic neuropathy, keratitis sicca, or salivary gland enlargement.

* Definite Sjögren's syndrome requires objective evidence of dryness of eyes/mouth and autoimmunity including a characteristic minor salivary gland biopsy (criteria IA, IB, and IC). Probable Sjögren's syndrome does not require a minor salivary gland biopsy but can be diagnosed by demonstrating decreased salivary function (criteria IA, IB-1, and IC). Reprinted from Fox and Saito (4), with permission.

San Diego criteria include patients with human immunodeficiency virus (HIV) or other retroviral infection, hepatitis B or C infection, lymphoma, sarcoidosis, autonomic neuropathy, primary fibromyalgia syndrome, amyloidosis, or other diseases that infiltrate the salivary and lacrimal glands.

Complaints of ocular dryness are much more common than objective evidence of KCS. Decreased volume of tears is detected by the *Schirmer test* in which strips of filter paper are placed in the lower conjunctival sac. A modification of this test (Schirmer II test) involves stimulating the nasolacrimal reflex by gently inserting a cotton swab into the nostril; the increase in tear flow is then measured on both the contralateral and ipsilateral eye (5). The qualitative integrity of the cornea and conjunctival epithelial layer can be assessed by Rose Bengal staining. These tests are easily performed in the office and allow the clinician to assess the correlation between symptoms and objective KCS. A marked discrepancy between symptoms and signs might suggest other causes of ocular discomfort, including blepharitis (inflammation of the eyelids, particularly in patients who use eye drops with preservatives), depression, and anxiety, that contribute to symptoms of dryness.

Salivary secretions are easily measured by whole saliva sialometry. The patient sucks on a piece of sugarless candy for 3 minutes and expectorates. If the expectorated volume indicates significant dryness, biopsy of a minor salivary gland may be performed. Biopsy is required to diagnose "definite" SS; the diagnosis of "probable" SS can be fulfilled without a biopsy and is generally preferred for routine clinical purposes.

The presence of autoantibodies such as antinuclear antibody (ANA) or rheumatoid factor provides evidence for a systemic autoimmune process. Using Hep-2 cells as a substrate, antibody titers ≥1:320 are considered positive and generally have a fine speckled pattern, due to the presence of anti-SS-A (Ro) and anti-SS-B (La) antibodies. Patterns such as anticentromere and antinucleolar antibody often suggest an associated disease, such as systemic sclerosis (scleroderma) in its early stage of evolution or forme fruste manifestation. The absence of these autoantibodies suggests other causes of sicca complex, such as lymphoma, sarcoidosis, hepatitis C, or retroviral infection.

Many patients have significant dry eye and dry mouth symptoms, yet fail to satisfy the criteria for sicca symptom complex. In particular, many patients with fibromyalgia or depression have sicca symptoms, but lack histologic abnormalities and autoantibodies. These patients need to be reassured that the sicca process is local, and that progression to an autoimmune process is unlikely.

EPIDEMIOLOGY

The incidence of primary SS reported in the literature varies from less than 1 in 1000 people to more than 1 in 100. Most of the estimates are based on retrospective chart reviews and are subject to referral bias as well as differences in classification criteria used to make the diagnosis. These differences are particularly important in interpreting clinical studies on the incidence of associated diseases (such as lymphoma, multiple sclerosis, and dementia) or the results of treatment with particular pharmacologic agents. Many of the current debates about the frequency of SS and demyelinating disorders, lymphoma incidence, and retroviral infections partly result from the lack of agreement on the diagnostic criteria.

Using the San Diego criteria, the prevalence of primary SS is estimated to be approximately 1 in 1250 individuals, based on a retrospective review of records of patients enrolled in a health maintenance organization (6). Another way to estimate the frequency of SS in the general population is to assess the frequency of antibodies to SS-B in blood donors. This frequency of anti-SS-B antibodies was about 1 in 2500 consecutive adult donors to the San Diego Blood Bank (7), and a similar frequency was noted among Canadian blood donors (8).

PATHOGENESIS

Essential features of SS include focal lymphoid infiltrates in the lacrimal and salivary glands (Fig. 22-1A). Under high magnification (Fig. 22-1C and D), lymphocytes can be seen in direct contact with glandular epithelial cells. Immunohistologic studies indicate that these are predominantly CD4 T cells with restricted antigen receptor (TCAR) and reactivity against SS-A associated peptides (9,10). Another important feature of the SS salivary gland biopsy is the expression of HLA-DR (ie, major histocompatibility complex class II) antigens on the glandular epithelial cells, in contrast to normal glandular epithelial cells, which lack HLA-DR expression. The presence of cell-surface HLA-DR allows these epithelial cells to present exogenous antigens and autoantigens to the CD4 T cells. Other histologic features of the salivary gland include the conversion of capillaries to "high endothelial venules," which are structures that promote the migration of lymphocytes from the circulation into the gland via specific cell-adhesion molecules. Also, higher magnification electron microscopic views of the basement membrane surrounding the blood vessels and ductal epithelial cells (Fig. 22-1D) do not show the electron-dense deposits indicating immune complex deposition. Taken together, these features emphasize the importance of cell-mediated glandular destruction, rather than antibody or immune complex–complement-mediated mechanisms.

There is an increased frequency of B-cell lymphomas, particularly involving the cervical lymph nodes and salivary glands, among SS patients. In addition, glandular swelling without frank neoplastic changes (pseudolymphoma) may occur. The B cells from salivary biopsies in these patients can produce autoantibodies (11,12), have preferential use of cer-

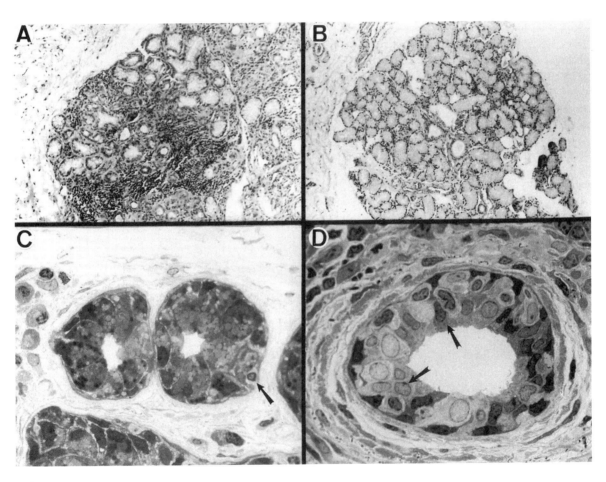

(Figure 22-1)
Biopsies of minor salivary gland from a normal person and from patients with Sjögren's syndrome (SS). A: Tissue from a patient with SS. A focal lymphocytic infiltrate is present in the center portion of the lobule. B: Tissue obtained at autopsy from an individual lacking evidence of any systemic autoimmune disease. C and D: Higher magnification views of lymphocytes (arrows) infiltrating acinar and ductal cells in an SS patient.

tain variable regions (especially the V-kappa III subgroup) (13), and may exhibit oligoclonal expansion detected by Southern blot methods (14-16). It is hypothesized that continued stimulation of local B cells by autoantigens or T cells leads to an increased risk of karyotypic changes and lymphoma in a multi-step process (17).

The actual mechanism of glandular destruction by CD4 T cells remains unknown, but may involve induction of granzyme A and perforin (18). These serine proteases are closely associated with lytic capacity of both CD4 and CD8 T cells (19). Recently, abnormalities in preprogrammed death (apoptosis) of lymphocytes due to upregulated bcl-2 have been proposed to contribute to the pathogenesis of SS (20,21). Also, decreases in the neural innervation of the glands may occur at an early stage of pathogenesis and prevent adequate function of the residual glandular elements (22).

Extraglandular Manifestations

Common symptoms in SS patients are fatigue and vague changes in cognitive function. The evaluation and treatment of these symptoms is often difficult because the etiology may be multifactorial. In general, fatigue and cognitive changes due to active vasculitis in SS patients are associated with elevation of acute phase reactants such as erythrocyte sedimentation rate (ESR), C-reactive protein (CRP), and immunoglobulin (IgG) levels. Also, objective abnormalities may be noted on electroencephalogram (EEG), magnetic resonance images (MRI), and neuropsychometric testing. In the absence of objective signs of active autoimmune disease, other causes of fatigue such as disrupted sleep patterns (ie, nonrestorative sleep), anxiety or depression, hypothyroidism, and medication side effects should be considered.

Central nervous system abnormalities in SS patients also can present as multiple sclerosis-like demyelinating lesions or thrombotic lesions, but these usually have focal abnormalities on neurologic exam. Peripheral neuropathies can result from large-vessel vasculitis (mononeuritis multiplex) or small-vessel occlusion with sensory neuropathies affecting the extremities (1).

Dermal manifestations may range from skin and vaginal dryness to vasculitis. Renal manifestations are not usually clinically significant in SS patients, although biopsies of patients may show a mild interstitial nephritis. Treatment of SS with drugs that exacerbate interstitial nephritis (ie, particular antibiotics and herbal medicines) may lead to significant renal problems. Gastrointestinal manifestations are frequent, particularly hiatal hernia symptoms and difficulty swallowing. These result from the decreased volume of saliva that normally facilitates swallowing and neutralizes gastric acidity.

Upper respiratory tract dryness is common and contributes to recurrent or persistent attacks of sinusitis in SS patients. The tenacious mucus secretions in the upper airways may contribute to bronchitis or pneumonia. Other pulmonary manifestations include lymphocytic interstitial pneumonitis and pleural effusions. Cardiac symptoms can include pericardial effusion, with a frequency similar to that seen in SLE patients.

DIFFERENTIAL DIAGNOSIS

There is an extensive differential diagnosis in patients who present with lacrimal or salivary gland enlargement or clinical symptoms of sicca (Table 22-2).

(Table 22-2)

Systemic diseases associated with enlarged lacrimal/salivary glands and/or glandular dysfunction

Infiltrative process
  Lymphoma
  Amyloidosis
  Hemochromatosis
  Sarcoidosis (Hereford's syndrome)
  Fatty infiltrates including hypercholesterolemia, hypertriglyceridemia, alcoholism
Infectious processes
  Human immunodeficiency virus (HIV) and human T-leukemia virus (HTLV-1/2)
  Hepatitis B and C
  Syphilis
  Trachoma
  Tuberculosis
Neuropathic dysfunction of the glands
  Multiple sclerosis
  Cranial neuropathies (seventh nerve)
    Bell's palsy
    Vasculitis
Autonomic neuropathy
  Idiopathic
  Drug-related
  Age-related
  Disease-related including diabetes mellitus and SLE

Infiltrative Diseases

Any process that replaces the lacrimal and salivary gland tissues, such as sarcoidosis, lymphoma, hemochromatosis, or amyloidosis, can result in dryness. In addition, glandular swelling can result from the deposition of fat in the glands associated with diabetes, alcoholism, pancreatitis, cirrhosis, and hypertriglyceridemia.

Infectious Diseases

Several infectious processes can mimic SS, including tuberculosis, trachoma, and syphilis. These possibilities must be considered in immunocompromised patients, and in patients from certain countries.

Sicca symptoms can develop in patients with retroviral infections due to human T-lymphotropic virus type 1 (HTLV-1) (particularly in endemic areas) and in individuals infected with HIV. Diffuse infiltrative lymphadenopathy syndrome (DILS) occurs in HIV-infected patients (23). It is more common in children (up to 10% of neonatal HIV cases), and occurs in approximately 0.5% of HIV-infected adults. Recognition of this syndrome is important both for safety (correct disposal of infected materials for protection of health care professionals) and for early therapy using antiviral medications. DILS patients differ from SS patients in the types of lymphocytes that infiltrate the salivary glands (ie, a predominance of CD8 T cells) and in the general absence of ANA (23). Patients with hepatitis B or C infection may develop autoimmune features, including sicca symptoms and mixed cryoglobulinemia (24). Again, prompt recognition of these patients is important for both patient care and correct disposal of hazardous materials. Furthermore, patients with sicca symptoms and autoantibodies in association with hepatitis C infection may have serious side effects more frequently when their hepatitis is treated with interferon-α (25).

Side Effects of Medications

Anticholinergic side effects occur in patients who receive a wide spectrum of medications for blood pressure, depression, muscle spasm, fibromyalgia, sleep disorders, and cardiac arrhythmia (Table 22-3). Frequently, older patients with mild sicca symptoms experience significant exacerbation of these symptoms due to these medications. Significant improvement may be achieved simply by using alternative drugs that do not cause these side effects.

Other Conditions Associated with Sicca Symptoms

Blepharitis and blepharospasm can mimic or exacerbate KCS. Blepharitis results from blockage or infection of the meibomian glands. It has been proposed that exotoxin(s) released by local bacteria can cause or contribute to KCS. This possibility should be considered in a Sjögren's patient who has increased symptoms but in whom KCS appears to have improved, according to examination by Rose Bengal or fluorescein staining. Blepharitis frequently occurs in SS patients who are using excessive amounts of ocular lubricant at night, which can block the lacrimal glands, and is sometimes exacerbated by artificial tears that contain preservatives. Using eyelid scrubs, avoiding lubricating gels, switching to a preservative-free tear solution, and taking oral doxycycline may prove helpful.

(Table 22-3)
Medications with anticholinergic side effects

Antihypertensives
  Clonidine and prazosin (alpha 1-blocker)
  Prazosin (alpha 2-blocker)
  Propranolol (beta blocker)
  Reserpine
  Methyldopa (Aldomet) and guanethidine
Antidepressants (tricyclics and monoamine oxidase
    inhibitors)
  Amitriptyline and nortriptyline
  Imipramine and desipramine
  Doxepin
  Phenelzine and tranylcypromine
  Amoxapine and trimipramine
Cardiac antiarrhythmic drugs
  Disopyramide
  Mexiletine
Parkinson's disease (anticholinergic agents)
  Trihexyphenidyl
  Benztropine
  Biperiden
  Procyclidine
Anti-ulcer agents
  Atropine-like drugs
  Metoclopramide and other drugs that decrease
    gastric motility
Muscle spasms
  Cyclobenzaprine
  Methocarbamol
Decongestants (over-the-counter cold remedies)
  Ephedrine
  Pseudoephedrine

Graft-versus-host disease (GVHD) after bone marrow transplantation results in lymphocytic infiltration and a sicca syndrome. Presumably, immune responses against foreign HLA antigens play a role in pathogenesis. Although the disease initially was considered to be similar to SS, studies of biopsy specimens from GVHD patients bear a closer resemblance to severe lichen planus.

Progressive dryness can develop in patients who have had radiation to the head and neck. This process may develop years after the initial radiation and may represent an induced form of autoimmune reaction against antigens liberated from the damaged tissue.

Sarcoidosis may present with glandular swelling and sicca symptoms, although anterior uveitis is a more common ocular manifestation. The presence of noncaseating granulomatous infiltrates, elevated angiotensin-converting enzyme (ACE), and hilar adenopathy on chest radiograph help distinguish sarcoidosis from SS.

Patients with multiple sclerosis have problems with dry eyes and dry mouth, probably due to interference with cholinergic innervation of their glands. However, in a subset of SS patients focal lymphocytic infiltrates in the brain tissue result in multiple sclerosis-like symptoms and abnormal brain scans on magnetic resonance imaging.

TREATMENT OF SICCA SYMPTOMS
Keratoconjuctivitis Sicca

Artificial tears are essential for the treatment of KCS. Artificial tears have at least two distinct components: the moisturizing component and the preservative. If the tears are helpful but do not last long enough, then a more viscous solution (eg, a higher concentration of hydroxymethylcellulose) or a different vehicle to concentrate the moisturizing element (eg, a polymer-like dextran) is indicated.

Reaction to a preservative in artificial tears can cause a burning sensation soon after installation. These reactions were much more frequent in the past when benzalkonium chloride and thimerosal were commonly used in artificial tears. These preservatives, although no longer used in artificial tears, are still widely used in other ophthalmologic preparations (particularly topical antibiotics) and may contribute to ocular irritation. Irritation of the eyelids in patients with blepharitis may be related to the preservatives present in some ocular lubricants used at night. Using excessive amounts of lubricant at night may also plug the meibomian glands.

If a particular artificial tear solution seems helpful but the benefit does not last long enough, punctal occlusion may be performed on a temporary or permanent basis. The puncta are the tiny openings at the medial aspect of the lower lids. Temporary blockage with collagen plugs provides an opportunity to evaluate the symptomatic benefit and to make sure that reflex tearing is not excessive (eg, tears running down the patient's cheeks). If helpful, permanent punctal occlusion can be done by electrocautery in the ophthalmologist's office, a quick procedure requiring only a topical anesthetic.

Xerostomia

Patients with residual salivary gland function may benefit from either local or systemic methods to stimulate flow. Gustatory stimulation with sugarless mints is often effective, as is chewing sugarless gum. However, sugarless gum may contain carbohydrates that have cariogenic potential in the presence of reduced salivary function. Some patients find that chewing on paraffin wax or a fruit pit provides adequate masticatory stimulation without increasing dental caries. Recent studies suggest that oral pilocarpine may be useful in stimulating saliva (19).

Low-grade oral yeast infections are common in SS patients (19). Predisposing factors include recent use of antibiotics or corticosteroids. Treatment is particularly difficult in patients with dentures, since continued excoriation of the mucosal surface occurs. Many topical antifungal drugs are available, but some oral preparations have only a small amount of the antifungal agent and a high concentration of glucose (to improve the taste), which contributes to dental decay if used for a long period. Nystatin, available as oral troches and as vaginal suppositories that can be sucked, is helpful if used for about 20 minutes twice daily for at least 6 weeks to prevent recurrence. Patients with very dry mouth may need to sip water periodically to help dissolve the troches. Clortrimazol (also available as troches) may be used in the same manner. To permit drug access to all intraoral mucosal sites, dentures should be removed while the tablets dissolve. Dentures also must be treated to remove traces of candida; patients should be referred to a dentist to discuss the method of disinfectant.

Angular cheilitis is treated by applying topical antifungal cream two to three times per day for several weeks.

SYSTEMIC MEDICATIONS

The overall approach to systemic therapy for patients with Sjögren's syndrome is similar to that for patients with SLE. Nonvisceral manifestations (arthralgias, myalgias, skin, fatigue) are generally treated with salicylates, nonsteroidal agents, and often hydroxychloroquine. Among the disease-modifying antirheumatic drugs, antimalarials (chloroquine and hydroxychloroquine) have proved useful in decreasing arthralgia, myalgia, and lymphadenopathy in SS patients (27). In a European study (28), hydroxychloroquine improved the erythrocyte sedimentation rate but did not increase tear flow volumes.

As in SLE, corticosteroids are given for visceral involvement including vasculitic skin lesions, pneumonitis, neuropathy, and nephritis. Drugs such as hydroxychloroquine, azathioprine, and methotrexate are used to help taper the corticosteroids. Cyclosporine may be used (29), but many SS patients tend to develop interstitial nephritis, which limits the usefulness of this drug. Cyclophosphamide is occasionally required for life-threatening illness. However, the increased frequency of lymphoma in SS patients (12) requires caution, and cyclophosphamide should be delivered as pulse therapy rather than daily oral administration.

SURGERY

Patients with Sjögren's syndrome have unique problems during the preoperative, perioperative, and postoperative periods. The usual preoperative instruction of "nothing by mouth" after dinner or midnight on the day prior to surgery poses a problem for SS patients. In the absence of normal saliva flow, patients can reduce discomfort by using artificial salivas during this time.

Operating rooms and recovery areas have extremely low humidity, which is compounded by nonhumidified oxygen leaking around a face mask. Therefore, SS patients are at increased risk for developing corneal abrasions during surgery and in the postoperative setting. Anesthetics decrease the blink reflex, which also contributes to this problem. Applying ocular lubricants before surgery and in the postoperative recovery suite reduces the chance of this complication.

Upper airway dryness in the SS patient may lead to mucus plug inspissation during the postoperative period, followed by obstructive pneumonia. The risk of this complication is reduced by using humidified oxygen and avoiding medications that excessively dry the upper airways (ie, agents used by anesthesiologists to control secretions). Adequate hydration and respiratory therapy after surgery help keep airways clear.

An additional problem for the anesthesiologist is the poor condition of teeth in SS patients, because teeth can be easily damaged during intubation. Not only can this lead to tooth loss and the risk of aspiration, but many of these patients have incurred great expense in obtaining partial dentures that attach to remaining teeth; any further tooth loss would greatly affect these devices.

In many surgical procedures, antibiotics are routinely given prophylactically, which greatly increases the risk for developing oral candidiasis in SS patients. Prophylactic use of topical oral antifungal drugs such as nystatin may help prevent this complication. Precautions regarding corticosteroid coverage are important, because patients remain relatively adrenal insufficient after an extended period on these agents.

Finally, assessment of an SS patient's fluid status may be relatively difficult during the postoperative period. Normal clinical clues such as the moisture in the ocular and oral membranes may be quite misleading. Furthermore, some SS patients have a tendency to develop interstitial nephritis, which prevents adequate urine concentration and fluid balance. This problem may be exacerbated by antibiotics such as aminoglycosides.

ROBERT I. FOX, MD, PhD

1. Fox R: Clinical features, pathogenesis and treatment of Sjögren's syndrome. Curr Opin Rheumatol 8:438-445, 1996.
2. Daniels TE: Labial salivary gland biopsy in Sjögren's syndrome. Arthritis Rheum 27:147-156, 1984
3. Vitali C, Bombardieri S, Moutsopoulos HM, Balestrieri G, et al: Preliminary criteria for the classification of Sjögren's syndrome—Results of a prospective concerted action supported by the European community. Arthritis Rheum 36:340-347, 1993
4. Fox RI, Saito I: Criteria for diagnosis of Sjögren's syndrome. Rheum Dis Clin North Am 20:391-407, 1994
5. Tsubota K: The importance of Schirmer test with nasal stimulation. Am J Ophthalmol 11:106-108, 1991
6. Fox RI, Howell FV, Bone RC, Michelson: Primary Sjögren's syndrome: clinical and immunopathologic features. Semin Arthritis Rheum 14:77-105, 1984
7. Fox RI, Chan EK, Kang H: Laboratory evaluation of patients with Sjögren's syndrome. Clin Biochem 25:213-222, 1992
8. Fritzler MJ, Pauls JD, Kinsella TD, et al: Antinuclear, anticytoplasmic, and anti-Sjögren's syndrome antigen A (SS-A/Ro) antibodies in female blood donors. Clin Immunol Immunopathol 36:120, 1985
9. Matsumoto I, Tsubota K, Satake Y, et al: Common T cell receptor clonotype in lacrimal glands and labial salivary glands from patients with Sjögren's syndrome. J Clin Invest 97:1969-1977, 1996.
10. Namekawa T, Kuroda N, Kato T, Yamamoto K, Murata H, Saitoh Y, Sumida T: Identification of SSA reactive T cells in labial salivary glands from patients with Sjogren's syndrome. J Rheumatol 20:92-99, 1995
11. Talal N, Asofsky R, Lightbody P: Immunoglobulin synthesis by salivary gland lymphoid cells in Sjögren's syndrome. J Clin Invest 19:19-27, 1979
12. Fox RI, Adamson TC III, Fong S, Robinson CA, Morgan EL, Robb JA, Howell FV: Lymphocyte phenotype and function of pseudolymphomas associated with Sjögren's syndrome. J Clin Invest 72:52-62, 1983

13. Fox RI, Chen PP, Carson DA, Fong S: Expression of a cross-reactive idiotype on rheumatoid factor in patients with Sjögren's syndrome. J Immunol 136:477-483, 1986

14. Fishleder A, Tubbs R, Hesse B, Levin H: Immunoglobulin-gene rearrangement in benign lymphoepithelial lesions. N Engl J Med 316:1118-1121, 1987

15. Freimark B, Fox RI: Immunoglobulin gene rearrangements in Sjögren's syndrome (Letter). N Engl J Med 317:1158, 1987

16. Schmid SL, Jackson MR: Making class II presentable. Nature 369:103-105, 1994

17. Pisa E, Pisa P, Kang H, Fox R: High frequency of t(14;18) translocation in salivary gland lymphomas from Sjögren's syndrome patients. J Exp Med 174:1245, 1991

18. Alpert S, Pisa E, Weissman I, Fox R: Expression of granzyme A in salivary gland biopsies from patients with Sjögren's syndrome. Arthritis Rheum, in press

19. Fox RI, Hugli TE, Lanier LL, Morgan EL, Howell F: Salivary gland lymphocytes in primary Sjögren's syndrome lack lymphocyte subsets defined by Leu 7 and Leu 11 antigens. J Immunol 135:207, 1985

20. Ogawa N, Dang H, Kong L, Anaya J, Liu G, Talal N: Lymphocyte apoptosis and apoptosis-associated gene expression in Sjögren's syndrome. Arthritis Rheum 39:1875-1886, 1996

21. Fox R: Pathogenesis of Sjögren's syndrome. Med Clin North Am (in press)

22. Konttinen YT, Hukkanen M, Kemppinen P, et al: Peptide-containing nerves in labial salivary glands in Sjögren's syndrome. Arthritis Rheum 35:815-820, 1992

23. Itescu S, Winchester R: Diffuse infiltrative lymphocytosis syndrome: a disorder occurring in human immunodeficiency virus-1 infection that may present as a sicca syndrome. Rheum Dis Clin North Am 18:683-697, 1992

24. Haddad J, Deny P, Munz-Gotheil C, Ambrosini JC: Lymphocytic sialadenitis of Sjögren's syndrome associated with chronic hepatitis C virus liver disease. Lancet 8:321-323, 1992

25. Muratori L, Lenzi M, Cataleta M, Giostra F, Cassani F, Ballardini G, Zauli D, Bianchi FB: Interferon therapy in liver/kidney microsomal antibody type 1-positive patients with chronic hepatitis C. J Hepatol 21:199-203, 1994

26. Daniels T, Fox P: Salivary and oral components of Sjögren's syndrome. Rheum Dis Clin North Am 18:571-589, 1992

27. Fox RI, Chan E, Benton L, Fong S, Friedlaender M, Howell FV: Treatment of primary Sjögren's syndrome with hydroxychloroquine. Am J Med 85:62-67, 1988

28. Kruize AA, Henre RJ, Kallenberg CG, et al: Hydroxychloroquine treatment for primary Sjögren's syndrome: a two-year, double-blind crossover trial. Ann Rheum Dis 52:360-364, 1993

29. Dalavanga YA, Detrick B, Hooks JJ, Drosos AA, Moutsopoulos HM: Effect of cyclosporin A (CyA) on the immunopathological lesion of the minor salivary glands from patients with Sjögren's syndrome. Ann Rheum Dis 46:89-92, 1990

23

VASCULITIS
A. EPIDEMIOLOGY, PATHOLOGY, AND PATHOGENESIS

The vasculitides are a heterogenous group of clinical syndromes characterized by inflammation of blood vessels (1-6). The precise definition of these disorders is complicated by the relative rarity of the vasculitis syndromes, discordant disease definitions, regional variations, and ethnic biases. For example, the incidence of Kawasaki disease, Behçet's syndrome, Takayasu arteritis, and thromboangiitis obliterans is increased in Japanese populations. The incidence of giant cell arteritis is greater in populations of northern European background, as well as in the northern latitudes. In contrast to the striking male dominance (80%) seen in the series of Behçet's syndrome in the Middle East, series from the USA generally report nearly equal incidence in men and women.

The age of onset of symptoms is quite variable in the vasculitides (Table 23A-1). Although the mean age of onset of several of the primary vasculitis syndromes, including polyarteritis nodosa, allergic granulomatosis and angiitis, Wegener's granulomatosis, and hypersensitivity vasculitis, is in the fifth decade of life, these diseases can present at both extremes of age. Kawasaki disease is seen almost exclusively in the pediatric-aged population. The incidence of Henöch–Schönlein purpura (HSP) has a bimodal distribution. The majority of cases occur in pediatric populations between the ages of 4 and 7 years. In contrast, the mean age at onset of HSP in adults is 45. Thromboangiitis obliterans and Takayasu arteritis tend to affect young adult populations. Giant cell arteritis is generally limited to populations beyond the sixth decade of life.

PATHOLOGY
There is considerable overlap in the patterns of pathologic involvement in the major vasculitis syndromes (Table 23A-2) (2-5,7). With the possible exception of hypercellular occlusive thrombii seen in thromboangiitis obliterans, pathologic findings are not diagnostic for a specific syndrome. In some cases, immunofluorescent studies may provide useful information. Both IgM and C3 may be demonstrated in early hypersensitivity vasculitis lesions. The presence of IgA and C3 in a small vessel vasculitis lesion is suggestive of the diagno-

(Table 23A-1)
*Epidemiology of the major vasculitides**

Vasculitides	Incidence per 1×10^6 (Range)	Mean Age at Onset (Yr)	Sex (% Male)	Ethnic Association
Polyarteritis nodosa	4 (2–18)	48±1.7	62	None
Allergic granulomatosis and angiitis	2.4 (2.4–4.0)	50±3.0	52-65	None
Wegener's granulomatosis	8.5 (0.7–8.5)	45±1.2	64	None
Kawasaki disease (Japan)	900 (< 5 yrs)	1.0–1.5 (0.1–11)§	60	Japanese
Kawasaki disease (US)	Asian 333 Black 234 White 127 (< 5 yrs)	2.9–3.8 (0.1–13)§	60	Asian African American
Hypersensitivity vasculitis	Less common†	47±2.0 (95% >16 yrs)	46	None
Henöch–Schönlein purpura	140 (3–140)	4.5–17 (0.2–adult; 71% <20 yrs)§	54	None
Beçhet's syndrome	Variable‡	27	66	E. Mediterranean, Japanese
Takayasu arteritis	2.6 (0.2–2.6)	26±1.2 (3–75; 92% <40 yrs)§	14	Asian
Giant cell arteritis	178 (150–250 in those >50 yrs)	69±0.5 (90% >60 yrs)	20	N. European
Thromboangiitis obliterans	Rare†	33 (11–45; 96% <40 yrs)§	80	Far Eastern, Middle Eastern, Asian

* Data are summarized from references 1, 3-6.
† Because of the relative rarity of the vasculitides and variations in disease definition, precise data on disease incidence is unavailable.
‡ The frequency of Behçet's disease is variable. Prevalence of 1/1000 has been reported in Japan, while prevalence of 1/300,000 has been reported in the US.
§ Reports the range in years of onset of disease.

*Pathologic parameters of the major vasculitides**

Vasculitides	Class of Vessel Involvement	Organ System Involvement	Vessel Wall Involvement	Histopathology of the Vessels		Renal and (Other) Pathology
				Cellular	Other	
Polyarteritis nodosa	Small and medium sized muscular arteries	Viscera, muscles, testes, nerves, renal (not pulmonary arteries)	Early lesion: media, full: transmural	Early: PMN Full: L,M,PMN Less: Eos,Gr	Fibrinoid necrosis, fibrin, thrombosis, ↓ internal elastic membrane, ↓ media, aneurysms	Segmental necrotizing GN, crescents, arteritis
Allergic granulomatosis and angiitis	Small and medium sized arteries, veins, venules	Lungs, viscera, cardiac, renal, nerves, muscle	Transmural	Early: Eos Full: Eos,L,M, PMN,Gr,GC	Less common: fibrinoid necrosis, thrombosis, aneurysms	Focal segmental necrotizing GN, crescents, vasculitis, interstitial Eos (Tissue Eos, necrotizing granuloma)
Wegener's granulomatosis	Small arteries and veins; also larger arteries, arterioles, venules and capillaries	Upper and lower respiratory, renal, skin, eye, heart, nervous system	Transmural	Early: PMN Full: L,M,PMN, Gr,GC Less: Eos	Fibrinoid necrosis, necrotizing granuloma, ↓ elastic membrane	Focal segmental necrotizing GN, crescents; less common: vasculitis and interstitial nephritis (Lung necrosis; necrotizing granuloma)
Kawasaki disease	Medium muscular arteries; rarely veins, large arteries	Cardiac; also iliac, renal, internal, mammillary	Panarteritis	Early: PMN,L,M Full: L,M,H	Thrombosis, aneurysm, endothelial proliferation, rare: fibrinoid necrosis	Renal: None (pericarditis, myocarditis, epicarditis, valvular involvement)
Hypersensitivity vasculitis	Postcapillary venules, arterioles, venule; rare: small arteries, veins	Skin; rare: viscera, heart, synovium	—	Early: PMN; L,M Full: PMN; L,M or PMN,L,M,Eos	Leukocytoclasis, fibrin, fibrinoid necrosis, RBC extravasation	Rare: interstitial nephritis (rare: myocarditis, hepatitis)
Henöch–Schönlein purpura	Precapillary arterioles, postcapillary venules, capillaries	Skin, GI, renal, synovium	—	Early: PMN Full: PMN,L,M Rare: Eos	Fibrinoid necrosis of arterioles, fibrin, RBC extravasation, thrombosis	Proliferation of mesangial cells, increased matrix, epithelial crescents
Behçet's syndrome	Small vessels; rare: large vessel, vasa vasorum	Oral, genital, other skin sites, eye, CNS, GI, synovium	—	Early: ?PMN Full: L,M	Early: leukocytoclasis; less common: fibrin, thrombosis, RBC extravasation	Rare: GN, immune complexes (thrombophlebitis, pustular skin lesions with PMN)
Takayasu arteritis	Large elastic arteries, selected muscular arteries	Aorta and major branches (arch), pulmonary artery	Early lesion: media, full: panarteritis	L,M,Gr, plasmacytoid Rare: GC	↓ media, musculoelastic lamellae; dissection, aneurysm, fibrosis	Renal: 2° ischemic and hypertensive changes (rare: pericarditis, myocarditis)
Giant cell arteritis	Large and medium muscular arteries; less common: aorta	Extra-cranial arteries of head and neck; less common: any other artery	Panarteritis dominant site: media	L,M,H,Gr,GC, Less: PMN,Eos	↓ elastic membrane, intimal proliferation, aneurysm, dissection, rare: necrosis	Renal: rare ischemic changes 2° to renal artery angiitis, (granulomatous hepatitis)
Thromboangiitis obliterans	Intermediate and small arteries and veins	Extremities: distal > proximal. Very rare: head, cardiac, viscera	Transmural	Early: PMN Full:L,M,H,PMN Rare: GC	Hypercellular occlusive thrombus, fibrosis, spares elastic membrane and vessel structure, no necrosis	Renal: none

* The information is summarized from references 3–5, 7. PMN = polymorphonuclear leukocytes, L = lymphocytes, M = monocyte, H = histiocytes, Eos = eosinophils, Gr = granuloma, GC = giant cells/multinucleated giant cells, GI = gastrointestinal, CNS = central nervous system, RBC = red blood cells, GN = glomerulonephritis. "↓" represents damage or destruction.

sis of HSP. The overlap between the pathologic changes in the vasculitides is especially evident in the kidney. Even though many of these diseases affect the kidney, the histologic pattern of involvement is generally nonspecific; consequently, the renal biopsy may not differentiate between these syndromes. The major vasculitis syndromes are defined by clinicopathologic parameters. Recent publications (1,2) emphasize the importance of combining clinical information with pathologic findings in establishing the diagnosis.

Vasculitis lesions tend to be both focal and segmental. The lesions are focal in the sense that not all vessels of a similar size will be affected by the pathologic process. The lesions are considered segmental because only certain portions, or segments, of an affected vessel may be involved with the pathologic process. For example, serial sections through a temporal artery biopsy may go from a normal vessel to a site of severe involvement in a space of several millimeters. Moreover, the pattern of inflammation within the vessel wall may not be uniform. Early lesions in both polyarteritis nodosa and Takayasu arteritis may be limited to the media. The pattern of inflammation in Takayasu arteritis may be patchy rather than diffuse. Finally, the entire circumference of the vessel may not be uniformly involved. Instead of involving the entire circumference, only a portion of the blood vessel wall may be affected, producing a sectorial pattern of inflammation. The focal, segmental, and even sectorial nature of vasculitis lesions is an important consideration in evaluating diagnostic biopsies. Evaluating a larger volume of tissue increases the likelihood of identifying an inflammatory lesion if present. The need to obtain an adequate sized biopsy specimen and to do serial step sections on temporal artery biopsies has been emphasized.

PATHOGENESIS

No single pathophysiologic process accounts for the spectrum of pathology observed in the vasculitides. Moreover, even within a specific vasculitis syndrome, different disease initiating events may lead to a final common pathway. The limitation of knowledge on the causes of vasculitis reflects, in part, the paucity of relevant animal models to study and the inherent difficulties in studying pathogenesis in clinical populations (8).

Immune Complexes

The concept that immune complexes mediate inflammatory vessel disease is based on systematic studies of the animal models of serum sickness and the Arthus reaction (3,9). The following elements must be present for the expression of vasculitis in these animal models: 1) increased vascular permeability; 2) deposition of circulating (or the in situ precipitation of) immune complexes below the level of the vascular endothelium; 3) the activation of complement; and 4) the attraction of polymorphonuclear leukocytes (PMN) to the vessel wall. Mechanisms leading to an increase in vascular permeability include the release of platelet activating factors, and vasoactive amines and other soluble mediators from platelets, mast cells, or basophils. The relevance of these mediators in the clinical expression of immune complex-mediated vasculitis, however, has not been established.

Indirect evidence suggests immune complex-mediated mechanisms of vasculitis may be pertinent in hypersensitivity vasculitis, HSP, cryoglobulinemia, and the hepatitis B virus-associated vasculitis. In these diseases, immunofluorescent studies may demonstrate the presence of antigen (bacterial, mycobacterial, or viral antigen), immunoglobulin, and C3 in biopsies of early vasculitis lesions.

Antibodies

The role of antibodies, other than those present in immune complexes, in the development of vasculitis is less well defined. Anti-neutrophil cytoplasmic autoantibodies (ANCA) are present in patients with systemic necrotizing vasculitis, including Wegener's granulomatosis, allergic granulomatosis, and angiitis and polyarteritis nodosa. A subset of these autoantibodies (c-ANCA) bind to specially preserved PMNs with a diffuse, granular cytoplasmic staining pattern (Fig. 23A-1). The c-ANCA binds to a serine proteinase (proteinase 3) found in the primary granules of the PMN. In vitro studies suggest a potential role for c-ANCA in the pathophysiology of necrotizing vasculitis (10). Under normal conditions the proteinase 3 is in an intracellular location and inaccessible to extracellular antibodies. However, after exposure to certain cytokines, granule constituents, including proteinase 3, are found on the cell surface of both PMNs and monocytes. The c-ANCA will interact with these activated cells, stimulating respiratory burst activity and degranulation. Polymorphonuclear leukocytes that have been activated with cytokines and stimulated with c-ANCA in vitro can damage endothelial cells. The role for this potential mechanism in the in vivo expression of necrotizing vasculitis requires additional investigation.

A potential causal role has been suggested for antibodies directed toward structures on the surface of endothelial cells. Antiendothelial cell antibodies have been demonstrated in a number of autoimmune and vasculitis diseases (11). In vitro, antiendothelial cell antibodies can damage endothelial cells by both antibody-dependent cellular cytotoxicity (ADCC) and complement activation mechanisms. Serum from patients with acute Kawasaki syndrome can lyse cytokine-activated allogenic endothelial cells in complement dependent in vitro study systems (12,13).

Endothelial Cells

Because the endothelium serves as the interface between the intra- and extra-vascular compartments, these cells are in-

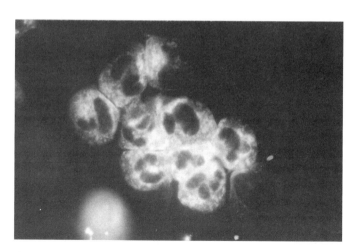

(Figure 23A-1)
Indirect immunofluorescence microscopy of alcohol-fixed neutrophils demonstrating the staining pattern produced by cytoplasmic antineutrophil cytoplasmic autoantibodies (c-ANCA). The granular pattern of cytoplasmic immunofluorescence of the c-ANCA is seen. (Original magnification ×400).

volved in a wide variety of physiologic regulatory functions such as vascular permeability, aggregation of vascular formed elements, adhesion of formed elements such as platelets and leukocytes, regulation of cell trafficking into the extra-vascular compartment, and regulation of coagulation. These endothelial cell regulatory functions are mediated, in part, by a number of secreted substances such as prostaglandin, adenosine nucleotide, and platelet activating factor.

In addition to these vascular regulatory functions, endothelial cells have the potential to regulate and modify immune responses. They can secrete a number of cytokines that may regulate immune responses at the vascular level (14). In vitro endothelial cells secrete low levels of interleukins 1 and 6 (IL-1 and IL-6). A marked increase in the production of these cytokines can be demonstrated following stimulation. The endothelial cells can also be stimulated to secrete IL-8, interferons, granulocyte-macrophage colony stimulating factor (CSF), granulocyte CSF, and macrophage CSF. These cytokines, locally secreted, could have a significant effect on vascular inflammatory responses. The endothelial cells can also express important cell-surface immunoregulatory molecules (Table 23A-3). The low level of basal major histocompatibiltiy complex (MHC) I expression on endothelial cells, which can be enhanced following a variety of stimuli, provides a potential ligand for cell-mediated cytotoxic responses. Although absent in the basal state, MHC II expression on endothelial cell surfaces can be stimulated by interferon γ. Such endothelial cells can effectively present antigen to CD4 T cells, stimulating a proliferative response. The endothelial cells induced ability to present antigen may play a central role in any potential mechanism of T cell mediated vasculitis. Endothelial cells also can express cell surface adhesion molecules. Such molecules play a important role in physiologic cell-to-cell interactions as they facilitate leukocyte egress from the intravascular space (15). The cell adhesion molecules may also play a potential role in the clinical expression of vasculitis. In the animal model of the Shwartzman reaction, the binding of the leukocyte adhesion molecule from the CD18 family of integrins to the intercellular adhesion molecule-1 (ICAM-1) on the endothelial cells plays a critical role in the expression of the hemorrhagic vasculitis (15). Antibodies to either CD18 or ICAM-1 markedly inhibit the develpment of the hemorrhagic vasculitis.

Lymphocytes

A role for lymphocyte-mediated responses has been suggested for the expression of Wegener's granulomatosis, Takayasu arteritis, and giant cell arteritis. Of these vasculitides, the role for antigen-driven T-cell responses is most clearly defined in the pathogenesis of giant cell arteritis (17-20). Studies of genetic factors of disease expression have generally demonstrated an over-representation of the HLA–DR4 haplotype in patient populations with giant cell arteritis. This association has been mapped to the HLA–DRB1 locus (17) In comparing the sequences of disease-associated and non-associated HLA–DRB1 genes, a sequence polymorphism within the hypervariable region 2 of the HLA–DRB1 gene spanning amino acid positions 28 to 31 is identified in patients with giant cell arteritis. Based on models of the HLA–DR molecule, this amino acid sequence defines a shallow pocket on the floor of the antigen binding cleft. This pocket may contribute to the interactions necessary for antigen binding in the cleft. The demonstration of a disease-associated sequence polymorphism in an antigen binding element of the HLA–DR molecule suggests that antigen selection and presentation in the context of an MHC II restricted response is a necessary element in the pathogenesis of giant cell arteritis.

Studies of the mononuclear cell profiles in the inflammatory lesions of temporal artery biopsies also support an antigen-driven response in the pathogenesis of giant cell arteritis (18,19). The CD4 T cells are the dominant cell phenotype in the arteritis lesions. Only a small percentage (<5%) of the infiltrating T cells demonstrate evidence of activation such as IL-2R expression. These cells demonstrate evidence of recent activation through the antigen receptor, and the majority of this small subset of activated T cells also produces interferon γ. Detailed analysis of T cell receptor (TCR) expression demonstrates only a small percentage of the CD4 T cells undergo clonal expansion. Clonally expanded CD4 with identical TCR patterns can be identified in anatomically distinct lesions from the same biopsy, and the clonally expanded T cells in the arteritis lesions are enriched rela-

(Table 23A-3)

*Endothelial cells: potential immunoregulatory functions**

Parameter	Expression	Potential Mechanism
MHC I	Basal: + Induced: TNF, IFN-γ, IFN-α/γ, infection	Ligand to CD8 which is present on a subset of T cells and LGL. May serve as target for cell-mediated cytotoxicity, regulation of T cells
MHC II	Basal: 0 Induced: IFN-γ ? antigen	Ligand to CD4 which is present on a subset of T cells. Endothelial cells can present antigen in MHC restricted fashion with resulting T cell proliferation
LFA-3	Basal: + Induced: ?	Ligand to CD2 on T cells and LGL. May provide signal to T cell that results in augmented IL-2 production
ICAM-1	Basal: + Induced: IL-1, TNF, IFN-γ, endotoxins	Ligand to CD18 family of leukocyte integrins which are present on lymphocytes, LGL, monocytes, and activated macrophages and PMN

* Information is summarized from references 14–16. MHC = major histocompatibility complex, TNF = tumor necrosis factor, IFN = interferon, LGL = large granular leukocyte, LFA = lymphocyte function associated, ICAM = intercellular adhesion molecule, PMN=polymorphonuclear leukocytes.

(Table 23A-4)

Cytokine expression in Wegener's granulomatosis and giant cell arteritis

	Serum Levels		
	Elevated	Normal	Expression
Wegener' granulomatosis	IL-2	IL-1	In renal tissue: TNF-α
	sIL-2R	IFN-γ	IL-1β
	IL-6	sCD4	IL-2R
	TNF-α	sCD8	
	IFN-α		
	sICAM-1		
	sVCAM-1		
	sE-selectin		
Giant cell arteritis	IL-6	TNF-α	In temporal artery: TNF-α
	sIL-2R		IL-1β
	sICAM-1		IL-2
			IL-6
			TGF-β
			IFN-γ

* IL = interleukin, IL-2R = interleukin 2 receptor, sIL-2R = soluble interleukin 2 receptor, IFN = interferon, TNF = tumor necrosis factor, sCD4 = soluble CD4, sCD8 = soluble CD8, sICAM-1 = soluble intercellular adhesion molecule 1, sVCAM-1 = soluble vascular adhesion molecule 1.

tive to the peripheral blood compartment. Moreover, activated macrophages producing IL-1 and IL-6 that are readily demonstrated in arteritis lesions could serve as efficient antigen presenting cells. These observations provide compelling evidence that a localized, antigen-driven immune response is important in the pathogenesis of giant cell arteritis. The putative giant cell arteritis associated antigen(s) remains to be identified.

Cytokines

Cytokine and soluble mediator expression has been studied in Wegener's granulomatosis and giant cell arteritis (Table 23A-4). The general pattern of pro-inflammatory cytokine expression in the setting of active vasculitis suggests a final common pathway for disease expression. Elevated levels of IL-6 and/or sIL-2R may correlate with disease activity. The pattern of cytokine expression, however, does not appear to define a specific vasculitis syndrome.

THOMAS R. CUPPS, MD

1. American College of Rheumatology Subcommittee on Classification of Vasculitis: The American College of Rheumatology 1990 Criteria for the Classification of Vasculitis. Arthritis Rheum 33:1065-1144, 1990
2. Jennette JC, Falk RJ, Andrassy K, et al: Nomenclature of systemic vasculitis: proposal of an international consensus conference. Arthritis Rheum 37:187-192, 1994
3. Cupps TR, Fauci AS: The vasculitides. In Smith LH (ed): Major Problems in Internal Medicine. Philadelphia, WB Saunders 21:1-211, 1982
4. Fauci AS, Haynes BF, Katz P: The spectrum of vasculitis. Clinical, pathologic, immunologic, and therapeutic considerations. Ann Intern Med 89:660-676, 1978
5. Systemic Vasculitides. Churg A, Churg J (eds). New York, Igaku-Shoin, 1991
6. Watts RA, Carruthers DM, Scott DGI: Epidemiology of systemic vasculitis: changing incidence or definition. Semin Arth Rheum 25:28-34, 1995
7. Lie JT, Members and Consultants of the American College of Rheumatology Subcommittee on Classification of Vasculitis: Illustrated histopathologic classification criteria for selected vasculitis syndromes. Arthitis Rheum 33:1074-1087, 1990
8. Cupps TR: Infections and vasculitis: mechanisms considered. In LeRoy EC (ed): Systemic Vasculitis, the Biologic Basis. New York, Marcel Dekker, 1992, pp 483-503
9. Reinisch CL, Moyer CF: Animal models of vasculitis. In Churg A, Churg J (eds): Systemic Vasculitides. New York, Igaku-Shoin, 1991, pp 31-40
10. Falk RJ, Terrell RS, Charles LA, Jennette JC: Anti-neutrophil cytoplasmic autoantibodies induce neutrophils to degranulate and produce oxygen radicals *in vitro.* Proc Natl Acad Sci USA 87:4115-4119, 1990
11. Brasile L, Kremer JM, Clarke JL, Cerilli J: Identification of an autoantibody to vascular endothelial cell-specific antigens in patients with systemic vasculitis. Am J Med 87:74-80, 1989
12. Leung DYM, Collins T, Lapiere LA, et al: Immunoglobulin M antibodies present in the acute phase of Kawasaki syndrome lyse cultured vascular endothelial cells stimulated by gamma interferon. J Clin Invest 77:1428-1435, 1986
13. Leung DYM, Geha RS, Newburger JW, et al: Two monokines, interleukin 1 and tumor necrosis factor, render cultured endothelial cells susceptible to lysis by antibodies circulating during Kawasaki syndrome. J Exp Med 164:1058-1972, 1985
14. Huges CCW, Savage COS, Pober JS: The endothelial cell as a regulator of T-cell function. Immunol Rev 117:85-102, 1990
15. Argenbright LW, Barton RW: Interactions of leukocyte integrins with intercellular adhesion molecule 1 in the production of inflammatory vascular injury in vivo. J Clin Invest 89:259-272, 1992
16. Sundy JS, Haynes BF: Pathogenic mechanisms of vessel damage in vasculitis syndromes. Rheum Dis Clin North Am 21:861-881, 1995
17. Weyand CM, Hicok KC, Hunder GG, Goronzy JJ: The HLA-DRB1 locus as a genetic component in giant cell arteritis. Mapping of a disease-linked sequence motif to the antigen binding site of the HLA-DR molecule. J Clin Invest 90:2355-2361, 1992
18. Weyand CM, Schonberger J, Oppitz U, et al: Distinct vascular lesions in giant cell arteritis share identical T cell clonotypes. J Exp Med 179:951-960, 1994
19. Weyand CM, Hicok KC, Hunder GG, Goronzy, JJ: Tissue cytokine patterns in patients with polymyalgia rheumatica and giant cell arteritis. Ann Intern Med 121:484-491, 1994
20. Weyand CM, Goronzy JJ: Giant cell arteritis as an antigen-driven disease. Rheum Dis Clin North Am 21:1027-1039, 1995

The clinical course of the different forms of systemic vasculitis may be brief or prolonged, benign or fatal (1,2). Classification criteria have been established for the major forms of vasculitis; considerable overlap exists among the vasculitic syndromes (3) (see Appendix I). When a patient is seen who has manifestations that overlap with more than one type of vasculitis or who does not easily fit into a specific category, the extent of involvement should be defined as carefully as possible and treatment decided accordingly.

TAKAYASU'S ARTERITIS
Clinical Manifestations

Takayasu's arteritis, a chronic vasculitis of the aorta and its branches, is most common in young women of Asian descent (4). It seldom starts after the age of 40 years. The proximal aorta and its branches tend to be involved to the greatest degree, but any part of the aorta may be affected. In the early phases, nonspecific symptoms such as malaise and arthralgias are frequent. Mild synovitis is noted in about 20% of patients. Erythema nodosum-like vasculitis lesions may occur over the legs. The disease progresses at a variable rate; after weeks or months, manifestations of vascular insufficiency become apparent and include coolness of one or more extremities, headaches, dizziness, amaurosis, or diplopia. Angina pectoris may develop due to narrowing of coronary artery ostia. The blood pressure may become difficult to detect because of narrowing of the subclavian artery or more distal vessels. Pain in the arms with sustained use may develop (arm claudication), and claudication in the legs may result from narrowing of the distal aorta or iliac vessels. Intra-abdominal and cerebral ischemia may develop due to narrowing of mesenteric or cervical vessels.

Asymmetrically reduced peripheral pulses are present in nearly all patients. Blood pressure differences of >10 mm Hg are found in most patients. Hypertension is present in 40% of patients secondary to renal artery stenosis, peripheral arterial obstruction, or rigidity of inflamed large vessels. Bruits may be audible over the carotid, subclavian, and other large arteries, and aortic valve insufficiency may be present due to aortic root dilation.

Laboratory Tests

A normochromic anemia, elevated erythrocyte sedimentation rate (ESR), and thrombocytosis are present during the inflammatory phase of the disease. Hyperglobulinemia occurs occasionally. The electrocardiogram may reveal an ischemic pattern, and widening of the thoracic aorta may be detected on chest radiography. Arteriography shows smooth, tapered narrowings, occlusions, or aneurysms of the aorta and its proximal branches (Fig. 23B-1).

Diagnosis

The diagnosis of Takayasu's arteritis should be suspected in young women with a history of a systemic inflammatory illness, altered arterial pulses, or bruits over large arteries. The diagnosis generally is confirmed by arteriography. Digital subtraction angiography with intravenous dye injection provides less distinct resolution of the vessel wall outlines and a more restricted survey of the arterial tree, but the technique may be adequate in some cases. Computed tomography and magnetic resonance angiography (MRA) studies show luminal narrowing and mural thickening in vessels and may be useful to support initial arteriographic findings and in follow-up monitoring. Because of the size of the vessels affected, biopsies are rarely obtained. Takayasu's arteritis tends to be chronic. The 15-year survival rate has been reported to be over 80% (5).

Differential diagnosis includes carotid artery dissection that is usually localized, early arteriosclerosis in patients with risk factors, heritable connective tissue disorders such as Ehlers–Danlos syndrome, and giant cell arteritis.

GIANT CELL ARTERITIS
Clinical Manifestations

Giant cell arteritis is also known as temporal arteritis or cranial arteritis. It affects individuals over 50 years of age and is more common in women. Individuals of northern European extraction are particularly susceptible, with incidence rates as high as 20–30 new cases annually per 100,000 persons over the age of 50 years (6). It affects the same population as the closely associated process of polymyalgia rheumatica.

The disease usually begins gradually and may be present for a number of weeks or months before its recognition. At times, the onset is abrupt and flu-like. Early symptoms include malaise, fatigue, fever (sometimes as high as 104°F), weight loss, and polymyalgia rheumatica. Common manifestations related to vascular involvement include headaches, tenderness of the scalp (especially over the temporal arteries), jaw claudication (fatigue and discomfort in the muscles of mastication during chewing), visual loss, diplopia, aortic arch syndrome, and cough or sore throat.

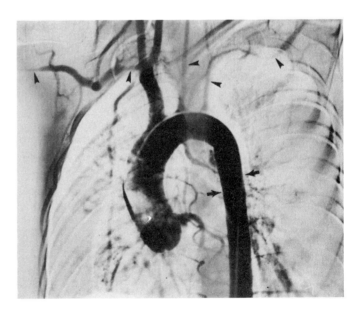

(Figure 23B-1)
Takayasu's arteritis. Aortogram showing slight narrowing of the descending aorta (arrows) and multiple narrowed segments of large thoracic and cervical arteries (arrow heads).

The temporal arteries may be erythematous, thickened, and tender (Fig. 23B-2). Occasionally, the occipital, facial, or postauricular arteries are similarly affected. Visual loss occurs in about 15% of patients and may be an early symptom (7). Vision loss usually results from retinal ischemia secondary to involvement of the ophthalmic or posterior ciliary arteries. It is abrupt and painless. However, amaurosis fugax may precede permanent blindness. Permanent visual impairment varies from a partial deficit of one eye to complete bilateral blindness. In patients with visual manifestations, the ophthalmologic examination may reveal ischemic optic neuropathy early, and optic atrophy after several weeks.

Clinical involvement of the aortic arch and its branches occurs in approximately 10%–15% of patients and may cause reduced blood pressure in one or both arms, arm claudication, or focal cerebral ischemia (7). Peripheral neuropathy occurs in a minority of patients, but involvement of the skin, intracranial vessels, kidneys, or lungs rarely occurs. Aortic aneurysm is a late complication in about 10% of patients and is often first detected 6–7 years after the initial diagnosis of giant cell arteritis (8).

Laboratory Tests

The ESR tends to be higher than in other vasculitis syndromes, averaging about 80–100 mm/hr (Westergren). Rarely, it may be normal, even when the disease is active.

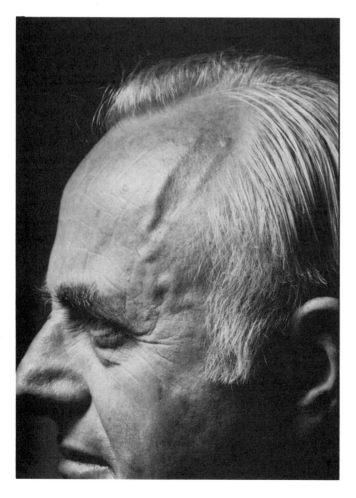

(Figure 23B-2)

Giant cell arteritis. Swollen tender left temporal artery which is more prominent than seen in most cases. Pulsations were present on palpation and the wall was thickened when compared to the right side.

Other acute-phase serum proteins such as C reactive protein are similarly elevated. Additional laboratory alterations include increased hepatic enzymes in 20%–30% of patients, and elevated levels of factor VIII and interleukin-6.

Diagnosis

Giant cell arteritis should be suspected in patients older than age 50 who develop a new type of headache, jaw claudication, fever, or polymyalgia rheumatica. Careful examination may reveal a thickened or tender temporal artery, new carotid artery bruits, or bruits over the axillary or brachial arteries. Biopsy of the most abnormal segment of the temporal arteries should be performed to confirm the diagnosis even when manifestations seem relatively typical. Positive biopsies show mural lymphocytes, macrophages, giant cells, and a disrupted elastic lamina. If a temporal artery is clearly inflamed, only a short piece of the abnormal part of the artery needs to be biopsied. However, because involvement tends to be patchy, a 3–6 cm segment should be obtained when the physical findings are indeterminate. The biopsied arterial segment should be examined at several levels. If the first side is negative, consideration should be given to biopsying the other temporal artery. A properly performed temporal artery biopsy will define the need for corticosteroid therapy in about 90% of cases.

Other forms of arteritis occasionally affect the temporal artery and cause clinical and pathologic findings compatible with giant cell arteritis, including Wegener's granulomatosis and polyarteritis nodosa (7). Takayasu's arteritis begins at an early age, less commonly involves branches of the external carotid artery, and has not been demonstrated to involve the temporal artery. Occasionally, amyloidosis affects temporal arteries or causes jaw or arm claudication.

POLYARTERITIS NODOSA
Clinical Features

Polyarteritis nodosa may affect any organ of the body, but skin, peripheral nerves, joints, intestinal tract, and kidneys are most commonly involved (9). The lungs are usually spared. Although the severity varies, polyarteritis nodosa is a serious and often progressive and fatal illness. Vasculitis similar to polyarteritis nodosa may be an occasional secondary or associated manifestation of other diseases such as rheumatoid arthritis (RA) and systemic lupus erythematosus (SLE).

Polyarteritis nodosa is uncommon; estimates of its incidence in the general population have ranged from about 5 to 10 per million persons per year. The disease is twice as common in men. It may be observed in children and the elderly, but it is more common in middle age.

Onset of disease may be gradual or abrupt. Constitutional symptoms such as fever and malaise are usually present. Cutaneous manifestations include palpable purpura, infarctive ulcers of varying sizes, and livedo reticularis. Joint pain is common, but synovitis is less frequent.

Multiple mononeuropathies are the most typical neurologic manifestation and occur in one-half or more of all patients. Sharp sudden pain or paresthesias in the distribution of a peripheral nerve are often the first symptoms, followed by weakness of the muscles supplied by that nerve. Several nerves may become involved progressively, resulting in a severe diffuse polyneuropathy.

Vascular nephropathy and segmental necrotizing glomerulonephritis may lead to renovascular hypertension. Gastrointestinal ischemia causes abdominal pain and findings of an acute abdomen. Occasionally, the cystic or appendiceal artery may be involved. Hematemesis or melena may result from vasculitis of the upper or lower gastrointestinal tract. Liver involvement causes transaminase elevations. Coronary arteritis may result in myocardial ischemia or congestive heart failure.

Laboratory Tests

As in most systemic vasculitides, tests show a normochromic, normocytic anemia, an elevated ESR and other acute-phase reactants, neutrophilic leukocytosis, and thrombocytosis. Serum complement is usually normal but may be reduced in patients with a pathogenesis involving immune complexes. Serum rheumatoid factor may be present in this latter group.

Hepatitis B surface antigen and antibody have been found in 15% or more of patients and may be present continuously or transiently. Hepatitis C and A also have been identified. Patients who are positive for hepatitis antigen or antibodies usually appear similar to those who are negative. Hepatic dysfunction is generally mild and does not parallel the severity or activity of the vasculitis. Urinalysis in those with glomerulonephritis shows red blood cells, red cell casts, and proteinuria. Renal insufficiency may develop.

Histologic examination of biopsy specimens reveals an acute inflammatory infiltrate with polymorphonuclear leukocytes and a variable number of macrophages, lymphocytes, and eosinophils (Fig. 23B-3). Fibroid necrosis is often present. Lesions in various stages of development may be present in the same specimen. Disruption of the elastic laminae results in arterial dilation or formation of an aneurysm.

Diagnosis

It is important to pursue the diagnosis aggressively and start therapy promptly to limit organ damage. Polyarteritis nodosa should be suspected in patients with unexplained fever, weight loss, fatigue, and multisystem findings. Evidence of vasculitis should be established whenever possible by biopsy of clinically involved tissues. Biopsy of the skin or

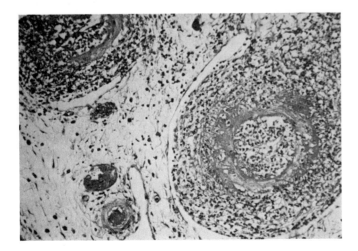

(Figure 23B-3)
Polyarteritis nodosa. Photomicrograph of small muscular artery showing acute inflammation, destruction of mural structures, and fibrinoid necrosis.

sural nerve generally yields small arteries, and of the muscle or testes, somewhat larger vessels. The chance of finding vasculitis in an organ without evidence of involvement is lower than when the organ is affected. A kidney biopsy may be considered in patients with abnormal urinary sediment or proteinuria.

Mesenteric arteriograms may be helpful when abdominal pain or elevated hepatic enzymes are present and a biopsy site cannot be readily identified. Typical angiographic changes include multiple arterial aneurysms and tapered narrowings and irregularities. However, similar changes may be present in other forms of vasculitis, including Wegener's granulomatosis, Churg–Strauss syndrome, vasculitis in SLE, or other illnesses such as infective endocarditis, atrial myxoma, and noninflammatory connective tissue disorders such as fibromuscular dysplasia.

Before the use of corticosteroids, the 5-year survival of polyarteritis was reported to be less than 15%. In recent years survival has improved; studies now indicate a 5-year survival of 60% or more (9). The prognosis of polyarteritis nodosa is worse in older persons and those with more extensive visceral or central nervous system involvement. Most deaths caused by polyarteritis nodosa occur within the first year of disease as a result of uncontrolled vasculitis or superimposed infections related to therapy (10).

CHURG–STRAUSS SYNDROME
Clinical Features

The Churg–Strauss syndrome, initially reported under the descriptive title allergic granulomatosis and angiitis, is uncommon (9,11). Involvement of the lungs helps distinguish it from polyarteritis nodosa. This condition occurs in patients with asthma or a history of allergy. It usually develops in middle age and affects men more commonly than women. In many patients, the disease follows a phasic pattern. Initially, an increase in allergic manifestations occurs, especially asthma, followed by eosinophilia and finally vasculitis.

Fever, malaise, and weight loss are common early manifestations. As the vasculitis develops, asthma may become less prominent. Cutaneous findings include petechiae, purpura, or ulcerations. Chest discomfort or shortness of breath may result from pulmonary lesions. Peripheral neuropathy, usually multiple mononeuropathies, is common. Abdominal symptoms include diarrhea, pain, or a mass due to ischemia or infarction of abdominal organs. Renal lesions tend to be less severe than in polyarteritis nodosa. Eosinophilic granulomatous involvement of the gastrointestinal and urinary tracts or prostate is a unique feature of this syndrome.

Laboratory Tests

Eosinophilia is present in essentially all patients but resolves in response to treatment. Serum complement is usually normal. Renal function may be diminished in patients with vascular nephropathy or glomerulonephritis. Urinalysis reveals proteinuria and red blood cell casts. Chest radiographs show patchy or nodular infiltrations or diffuse interstitial disease.

Biopsy of involved tissues shows angiitis and extramural necrotizing microgranulomas, usually with eosinophilic infiltrates. The vascular infiltration includes eosinophils and may be granulomatous or nongranulomatous. Veins may be affected as well as arteries.

Diagnosis

The syndrome should be suspected in patients with worsening asthma who develop fever and evidence of a systemic illness. The diagnosis should be confirmed by biopsy of involved tissues. Abdominal angiograms may show findings similar to those in polyarteritis nodosa.

The mortality rate is lower than that in polyarteritis nodosa, and remission is seen in some cases. This syndrome needs to be differentiated from Loffler's syndrome, hypersensitivity vasculitis, and Wegener's granulomatosis.

WEGENER'S GRANULOMATOSIS
Clinical Findings

Wegener's granulomatosis is an uncommon vasculitis that occurs in young or middle-aged adults and is slightly more common in men (12,13). It is often considered a triad of necrotizing granulomatous vasculitis of the tissues of the upper respiratory tract, the lower respiratory tract, and focal segmental glomerulonephritis. However, limited forms occur that may affect only one of these areas, and other tissues also may be involved. Small arteries and veins are the predominant vessels affected.

Patients often present with nonspecific findings of fever, malaise, weight loss, arthralgias, myalgias, and chronic rhinitis or worsening sinusitis. Pain over the sinus areas and purulent or bloody nasal discharge are typical upper respiratory symptoms. Nasal or oral mucosal ulcerations are early findings. Destructive changes lead to a saddle-nose deformity.

Pulmonary involvement may be asymptomatic or may cause chest pain, shortness of breath, bloody or purulent sputum, and hemorrhage. Tracheal lesions and especially subglottic involvement may produce stenosis. Eye symptoms include episcleritis, uveitis, and proptosis due to orbital granulomas. Cranial nerve deficits may be the result of granulomatous inflammation in or near the upper airways.

Cutaneous findings include nodules, purpura, and ulcerations. Arthritis is infrequent and usually transient.

Laboratory Tests

Patients with renal involvement have proteinuria, hematuria, and red blood cell casts. Chest radiographs show nodules and infiltrations that often cavitate.

Serum antibodies that react with cytoplasmic components of neutrophils (c-ANCA) are present in approximately 80% of patients, especially those with active multisystem disease (14). The test is positive most commonly in those with widespread systemic disease and less frequently in limited forms and inactive disease. Antibodies to perinuclear cytoplasmic particles (p-ANCAs) are present in a minority of patients with Wegener's granulomatosis, but are more common in microscopic polyangiitis. ANCAs are found in a minority of patients with polyarteritis nodosa and other forms of vasculitis.

Histologic examination of involved specimens shows a necrotizing granulomatous inflammatory process with involvement of small arteries and veins. In some inflammatory lesions, especially of the upper airway structures, vasculitis is not a prominent feature, and it may not be found in biopsy specimens of limited size. Purpuric skin lesions may show leukocytoclastic vasculitis.

Diagnosis

The diagnosis should be suspected in patients with progressive upper or lower respiratory tract manifestations and nasal or oral ulcerations. The presence of serum c-ANCA makes the diagnosis likely. Biopsy of involved tissues should be performed to confirm the diagnosis.

Septic processes, especially fungal and mycobacterial infections, should be excluded. Angiocentric T-cell lymphomas (lymphomatoid granulomatosis) produce somewhat similar destructive lesions. Patients with Churg—Strauss syndrome may present with a similar triad of organ involvement.

VASCULITIS ASSOCIATED WITH RHEUMATIC DISEASES
Clinical Findings

Blood vessels are involved in many connective tissue disorders. Perivascular leukocyte cuffing without damage to the vessel or tissue ischemia is part of the disease process, but it is not considered vasculitis by itself. Proliferation of the blood vessel intima (obliterative endarteritis) with little evidence of active inflammation may develop and cause tissue ischemia. This bland thickening of the intima is often seen in systemic sclerosis and results in ulcers or infarction of the distal finger pads. Somewhat similar changes may occur in RA and other connective tissue disorders producing dermal infarctions at the fingernail folds and elsewhere.

In a small proportion of patients with RA, SLE, and other connective tissue disorders, necrotizing vasculitis develops during the course of disease (15). The vessels involved may be small, medium-sized muscular arteries, or even larger arteries that show histologic changes indistinguishable from polyarteritis nodosa.

Patients with RA who develop necrotizing vasculitis are more likely to be male and to have erosive joint disease, rheumatoid nodules, and high titers of serum rheumatoid factor. At the time of active vasculitis, serum complement is reduced and immune complexes appear in the serum. Frequent manifestations include skin infarctions over the lower extremities and multiple mononeuropathies. Mesenteric ischemia may occur. Renal disease is very rare. Patients with SLE who develop necrotizing vasculitis typically have livedo reticularis, Raynaud's phenomenon, cutaneous lesions, and digital gangrene.

Diagnosis

Vasculitis should be suspected in patients with a connective tissue disorder whose symptoms rapidly become worse (especially systemic symptoms such as fever) and who develop skin lesions, neuropathy, or abdominal pain.

Electromyograms help elucidate the type of neuropathy. Skin or sural nerve biopsies aid in documenting the presence of vasculitis. Mesenteric angiograms help clarify the nature of abdominal pain when present, gastrointestinal bleeding secondary to bowel ischemia, or both.

CENTRAL NERVOUS SYSTEM VASCULITIS
Clinical Features

Many forms of vasculitis affect the central nervous system (CNS); however, when vasculitis occurs without any associated disease, it is designated primary vasculitis of the central nervous system. Primary CNS vasculitis is uncommon. It occurs at all ages with onset common between 40 and 50 years of age. It appears to be somewhat more frequent in men (16). Very little is known of its pathogenesis, but about 25% of cases have been associated with lymphoreticular neoplasms. It has also been associated with herpes zoster, human T lymphotrophic virus type III, and human immunodeficiency virus (HIV) infection.

The course of primary CNS vasculitis is variable. It may be fatal within weeks or chronically progressive over 1 or more years. Early symptoms are confusion, headache, and progressive impairment of intellectual functioning. Focal neurologic deficits, seizures, and cranial nerve involvement occur frequently. In occasional instances, spinal cord vessels also become involved.

Laboratory Tests

The hemoglobin level, leukocyte count, and ESR are generally normal. Cerebrospinal fluid may show an increased opening pressure, mild pleocytosis, and mildly increased protein concentration. Magnetic resonance imaging of the head demonstrates multiple lesions. Cerebral angiograms typically show intermittent narrowing and dilation of small and medium-sized intracranial blood vessels. Vessels in one region, such as the base of the brain, may be affected more prominently. In other cases, generalized intracerebral involvement is present.

Diagnosis

Diagnosis is often difficult. CNS vasculitis should be considered in patients who present with progressive headaches, impaired mental function, and multifocal neurologic deficits, especially if there is a history of herpes zoster infection, lymphoma, or illicit drug use. In these cases, angiograms should be performed to detect smooth-walled tapered areas and aneurysms. However, angiograms are not always definitive. Arterial spasm (related to either the procedure or intracranial hemorrhage) and other diseases may produce similar changes. Normal appearance on angiograms is rare in CNS vasculitis but does not exclude the diagnosis.

Brain and leptomeningeal biopsy, while not a simple procedure, is definitive when positive and should be considered when the diagnosis seems likely. Histologically, the most common finding is a granulomatous vasculitis. Because the vessels are involved in a patchy distribution, small biopsy specimens obtained via burr holes may not include an involved artery. Patients diagnosed by angiograms alone constitute a less well-defined group.

Conditions that produce similar findings to CNS vasculitis include Cogan's syndrome (nonsyphilitic interstitial keratitis and vestibular dysfunction), Behçets syndrome, SLE, polyarteritis nodosa, and antiphospholipid syndrome.

HYPERSENSITIVITY VASCULITIS
Clinical Findings

This category includes cases of vasculitis of small vessels, especially arterioles and venules, secondary to an immune response to exogenous substances. Reactions to drugs are the most common cause (17).

Onset is usually abrupt and occurs after exposure to the etiologic agent. Palpable purpura is the most common clinical manifestation (Fig. 23B-4). Cutaneous ulcerations may

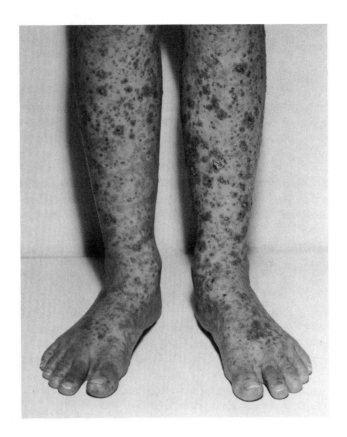

(Figure 23B-4)
Hypersensitivity vasculitis. Extensive palpable purpuric lesions over legs. Some lesions became confluent, and superficial ulcerations developed.

develop, transient arthralgias are frequent, and systemic symptoms may be present. The severity of the illness varies considerably from a few scattered purpuric spots to an extensive, prolonged, systemic process.

Laboratory Findings

The laboratory alterations are usually nonspecific and may be limited in mild cases. The ESR is usually elevated. Serum complement, especially C4, may be reduced during the acute phase, and eosinophilia may be present.

Biopsy of cutaneous lesions shows leukocytoclastic vasculitis of arterioles and postcapillary venules and neutrophils, nuclear fragments secondary to karyorrhexis, perivascular hemorrhage, and fibrinoid deposits. Eosinophils are often present. In a minority of cases, lymphocytic infiltrations predominate. Microhematuria occurs, but renal failure is uncommon.

Diagnosis

Hypersensitivity vasculitis is diagnosed by biopsy with the finding of cutaneous vasculitis and, on occasion, identification of a potential inciting agent. Manifestations usually appear abruptly. All lesions tend to be at approximately the same stage of development and generally resolve after a period of days or weeks.

The clinical definition of this syndrome has been difficult because a responsible agent cannot be identified in many patients who have compatible clinical and biopsy findings. In some patients, symptoms persist and the disease becomes chronic, especially with cutaneous involvement, even though there is no apparent continuous exposure to a sensitizing substance. These observations raise questions about other possible pathogenic mechanisms. Furthermore, clinical manifestations in hypersensitivity vasculitis are not distinctive, and similar clinical pictures may be associated with a variety of other disorders such as Henöch–Schönlein purpura, rheumatic disorders, cryoglobulinemia, and infections. Microscopic polyangiitis and cutaneous polyarteritis nodosa may be difficult to distinguish from hypersensitivity vasculitis, other than the chronic course in the former. Other less common forms of vasculitis, such as hypocomplementemic urticarial vasculitis, and infections such as bacterial endocarditis, also need to be differentiated from hypersensitivity vasculitis.

MICROSCOPIC POLYANGIITIS
Clinical Manifestations

Microscopic polyangiitis, also called microscopic polyarteritis, is a systemic necrotizing vasculitis that involves small vessels including arterioles, capillaries, and venules. Men are affected more often than women. The average age at onset is about 50 years. This condition is uncommon and its actual incidence is unknown. Typical manifestations include glomerulonephritis, pulmonary hemorrhage or infiltration, musculoskeletal pains (sometimes with synovitis), purpura, peripheral neuropathy, and abdominal pain.

The illness may begin gradually or abruptly. Systemic symptoms such as malaise, fatigue, and fever are usually present. Most patients have some renal insufficiency at the time of diagnosis, and renal function often progressively deteriorates. Pulmonary hemorrhage caused by capillaritis occurs in one-third of cases and produces hemoptysis, dyspnea, and anemia. Diffuse interstitial lung changes and infiltrations may occur. Gastrointestinal pain or bleeding caused by mesenteric vascular ischemia can develop. Mononeuritis multiplex or polyneuropathy develops in 20% of patients, and episcleritis is present in approximately 30%.

Relapses may be seen during the course of the disease, which can be exacerbations of earlier findings or new manifestations. Most relapses include cutaneous rash and arthralgias.

Laboratory Tests

Changes due to the inflammation are present, including anemia, elevated erythrocyte sedimentation rate, and other acute phase reactants. Serum rheumatoid factor is found in some cases. The presence of serum perinuclear-antineutrophil cytoplasmic antibodies (p-ANCA) is an important diagnostic finding; they are found in two-thirds or more of cases. The majority of these antibodies are directed against myeloperoxidase (anti-MPO).

Diagnosis

Microscopic polyangiitis should be suspected in middle-aged men who present with findings of a systemic inflammatory illness and subacute progressive renal insufficiency. Multisystem involvement suggests vasculitis. The diagnosis is essentially confirmed if renal biopsy shows focal pauci-immune segmental necrotizing glomerulonephritis with extracapillary proliferation forming crescents. Chest radiographs in patients with pulmonary hemorrhage show infiltrations or alveolar shadowing in the absence of pulmonary edema or infection. Biopsy of purpuric lesions or other affected organs usually shows leukocytoclastic vas-

culitis. The presence of p-ANCA strongly supports the diagnosis, but the test is not as sensitive nor as specific as c-ANCA is in Wegener's granulomatosis. Visceral angiography is not generally helpful, even in patients with abdominal involvement, because vessels affected are generally too small to be visualized. Microscopic polyangiitis is distinguished from polyarteritis nodosa by the predominant involvement of small vessels, prominent glomerulonephritis, pulmonary manifestations, and p-ANCA (18). Goodpasture's syndrome, which also presents with a pulmonary–renal syndrome, is distinguished from microscopic angiitis by the absence of vasculitis and multisystem involvement and the presence of serum antibasement membrane antibodies.

CRYOGLOBULINEMIA
Classification

Cryoglobulins are immunoglobulins that have the property of reversibly precipitating at reduced temperatures. Cryoglobulins are present in a variety of autoimmune, neoplastic, and infectious disorders. They may be grouped into two general categories (Table 23B-1).

Type I cryoglobulins consist of a single monoclonal protein and are generally associated with multiple myeloma, macroglobulinemia, and less common other neoplastic proliferations of lymphocytes. These cryoglobulins generally are readily detectable as monoclonal components on electrophoresis of serum. They often produce no symptoms but occasionally cause Raynaud's phenomenon, livedo reticularis, purpura, or ischemic ulcers due to hyperviscosity and plugging of small vessels in the acral parts of the body when cooled. Vasculitis is rare. In several large series of patients with cryoglobulinemia, monoclonal cryoproteins constitute

(Table 23B-1)
Clinical associations of cryoglobulinemia

Monoclonal cryoglobulins
    Multiple myeloma (IgG, IgA), macroglobulinemia (IgM), lymphoproliferative disorders, angioimmunoblastic lymphadenopathy
Mixed cryoglobulins
    Essential mixed cryoblulinemia
    Connective tissue diseases
        Systemic lupus erythematosus, rheumatoid arthritis, polyarteritis nodosa, Sjögren's syndrome, systemic sclerosis, etc.
    Infections
        Viral: hepatitis A, B, C, infectious mononucleosis, cytomegalovirus
        Bacterial: subacute bacterial endocarditis, post-streptococcal glomerulonephritis, leprosy, syphilis, Lyme disease, intestinal bypass disorder
        Parasitic: schistosomiasis, echinococcosis, toxoplasmosis, malaria, kalar-azar
    Lymphoproliferative disease
        Macroglobulinemia, chronic lymphocytic leukemia, lymphoma, angioimmunoblastic lymphadenopathy
    Miscellaneous
        Chronic liver disease, proliferative glomerulonephritis, sarcoidosis

about one-third of those encountered. The frequency of immunoglobulin types seen in this group of patients is the same as the frequency of all immunoglobulins that produce tumors: IgG is most frequent, IgM less common, and IgA least frequent.

Type II cryoglobulins consist of more than one class of immunoglobulin. They are common, constituting about two-thirds of the cryoglobulins seen in the Western world. Type II cryoglobulinemia appears as a primary disease (essential or primary mixed cryoglobulinemia) or as a manifestation of some other underlying disease. Mixed cryoglobulins generally contain IgM molecules together with IgG, although other combinations are found. One component, usually IgM, has antiglobulin activity (rheumatoid factor) and is the reason for the complex formation and the cryoprecipitation. They may also contain other antigens such as hepatitis B virus, other infecting agents, and nuclear and complement proteins. These cryoglobulins are more difficult to detect because they precipitate more slowly and tend to be present in small quantities (50–500 mg/dL).

Mixed cryoglobulins have been further subdivided into those in which one component is monoclonal, usually the IgM, and those in which all components are polyclonal. This division appears to have little clinical or prognostic significance in patients whose cryoglobulins are associated with nonmalignant disorders.

Pathophysiology

The frequent association with chronic infections and the presence of proteins from infecting agents in the cryoprecipitates have suggested that IgG antibodies complexed with an infecting agent (antigen) induce the production of IgM anti-antiglobulins. When infections resolve, the cryoglobulins and antiglobulins are no longer formed.

Mixed cryoglobulins have all the properties of an immune complex. They activate the complement sequence and, when deposited in small peripheral blood vessels, cause vasculitis through complement-mediated inflammation. It is uncertain why some patients have symptoms and others do not, and why there are differences in severity and organ involvement. Determining factors may be related to the nature of the antigen or antibody raised, the size of the complexes, the function of the reticuloendothelial system, the ability of activate complement, or endothelial cell–immune complex interactions.

Clinical Features

Cutaneous lesions are most common and include palpable purpura, urticaria, and ulcers. Other features include Raynaud's phenomenon, arthralgias, glomerulonephritis, peripheral neuropathy, hepatomegaly, splenomegaly, and lymphadenopathy. Thyroiditis, Sjögren's syndrome, pneumonitis, and pericarditis may be present.

The course may be mild or prolonged and is influenced by the organs involved and any associated underlying disease. Progressive glomerulonephritis is often the most serious manifestation (19). In some patients with primary mixed cryoglobulinemia, cirrhosis or a lymphoproliferative disorder eventually develops.

Laboratory Tests

Serum gammaglobulins are often elevated, rheumatoid factor is present, and complement levels are decreased. Hepatitis B and C viruses frequently have been associated with mixed

cryoglobulinemia (20). Hepatitis A and other agents, including Epstein–Barr virus, cytomegalovirus, and HIV, have also been found and suggest a viral-related pathogenesis.

Serum containing cryoglobulins becomes opalescent and forms a visible precipitate when incubated at 0–4°C. The quantity of cold-insoluble proteins can be determined either by means of a cryocrit or more accurately by isolating the cryoglobulin and measuring the amount of precipitate formed. Further characterization of the protein type can be carried out by immunoelectrophoresis or immunoglobulin quantitation. In searching for cryoglobulins, it is important to draw the blood in a warm syringe, allow it to clot, separate the serum at 37°C, and then incubate the serum in the cold for several days.

Diagnosis

Serum should be tested for cryoglobulins in patients with vasculitis and those with connective tissue disorders, infections, and neoplasms, especially when cutaneous or renal involvement or evidence of vasculitis develops. Analysis of the cryoglobulin components may elucidate the nature of the disease and help in the decisions regarding therapy.

GENE C. HUNDER, MD

1. Churg A, Churg J (eds): Systemic Vasculitides. New York, Igaku-Shoin, 1991, pp 389
2. Hunder GG: Vasculitis. Rheum Dis Clin North Am 21:861-1164, 1995
3. American College of Rheumatology Subcommittee on Classification of Vasculitis: The American College of Rheumatology 1990 Criteria for the Classification of Vasculitis. Arthritis Rheum 33:1065-1144, 1990
4. Kerr GS, Hallahan CW, Giordano J, et al: Takayasu arteritis. Ann Intern Med 120:919-929, 1994
5. Ishikawa K, Maetani S: Long-term outcome for 120 Japanese patients with Takayasu's disease: clinical and statistical analyses of related prognostic factors. Circulation 90:1855-1860, 1994
6. Salvarani C, Gabriel SE, O'Fallon WM, Hunder GG: The incidence of giant cell arteritis in Olmsted County, Minnesota: apparent fluctuations in a cyclic pattern. Ann Intern Med 23:192-194, 1995
7. Lie JT: Aortic and extracranial large vessel giant cell arteritis: a review of 72 cases with histopathologic documentation. Sem Arthritis Rheum 24:422-431, 1995
8. Evans JM, O'Fallon WM, Hunder GG: Increased incidence of aortic aneurysm and dissection in giant cell arteritis: a population-based study. Ann Intern Med 122:502-507, 1995
9. Lhote F, Guillevin L: Polyarteritis nodosa, microscopic polyangiitis, and Churg-Strauss syndrome: clinical aspects and treatment. Rheum Dis Clin North Am 21:911-947, 1995
10. Fortin PR, Larson MG, Watters AK, Yeadon CA, Choquette D, Esdaile JM.: Prognostic factors in the polyarteritis nodosa group: a review of 45 cases. J Rheumatol 22:78-84, 1995
11. Guillevin L, Shote F, Grayraud M, Cohen P, Jarrousse B, Lortholary O, Thibult N, Casassus P: Prognostic factors in polyarteritis nodosa and Churg-Strauss syndrome. A prospective study in 342 patients. Medicine 75:17-28, 1996
12. Hoffman GS, Kerr GS, Leavitt RY, Hallahan CW, Lebovics RS, Travis WD, Rottem M, Fauci AS: Wegener granulomatosis: an analysis of 158 patients. Ann Intern Med 116, 488-498, 1992
13. Duna GF, Galperin C, Hoffman GS: Wegener's granulomatosis. Rheum Dis Clin North Am 21:949-986, 1995
14. Jennette JC, Falk RJ: Disease associations and pathogenic role of antineutrophil cytoplasmic autoantibodies in vasculitis. Curr Opin Rheumatol 4:9-15, 1992
15. Bacon PA, Carruthers DM: Vasculitis associated with connective tissue disorders. Rheum Dis Clin North Am 21:1077-1096, 1995
16. Calabrese LH, Duna G: Evaluation and treatment of central nervous system vasculitis. Curr Opin Rheumatol 7:37-44, 1995
17. Michel BA, Hunder GG, Bloch DA, Colabrese LH: Hypersensitivity vasculitis and Henoch-Schonlein purpura: a comparison between the two disorders. J Rheumatol 19:721-728, 1992
18. Guillevin L, Lhote F: Distinguishing polyarteritis from microscopic polyangiitis. Curr Opin Rheumatol 7:20-24, 1995
19. D'Amico G, Fornasier A: Cryoglobulinemic glomerulonephritis: a membranoproliferative glomerulonephritis inducedby hepatitis C virus. Am J Kid Dis 25:361-369, 1995
20. Gumber SC, Chopra S: Hepatitis C: a multifaceted disease: review of extrahepatic manifestations. Ann Intern Med 123:615-620, 1995

The cornerstone for successful treatment of vasculitis is making an accurate diagnosis as quickly as possible, recognizing the prognosis, and anticipating the effects of disease and treatment on other concurrent illnesses (1).

The severity of disease, anatomic distribution of involvement, rate of progression, and preexisting conditions should determine the aggressiveness of therapy. With the exception of acute Kawasaki syndrome, in which salicylates and high-dose intravenous immunoglobulin are indicated, therapy for all other forms of severe systemic vasculitis should begin with high-dose corticosteroids (eg, prednisone 1 mg/kg/day). Whether corticosteroids should be given as a single morning dose, in two or three split doses, or as a large intravenous pulse or bolus (such as methylprednisolone 1 gram), or whether a cytotoxic agent should be used at the onset requires considering the status of each patient. For example, most patients with giant cell arteritis improve dramatically after corticosteroid therapy alone, whereas most patients with generalized Wegener's granulomatosis and associated glomerulonephritis progress to renal failure and death if not treated with a cytotoxic agent such as cyclophosphamide (2).

TAKAYASU'S ARTERITIS

About 20% of patients with Takayasu's arteritis have a monophasic, self-limiting illness that does not require treatment. Most of these individuals are diagnosed during routine examination at which pulse deficits, asymmetries, or bruits are recognized. Subsequent vascular imaging studies reveal typical patterns of stenoses and or aneurysms of the aorta and its primary branches. Other patients are diagnosed because they develop symptoms of claudication or other ischemic events and constitutional symptoms. Patients that have symptoms or serologic markers of active disease, such as elevated erythrocyte sedimentation rate (ESR), usually respond to corticosteroid therapy (eg, prednisone 1 mg/kg/day), and some may be successfully tapered off without disease relapse (3). Cytotoxic agents are beneficial in patients who fail to respond or who relapse upon tapering corticosteroids (4,5).

Among the most difficult management problems in Takayasu's arteritis is recognition and treatment of clinically silent progressive disease. Active disease in asymptomatic individuals has been identified by periodic arteriographic studies and bypass graft surgeries that have revealed new sites of stenosis or aneurysm. These observations indicate that clinical findings and inflammatory markers such as ESR or von Willebrand factor antigen are not sufficiently sensitive or specific to identify all patients with active disease (3,4).

Vascular bypass procedures have successfully diminished morbidity and mortality in carefully selected patients with cerebral, coronary, or peripheral ischemic vascular disease and renal artery stenosis with hypertension (6). Less often, dilation of the aortic root may lead to severe aortic regurgitation, requiring an aortic graft and aortic valve replacement. The usual limitations of vascular surgery are further complicated by the possibility of active arteritis leading to occlusion at the graft origin or insertion. As many as one-third of bypass procedures require revision at some time (3,6). Several questions about vascular surgery in Takayasu's arteritis remain unanswered (6-8). Do the limitations in detecting active disease justify pre- and postoperative corticosteroid therapy for all patients? Should patients with anatomically severe but asymptomatic lesions have prophylactic surgery (eg, bilateral common carotid occlusion), or should the clinician temporize until ischemic symptoms occur? Is there a difference in long-term graft patency between autologous vein or artery and synthetic graft materials? Does long-term anticoagulation with antiplatelet agents or warfarin affect graft patency? Is transluminal angioplasty comparable to bypass surgery for some specific lesions?

Hypertension and its treatment are critical aspects of care for patients with Takayasu's arteritis. In some series, especially those from Asia, hypertension is among the most common presenting manifestations and may affect up to 90% of patients. It is one of the leading causes of morbidity and mortality in this disorder. Inadequately treated hypertension contributes more often to cerebrovascular, cardiovascular, and renovascular organ failure than primary vascular stenotic lesions. Whenever feasible, anatomic correction of aggravating or causative lesions (eg, renal artery stenosis) should be attempted. Marked improvement or "cure" of renovascular hypertension is well documented in this setting. Hypertension complicating pregnancy in a patient with Takayasu's arteritis represents a special problem. It is the leading risk factor for poor outcome for both mother and fetus. To date, there is no proof that pregnancy itself enhances vascular inflammation.

Mortality has been reported to range from as little as 3% up to 35% in the first 5 years of onset (4). This great variation is probably due to differences in study methodology, as well as variable access to medical and surgical treatment in different parts of the world. Morbidity from disease and treatment has been estimated to cause partial or complete disability in up to 75% of patients (3).

GIANT CELL ARTERITIS

Corticosteroids continue to be the most effective treatment for giant cell arteritis. Prednisone (0.7–1 mg/kg/day) reduces symptoms within 2 days and often eliminates symptoms within a week. One month after clinical and laboratory parameters, particularly ESR, have returned to normal, tapering can begin. Unfortunately, the ESR does not always normalize, even with disease control, so it should not be relied on as the only measure. Occasional patients either may not achieve complete remission or may not be able to be tapered off steroids. Cytotoxic or immunosuppressive agents have been recommended for such individuals by some authors, but the utility of these agents, as demonstrated in controlled comparative trials, has not been addressed (9).

Treatment and follow-up of giant cell arteritis has been influenced by an increasing appreciation of extracranial large-vessel involvement and potential sequelae. Examples include aortic dissection, renal artery stenosis and hypertension, coronary artery disease, and subclavian, iliac, or femoral artery stenosis. Because these patients are elderly, there has been a tendency to assume that disease in extracranial large vessels was probably secondary to atherosclerosis, which in fact may be a coincidental finding. Nonetheless, histologic proof of large-vessel inflammation has been documented in 15%–75% of cases. Consequently, patients suspected of having giant cell arteritis should have a careful evaluation of large vessels, much like that done for Takayasu's arteritis. Recognition of abnormalities has implications for medical and possibly surgical therapies.

Evidence that as many as 40% of patients with polymyalgia rheumatica may have histologic evidence of giant cell arteritis has continued to fuel controversy over whether all patients with polymyalgia rheumatica should be treated with high-dose corticosteroids. This issue is not likely to be resolved soon. However, the clinical overlap of these disorders does obligate careful vascular evaluations of patients with presumed polymyalgia rheumatica.

POLYARTERITIS NODOSA AND MICROSCOPIC POLYANGIITIS

Untreated, these quite similar diseases have been estimated to have a 5-year mortality rate in excess of 85%. Factors that impart a poor prognosis in individual cases include glomerulonephritis, gastrointestinal ischemia, cardiac involvement, and cerebral vasculitis. Treatment with high-dose corticosteroids has decreased 5-year mortality to about 30%–45% (10–11). When corticosteroids have been used in conjunction with an immunosuppressive/cytotoxic agent (usually cyclophosphamide, and less often azathioprine, about 2 mg/kg/day) relapses were less frequent (11) than noted with corticosteroid therapy alone. The additional use of plasmapheresis does not appear to provide any distinct advantages (10). When cyclophosphamide is used, it is uncertain whether daily oral or monthly pulse intravenous therapy are superior in relative efficacy. A reasonable approach to treatment in patients with normal renal function and no critical organ ischemia is to initiate therapy with only corticosteroids. If improvement does not follow within days, if deterioration occurs, or if renal, cardiac, intestinal, or central nervous system disease becomes apparent, therapy with a cytotoxic agent should be added.

The treatment recommendations for these disorders assume that infectious causes of vasculitis, which may have similar or identical patterns, have been evaluated and ruled out. Examples include endocarditis (bacterial or fungal), the hepatitis viruses (particularly B and C), HIV, and less often cytomegalovirus. If vasculitis was one of the manifestations of a viral infection, antiviral therapy should be a part of the treatment. In some cases, with mild disease, antiviral therapy alone may be sufficient.

CHURG–STRAUSS SYNDROME

Churg–Strauss syndrome is much less common than polyarteritis nodosa or microscopic polyangiitis. Consequently, information about its therapy is anecdotal. Some authors believe Churg–Strauss syndrome is more responsive to corticosteroids than polyarteritis or microscopic polyangiitis. The same principles for individualizing therapy and for adding a cytotoxic agent, as noted for polyarteritis nodosa and microscopic polyangiitis apply.

WEGENER'S GRANULOMATOSIS

Survival in Wegener's granulomatosis has been improved by aggressive therapy combining prednisone and daily cyclophosphamide, as well as by recognizing milder, more indolent forms of disease without renal involvement (about 20% of patients). Although combined drug therapy has been life-saving for many patients, it has become clear that for limited indolent disease, such treatment may carry excessive risk. Palliation of limited disease is often achieved with corticosteroid therapy alone, but disease progression and relapses are common.

For patients with severe, life-threatening disease, corticosteroids and daily low-dose cyclophosphamide (2 mg/kg and in extreme situations up to 4 mg/kg) remain the treatment of choice (2,12). However, toxicity is distressing and has led to trials of high-dose intravenous cyclophosphamide and studies of other agents such as methotrexate. Preliminary results indicate that pulse cyclophosphamide and corticosteroids may provide substantial initial improvement, but this combined therapy is not as effective as daily low-dose cyclophosphamide in maintaining improvement (12). Methotrexate therapy is a reasonable treatment option for selected patients with Wegener's granulomatosis (13,14). Other attempts to identify less toxic therapies for milder forms of disease include trials of daily trimethoprim–sulfamethoxazole (15). The results of these studies are controversial. Several small studies have sought to evaluate the immunosuppressive potential of high-dose intravenous immunoglobulin in Wegener's granulomatosis. In a recent trial involving 15 patients, 40% experienced some improvement of minor disease manifestations; however, none of the patients achieved remission (16).

The most serious and common complication of intense immunosuppressive therapy is severe infection, especially *Pneumocystis carinii* pneumonia (2,17). Pneumocystis infections commonly develop during the period of intensive therapy, suggesting that chemoprophylaxis is prudent, especially during cyclophosphamide therapy.

Because delayed treatment of disease exacerbations enhances risks of poor outcome, there has been much interest in early treatment based on markers of impending relapse. The antibody to the neutrophil antigen proteinase 3, one of a family of antineutrophil cytoplasmic antibodies (ANCA), has been evaluated for its utility as a surrogate marker for active Wegener's granulomatosis. Although ANCA titer changes have been shown to correlate with disease activity in at least two-thirds of patients, variability in individual cases and prognostic utility have been disappointing in a substantial minority of patients. Most authorities agree that changes in ANCA titers should *not* be the principal element in guiding changes in therapy.

Wegener's granulomatosis is an excellent example of the necessity for a multidisciplinary team approach to achieve the best possible outcome. Chronic otitis media may require tympanotomy and drainage tubes; hearing loss may progress to the need for hearing aids. Nasal and sinus disease may be complicated by chronic crusting, mucopurulent discharge, and secondary infection that may require daily irrigation and occasionally debridement or surgery. The development of subglottic stenosis may necessitate dilatation, intralesional corticosteroid injections, tracheostomy, or even extensive reconstructive surgery. Retro-orbital pseudotumor and lacrimal duct obstruction may demand ophthalmic surgery, as well as medical treatment. Finally, complications of aggressive immunosuppressive therapy, including infections, hemorrhagic cystitis, or bladder cancer from cyclophosphamide, may require special expertise for management.

CENTRAL NERVOUS SYSTEM VASCULITIS

Recent findings have stressed the clinical heterogeneity, variable prognosis, and limitations of neuroimaging studies, including angiography, in providing a definitive diagnosis of central nervous system (CNS) vasculitis. Even the histopathologic finding of vasculitis on brain biopsy is not definitive until infectious, malignant, and drug-induced (especially cocaine) causes have been ruled out (18,19). Each underlying cause obviously requires different therapies. Based only on uncontrolled empiric experience, it is generally recommended that primary CNS vasculitis be treated with high-dose prednisone (1–2 mg/kg/day) for 4–6 weeks, which is often given in combination with oral cyclophosphamide (2 mg/kg). After a response has been achieved, prednisone should be tapered over a period of several months; if cyclophosphamide was given, the drug should be continued for at least 12 months after all signs of disease have resolved. Other forms of vasculitis involving the central nervous system, in particular postpartum cerebral angiopathy and benign CNS angiopathy, are treated with high-dose corticosteroids for several weeks with tapering over 4–6 months. A calcium channel blocker may be beneficial.

HYPERSENSITIVITY VASCULITIS

Patients with other forms of vasculitis for whom prognosis is dependent on organ involvement other than the skin may present with cutaneous lesions identical to hypersensitivity vasculitis (eg, microscopic polyangiitis, cryoglobulinemia and vasculitis, Churg–Strauss syndrome, Wegener's granulomatosis, and vasculitis associated with HIV, hepatitis, or malignancy). Thus, when confronted with cutaneous lesions of a vasculitic nature, the clinician is obligated to search for more serious forms of illness. In acute hypersensitivity vasculitis, visceral involvement is usually less common and less severe than in polyarteritis nodosa, Wegener's granulomatosis, or Churg–Strauss syndrome. Consequently, a more cautious therapeutic approach is advised. If illness is mild and a drug reaction is suspected, the likely causative medication should be discontinued. If the patient has had a self-limiting or treatable infection, cautious follow-up (with or without antibiotic therapy) may be adequate. However, in the setting of visceral ischemia or glomerulonephritis, it is prudent to prescribe daily corticosteroids. Sustained resolution of abnormalities should lead to a slow taper and discontinuation of steroids over 4-8 weeks.

CRYOGLOBULINEMIA

In patients with secondary forms of cryoglobulinemic vasculitis related to malignancy, infections, or inflammatory disorders, treatment should be directed at the primary disease process. Treatment of patients with essential or viral-associated mixed cryoglobulinemia depends on the severity of disease. Supportive treatment of symptoms alone may be adequate for the typical patient with mild purpura and arthralgias. Patients with progressive renal disease or neuropathy require a more aggressive therapeutic approach

that may include high-dose corticosteroids, immunosuppressive agents, and plasmapheresis. Anti-viral therapy (vidarabine or interferon α for hepatitis B-associated cryoglobulinemia and vasculitis has been palliative for most patients; in one study over 50% of patients achieved long-term remissions (20,21). When therapy has been effective, the need for broad-spectrum immunosuppressive agents has markedly decreased. Unfortunately, the results for hepatitis C have been less encouraging. Although more than 50% of patients treated with interferon α improve, relapses are common when therapy is discontinued (21). Interferon α cannot be given indefinitely because of the high frequency of toxicity.

LONG-TERM THERAPY

Because most systemic vasculitides are not cured, realistic goals include diminishing morbidity from disease and treatment, while hoping that the underlying process will undergo an extended treatment-induced remission or will be self-limited. Examples of vasculitides that may be monophasic are the hypersensitivity vasculitides, Henöch–Schönlein purpura, polyarteritis nodosa/microscopic polyangiitis, giant cell arteritis of the elderly, and Takayasu's arteritis. However, many individuals with polyarteritis nodosa/microscopic polyangiitis, giant cell arteritis, Takayasu's arteritis, Wegener's granulomatosis, Churg–Strauss syndrome, and Behçet's disease who achieve remission later relapse after a brief interval or sometimes even after more than 10 years of treatment-free sustained remission (2,3). These patients do not possess any clinical or serologic markers that predict risk of recurrence. Thus, regardless of how well a patient with these disorders has fared over time, the physician is obligated to maintain surveillance.

The clinician embarking on corticosteroid therapy should consider the effects of treatment on intravascular volume, blood pressure, glucose metabolism, and electrolyte balance. Caution is especially important in elderly patients and those with preexisting hypertension, cardiac disease, or diabetes mellitus. When treatment is indicated for systemic vasculitis, high doses should be maintained until all manifestations of active disease have abated. Tapering corticosteroids should follow after about 1 month, although there is no consensus of opinion about strategies for tapering corticosteroids. One approach is to reduce prednisone to alternate day doses so that within 2–3 months (in the absence of relapse or exacerbations) a dose of about 1 mg/kg every other day is achieved. During the subsequent 2–3 months, tapering of the alternate-day schedule continues until therapy is discontinued. However, waxing and waning of disease may force alterations in these guidelines. The immunologic defects induced by corticosteroids are dependent on dose, frequency, and duration of treatment. As each factor increases, the incidence of opportunistic infections and other side effects increases. The use of alternate-day prednisone (single morning dose) is associated with less toxicity than daily treatment. However, even when alternate-day prednisone dosing can be achieved, the risk of osteoporosis and fracture is great. All patients who receive long-term corticosteroids should be placed on bone conservation therapy.

In some vasculitides that respond to corticosteroids, relapses become so common that continuous prednisone therapy may begin to produce more morbidity than the underlying illness. Cytotoxic therapy should be considered in such cases to enhance the likelihood of remission as well as for steroid-sparing effects. Cyclophosphamide has been the most thoroughly studied cytotoxic agent for treatment of vasculitis. Although this agent may be life-saving and may be the best-known means of achieving remission in severe systemic vasculitides, it may also cause substantial morbidity and even mortality. Its use requires close vigilance of bladder and bone marrow effects, titration of doses, high oral fluid intake to dilute cyclophosphamide-derived bladder toxins (such as acrolein), and urologic consultation for any sign of bladder toxicity. It is this experience that has led to investigation of alternative cytotoxic therapies, such as weekly methotrexate (13,14).

GARY S. HOFFMAN, MD

1. Hoffman GS, Kerr GS: Recognition of systemic vasculitis in the acutely ill patient. In Mandell BF(ed): Management of Critically Ill Patients with Rheumatologic and Immunologic Diseases. Marcel Dekker, Inc., 1994, pp. 279-308

2. Hoffman GS, Kerr GS, Leavitt RY, et al: Wegener's granulomatosis: an analysis of 158 patients. Ann Intern Med 116:488-498, 1992

3. Kerr GS, Hallahan CW, Giordano J et. al. Takayasu's arteritis. Ann Intern Med 120:919-29. 1994

4. Hoffman GS : Treatment of resistant Takayasu's arteritis. Rheum Dis Clinics N Am 21:73-80. 1995

5. Hoffman GS, Leavitt RY, Kerr GS, et al: Treatment of Takayasu's arteritis with methotrexate. Arthritis Rheum 37:578-582, 1994

6. Giordano JM, Leavitt RY, Hoffman GS, et al: Experience with surgical treatment of Takayasu's disease. Surgery 109:252-258, 1991

7. Tyagi S, Singh B, Kaul UA, et al: Balloon angioplasty for renovascular hypertension in Takayasu's arteritis. Am Heart J 125:1386-1393, 1993

8. Rao SA, Mandalam KR, Rao VR, et al: Takayasu's arteritis: initial and longterm followup in 16 patients after percutaneous transluminal angioplasty of the descending thoracic and abdominal aorta. Radiology 189:173-179, 1993

9. Wilke WS, Hoffman GS: Treatment of glucocorticoid-resistant giant cell arteritis. Rheum Dis Clin N Am 21:59-71, 1995

10. Guillevin L, Lhote F, Cohen P, et al: Corticosteroids plus pulse cyclophosphamide and plasma exchanges versus corticosteroids plus pulse cyclophosphamide alone in the treatment of polyarteritis nodosa and Churg–Strauss syndrome patients, with factors predicting poor prognosis. Arthritis Rheum 38:1638-1645, 1995

11. Guillevin L, Jarrousse B, Lok C, et al: Longterm followup after treatment of polyarteritis nodosa and Churg–Strauss angiitis with comparison of steroids, plasma exchange, and cyclophosphamide to steroids and plasma exchange. A prospective randomized trial of 71 patients. J Rheumatol 18:567-574, 1991

12. Hoffman GS, Leavitt RY, Fleisher TA, et al: Treatment of Wegener's granulomatosis with intermittent high-dose intravenous cyclophosphamide. Am J Med 89:403-410, 1990

13. Hoffman GS, Leavitt RY, Kerr GS, Fauci AS: The treatment of Wegener's granulomatosis with glucocorticoids and methotrexate. Arthritis Rheum 35:6112-6118, 1992

14. Sneller MC, Hoffman GS, Talar-Williams C, et al: An analysis of 42 Wegener's granulomatosis patients treated with methotrexate and prednisone. Arthritis Rheum 38:608-613, 1995

15. DeRemee RA: The treatment of Wegener's granulomatosis with trimethoprim/sulfamethoxazole: illusion or vision? Arthritis Rheum 31:1068-1072, 1988

16. Richter C, Schnabel A, Cernok E, et al: Treatment of anti-neutrophil cytoplasmic antibody (ANCA)-associated systemic vasculitis with high dose intravenous immunoglobulin. Clin Exp Immunol 101:2-7,1995

17. Ognibene FP, Shelhamer JH, Hoffman GS, et al: Pneumocystis carinii pneumonia: A major complication of immunosuppressive therapy in patients with Wegener's granulomatosis. Am J Respir Crit Care Med 151:795-799, 1995

18. Calabrese LH, Duna GF: Evaluation and treatment of central nervous system vasculitis. Curr Opin Rheumatol 7:37-44, 1995

19. Merkel PA, Koroshetz WJ, Irizarry MC, Cudkowicz ME: Cocaine-associated cerebral vasculitis. Sem Arthritis Rheum 25:172-83, 1995

20. Guillevin L, Lhote F, Leon A, et al: Treatment of polyarteritis nodosa related to hepatitis B virus with short term steroid therapy associated with antiviral agents and plasma exchanges. A prospective trial in 33 patients. J Rheumatol 20:289-98, 1993

21. Misiani R, Bellavita P, Fenili D, et al: Interferon alpha-2a therapy in cryoglobulinemia associated with hepatis C virus. N Engl J Med 330:751-756, 1994

24 POLYMYALGIA RHEUMATICA

The initial description of polymyalgia rheumatica was by Bruce, who used the name "senile rheumatic gout" (1). During the 1950s, when the syndrome was described repeatedly, it was thought to be related to rheumatoid arthritis. In 1957, Barber concluded that the condition was a separate clinical entity within the rheumatoid group of diseases and suggested the name polymyalgia rheumatica. Myalgic symptoms similar to polymyalgia rheumatica were also recognized in several early reports on temporal arthritis. In the beginning of the 1960s, it was found that several patients with polymyalgia rheumatica had histologically verified giant cell arteritis in temporal artery biopsies. An attractive hypothesis was formed suggesting that temporal arteritis and polymyalgia rheumatica are two expressions of underlying generalized giant cell arteritis.

EPIDEMIOLOGY

Polymyalgia rheumatica is almost exclusively reported in whites. It is much more common among people of northern European descent than among southern Europeans. The disease is very rare among blacks and Asians. The incidence increases with higher age, and the disease is rarely diagnosed in those below the age of 50.

Polymyalgia rheumatica is roughly twice as common in women as in men. In a recent survey from Gothenburg, Sweden, the annual incidence was found to be 17 per 100,000; for the population over 50 years of age it increased to 50 per 100,000 inhabitants (2).

CLINICAL PRESENTATION

Almost all patients display systemic symptoms. Fever is the most frequent symptom; weight loss and malaise are also common. The onset may sometimes be so acute that the patient can tell the exact date when the illness began, although it is often more insidious. The majority of all patients note muscular symptoms at the onset of disease. The muscles of the neck and shoulders, especially, are involved early, and a mistaken diagnosis of frozen shoulder or cervical myelopathy may be made at an early stage of disease. During the subsequent disease course, muscular involvement becomes more widespread. Eventually patients have symptoms from all proximal muscle groups, including the brachial-cervical region, hip, and thigh.

Morning stiffness is a characteristic complaint. Unlike patients with rheumatoid arthritis, in whom symptoms arise from small joints and cause difficulty performing tasks such as buttoning clothes, patients with polymyalgia rheumatica localize their symptoms to the proximal muscles and joints and complain of difficulty in performing such activities as getting out of bed, rising from a chair, climbing into a train, cleaning windows, or combing hair. In one-third of patients, aching and stiffness is so severe that self care becomes difficult.

Despite these distressing clinical symptoms, objective findings are rare. The fact that patients localize their symp-

toms to the muscles would suggest a muscular disease. Physical examination, however, only reveals muscle tenderness; atrophy is rarely found. Synovial biopsy specimens from large joints reveal mild, nonspecific synovitis. Abnormal uptake on joint scintigrams, mainly from the shoulders have been observed, but objective signs of synovitis are rare.

There are no specific laboratory tests for polymyalgia rheumatica. A highly elevated erythrocyte sedimentation rate (ESR) is the rule, usually above 50 mm/hour. In addition, increased levels of fibrinogen, haptoglobin, and platelets are a characteristic finding. Another commonly used indicator of inflammatory reaction is elevation of C-reactive protein levels. Anemia and abnormal liver function tests are also observed often.

Diagnosis is based on clinical criteria. These include pain and stiffness in at least two large muscle groups (ie, neck and shoulders-upper arms, hips, and thighs) with a duration of symptoms of more that two weeks, and without clinical or laboratory evidence of infection, rheumatoid arthritis, systemic lupus erythematosus, periarteritis nodosa, or malignancy. Furthermore, an elevated ESR and age greater than 50 years are also required, as well as rapid and lasting relief of symptoms after institution of corticosteroid therapy (3).

PATHOGENESIS

The cause of polymyalgia rheumatica is unknown and the association with giant cell arteritis is still a matter of controversy. An infectious process is suggested by the fever, leukocytosis, elevated ESR, and generalized illness of the patients, but no organisms have ever been isolated. The predominance in the white population, familial aggregation and the association with HLA–DR4 antigen favor a genetic predisposition (4). There is controversy as to whether polymyalgia rheumatica and giant cell arteritis are expressions of the same disease or are two different, partly overlapping diseases. In view of the clinical similarities between polymyalgia rheumatica patients with and without signs of arteritis in a temporal artery biopsy, many authors favor the concept that polymyalgia rheumatica is an expression of underlying giant cell arteritis. Others believe that a single causative factor is responsible for the two conditions, sometimes expressing itself as polymyalgia rheumatica and sometimes as giant cell arteritis (5). More than 90% of temporal artery specimens from giant cell arteritis patients with signs of cranial symptoms (headache, scalp tenderness) show a granulomatous inflammatory reaction concentrated around the inner half of the media and centering on a disrupted internal elastic lamina.

Polymyalgia rheumatica is diagnosed primarily by the clinical presentation of muscle pain and stiffness in the proximal portions of the extremities and torso, by increased ESR, and by the clinical response to glucocorticoids. Recently it has been shown that tissue samples from patients with polymyalgia rheumatica who had no histologic evidence of inflammation contained inflammatory cytokines, suggesting vascular disease (6). Recent studies have also shown morphologic similarities in terms of vessel wall atrophy and calcifications in noninflamed vascular segments in patients with polymyalgia rheumatica and giant cell arteritis (7).

TREATMENT

The aims of treatment are to relieve the patient of troublesome symptoms and prevent vascular complications from an underlying vasculitis. Corticosteroids are the drug of choice. Nonsteroidal anti-inflammatory drugs may give partial relief of polymyalgia rheumatica symptoms, but have not been shown to prevent vascular complications. Thus, there is a consensus for the use of short-acting corticosteroids, such as prednisolone, in this disease. The recommendations on the initial dose of prednisolone vary depending on the condition of the patient as well as the suspicion that underlying giant cell arteritis may be present. For patients with polymyalgia rheumatica without any signs of overt giant cell arteritis, 15 to 30 mg/day is often recommended; however, the starting dose of prednisolone must be chosen with respect to the condition of the patient. In patients starting with a higher daily dose than 15 mg, the dose can be reduced weekly by 5 mg until a dose of 15 mg is reached. Dose reduction necessitates careful monitoring, and the patient must report recurrence of symptoms. The ESR should be assessed every second to third week. Dose reduction below the level of 15 mg/day of prednisolone can be achieved in steps of 2.5 mg every month. A maintenance dosage of prednisolone of 2.5 mg to 7.5 mg is usually reached within 6 to 12 months.

The duration of the treatment varies according to the patient. No laboratory test can predict when therapy should be discontinued. After approximately 6–12 months without any symptoms of disease and with a normal ESR on a maintenance dose of 2.5 mg of prednisolone, treatment may be stopped. Approximately 50% of patients remain free from symptoms, while the rest will relapse during the following months. If clinical relapse is detected early, restarting treatment with 10–15 mg of prednisolone is usually sufficient. Corticosteroids relieve the symptoms of polymyalgia rheumatica, but there is no evidence to suggest they shorten the duration of the disease.

The most commonly reported adverse effects of corticosteroids are vertebral crush fractures, hip fractures, diabetes mellitus, peptic ulcers, and cataracts. The prevalence of these complications varies widely in available studies. In addition, these conditions are common in the elderly population, making it difficult to attribute such events to corticosteroid treatment. In order to minimize adverse events, the drug should be administered in a single dose in the morning using the lowest possible dose that will keep the patient free of symptoms. There are conflicting data on the role of methotrexate as a corticosteroid-sparing agent in polymyalgia rheumatica (8,9).

PROGNOSIS

Similar to biopsy-proven giant cell arteritis (10), polymyalgia rheumatica without any histologic evidence of giant cell arteritis in a temporal artery biopsy has recently been shown to be statistically associated with increased cardiovascular mortality.

BENGT-ÅKE BENGTSSON, MD, PhD

1. Bruce W: Senile rheumatic gout. Br Med J 2:811-813, 1888
2. Schaufelberger C, Bengtsson BÅ, Andersson R: Epidemiology and mortality in 220 patients with polymyalgia rheumatica. Br J Rheumatol 34:261-264, 1995
3. Bengtsson BÅ, Malmvall BE: Giant cell arteritis. Acta Med Scand (Suppl 658:1-102, 1982
4. Cid MC, Ercilla G, Vilaseca J, et al: Polymyalgia rheumatica: a syndrome associated with HLA-DR4 antigen. Arthritis Rheum 31:678-681, 1988
5. Hunder GG: More on polymyalgia rheumatica and giant cell arteritis. West J Med 141:68-70, 1984
6. Weyand CM, Hicok KC, Hunder GG, Goronzy JJ: Tissue cytokine pattern in patients with polymyalgia rheumatica and giant cell arteritis. Ann Intern Med 121:484-491, 1994
7. Nordborg E, Bengtsson BÅ, Nordborg C: Temporal artery morphology and morphometry in giant cell arteritis. APMIS 99:1013-1023, 1991
8. Ferraccioli G, Salaffi F, De Vita S, Casatta L, Bartoli E: Methotrexate in polymyalgia rheumatica: preliminary results of an open, randomized study. J Rheumatol 23:624-628, 1996
9. van der Veen MJ, Dinant HJ, van Booma-Frankfort C, van Albada-Kuipers A, Bijlsma JWJ: Can methotrexate be used as a steroid sparing agent in the treatment of polymyalgia rheumatica and giant cell arteritis? Ann Rheum Dis 55:218-223, 1996
10. Nordborg E, Bengtsson BÅ: Death rates and causes of death in 284 consecutive patients with giant cell arteritis confirmed by biopsy. Br Med J 299:594-595, 1990

25 BEHÇET'S DISEASE

Behçet's disease is an inflammatory condition of multiple organ systems in which recurrent oral and genital ulcers are the most typical signs (1,2) (Table 25-1). Less common clinical features include cerebral vasculitis, arterial aneurysms, deep vein phlebitis, aseptic meningitis, and discrete bowel ulcers. Because there are no specific pathologic or serologic tests, the diagnosis is often difficult and only about one-half of the patients referred to specialists with a diagnosis of Behçet's disease turn out to have the disease.

CLINICAL FEATURES

All the clinical events are episodic, occur over several years, and seldom are all in place at one time. Multiple oral aphthous ulcers are a cardinal feature, precede other signs in nearly all patients, and recur as rounded, painful "canker sores" at any site in the oral, lingual, and naso-pharyngeal mucosa. A typical aphtha evolves from a papule to a red-rimmed ulcer with central exudation, then to a clean ulcer before healing in days to weeks. Residual scarring is uncommon. The patient has oral ulcers 50% to 100% of the time. Similar ulcers on the vulva, cervix, scrotum, and penis are less prevalent than oral ulcers, but may erupt two or three times each year (Fig. 25-1).

Uveitis may develop within months of onset but usually appears after several years of the aphthous ulcers. Hypopyon (pus in the anterior chamber of the eye) is an extreme form of anterior uveitis and was prominent in early reports (3). More usual is a painless blurring of vision in one or both eyes due to some combination of anterior and posterior uveitis and retinal vasculitis (4). Patients report "spots" in their vision. Ophthalmologists use fundoscopy and slit lamp to detect cellular infiltrations in the media and/or actual retinal vasculitis with areas of infarction. Usually the eye disease becomes bilateral, involves the anterior and posterior uvea as well as the retina, and can lead to blindness within a few years. Scleritis, conjunctivitis, and lid lesions do not qualify as Behçet's-related eye disease.

Cutaneous lesions are found when patients are carefully examined (5). The most common lesions are recurring papules and pustules several millimeters in diameter on the upper trunk and thighs. While typical erythema nodosum is uncommon, nodose lesions with pustular tips are not rare. The pathergy response (Table 25-1) is an erythematous papule or pustule arising 24–48 hours after a skin injection or needle prick. Standardization of this test has been elusive. It is variously stated that the lesion should exceed 2 or 5 mm in diameter and appear 24 or 48 hours after forearm skin is pricked obliquely to a depth of 0.5 to 1 cm by a 22- or a 25-gauge needle (1,2,6). While some version of this test is said to be positive in most patients from the Middle and Far East, it is less often positive in patients seen in North America or East India.

About one-half of all patients experience synovitis in large joints, usually during exacerbations (7). The arthritis may involve knees, ankles, wrists, and tendon entheses in a recurring but rarely destructive process. Synovial fluid cell counts are inflammatory (5,000–25,000/mm^3) with a predominance of polymorphonuclear (PMN) leukocytes. Synovial biopsies

(Table 25-1)
International criteria for classification of Behçet's disease (1) *

Approximate Prevalence (percent)	Criteria	Description
100	Recurrent oral ulceration, aphthous	Recurring at least three times in a year
80	Recurrent genital ulceration, aphthous	Scrotal, penile, vulvar, or cervical
60–70	Eye inflammation	Anterior or posterior uveitis, or retinal vasculitis
60–80	Skin inflammation	Pseudofolliculitis, papulopustular or acne form lesions or erythema nodosum-like
Variable	Pathergy skin test	Erythematous papule >2 mm at entry site of disposable 20- or 22-gauge needle, penetrated obiquely to depth of about 5 mm, read at 48 hours

* All lesions should be verified by a physician, and eye inflammation should be verified by an ophthalmologist.

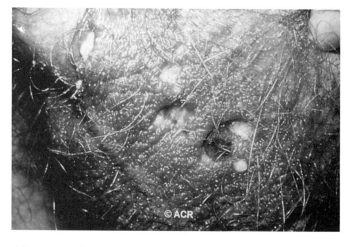

(Figure 25-1)
Scrotal ulcers in a patient with Behçet's disease. Reprinted from Clinical Slide Collection on the Rheumatic Diseases, with permission of American College of Rheumatology.

have shown infiltrates of PMN or mononuclear cells. Although Behçet's disease is not associated with HLA-B27, sacroiliitis can be detected in those Behçet's patients who have the HLA-B27 antigen. Central nervous system inflammation can present as aseptic meningitis with headache, fever, and stiff neck associated with cerebrospinal fluid (CSF) pleocytosis. This may present as an isolated event or, more ominously, in association with stroke (8). The CSF cell counts during episodes are elevated (above $5/mm^3$) but usually less than $100/mm^3$.

In the acute stage, PMN cells predominate, but after a few days lymphocytes outnumber them. The CSF protein can be normal or slightly elevated, while oligoclonal bands (IgA, IgM) and elevated immunoglobulin suggest either local production of antibodies or a breach in the blood–brain barrier. When Behçet's vasculitis occurs in the brain, CSF pleocytosis accompanies it. Patients experience sudden focal neurologic deficits from ischemic vasculitis in the brain stem. Lesions of the corticospinal tracts of the brain stem or cord can result in hemiparesis or quadriparesis often associated with cerebellar ataxia or pseudobulbar palsy. Magnetic resonance imaging (MRI) in acute phases reveals areas of increased signal in the brain stem, periventricular white matter, and basal ganglia. Neurologic deficits may remain even when MRI shows reduced lesional size after treatment. Cerebral angiography is seldom indicated, as the vessels involved are usually too small to show abnormalities. A distinctive syndrome of cerebral venous thrombosis is suspected when a patient presents with non-meningitic headache and elevated CSF pressure, eg 400-500 mm (9). The site of venous occlusions is seen on digital subtraction angiography or MRI.

About 20% of patients have deep vein phlebitis. Phlebitis affecting leg veins can ascend to the inferior vena cava. Syndromes of superior vena caval occlusion and Budd–Chiari syndrome are reported, but superficial phlebitis that can cause nodules on the extremities is more common. Pulmonary embolism is rare. Arterial pseudo-aneurysms are more common than ischemic occlusions. These aneurysms arise from areas of panarteritis and, when resected, can recur at the anastomosis. The intimal and medial layers are replaced by vasculitic inflammation. Clinical signs may be sudden, such as ominous hypotension due to rupture, but extremity and iliac aneurysms can be detected as a pulsating mass.

In the pulmonary circulation, a virtually pathognomonic presentation is pulmonary artery–bronchus fistula presenting as sudden, severe hemoptysis (10). This syndrome is more common in men than in women. Recognition of this lesion, as with other vasculitic aneurysms, can be life saving. Pulmonary embolism may be erroneously diagnosed, as the V–Q scan misleads; however, radiographs show perihilar radiologic opacities, and high-resolution computed tomography scan is almost as helpful as pulmonary arteriography (10). Patients having prominent venous or arterial phases of Behçet's vasculitis are susceptible to phlebitis or aneurysm developing at the sites of vessel trauma, such as venous or arterial puncture sites.

Gastrointestinal involvement can manifest as discrete mucosal ulcerations, especially in the terminal ileum, cecum, and ascending colon (11). Patients present with abdominal pain, bleeding, or perforation. Differentiation from Crohn's disease is often difficult. Although the endoscopist may not obtain adequate tissue for diagnostic pathology, specimens resected are free of granulomatous colitis. In a Japanese series of patients, recurrence after resection was usual, but rigorous immunotherapy was not given (11). Nephritis is rare, but secondary amyloidosis can complicate Behçet's disease, when treatment is not optimal.

PATHOLOGY AND IMMUNOPATHOGENESIS

The cause of Behçet's disease is unknown. Pathologic examination of evolving oral ulcers reveals emigration of T lymphocytes and plasma cells from dermal blood vessels into the epidermis. Degeneration at the dermo-epidermal junction leads to necrosis and slough, forming an aphthous ulcer (12). Histology of the vulvar ulcers is equally nonspecific, but vasculitis is sometimes seen. At most other sites of Behçet's disease, an immune-mediated vasculitis is found. Deposits of IgM and C3 can be identified in dermal vessels. Leukocytoclastic vasculitis is likely when palpable purpura is present and nodose lesions may contain dermal round cell or neutrophilic infiltrates (5). Frank necrotizing vasculitis has been reported in skin, genital, and visceral lesions.

At autopsy, cerebral lesions of patients succumbing to central nervous system disease show perivascular infiltrates, whereas late lesions reveal gliosis and demyelination (13). Old lesions resemble plaques of multiple sclerosis. Most of the inflammatory cells in affected eyes are CD4 lymphocytes. The CSF in active central nervous system disease has an elevated lymphocyte count (8), and nonspecific elevations of IgA, IgG, and IgM. With successful treatment, the cell count and protein abnormalities disappear. Arterial pseudo-aneurysms result from a panarteritis. Little is known about the pathogenesis of the venous occlusions. Presumably they are vasculitic with superimposed thrombus formation. Bowel lesions, when examined in resected specimens, show vasculitis.

Acute phase reactants are sometimes elevated in active disease; however, uveitis can be active when the serum and erythrocyte sedimentation rate are normal. Circulating immune complexes are detected in most patients. Lymphocyte typing reveals regional variation and, in Northern Caucasians, are unnecessary. HLA–B51, a "split" of HLA–B5, is more common in Japanese (14) and Eastern Mediterranean patients than in controls. No consistent HLA association has been found in English, North American, or East Indian patients. Cellular and humoral immunity are normal in Behçet's disease patients, but in preactive phases, CD4 lymphocytes are reduced in number and function (15). A rationale for the use of colchicine has been the observation that supernatants of patients' lymphocytes have enhanced neutrophil potentiating activity as compared with controls. Putative antigens that have been considered, but not confirmed, as pathogens are oral streptococci and herpes viruses. Increased frequencies of circulating CD8 T lymphocytes expressing a γδ T cell receptor suggest exposure to a microbial antigen (16).

DIFFERENTIAL DIAGNOSIS

Crohn's disease, especially of the colon, has features that overlap with Behçet's, including aphthous ulceration, uveitis, and skin lesions. In Crohn's disease, the bowel is more extensively involved, and pathology reveals a granulomatous enteritis. Cicatricial or mucous membrane pemphigoid and lichen planus are often mistaken for Behçet's disease, but biopsy and experienced dermatologic consultation will correct this. Patients with hypereosinophilic syndrome can present with oral–genital ulceration, but the eosinophilia settles the issue. Recurrent oral and genital ulcers can be troublesome in myelodysplastic syndrome and in acquired immune deficiency due to human immunodeficiency virus. A patient should not be diagnosed with Behçet's disease when oral and genital ulcers are the only findings. Many referred patients have an entity best described as "pseudo-Behçet's syndrome" (17). Clues to the diagnosis include multiple previous procedures and operations, visits to many diagnostic centers, chronic use of opiate analgesics for prominent painful symptoms, and perceived or even factitial mucosal or skin "lesions."

TREATMENT

Corticosteroids have a palliative effect and are used topically, (for example, triamcinolone) in a gel for application in the mouth. Colchicine (0.6–1.2 mg/day) can reduce the severity and frequency of mucosal and eye lesions. Thalidomide (50–200 mg/day) suppresses resistant severe oral and genital ulceration (18), but its use is very limited as it requires federal approval and carries risks of phocomelia and axonal neuropathy.

Retinal, central nervous system, and arterial disease may be treated with chlorambucil (8). One method is to use 0.1 mg/kg/day for several months until the disease is controlled, then taper to lower levels until it is discontinued after six months of remission. An ophthalmologist should monitor the visual acuity and the activity level of the uveitis or retinal vasculitis. Acute central nervous system and pulmonary vasculitis may be treated with intravenous methylprednisone and bolus cyclophosphamide. Concurrent prednisone is not needed for eye disease, but when it is already in place, such as with cerebral vasculitis, it can be tapered and withdrawn over a few months after starting chlorambucil. Central nervous system vasculitis patients taking chlorambucil cease having recurrences and almost always stay in prolonged remission after the drug is stopped. Recurrent retinal vasculitis, on the other hand, may well require treatment for relapses over a period of three or more years. Chlorambucil use is associated with the increased risk of infections, and patients should be told to expect amenorrhea or aspermia resulting from prolonged treatment (>1 year). Alternative methods of chlorambucil such as short-term high-dose also appear to control disease effectively (19). Azathioprine is less effective than chlorambucil. Cyclosporine begun in a dose of 5 mg/kg/day also suppresses eye and mucosal disease (20). However, cessation of cyclosporine allows the disease to relapse, unlike chlorambucil therapy. The risks of neoplasia from the above regimens of chlorambucil are not great in the first decade of follow-up (21).

J. DESMOND O'DUFFY, MB

1. International Study Group for Behcet's Disease: Criteria for diagnosis of Behçet's disease. Lancet 335:1078-1080, 1990

2. Pande I, Upal SS, Kailash S, Kumar A, Malaviya AN: Behçet's disease in India: A clinical, immunological, immunogenetic and outcome study. Br J Rheumatol 34:825-830, 1995

3. Behçet H: Über rezidivierende, aphthose, durch ein Virus verursachte Geschwüre am Mund am Auge und an den Genitalien. Dermatologische Wochenschrift 105:1152-1157, 1937

4. BenEzra D, Cohen E: Treatment and visual prognosis in Behçet's disease. Br J Ophthalmol 70:589-5925, 1986

5. Su WPD., Chun SI, Lee S, et al: Erythema nodosum-like lesions in Behçet's syndrome. A histopathologic study of 30 cases. In O'Duffy J.D., Kokmen E. (eds.): Behcet's Disease: Basic and Clinical Aspects. New York, Marcel Dekker, Inc, pp 229-240,1991

6. Friedman-Birnbaum R, Bergman R, Aizen E: Sensitivity and specificity of pathergy test results in Israeli patients with Behçet's disease. Cutis 45:261-264,1990

7. Yurkadul S, Yazici H, Tuzun Y, et al: The arthritis of Behçet's disease: A prospective study. Ann Rheum Dis 42:505-515, 1983

8. O'Duffy JD, Robertson DM, Goldstein NP: Chlorambucil in the treatment of uveitis and meningoencephalitis of Behçet's disease. Am J Med 76:75-84,1984

9. Wechsler B, Dell'Isola B, Vidailhet M, Dormont D, Piette J, Bletry O, Godeau P: MRI in 31 patients with Behçet's disease and neurological involvement: Prospective study with clinical correlation. J Neuro Neurosurg Psych 56:793-798,1993

10. Erkan F, Cavdar T: Pulmonary vasculitis in Behçet's disease. Am Rev Respir Dis 146:232-239,1992

11. Iida M, Kobayashi H, Matsumoto T, Okada M, Fuchigami T, Yao T, Fujishima M: Postoperative recurrence in patients with intestinal Behçet's disease. Dis Colon Rectum 37:16-21,1994

12. Lehner T: Progress report: Oral ulceration in Behçet's syndrome. Gut 18:491-511,1977

13. McMenemey WH, Lawrence BJ: Encephalomyelopathy in Behçet's disease: Report of necropsy findings in two cases. Lancet 2:353-358,1957

14. Mizuki N, Ohno S,et al: Microsatellite polymorphism between the tumor necrosis factor and HLA-B genes in Behçet's disease. Human Immunol 43, 129-135,1995

15. Sakane T, Kotani H, Takada S, Tsunematsu T: Functional aberration of T cell subsets in patients with Behçet's disease. Arthritis Rheum 25:1343-1351,1982

16. Fortune F, Walker J, Lehner T: The expression of T cell receptor and the prevalence of primed, activated, and IgA-bound T cells in Behçet's disease. Clin Exp Immunol 82:326-332,1990

17. Levine JA, O'Duffy JD: Pseudo-Behçet's syndrome. A description of twenty-three cases. In Behçet's Disease. P Godeau, B. Wechsler (eds). Excerpta Medica, Amsterdam, International Congress Series 1037, 1993

18. Gardner-Medwin JMM, Smith NJ, Powell RJ: Clinical experience with thalidomide in the management of severe oral and genital ulceration in conditions such as Behçet's disease: Use of neurophysiological studies to detect thalidomide neuropathy. Ann Rheum Dis 53:828-832,1994

19. Tessler HH, Jennings T: High-dose short-term chlorambucil for intractable sympathetic ophthalmia and Behçet's disease. Br J Ophthalmol 74:353-357,1990

20. Masuda K, Urayama A, Kogure M, et al: Double-masked trial of cyclosporine versus colchicine and long-term open study of cyclosporine in Behçet's disease. Lancet 1:1093-1095,1989

21. Matteson EL, O'Duffy JD: Treatment of Behcet's disease with chlorambucil. In O'Duffy J.D., Kokmen E. (eds): Behcet's Disease: Basic and Clinical Aspects. New York, Marcel Dekker, Inc., pp 575-580, 1991

Relapsing polychondritis is a relatively uncommon disorder characterized by widespread, progressive inflammation and destruction of cartilaginous structures and connective tissues. Common clinical features are auricular, nasal, and respiratory tract chondritis with involvement of organs of special sense, such as the eyes and audiovestibular apparatus. Polyarthritis and vascular involvement are also common (1,2). Pearson et al (3) first used the term *relapsing polychondritis* to described the episodic nature of the disease, and it is the widely accepted terminology. The etiology is unknown, but it is considered to be an autoimmune disorder with evidence of cellular and humoral response to cartilaginous structures, including collagen types II, IX, and XI (4,5). The disease occurs in all age groups with peaks between 40 and 50 years. Both genders are affected equally (6), although women more often have serious airway involvement (7).

CLINICAL FEATURES

The clinical features of relapsing polychondritis are summarized in Table 26-1. Auricular chondritis, the most common presenting symptom, is characterized by sudden onset of pain and swelling with redness and warmth of the cartilaginous portion of the external ear. The lobule is spared. The inflammation may subside spontaneously or with treatment. With repeated attacks, the involved external ear becomes soft and floppy (Fig. 26-1). Sudden onset of hearing loss and vertigo may occur due to involvement of the audiovestibular structures or vasculitis of the internal auditory artery.

Polyarthritis is the second most common presenting symptom at onset. Typically, the arthropathy is migratory, asymmetric, and nonerosive, and it involves large and small joints of the peripheral or axial skeleton.

Chondritis of the respiratory tract may result in collapse of nasal cartilage causing saddle nose deformity. Involvement of the laryngeal and tracheobronchial tract may result in hoarseness, choking sensation, tenderness over the thyroid cartilage, cough, stridor, or wheezes. Major airway collapse causes respiratory obstruction with high morbidity and mortality, requiring emergency recognition and treatment (7). Secondary infections of the upper and lower respiratory tracts are also common in patients with severe airway involvement.

Ocular inflammation frequently occurs. Common presentations are scleritis/episcleritis (Fig. 26-2), conjunctivitis, iritis/chorioretinitis, and keratitis. Less common are optic neuritis, scleromalacia, retinal detachment, proptosis, exophthalmos, extra-ocular muscle palsy, and glaucoma (8).

Cardiovascular involvement in relapsing polychondritis includes aortic insufficiency, mitral regurgitation, pericarditis, and cardiac ischemia. Two fatalities due to cardiovascular complications have been described: one results from complete heart block, acute aortic insufficiency, and cardiovascular collapse (9) and one is caused by aortic valve rupture (10). Vascular involvement of large vessels may present as an aneurysm (eg, aorta and subclavian artery) or as thrombosis due to vasculitis or coagulopathy. Leukocytoclastic vasculitis indicates small-vessel involvement.

(Table 26-1)
Clinical manifestations of relapsing polychondritis

Manifestation	Frequency (%)	
	At Onset	Cumulative
Auricular chondritis	40	85
Nasal chondritis	25	59
Saddle nose deformity	18	29
Arthritis	37	62
Ocular symptoms	20	52
Laryngotracheal-bronchial symptoms	24	49
Laryngotracheal stricture	15	23
Hearing loss	9	32
Vestibular dysfunction	0	17
Systemic vasculitis	3	12
Valvular dysfunction	0	8
Cutaneous lesions	12	27
Aneurysm	0	6

* Data modified from Luthra et al (1) and Herman (2).

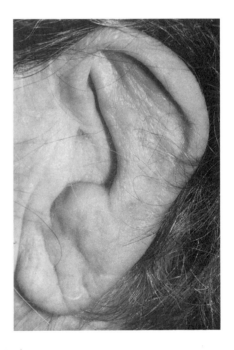

(Figure 26-1)
Floppy appeerence of external ear due to chronic chondritis.

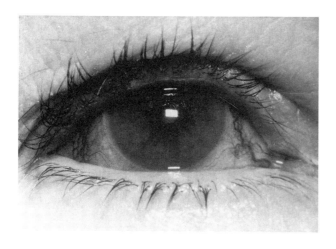

(Figure 26-2)
Episcleritis and scleritis with engorged, tortuous blood vessels.

Various mucocutaneous lesions are seen, including erythema nodosum, panniculitis, livedo reticularis, urticaria, cutaneous polyarteritis nodosa, and aphthous ulcers. Renal involvement is uncommon in relapsing polychondritis, but can occur as segmental, proliferative, and crescenteric glomerulonephritis (11).

Acute or subacute disorders of cranial nerves II, III, IV, VI, VII, and VIII may occur, causing ocular palsy, optic neuritis, facial palsy, hearing loss, and vertigo. Other neurologic complications are hemiplegia, chronic headache, ataxia, seizure, confusion, dementia (12), and meningoencephalitis (13).

ASSOCIATED DISORDERS

More than 30% of patients with relapsing polychondritis also have an autoimmune, rheumatologic, or hematologic disorder (6). Diseases that have been associated with relapsing polychondritis are systemic lupus erythematosus (SLE), rheumatoid arthritis, Sjögren's syndrome, systemic vasculitis, systemic sclerosis, overlap connective tissue disease, Behçet's syndrome, essential mixed cryoglobulinemia, thyroid disease, inflammatory bowel disease, spondyloarthropathies (ie, Reiter's syndrome, psoriatic arthritis), dysmyelopoietic syndrome, diabetes mellitus, and malignancy, including Hodgkins and non-Hodgkins lymphoma, chronic myelomonocytic leukemia, and carcinoma of various organs (6,14). In most instances, the associated disorder precedes the onset of relapsing polychondritis by several months or years (6).

DIAGNOSIS

Abnormal results of laboratory tests are generally nonspecific. Most patients have anemia typical of chronic disease, mild leukocytosis, or thrombocytosis. Elevated erythrocyte sedimentation rate and hypergammaglobulinemia are common (6). Urinalysis is typically normal, but proteinuria or cellular sediments can be seen in patients with renal involvement. Common serologic findings are rheumatoid factors (10% to 20% of patients) and antinuclear antibodies (15% to 25% of patients). Anti-native DNA has been reported, but these patients may have coexisting SLE. Serum complement levels are usually normal or increased. Cryoglobulin can be found in a small number of patients, and autoantibodies to collagen types II, IX, and XI have been reported (5).

Biopsy is not necessary because the diagnosis of relapsing polychondritis is based on clinical features. McAdam et al proposed the following diagnostic criteria: bilateral auricular chondritis, nonerosive and seronegative inflammatory polyarthritis, nasal chondritis, ocular inflammation, respiratory tract chondritis, and cochlear or vestibular dysfunction. At least three of these proposed criteria are required to make a definite diagnosis of relapsing polychondritis (6). If the clinical presentation is uncertain, chondritis due to other causes must be excluded, especially infectious disorders. Biopsy and cultures or other tests are necessary to exclude syphilis, leprosy, fungal invasion, or other bacterial infections.

Narrowing or stricture of the tracheobronchial tract can be identified with tomographic radiologic imaging and computed tomography (CT) (15). CT scan is safe, rapid, and accurate and is the procedure of choice. Typical findings include a narrowed lumen due to wall thickening and collapse of the supporting cartilaginous structures.

Other investigations should be considered, such as pulmonary function tests (16), particularly in patients with chronic cough or dyspnea. Echocardiography, cardiac catheterization, and angiography should be done in patients with prominent symptoms and signs of cardiovascular involvement.

TREATMENT

Nonsteroidal anti-inflammatory drugs may be adequate for patients with mild polychondritis limited to arthralgia and nasal or auricular chondritis. Patients with more severe disease—scleritis/uveitis and systemic symptoms—need corticosteroid treatment. Doses of 30 to 60 mg prednisone (or equivalent drug) and an immunosuppressive agent such as azathioprine or cyclophosphamide should be initiated. The corticosteroid dosage can be tapered once therapeutic response occurs. Cyclosporin A has been used in refractory patients with good response (17).

Acute airway obstruction unresponsive to oral corticosteroids has been successfully treated with intravenous pulse methylprednisolone (18). A patient with renal disease had improved kidney function after monthly treatments with pulse intravenous cyclophosphamide for 6 months (19). A combination of oral prednisone, dapsone, and cyclophosphamide has been used with variable responses. Acute airway obstruction may require tracheostomy, and stents are necessary in patients with tracheal collapse (20). Surgical intervention is indicated for patients with severe cardiac valvular involvement or a large-vessel aneurysm. Infections during corticosteroid and immunosuppressive therapy demand aggressive measures to identify the agent and initiate prompt treatment.

PROGNOSIS AND SURVIVAL

The survival rate for patients with relapsing polychondritis is 74% at 5 years and 55% at 10 years (21). Common causes of death are infections and cardiovascular disease with either systemic vasculitis or rupture of large-vessel aneurysms. Airway obstruction with or without superimposed infections was the cause of death in 10% and 28% of cases in two series (6,21). Only 48% of the fatalities were considered to be related to relapsing polychondritis in a recent study by Michet et al (21), compared with 86% in an earlier study by McAdam et al (6). This difference was thought to be due to age, since patients in the Michet et al study were older. Malignancy is an uncommon cause of death.

VALEE HARISDANKUL, MD, PhD

1. Luthra HS, Michet CJ Jr: Relapsing polychondritis. In Klippel JH, Dieppe P (eds): Rheumatology. London, Mosby, 1994, pp 6.31.1-4

2. Herman JH: Polychondritis. In Kelly WN, Harris ED, Ruddy S, Sledge CB (eds): Textbook of Rheumatology, 4th ed. Philadelphia, WB Saunders, 1993, pp 1400-1411

3. Pearson CM, Kline HM, Newcomer VD: Relapsing polychondritis. N Engl J Med 263:51-58, 1960

4. Herman JH, Dennis MV: Immunopathologic studies in relapsing polychondritis. J Clin Invest 52:549-558, 1973

5. Alsalameh S, Mollenhauer J, Scheuplein F, Stross H, Kalden JR, Burkhardt H, Burnester GR: Preferential cellular and humoral immune reactivities to native and denatured collagen types IX and XI in a patient with fatal relapsing chondritis. J Rheumatol 20:1419-1424, 1993

6. McAdam LP, O'Hanlan MA, Bluestone R, Pearson CM: Relapsing polychondritis: prospective study of 23 patients and a review of the literature. Medicine 55:193-215, 1976

7. Eng J, Sabanathan S: Acute complications in relapsing polychondritis. Ann Thoracic Surgery 51:686-692, 1991

8. Chen CJ, Harisdangkul V, Parker JL: Transient glaucoma associated with anterior diffuse scleritis in relapsing polychondritis. Glaucoma 4:109-111, 1982

9. Bowness P, Hawley IC, Morris T, Dearden A, Walport MJ: Complete heart block and severe aortic incompetence in relapsing polychondritis: clinicopathologic findings. Arth Rheum 34:97-100, 1991

10. Marshall DA, Jackson R, Capell HA: Early aortic valve cusp rupture in relapsing polychondritis. Ann Rheum Dis 51:413-415, 1992

11. Chang-Miller A, Okamura M, Torres VE, Michet CJ, Wagoner RD, Donadio JV, Offord KP, Holley KE: Renal involvement in relapsing polychondritis. Medicine 66:207-217, 1987

12. Sundaram MBM, Rajput AH: Nervous system complications of relapsing polychondritis. Neurology 33:513-515, 1983

13. Hanslik T, Wechsler B, Piette JC, Vidailhet M, Robin PM, Godeau P: Central nervous system involvement in relapsing polychondritis. Clin Experimental Rheum 12:539-541, 1994

14. Shirota T, Hayashi O, Uchida H, Tonozaka N, Sakai N, Itoh H: Myelodysplastic syndrome associated with relapsing polychondritis: unusual transformation from refractory anemia to chronic myelomonocytic leukemia. Ann Hematology 67:45-47, 1993

15. Davis, SD, Berkmen YM, King T: Peripheral bronchial involvement in relapsing polychondritis: demonstration by thin-section CT. Amer J Roentgen 153:953-954, 1989

16. Krell WS, Staats BA, Hyatt RE: Pulmonary function in relapsing polychondritis. Am Rev Respir Dis 133:1120-1123, 1986

17. Svenson KLG, Holmdahl R, Klareskog L, Wibell L, Sjoberg O, Klintmalm GBG, Bostrom H: Cyclosporin A treatment in a case of relapsing polychondritis. Scand J Rheumatol 13:329-333, 1984

18. Lipnick RN, Fink CW: Acute airway obstruction in relapsing polychondritis: treatment with pulse methylprednisolone. J Rheumatol 18:98-99, 1991

19. Stewart KA, Mazanec DJ: Pulse intravenous cyclophosphamide for kidney disease in relapsing polychondritis. J Rheumatol 19:498-500, 1992

20. Dunne JA, Sabanathan S: Use of metallic stents in relapsing polychondritis. Chest 105:864-867, 1994

21. Michet CJ, McKenna CH, Luthra HS, O'Fallon WM: Relapsing polychondritis: survival and predictive role of early disease manifestations. Ann Intern Med 104:74-78, 1986

27 ANTIPHOSPHOLIPID SYNDROME

Antiphospholipid syndrome (APS) is a disorder of recurrent arterial or venous thromboses, pregnancy losses, and/or thrombocytopenia associated with persistently positive results of anticardiolipin or lupus anticoagulant tests (1) (Table 27-1). The disorder may occur in association with systemic lupus erythematosus or other autoimmune diseases, or it may occur alone (primary antiphospholipid syndrome). Clinical and laboratory features of APS appear to be the same in the presence or absence of an autoimmune disorder (2).

Although the disorder has been described most frequently in adults, children can be affected. An apparent female predominance may be explained by pregnancy wastage being a prominent presenting feature of the disorder. The occurrence of APS in more than one family member is relatively uncommon, but relatives of affected patients are often positive for anticardiolipin or lupus anticoagulant tests without clinical complications (3). Some authorities suggest an association of APS with the C4 null haplotype (4).

ETIOLOGY AND PATHOGENESIS

Only some patients with antiphospholipid antibodies experience clinical complications, suggesting that other factors related to either antibody specificity or host susceptibility may be involved. A number of studies in experimental animals suggest that these antibodies may be involved in disease pathogenesis. For example, mice passively immunized with human anticardiolipin antibodies suffer pregnancy wastage or fetal resorptions (5,6). In other studies, mice infused with either purified immunoglobulins or affinity purified anticardiolipin antibodies from patients with APS developed increased thrombus size and delayed thrombus disappearances (7).

(Table 27-1)
Clinical and laboratory features of antiphospholipid syndrome[*]

Clinical	Laboratory
Major features	
Venous thrombosis	Lupus anticoagulant
Arterial thrombosis	antibodies
Thrombocytopenia	Anticardiolipin antibodies
Other proposed features	(medium-to-high positive
Endocardial valvular	IgG, IgM, or IgA)
vegetations	
Livedo reticularis	
Migraine headaches	
Transverse myelopathy	
Chorea	
Leg ulcers	

[*] A diagnosis of APS should be based on a history of one major clinical feature (preferably not explainable by any other predisposing condition) and a positive laboratory test that has remained positive for several weeks to months.

How antiphospholipid antibodies induce thrombosis is unknown. Several investigators have shown that these antibodies inhibit select reactions in the coagulation cascade catalyzed by negatively charged phospholipids. The reactions include factor X activation, prothrombin–thrombin conversion, protein C activation, and inactivation of factor Va by activated protein C. Inhibition of protein C activation or neutralization of factor Va inactivation by antiphospholipid antibodies would induce a "pro-thrombotic state" in affected individuals (8). Anticardiolipin antibodies cross-reactive with phosphatidylserine have also been demonstrated to bind and activate platelets (9), a process that might also induce thrombosis. Other postulated mechanisms include enhancement of thromboxane synthesis by platelets, inhibition of prostacyclin synthesis, and stimulation of tissue factor production by endothelial cells.

The role of β_2 glycoprotein 1 (β_2GP1), a plasma protein, in antiphospholipid antibody-mediated thrombosis is of considerable interest (10). β_2GP1 binds negatively charged molecules, including phospholipids, and is thought to be a "natural anticoagulant" by its ability to inhibit coagulation reactions that are catalyzed by negatively charged phospholipids, such as prothrombin–thrombin conversion (10). β_2GP1 markedly enhances binding of antiphospholipid antibodies to cardiolipin in enzyme-linked immunosorbent assays (ELISA), a reaction variously attributed to anticardiolipin antibodies binding β_2GP1 directly (10,11), a β_2GP1–phospholipid complex, or "new" epitopes on phospholipid in phospholipid–β_2GP1 complexes (12,13). Immunization of mice with β_2GP1 results in production of antibodies specific for both β_2GP1 and cardiolipin (14). However, anticardiolipin antibodies are also induced by phospholipid-binding proteins other than β_2GP1, including human IgG antiphospholipid antibodies. Presently, many authorities believe that antiphospholipid antibodies may induce thrombosis by neutralizing the anticoagulant effects of β_2GP1 (11).

CLINICAL FEATURES

Occurrence of one clinical complication of APS need not mean that the patient will be subject to others. For example, some women with recurrent pregnancy losses never have thrombosis and vice-versa.

Thrombosis

Blood vessels of all sizes in the venous and arterial circulation appear subject to thrombosis. Events are usually sporadic and appear unrelated to antibody levels, which often remain high for several years. In the majority of patients, recurrent events are confined to either the arterial or the venous circulation, suggesting that factors influencing arterial and venous thrombosis may differ. Because of the variety of vascular sites affected, clinical presentations may vary. Deep-vein thrombosis is the most frequent site affected in the venous circulation, but thrombosis has also been de-

PRIMER ON RHEUMATIC DISEASES 313

scribed in the pulmonary vessels, inferior vena cava, renal, hepatic (Budd–Chiari syndrome), and sagittal veins (15). Stroke or transient ischemic attacks are the most common presentations of arterial thrombosis, but myocardial, adrenal, and gastrointestinal infarction, as well as gangrene of the extremities, have been described.

Some patients experience thrombosis at multiple sites, either simultaneously or over a short period of time, often with life-threatening consequences. The term "catastrophic antiphospholipid syndrome" has been used to describe this presentation (16). Thrombotic thrombocytopenic purpura and diffuse intravascular coagulation should be excluded.

Pregnancy Loss

Pregnancy loss can occur at any stage of gestation, although fetal death in the second or third trimester is characteristic. The cause of fetal death is believed to be placental vessel thrombosis resulting in infarction (17); alternatively, antibody cross-reactivity with phosphatidylserine on membranes of trophoblastic tissue may mediate placental damage (18). The aborted fetus is usually small for date but is often otherwise normal. Few cases have been reported of vascular thrombosis in neonates born to anticardiolipin-positive mothers.

Thrombocytopenia

Patients with APS occasionally present with thrombocytopenia alone (19). More frequently, however, mild to moderate thrombocytopenia (platelet counts in the range of 100,000–150,000/mm³) accompanies some other clinical complica- tion. Thrombocytopenia does not always protect patients from thrombosis, but anticoagulation therapy in this setting is risky.

Minor Features

Other clinical and laboratory features are reported in APS, although their frequency and clinical significance are unclear. These include cardiac valvular vegetations (Libman–Sachs endocarditis) and valvular insufficiency, livedo reticularis, leg ulcers, migraine headaches, and a variety of neurologic complications, including chorea and transverse myelopathy (20). Some patients have Coombs' positive tests occasionally associated with hemolytic anemia (19).

DIFFERENTIAL DIAGNOSIS

None of the clinical or laboratory features of APS are confined to that disorder. A diagnosis of APS should be considered in the following circumstances: unexplained arterial or venous thrombosis, thrombotic involvement of unusual sites (eg, renal or adrenal veins), thrombosis in a patient younger than 50 years, recurrent thrombotic events, second or third trimester losses, and more than one APS event in the same individual. Confirmation should rely on an unequivocally positive test for lupus anticoagulant or medium to high titer of anticardiolipin antibodies (preferably IgG isotype) (Table 27-1).

Other diagnoses that should be considered in patients with unexplained venous thrombosis include factor V Leiden (activated protein C resistance), protein C, protein S, or antithrombin III deficiency; dysfibrinogenemias; abnormalities of fibrinolysis; nephrotic syndrome; polycythemia vera; Behçet's syndrome; paroxysmal nocturnal hemoglobinuria; and side effect of oral contraceptives. In patients with arter-

ial occlusion, considerations should include hyperlipidemias, diabetes mellitus, hypertension, vasculitis, sickle cell disease, homocystinuria, and Buerger's disease.

Antiphospholipid syndrome accounts for only a small fraction of pregnancy losses. Other causes of pregnancy wastage include fetal chromosomal abnormalities, anatomic anomalies of the maternal reproductive tract, and maternal disorders such as endocrine, infectious, autoimmune, and drug-induced disease (21).

LABORATORY TESTS

Both anticardiolipin and lupus anticoagulant tests should be ordered for patients suspected of having APS, since one test can be positive without the other. Anticardiolipin tests use a standardized ELISA technique (22). Results are reported according to isotype (IgG, IgM, or IgA) and level of positivity in GPL (for IgG), MPL (for IgM), or APL (for IgA) units. Because of interlaboratory variations in test results, it has been suggested that anticardiolipin levels be also reported semi-quantitatively as high (>80 units), medium (20–80 units), or low (10–20 units). A medium-to-high positive IgG anticardiolipin is most specific for diagnosis of APS.

The lupus anticoagulant test is attributable to prolongation of clotting times by antiphospholipid antibodies in vitro (23). However, other causes of prolonged clotting times include deficiencies of coagulation factors and clotting factor inhibitors (eg, antiprothrombin, antifactor VIII). The lupus anticoagulant is identified by the following criteria: 1) prolonged partial thromboplastin time (PTT), Russell viper venom time, or kaolin clotting time; 2) correcting the test by mixing patient and normal plasma (to exclude a coagulation factor deficiency); and 3) normalization of the test by addition of freeze-thawed platelets or phospholipids to the patient plasma (a phenomenon seen only with the lupus anticoagulant). The lupus anticoagulant test cannot be performed reliably in patients on oral anticoagulants or heparin.

TREATMENT
Thrombosis

Patients with venous or arterial thrombosis are often subject to recurrence, and prophylaxis with oral anticoagulants is necessary. Recent studies suggest that a target international normalized ratio of 3.0 is usually effective in preventing thrombosis (24). Some authorities include half an adult aspirin daily with warfarin for arterial thrombosis prophylaxis, but this increases the risk of bleeding. Patients who suffer thrombotic recurrences despite adequate anticoagulation with warfarin may be treated with twice daily subcutaneous heparin at doses sufficient to achieve a PTT of 1.5 to 2 times normal or with immunosuppressive therapy (cyclophosphamide, administered daily or as monthly intravenous pulses). However, these therapies are of varying benefit. High doses of prednisone (tapered over a few months), intravenous cyclophosphamide pulses, and heparin followed by warfarin have been used in patients with catastrophic APS, but the efficacy of this regimen is unproven (15).

Pregnancy Wastage

Pregnancy outcome can be markedly improved in women with APS using subcutaneous heparin at doses of 5000 to 10,000 units, twice daily, plus one low-dose aspirin (60–80 mg) daily (25). Since osteoporosis is a consequence of prolonged heparin therapy, vitamin D and calcium should also be prescribed. Thrombocytopenia and, rarely, thrombosis are idiosyncratic side effects of heparin therapy. If pregnancy loss occurs despite heparin, 4- or 5-day pulses of intravenous gamma globulin (0.4 gm/kg/day) given monthly plus one low-dose aspirin daily is an effective, safe, but expensive alternative (25,26). Prednisone at doses of 20–60 mg plus low-dose aspirin daily have been used successfully in preventing pregnancy losses, but this alternative is recommended only when other regimens have failed, and patients must be made fully aware of (and accept) the risks of prolonged, high-dose corticosteroid therapy.

Children born to mothers with APS have developed normally, and parents can be assured that the child's risk of developing APS is probably small.

PROGNOSIS

The risk of recurrent thrombosis in patients treated appropriately with oral anticoagulants is small. Since no treatment has proved uniformly successful in patients with catastrophic APS (15,16) or in patients with recurrences despite adequate anticoagulation therapy, prognosis should be guarded in those instances.

The risks of thrombosis in women who have a history only of pregnancy losses and in patients with anticardiolipin or lupus anticoagulant antibodies who have no clinical symptoms are unknown.

E. NIGEL HARRIS, MD

1. Harris EN: Syndrome of the black swan. Br J Rheumatol 26:324-326, 1987

2. Vianna JL, Khamashta MA, Ordi-Ros J, et al: Comparison of the primary and secondary antiphospholipid syndrome: a European multicenter study of 114 patients. Am J Med 96:3-9, 1994

3. Goldberg SN, Greco TP: A family study of anticardiolipin antibodies and associated clinical correlations. Am J Med 69:473-479, 1995

4. Wilson WA, Scopelitis E, Michalski JP, Pierangeli SS, Silvera LH, Elston RC, Harris EN: Familial anticardiolipin antibodies and C4 deficiency genotypes that coexist with MHC DQB1 risk factors. J Rheum 22:227-235, 1995

5. Branch DW, Dudley DJ, Mitchell MD: Immunoglobulin G fractions from patients with antiphospholipid antibodies cause fetal death in BALB/C mice: a model for autoimmune fetal loss. Am J Obstet Gynecol 163:120-126, 1990

6. Blank M, Tincani A, Shoenfeld Y: Induction of experimental antiphospholipid syndrome in naive mice with purified IgG antiphosphatidylserine antibodies. J Rheumatol 21:100-104, 1994

7. Pierangeli SS, Liu XW, Barker JH, Anderson G, Horns EN: Induction of thrombosis in a mouse model by IgG, IgM and IgA immunoglobulins from patients with the antiphospholipid syndrome. Thromb Haemostas 74:1361-1367, 1995

8. Harris EN: Antiphospholipid syndrome. In Klippel JH, Dieppe PA (eds): Rheumatology. London, Mosby-Year Book Europe, 1994, p 32.1.6

9. Smirnov MD, Triplett DT, Comp PC, Esmon NL, Esmon CT: On the role of phosphatidylethanolamine in the inhibition of protein C activity by antiphospholipid antibodies. J Clin Invest 95:309-316, 1995

10. Campbell AL, Pierangeli SS, Wellhausen S, Harris EN: Comparison of the effect of anticardiolipin antibodies from patients with the antiphospholipid syndrome and with syphilis on platelet activation and aggregation. Thromb Haemostas 73:529-534, 1995

11. Roubey RAS: Autoantibodies to phospholipid-binding plasma proteins: a new view of lupus anticoagulants and other "antiphospholipid" autoantibodies. Blood 84:2854-2867, 1994

12. Matsuura E, Igarashi Y, Yasuda T, Triplett DA, Koike T: Anticardiolipin antibodies recognize beta(2)-glycoprotein 1 structure altered by interacting with an oxygen modified solid phase surface. J Exp Med 179:457-462, 1994

13. Borchman D, Harris EN, Pierangeli SS, Lamba OP: Interactions and molecular structure of cardiolipin and β_2-glycoprotein (β_2-GP1). Clin Exp Immunol 102:373-378, 1995

14. Gharavi AE, Sammaritano LR, Wen J, Elcon OP: Induction of antiphospholipid autoantibodies by immunization with β_2 glycoprotein 1. J Clin Invest 90:1105-1109, 1992

15. Lockshin MD: Antiphospholipid antibody syndrome. Rheum Dis Clin N Am 20:45-60, 1994

16. Asherson RA: The catastrophic antiphospholipid syndrome. J Rheumatol 19:508-512, 1992

17. Out HJ, Kooijman CD, Bruinse HW, Derksen RH: Histopathological findings in placental from patients with intra-uterine fetal death and anti-phospholipid antibodies. Eur J Obstet Gynecol Reprod Biol 41:179-186, 1991

18. Lyden TW, Vogt E, Ng A-K, Johnson PM, Rote NS: Monoclonal antiphospholipid antibody reactivity against human placental trophoblast. J Reprod Immunol 22:1-14, 1992

19. Deleze M, Alarcon-Segovia D, Oria CV: Hemocytopenia in systemic lupus erythematosus: relationship to antiphospholipid antibodies. J Rheumatol 16:926-930, 1989

20. Asherson RA, Cervera R: The antiphospholipid syndrome: a syndrome in evolution. Ann Rheum Dis 51:147-150, 1992

21. Pridham DD, Cook CL: Habitual abortion. In Harris EN, Exner T, Hughes GRV, Asherson RA (eds): Phospholipid Binding Antibodies. Boca Raton, FL, CRC Press, 1991, pp 271-306

22. Harris EN, Pierangeli SS, Birch D: Anticardiolipin wet workshop report: 5th International Symposium on Antiphospholipid Antibodies. Am J Clin Pathol 101:616-624, 1994

23. Triplett DA: Antiphospholipid antibodies and thrombosis: a consequence, coincidence, or cause? Arch Pathol Lab Med 117:78-88, 1993

24. Khamashta MA, Cuadrado MJ, Mujic F, Taub NA, Hunt BJ, Hughes GRV: The management of thrombosis in the antiphospholipid-antibody syndrome. N Engl J Med 332:993-997, 1995

25. Branch DW, Silver RM, Blackwell JL, Reading JC, Scott JR: Outcome of treated pregnancies in women with antiphospholipid syndrome: an update of the Utah experience. Obstet Gynecol 80:614-620, 1992

26. Spinatto JA, Clark AL, Pierangeli SS, Harris EN: Intravenous immunoglobulin therapy for the antiphospholipid syndrome in pregnancy. Am J Obstet Gynecol 172:690-694, 1995

ADULT STILL'S DISEASE

The clinical features of adult Still's disease resemble the systemic form of juvenile rheumatoid arthritis. The disorder is rare, affects both genders equally, and exists worldwide. The majority of cases are 16–35 years of age (1).

CLINICAL, LABORATORY AND RADIOGRAPHIC FINDINGS

The clinical manifestations and laboratory findings of adult Still's disease (2,3) are summarized in Table 28-1. Usually the initial symptom is sudden onset of a high spiking fever. The fever spikes once daily (rarely, twice daily), usually in the evening, and the temperature returns to normal in 80% of patients untreated with antipyretics. Arthralgia and severe myalgia are universal. Arthritis is almost universal but may be mild and overlooked by a physician whose attention is drawn to more dramatic manifestations. Initially the arthritis affects only a few joints but may then evolve into polyarticular disease. The most commonly affected joints are the knee (84%) and wrist (74%). The ankle, shoulder, elbow, and proximal interphalangeal joints are involved in one-half and the metacarpophalangeals in one-third of patients. Involvement of the distal interphalangeal joints in one-fifth of patients is notable (2,4-7).

Still's rash, present in more than 85% of patients, is almost pathognomonic. The rash is salmon pink, macular or maculopapular, frequently evanescent, and often occurs with the evening fever spike. Because the rash may not be noticed by the patient, a check during evening rounds can lead to the detection of this almost diagnostic finding. The rash is most common on the trunk and proximal extremities, but is present on the face in 15% of patients. It can be precipitated by mechanical irritation from clothing, rubbing (Koebner's phenomenon), or a hot bath. The rash may be mildly pruritic.

An elevated erythrocyte sedimentation rate is universal. Leukocytosis is present in 90% of cases, and in 80% the white blood cell count is 15,000/mm³ or more. The liver function tests may be elevated in up to three-quarters of patients (2,7-9). Anemia, sometimes profound, is common. Rheumatoid factor and antinuclear antibody tests are generally negative and, if present, are of low titer. Synovial and serosal fluids are inflammatory, with a predominance of neutrophils (2,7).

Radiographic findings at presentation are nonspecific. Early in the disease course, soft-tissue swelling and periarticular osteoporosis may be found. With time, cartilage narrowing or erosion develop in most patients. Characteristic radiographic findings are typically found in the wrist, including nonerosive narrowing of the carpometacarpal and intercarpal joints, which progresses to bony ankylosis (2,6,10,11).

DIAGNOSIS

Although several sets of diagnostic criteria have been proposed (4,7,12), the criteria of Cush et al (4) are a practical guide (Table 28-2). It is important to note that most patients do not present with the full-blown syndrome. Fever is the most common first manifestation, and other features develop over a period of a couple of weeks or occasionally months. A patient with high daily fever spikes, severe myalgia, arthralgia, arthritis, Still's rash, and leukocytosis (frequently in combination with other manifestations outlined in Table 28-1) is unlikely to have anything other than adult Still's disease. Thus, this diagnosis should top the differential diagnosis list (Table 28-3). Most other diagnoses can be excluded on clinical grounds or by simple diagnostic tests. Recently, a markedly elevated serum ferritin has been proposed as being highly suggestive of Still's disease (12,13).

ETIOLOGY

The etiology of adult Still's disease is unknown. Studies of linkage to HLA antigens have been inconclusive (2,6). Immune complexes have been suggested as playing a pathogenic role (6), but this has not been confirmed (2). The principal hypothesis is that Still's disease results from a virus or other infectious agent, but study results lack consistency (14). Pregnancy or use of female hormones have not been associated with the development of Still's disease (15). The possible role of stress as an inducing phenomenon has been raised (15).

DISEASE COURSE AND OUTCOME

Approximately one-fifth of patients with Still's disease experience long-term remission within 1 year. One-third of patients have a complete remission followed by one or more relapses. The timing of relapse is unpredictable, although relapse tends to be less severe and of shorter duration than the initial episode (2,4,6). The remaining patients have a chronic disease course. The principal problem is chronic arthritis, and some patients with severe involvement of the hips and, to a lesser extent, the knees have required total joint replacement (2,4,7,9).

The presence of polyarthritis (four or more joints involved) or root joint involvement (shoulders or hips) has been identified as a marker for a chronic disease course in a number of studies (2,4,9). A prior episode in childhood (which occurs in about one in six patients) and a need for more than 2 years of therapy with systemic corticosteroids may also be markers of poor prognosis (4).

Overall, the prognosis is good. A recent controlled study noted that an average of 10 years after diagnosis, patients with adult Still's disease had significantly higher levels of pain, physical disability, and psychologic disability than their unaffected siblings of the same gender. However, the levels of pain and disability in patients with adult Still's disease were lower than in other chronic rheumatic diseases. Educational attainment, occupational prestige, social functioning, and family income did not differ between the Still's patients and the controls (16). The results suggest that pa-

(Table 28-1)
*Clinical manifestations and laboratory tests in adult Still's disease**

Characteristic[†]	No. Patients Positive/Total No.	Percentage
Clinical Manifestations		
Female	145/283	51
Childhood episode (≤15 years)	38/236	16
Onset 16–35 years	178/233	76
Arthralgia	282/283	100
Arthritis	249/265	94
Fever ≥39°C	258/266	97
≤39.5°C	54/62	87
Sore throat	57/62	92
JRA rash	248/281	88
Myalgia	52/62	84
Weight loss ≥10%	41/54	76
Lymphadenopathy	167/264	63
Splenomegaly	138/265	52
Abdominal pain	30/62	48
Hepatomegaly	108/258	42
Pleuritis	79/259	31
Pericarditis	75/254	30
Pneumonitis	17/62	27
Alopecia	15/62	24
Laboratory Tests		
Elevated ESR	265/267	99
WBC ≥10,000/mm^3	228/248	92
≥15,000/mm^3	50/62	81
Neutrophils ≥80%	55/62	88
Serum albumin <3.5 gm/dl	143/177	81
Elevated hepatic enzymes[‡]	169/232	73
Anemia (hemoglobin ≥10 gm/dl	159/233	68
Platelets ≥400,000/mm^3	37/60	62
Negative antinuclear antibody test	256/278	92
Negative rheumatoid factor	259/280	93

* Data from Pouchot et al (2), including patients reviewed by Ohta et al (J Rheumatol 1987;14:1139-1146). Data for fever ≥39.5°C, sore throat, myalgia, weight loss, abdominal pain, pneumonitis, alopecia, WBC ≥15,000/mm^3, neutrophils, and platelets are from Pouchot et al (2) only, as these data were likely underreported in early studies.
† JRA = juvenile rheumatoid arthritis; ESR = erythrocyte sedimentation rate; WBC = white blood cells.
‡ Any elevated liver function test.

tients with Still's disease are remarkably resilient in overcoming handicaps. However, premature death may be slightly increased above normal. Causes of fatality include hepatic failure, disseminated intravascular coagulation, amyloidosis, and sepsis, all of which are likely due to the Still's disease (2–4,7,9).

(Table 28-2)
*Criteria for the diagnosis of adult Still's disease**

A diagnosis of adult Still's disease requires the presence of all of the following:
  Fever ≥39°C (102.2°F)
  Arthralgia or arthritis
  Rheumatoid factor <1:80
  Antinuclear antibody <1:100
In addition, any two of the following are required:
  White blood cell count ≥15,000 cells/mm^3
  Still's rash
  Pleuritis or pericarditis
  Hepatomegaly or splenomegaly or generalized lymphadenopathy

* From Cush et al (4).

TREATMENT
Acute Disease

Approximately one-fourth of patients respond to nonsteroidal anti-inflammatory drugs (NSAIDs) alone. This group of patients usually has a good prognosis. Enteric-coated aspirin has been the most commonly used NSAID, and high doses are often required. The dose should be titrated so that the serum salicylate level is between 15 and 25 mg/dl. A second NSAID, most commonly indomethacin, is sometimes required in addition to aspirin. Response may be slow (2).

A major concern with NSAID therapy has been hepatotoxicity. Liver function test abnormalities, a common finding on presentation, are likely an integral part of the disease and

(Table 28-3)
Differential diagnosis of adult Still's disease

Granulomatous disorders
  Sarcoidosis
  Idiopathic granulomatosis hepatitis
  Crohn's disease
Vasculitis
  Serum sickness
  Polyarteritis nodosa
  Wegener's granulomatosis
  Thrombotic thrombocytopenic purpura
  Takayasu's arteritis
Infection
  Viral infection (eg, hepatitis B, rubella, parvovirus, Coxsackie virus, Epstein–Barr, cytomegalovirus, HIV)
  Subacute bacterial endocarditis
  Chronic meningococcemia
  Gonococcemia
  Tuberculosis
  Lyme disease
  Syphilis
  Rheumatic fever
Malignancy
  Leukemia
  Lymphoma
  Angioblastic lymphadenopathy
Connective tissue disease
  Systemic lupus erythematosus
  Mixed connective tissue disease

usually return to normal despite continued NSAID therapy (2). However, frequent monitoring of liver function, even after hospital discharge, is mandatory for patients receiving NSAIDs. NSAIDs may also increase the risk of intravascular coagulopathy.

Patients who fail to respond to NSAIDs and those with severe disease require systemic corticosteroids. Severe disease includes pericardial tamponade, myocarditis, severe pneumonitis, intravascular coagulopathy, rising values on liver function tests during NSAID treatment, and individuals who do not respond to NSAIDs. Generally, prednisone in a dose of 0.5–1.0 mg/kg/day is needed initially, but relapse can occur with tapering (2). Intravenous pulse methylprednisolone has been used for life-threatening acute disease (17,18).

Chronic Disease

No controlled studies of second-line agents for the treatment of Still's disease have been published. The most common cause of chronicity is arthritis. Intramuscular gold, hydroxychloroquine, sulfasalazine, and penicillamine have been used to control the arthritis, and anecdotal reports suggest these drugs are beneficial (2).

Immunosuppressive agents including azathioprine and cyclophosphamide have been used in resistant cases. Recently, low-dose weekly methotrexate in doses similar to those used in adult rheumatoid arthritis has been used to control both chronic arthritis and chronic systemic disease (19–21). While methotrexate is potentially hepatotoxic, it seems likely that this agent will be used increasingly. Mild chronic systemic disease (eg, fatigue, fever, rash, serositis) may also respond to hydroxychloroquine. A decade after disease onset, approximately one-half of patients still require second-line agents, and one-third of these require low-dose corticosteroids (16).

Adult Still's disease affects primarily young adults at a time when they are completing their education, starting a career, or starting a family, which can make it particularly devastating. Physiotherapists, occupational therapists, psychologists, or arthritis support groups may all be needed to care for individual patients. A knowledgeable, caring physician can make a tremendous difference. It is important to realize that Still's disease can remit even years after onset and that the vast majority of patients are leading remarkably full lives a decade after the onset of the disease.

JOHN M. ESDAILE MD, MPH

1. Magadur-Joly G, Billaud E, Barrier JH, Pennec YL, Masson C, Renou P, Prost A: Epidemiology of adult Still's disease: estimate of the incidence by a retrospective study in west France. Ann Rheum Dis 54:587-590, 1995
2. Pouchot J, Esdaile JM, Sampalis J, et al: Adult Still's disease: manifestations, disease course, and outcome in 62 patients. Medicine 70:118-136, 1991
3. Ohta A, Yamaguchi M, Tsunematsu T, et al: Adult Still's disease: a multicenter survey of Japanese patients. J Rheumatol 17:1058-1063, 1990
4. Cush JJ, Medsger TA Jr, Christy WC, Herbert D, Cooperstein LA: Adult-onset Still's disease: clinical course and outcome. Arthritis Rheum 30:186-194, 1987
5. Del Paine DW, Leek JC: Still's arthritis in adults: disease or syndrome? J Rheumatol 19:431-435, 1983
6. Elkon KB, Hughes GRV, Bywaters EGLet al: Adult-onset Still's disease: twenty-year follow-up and further studies of patients with active disease. Arthritis Rheum 25:647-654, 1982
7. Reginato AJ, Schumacher HR Jr, Baker DG, O'Connor CR, Ferreiros J: Adult onset Still's disease: experience in 23 patients and literature review with emphasis on organ failure. Seminars Arthritis Rheum 17:39-57, 1987
8. Esdaile JM, Tannenbaum H, Lough JO, Hawkins D: Hepatic abnormalities in adult Still's disease. J Rheumatol 6:673-679, 1979
9. Wouters JGW, van de Putte LBA: Adult-onset Still's disease: clinical and laboratory features, treatment and progress of 45 cases. Q J Med 61:1055-1065, 1986
10. Medsger TA Jr, Christy WC: Carpal arthritis with ankylosis in late onset Still's disease. Arthritis Rheum 19:232-242, 1976
11. Bjorkengren AG, Pathria MN, Sartoris DJ, Terkeltaub R, Esdaile JM, Weisman M, Resnick D: Carpal alterations in adult-onset Still's disease, juvenile chronic arthritis and adult-onset rheumatoid arthritis: a comparative study. Radiology 165:545-548, 1987
12. Yamaguchi M, Ohta A, Tsunematsu T, et al: Preliminary criteria for classification of adult Still's disease. J Rheumatol 19:424-430, 1992
13. Van Reeth C, Le Moel G, Lasne Y, Revenant M-C, Agneray J, Kahn M-F, Bourgeois P: Serum ferritin and isoferritins are tools for diagnosis of active adult Still's disease. J Rheumatol 21:890-895, 1994
14. Newkirk MN, Lemmo A, Commerford K, Esdaile JM, Brandwein S: Aberrant cellular localization of rubella viral genome in patients with adult Still's disease. Autoimmunity 16:39-43, 1993
15. Sampalis JS, Medsger TA Jr, Fries JF, et al: Risk factors for adult Still's disease. J Rheumatol 23:2049-2054, 1996
16. Sampalis JS, Esdaile JM, Medsger TA Jr, et al: A controlled study of the long-term prognosis of adult Still's disease. Am J Med 98:384-388, 1995
17. Kharaishi M, Fam AG: Treatment of fulminant adult Still's disease with intravenous pulse methylprednisolone therapy. J Rheumatol 18:1088-1090, 1991
18. Bisagni-Faure A, Job-Deslandre C, Menkès CJ: Treatment of Still's disease with bolus methylprednisolone. Rev Rhum Mal Osteoartic 59:228-232, 1992
19. Aydintug AO, D'Cruz D, Cervera R, Khamashta MA, Hughes GR: Low dose methotrexate treatment in adult Still's disease. J Rheumatol 19:431-435, 1992
20. Kraus A, Alarcon-Segovia D: Fever in adult onset Still's disease: response to methotrexate. J Rheumatol 18:918-920, 1991
21. Bourgeois P, Palazzo E, Belmatoug N, Kahn M-F: Low dose methotrexate in adult Still's disease: second-line treatment or steroid-sparing? Arthritis Rheum 32(suppl):S60, 1989

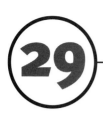

REFLEX SYMPATHETIC DYSTROPHY AND TRANSIENT REGIONAL OSTEOPOROSIS

REFLEX SYMPATHETIC DYSTROPHY

The symptom complex of reflex sympathetic dystrophy (RSD) is characterized by severe limb pain, swelling, and autonomic dysfunction. Weir Mitchell first described this condition, which he termed *causalgia*, in 1864 after observing that some soldiers recovering from gunshot wounds complained of persistent burning pain in their extremities (1). Several other designations have been applied to this syndrome, including Sudeck's atrophy, algodystrophy, and shoulder–hand syndrome, but reflex sympathetic dystrophy is the preferred term.

Clinical Features

The predominant and most disabling feature of RSD is pain (2). It is an intense, deep, chronic burning sensation exacerbated by movement, dependent posture, and emotional stress. The pain does not follow a dermatomal pattern or specific nerve distribution and is out of proportion to the inciting injury or event. Typically, patients complain of allodynia (pain induced by a non-noxious stimulus) and hyperalgesia (lowered pain threshold and enhanced pain perception). Most patients guard the affected limb from any stimulus and resist even the slightest movement, making physical examination difficult.

The pain is often accompanied by local edema and vasomotor changes. Initially, the extremity may be warm, red, and dry, but later it can become cyanotic, cool, pale, and hyperhidrotic. Cyanosis, mottling, and livedo reticularis can be observed in the contralateral extremity. Some patients develop motor abnormalities such as weakness, muscular incoordination, tremor, and muscle spasms. Dystrophic changes may produce shiny-looking, thin skin, and the nails may become brittle and exhibit altered growth patterns. Some patients eventually develop contractures, especially of the palmar fascia and tendon sheaths of the hands. RSD can affect more proximal joints, such as the knee or shoulder, and occur in several areas. Some patients have recurrent episodes.

Steinbrocker described three clinical stages of RSD (3). Stage 1 (acute) lasts 3–6 months and is characterized by pain, hypersensitivity, swelling, and vasomotor changes that lower (or raise) the temperature in the extremity, giving it a dusky purple appearance and causing dependent rubor. Sudomotor changes frequently occur, causing hyperhidrosis and hypertrichosis. Stage 2 (dystrophic) is characterized by persistent pain, disability, and atrophic skin changes. Stage 3 (atrophic) is marked by atrophy of subcutaneous tissues and, often, contractures. Not all patients follow this pattern of clinical progression, however (4).

Reflex sympathetic dystrophy has been observed in every race and all geographic locations, but the lack of uniform diagnostic criteria precludes accurate epidemiologic analysis (5). It is seen most commonly in patients 40–60 years of age, but RSD can occur in children and elderly persons. Major or minor trauma (as trivial as stubbing a toe) is the most common precipitating factor, followed by peripheral nerve injury including entrapment neuropathies. RSD is also associated with radiculopathies, stroke, hemiplegia, arthroscopy, neoplasm, arterial or venous thrombosis, and use of certain medications such as antituberculous drugs and barbiturates.

Diagnosis

Making the diagnosis of reflex sympathetic dystrophy may be difficult. The clinical manifestations are diverse, and many patients manifest atypical and incomplete presentations. The diagnosis is largely based on recognizing the distinctive array of signs and symptoms in the setting of preceding trauma or an associated medical condition and ruling out other causes (Table 29-1). Although there are no defining laboratory abnormalities, some studies can help support the diagnosis. Plain radiographs of the involved extremity may show patchy osteopenia, termed Sudek's atrophy by radiologists. Unfortunately, this is an inconsistent finding that can also occur following disuse or immobilization. Thermography can detect slight temperature differences between the involved and contralateral extremity (Fig. 29-1), but the test lacks specificity.

Three-phase bone scan is specific for RSD, but estimates of sensitivity vary from 50% to 90% (6,7). The first two phases

(Table 29-1)
Differential diagnosis of reflex sympathetic dystrophy

Chronic arterial insufficiency
Raynaud's disease
Thromboembolism
Infection
 Cellulitis
 Osteomyelitis
 Septic arthritis
Erythromelalgia
Trauma/fracture
Arthritis
 Atypical rheumatoid arthritis
 Crystalline arthropathies
 Osteoarthritis
 Reiter's syndrome
Rotator cuff tears or tendinitis
Osteonecrosis
Cerebrovascular disease
Psychosomatic illness

may demonstrate asymmetric blood flow and pooling, but the delayed image (third phase) is more typically abnormal with enhanced uptake in the peri-articular structures of the involved extremity (Fig. 29-2). The results of autonomic function test (eg, resting sweat output and quantitative sudomotor axon reflex test) may be abnormal in patients with RSD (8).

Pathogenesis

The mechanisms that lead to the development of RSD are not well understood, but numerous theories have been proposed. Current hypotheses are based on two different mechanisms: altered sympathetic outflow and regional inflammation (9). The presence of vasomotor instability and reports of dramatic improvement following sympathetic nerve blockade have led to the speculation that altered sympathetic outflow may mediate at least some of the features of RSD. Abnormal synapses between damaged afferent sensory nerves and efferent sympathetic nerves may permit mechanical and chemical cross-talk, resulting in overactivity of sympathetic nerves. Peripheral-central mechanisms have also been proposed.

In one model, mechanoreceptors stimulated at the site of injury trigger excessive repetitive excitation of the internuncial neurons in the spinal column. Activation of adjacent motor and sympathetic efferent nerves promote increased blood flow and vasomotor abnormalities in the affected extremity resulting in hyperalgesia, edema, color changes, and patchy osteopenia (3). Continued sensory input from the periphery promotes additional excitation in the spinal column,

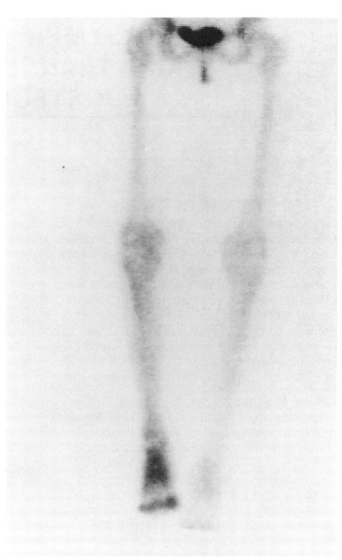

(Figure 29-2)
Bone scan of the same patient in Fig. 29-1 (anterior view). Increased radionuclide uptake is present in the right leg and is highest in the peri-articular tissues of the right foot.

setting up a reverberating circuit of pain and response. This sequence may be amplified by sympathetic fibers and this has been labeled "sympathetically mediated pain" (10).

The view that sympathetic dysfunction is responsible for RSD has been recently challenged (11). Some evidence suggests that sympathetic nerve blocks produce a significant placebo response, and , moreover, controlled studies demonstrating efficacy are not available. Drummond et al demonstrated that plasma levels of norepinephrine are lower on the affected side than in the uninvolved limb in patients with RSD, which suggests that autonomic disturbances are not related to sympathetic overactivity (12). Alternatively, it has been proved that RSD is a regional inflammatory response that is modulated by the peripheral and central nervous system (neurogenic inflammation) (13). In this model, injured nerve endings release mediators such as substance P and calcitonin gene-related peptide, which have pro-inflammatory actions and may interfere with neural pathways. Other authors have suggested that RSD is not a single syndrome but a heterogeneous group of disorders with multiple etiologies and pathogenic mechanisms (14).

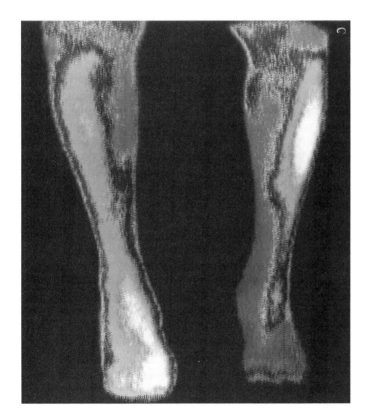

(Figure 29-1)
Thermography of the lower limbs in a 70-year-old woman with reflex sympathetic dystrophy of the right foot (anterior view). Note intense hyperthermia in the right foot with the highest temperatures dorso-medially.

Treatment

A variety of approaches have been used to treat RSD. It is essential to initiate therapy early, since the changes that occur in the later stages of RSD are often irreversible. The major goals of therapy are pain control, early joint mobilization, prevention of contractures and capsular retraction, and treatment of associated depression or anxiety (15).

Pain control is an essential component of therapy and frequently requires the use of narcotic analgesics. Physiotherapy should be initiated promptly to mobilize the affected extremity and lessen local edema. Passive and active range-of-motion exercises, tissue massage, heat baths, and, in some cases, transcutaneous electrical nerve stimulation (TENS) can be helpful. Other conditions that may be additional sources of discomfort (eg, carpal tunnel syndrome) or biomechanical problems (eg, metatarsalgia resulting from altered gait) should be addressed with the use of splints or assistive devices. Modification of the home or work environment may be required to lessen pain and permit maximum function.

Oral corticosteroids have proved very effective in the treatment of RSD, especially in patients with abnormal findings on bone scan (17). The initial dose of prednisone is 60–80 mg/day given in four divided doses for 2 weeks, then tapered and discontinued by the third or fourth week. Some patients require long-term low-dose prednisone (5–10 mg/day) to control symptoms. Calcitonin and intravenous regional ketanserin provide sustained pain relief for some patients (5).

Sympathetic nerve blockade has long been a popular treatment for RSD, although controlled studies demonstrating long-term efficacy have not been performed, and a strong placebo response is well documented (13). Therapeutic blocks are performed by injecting a local anesthetic into the lumbar sympathetic ganglia for lower extremity RSD and into the cervical sympathetic ganglia for upper extremity involvement. Regional blocks can be performed with the Bier block technique, which involves isolating the affected limb with a pneumatic tourniquet, injecting guanethidine, reserpine, or bretylium, and then releasing the tourniquet after 10–20 minutes. Usually a series of blocks are performed and the therapeutic effects monitored. If the response to regional block is transient, surgical sympathectomy can be performed. In rare instances, amputation is required to control pain, eradicate infection, or improve function; however, recurrence of RSD in the stump is common (17).

TRANSIENT REGIONAL OSTEOPOROSIS

The syndrome of transient regional osteoporosis manifests as monarticular or oligoarticular pain in young and middle-aged individuals, accompanied by striking osteopenia of the involved joint on plain radiographs. Some authors consider this entity a variant of RSD, but several features differ (18). Neuropathic pain, upper extremity involvement, and preceding trauma are unusual in transient regional osteoporosis. The syndrome has predilection for hip joint involvement, and neither vasomotor instability nor dystrophic changes are typical of this disorder. Although more common in men, transient regional osteoporosis does occur in women, particularly in pregnant women during the second and third trimester (19).

Diagnosis of transient regional osteoporosis is based on the presence of joint pain, diminished joint mobility, and localized osteopenia on radiographs. Bone scans reveal increased radionuclide uptake in the involved joint. Treatment is conservative and consists of non-weight bearing and analgesics. In contrast to RSD, this syndrome does not benefit from corticosteroids. Most patients recover completely in several weeks, and permanent joint damage is rare. However, a significant percentage of patients have recurrent episodes.

CHRISTOPHER T. RITCHLIN, MD

1. Mitchell SW, Morehouse GR, Keen WW: Gunshot wounds and other injuries of nerves. Philadelphia, Lippincott, 1864

2. Schwartzman RJ: Reflex sympathetic dystrophy and causalgia. Neurol Clin 10:953-973, 1992

3. Steinbrocker O, Argyros TG: The shoulder-hand syndrome: present status as a diagnostic and therapeutic entity. Med Clin North Am 42:1533-1553, 1958

4. Veldman PHJM, Reynen HM, Arntz IE, Goris RJ: Signs and symptoms of reflex sympathetic dystrophy: prospective study of 829 patients. Lancet 342:1012-1016, 1993

5. Raice E: Reflex sympathetic dystrophy. Br Med J 310:1645-1649, 1995

6. Kozin F, Geriant HK, Bekerman C, McCarty D: The reflex sympathetic dystrophy syndrome: II recognition and scintigraphic evidence of biraterality and of periarticular accentuation. Am J Med 60:332-338, 1976

7. Werner R, Davidoff G, Jackson DM, Cremer S, Ventocilla C, Wolf L: Factors affecting the sensitivity and specificity of the three-phase technetium bone scan in the diagnosis of reflex sympathetic dystrophy syndrome in the upper extremity. J Hand Surg 14A:520-523, 1989

8. Chelimsky TC, Low PA, Naessens JM, Wilson PR, Amadio PC, O'Brien PC: Value of autonomic testing in reflex sympathetic dystrophy. Mayo Clin Proc 70:1029-1040, 1995

9. Bonica JJ: Causalgia and other reflex dystrophies. In Bonica JJ (ed): The management of pain, 2nd ed. Philadelphia, Lea & Febiger, 1990, pp 220-243

10. Roberts J: A hypothesis on the physiologic basis for causalgia and related pains. Pain 24:297-311, 1986

11. Oyen WJG, Arntz IE, Claessens RM, Van der Meer JW, Corstens FH, Goris RJ: Reflex sympathetic dystrophy of the hand: an excessive inflammatory response. Pain 55(2):151-157, 1993

12. Drummond PD, Finch PM, Smythe GA: Reflex sympathetic dystrophy: the significance of differing plasma catecholamine concentrations in affected and unaffected limbs. Brain 114:2025-2036, 1991

13. Schott, GC: An unsympathetic view of pain. Lancet 245:634-636, 1995

14. Ochoa, JL, Verdugo, RJ: Reflex sympathetic dystrophy: a common clinical avenue for somatoform expression. Neurologic Clinics 13(2):351-363, 1995

15. Doury P, Dequeker J: Algodystrophy/reflex sympathetic dystrophy syndrome. In Klippel JH, Dieppe PA (eds): Rheumatology. London, Mosby, 1994, pp 7.38.1-7.38.6

16. Kozin F, Ryan L, Carerra GF, Soin JS, Wortmann RL: The reflex sympathetic dystrophy syndrome: III. Scintographic studies, further evidence for the therapeutic efficacy of systemic corticosteroids and proposed diagnostic criteria. Am J Med 60:23-30, 1981

17. Dielissen PW, Classen A, Veldman P, Goris R: Amputation for reflex sympathetic dystrophy. J Bone and Joint Surg 77:270-273, 1995

18. Lakhanpal S, Ginsburg WW, Luthra HS, Hunder GG: Transient regional osteoporosis: a study of 56 cases and review of the literature. Ann Intern Med 106:444-450, 1987

19. Brodell JD, Burns JE, Heiple KG: Transient osteoporosis of the hip of pregnancy. J Bone and Joint Surg 71:1252-1257, 1989

NEUROPATHIC ARTHROPATHY

The concept of an association between neurologic lesions and arthritis was first introduced by Jean-Martin Charcot in 1868 (1). The term *neuropathic arthropathy* refers to severe degenerative arthritis in the setting of neurologic damage to the involved joint or limb. The terms neurotrophic arthropathy, Charcot arthropathy, and neuroarthropathy are used synonymously.

EPIDEMIOLOGY

Accurate figures on the incidence and prevalence of neuropathic arthropathy in the general population are difficult to ascertain. The presence of sensory neuropathy is the only established risk factor for developing neuropathic arthropathy. Although motor function is usually preserved in the affected limb, neuropathic arthropathy has been reported after vigorous physical therapy in patients with severe weakness (2). Either central (upper motor neuron) lesions or peripheral (lower motor neuron lesions) may produce neuropathic arthropathy.

The neurologic diseases associated with neuropathic arthropathy have changed with time (Table 30-1). In the pre-penicillin era, neuropathic arthropathy was commonly associated with tabes dorsalis from tertiary syphilis. Diabetes is currently the most common cause of neuropathic arthropathy. Syringomyelia and spinal cord injuries are also frequently implicated in cases of neuropathic arthropathy. Less commonly encountered causes of neuropathic arthropathy include inflammatory or neoplastic lesions of the spinal cord or peripheral nerves, meningomyelocele, congenital neurologic abnormalities, and alcoholism. Rarely,

(Table 30-1)
Neurologic conditions associated with neuropathic arthropathy

Diabetes mellitus
Syringomyelia
Brain or spinal cord trauma
Meningomyelocele
Nerve trauma
Syphilis
Multiple sclerosis
Charcot–Marie–Tooth disease
Riley-Day syndrome
Pernicious anemia
Congenital insensitivity to pain
Alcoholism
Amyloidosis
Thalidomide exposure
Polyneuropathy of Dejerine–Sottas
Arnold–Chiari malformation
Leprosy
Yaws

cases occur in which no neurologic abnormality is identifiable (2).

CLINICAL FEATURES

Neuropathic arthropathy typically presents as an acute or subacute monarthritis with swelling, erythema, and variable amounts of pain in the affected joint. The two most constant clinical features of neuropathic arthropathy are the presence of a significant sensory neuropathy and a degree of pain that is less than would be expected considering the degree of joint destruction evident on radiographs. There is variability in the speed of onset, the rate of progression, and the balance between bone destruction and bony overgrowth in neuropathic arthropathy. When slowly progressive, neuropathic arthropathy often resembles osteoarthritis. When rapidly progressive and acute in onset, it mimics osteomyelitis. Initial examinations show swelling, erythema, joint effusions, and variable amounts of tenderness. With time, the neuropathic joint becomes deformed, with large effusions, palpable osteophytes, and loss of range of motion. Signs of inflammation may be present. Well-described clinical subsets of neuropathic arthropathy include neuropathic arthropathy of the diabetic foot and acute neuropathic arthropathy.

The Diabetic Foot

Symptomatic diabetic neuropathy occurs in as many as 13% of patients with diabetes (3). However, the estimated prevalence of neuropathic arthropathy among diabetics is 1 in 1680 (4). The joints of the foot are most commonly involved (5). Sixty percent of patients have involvement of the tarsometatarsal joint, 30% the metatarsophalangeal joints, and 10% have involvement of the tibiotalar joints. Patients present with a swollen midfoot or ankle, and variable degrees of erythema, warmth, and pain. Involvement of the midfoot may ultimately result in reversal of the curve of the metatarsal arch and "rocker bottom" deformity. The possibility of osteomyelitis or soft tissue infection in the feet must always be considered in diabetic patients.

Acute Neuropathic Arthropathy

This disorder usually occurs in the diabetic foot and may be preceded by minor trauma, such as an ankle sprain (6). It is characterized by the abrupt onset of swelling, often associated with marked warmth and erythema over the involved area. Pain is often present and may be severe. Dramatic radiographic changes and deformities may develop over a period of weeks.

Neuropathic arthropathy associated with diseases other than diabetes often has a different pattern of joint involvement. Approximately 5%–10% of patients with tabes dorsalis develop neuropathic arthropathy, commonly involving the knee, hip, ankle, and lumbar spine. Up to 25% of patients with syringomyelia develop neuropathic arthropathy, which typically affects the glenohumeral or other upper extremity joints. The pattern of neuropathic arthropathy in spinal cord trauma depends on the level of injury.

DIAGNOSIS

The diagnosis of neuropathic arthropathy can be made clinically. Helpful diagnostic tests include plain radiographs, bone scans, indium 111–labeled white blood cell (WBC) scans, and synovial fluid analysis. The differential diagnosis of neuropathic arthropathy includes osteomyelitis and other deep tissue infections, calcium pyrophosphate dihydrate (CPPD) deposition disease, Milwaukee shoulder/knee syndrome, osteonecrosis, and post-traumatic osteoarthritis.

Plain radiographs are extremely helpful in making a diagnosis of neuropathic arthropathy (2). Early features include demineralization, joint space narrowing, and osteophyte formation. Later features are bone fragmentation, periarticular debris formation, and joint subluxation (Fig. 30-1). Bone absorption, bone shattering, sclerosis, and massive soft tissue swelling are seen in some patients. Neuropathic joints are often described radiographically as "disorganized," with features of chaotic bony destruction and repair. The presence of sharply defined articular surfaces in neuropathic arthropathy is helpful in differentiating radiographic changes of neuropathic arthropathy from those of infection, where involved bone surfaces are indistinct. In diabetic neuropathic arthropathy, destruction with prominent fragmentation and loose body formation typically occurs in the tarsal bones, while absorptive changes may predominate in the metatarsals and forefoot (Fig. 30-2). Tarsometatarsal involvement is referred to as Lisfranc fracture–dislocation. In the spine, multilevel thoracic and lumbar involvement is common. Ankylosis, although rare in neuropathic arthropathy, can occur.

Bone scintigraphy with technetium 99m-MDP, and indium 111–labeled WBC scans may be useful diagnostic tests

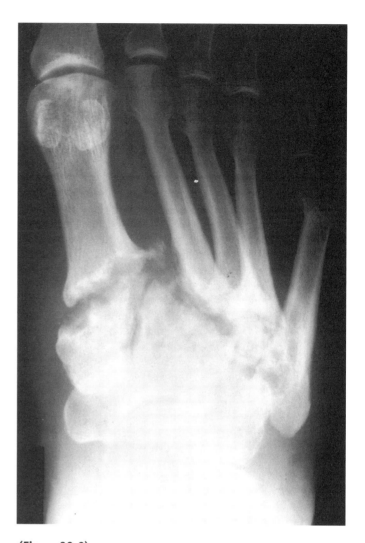

(Figure 30-2)
Neuropathic arthropathy in the diabetic foot. There is involvement of both the metatarsophalangeal joints and the midfoot. The typical combination of both resorptive and reparative processes results in a disorganized appearance.

in neuropathic arthropathy. Increased uptake of radiolabeled technetium and gallium occurs in neuropathic arthropathy. Unfortunately, uncomplicated neuropathy as well as infection are associated with increased blood flow to the affected area on bone scan. Thus, bone and gallium scans are not useful in differentiating infection from neuropathic arthropathy. In contrast, increased uptake of indium 111–labeled WBC occurs in osteomyelitis but not in neuropathic arthropathy (7). Magnetic resonance imaging may be helpful to rule out osteomyelitis, and classic findings of neuropathic arthropathy may be present (7).

Synovial fluid is typically noninflammatory. Fifty percent of synovial fluids from affected joints are hemorrhagic or xanthochromic. Effusions may be very large. CPPD crystals and basic calcium phosphate crystals have been identified in these joint effusions, but whether these crystals are markers of severe joint destruction or contribute to the pathogenesis of neuropathic arthropathy remains to be determined.

PATHOLOGY

The pathologic changes in neuropathic arthropathy are similar to those of advanced osteoarthritis with cartilage de-

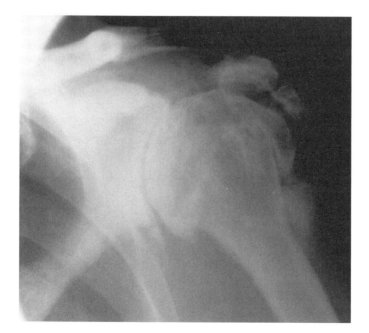

(Figure 30-1)
Neuropathic arthropathy in a shoulder of a patient with syringomyelia. Note the demineralization, bone fragmentation, loose body formation, and joint space narrowing.

struction, bone eburnation, osteophytosis, and loose body formation. The presence of "detritic synovitis," defined as fragments of cartilage and bone embedded in the synovium, is characteristic of neuropathic arthropathy, but it is also seen in severe osteoarthritis and other conditions (2). As reflected radiographically, neuropathic arthropathy can cause exuberant bone and cartilage overgrowth as well as joint destruction. Usually both processes are seen, but one process often predominates.

PATHOPHYSIOLOGY

Two major theories have been proposed to explain the development of neuropathic arthropathy. Charcot postulated that joint denervation produced physiologic changes, such as increased blood flow, which promoted metabolic alterations in cartilage and bone leading to joint degeneration. Virchow proposed that repeated episodes of minor trauma to joints that were unprotected by the response to pain facilitated damage through further trauma and inadequate repair. Experimental data exist to support both Charcot's and Virchow's theories. Charcot's hypothesis is supported clinically by reports of neuropathic arthropathy developing after revascularization procedures in diabetes and in patients on bedrest who could not have sustained trauma (8). Some clinical observations fit best with Virchow's theory. For example, fractures often accelerate or initiate neuropathic arthropathy (9), and acute neuropathic arthropathy is commonly seen after minor trauma (6). Certainly, these theories may not be mutually exclusive, and both mechanisms may contribute to the development of neuropathic arthropathy.

MANAGEMENT

There are no specific therapies for neuropathic arthropathy. The prognosis of patients with neuropathic arthropathy is variable, and depends on the severity of the condition and the response to therapeutic or surgical intervention.

Standard management strategies include joint immobilization and elevating the involved limb. Orthotics and joint protection devices can be particularly helpful with foot involvement. Rarely, the underlying neurologic problem is amenable to treatment. Agents such as amitriptyline can improve pain in neuropathic arthropathy. Good diabetic control may also ameliorate existing neuropathic arthropathy (10). Pulsed electromagnetic field therapy has been used with mixed results.

Surgical treatments such as arthrodesis may be helpful in reducing pain. The spine is particularly amenable to fusion, but patients with foot or knee involvement may also benefit from this procedure (11). Care must be taken to avoid nonunion and refracture. Exostectomy may restore some motion and decrease joint pain, and has been particularly useful in patients with severe rocker bottom deformities (12). Traditionally, total joint replacement was considered risky because of a high rate of prosthesis failure. With current techniques, however, joint replacement may be effective for selected patients (13). Indications include refractory pain and mild neurologic disease. Results are improved with correction of severe bone loss by generous bone grafting and careful ligamentous repair. Rarely, amputation of the affected joint is required.

Prevention is perhaps the best therapy. Prompt attention to any minor trauma to the diabetic foot or ankle may prevent the development of neuropathic arthropathy. Good control of blood glucose levels in diabetics decreases the incidence of neuropathy and thereby reduces the risk of neuropathic arthropathy.

ANN K. ROSENTHAL, MD

1. Gupta R: A short history of neuropathic arthropathy. Clin Orth Rel Res 296:43-49, 1993

2. Resnick D: Neuropathic osteoarthropathy. In Resnick D (ed), Diagnosis of Bone and Joint Disorders (3rd ed). Philadelphia: WB Saunders Company, 1995, pp 3413-3442

3. Dyck PJ, Karnes J, O'Brien PC: Diagnosis, staging, and classification of diabetic neuropathy and associations with other complications. In Dyck PJ, Thomas PK, Asbury A, Winegrad A, Porte D (eds): Diabetic Neuropathy. Philadelphia, WB Saunders Company 1987, pp 36-44

4. Horowitz SH: Diabetic neuropathy. Clin Orth Rel Res 296:78-85,1993

5. Scartozzi G, Kanat IO: Diabetic neuroarthropathy of the foot and ankle. J Am Pod Assoc 80:298-303, 1990

6. Slowman-Kovacs SD, Braunstein EM, Brandt KD: Rapidly progressive Charcot arthropathy following minor joint trauma in patients with diabetic neuropathy. Arthritis Rheum 33:412-417,1990

7. Seabold JE, Flickinger FW, Kao SCS, Gleason TJ, Kahn D, Nepola JV, Marsh JL : Indium-111 leukocyte/technetium-99m-MDP bone and magnetic resonance imaging: difficulty of diagnosing osteomyelitis in patients with neuropathic osteoarthropathy. J Nucl Med 31:569-556, 1990

8. Edelman SV, Kosofsky EM, Paul RA, Kozak GP: Neuro-osteopathy (Charcot's joint) in diabetes mellitus following revascularization surgery. Three case reports and a review of the literature. Arch Intern Med 147:1504-1508, 1987

9. Johnson JTH: Neuropathic fractures and joint injuries: pathogenesis and rationale of prevention and treatment. J Bone Joint Surg 49A:1-30, 1967

10. Eynmontt MJ, Alavi A, Dalinka MK, Kyle GF: Bone scintigraphy in diabetic osteoarthropathy. Radiology 140:475-477, 1981

11. Drennan DB, Fahey JJ, Maylahn RJ: Important factors in acheiving arthrodesis of the Charcot knee. J Bone Joint Surg 53A: 1180-1193, 1971

12. Brodsky JW, Rouse AM: Exostectomy for symptomatic bony prominences in diabetic Charcot feet. Clin Orthop Rel Res 296:21-26, 1993

13. Soudry M, Binazzi R, Johanson NA, Bullough PG, Insall JN: Total knee arthroplasty in Charcot and Charcot-like joints. Clin Orthop Rel Res 296:199-204, 1993

SARCOIDOSIS

Sarcoidosis is a systemic, chronic, granulomatous disease of unknown etiology that chiefly strikes individuals 20–40 years of age (1–3). Although it most notably involves the lungs, sarcoidosis can affect nearly any organ system and mimic rheumatic diseases capable of causing fever, arthritis, uveitis, myositis, and rash.

PATHOGENESIS

Although the cause of sarcoidosis is unknown, the host immune response clearly plays a central role in pathogenesis (4–6). The disease is characterized by disseminated non-caseating granulomas. The sarcoid granuloma contains a central follicle of tightly packed epithelioid cells and multi-nucleated giant cells surrounded by lymphocytes, macrophages, monocytes, and fibroblasts. In the lung, the initial inflammation is an alveolitis composed chiefly of activated CD4 (helper) T cells whose cytokines recruit other cells to help form the granulomas (4). Alveolar T cells also preferentially express specific antigen receptors, which suggests T-cell response to a specific stimulus such as an organism or self-antigen (7). The character and intensity of the alveolitis is reflected in bronchoalveolar lavage fluid, which typically shows an increase in the lymphocytes and a high CD4/CD8 T-cell ratio.

Granulomas are widely distributed in sarcoidosis, occurring in the lung (86% of patients), lymph nodes (86%), liver (86%), spleen (63%), heart (20%), kidney (19%), bone marrow (17%), and pancreas (6%) (1,8). Granulomas compress tissues and mediate disease by secreting cytokines that provoke constitutional symptoms, recruiting inflammatory cells whose products injure local tissues, and elaborating growth factors that cause fibrosis (3,5,9). In addition, activated monocytes in granulomas convert vitamin D precursors to 1,25 dihydroxyvitamin D, which can increase intestinal absorption of calcium and cause hypercalcemia (10).

The peripheral blood reveals the dichotomy of depressed cellular immunity and enhanced humoral immunity (8). Depressed cellular immunity is evidenced by lymphopenia, a low helper/suppressor T-cell ratio (0.8/1 in sarcoidosis patients versus 1.8/1 in healthy controls), and cutaneous anergy (affecting 70% of patients). In contrast, activated humoral immunity is manifested by polyclonal gammopathy and autoantibody production. Approximately 20%–30% of patients have rheumatoid factor or antinuclear antibodies.

CLINICAL FEATURES

Sarcoidosis is most common in African Americans and northern European Caucasians. The prevalence among African Americans (40 per 100,000) is 8 times higher than that among white Americans (3,6). Women are slightly more often affected than men.

Patients with sarcoidosis commonly present with one of four problems: pulmonary symptoms (40%–45%), asymptomatic hilar adenopathy detected on chest roentgenogram (5%–10%), constitutional symptoms (25%), or extrathoracic inflammation (25%), which may include rheumatic manifestations (3,8).

Pulmonary Involvement

Respiratory symptoms are the most common presenting complaints and include dry cough, dyspnea, and nonspecific chest pain. Hemoptysis, rare at initial presentation, may become recurrent, massive, and even fatal in patients who develop mycetomas in pulmonary cysts (3). Pleural effusions are rare in sarcoidosis.

Regardless of initial symptoms, more than 90% of patients with sarcoidosis have abnormal findings on chest radiographs. Four types are recognized: type 0 is no abnormalities and occurs in fewer than 10% of patients; type I is most common (43%) and shows enlargement of hilar, mediastinal, and, often, right paratracheal lymph nodes; type II (24%) exhibits the adenopathy found in type I plus pulmonary infiltrates and is most common in patients presenting with symptomatic respiratory disease; and type III (13%) demonstrates infiltrates without adenopathy (3). This classification has prognostic significance. Approximately 80% of patients with type I chest films remit within 2 years (3). In contrast, only 30%–50% of patients with type II and fewer than 20% of patients with type III remit.

Constitutional Symptoms

Fever, weight loss, fatigue, and malaise are the presenting symptoms in 25% of patients. Fever is frequently associated with hepatic granulomas.

Rheumatologic Manifestations

Arthritis occurs in 10%–15% of patients with sarcoidosis (11–15). Two patterns of joint disease are recognized, classified by whether the arthritis occurs early (within the first 6 months after disease onset) or late in the course. The first form, in which arthritis is part of the initial presentation, is most common. The arthritis often begins in one or both ankles and may occasionally spread in additive fashion to involve the knees, proximal interphalangeal joints, metacarpophalangeal joints, wrists, and elbows. The axial skeleton is spared. Typically, 4–6 joints are involved, and monarthritis in this early phase is unusual. Periarticular swelling is more common than frank joint effusion, although when effusions occur, synovial fluid is usually noninflammatory. Tenosynovitis and heel pain may also occur. The pain is often periarticular and much more severe than the few objective signs of inflammation would suggest. Erythema nodosum is strikingly associated with early arthritis, occurring in 66% of patients. The syndrome of acute arthritis, erythema nodosum, and bilateral hilar adenopathy (Lofgren's syndrome) has an excellent prognosis with a 90% remission rate. Radiographs of sarcoidosis patients with acute arthritis almost never show bony or cartilaginous changes. The duration of acute arthritis averages several weeks, but may be as short as a few days or as long as 3 months. Few patients have repeated attacks of arthritis. Because hyperuricemia is common in sarcoidosis, patients with monarthritis, tenosynovitis, and recurrent musculoskeletal symptoms may be misdiagnosed as having gout.

The second form of arthritis begins 6 months or more after the onset of sarcoidosis (11). Late joint disease is generally less severe and less widespread. The knees are the most commonly involved joints, followed by the ankles and proximal interphalangeal joints. The average number of joints involved is 2–3; monarthritis can occur. Synovial effusions are noninflammatory or mildly inflammatory, as evidenced by synovial fluid white blood cell (WBC) counts of 250–6200/mm³ with 56%–100% mononuclear cells (15). Synovial histology is often less inflammatory than in rheumatoid arthritis, but occasionally reveals granulomas. In contrast to early arthritis, late disease is associated with chronic cutaneous sarcoidosis, but not with erythema nodosum. Late arthritis can be either transient or chronic. The chronic form often manifests itself by *dactylitis*, a sausage-like swelling of a digit, frequently with overlying cutaneous sarcoidosis. Typically, activities of daily living are not greatly impaired and pain is not intense. Radiographic changes are uncommon, but destructive and cystic changes can occur and are most often noted in the middle and distal phalanges of the hand (Fig. 31-1). Cystic lytic lesions in the middle portion of the phalanx are typical. Less obvious but also characteristic are diffuse trabecular changes, giving the bone a honeycomb appearance. These radiographic findings occur most frequently in patients with dactylitis, but occasionally they occur in patients without arthritis.

Several other rheumatologic manifestations may accompany sarcoidosis (Table 31-1). Sarcoidosis of the larynx, nasal turbinates, and nasal cartilage resembles Wegener's granulomatosis. Eye disease eventually develops in 22% of patients with sarcoidosis, most commonly uveitis (16). Patients may also develop lachrymal gland enlargement, conjunctival nodules, keratoconjunctivitis (similar to that seen in Sjögren's syndrome), and proptosis (similar to that seen in Wegener's granulomatosis). Clinically evident sarcoidosis of the skeletal muscles resembles polymyositis, characterized by slowly progressive proximal weakness, elevated creatine phosphokinase, and a myopathic pattern on elec-

tromyography. Muscle biopsy may reveal granulomatous myositis. Muscle involvement can also be asymptomatic. Mononeuritis multiplex, facial nerve palsy, and parotid gland enlargement are other signs common to both sarcoidosis and other rheumatologic diseases (Table 31-1).

Other Extrathoracic Manifestations

Peripheral lymphadenopathy, one of the most common manifestations of sarcoidosis, occurs in 75% of patients. Typically, the lymph nodes are nontender, range in size from 1–5 cm, and involve at least the cervical and often the axillary, epitrochlear, and inguinal regions (1–3). Skin involvement occurs in one-third of patients and serves as a marker for prognosis (3). Erythema nodosum appears early and is associated with an excellent prognosis. Papules, nodules, plaques, and scaling lesions, which can disfigure, are associated with chronic sarcoidosis. Sarcoidosis causing violaceous plaques over the cheeks, nose, and ears is called *lupus pernio*. Most patients (86%) have hepatic granulomas, but only 20% have hepatomegaly or elevated liver enzymes (especially alkaline phosphatase). Jaundice, intrahepatic cholestasis, postnecrotic cirrhosis, and portal hypertension without cirrhosis have been reported. Neurosarcoidosis, which occurs in 5% of patients, is rarely the sole presenting sign (3,17). Central nervous system manifestations include basilar meningitis, hydrocephalus, intracranial mass lesions, seizures, and neuroendocrine disorders, such as hypopituitarism and diabetes insipidus. Heart involvement leads to tachyarrhythmias, cardiomyopathy, or sudden death. Cor pulmonale complicates severe pulmonary disease. Renal

(Table 31-1)
Rheumatic manifestations of sarcoidosis

Manifestation	Frequency in Sarcoidosis (% of Patients)	Differential Diagnosis
Arthritis	15	Rheumatoid arthritis, rheumatic fever, systemic lupus erythematosus, gonococcal arthritis, gout, spondyloarthropathies
Parotid gland enlargement	5	Sjögren's syndrome
Upper airway disease (sinusitis, laryngeal inflammation, saddle-nose deformity)	3	Wegener's granulomatosis
Uveitis	19	
Anterior	18	Spondyloarthropathies
Posterior	7	Behçet's disease
Keratoconjunctivitis	5	Sjögren's syndrome
Proptosis	1	Wegener's granulomatosis
Myositis	4	Polymyositis
Mononeuritis multiplex	1	Systemic vasculitis
Facial nerve palsy	2	Lyme disease

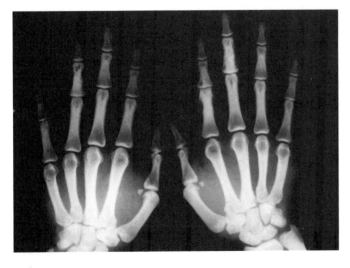

(Figure 31-1)
Radiograph of hands of a patient with chronic sarcoidosis. Note punched-out lesions on phalanges and soft tissue swelling.

manifestations of sarcoidosis include membranous glomerulonephritis, nephrocalcinosis, renal calculi, and renal insufficiency, with or without hypercalcemia (2). In the absence of massive hemoptysis, anemia is not a prominent feature of sarcoidosis. Leukopenia (WBC <4000/mm^3) occurs in 28% of patients, mild eosinophilia (>5% eosinophils) in 34%, and hypercalcemia in 19%. Serum angiotensin-converting enzyme (ACE) is elevated in 60% of patients with sarcoidosis, as it is in tuberculosis, lymphoma, diabetes, hyperthyroidism, Whipple's disease, Gaucher's disease, and other disorders (3,8).

DIAGNOSIS AND MANAGEMENT

No single finding or laboratory test establishes the diagnosis of sarcoidosis. Therefore, the diagnosis depends on a compatible clinical picture, histologic evidence of noncaseating granulomas, and exclusion of other possible causes. Biopsy is not necessary for an asymptomatic patient 20–40 years old with classic radiographic findings of paratracheal and bilateral symmetric hilar lymphadenopathy, because such a patient is exceedingly unlikely to have any other disorder. In symptomatic patients, however, other causes must be excluded, especially infections or lymphoma. When a patient does not have specific skin or conjunctival lesions, transbronchial lung biopsy is usually the preferred diagnostic test, as it is positive in nearly 90% of sarcoidosis patients with abnormal findings on chest radiographs and in two-thirds of those with a normal findings.

Skin anergy is typical but not diagnostic. The Kveim–Siltzbach test is performed by intradermal injection of a heat-treated suspension of sarcoidosis spleen extract, followed by a biopsy 4–6 weeks later. In approximately three-fourths of patients with sarcoidosis, evidence of a granulomatous inflammatory reaction is detected. However, the biopsy may have a 5% false-positive rate. Cells in the sarcoid granuloma produce ACE and 1,25 dihydroxy vitamin D. Accordingly, up to two-thirds of patients have elevated serum ACE levels, and the vast majority have hypercalcemia or hypercalciuria.

Most patients with sarcoidosis do well. Many, especially those with a type I chest film, remit spontaneously. However, 25% of patients develop pulmonary disability, and 10% die from progressive sarcoidosis. Markers for chronic symptomatic disease are advanced disease on radiograph, lupus pernio, and cardiac or neurologic involvement.

Treatment depends on the specific manifestations. Asymptomatic hilar adenopathy requires no therapy. Many patients with early or late sarcoid arthritis respond to nonsteroidal anti-inflammatory drugs, including salicylates (11,14,15). Colchicine can be effective, especially for acute sarcoidosis arthropathy. Mucocutaneous sarcoidosis often improves with chloroquine (3). Corticosteroids are indicated for severe lung disease, liver disease, hypercalcemia, cardiac inflammation, posterior uveitis, neurosarcoidosis, and severe sarcoidosis of other organs (3,18). The initial prednisone dose is 40 mg/day in divided daily doses, which more effectively control fever. The dose is then tapered 5 mg every 2 weeks to a 15 mg/day dose and maintained at that level for 4–8 months to make certain that the improvement has plateaued. If possible, prednisone can then be tapered off completely (18,19). The efficacy of immunosuppressive drugs is not established. Methotrexate may be corticosteroid-sparing in patients with chronic disease (20). Assessing treatment response depends chiefly on careful clinical examination, supplemented by changes in key tests such as chest radiographs and pulmonary function tests. Bronchoalveolar lavage fluid analysis, serum ACE levels, and gallium lung scanning have been useful in research, but have not yet altered patient management (3).

DAVID B. HELLMAN, MD

1. Longcope WT, Freiman DG: A study of sarcoidosis based on a combined investigation of 160 cases including 30 autopsies from the Johns Hopkins Hospital and Massachusetts General Hospital. Medicine 31:1-132, 1952

2. Mayock RL, Bertrand P, Morrison CE, Scott JH: Manifestations of sarcoidosis: analysis of 145 patients, with a review of nine series selected from the literature. Am J Med 35:67-89, 1963

3. Bascom RA, Johns CJ: The natural history and management of sarcoidosis. In Stollerman GH, Harrington WJ, Lamont JT, Leonard JJ, Siperstein MD (eds): Advances in Internal Medicine 1986, pp 213-241 vol. 31. Chicago, Yearbook Medical Publishers.

4. Keogh BA, Hunninghake GW, Line BR, Crystal RG: The alveolitis of pulmonary sarcoidosis: evaluation of natural history and alveolitis-dependent changes in lung function. Am Rev Respir Dis 128:256-265, 1983

5. Crystal RG, Roberts WC, Hunninghake GW, Gadek JE, Fulmer JD, Line BR: Pulmonary sarcoidosis: a disease characterized and perpetuated by activated lung T-lymphocytes. Ann Intern Med 94:73-94, 1981

6. Thomas PD, Hunninghake GW: Current concepts of the pathogenesis of sarcoidosis. Am Rev Respir Dis 135:747-760, 1987

7. Forman JD, Klein JT, Silver RF, Liu MC, Greenlee BM, Moller DR: Selective activation and accumulation of oligoclonal Vβ-specific T cells in active pulmonary sarcoidosis. J Clin Invest 94:1533-1542, 1994

8. Ainslie GM, Benatar SR: Serum angiotensin converting enzyme in sarcoidosis: sensitivity and specificity in diagnosis: correlations with disease activity, duration, extra-thoracic involvement, radiographic type and therapy. Q J Med 55:253-270, 1985

9. McFadden RG, Vickers KE, Fraher LJ: Lymphocyte chemokinetic factors derived from human tonsils: modulation by 1,25-dihydroxyvitamin D3 (calcitriol). Am J Respir Cell Mol Biol 4:42-49, 1991

10. Mason RS, Frankel T, Chan Y, Lissner D, Posen S: Vitamin D conversion by sarcoid lymph node homogenate. Ann Intern Med 100:59-61, 1984

11. Gumpel JM, Johns CJ, Shulman LE: The joint disease of sarcoidosis. Ann Rheum Dis 26:194-205, 1967

12. Spilberg I, Siltzbach LE, McEwen C: The arthritis of sarcoidosis. Arthritis Rheum 12:126-137, 1969

13. Kaplan H: Sarcoid arthritis: a review. Arch Intern Med 112:924-935, 1963

14. Glennas A, Kvien TK, Melby K, Refvem OK, Andrup O, Karstensen B, Thoen JE: Acute sarcoid arthritis: occurrence, seasonal onset, clinical features and outcome. Br J Rheumatol 34:45-50, 1995

15. Palmer DG, Schumacher HR: Synovitis with non-specific histological changes in synovium in chronic sarcoidosis. Ann Rheum Dis 43:778-782, 1984

16. Jabs DA, Johns CJ: Ocular involvement in chronic sarcoidosis. Am J Ophthalmol 102:297-301, 1986

17. Chapelon C, Ziza JM, Piette JC, Levy Y, Raguin G, Wechsler B, Bitker MO, Bletry O, Laplane D, Bousser MG, Godeau P: Neurosarcoidosis: signs, course and treatment of 35 confirmed cases. Medicine 69:261-276, 1990

18. Hunninghake GW, Gilbert S, Pueringer R, Dayton C, Floerchinger C, Helmers R, Merchant R, Wilson J, Galvin J, Schwartz D: Outcome of the treatment for sarcoidosis. Am J Respir Crit Care Med 149:893-898, 1994

19. Johns CJ, Zachary JB, Ball WC Jr: A ten-year study of corticosteroid treatment of pulmonary sarcoidosis. Johns Hopkins Med J 134:271-283, 1974

20. Lower EE, Baughman RP: Prolonged use of methotrexate for sarcoidosis. Arch Intern Med 155:846-851, 1995

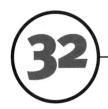

32 DEPOSITION AND STORAGE DISEASES

This chapter covers a number of unusual arthropathies that are caused by deposition of normal material such as metal ions, or storage of abnormal material such as lipids (1). Hemochromatosis, ochronosis, and Wilson's disease are characterized by cellular deposition of the normal metal ions: iron, calcium, and copper, respectively. Gaucher's, Fabry's, and Farber's disease, and multicentric reticulohistiocytosis result from cellular storage of abnormal lipids. Rheumatic changes are only one manifestation of these systemic disorders. In contrast, arthritis evolves as a predominant feature in hemochromatosis, ochronosis, Gaucher's disease, and multicentric reticulohistiocytosis.

HEMOCHROMATOSIS

Idiopathic hemochromatosis is an inherited disorder characterized by excessive body iron stores and the deposition of hemosiderin, which cause tissue damage and organ dysfunction (2). The disorder rarely appears before age 40 unless there is a family history, and men are affected 10 times more frequently than women, who are protected by menstruation. Increased intestinal iron absorption and visceral deposition can lead to the classic features of hepatic cirrhosis, cardiomyopathy, diabetes mellitus, pituitary dysfunction (including hypogonadism), sicca syndrome, and skin pigmentation mostly of melanin. Arthropathy is also a common and disabling complication (3).

Idiopathic hemochromatosis is an autosomal recessive disorder with the gene located near the HLA–A locus on chromosome 6 (4). Although A3 and B7 appear to be common antigens, homozygous and heterozygous patterns are consistent only within individual pedigrees without crossover. The expression of hemochromatosis with arthritis is most common in homozygotes who show the heaviest iron overload (5).

Prolonged excessive iron ingestion, such as in the South African Bantu, and repeated blood transfusion in chronic hypoproliferative anemia and thalassemia, may also result in iron deposition. Without tissue damage this disorder is known as *hemosiderosis*. With tissue damage it is called secondary hemochromatosis. The iron deposition in macrophages in secondary hemochromatosis is associated with less tissue damage and end-organ dysfunction compared to the idiopathic form.

Chronic progressive arthritis, predominantly affecting the second and third metacarpophalangeal (MCP) and proximal interphalangeal (PIP) joints and resembling rheumatoid arthritis, is the presenting feature in about one-half of the cases (Fig. 32-1). Involvement of the MCP joints is typically the most common rheumatologic feature at the time of diagnosis (5). The dominant hand may be solely or more severely affected. The finger joints and wrists are mildly tender with limited motion. Larger joints such as the shoulders, hips, and knees may also be affected. Hemochromatotic arthritis of the hips or shoulders may, at times, be rapidly progressive. True morning stiffness is not a feature.

The detection of an osteoarthritis-like disease that involves MCP and wrist joints, particularly in men during the fourth and fifth decades of life, should signal the possibility of underlying hemochromatosis. Arthropathy may be seen in individuals as young as age 26 before any other manifestations of the disease develop.

The radiologic changes of hemochromatosis resemble osteoarthritis, except that in hemochromatosis there is less osteophytosis. Ulnar styloid erosion may suggest rheumatoid disease, but the irregular joint narrowing and sclerotic cyst formation are more indicative of a degenerative process. Although the distal interphalangeal joints may be affected, the carpometacarpal joint changes of generalized osteoarthritis are not a feature. Somewhat similar MCP changes can occur in calcium pyrophosphate dihydrate crystal deposition without hemochromatosis. Hip joint involvement has been striking in most series. Some degree of diffuse osteoporosis may be present, presumably due to hypogonadism, but a direct effect of iron on bone is also possible. Chondrocalcinosis is characteristic of the arthropathy and is a late complication in about 50% of patients; it may be the sole abnormality (5). The hyaline cartilage of the shoulder, wrist, hip, and knee, and the fibrocartilage of the triangular ligament of the wrist and symphysis pubis may be affected. Superimposed attacks of calcium pyrophosphate dihydrate crystal synovitis

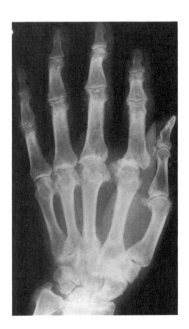

(Figure 32-1)

Radiograph of hand with hemochromatosis. Note the joint space narrowing, cystic subchondral lesions, joint space irregularity, mild subluxation, bony sclerosis, and small osteophytes in the metacarpophalangeal joints. Chondrocalcinosis is present in the ulnar carpal joint, and soft tissue has calcified around the interphalangeal joint of the thumb. Courtesy of Dr. HR Schumacher, Jr.

occur in these cases. The finding of chondrocalcinosis should always suggest the possibility of hemochromatosis.

Yersinia septic arthritis or septicemia is an unusual complication that may occur in patients with hemochromatosis because of a microbial requirement for an iron-rich environment. Hepatitis B and C viral infection may accelerate liver damage in patients with hemochromatosis (6).

Synovial fluid has good viscosity, with leukocyte counts below $1000/mm^3$. During acute episodes of pseudogout, synovial fluid leukocytosis with calcium pyrophosphate crystals can be found. Except for such episodes, the erythrocyte sedimentation rate is usually normal. With chronic liver disease, rheumatoid factor tests may be positive.

The diagnosis may be suspected by a raised serum iron and high ferritin concentration with increased saturation of the plasma iron-binding protein transferrin (1). These indices may not always be raised in the early stages of primary hemochromatosis. Needle biopsy of the liver provides the most definitive evidence of iron overload in hemochromatosis; the biopsy may also show fibrosis, cirrhosis, or hepatoma.

In idiopathic hemochromatosis, iron deposits affect parenchymal hepatic cells, whereas reticuloendothelial cells are most affected in secondary forms. Synovial biopsy in hemochromatosis shows iron deposition in the type B lining cells of synovium, whereas in rheumatoid arthritis, traumatic hemarthrosis, hemophilia, and villonodular synovitis, deposits form in the deeper layers or in the phagocytic type A lining cells. Hemosiderin deposits may also be found in the chondrocytes. Further evidence of iron may be found in biopsies of skin and intestinal mucosa, or in bone marrow, buffy coat, or urine sediment. The amount of iron excreted in the urine after administration of the iron-chelating agent deferoxamine correlates with the presence of parenchymal hepatic iron in hemochromatosis. Where available, direct noninvasive magnetic measurement of hepatic iron stores provides a quantitative method for early detection of iron overload or rapid evaluation of treatment.

The pathogenesis of the arthritis is unknown, as degenerative joint changes do not necessarily develop in relation to synovial iron. The low frequency of chondrocalcinosis in patients with hemophilia and rheumatoid arthritis weighs against synovial hemosiderin as a cause of chondrocalcinosis. It is speculated that ionic iron might inhibit pyrophosphatase activity and lead to a local concentration of calcium pyrophosphate in the joint. The deposition of calcium in cartilage appears to predispose to inflammatory and degenerative joint disease (3).

Following the diagnosis of hemochromatosis, it is imperative to obtain biochemical screening of at least first-degree relatives of the patient for medical preventive reasons. Screening is best done by measuring serum iron and serum iron-binding transferrin (7). Although HLA typing is useful in predicting the risk of disease in healthy relatives, it gives no indication of iron stores.

Aggressive phlebotomy therapy can prevent or reverse much organ damage. Weekly phlebotomies are generally needed until iron is depleted and mild anemia is present. Venesection may not prevent the progression of arthritis in hemochromatosis, but in some cases arthritis may improve after this therapy. Iron-chelating therapy with intravenous deferoxamine is generally effective, but impractical because of the expense and the need for intravenous administration.

New oral iron chelators are being tested. Their long-tem efficacy is uncertain and they are not without side effects.

Arthritis symptoms may be controlled by nonsteroidal anti-inflammatory drugs such indomethacin, but agents requiring hepatic metabolism, such as diclofenac or nabumetone should probably be avoided. Prosthetic hip, knee, and shoulder arthroplasties can be performed when required.

ALKAPTONURIA (OCHRONOSIS)

Alkaptonuria, a rare disorder transmitted by recessive mode of inheritance, results from a complete deficiency of the enzyme homogentisic acid oxidase (8). In six reported pedigrees it has been mapped to chromosome 3q (9). This deletion causes accumulation of homogentisic acid, a normal intermediate in the metabolism of phenylalanine and tyrosine, which is excreted in the urine. Alkalinization and oxidation of this acid cause the urine to turn black. The homogentisic acid retained in the body is deposited as a pigmented polymer in the cartilage and, to a lesser degree, in skin and sclerae. The darkening of tissue parts by this pigment is designated *ochronosis.*

The pigment, which is found in the deeper layers of the articular cartilage, is bound to collagen fibers, causing this tissue to lose its normal resiliency and become brittle and fibrillated. The erosion of this abnormal cartilage leads to denuding of subchondral bone and the penetration of tiny shards of pigmented cartilage into the bone, synovium, and joint cavity (10). It is likely that these pigmented cartilage fragments become a nidus for the formation of osteochondral bodies.

A progressive degenerative arthropathy develops, with symptoms usually beginning in the fourth decade of life. Features include arthritis of the spine (ochronotic spondylosis) and arthritis of the larger peripheral joints, with chondrocalcinosis, formation of osteochondral bodies, and synovial effusions (ochronotic peripheral arthropathy).

Initially, the spinal column is affected with pigment found in the annulus fibrosus and nucleus pulposus of the intervertebral discs (Fig. 32-2). Later the knees, shoulders, and hips deteriorate; the small peripheral joints are spared. In adults, the first sign of spondylosis may be an acute disc syndrome. Eventually, the condition resembles ankylosing spondylitis, with progressive lumbar rigidity and loss of stature.

Stiffness and loss of joint mobility are the predominant complaints, while pain is less prominent. Knee effusions, crepitus, and flexion contractures are common, but other signs of articular inflammation are ordinarily lacking. Fragments of darkly pigmented cartilage can occasionally be found in the joint fluid. Osteochondral bodies, which form in response to the deposition of cartilaginous fragments in the synovium, are often palpable in and around the knee joint and may reach several centimeters in diameter.

Nonarticular features of ochronosis include bluish discoloration and calcification of the ear pinnae, triangular pigmentation of the sclerae, and pigmentation over the nose, axillae, and groin. Prostatic calculi are common in men, and cardiac murmurs may develop from valvular pigment deposits.

The earliest features visible on roentgenograms are multiple vacuum discs of the spine. Eventually, the entire spine shows calcification of the discs with narrowing, collapse, and fusion. Chondrocalcinosis may affect the symphysis pu-

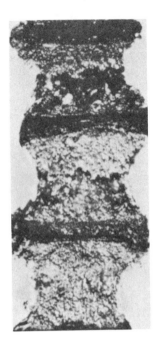

(Figure 32-2)
Part of a lumbar vertebral column of a 49-year-old woman with alkaptonuria who died of renal failure (ochronotic nephrosis). Blackened intervertebral discs are thin and focally calcified. This patient had incapacitating pain since age 36, with progressive limitation of back motion. Microscopic examination of the discs, which splintered easily, revealed nonrefractile granular pigment. Reprinted from Cooper J, Moran TJ: Studies on ochronosis. I. Report of case with death from ochronotic nephrosis. Arch Pathol 61:46-53, 1957, with permission.

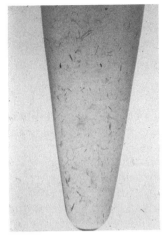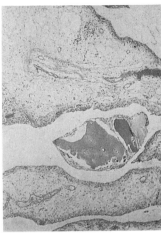

(Figure 32-3)
Ochronosis: synovial fluid and synovium (gross and microscopic). On the left, the synovial fluid reveals numerous dark particles and shards having the appearance of ground pepper. On the right, a low power microscopic view of the synovium shows fragments of darkly pigmented cartilage (H&E). Reprinted from J Rheumatol 1:45-53, 1974, with permission.

bis, costal cartilage, and ear helix. In contrast to ankylosing spondylitis, the sacroiliac and apophyseal joints are not affected. The roentgenographic appearance of the peripheral joints resembles that in primary osteoarthritis with loss of cartilage space, marginal osteophytes, and eburnation of the subchondral bone. Unlike primary osteoarthritis, however, degeneration of the shoulders and hips is more severe, and osteochondral bodies are seen.

The diagnosis of alkaptonuria is suspected when the patient gives a history of passing dark urine, or when fresh urine turns black on standing or on alkalinization. In individuals lacking this history, the diagnosis is made only after the detection of a false-positive test for diabetes mellitus or the onset of arthritis. Dark pigmented synovia may be seen on arthroscopy. Although a specific enzymatic method permits quantitation of homogentisic acid in urine and blood, no method is available to identify disease carriers.

Synovial fluid is usually clear, yellow, and viscous and does not darken with alkalinization. At times the fluid may be speckled with many particles of debris resembling ground pepper (Fig. 32-3). Leukocyte counts of a few hundred cells are predominantly mononuclear. Occasionally, the cytoplasm of mononuclear and polymorphonuclear cells contains dark inclusions of phagocytosed ochronotic pigment. Centrifugation and microscopic examination of synovial fluid sediment may show fragments of pigmented cartilage. Effusions may contain calcium pyrophosphate dihydrate crystals and show no inflammation. Pigmented cartilage fragments are embedded in synovium and are often surrounded by giant cells (8,10).

No effective treatment is available for the underlying metabolic disorder. Large amounts of ascorbic acid might prevent deposition of ochronotic pigment, but long-term effects of this therapy are unknown. Surgical removal of osteochondral loose bodies from the knee joint is warranted when these interfere with motion. Prosthetic joint replacement may be helpful.

WILSON'S DISEASE

Wilson's disease (hepatolenticular degeneration) is a rare metabolic disorder in which deposition of copper leads to dysfunction of the liver, brain, and kidneys. It is inherited as an autosomal recessive trait, and becomes symptomatic for individuals aged 6 to 40 years. A defective gene and related mutations provides some explanation for the wide phenotypic variation seen in Wilson's disease (11).

Total body copper is increased. The accumulation of copper in the liver leads to cirrhosis; in the cornea, to characteristic Kayser–Fleischer rings; in the basal ganglia, to lenticular degeneration and movement disorders; and in the kidneys, to renal tubular damage. An arthropathy may develop in as many as 50% of affected adults; arthritis is rare in children. Patients usually develop hepatic or neurologic symptoms in childhood or adolescence. Liver disease is the most common presentation between ages 8 and 16, with symptoms of jaundice, nausea, vomiting, and malaise. Acute hepatic failure may rarely develop. Neurologic symptoms are rare before age 12. Dysarthria and decreased coordination of voluntary movements are the most common complaints. Other presenting symptoms include acute hemolytic anemia, arthralgias, renal stones, and renal tubular acidosis.

The arthropathy is characterized by mild premature osteoarthritis of the wrists, MCP joints, knees, or spine. Occasionally, joint hypermobility also may be found. Ossified bodies of the wrists may be associated with subchondral cysts. Chondromalacia patellae, osteochondritis dissecans, or chondrocalcinosis of the knee may be associated with mild knee effusions. The arthropathy tends to be mild in patients treated early in life, but it may be more severe in patients with untreated disease of longer duration. A few patients show acute or subacute polyarthritis resembling rheumatoid arthritis. These seropositive cases are possibly a result of penicillamine therapy.

Synovial biopsies show hyperplasia of synovial lining cells with mild inflammation. Neither calcium pyrophosphate nor copper are seen by standard methods. Limited data are available concerning morphologic changes in joints. Microvilli formation, intimal cell hyperplasia, chronic inflammatory infiltrates, and vascular changes have been reported in synovium. Joint fluids have a low leukocyte count.

Radiologic features may include subchondral cysts, joint space narrowing, sclerosis, marked osteophyte formation, and multiple calcified loose bodies, especially at the wrist. Unlike hemochromatosis, involvement of the hip and MCP joints is uncommon. Periostitis at the femoral trochanters and other tendinous insertions, periarticular calcifications, and chondrocalcinosis have been reported. Changes in the spine are seen mainly in the midthoracic to lumbar areas and include squaring of the vertebral bodies, intervertebral joint space narrowing, osteophytes, and osteochondritis.

Skeletal manifestations of Wilson's disease include generalized osteoporosis in as many as 50% of patients. The osteoporosis is usually asymptomatic, unless spontaneous fractures occur (12). Osteomalacia, Milkman pseudofractures, and renal rickets have been reported. Some cases are from areas where nutritional deficiencies may also affect skeletal abnormalities.

Although Kayser–Fleischer corneal rings are pathognomonic of Wilson's disease, the diagnosis is established by laboratory investigations. Low serum copper and decreased serum ceruloplasmin levels occur in most cases, and in symptomatic patients urinary copper excretion is increased. Biliary excretion of copper is also markedly decreased. Microchemical evidence of copper deposition may be obtained from needle biopsy of the liver, but histochemical methods are unreliable. In doubtful cases, specialized studies with radioactive copper may be necessary.

The pathogenesis of the arthropathy is unclear, and its presence does not correlate with neurologic, hepatic, or renal disease. Although chondrocalcinosis has been observed in patients with Wilson's disease, light and transmission electron microscopy have failed to detect crystals containing calcium in synovial fluids or in cartilage and synovial biopsies. Copper has been found in the articular cartilage by elemental analysis of a few patients with Wilson's disease and could theoretically cause tissue damage mediated by oxygen-derived free radicals (12). Although the arthropathy is generally milder than that seen in hemochromatosis, its cause may be similar and it may involve deposition of calcium pyrophosphate dihydrate and the development of chronic arthritis.

Copper chelation with penicillamine, along with dietary copper restriction, is the treatment of choice. The role of liver transplantation is uncertain. Whether penicillamine can control the arthropathy is unclear, but contemporary series suggest that the arthropathy is milder in patients with earlier diagnoses and more intensive chelation therapy. Side effects from penicillamine reported in patients with Wilson's disease rarely include acute polyarthritis, polymyositis, or a syndrome resembling systemic lupus erythematosus. Otherwise, symptomatic measures suffice to control arthritis symptoms.

GAUCHER'S DISEASE

Gaucher's disease is a lysosomal glycolipid storage disease in which glucocerebroside accumulates in the reticuloendothelial cells of the spleen, liver, and bone marrow (13). It is an autosomal recessive disorder caused by subnormal activity of the hydrolytic enzyme glucocerebrosidase. The gene for Gaucher's disease is located on chromosome 1 in the q21 region. All the cells of the body are deficient in glucocerebroside activity in Gaucher's disease, but it is the glycolipid-engorged macrophages that account for all the nonneurologic features of the disease.

Fortunately, the most severe forms of Gaucher's disease are extremely rare, whereas milder forms are encountered frequently, particularly in the Jewish population. Gaucher's disease has been classified into clinical subdivisions. Type 1, the most common form, is the adult or chronic type that accounts for more than 99% of cases. It is a common familial disorder in Ashkenazi Jews, whereas other types occur in all ethnic groups. It is defined by the lack of neurologic involvement, and affected adults present with accumulation of glucocerebroside in the reticuloendothelial system causing organomegaly, hypersplenism, conjunctival pingueculae, skin pigmentation, and osteoarticular disease. It has the best prognosis, but may be mistaken for juvenile rheumatoid arthritis. Some patients with type 1 disease have few or no clinical manifestations. In these cases the condition may be discovered only when bone marrow is examined for some other reason, or if mild thrombocytopenia is investigated. Type 2, infantile, is a fulminating disorder with severe brain involvement and death within the first 18 months of life. Type 3, the intermediate or juvenile form, begins in early childhood and shows many features of the chronic form, with or without central nervous system dysfunction.

Skeletal involvement is characteristic of type 1 and to a lesser extent type 3, but not type 2 disease. Musculoskeletal involvement occurs in the adult and juvenile forms, but it is rarely the first symptom. Patients usually present with lymphadenopathy, hepatosplenomegaly, or signs and symptoms of hypersplenism. Nevertheless, rheumatic complaints may appear early in the disease course. Pain in the hip, knee, or shoulder is caused by disease of adjacent bone. In young individuals, the most common complaint is chronic aching around the hip or proximal tibia. This may last a few days but is usually recurrent. Another complaint is excruciating pain (bone crisis) involving the femur and tibia with tenderness, swelling, and erythema. Monarticular hip or knee degeneration is typical, and unexplained migratory polyarthritis sometimes occurs. Bony pain tends to lessen with age.

Other skeletal features include pathologic long bone fractures, vertebral compression, and osteonecrosis of the femoral or humeral heads or proximal tibia. The osteonecrosis can develop slowly, or rapidly with bone crisis. These crises usually affect only one bone area at a time. Because acute-phase reactants and bone scans are usually positive, the clinical picture of acute osteomyelitis is mimicked (pseudo-osteomyelitis). Surgical drainage in these cases commonly leads to infection and chronic osteomyelitis. Due to this increased susceptibility to infection, conservative management of bony lesions is recommended.

Asymptomatic radiologic areas of rarefaction, patchy sclerosis, and cortical thickening are common. Osteonecrosis of bone, particularly of the hips and pathologic fractures of the femur and vertebrae are the most serious and deforming features of Gaucher's disease. Involvement of the femur is thought to be a barometer of bone symptoms. Widening of the distal femur with the radiologic appearance of an Erlenmeyer flask is a frequent finding, but flaring of the bones can occur in the tibia and humerus as well.

When bone pain or other articular symptoms appear, the serum acid phosphatase and the angiotensin-converting enzymes are usually elevated. However, the most reliable method for diagnosing Gaucher's disease is the determination of leukocyte β-glucosidase. Diagnosis has been confirmed in the past by examination of bone marrow aspirate for the Gaucher cell, a large lipid storage histiocyte. This cell should be differentiated from globoid cells of another lysosomal storage disorder, Krabbe's disease (galactocerebrosidosis). Bone biopsy is not recommended because of the risk of secondary infection. Needle biopsy of the liver for assay of glucocerebroside may be performed, but washed leukocytes and extracts of cultured skin fibroblasts are easily obtained for glucocerebrosidase testing. These assays may also be used to detect heterozygous carriers. Amniocentesis has been used for the prenatal detection of diseased fetuses. When the diagnosis is established, genetic counseling for family members or prospective parents is recommended. Although enzyme assays are useful for genetic screening, DNA analysis using the polymerase chain reaction are much more precise (14).

Until recently, therapy of Gaucher's disease was mostly symptomatic, based on control of pain and infection. In adults, splenectomy may control hypersplenism, but bone disease may then accelerate. Partial splenectomy has been recommended as protection against post-splenectomy infection, and for its hepatic- and bone-sparing effect. Arthroplasty and complete joint replacement is often necessary, but loosening of prostheses occurs more often than in other disorders. Bleeding can be an operative problem.

With the commercial availability of replacement enzyme, the modified glucocerebroside (Ceredase), effective treatment of Gaucher's disease has become a reality (15). Periodic intravenous infusions of the enzyme over many months result in regression of the features of Gaucher's disease (13,15). Allogeneic bone marrow transplantation may be an option in advanced disease if an HLA-identical donor is available.

FABRY'S DISEASE

Fabry's disease is a lysosomal lipid storage disease in which glycosphingolipids accumulate widely in nerves, viscera, skin, and osteoarticular tissues (16). It is a sex-linked inherited disease caused by a deficiency of the enzyme α-galactosidase A. The gene and its mutations responsible for expression of this enzyme have been localized to the middle of the long arm of the X chromosome.

As a slowly progressive disorder predominately affecting men, clinical features are widespread and nonspecific; thus, diagnosis is often missed or delayed. In childhood the deposition is particularly marked in and around blood vessels, giving rise to the characteristic rash of dark blue or red angiokeratomas or telangiectases around the buttocks, thighs, and lower abdomen. When diffuse, it is referred to as *angiokeratoma corporis diffusum* and is almost always associated with hypohidrosis.

The kidneys are the main target organ and proteinuria gradually develops in childhood or adolescence with abnormal urinary sediments including birefringent lipid crystals (Maltese crosses). Progressive renal disease leads to renal failure. Cardiovascular and cerebrovascular deposition of the sphingolipid parallels the renal disease, with vascular insufficiencies or sudden death. Ocular changes are severe. A characteristic corneal opacity seen by slit lamp examination occurs early and can be helpful in diagnosis even in heterozygous women.

Some patients experience the insidious development of polyarthritis with degenerative changes and flexion contractures of the fingers, particularly of the distal interphalangeal joints. Foam cells have been described in the synovial vessels and connective tissues. Radiographs may show infant-like opacities of bone and osteoporosis of the spine. Osteonecrosis of the hip and talus have been described. Eighty percent of children or young adults undergo painful crises of burning paresthesias of the hands and feet and later of whole extremities. These attacks are associated with fever and elevations of the erythrocyte sedimentation rate.

Genetic counseling should be offered to affected families. Measurement of α-galactosidase to α-galactosidase activity ratios in leukocytes and fibroblasts provide reasonable discrimination between carriers and non-carriers. Identification by DNA studies is reserved for subjects showing equivocal results.

Treatment is not satisfactory. Anti-platelet medication may suppress vascular damage. Burning paresthesias may benefit from phenytoin or carbamazepine. Without dialysis or transplantation most affected men develop renal failure before age 50.

FARBER'S DISEASE

Farber's disease is a lysosomal lipid storage disease in which a glycolipid ceramide accumulates widely in many tissues including the skin and musculoskeletal system (17). It is an autosomal recessive disorder caused by a deficiency of the enzyme acid ceramidase. Affected children show disease manifestations by the age of four months and die before the age of four years.

A hoarse cry from thickened vocal cords or swollen painful joints may be the first features. The appearance of tender, subcutaneous nodules follows, and the early occurrence of nodules correlates with shortened survival. All the extremities may be swollen and tender, but this gives way to more localized joint swelling with nodules around the fingers, wrists, elbows, and knees. Joint contractures develop later and especially affect the fingers and wrists. The gastrointestinal, cardiovascular, and nervous systems gradually become involved. Death usually results from respiratory disease. Diagnosis can be confirmed by demonstrating a deficiency of acid ceramidase both in leukocytes and fibroblasts.

LIPOCHROME HISTIOCYTOSIS

Lipochrome histiocytosis is an extremely rare lysosomal storage disease associated with pulmonary infiltrates, splenomegaly, hypergammaglobulinemia, polyarthritis, and increased susceptibility to infection (18). The disorder is familial. Histiocytes show lipochrome pigment granulation, and peripheral blood leukocytes exhibit impaired activity.

MULTICENTRIC RETICULOHISTIOCYTOSIS

Multicentric reticulohistiocytosis is a rare dermatoarthritis of unknown cause characterized by the cellular accumulation of glycolipid laden histiocytes and multinucleated giant cells in skin and joints. The most common presentation is a painful destructive polyarthritis resembling rheumatoid arthritis, for which affected persons may be mistakenly treated. The joint manifestations precede the appearance of skin lesions in most patients, but the appearance and location of the skin nodules are not entirely characteristic of rheumatoid arthritis (Fig. 32-4). Although a self-limited form may be seen in childhood, adult multicentric reticulohistiocytosis predominantly affects middle-aged women. The onset is insidious and is characterized by polyarthritis, skin nodules, and in many cases xanthelasma. Small papules and bead-like clusters around the nail folds are characteristic, with nodulation of the skin of the face and hands. Skin nodules are yellowish, purple, or brown in color and are of varying size, occurring over the hands (Fig 32-4), elbows, face, and ears. Oral, nasal, and pharyngeal mucosa involvement is seen in one-fourth of patients, sometimes with ulceration. Various visceral sites may also be affected.

Symmetric polyarthritis resembles rheumatoid disease when PIP joints are affected, and psoriatic arthritis when involvement of distal interphalangeal joints predominates. Tenosynovial involvement may also occur. Remission of polyarthritis may be seen after many years of progressive disease.

Early radiographs show "punched out" bony lesions resembling gouty tophi, followed by severe joint destruction. Spinal involvement with erosions and subluxations including atlantoaxial damage may occur.

No specific laboratory abnormality has yet been demonstrated, and the diagnosis is established by examination of biopsies of affected tissues. Both the skin and synovium (Fig. 32-5) are infiltrated by large, multinucleated giant cells. The cytoplasm has a ground glass appearance and stains positively for lipids and glycoproteins with periodic acid-Schiff stain (PAS positive). Definitive analysis of these cell contents has not been made, but it is probably a glycolipid. Triglycerides, cholesterol, and phosphate esters appear to be present in the lesion, suggesting either that histiocytes are stimulated to produce these substances or that this is a form of lipid storage disease. These histiocytes also elaborate cytokines that contribute to synovial cell proliferation. Syn-

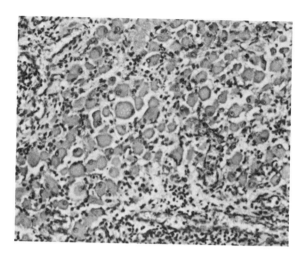

(Figure 32-5)

Photomicrograph of synovium (knee) from a 54-year-old woman with multicentric reticulohistiocytosis shows numerous histiocytes and multinucleated giant cells that contain large amounts of periodic acid–Schiff (PAS)–positive material. Reprinted from McCarty DJ, Koopman WJ: Arthritis and Allied Conditions. Philadelphia, Lea & Febiger, 1993.

ovial fluid leukocyte counts range from 220 to 79,000 cells/mm^3, with mononuclear cells predominating. Scanning the synovial fluid Wright-stained smear or wet preparation may reveal giant cells or large, bizarre macrophages.

There is no known cause or familial association. Although the pathogenesis is unknown, hidden malignancy and tuberculosis have been implicated. Rheumatoid factor does not occur. Some patients develop positive reactions to tuberculin (PPD positive). There are case descriptions with associated Sjögren's syndrome and polymyositis. Multicentric reticulohistiocytosis has also been implicated with a variety of malignancies (19). Death due to the disease itself has not been reported, but patients may be left with severe joint disability.

Spontaneous remission of skin and arthritis occurs in some cases, especially in childhood. In the remainder, corticosteroids or topical nitrogen mustard may improve the skin lesions, and cyclophosphamide may control both skin and joint disease in severe cases (20).

DUNCAN A. GORDON, MD

1. Rooney PJ: Hyperlipidemias, lipid storage disorders, metal storage disorders and ochronosis. Curr Opin Rheumatol 3:166-171, 1991

2. Conrad ME, Umbreit JN, Moore EG, et al: Hereditary hemochromatosis: a prevalent disorder of iron metabolism with an elusive etiology. Am J Hematol 47:218-224, 1994

3. Adams PC, Speechley M: The effect of arthritis on the quality of life in hereditary hemochromatosis. J Rheumatol 23:707-710, 1996

4. Worwood M, Dorak MT, Raha-Chowdhury R, et al: Genetics of hemochromatosis. Adv Exp Med Biol 356:309-318, 1994

5. Mathews JL, Williams HJ: Arthritis in hereditary hemochromatosis. Arthritis Rheum 30:1137-1141, 1987

6. Piperno A, Fargion S, D'Alba R, et al: Liver damage in Italian patients with hereditary hemochromatosis is highly influenced by hepatitis B and C virus infection. J Hepatol 16:364-368, 1992

7. Adams PC, Gregor JC, Kertesz AE, et al: Screening blood donors for hereditary hemochromatosis: decision analysis model based on a 30-year database. Gastroenterol 109:177-188, 1995

8. Schumacher HR, Holdsmith DE: Ochronotic arthropathy. I. clinicopathologic studies. Semin Arthritis Rheum 6:207-246, 1977

9. Janocha S, Wolz W, Sorsen S, et al: The human gene for alkaptonuria maps to chromosome 3q. Genomics 19:5-8, 1994

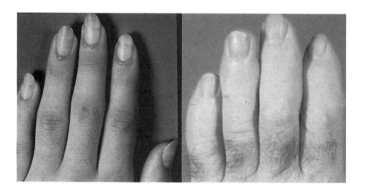

(Figure 32-4)

The fingers of a 16-year-old girl on the left reveal multiple, reddish–brown, tender papulonodules that are periungual in distribution. On the right is the hand of another patient with multiple nodules in the fingers. These nodules are firm, can fluctuate in size, and may disappear spontaneously. Reprinted from the Revised Clinical Slide Collection on the Rheumatic Diseases, with permission of the American College of Rheumatology.

10. Gaines JJ, Tom GD, Kahn KN: The ultrastructural and light microscopic study of the synovium in ochronotic arthropathy. Hum Pathol 18:1160-1164, 1987

11. Thomas GR, Forbes JR, Roberts EA, et al: The Wilson disease gene: spectrum of mutations and their consequences. Nature Genetics 9:210-217, 1995

12. Memerey KA, Eider W, Brewer GJ, et al: The arthropathy of Wilson's disease: clinical and pathologic features. J Rheumatol 13:331-337, 1988

13. Beutler E: Gaucher's disease—current concepts. N Engl J Med 325:1354-1360, 1991

14. Mistry PK, Smith SJ, Ali M, et al: Genetic diagnosis of Gaucher's disease. Lancet 339:889-892, 1992

15. Grabowski GA, Barton NW, Pastores G, et al: Enzyme therapy in type 1 Gaucher disease: comparative efficacy of mannose-terminated glucocerebrosidase from natural and recombinant sources. Ann Intern Med 122:33-39, 1995

16. Anon: Anderson-Fabry Disease (editorial). Lancet 336:24-25, 1990

17. Chanoki M, Ishii M, Fukaik, et al: Farber's lipogranulomatosis in siblings: light and electron microscopic studies. Br J Dermatol 121:779-785, 1989

18. Rodey GE, Park BH, Ford DK, et al: Defective bacteriocidal activity of peripheral blood leukocytes in lipochrome histiocytosis. Am J Med 49:322-327, 1970

19. Kenik JG, Fok F, Hueter CJ, et al: Multicentric reticulohistiocytosis in a patient with malignant melanoma; a response to cyclosphosphomide and a unique cutaneous feature. Arthritis Rheum 33: 1047-1051, 1990

20. Franck N, Amor B, Ayral X, et al: Multicentric reticulohistiocytosis and methotrexate. J Am Acad Dermatol 33:524-525, 1995

ARTHROPATHIES ASSOCIATED WITH HEMATOLOGIC AND MALIGNANT DISORDERS

HEMOPHILIC ARTHROPATHY

Hemophilia is an inherited, X-linked, recessive disorder of blood coagulation found almost exclusively in males. Female heterozygotes are generally asymptomatic carriers of the disease. Hemophilia A (classic hemophilia) is caused by Factor VIII deficiency, whereas Hemophilia B (Christmas disease) is caused by Factor IX deficiency.

Factor VIII is a 265 kD coagulant protein that activates factor X by proteases in the intrinsic coagulation pathway and circulates bound to von Willebrand protein. The gene for factor VIII has been mapped to the X chromosome facilitating prenatal diagnosis and carrier detection. Approximately one in 10,000 males is born with deficiency of factor VIII, which results in the disorder characterized by bleeding into soft tissues, muscles, and joints. Factor levels of 5% or less are virtually always associated with spontaneous hemarthrosis. Factor levels of greater than 5% generally require trauma to produce bleeding. Infrequently, female heterozygotes have low factor VIII levels due to random inactivation of X chromosomes in factor VIII-producing tissues. These carriers may have abnormal bleeding with major surgery, menses, or trauma. Rarely, true female hemophiliacs may occur from consanguinity within families with hemophilia A. Spontaneous bleeding to muscle or soft tissues may result in large bloody collections or pseudotumors, producing muscle necrosis and compartment syndromes. Compressive femoral neuropathy may result from retroperitoneal hematoma.

Factor IX is a 55 kD proenzyme that is converted to an active protease by factor IXa or by the tissue factor–VIIa complex. Factor IX, in combination with activated factor VIII, subsequently activates factor X. The factor IX gene has been cloned and localized to the X chromosome. Deficiency of factor IX occurs in approximately 1 in 100,000 male births, producing a clinical picture indistinguishable from factor VIII deficiency. Other factor deficiencies such as those of factors XI, VII, V, X, and II are rarely associated with hemarthrosis.

Hemarthrosis, the most common bleeding manifestation, occurs in up to two-thirds of patients with hemophilia (1). Hemarthrosis occurs spontaneously or with minor trauma, the onset includes stiffness, pain, warmth, and swelling. The age of onset and frequency of hemarthrosis is determined by the level of factor deficiency. The knee, elbow, and ankle are the most frequently affected joints. Subacute and chronic arthropathy develops with persistent synovial thickening, pain, and deformity, even in the later stages when hemarthrosis is less common. Late manifestations also include chronic joint contracture and degenerative joint disease, particularly of the knees. Septic arthritis is a rare complication of hemophilic arthropathy, although it may become more prevalent with the high prevalence of human

immunodeficiency virus (HIV) infection in hemophiliacs (2). Chronic arthritis appears to be more frequent in classic hemophilia than in Christmas disease, although hemarthrosis is equally prevalent.

Since the 1960s the widespread availability of plasma products concentrated with factor VIII has revolutionized the care of patients with hemophilia by reducing the severity of bleeding episodes and joint deformity, and by permitting surgical procedures. Tragically, over the last decade these products have also led to the proliferation of HIV infection, viral hepatitis, and chronic liver disease among hemophiliacs. Currently, more hemophiliacs die of acquired immunodeficiency syndrome (AIDS) than any other cause. Increased morbidity with concomitant HIV infection may also result from reduced muscle tone and bulk (3). Purification of factor VIII concentrates with monoclonal anti-factor VIII antibody and heat lyophilization has markedly increased the safety of factor VIII therapy. Recombinant factor VIII is now available and should completely eliminate the risk of infectious complications. Hemophiliacs who have received multiple transfusions may develop IgG antibodies (inhibitors) to factor VIII, which prevents effective replacement therapy or plasmapheresis.

The pathogenesis of hemophilic arthropathy is incompletely understood, but it may result from excessive iron deposition in synovial membrane and cartilage. Because prothrombin and fibrinogen are absent within joints, blood remains as a liquid . Plasma gradually resorbs and the remaining red cells are phagocytized by synovial lining cells and macrophages. Hemosiderin is found in synovial lining cells and may be toxic to them, resulting in chronic proliferation of the synovium or pannus composed of few lymphocytes, but primarily fibrous tissue (Fig. 33-1). Although circulating immune complexes and decreased total serum complement have been found in some patients, a specific immune response does not appear to be involved. Moreover, no single HLA haplotype appears to relate to either the presence of hemophilia or hemophilic arthropathy (4).

Radiographic findings include findings typical of degenerative arthritis: joint space narrowing, subchondral sclerosis, and subchondral cyst formation (Fig. 33-2). The extensive iron deposition in synovium leads to increased soft tissue density around joints. In children, radiographic features include epiphyseal irregularities, widening of the femoral intracondylar notch, squaring of the inferior patella, and enlargement of the proximal radius in the elbow. Magnetic resonance imaging may be useful even in late-stage joints to help detect significant synovial hypertrophy (5).

Treatment of acute hemarthrosis includes prompt treatment with factor VIII concentrate or recombinant form. Adjunctive therapy includes rest, ice packs, and analgesics fol-

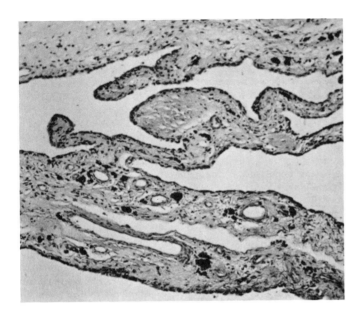

(Figure 33-1)
Photomicrograph of synovium obtained from the knee of a 76-year-old man with classic hemophilia (factor VIII deficiency) who had repeated episodes of hemarthrosis and developed severe osteoarthritis. Note heavy deposits of iron-containing pigment (hemosiderin in lining cells and deeper portions of the synovium. Reprinted from Koopman WJ (ed): Arthritis and Allied Conditions. Philadelphia, Lea & Febiger, 1993, with permission.

lowed by physical therapy. Aspiration is generally avoided unless the joint is unusually tense or sepsis is suspected, and then should be done following factor VIII replacement. Corticosteroids, whether intra-articular or systemic, do not seem to be effective. The subacute synovitis that develops later may be treated with nonsteroidal anti-inflammatory drugs, which appear to be safe in hemophilic arthropathy. D-penicillamine may be effective in chronic hemophilic arthropathy. Surgical or radiation synovectomy may reduce the frequency of hemarthrosis (6). Joint replacement appears to be an effective approach for end-stage disease (7,8).

HEMOGLOBINOPATHY-ASSOCIATED ARTHROPATHY
Sickle-cell Disease

The sickle cell hemoglobinopathies that produce musculoskeletal complications include sickle cell anemia (S-S) and the compound heterozygous states including sickle β-thalassemia, S-thalassemia sickle C disease (S-C), and sickle D disease (S-D). With deoxygenation, sickle cell hemoglobin (HbS) polymerize and red blood cells containing HbS change from a biconcave disc to an elongated crescent-shaped sickle cell. Sickle cells lack the deformability of normal red cells and may cause obstruction in the microcirculation, leading to further tissue hypoxia and sickling. The musculoskeletal complications of the sickle cell hemoglobinopathies include painful crises, dactylitis, osteonecrosis, gout, and osteomyelitis.

Painful crises are the most common musculoskeletal complication. Recurrent painful crises particularly affect the abdomen, chest, back, and joints. Precipitants include viral or bacterial infection, dehydration, and acidosis. Juxta-articular areas of long bones are the most frequent sites of involvement. Localized swelling may occur, especially in the anterior tibial area. The duration of painful crises is variable, but

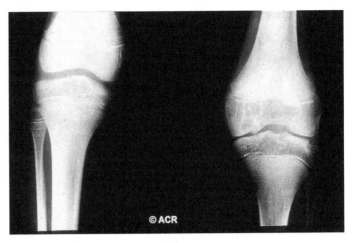

(Figure 33-2)
A posteroanterior projection of the knees of a young patient with hemophilic arthropathy. The knee on the right shows overgrowth of the epiphyseal centers of ossification. The subchondral bone of the adjacent margins is irregular with areas suggestive of erosion or breakdown. Widening of the intercondylar tibial notch is characteristic. Reprinted from clinical slide collection on the Rheumatic Diseases with permission of the American College of Rheumatology.

is usually no longer than 2 weeks. Treatment consists of supportive therapy, including intravenous hydration, oxygen, folate supplementation, and analgesics.

Joints may be directly involved in sickle cell crises, producing a painful arthritis of large joints with small effusions. Synovial fluid is typically non-inflammatory with a predominance of mononuclear cells. The mechanism of sickle cell arthropathy may be the result of reaction to juxta-articular bone infarcts or synovial ischemia and infarction. In one unusual case of inflammatory arthritis, electron microscopy of synovial fluid revealed crystal-like arrays of sickled hemoglobin tactoids in erythrocytes that were enfolded and phagocytized by the cells of the synovial fluid, suggesting that sickled cells may sometimes provoke an inflammatory response (9). Treatment of arthritis associated with sickle cell disease is identical to that of painful crises.

Osteonecrosis of the femoral head occurs in up to one-third of patients with S-S. Osteonecrosis of the humeral head occurs in up to 26% of patients. Osteonecrosis is generally thought to result from local hypoxia due to veno-occlusion by sickled cells, although one recent study suggested that it may be due to a septic process involving the presence of bacteria in necrotic bone (10). In the spine, bony infarcts result in the characteristic biconcave or "fishmouth" vertebrae. Radiographic findings may include juxta-articular osteopenia and bone infarcts (Fig. 33-3). Treatment of osteonecrosis of the hip consists of total hip arthroplasty, although failure (particularly due to acetabular loosening) may occur as the result of marrow hyperplasia and intramedullary sclerosis (11).

Dactylitis may occur in children with sickle cell disease (either S-S, S-C, or S-thalassemia) and is due to vaso-occlusions in the bones of the hands and feet (the so-called "hand–foot" syndrome) resulting in an acute, painful, non-pitting swelling of the hands and feet (Fig. 33-4) The average age at the time of diagnosis is 18 months, and dactylitis may be the presenting manifestation. Fever and leukocytosis are frequent and may be a source of diagnostic confusion. Roentgenographic features include periosteal new bone formation or intramedullary densities in the phalanges, metacarpals, and metatarsals. Symptoms usually resolve

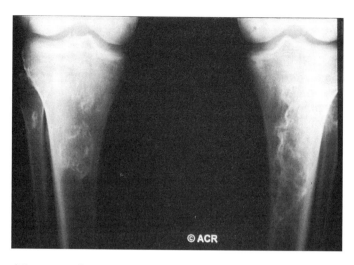

(Figure 33-3)
Sickle cell anemia knees. This posteroanterior projection of both knees demonstrates moderate osteopenia and coarse trabeculae. The medullary cavity is widened throughout with atrophy of the cortices. Small bone infarcts are seen in the femoral shafts. The joints are normal. Reprinted from the Revised Clinical Slide Collection on the Rheumatic Diseases, with permission of the American College of Rheumatology.

within a week, although recurrences are common. Necrosis of the epiphysis may lead to digital shortening.

Osteomyelitis occurs with increased frequency (as much as 300-fold) in individuals with S-S disease, probably due to the combination of bone infarction and impaired host defenses. *Salmonella* osteomyelitis accounts for approximately 50% of the cases, although the reason for this organism's predominance is not known. Treatment with appropriate antibiotics generally leads to resolution, although there may be recurrences.

Gout is a rare complication of sickle cell disease (12). Presumably, increased synthesis of nucleic acids occurs as a result of the erythropoietic response to hemolysis, with subsequent catabolism of the nucleic acid to urate. Renal damage during the third decade resulting from infarction and/or ischemia leads to sustained hyperuricemia.

Thalassemia

The thalassemias are a group of congenital disorders characterized by defects in the synthesis of one or more of the subunits of hemoglobin. Only β-thalassemia is associated with musculoskeletal complications. Patients with β-tha-

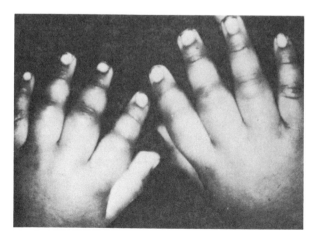

(Figure 33-4)
Sickle cell dactylitis or "hand–foot" syndrome.

lassemia have normal β chains of hemoglobin, but they are produced in diminished or sometimes undetectable amounts. β-thalassemia trait (or minor) is a relatively common entity that is rarely associated with clinical manifestations. β-thalassemia major (also known as Cooley's anemia), by contrast, is one of the most severe forms of congenital hemolytic anemia. Individuals with this form of the disease are typically transfusion-dependent and infrequently survive into adulthood.

Musculoskeletal complications of β-thalassemia major may result from expansion of the erythroid marrow and may include osteoporosis, pathologic fractures, and epiphyseal deformities. Thalassemia minor has been associated with recurrent asymmetric arthritis, with episodes lasting less than 1 week (13). A more persistent, nonerosive synovitis without joint effusions has also been described. Synovial fluid is noninflammatory in thalassemia minor. No synovial pathology is evident by light microscopy, although electron microscopy reveals multilamination of vascular basement membrane and large amounts of thin fibrils surrounding connective tissue cells (14). As with the bone abnormalities associated with thalassemia major, the arthritis associated with thalassemia minor may be due to para-articular bone thinning from chronic marrow expansion.

MYELOMA-ASSOCIATED DISORDERS

Multiple myeloma, one of the most common plasma cell dyscrasias, is frequently associated with bone involvement in the form of lytic lesions, osteoporosis, and pathologic fractures. Approximately 15% of patients have associated amyloidosis of the light chain type, which is rarely occurs with a symmetric small joint arthropathy simulating rheumatoid arthritis (see Chapter 34, Amyloidoses). Classically, amyloid infiltration in the synovium of the shoulders produces the so-called "shoulder pad sign." Bone pain, particularly in the back or chest wall, occurs in as many as 60% of patients with multiple myeloma. Up to one-third of patients can present with generalized bone loss due to the combined activity of cytokines (osteoclast activating factors) secreted by myeloma cells such as interleukin-1, tumor necrosis factor, and lymphotoxin. The distinction between idiopathic osteoporosis may be difficult initially, although serum protein electrophoresis, immunoelectrophoresis, and determination of Bence–Jones proteinuria will usually allow detection of multiple myeloma. Because bone lesions in most patients are lytic rather than blastic, radioisotope bone scans rarely identify lesions and are therefore less useful than plain radiography.

Osteosclerotic myeloma is a rare form of the disease associated with sclerotic rather than lytic bone lesions and a more indolent course. A severe neuropathy is a frequent accompaniment. POEMS syndrome is a rare, related systemic disorder characterized by the combination of *p*olyneuropathy, *o*rganomegaly, *e*ndocrinopathy, *M*-protein and *s*kin changes (15). The skin changes consist of thickening, abnormal pigmentation, and in some cases, a scleroderma-like appearance. Fever, weight loss, and thrombocytosis are also frequently seen.

WALDENSTROM'S MACROGLOBULINEMIA

Waldenstrom's macroglobulinemia is a lymphoproliferative disorder with associated serum monoclonal IgM. It is associated with lymphadenopathy, hepatosplenomegaly, and hyperviscosity syndrome. Unlike myeloma, Waldenstrom's is not associated with bone lesions or hypercalcemia. Purpuric skin lesions may be seen, and associated light-chain amyloidosis may occur.

CANCER AND ARTHRITIS

Malignancies are associated with a number of connective tissue diseases, notably dermatomyositis and various solid tumors, Sjögren's syndrome and lymphoma, scleroderma with adenocarcinoma of the lung, and following treatment with cytotoxic agents. These conditions and hypertrophic pulmonary osteoarthropathy (a syndrome associated with solid tumors) are covered elsewhere in the *Primer*. This section will cover hematologic malignancies and malignancies associated with diffuse articular symptoms.

Carcinoma polyarthritis

Rarely, arthritis may be associated with metastatic cancer or occult malignancy. In the case of metastatic disease, the arthritis is usually monarticular (often the result of metastasis to the joint or periarticular bone), whereas polyarthritis has been associated with occult malignancy of the breast and lung. In the latter condition, abrupt onset, sparing of the small joints of the hands and wrists, and absence of rheumatoid factor serve to distinguish it from rheumatoid arthritis. Polymyalgia rheumatica is sometimes misdiagnosed in this setting.

Leukemia

Leukemias are neoplasms of hematopoietic cells that develop in the bone marrow before spreading to peripheral blood, spleen, lymph nodes, and eventually to other tissues. The acute leukemias are characterized by the clonal proliferation of immature hematopoietic cells. Although joint symptoms are uncommon in adults with acute leukemia, up to 60% of children with acute lymphoblastic leukemia develop arthralgia and arthritis. In fact, arthritis may be a presenting feature in children [16]. The arthritis is typically an asymmetric polyarthritis involving large joints such as the knees, shoulders, and ankles, which may predate peripheral blood abnormalities. The occasional presence of rheumatoid factor and antinuclear antibodies can cause confusion. Nocturnal bone pain, hematologic abnormalities, and occasional radiographic abnormalities such as periosteal elevation should suggest the possibility of leukemia.

Leukemic arthropathy may be due to direct infiltration into the synovium, para-articular periostitis, intra-articular hemorrhage, or rarely crystal-induced synovitis. Immunocytologic analysis of joint fluid can establish the diagnosis of leukemic arthritis in the early stages [17,18]. Treatment of the underlying malignancy generally results in resolution of the arthritis.

Lymphoma

Symptomatic skeletal involvement is uncommon with the lymphomas, although bone lesions may be found at autopsy in up to 50% of cases. Polyarthralgia may be associated with lymphoma, although this is rarely a presenting manifestation. Cutaneous T-cell lymphoma is infrequently associated with polyarthritis simulating rheumatoid arthritis.

ANGIOIMMUNOBLASTIC LYMPHADENOPATHY

Angioimmunoblastic lymphadenopathy is a lymphoproliferative disorder characterized by lymphadenopathy, hepatosplenomegaly, and urticaria or maculopapular skin eruption with constitutional signs of fever and weight loss [19]. Coombs-positive hemolytic anemia, and polyclonal hypergammaglobulinemia are also common features. Serositis (pleural and pericardial) and polyarthritis are less frequently associated. The polyarthritis is typically noninflammatory and nonerosive [20]. Serum rheumatoid factor and antinuclear antibodies are generally absent. Nevertheless, the condition may be confused with autoimmune diseases such as rheumatoid arthritis, adult Stills disease, or systemic lupus erythematosus. The diagnosis is confirmed by lymph node biopsy that shows a distinctive appearance of a proliferation of small blood vessels and replacement of normal lymph node architecture by a combination of plasma cells, immunoblasts, and eosinophils. Treatment consists of combination therapy with corticosteroids and cytotoxic agents. Approximately 35% of patients with angioimmunoblastic lymphadenopathy will develop B-cell lymphoma despite therapy.

ROBERT W. SIMMS, MD

1. Steven MM, Yogarajah S, Madhok R, Forbes CD, Sturrock RD: Hemophilic arthritis. J Med 58:181-197, 1986
2. Gregg-Smith S, Pattison R, Dodd C, Giangrande P, Duthie R: Septic arthritis in hemophilia. J Bone Joint Surg [Br] 75:368-370, 1993
3. Bale J, Contant C, Garg B, Tilton A, Kaufman D, Wasiewski W: Neurologic history and examination results and their relationship to human immunodeficiency virus type I serostatus in hemophilic subjects: results from the hemophilia growth and development study. Pediatrics 91:731-741, 1993
4. Steven MM, Sturrock RD, Forbes CD, Dick HM: HLA antigens in hemophilic arthritis: a family study. Disease Markers 4:239-242, 1986
5. Nuss R, Kilcoyne R, Geraghty S, Wiedel J, Manco-Johnson M: Utility of magnetic resonance imaging for management of hemophilic arthropathy in children. J Pediatr 123:388-392, 1993
6. Kasteren MV, Novakova I, Boerboom A, Lemmens J: Long term follow up of radiosynovectomy with yttrium-90 silicate in hemophilic hemarthrosis. Ann Rheum Dis 52:548-550, 1993
7. Nelson IW, Sivamurugan S, Latham PD, Matthews J, Bulstrode CJ: Total hip arthroplasty for hemophilic arthropathy. Clin Orthop Rel Res 276:210-213, 1992
8. Teigland JC, Tjonnfjord GE, Evensen SA, Charania B: Knee arthroplasty in hemophilia. Five to twelve year follow-up of 15 patients. Acta Orthop Scand 64:153-156, 1993
9. Mann D, Schumacher HR, Jr: Pseudoseptic inflammatory knee effusion caused by phagocytosis of sickled erythrocytes after fracture into the knee joint. Arthritis Rheum 38:284-287, 1995
10. Shah A, Mukherjee A, Moreau P: Nine knee arthroplasties for sickle cell disease. Acta Orthop Scand 150:152, 1993
11. Moran M, Huo M, Garvin K, Pelicci P, Salvati E: Total hip arthroplasty in sickle cell disease. Clin Orthop 140-148, 1993
12. Reynolds MD: Gout and hyperuricemia associated with sickle-cell anemia. Semin Arthritis Rheum 12:404-413, 1983
13. Gerster JC, Dardel R, Guggi S: Recurrent episodes of arthritis in thalassemia minor. J Rheumatol 11:352-354, 1984
14. Schumacher HR, Dorwart BB, Bond J, Alavi A., Miller W: Chronic synovitis with early cartilage destruction in sickle cell disease. Ann Rheum Dis 36:413-419, 1977
15. Fam A, Rubenstein J, Cowan D: POEMS syndrome. Arthritis Rheum 29:233-241, 1986
16. Saulsbury FT, Sabio H: Acute leukemia presenting as arthritis in children. Clin Pediatr 24:625-628, 1985
17. Brooks PM: Rheumatic manifestations of neoplasia. Curr Opin Rheumatol 4:90-93, 1992
18. Harden EA, Moore JO, Haynes BF: Leukemia-associated arthritis: identification of leukemic cells in synovial fluid using monoclonal and polyclonal antibodies. Arthritis Rheum 27:1306-1308, 1984
19. Steinberg AD, Seldin MF, Jaffee ES, et al: NIH Conference: angioimmunoblastic lymphadenopathy with dysproteinemia. Ann Intern Med 108:575-584, 1988
20. McHugh NJ, Campbell GJ, Laudreth JJ, et al: Polyarthritis and angioimmunoblastic lymphadenopathy. Ann Rheum Dis 46:555-558, 1987

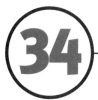

THE AMYLOIDOSES

For more than a century, pathologists have described organs infiltrated with a homogeneous eosinophilic material that stains with iodine and binds the organic dye, Congo red. Based on the staining with iodine and sulfuric acid, Virchow designated all such deposits as "amyloid" (in his era, cellulose-like), which has been retained despite the recognition that chemically, carbohydrate represents only a small proportion of the deposit. Over the past 25 years, the idea that a single amyloid substance appears during the course of a number of several diseases has been replaced by a body of data showing there are many amyloidoses. Each one represents a different protein and is specific for each disease, with the resulting organ compromise related to the location, quantity, and rate of deposition (1).

The main reason these disorders were assigned to rheumatology is the historic association of long-standing inflammatory joint disease with amyloid deposition in the kidneys, liver, and spleen. The clinical presentation of amyloid as arthropathy is infrequent, occurring primarily in three settings: AL, the amyloid associated with immunoglobulin L-chain deposition, $A\beta_2m$, the amyloid derived from β_2 microglobulin in patients with chronic renal failure, and in occasional patients with ATTR, the transthyretin (TTR) associated familial disease.

AMYLOIDS

All the amyloids appear as homogeneous, hyaline, eosinophilic material on hematoxylin and eosin staining. They demonstrate apple green–positive birefringence with polarized light after Congo red staining, have a fibrillar structure on electron microscopy, and stain positively with antibody specific for P component. Thirteen discrete fibril precursors have been identified in human diseases during the past two decades (Table 34-1). Several other conditions have been noted in which Congophilic material has been found in tissues, but the nature of the protein(s) has not yet been established chemically. At least two additional molecules, apolipoprotein AII and insulin, have been seen only in deposits in animals with amyloid.

What makes any protein amyloidogenic is uncertain. All the precursors except the cellular form of the prion protein and lysozyme (the precursor in the Ostertag form of hereditary renal amyloidosis) have substantial β-pleated sheet structure, but that in itself is insufficient. The fibril subunits are derived from precursors that are from 3.5 to 30 kD, apparently reflecting certain size constraints. A variety of pathogenic modes are involved. Increased production of a precursor, either locally or systemically, as a result of a prolonged normal stimulus to the synthesizing cell, or monoclonal proliferation of a cell producing the amyloidogenic protein may be responsible. There may be decreased excretion of the precursor, as in the amyloid of chronic renal failure. Structural abnormalities of a normal protein secondary to a germline mutation may also predispose to fibril formation. Finally, it is possible that a defect may exist in an as yet undefined process responsible for the normal degradation and disposition of either single proteins or a group of proteins with amyloidogenic properties when present at levels only slightly higher than normal.

The diagnosis of any form of amyloidosis is made pathologically by demonstrating material that is homogeneous in conventional histology, stains with Congo red with a char-

(Table 34-1)
The chemical classification of the amyloidoses as suggested by the Committee on Nomenclature at the VIth International Symposium on Amyloidosis, August 5–8, 1990, Oslo, Norway.

Amyloid Protein	Precursor Protein	Clinical Syndrome
AL	Immunoglobulin L-chain	Primary amyloid, multiple myeloma
AH	Immunoglobulin H-chain	Primary amyloid, multiple myeloma
AA	Apo-SAA	Inflammation associated with familial Mediterranean fever, Muckle–Wells
ATTR	Transthyretin (TTR)	Familial amyloidotic polyneuropathy, senile systemic amyloidosis, isolated vitreous amyloid
AGEL	Gelsolin	Familial amyloidotic polyneuropathy—Finnish lattice corneal dystrophy
AApoAI	Apolipoprotein A-I	Familial amyloidotic polyneuropathy Van Allen
$A\beta_2m$	β_2 microglobulin	Dialysis-associated amyloidosis
AÃ	Ã-protein precursor	Alzheimer's disease, Down's syndrome, HCHWA* (Dutch)
ACys	Cystatin C	HCHWA* (Iceland)
ACal	Calcitonin	Medullary carcinoma of the thyroid
AIAPP	Islet amyloid polypeptide	Insulinoma, type II diabetes mellitus
AANF	Atrial natriuretic factor	Isolated atrial amyloid
AScr	Scrapie (prion) protein	Creutzfeldt–Jakob, Gerstmann–Straussler–Scheinker syndrome
AFibrin	Alpha chain fibrinogen	Hereditary renal amyloid
ALys	Lysozyme	Hereditary non-neuropathic systemic amyloidosis (Ostertag type)

* HCHWA = hereditary cerebral hemorrhage with amyloidosis.

(Table 34-2)

The results from a series of publications describing various sampling sites for biopsy in patients with documented amyloid deposition. Where data were supplied concerning the form of amyloid they are included in the table.

Tissue	Positive	Amyloid Protein		
		AL	AA	FA
Gingiva	19/26			
	11/19	7/10	4/9	
	6/32			
Marrow		39/80		
Rectal	47/62	5/5	19/27	14/18
			*6/115	
			*2/47	
	24/31	24/31		
Subcutaneous	2/47		*2/47	
fat	28/32	18/19	4/6	6/7
	9/12	2/3	7/9	
	70/83	46/52	12/18	12/13
		20/28		
Renal	21/24			
		29/30		
Hepatic	13/27			

* RA patients only
FA = Familial amyloid
These data compiled from studies published since late 1940s.
Denominators represent total number of patients documented.

acteristic birefringence when viewed under polarized light, binds metachromatic dyes such as thioflavine T, and is fibrillar in its ultrastructural appearance. Biopsy tissues from clinically affected organs have a high yield of amyloid, but sampling of more accessible tissues, notably the rectum and subcutaneous fat, may also have a good return with lower risk (2) (Table 34-2). Japanese researchers have found tissue obtained from the gastric mucosa on upper endoscopy a good site to sample.

Each form of amyloid is defined by the nature of the fibril protein (Table 34-1). It is now possible to stain pathologic specimens with antibodies specific for many of the precursors, thereby establishing the nature of the deposits and the character of the responsible disease (3).

Several molecules are associated with all forms of amyloid deposition. Although some of them may be intrinsically fibrillogenic, none have been found as the sole component of any human amyloid deposit. The first of these to be described was the P-component, a salt-soluble molecule with the electron microscopic appearance of a pentagon, hence the designation P-component (4). An antiserum to the P-component can be used in addition to Congo red staining to confirm the nature of the tissue material as an amyloid. The P-component is derived from a serum precursor (serum amyloid P-component, or SAP) that behaves as an acute-phase reactant in the mouse but not in humans. It shares structural features with C-reactive protein and has been grouped with the latter and several other proteins as members of the pentraxin (each functional molecule having five subunits) family. The role of the P-component in the pathogenesis of amyloid deposition is unclear, but recent studies have shown that intravenously injected purified P-component binds to deposited fibrils in tissues. Based on this observation, radiolabeled P-component has been used experimentally as a reagent for gamma scanning to determine the presence and extent of deposits in patients with clinical disease (5).

A second molecule that appears to be common to all amyloids is apolipoprotein E (Apo E). Its role is also unclear, but an allele, Apo E4, is in statistically significant linkage dysequilibrium with sporadic cases of Alzheimer's disease. It has not been determined if the Apo E found in the deposits is actually E4 or another allele. Studies in patients with familial Mediterranean fever who have type AA amyloid (see below) or familial amyloidotic polyneuropathy with TTR amyloid indicate that the degree of deposition is not related to the presence of the Apo E4 allele. Thus it is likely that the Apo E found in the deposits is not exclusively of the E4 type.

A third common component of most or all deposits is heparan sulfate proteoglycan (HSPG), a normal constituent of basement membranes (6). Its role in the process of fibrillogenesis or deposition is unclear. However, the administration of low-molecular weight analogs of HSPGs have an inhibitory affect on the development of experimental murine AA amyloid produced in the course of an inflammatory response. These observations have led to the investigation of these compounds as potential therapeutic agents for all forms of amyloid.

Other basement membrane components such as laminin have been found in some amyloid deposits, but their universality and specificity have not been established beyond doubt.

Several molecules have been regularly identified in the deposits of Alzheimer's disease including α_1-antichymotrypsin, the tau protein, and a protein called NAC (nonamyloid component). NAC has also been found to have some intrinsic fibrillogenic tendency. The role these molecules play in any form of amyloid is not yet established.

CLINICAL FEATURES
AL Amyloid

Although the most common clinical form of amyloid deposition in the United States is probably the β-protein plaque of Alzheimer's disease, the systemic disorder most likely to come to the attention of rheumatologists is AL disease, either in the form of primary amyloidosis or in the course of multiple myeloma (7). The usual presentation is renal disease with proteinuria or renal failure. The renal disease may be massive, occurring as full-blown nephrotic syndrome, or relatively mild. True nephropathic proteinuria must be distinguished from the excretion of large amounts of free monoclonal L-chains, sometimes described in light chain myeloma. The latter is usually associated with renal disease such as myeloma kidney, with the dominant urine protein being the monoclonal L-chain responsible for the formation of the characteristic tubular casts. In amyloid nephropathy, the monoclonal component is usually minor in the glomerular leakage pattern of proteinuria. The amount of urinary protein may diminish with the onset of renal insufficiency. Occasionally, renal tubular disorders precede renal failure. Both concentration and acidification defects have been described. Hypertension can occur, and the kidneys may be normal in size, small, or enlarged. The latter usually occurs early in the disease. As in all forms of proteinuric nephropathy, intravenous urography should be carried out with care, if at all.

The second most common presentation of AL disease is that of cardiomyopathy. Echocardiography has made its detection relatively straightforward, showing noncompliant hemodynamics, thickening of the interventricular septum and valve leaflets, and the presence of "sparkling" of the ventricular echos in advanced disease (8). The earliest abnormality appears to be diastolic dysfunction with a change in the flow patterns from the normally dominant early filling to a state in which the atrial component is major. This change also occurs during the course of normal aging and thus may not be diagnostic in elderly patients. An echocardiographic pattern reflecting "pseudonormalization" may be seen before the appearance of the restrictive picture.

The presence of cardiac amyloid can be definitively established by endomyocardial biopsy followed by staining with the appropriate immunohistochemical reagents to identify monoclonal L-chain or TTR deposition. Radioactive technetium scanning has been advocated as a diagnostic screen for cardiac amyloid deposition, but the results have been inconsistent. Coronary deposition of AL and AA have been noted, but myocardial deposits of AA are rare. Both digoxin and nifedipine toxicity have been reported in patients with cardiac amyloid deposition. Evidence suggests that the two drugs are bound to the fibrils and their effective concentrations disproportionately increased in the myocardial deposits.

About 20% of patients with AL amyloid have a dominant neuropathic presentation. Symptoms are sensorimotor with the first manifestation frequently carpal tunnel syndrome, but lower extremity involvement also occurs. Biopsy of an involved nerve may reveal amyloid deposition; however, recent studies have suggested that clinically uninvolved sural nerve biopsy is not a high-yield procedure (9). Carpal tunnel syndrome is only rarely associated with AL disease in the absence of other symptoms, although it may be the presenting complaint and precede other manifestations by a significant time period. TTR amyloid is the most common form of isolated carpal tunnel amyloid deposition and may occur in the absence of other clinically significant organ involvement. However, analyses of patients requiring carpal tunnel release because of symptomatic median nerve compression, in the absence of systemic disease, suggest that any form of amyloid is found only in 2%–3% of the patients (10).

Periarticular amyloid deposition presenting as a pseudoarthritis has been reported in AL disease (11). However, joint effusions may also be present with amyloid fibrils found in fluid obtained by arthrocentesis. A soft tissue "shoulder pad sign" may be the major physical finding.

A potentially fatal complication of AL disease is an acquired deficiency of clotting factor X (12). In vivo studies carried out in a patient with such a defect suggested that the factor was bound to the fibrils in the deposits. However, analysis of amyloid deposits from another patient failed to identify factor X associated with the fibrils, nor could in vitro binding to fibrils be demonstrated. Thus, although factor binding to fibrils seems likely, it has not yet been definitively demonstrated.

Organ failure produced by extensive amyloid deposition is treated by supportive measures. Patients with end-stage renal disease have undergone dialysis and renal transplantation with reasonable responses. If precursor synthesis is not abrogated, however, the transplanted organ will show evidence of disease within 4 years.

Limited randomized prospective trials of melphalan and prednisone in regimens similar to those used in the treatment of multiple myeloma, with and without added colchicine, have been performed (13,14). Preliminary findings suggest enhanced survival in the patients receiving melphalan and prednisone with no effect of the added colchicine. The data suggest that, in the absence of a clear contraindication, all patients with renal failure should be offered treatment with these agents.

Preliminary studies have shown early promising results from intensive chemotherapy followed by autologous peripheral stem cell rescue in AL disease. The approach has been patterned on similar large-scale trials in multiple myeloma and reflects the view that in AL without myeloma, the clone producing the amyloidogenic protein is smaller and has a lesser proliferative potential than those seen in patients whose disease fulfills the diagnostic criteria for multiple myeloma.

Certain anthracycline compounds may inhibit the process of fibrillogenesis per se, without affecting the proliferative capacity of the immunoglobulin-producing cells. The mechanism of the inhibition is unknown, but ongoing clinical and laboratory trials suggest promising results (G. Merlini, personal communication).

The chemical features of immunoglobulin light chains that render them amyloidogenic have been under intense investigation from the time that they were identified as amyloid precursors. Fibrils from the deposits of 60 patients with AL have been obtained by the distilled water extraction procedure in sufficient quantity to establish the subunit size, L-chain class and subclass, and in many cases partial or full amino acid sequence (15). Lambda chains are the precursor more than twice as frequently as kappa chains. Fibrils belonging to all L-chain V-region subclasses have been identified. In comparison with all human L-chains that have been sequenced, serum and urine L-chains and fibrils from patients with AL disease have statistically significant increases in the proportion of proteins belonging to the V lambda VI and V kappa I subclasses. Most deposits contain L-chain fragments beginning with a normal amino terminus. Fewer than 10% contain only intact L-chains. About one quarter contain both intact chains and one or more fragments, while 10% contain fragments 12 kD or smaller. The last observation suggests why 10%–15% of AL tissue deposits may not stain with commercially available antisera specific for L-chain constant region determinants. These data are most consistent with some form of proteolysis playing a major role in the pathogenesis of disease. However, biosynthetic experiments suggest a possible role for the synthesis of abnormal chains in addition to the production of free monoclonal L-chains of the same class as the deposited protein in all patients, including the 10%–20% who show no monoclonal L-chains in the serum or urine. The aberrant products maybe smaller, based on fragment synthesis or intracellular degradation, or larger, as a result of glycosylation. In 80%–90% of patients, serum and urine immunoelectrophoresis reveals the Ig precursor.

Recent analyses comparing amyloidogenic and nonamyloidogenic L-chains suggest that certain substitutions at particular positions may result in more amyloidogenic structures. Further studies are necessary to refine these models and improve their predictiveness.

β₂-Microglobulin Amyloid

The second form of amyloid deposition associated with a significant articular presentation is the deposition of β_2-microglobulin in patients with chronic renal disease (16). Originally, all of the reported patients presenting with the syndrome of joint pain, carpal tunnel syndrome, and osteonecrosis had been on dialysis, usually for periods longer than 7 years. More recently, the condition has been reported after shorter periods of renal support, and at least one case has been identified in which the patient had not been dialyzed. In each case, when examined, the deposited protein was found to be β_2m, the 12.5-kD polypeptide component of class I proteins of the major histocompatibility complex. Studies of fibrils extracted from the deposits reveal that the subunit is an intact polypeptide, of normal amino acid sequence, either as monomer or dimers. Recently, it has been suggested that nonenzymatic glycation may play a role in the process of fibrillogenesis of this precursor. Subcutaneous fat aspiration does not seem to be as useful in this form of systemic deposition.

AA Amyloid

The third rheumatologically associated form of amyloid deposition is that found in patients with rheumatoid arthritis (RA) and familial Mediterranean fever consisting of the AA (Amyloid A) protein. The AA protein was initially discovered as the main component of amyloid deposits. The fibril was found to have a serum precursor, SAA (serum amyloid A) (17). SAA has a polypeptide weight of 12.5 kD but circulates as an apoprotein of high-density lipoprotein (HDL) in a molecular complex of about 250 kD and appears to play a role in cholesterol metabolism. It behaves as an acute-phase reactant in all species in which it has been studied. It is synthesized primarily in the liver in response to elevated levels of the cytokine interleukin (IL)-6, which in turn responds to IL-1 and tumor necrosis factor. The fibril subunit has a normal sequence with a molecular size of 7.5 kD, although a range of polypeptides has been found in various preparations.

Humans may be polymorphic in their ability to degrade SAA to small peptides, with some individuals being incapable of completely digesting the increased substrate load present during the course of inflammation. Digestion is incomplete and the 7.5 kD intermediate product is fibrillogenic. While reasonable, the hypothesis has not been rigorously tested.

Older autopsy studies indicated that as many as one-quarter of patients with RA had significant tissue amyloid deposits, with the severity of the deposition correlated with the extent and duration of disease (18). More recent analyses by rectal biopsy or subcutaneous fat aspiration have shown that about 5% have detectable deposits with perhaps one-third of these displaying clinical disease, usually renal or hepatic deposition. Frequencies from some countries appear to be somewhat higher. Amyloid renal disease was the cause of 10% of the deaths in RA patients during a 10-year period when 35% of the initial 1000 patients died from all causes.

In much of the world, AA deposition is common in the course of chronic infectious diseases such as leprosy, tuberculosis, and osteomyelitis. The frequency in the course of noninfectious inflammatory diseases such as juvenile rheumatoid arthritis is higher in Europe (5%–10%) than it is in the United States (1%).

Investigations of the genetic predisposition toward AA deposition have been encouraged by the discovery that the amyloid found in some well-defined groups of patients with the apparently autosomal recessive disorder familial Mediterranean fever was the AA protein. Virtually all Sephardic Jews and many Turks who display the clinical features of the disease (ie, episodes of fever, arthralgias, abdominal or pleuritic inflammation) develop renal amyloidosis, usually by the end of the second decade of life. Ashkenazi Jews, Armenians, and other groups display the episodic inflammatory disease but do not develop amyloid. Hence two discrete events may be involved. The gene responsible for the first, inherited in an autosomal recessive manner, is found on chromosome 16. Its function has not yet been determined, but it presumably leads to a low threshold for triggering an inflammatory response or an inability to terminate the response. The second event, perhaps related to an inability to process the SAA produced in the course of the inflammation or the production of a dominant amyloidogenic isoform, is associated with renal amyloid deposition. Fortunately, it has now been established that daily colchicine administration can abort both the acute episodes and the development of amyloid in susceptible individuals, if it is administered before renal disease develops.

Aging and Amyloid

Five different anatomic sites of amyloid deposition have been associated with aging, apparently without predisposing disease. The fibril precursors have been identified in all of them, the beta protein of Alzheimer's disease (in the brain), islet-associated polypeptide (in the pancreas) associated with type II diabetes mellitus, atrial natriuretic factor, the fibril of isolated atrial amyloid, and transthyretin, the fibril precursor of senile systemic (cardiac) amyloid. The precursor of human aortic amyloid has recently been identified as Apo AI (P. Westermark, personal communication). Mutant forms of the β protein, transthyretin and Apo AI have also been associated with more severe, autosomal dominant forms of amyloid deposition in tissue sites similar to those seen in the late onset conditions (20). Abnormal accumulation of β-amyloid protein and β-amyloid precursor protein have been identified in the rimmed vacuoles in muscle from patients with inclusion body myositis. While beta protein deposition has only been found to be significant in the brain, the mutant TTRs and Apo AI produce severe sensorimotor and autonomic neuropathy, vitreopathy, and nephropathy. Some patients with the latter have come to the attention of rheumatologists when they present with Charcot joints. In addition, the TTR patients also develop cardiomyopathy.

Familial Amyloidosis

Other rare familial autosomal dominant forms of amyloidosis have been associated with 1) the deposition of a mutant form of gelsolin, an actin-binding protein, found in the Finnish form of amyloidotic neuropathy and lattice corneal dystrophy, and 2) a mutation in the gene encoding cystatin C, a lysosomal proteinase inhibitor found deposited in the cerebral blood vessels of Icelandic kindreds with hereditary cerebral hemorrhage with amyloid. Two familial forms of amyloid in which precursors recently have been identified are nephropathic. One is associated with a mutation in the αI chain of fibrinogen and the other is caused by a mutation in lysozymes found in families with the Ostertag form of renal amyloidosis.

SUMMARY

What may one conclude after inspecting the family of amyloid fibrils, their precursors, and the diseases in which they occur? Many of the proteins contain within their structures a sequence of amino acids that have the capacity in vitro to associate either with the same or another sequence in adjacent molecules to form fibrils that are no longer soluble under physiologic conditions. It is likely that these stretches of sequence are constrained by the internal environments of the molecules in which they are embedded. It has been suggested that the intact proteins can exist in fibrillogenic or nonfibrillogenic conformations (20). If the constraints are lessened, removed (eg, by mutation, by proteolytic nicking, by the incorporation of an oligosaccharide), or made less relevant by a local increase in concentration, the number of molecules having the fibrillogenic conformation may increase and begin a process of nucleation that results in fibril formation. It is possible that most or all tissues have a complement of proteases capable of disposing of small amounts of such structures. When the capacity is exceeded by an increased substrate load or is reduced by other physiologic or pathologic processes, the fibrils accumulate with resultant organ compromise. It is only by understanding these phenomena that rational approaches to therapy of these conditions will be possible.

JOEL BUXBAUM, MD

1. Kisilevsky R, Gauldie J, Benson MD, et al (eds): Amyloid and Amyloidosis 1993. New York, London, Parthenon, 1994

2. Gertz MA, Li CY, Shirahama T, Kyle RA: Utility of subcutaneous fat aspiration for the diagnosis of systemic amyloidosis (immunoglobulin light chain). Arch Intern Med 148:929-933, 1988

3. Gallo GR, Feiner HD, Chuba JV, Beneck D, Marion P, Cohen DH: Characterization of tissue amyloid by immunofluorescence microscopy. Clin Immunol Immunopathol 39:479-488, 1986

4. Hind CRK: Amyloidosis and Amyloid P Component. New York, John Wiley & Sons, 1989

5. Hawkins PN, Cavender JP, Pepys MB: Evaluation of systemic amyloidosis by scintigraphy with 125I-labeled serum amyloid P component. N Engl J Med 323:508-513, 1990

6. Young ID, Willmer JP, Kisilevsky R: The ultrastructural localization of sulfated proteoglycans is identical in the amyloids of Alzheimer's disease, AA, AL, senile cardiac and medullary carcinoma associated amyloidosis. Acta Neuropathol (Berlin) 78:202-208, 1989

7. Kyle RA, Gertz MA: Primary systemic amyloidosis: clinical and laboratory features in 474 cases. Semin Hemat 32:45-59, 1995

8. Simons M, Isner JM: Assessment of relative sensitivities of noninvasive tests for cardiac amyloidosis in documented cardiac amyloidosis. Am J Cardiol 68:425-427, 1992

9. Simmons Z, Blaivas M, Aguilera AJ, Feldman EL, Bromber MB, Towfighi J: Low diagnostic yield of sural nerve biopsy in patients with peripheral neuropathy and primary amyloidosis. J Neurol Sci 120:60-63, 1993

10. Bjerrum OW, Rygaard-Olsen C, Dahlerup B, Bang FB, Haase J, Jantzen E, Overgaard J, Sehested PC: The carpal tunnel syndrome and amyloidosis. A clinical and histological study. Clin Neurol Neurosurg 86:29-32, 1984

11. Wiernik P: Amyloid joint disease. Medicine 51:465-479, 1972

12. Greipp PR, Kyle RA, Bowie EJ: Factor-X deficiency in amyloidosis: a critical review. Am J Hematol 11:443-450, 1981

13. Kyle RA, Gertz MA, Garton JP, Greipp PR, et al: Amyloid and Amyloidosis. New York, Parthenon Publishing, New York, 1994, p 648

14. Skinner M, Anderson JJ, Simms R, et al: Treatment of 100 patients with primary amyloidosis: a randomized trial of melphalan, prednisone and colchicine versus colchicine only. Am J Med 100:290-298, 1996

15. Buxbaum J: Mechanisms of disease: Monoclonal immunoglobulin deposition. Amyloidosis, light chain deposition disease, and light and heavy chain deposition disease. Hematol Oncol Clin N Am 6:323-346, 1992

16. Gejyo F, Yamada T, Odani S, et al: A new form of amyloid protein associated with chronic hemodialysis was identified as B2-microglobulin. Biochem Biophys Res Commun 129:701-706, 1985

17. Sipe JD: Amyloidosis. Ann Rev Biochem 61:947-975, 1992

18. Husby G: Amyloidosis and rheumatoid arthritis. Clin Exp Rheumatol 3:173-180, 1985

19. Jacobson DR, Buxbaum JN: Genetic aspects of amyloidosis. Adv Hum Genet 20:69-123, 1991

20. Kelly JW, Lansbury PT Jr: A chemical approach to elucidate the mechanism of transthyretin and beta-protein amyloid fibril formation. Amyloid. Int J Exp Clin Invest 1:186-205, 1994

35 NEOPLASMS OF THE JOINT

Neoplasms of the joint are uncommon. They may arise from any anatomic structure of a joint, as well as from extrinsic structures that may impinge on the confines of the joint. In addition to true neoplasms, tumor simulators must also be considered in the differential diagnosis of masses arising about joints.

BENIGN SOFT TISSUE TUMORS

Lipoma

Lipoma is the most common benign soft tissue tumor (1), and the extremity is a frequent site. Characteristically, lipomas are soft, compressible, asymptomatic, and mobile. A key feature is the long history and slow growing nature of the mass. They are uncommon in the hands or feet, and are rarely seen in children. Synovial lipomas are often solitary, intra-articular, and subsynovial structures that are responsible for nondescript symptoms. They show a predisposition for the knee. Lipoma arborescens is also a monarticular lesion characterized by villous lipomatosis of the synovium. It is associated with chronic conditions of the joint such as rheumatoid arthritis and osteoarthritis (OA).

Plain radiography may demonstrate a soft tissue mass, sometimes with evidence of central osseous metaplasia. Computed tomography (CT) imaging is virtually diagnostic, showing a homogeneous, low density, and clearly marginated soft tissue lesion. Fibrous septation or a capsule are occasionally seen, and intravenous contrast injection does not produce enhancement of the tumor.

Treatment usually involves surgical excision with a narrow margin. One entity, the intramuscular lipoma, has a tendency to pervade adjacent muscles. This pervasive character may be one reason for the small risk of recurrence following excision.

Hemangioma

Vascular tumors are common lesions that affect all age groups (1). The most common hemangioma has capillary and cavernous subtypes that form part of a spectrum with significant overlap. Most lesions are asymptomatic in early life but become noticeable in early adulthood. Hemangiomas affecting joints are uncommon, but usually involve the synovium when present. Synovial hemangiomatosis is classically unilateral with a predilection for the knee. Patients present with pain, swelling, and decreased range of motion. Synovial lesions can be pedunculated, which may cause symptoms of locking or painful impingement, or diffuse, which may present with pain, repeated hemarthroses, and synovitis similar to hemophilia. Articular cartilage degeneration is one important sequel of hemosiderin deposition that accompanies repeated hemarthroses.

Hemangiomas are occasionally associated with distinct syndromes. Those pertinent to joints include the Klippel–Trenaunay–Weber syndrome (2) of varicose veins, soft tissue and bony hypertrophy, and cutaneous hemangiomas; Maffucci's syndrome of multiple enchondromas and soft tissue hemangiomas (3) and synovial hemangiomatosis in association with the Nevus of Ota (4). Hemangiomas may also be associated with osteomalacia and massive osteolysis. It is not uncommon for deep or synovial hemangiomas to be associated with regional cutaneous hemangiomas. Some authors suggest that patients with joint symptoms and overlying cutaneous hemangiomas should be investigated for the possibility of intra-articular vascular malformations (4).

Radiographically, calcification may appear as a nonspecific fluffiness, phleboliths, or metaplastic calcification. Cortical erosion, cortical hyperostosis, and periosteal new bone formation have also been described. Angiography is an excellent technique for determining the extent of the tumor, degree of vascularity, and the major arterial sources. Magnetic resonance imaging, particularly with contrast enhancement, is able to demonstrate similar features and adds further information regarding the tissue layers that may be involved.

Complete excision can be difficult with large hemangiomas. Embolization may be combined with surgical excision. When employed alone, embolization is often unsuccessful due to development of collateral channels. Pedunculated synovial hemangiomatoses are easily excised, but the diffuse variety often requires synovectomy.

Hemangiopericytoma

Hemangiopericytoma is a soft tissue tumor with benign and malignant forms that arises from the mesenchymal cells (Zimmerman cells) of the capillary wall (1). It is a slowly growing, firm, painless mass that usually occurs in the deeper tissues of the thigh and may mimic the various bursae about the knee. It is extremely vascular; angiography demonstrates a peripheral distribution of the plexiform network of vessels that characterizes this tumor. Other features seen on angiogram include a lobular nature, tumoral vascularization, and a heterogeneous blush.

Management of this lesion includes wide excision and obliteration of the feeding vessels. Careful histologic examination is required to exclude the possibility of malignancy.

Neuromas

Neuromas may also present as masses arising from joints. Often painful, neuromas may be single or multiple. They may be associated with von Recklinghausen's disease, or may arise spontaneously or as a result of trauma. Digital neuromas are common in the foot (Morton's neuroma) and are often found between the third and fourth metatarsal heads on the plantar surface. An iatrogenic cause for neuromas is recognized in patients where operative incisions such as arthroscopy portals have injured cutaneous nerves.

Symptoms include a painful or sensitive nodule with dysesthesia along the distribution of the cutaneous nerve when manipulated. A positive Tinel's sign may be elicited. Excision of the neuroma will remove symptoms in the majority of patients. In some patients, pain will persist.

Synovial Chondromatosis

Synovial chondromatosis is an idiopathic condition characterized by the formation of cartilage in the synovium (5). This monarticular condition commonly affects middle-aged men, and involves large joints such as the knee, hip, and elbow. Symptoms include pain, decreased range of joint motion, and occasional joint instability. Secondary OA may result from mechanical injury to the articular cartilage.

The synovium is hyperplastic with a villonodular appearance. Cartilaginous nodules are found within the synovial lining; they are believed to arise from chondral metaplasia. Detachment of the nodule from the synovium sees further growth of the loose body, as the cartilage derives its nutrient from synovial fluid. Large nodules may be palpable as mobile intra-articular loose bodies, or sometimes may penetrate the joint capsule and continue to grow in the juxta-articular soft tissue.

Radiographs of affected joints may show an intra-articular conglomeration of radiodense objects ranging from minute flecks to fairly sizable bodies (Fig. 35-1). If mineralization of the cartilage has not occurred, soft tissue shadows may be visible. Arthrography will demonstrate the multitude of radiolucent nodules and, when combined with CT imaging, the extent of the disease including the degenerative changes in the joint may be easily appreciated.

Management includes surgical removal of all loose bodies and synovectomy. Persistent joint stiffness or pain may be a problem, particularly if secondary degenerative joint changes are present.

Soft Tissue Chondromatosis

Rarely, chondromas may form in soft tissues about joints (5). As with synovial chondromatosis, middle-aged men are usually affected. The tumors are very slow growing and usually occur in the hands or feet. Histologically, this tumor is composed of mature hyaline cartilage as well as less mature proliferative cells with mitotic figures, a characteristic that may be mistaken for malignancy. As with most carti-

laginous tumors, stippled calcification may be detected on radiography. Soft tissue chondromas are easily shelled out at surgery.

Fibromatosis

Fibrous tumors arise from the fibrous aponeuroses closely related to the small joints of the hands and feet. Several forms are recognized, including juvenile aponeurotic fibromas, infantile dermal fibromatosis, and aggressive infantile fibromatosis (1,6). Painless, slowly growing masses of varying size are noted, with juvenile aponeurotic fibromas characteristically appearing on the palmar or plantar surface and infantile dermal fibromatosis occurring on the dorsal surface. Aggressive infantile fibromatosis may occur on any part of the extremity. There is a slight male predominance.

The lesions consist of interlacing bundles of spindle-shaped cells and collagen, which have an infiltrative quality. Variable mitotic activity together with the infiltrative nature of these lesions may cause them to be mistaken for fibrosarcoma.

Magnetic resonance imaging (MRI) is the most helpful technique for identifying the mass and assessing its relationship to other structures. Recurrence is common after surgery because of the infiltrative pattern of growth.

MALIGNANT SOFT TISSUE TUMORS

Soft tissue sarcomas are uncommon neoplasms accounting for less than 1% of all cancers. They occur over a wide age range, but show a predilection for late adult life. The extremities, particularly the lower limbs, are common sites for soft tissue sarcomas. Most soft tissue sarcomas share a common biologic behavior. They are well circumscribed, firm, and often painless rapidly growing masses. Their occurrence around joints may be mistaken for more common cysts (Baker's cyst) or bursae (pes anserine). Metastases occur in up to 40% of cases and is often the preterminal event.

Malignant Fibrous Histiocytoma

Malignant fibrous histiocytoma is the most common soft tissue sarcoma (7,8). Its etiology remains unclear, although evidence suggests a histiocytic and fibroblastic origin. Several forms of this tumor have been described, including storiform–pleomorphic, myxoid, giant cell, angiomatoid, and inflammatory.

Liposarcoma

Liposarcoma is the second most prevalent soft tissue sarcoma, occurring in slightly younger patients (fifth decade) than malignant fibrous histiocytoma (9). Like malignant fibrous histiocytomas, liposarcomas may be subclassified by histology into several subtypes: well-differentiated, round cell, poorly differentiated, and pleomorphic. The cell of origin is the lipoblast, although in the poorly differentiated form this may be difficult to diagnose. Liposarcomas arise de novo and not from pre-existing lipomas.

Synovial Sarcoma

Synovial sarcoma is relatively uncommon. It occurs predominantly in young adults, is often painful, and arises in close proximity to joints, tendons, or bursae (10). In addition, there may be a long premorbid history dating back several years. It is regarded as a high-grade tumor. Histologically, there are two main types: a monophasic subtype is charac-

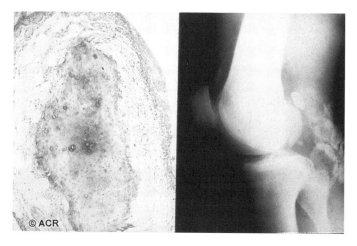

(Figure 35-1)

Synovial chondromatosis: knee. **Left:** *A mass of hyaline cartilage lies within the fibroadipose tissue of synovial membrane.* **Right:** *Multiple, rounded calcified masses appear in the posterior aspect of the knee. The calcified masses are stippled in some areas and elsewhere have a radiolucent center. Reprinted from Revised Clinical Slide Collection on the Rheumatic Diseases, with permission of the American College of Rheumatology.*

terized by interlacing sheets and bundles of spindle-shaped cells; and a biphasic subtype, which has in addition to the spindle-shaped cells, epithelioid cell groups that cluster together to form pseudoglandular structures. Plain radiographs may demonstrate tumoral calcification.

Fibrosarcoma

Following the description of malignant fibrous histiocytoma, fewer cases of fibrosarcoma have been diagnosed (11). This tumor can occur in relation to fibrous structures around the joint such as tendons, ligaments, and fibrous aponeuroses. It frequently invades surrounding structures and a well-differentiated tumor may closely resemble fibromatosis. Fibrosarcoma of childhood appears to be a different entity, occurring more often in boys before the age of two years. The distal extremities are more commonly affected. Fibrosarcoma of childhood usually carries a better prognosis.

Rhabdomyosarcoma

Rhabdomyosarcoma is a soft tissue sarcoma arising from skeletal muscle (12). It is the most prevalent soft tissue sarcoma in the pediatric age group. In children, the primary sites are the head and neck or urogenital system. In adults, the muscles of the extremities are more commonly affected. There are different histologic types including embryonal, alveolar, and pleomorphic. The embryonal subtype is usually seen in young children, alveolar is more frequently encountered in older children and young adults, and pleomorphic, which is the least common variety, predominates in adults. Unlike the other soft tissue sarcomas, rhabdomyosarcomas are poorly circumscribed and extremely invasive. The prognosis is poor.

DIAGNOSIS AND MANAGEMENT OF SOFT TISSUE SARCOMAS

The key imaging study for localizing soft tissue sarcomas is MRI (13). However, most sarcomas have a similar appearance on MRI, making histiotypic differentiation difficult. Diagnosis therefore depends on histologic examination of biopsy material. Computed tomography scanning can determine adjacent bone involvement; this may be supplemented with radioisotope scans, which give added information on metastatic spread. Chest radiographs and CT scans are mandatory studies for clinical staging of the sarcoma.

Resection with limb-preserving wide surgical margins is the accepted form of treatment for local disease (14). When combined with radiation therapy, treatment yields recurrence rates that are less than 15% (15). The use of chemotherapy has been disappointing. Pulmonary metastasectomy provides an encouraging alternative for controlling pulmonary disease.

BENIGN TUMORS OF BONE
Osteochondromas

Osteochondromas are cartilage-capped projections of bone that arise from the growth plate of bones (5). They are connected via a narrow stalk (pedunculated) or a broad base (sessile). The origin of these lesions is from aberrant growth of cartilage cell rests in the metaphysis. They may be solitary or multiple (diaphyseal aclasis), usually involving the long bones. The knee is the most common site for such growths. Lesions are usually noticed around the adolescent growth spurt. With increased age, osteochondromas grow away from the epiphysis. Unless traumatized or causing mechanical impingement, most osteochondromata remain asymptomatic. Tethering of major nerves may cause neurologic compromise; displacement of major vessels such as the popliteal, may cause a pseudoaneurysm. Rapid increases in size or pain should be investigated for the possibility of malignant change.

Radiographic features of osteochondromata include a continuation of the cortex and trabecular bone from host bone into the body of the osteochondroma. Stippled calcification may indicate the extent and thickness of the cartilage cap. Bony erosions or irregularities on the bossed surface of the osteochondroma suggest malignant change. Magnetic resonance images clearly delineate the cartilage cap, allowing an assessment of its thickness to be made. Cartilage caps thicker than 1 cm should be carefully examined for malignant change. Isotope scans are usually unhelpful, because they universally show an increase in activity commensurate with growing bone.

Limited excision of symptomatic lesions is sufficient, but more extensive resections are required if malignant change is suspected.

Enchondromas

Enchondromas are abnormal growths of cartilage arising within the medulla of tubular bones (5). They affect the short bones of the hands or feet and, when multiple (Ollier's disease) can cause significant deformity of bone and joints. Like osteochondromata, enchondromas become more prominent with age. They may be asymptomatic or may cause symptoms of joint instability or pain, particularly if there is an associated pathologic fracture. Malignant change, heralded by increasing pain or size, is possible but usually uncommon.

Radiographs demonstrate an expansile, centrally placed lesion with the characteristic calcific stippling of a cartilage tumor. Endosteal scalloping may occur and, if associated with symptoms, should be scrutinized for malignant change. Simple curettage and bone grafting will suffice in most cases.

Periosteal Chondromas

Periosteal chondromas arise from cartilage metaplasia in the periosteum (5). Unlike osteochondromata and enchondromas, these lesions tend to occur later (third to fifth decades). They have a predilection for the hands and feet, but also occur in the proximal long bones. Periosteal chondromas are usually found incidentally, as very few have symptoms. They may be palpable in the hands and feet as a smooth prominence on the surface of bone.

Diagnosis is aided by plain radiography, demonstrating scalloping and/or thickening of the underlying cortex and periosteal buttressing on either side of the lesion. Calcific stippling may be seen in the cartilage.

Articular Chondromas

Articular chondromas (dysplasia epiphysealis hemimelica or Trevor's disease) are rare. Like osteochondromata or enchondromas, they represent aberrant cartilage formation (16). They involve single or multiple epiphyses on one side of the body and are more frequently found in the distal epiphyses of the femur and tibia as well as the talus. These tumors usually result in joint deformity, restricted range of motion, pain, and secondary degenerative joint disease.

The radiographic features are asymmetric enlargement or a lobular mass arising from the epiphysis, with associated central calcific stippling.

The involvement of articular cartilage and the associated deformity predisposes the patient to unsatisfactory joint function even after surgery. Postoperative degenerative joint disease, deformity, or even ankylosis is not uncommon.

Chondroblastoma

Chondroblastoma is a rare, benign epiphyseal lesion of cartilaginous origin that arises in children or young adults (5). The knee is the usual site for these tumors. Pain is the most consistent symptom and is often referred to the adjacent joint. Examination is unremarkable. Eccentric destruction of epiphyseal bone with a sharply demarcated sclerotic border is typically seen on radiographs. The tumor can be mistaken for giant cell tumor, and this erroneous diagnosis may also be compounded by finding a variable number of multinucleated giant cells. The nuclei of these cells resemble chondroblasts, and a chondroid matrix is present. Lace-like calcification of the chondroid matrix ("chicken wiring") is characteristic. Thorough intralesional curettage with phenolation and bone grafting is adequate treatment.

Osteoid Osteoma

Osteoid osteomas may occur in the metaphysis or epiphysis. The resulting soft tissue swelling or sympathetic joint effusion may suggest an intra-articular abnormality. Pain, particularly at night, is a key feature.

The classic radiographic features of an extra-articular lesion include an intensely sclerotic lesion with a central lucency (nidus) and thickening of the overlying cortical bone (Fig. 35-2). Epiphyseal lesions, however, may demonstrate far less sclerosis, and the lucent nidus may be the main feature. Isotope scans are strongly positive in either case. Computed tomography scanning is an excellent modality for visualizing osteoid osteoma and for localizing the nidus.

Definitive treatment involves surgical removal of the cherry red nidus of granulating tissue. More recently, interest has been shown in the medical management of this lesion with prostaglandin antagonists.

Giant Cell Tumor of Bone

Giant cell tumor of bone is an aggressive tumor of uncertain etiology (5,17). Proliferation and overactivity of giant cells and osteoclasts are thought to mediate the extensive osseous lysis. It occurs in young adults (third to fifth decades) and is most commonly located at the knee. Progressively increasing pain is the main symptom, which is related to weight bearing-activities. Advanced disease is accompanied by unremitting pain that is unresponsive to non-narcotic analgesics. Sudden exacerbation of symptoms may signal pathologic fracture. A soft tissue mass is less common but may occur as the tumor erodes through the cortex into the adjacent soft tissue.

Plain radiography demonstrates a poorly marginated lytic lesion that extends up to and sometimes through subchondral bone. The lesion does not mineralize and shows little in the way of periosteal reaction. A pathologic fracture may be visible. Computed tomography scanning or MRI are useful techniques for demonstrating the intraosseous and soft tissue extent of the lesion.

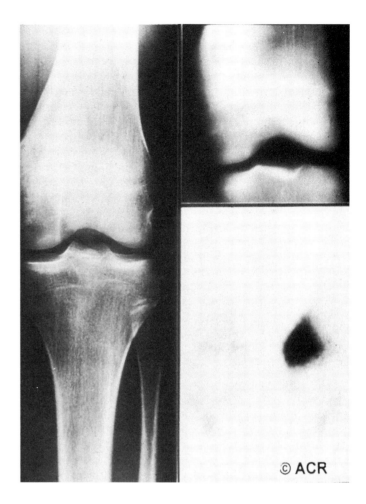

© ACR

(Figure 35-2)
Osteoid osteoma: knee. Left: An anteroposterior view of the knee demonstrates a small area of lucency in the medial aspect of the distal femur. Upper right: A tomogram of the knee clearly demonstrates the area of radiolucency with a calcified central nidus and an area of surrounding sclerosis. Lower right: A bone scan demonstrates intense uptake in the left distal medial femur. Osteoid osteomas are many times not detected by a plain roentgenogram, and tomography or a bone scan may be needed for further evaluation. Reprinted from the Revised Clinical Slide Collection on the Rheumatic Diseases, with permission of the American College of Rheumatology.

In most cases, thorough curettage of the tumor followed by the application of phenol to the bone surface and refilling of the cavity with bone cement reduces the risk of local recurrence. This technique also permits early weight-bearing activity. Prosthetic or allograft replacement may be required if the articular surface cannot be salvaged or if there has been a widely displaced pathologic fracture.

MALIGNANT BONE TUMORS
Osteosarcoma

Osteosarcoma is the most commonly seen primary malignant tumor of bone in children (5). It has a peak incidence in the second to third decades and shows a male preponderance. The main site for osteosarcomas is the growing end of long bones, particularly the knee. There are several histologic subtypes, including osteoblastic, fibroblastic, and chondroblastic. Osteosarcoma may also be classified according to its site (intramedullary or central, periosteal, parosteal) which has been shown to have implications for biologic behavior. The diagnosis hinges on identifying osteoid production by neoplastic cells. Major symptoms are pain, and/or a mass near a joint. Attention may be brought to the lesion following minor trauma, which in the past gave rise to the erroneous assumption that trauma was an etiologic factor. Close proximity to a joint, extension into the joint, or pathologic fracture may be associated with a joint effusion and decreased range of motion.

Plain radiography demonstrates a mixed sclerotic-lytic lesion situated in the metaphysis of the bone (Fig. 35-3), often with an extension into the epiphysis if the growth plate has closed. If open, the growth plate may form a natural barrier against spread into the epiphysis. There is usually a significant soft tissue component, and a periosteal reaction is common. The periosteal reaction may be limited to the junction of periosteum and cortex (Codman's triangle) or may occur throughout the entire length of elevated periosteum with radiopaque spicules passing perpendicularly from the bone to the periosteum (sun ray spicules). Magnetic resonance imaging is ideal for demonstrating the intraosseous extent of the tumor and the associated tissue edema. It also accurately delineates the soft tissue component and the intra-articular extension of the tumor if present. Both features are vital for preoperative surgical planning. Further clinical staging of the tumor includes a bone scan to screen for other osseous lesions, as well as to use as a baseline for assessing response to chemotherapy. Chest radiographs and CT scans are performed to exclude or diagnose pulmonary metastases. Pretreatment biopsy is essential for confirming the diagnosis and for comparisons with postchemotherapy tissue.

The management of osteosarcoma includes preoperative chemotherapy, wide surgical resection, and postoperative chemotherapy (18). Reconstruction with prostheses or biologic materials is used in limb-sparing procedures. Amputation is still an option when satisfactory limb function or adequate local control cannot be expected after removal of the tumor. The 5-year survival rate for adequately treated osteosarcoma is approximately 75%.

Parosteal Osteosarcoma

Parosteal osteosarcoma is a low-grade variant of osteosarcoma that arises from the surface of bone (5). It is typically situated in the posterior aspect of the distal femur and presents as a slowly growing mass in the popliteal fossa. There are few symptoms; in fact, it may be an incidental finding after examination for some other condition. By the time the tumor becomes palpable, it is moderately large. Grossly, the tumor arises from the cortex and grows into the soft tissue with only a small proportion of cases showing medullary involvement. The tumor may closely surround the bone of origin, leaving only a thin gap between it and the underlying host bone. A soft tissue component is unusual and may signify dedifferentiation.

Plain radiography demonstrates a densely sclerotic exophytic cortical lesion. There may be a thin separation between the mass and the underlying bone. Computed tomography scans are valuable for demonstrating the extent of osseous involvement, and the characteristic thin space between mass and cortex can be easily seen. Careful inspection of CT and MRI images are required to identify an area (preferably soft tissue component) that may be suitable for biopsy.

The management of parosteal osteosarcoma is wide surgical resection and reconstruction. Chemotherapy is included if there is evidence of dedifferentiation or distant spread.

Chondrosarcoma

Chondrosarcoma is the third most prevalent primary malignancy of bone (5). It may also arise from sarcomatous change of a benign cartilaginous tumor such as osteochondroma or enchondroma. Chondrosarcoma occurs in an older age group than osteosarcoma. The common sites for primary chondrosarcoma include the proximal and distal femur, the proximal tibia, and the proximal humerus. The major symptom is continuing pain; occasionally a mass is seen. Histologically, chondrosarcoma is identified by the disorganized synthesis and arrangement of cartilage matrix, the presence of multinucleated chondrocytes, and mitotic figures. Differentiation between well-differentiated low-grade chondrosarcoma and enchondroma can be extremely difficult. Clinical symptoms and radiologic information are required for diagnosis.

Plain radiographs often show a lytic lesion with central mineralization. There may be expansion of bone or scalloping of the endosteum. Perforation of the cortex is a strong indication of malignancy. A soft tissue component may be identified by the presence of extraosseous calcification. Magnetic resonance imaging scans are very helpful. Other clinical staging may be done as for the malignant tumors described above.

TUMOR SIMULATORS
Synovial Cysts

Synovial cysts or ganglion cysts arise from the synovial lining of tendon sheaths or from the joint itself. Etiologic processes include trauma, inflammation, and degeneration. Cysts may be firm or hard, with or without pain. They may vary in size and disappear completely, only to return at a later time. Some, such as Baker's cysts, may grow to enormous

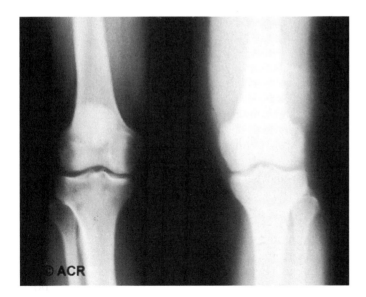

(Figure 35-3)
Osteosarcoma: femur. An anteroposterior standing view shows sclerosis in the left distal femur and soft-tissue calcification, findings compatible with an osteosarcoma. Reprinted from the Revised Clinical Slide Collection on the Rheumatic Diseases, with permission of the American College of Rheumatology.

sizes. Well known sites for these cysts include the popliteal fossa, the superior tibiofibular joint, dorsal and volar carpal joints, dorsal tarsus, and lateral aspect of the knee joint.

Ultrasound, CT scanning, and MRI can all demonstrate the homogeneous fluid-filled cyst. Computed tomography scans and MRI images are particularly useful for determining the extent and the possible location of the source of the cyst. This is important because recurrence is common unless the neck of the cysts is followed to its source and repair of the capsular rent is performed.

Aneurysms

Popliteal aneurysms are the most common aneurysms in the extremity and can be mistaken for a popliteal cysts or tumor. Pain or a mass is the usual presenting complaint. The patient's history may suggest peripheral vascular disease, including intermittent claudication, rest pain, or cold intolerance. A pulsatile mass and bruit on examination is usually indicative of an aneurysm, although a transmitted pulse through a tumor may sometimes mimic this.

Angiography is diagnostic. Sonography, Doppler studies, MRI imaging, and contrast CT scans may help to exclude a tumor.

Myositis Ossificans

Trauma to soft tissue may induce localized myositis ossificans, a heterotopic formation of bone and cartilage (5). Its appearance near joints or in relation to the joint capsule may mimic osteoblastic tumors. Occasionally, myositis ossificans may arise without trauma, in paraplegic or head injury patients. The mass evolves through various stages. In the early phase, the mass may be painful, doughy, and warm. Later it may become firmer, larger, and fixed to surrounding structures. Biopsy of the tissue may show an exuberant osteoblastic response that can be mistaken for osteosarcoma. Finally, with maturation of the lesion, a cortical shell develops around the mass as it stops growing. Over time, it may shrink and develop all the histologic features of normal mature bone. One feature that differentiates myositis ossificans from osteosarcoma is the maturation of bone at the periphery of the lesion, which is unusual in osteosarcoma. Serial radiographs are required to document the evolution of this condition.

Pigmented Villonodular Synovitis

Pigmented villonodular synovitis is a proliferative disorder of unclear etiology (19). Controversy remains over whether there is an inflammatory or neoplastic origin (20). It is characterized by a localized or diffuse proliferation of synovium, which may spread to involve the subchondral bone. There may be a sizeable soft tissue component that, when present beyond the confines of the joint capsule, may mimic a soft tissue tumor. The small joints of the hands and feet are commonly involved, while the knee joint is the most likely large joint to be affected. Pigmented villonodular synovitis is typically monarticular, although multiple joint involvement is seen. It may be localized as a solitary gray-yellow nodule or polyp, or as a diffuse villous process of the synovium. Histologically, there is marked stromal proliferation, a fibroblastic reaction, multinucleated giant cells, foam cells, and hemosiderin deposition.

Radiographically, a soft tissue mass is seen, often in association with bony erosions or sclerotic cyst formation. Early

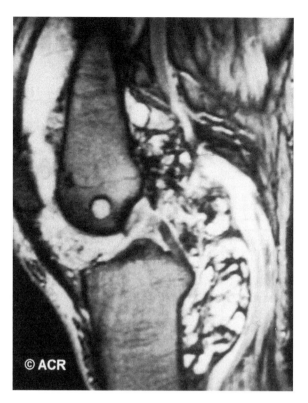

(Figure 35-4)

Pigmented villonodular synovitis: knee. The T2-weighted sagittal image (MRI) shows an extensive multilobulated mass in a patient known to have pigmented villonodular synovitis. The mass extends posteriorly and anteriorly, and contains a considerable volume of fluid, which has a signal of high intensity (white). There is cystic change in the distal femoral condyle. Reprinted from the Revised Clinical Slide Collection on the Rheumatic Diseases, with permission of the American College of Rheumatology.

in the disease, cyst formation is present without articular changes. Magnetic resonance images clearly demonstrate a lobulated mass, joint effusion, bone erosions and hemosiderin-laden tissue (Fig. 35-4). This is the preferred imaging technique prior to biopsy confirmation.

PETER F. M. CHOONG, MD
DOUGLAS J. PRITCHARD, MD

1. Enzinger FM, Weiss SW (eds): Soft Tissue Tumors, 3rd ed. St. Louis, Mosby, 1995
2. Milikow E, Easch T: Hemangiomatosis, localized growth disturbance and intravascular coagulation disorder presenting with an unusual arthritis resembling hemophilia. Radiology 97:387-388, 1970
3. Lewis RJ, Ketcham AS: Maffucci's syndrome: functional and neoplastic significance. Case report and review of the literature. J Bone Joint Surg 55A:1456-1479, 1973
4. Choong P, Baker C: Arthrocutaneous hemangiomatosis with destructive arthritis. Aust NZ J Surg 60:725-729, 1990
5. Dahlin DC, Unni KK (eds): Bone Tumors. General Aspects and Data on 8,542 Cases, 3rd ed. Springfield, Thomas, 1986
6. Dehner LP, Askin FB: Tumors of fibrous tissue origin in childhood. A clinico-pathologic study of cutaneous and soft tissue neoplasms in 66 children. Cancer 38:888-900, 1976
7. Rooser B, Willen H, Gustafson P, Alvergard TA, Rydholm A: Malignant fibrous histiocytoma of soft tissue. A population based epidemiologic and prognostic study of 137 patients. Cancer 67:499-505, 1991
8. Pritchard DJ, Reiman HM, Turcotte RE, Ilstrup DM: Malignant fibrous histiocytoma of the soft tissues of the trunk and extremities. Clin Orthop 289:58-65, 1993
9. Springfield D: Liposarcoma. Clin Orthop 289:50-57, 1993

10. Wright PH, Sim FH, Soule EH, Taylor WF: Synovial sarcoma. J Bone Joint Surg 64A:112-122, 1982

11. Pritchard DJ, Soule EH, Taylor WF, Ivins JC: Fibrosarcoma: A clinico-pathologic and statistical study of 199 tumors of the soft tissues of the extremities and trunk. Cancer 33:888-897, 1974

12. Hays DM: Rhabdomyosarcoma. Clin Orthop 289:36-49, 1993

13. Sundaram M, McLeod RA: MR imaging of tumor and tumor-like lesions of bone and soft tissue. Am J Radiology 155:817-824, 1990

14. Rosenthal HG, Terek RM, Lane JM: Management of extremity soft tissue sarcoma. Clin Orthop 289:66-72, 1993

15. O'Connor MI, Pritchard DJ, Gunderson LL: Integration of limb-sparing surgery, brachytherapy and external-beam irradiation in the treatment of soft-tissue sarcomas. Clin Orthop 289:73-81, 1993

16. Kettelkamp DB, Campbell CJ, Bonfiglio M: Dysplasia epiphysealis hemimelica. J Bone Joint Surg 48A:746-766, 1966

17. Manaster BJ, Doyle AJ: Giant cell tumors of bone. Radiol Clin of North Am 31:299-323, 1993

18. Damron TA, Pritchard DJ: Current combined treatment of high-grade osteosarcomas. Oncology 9:327-343, 1995

19. Rao AS, Vigorita VJ: Pigmented villonodular synovitis (giant cell tumor to tendon sheath and synovial membrane): a review of either-one cases. J Bone Joint Surg 66A:76-94, 1984

20. Choong PFM, Willen H. Nilbert M, Mertens F, Mandahl N, Carlen B, Rydholm A: Pigmented villonodular synovitis. Monoclonality and metasta-sis—a case for neoplastic origin? Acta Orthop Scand 66:64-68, 1995

ARTHROPATHIES ASSOCIATED WITH ENDOCRINE DISEASE

36

Hormones produced by organs of the endocrine system influence pathophysiologic mechanisms that contribute to the development of a variety of musculoskeletal disorders. Clinicians should be aware of these interactions in several different settings. First, patients with an underlying endocrine disorder may initially present with a musculoskeletal problem. Second, patients with established endocrine disorders are not cured by hormonal replacement or suppression; in fact, they develop predictable sequelae affecting the musculoskeletal system. Finally, many of the endocrine and rheumatic diseases share similar immunopathogenesis and genetic predispositions. As a consequence, expressions of rheumatic diseases may change in response to hormone fluctuations, and co-occurrences of rheumatic and endocrine disorders are recognized (1).

COMMON MUSCULOSKELETAL DISORDERS SEEN WITH ENDOCRINE DISEASE

Endocrine diseases are associated with—if not causal of—a variety of musculoskeletal disorders (Tables 36-1 and 36-2). Carpal tunnel syndrome occurs in pregnancy, diabetes, and hypothyroidism (2). In pregnancy, the cause may be related to a temporary excess of sex hormones, similar to the appearance of this syndrome in women using high estrogen-content birth control pills. Depending on the trimester, treatment with wrist splints and even a glucocorticoid injection may be preferable to the usually curative surgical ap-

proach in this self-limited neuropathy. A patient with hypothyroidism can expect a similarly rapid resolution of carpal tunnel syndrome with thyroid hormone replacement. Conversely, diabetes often has both intraneural and extraneural components to the syndrome. Many patients only partially respond to surgical resection of the flexor retinaculum of the wrist.

Pseudogout is associated with several endocrinopathies. Primary hyperparathyroidism appears to have a higher incidence of pseudogout at any age (3). Patients with hypothyroidism and joint effusions often have calcium pyrophosphate dihydrate crystals in the synovial fluid. Curiously, however, even complete correction of the underlying endocrine disorder rarely alters the course of the pseudogout. Diffuse idiopathic skeletal hyperostosis (DISH) is associated with Type II diabetes (adult onset) (4). Although DISH may be found in some cases of acromegaly

(Table 36-1)
*Nonspecific musculoskeletal manifestations of endocrine disease**

Sign or Symptom	Diseases
Carpal tunnel syndrome	Hypothyroidism
	Diabetes
	Pregnancy
	Acromegaly
Pseudogout	Hyperparathyroidism
	Hypothyroidism
Diffuse idiopathic skeletal hyperostosis	Type II diabetes
Osteonecrosis	Cushing's syndrome
	Hypothyroidism
Weakness with normal CK	Acromegaly
	Cushing's syndrome
	Hyperthyroidism
With elevated CK	Hypothyroidism
Osteoporosis	Hyperparathyroidism
	Hyperthyroidism

* CK = Creatine kinase

(Table 36-2)
*Musculoskeletal sequelae of endocrine disease**

Endocrine Disease	Rheumatic Manifestation
Diabetes	Limited joint mobility
	Neuropathic arthropathy
	DISH
	Trigger finger (flexor tenosynovitis)
	Dupuytren's contracture
Hyperthyroidism	Acropachy
	Muscle weakness
	Osteoporosis
Hypothyroidism	Muscle weakness with elevated CK
	Fibromyalgia
	Arthritis—CPPD
	Arthritis—inflammatory
	Carpal tunnel syndrome
	Osteonecrosis
Hyperparathyroidism (primary)	Pseudogout
	Osteoporosis
	Muscle weakness
Cushing's syndrome	Muscle weakness
	Osteoporosis
	Osteonecrosis
Acromegaly	Carpal tunnel syndrome
	Back pain
	Osteoarthritis

* DISH = diffuse idiopathic skeletal hyperostosis; CK=creatine kinase; CPPD = calcium pyrophosphate dihydrate.

with back pain, it is not clear that the overall incidence is increased in this disorder.

Osteonecrosis most commonly occurs in patients receiving exogenous glucocorticoids, but may also complicate endogenous Cushing's disease. Osteonecrosis may be associated with hypothyroidism, although the mechanisms remain less clear (5). Injury to the endothelium and hyperlipidemia are thought to be potential contributing factors in hypothyroidism and Cushing's syndrome.

Proximal muscle weakness is a common presenting symptom of endocrine diseases, including Cushing's syndrome, hyperthyroidism, and acromegaly. Muscle enzyme tests such as serum creatine kinase (CK) are characteristically normal; however, hypothyroidism may have muscle weakness with extremely elevated CK levels (6). When associated with skin and eyelid abnormalities, myxedema (hypothyroidism) can easily be confused with dermatomyositis.

Although estrogen deficiency is a major contributing factor for osteoporosis, both hyperparathyroidism and hyperthyroidism may also cause osteoporosis. Primary hyperparathyroidism causes net increased bone resorption over bone formation, especially in postmenopausal women (7). Careful attention to even mild increases in serum calcium should be emphasized in all patients with osteoporosis. Similarly, chronic hyperthyroid states, including thyroid replacement therapy, may result in net bone loss through increased bone resorption (8). In general, clinicians should use the minimum thyroid dose required to achieve the desired effect. Bone density determinations should be considered in all patients on long-term thyroid replacement therapy.

MUSCULOSKELETAL SEQUELAE OF ENDOCRINE DISEASE
Diabetes Mellitus

Diabetes mellitus has a variety of microvascular abnormalities that affect virtually all tissues, especially bone, nerve, muscle, tendon, and skin. Collagen accumulation in the skin and tendons produces progressive stiffness and flexion deformities of the proximal interphalangeal and metacarpal phalangeal joints (diabetic cheirarthropathy or diabetic hand syndrome) (9). This condition occurs in both the juvenile (Type I) and adult onset (Type II) forms of diabetes and may reflect microvascular abnormalities in other organs such as the kidney and eye. Additionally, both flexor tenosynovitis causing trigger fingers and Dupuytren's contractures of the palmar fascia are more common in diabetes (10).

Neuropathic arthritis (Charcot joints) can involve the ankle and tarsus in patients with diabetes (11). With the dramatic reduction of late stage syphilis, neuropathic arthropathy in the feet is almost pathognomonic for diabetes. A peripheral neuropathy is essential for the development of this destructive arthritis; it accounts for the reduced pain level despite obvious deformities. Foreign bodies can lodge, undetected, in the feet of patients with diabetic neuropathy.

A peculiar osteolysis of bone, usually involving the metatarsals and phalanges and occasionally complicated by osteomyelitis, can occur in the absence of severe neuropathy, vasculopathy, or infection. Plain radiographs of the feet and ankles should be taken when a patient with diabetes presents with foot symptoms.

Hyperthyroidism

Hyperthyroidism due to Graves' disease may have several specific extra-thyroidal manifestations involving the skin, eyes, and musculoskeletal system. Thyroid acropachy is a unique soft tissue syndrome associated with periostitis of the metacarpal bones, resulting in diffusely swollen fingers and clubbing, along with pretibial myxedema and exophthalmos. The syndrome may occur even when a euthyroid state has been achieved (12).

Hypothyroidism

A wide spectrum of rheumatic complaints occurs in patients with hypothyroidism. A fibromyalgia-like symptom complex with muscle aches and tender points may be seen early; replacement therapy with thyroid hormone virtually eliminates the complaints and distinguishes it from classic fibromyalgia. An inflammatory arthritis that may be difficult to separate from rheumatoid arthritis (RA), especially if the rheumatoid factor test is positive, may be seen (13). The arthritis predominantly involves the small joints of the hands and appears to differ from the viscous noninflammatory effusions observed in large joints of patients with hypothyroidism. In general, the arthritis completely resolves with normalization of the thyroid hormone levels.

Acromegaly

Acromegaly has prominent, distinct connective tissue manifestations related to excess tissue proliferation. The effects of growth hormone and the somatomedins on the acral and other soft tissues often go undetected for many years, resulting in dramatic musculoskeletal problems when they are finally diagnosed. There are prominent changes in the hands, feet, and face. Carpal tunnel syndrome results from intrinsic and extrinsic compression of the median nerve.

Radiographs of the hands or feet reveal widened joint spaces, abnormal distal phalangeal tufts, and characteristic soft tissue hypertrophy. Over many years, the hypertrophied articular cartilage, which accounts for the initial widened joint space seen on radiographs, is injured and actually can result in osteoarthritis with joint space loss after several decades of the disease (14). The combination of joint disease and muscle weakness of the paraspinal muscles probably accounts for the common back pain complaints in these patients.

Hyperparathyroidism

Primary hyperparathyroidism was traditionally associated with a severe osteoclast-mediated bone disease called osteitis fibrosa cystica. The earlier detection of hyperparathyroidism with automated testing of serum calcium has resulted in a shift to osteoporosis as the most common metabolic bone disease. Although osteitis fibrosa cystica and its associated arthropathy have become distinctly rare in patients with primary hyperparathyroidism, it is still observed in certain patients with renal osteodystrophy and secondary hyperparathyroidism (15).

SEX HORMONES AND AUTOIMMUNE DISEASES

The influences of sex hormones on the immune system and inflammatory pathways play a critical role in many aspects of rheumatic disease. In most rheumatic diseases, an imbalance between the sexes is evident. For instance, RA, systemic lupus erythematosus (SLE), and fibromyalgia usually occur in women, whereas ankylosing spondylitis and gout are typically present in men.

Pregnancy has a powerful effect on several of the rheumatic diseases. Reasons for the onset of a new rheumatic disease such as SLE, and the remission associated with RA during pregnancy continue to be debated. In RA, the critical inter-relationships of the sex hormones and cortisol with HLA genes of both the biologic parents need to be defined in this complex system (16). Women with SLE who become pregnant can expect a variable effect on disease activity; however, an exacerbation of the disease during the last trimester and early postpartum period is common (17). The effect of pregnancy on other autoimmune diseases is less predictable, probably because of the relatively small numbers. However, the first appearance of a variety of connective tissue disorders, including SLE, systemic sclerosis, and polymyositis, during pregnancy has been well described.

HORMONAL THERAPY OF CONNECTIVE TISSUE DISEASE

The numerous effects of hormones on the immune response and the control of the connective matrix synthesis and degradation has resulted in the development of hormones as therapeutic agents. Although glucocorticoids are the prototypic hormone used in management of the rheumatic diseases, ongoing studies are examining the effects of using androgens including dehydroepiandrosterone (DHEA) and prolactin inhibitors for treatment of SLE, human chorionic gonadotropin for ankylosing spondylitis, growth hormone for fibromyalgia, relaxin for systemic sclerosis, and 1,25 dihydroxyvitamin D for psoriatic arthritis.

JAMES L. MCGUIRE, MD
RONALD F. VAN VOLLENHOVEN, MD, PhD

1. Vianna JL, Haga HJ, Asherson RA, et al: A prospective evaluation of antithyroid antibody prevalence in 100 patients with systemic lupus erythematosus. J Rheumatol 18:1193-1195, 1991

2. Frymoyer JW, Bland J: Carpal tunnel syndrome in patients with myxedematous arthropathy. J Bone Joint Surg 55A: 78-82, 1973

3. Alexander GM, Dieppe PA, Doherty M, Scott DGI: Pyrophosphate arthropathy: a study of metabolic associations and laboratory data. Ann Rheum Dis 41:377-381, 1982

4. Resnick D, Shapiro RF, Wiesner KE, et al: Diffuse idiopathic skeletal hyperostosis (DISH): ankylosing hyperostosis of Forestier and Rotes-Querol. Semin Arthritis Rheum 7:153-187, 1978

5. Seedat YK, Randeree M: Avascular necrosis of the hip joint in hypothyroidism. S Afr Med J 49:2071, 1975

6. Hochberg MC, Edwards CQ, Barnes HV, Arnett FC, Koppes GM: Hypothyroidism presenting as a polymyositis-like syndrome. Arthritis Rheum 19:1363-1366, 1976

7. Pak CYC, Stewart A, Kaplan R, et al: Photon absorption metric analysis of bone density in primary hyperparathyroidism Lancet 2:7-8, 1975

8. Mundy GR, Shapiro JL, Banelin JG, et al: Direct stimulation of bone resorption by thyroid hormone. J Clin Invest 58:529-534, 1976

9. Starkman HS, Gleason RE, Rand LI, Miller DE, Soeldner JS: Limited joint mobility (LJM) of the hand in patients with diabetes mellitus: relation to chronic complications. Ann Rheum Dis 45:130-135, 1986

10. Mackenzie AH: Final diagnosis in 63 patients presenting with multiple palmar flexor tenosynovitis (MPFT). Arthritis Rheum 18:415, 1975 (abstract)

11. Sinha S, Munichodoppa CS, Kozak GP: Neuropathic (Charcot) joints in diabetes mellitus (clinical study of 101 cases). Medicine 51:191-210, 1972

12. Gimlette TMD: Thyroid achropathy. Lancet 1:22-24, 1960

13. le Riche NGH, Bell DA: Hashimoto's thyroiditis and polyarthritis: a possible subset of seronegative polyarthritis. Ann Rheum Dis 43:594-598, 1984

14. Holt PJL: Locomotor abnormalities in acromegaly. Clin Rheum Dis 7:689-709, 1981

15. Rubin LA, Fam AG, Rubenstein J, Campbell J, Saiphoo C: Erosive azotemic osteoarthropathy. Arthritis Rheum 27:1086-1094, 1984

16. Nelson JL: Maternal-fetal immunology and autoimmune disease: is some autoimmune disease auto-alloimmune or allo-autoimmune? Arthritis Rheum 39:191-194, 1996

17. Fine LG, Barnett EV, Danovitch GB: Systemic lupus erythematosus in pregnancy. Ann Intern Med 94:667-677, 1981

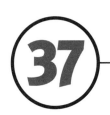

MUSCULOSKELETAL MANIFESTATIONS OF HYPERLIPOPROTEINEMIA

Patients attending lipid clinics have more musculoskeletal complaints than controls (1,2), although other studies have not confirmed this association (3,4). In a study of more than 1000 randomly selected Scandinavian men aged 50 to 60, there was no increased frequency of musculoskeletal complaints among those with either type II or type IV hyperlipoproteinemia compared with those whose lipoprotein levels were normal (3). In another study from England, only three of 166 patients with hyperlipoproteinemia (two with type II, one with type IV) had transient nondeforming polyarthritis and 8 patients (all with type IV) had gout (4). The authors of this study concluded that noncrystalline causes of musculoskeletal symptoms in patients with hyperlipoproteinemia were uncommon.

However, a recent study indicates that musculoskeletal symptoms may be the initial manifestation of metabolic disease. Musculoskeletal complaints were significantly more common in patients with various types of hyperlipidemia than in controls, and these symptoms antedated the diagnosis of hyperlipidemia in 62% of the cases (1). Awareness of these clinical manifestations may lead to earlier diagnosis and treatment with a reduction of morbidity and mortality.

TYPE II HYPERLIPOPROTEINEMIA

Type II hyperlipoproteinemia (also known as familial hypercholesterolemia) is defined by the presence of significantly elevated serum cholesterol levels and increased low-density lipoproteins (LDL), which are associated with accelerated atherosclerosis. Type IIa is inherited as an autosomal dominant trait, occurring in 1–2/1000 people (5). Total serum cholesterol levels are as high as 550 mg/dl, and clinical manifestations of coronary artery disease may be seen in the second decade of life. The homozygous form, type IIb, is rare, with a prevalence estimated at 1/1,000,000 (5). These patients may have serum cholesterol levels exceeding 1000 mg/dl. Both forms of type II hyperlipoproteinemia cause tendinous, tuberous, and periosteal xanthomas. In type IIb, xanthomas often develop in early childhood (6,7) and tend to appear over extensor surfaces, commonly the Achilles tendon, dorsum of the wrist, knee, elbow, and gluteal area. Other manifestations of hypercholesterolemia such as xanthelasma and arcus cornea are also seen in these patients.

A migratory, episodic polyarthritis with an abrupt onset has been described in patients with type II hyperlipoproteinemia (7–9). The arthritis occurs in over one half of the patients with homozygous disease and in 4% of those with heterozygous disease, according to one study (7). In a subsequent study of 73 heterozygotes, 40% had at least one episode of articular symptoms, primarily either Achilles tendon pain or Achilles tendinitis (10). These episodes are associated with inflammatory clinical findings and elevated levels of acute-phase reactants. The musculoskeletal manifestations of these patients share many features with acute rheumatic fever, a diagnosis often confused with the arthritis related to hyperlipoproteinemia. The episodes of arthritis can be recurrent and can affect large or small joints in either the lower or upper extremities. Synovial fluid in these patients has generally not revealed markedly inflammatory features.

Acute tendinitis and tenosynovitis of the Achilles tendon is often present in patients with type II hyperlipoproteinemia (6,9). Achilles tendinitis may antedate the presence of xanthomas by several years (9).

TYPE IV HYPERLIPOPROTEINEMIA

Type IV hyperlipoproteinemia (also known as familial hypertriglyceridemia) is characterized by elevation of triglycerides in association with increased very-low-density lipoproteins and serum triglyceride levels that may exceed 1000 mg/dl. This condition, which is inherited as an autosomal dominant trait, is often associated with obesity, hypertension, diabetes mellitus, and increased serum uric acid levels (5).

Arthralgias in large and small joints, without inflammatory findings, have been described in patients with type IV hyperlipoproteinemia that were not attributable to rheumatoid arthritis or gout (11,12). In contrast to type II hyperlipoproteinemia, joint manifestations in patients with type IV hyperlipoproteinemia tend to be bilateral and not episodic. Radiographs of symptomatic joints do not show erosive changes, but one-half of these patients have periarticular cystic changes (Fig. 37-1) (12). In some patients with type IV hyperlipoproteinemia, the degree of articular symptoms seems to parallel the serum triglyceride level. Many of

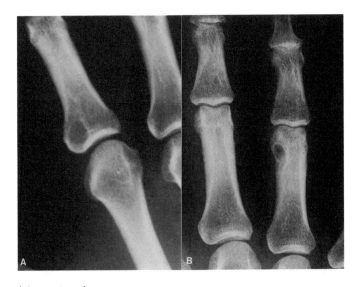

(Figure 37-1)
Periarticular bone cysts are seen in the hands of two patients (panels A and B) with type IV hyperlipoproteinemia.

(Table 37-1)
Classification of hyperlipidemia+

Phenotype	Lipoprotein Abnormality	Lipid Abnormality	Musculoskeletal Manifestations
Type I	Chylomicrons increased	Markedly increased triglycerides	Eruptive xanthomas
Type IIa	LDL increased	Increased cholesterol	Tendinous, tuberous xanthomas; migratory, episodic polyarthritis; Achilles tendinitis
Type IIb	LDL and VLDL increased	Increased cholesterol and triglycerides	Tendinous, tuberous xanthomas; migratory, episodic polyarthritis; Achilles tendinitis
Type III	Chylomicrons and VLDL remnants increased	Increased cholesterol; increased- to markedly increased triglycerides	Tendinous, tuberous, and plane xanthomas
Type IV	VLDL increased	Increased triglycerides	Eruptive tendinous and tuberous xanthomas; arthralgias
Type V	Chylomicrons and VLDL increased	Increased cholesterol, markedly increased triglycerides	Eruptive xanthomas

+ Modified from Fredrickson et al (13) with permission. LDL = low-density lipoprotein; VLDL = very-low-density lipoprotein.

these patients have abnormalities in glucose tolerance (12). When synovial fluid analysis has been performed, the fluid was found to be mildly inflammatory but without evidence of monosodium urate crystals (12).

XANTHOMAS

Xanthomas may be seen in all types of hyperlipoproteinemias (Table 37-1). Tendinous and tuberous xanthomas occur in types II, III, and IV hyperlipoproteinemia (5,13). Type III hyperlipoproteinemia may also present with xanthomas on the palms of the hands (xanthoma striata palmaris) (13). Eruptive xanthomas over the back, buttocks, knees, and shoulder occur in types I and IV and occasionally type V hyperlipoproteinemia (5,13). A lytic lesion of the proximal femur has been reported in a patient with type V hyperlipoproteinemia (14). Histologic examination revealed the bone marrow was infiltrated by foamy histiocytes surrounded by granulomatous reaction; there was no apparent evidence of malignancy.

TOM MASON, MD

1. Klemp P, Halland AM, Majoos FL, Steyn K: Musculoskeletal manifestations in hyperlipidaemia: a controlled study. Ann Rheum Dis 52:44-48, 1993
2. Wysenbeek AJ, Shani E, Beigel Y: Musculoskeletal manifestations in patients with hypercholesterolemia. J Rheumatol 16:643-645, 1989
3. Welin L, Larsson B, Svardsudd K, Tibblin G: Serum lipids, lipoproteins and musculoskeletal disorders among 50- and 60-year-old men. Scand J Rheum 7:7-12, 1977
4. Struthers GR, Scott DL, Bacon PA, Walton KW: Musculoskeletal disorders in patients with hyperlipidemia. Ann Rheum Dis 42:519-523, 1983
5. Bilheimer DW: Disorders of lipid metabolism. In Kelley WN (ed): Textbook of Internal Medicine, vol. 2. Philadelphia, J.B. Lippincott, 1989, pp 2258-2269
6. Shapiro JR, Fallat RW, Tsang RC, Glueck CJ: Achilles tendinitis and tenosynovitis. Am J Dis Child 128:486-490, 1974
7. Khachadurian AK: Migratory polyarthritis in familial hypercholesterolemia (type II hyperlipoproteinemia). Arthritis Rheum 11:385-393, 1968
8. Rooney PJ, Third J, Madkour MM, Spencer D, Dick WC: Transient polyarthritis associated with familial hyperbetalipoproteinaemia. Q J Med 47:249-259, 1978
9. Glueck CJ, Levy RI, Fredrickson DS: Acute tendinitis and arthritis. A presenting symptom of familial type II hyperlipoproteinemia. JAMA 206:2895-2897, 1968
10. Mathon G, Gagne C, Brun D, Lupien P-J, Moorjani S: Articular manifestations of familial hypercholesterolaemia. Ann Rheum Dis 44:599-602, 1985
11. Goldman JA, Glueck CJ, Abrams NR, Steiner P, Herman JH: Musculoskeletal disorders associated with type-IV hyperlipoproteinemia. Lancet ii:449-452, 1972
12. Buckingham RB, Bole GG, Bassett DR: Polyarthritis associated with type IV hyperlipoproteinemia. Arch Intern Med 135:286-290, 1975
13. Fredrickson DS, Levy RI, Lees RS: Fat transport in lipoproteins: an integrated approach to mechanisms and disorders. New Engl J Med 276:34-44, 94-103, 148-156, 215-225, 273-281, 1967
14. Siegelmann SS, Schlossberg I, Becker NH, Sachs BA: Hyperlipoproteinemia with skeletal lesions. Clin Orthop 87:228-232, 1972

MUSCULOSKELETAL PROBLEMS IN DIALYSIS PATIENTS

Patients treated with prolonged hemodialysis are now surviving longer and are increasingly developing musculoskeletal problems. Renal osteodystrophy, crystal deposition, and β_2 microglobulin amyloidosis are presently recognized as the major etiologic factors.

RENAL OSTEODYSTROPHY
Secondary Hyperparathyroidism

Hyperparathyroid disease is the most frequent form of osteodystrophy in hemodialysis patients (1). The predominant findings in uremic hyperparathyroidism are hyperhospatemia, deficient generation of 1,25-dihydroxyvitamin D by the kidney, and low calcium intake and absorption (2). Monoclonal proliferation of parathyroid cells may be one explanation for the failure of medical management (3). Preventive treatments include the use of high calcium concentrations in the dialysate and control of phosphatemia by dietary phosphorus restriction and the use of phosphorus binders, such as calcium carbonate with meals. Further enrichment of the diet with calcium supplements between meals, and vitamin D derivatives may also be necessary. The use of aluminum-containing phosphate binders is now drastically restricted because of the risk of aluminum intoxication. Serum immunoreactive 1-84 parathyroid hormone (PTH) should be maintained at a concentration of 1.5 to 3 times the upper value of normal, to avoid adynamic bone disease.

Secondary hyperparathyroidism is usually asymptomatic but may be the source of bone pain, polyarthralgia, or enthesopathy. Serum alkaline phosphatase activity, pyridinoline, osteocalcin and immunoreactive 1-84 PTH concentrations are increased. Serum phosphate levels are usually elevated, whereas the level of serum calcium is variable. The most characteristic radiologic feature is subperiostal resorption of bone, which is seen most clearly on the radial border of the middle phalanges (Fig. 38-1). Bone resorption may also lead to acroosteolysis of the phalangeal tufts, widening of the acromioclavicular and sacroiliac joints or of the pubic symphysis, and small articular erosions. The frequency of these erosions increases with dialysis duration (3), but they do not correlate with symptoms (4) and are not always related to hyperparathyroidism. More advanced hyperparathyroidism may be responsible for painful erosions at the sites of tendon attachment, which bear a high risk of tendon rupture. The skull may be affected and exhibit a "pepperpot" appearance. Osteosclerosis of the spine may be observed, with vertebral bodies showing a "rugger jersey" appearance, due to resorption of bone from the central portion. Brown tumors are rare and must be differentiated from amyloid erosions. Extraskeletal calcifications can develop, particularly in the eye, periarticular tissues, and small blood vessels or skin, leading to pruritus.

Secondary hyperparathyroidism can be treated by 1α hydroxylated vitamin D derivatives, provided that calcium and phosphorus serum levels can be controlled, and no extensive soft tissue or vascular calcifications develop. Pulse intravenous administration of these sterols has been reported as particularly effective, due to direct negative effect on PTH secretion obtained by high concentrations. When hyperparathyroidism is too advanced or resists medical management, subtotal parathyroidectomy is indicated.

Aluminum-Induced Bone Disease

Aluminum-induced bone disease follows intoxication with high aluminum content in the dialysate solution and/or prolonged ingestion of aluminum-containing phosphate binders. Affected patients typically experience bone pain, proximal muscle weakness, and pathologic fractures, particularly of first ribs (5,6). Serum calcium level are normal or elevated, especially if the patient is treated with vitamin D. Serum alkaline phosphatase activity and intact PTH

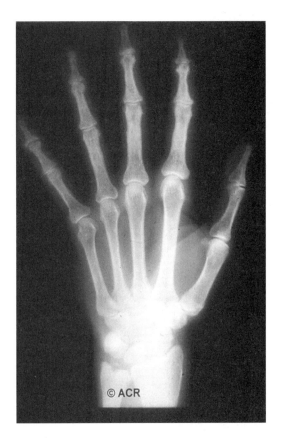

© ACR

(Figure 38-1)
This roentgenogram demonstrates moderately severe osteopenia in the hand of a patient with hyperparathyroidism. Subperiosteal bone resorption is marked at the radial aspect of the middle phalanges (usually the index and middle fingers are most involved). Note that the distal phalanges of the thumb and index finger exhibit subperiosteal bone resorption and acrolysis. Reprinted from the Revised Clinical Slide Collection on the Rheumatic Diseases, with permission of the American College of Rheumatology.

concentrations are normal or low. Aluminum serum levels are elevated either spontaneously or after deferoxamine mesylate infusion. Bone histology demonstrates heavy staining for aluminum of the mineralization front, decreased cellular activity, and either increased or normal osteoid, respectively, characterizing the two histologic forms of the disease: osteomalacia and adynamic bone disease (7). Elimination of the source of aluminum and treatment with deferoxamine mesylate can cure this disabling osteopathy.

Adynamic Bone Disease

Adynamic bone histology may develop in the absence of aluminum intoxication (1). It is the most frequent type of osteodystrophy in continuous ambulatory peritoneal dialysis patients. The major cause appears to be overtreatment of hyperparathyroidism. The condition may be associated with an increased incidence of fractures.

MUSCULAR INVOLVEMENT

Muscular cramps are common during hemodialysis and are thought to be due to extracellular volume contraction (8). A proximal myopathy may affect dialysis patients, due to aluminum intoxication or abnormal vitamin D metabolism and, very rarely, to excessive phosphorus binding causing hypophosphatemia. Hyperparathyroidism may be responsible for arterial calcification and muscular infarctions.

DISORDERS OF MICROCRYSTALLINE ORIGIN

Periarticular calcifications are common and are related to hyperphosphatemia, high serum calcium–phosphorus products, and secondary hyperparathyroidism. Such calcifications are composed of calcium phosphate (mainly apatite) crystals. They are usually asymptomatic, but apatite can induce acute articular, or more frequently, periarticular inflammatory episodes. Despite careful search for crystals and infectious agents, some acute joint and bursal effusions remain unexplained. Occasionally, calcium deposits grow into pseudotumoral masses. Apatite deposition in dialysis patients may lead to joint erosions (9) and a destructive arthropathy of the spine (10).

Calcium oxalate crystal deposition can occur at various sites, including bone, synovium, and cartilage, and is one cause of synovial calcification or chondrocalcinosis in dialysis patients. This has been mainly observed in patients whose diets are supplemented with vitamin C, a precursor of oxalate (11). Gout and calcium pyrophosphate crystal deposition disease are rare despite the frequency of hyperuricemia and gout before dialysis (5) and the presence of secondary hyperparathyroidism.

BONE AND JOINT INFECTIONS

Bone and joint infections are well documented complications of hemodialysis and require urgent management with appropriate antibiotics. Immune defenses of patients treated with hemodialysis are impaired, and the arteriovenous fistula is a potential source of hematogenous spread. Intra- or periarticular corticosteroid injections are also an important source of infection and should be avoided in these patients. Unusual infections can include listeriosis associated with secondary iron overload after transfusions.

DIALYSIS ARTHROPATHY AND β_2 MICROGLOBULIN AMYLOID

The deposition of β_2 microglobulin amyloid in articular and periarticular tissues of dialysis patients has been well documented in the last decade (12-14). Carpal tunnel syndrome, a prominent feature, is usually bilateral and severe enough to require surgery. A chronic, grossly symmetric arthropathy is also frequently observed and includes chronic arthralgias, particularly of the shoulders, chronic joint swelling with non-inflammatory effusions, recurrent hemarthrosis, Baker's cysts, and finger tendon tenosynovitis. Large subchondral bone erosions, predominantly of the hip at sites of synovium attachment or reflexion, may lead to pathologic fracture of the femoral neck. Shoulder pain may be related to amyloid thickening of the rotator cuff tendons or subacromial bursa, which can lead to a chronic impingement syndrome. Destructive arthropathy involves the spine—and may lead to spinal cord or nerve root compromise—and/or large joints of the limbs. Some patients may even develop a pseudo-rheumatoid arthropathy, with grossly symmetric amyloid infiltration and morning stiffness of short duration. The diagnosis can be suspected on ultrasound demonstration of thickening of the rotator cuff tendon (15) and is established by examination of synovial fluid (16), as well as by biopsy. Systemic deposits are rare but may be responsible for intestinal hemorrhage or cardiac dysfunction. Lack of β_2 microglobulin catabolism by the kidney and unsatisfactory elimination of the molecule through dialysis membranes are important in the pathogenesis of the disorder. β_2 microglobulin modified with advanced glycation products has been identified in deposits and shown to stimulate monocyte chemotaxis and macrophage secretion of tumor necrosis factor and interleukin-1 (17). β_2 microglobulin amyloid deposits have been observed even before the start of dialysis therapy (18), but the frequency of dialysis arthropathy increases with the patient age and length of survival; up to 65% of individuals who have received 10 or more years of maintenance hemodialysis using standard cuprophane membranes (which are impermeable to β_2 microglobulin) may be affected. The use of more permeable membranes may delay the onset of the disease, but thus far has been unable to totally prevent its development. Kidney transplantation halts disease progression, even though deposits persist, and improves the joint symptoms dramatically, probably as a consequence of steroid treatment (19).

THOMAS BARDIN, MD

1. Sherrard DJ, Hercz G, Pei Y, et al: The spectrum of bone disease in end-stage renal failure. An evolving disorder. Kidney Intern 43:436-442, 1993

2. Hruska KA, Teitelbaum SL: Renal osteodystrophy. N Engl J Med 333:166-174, 1995

3. Arnold A, Brown MF, Urena P, Gaz RD, Sarfati E, Druëke T: Monoclonality of parathyroid tumors in chronic renal failure and in parathyroid hyperplasia. J Clin Invest 95:2047-2053, 1995

4. Rubin LA, Fam AG Rubinstein, et al: Erosive azotemic osteoarthropathy. Arthritis Rheum 27:1086-1094, 1984

5. Chou CT, Wasserstein I, Schumacher HR, et al: Musculoskeletal manifestations in hemodialysis patients. J Rheumatol 12:1149-1153, 1985

6. Hodsman AB, Sherrard DJ, Wong EG, et al: Vitamin D restaint osteomalcia in hemodialysis patients lacking secondary hyperparathyroidism. Ann Intern Med 94:629-637, 1981

7. Kriegshouser JS, Swee RG, McCarty JT, et al: Aluminum toxicity in patients undergoing dialysis: radiological findings and prediction of bone biopsy results. Radiology 164:399-403, 1987

8. Mulutinovitch J, Graefe V, Follete WC, et al: Effect of hypertonic glucose on the muscular cramps of hemodialysis. Ann Intern Med 90:926-928, 1979

9. Schumacher HR, Miller JL, Ludivico C: Erosive arthritis associated with apatite crystal deposition. Arthritis Rheum 24:31-37, 1981

10. Kuntz D, Naveau B, Bardin T, et al: Destructive spondylarthropathy in hemodialyzed patients: a new syndrome. Arthritis Rheum 27:369-375, 1984

11. Reginato AJ, Kurnik B: Calcium oxalate and other crystals associated with kidney diseases and arthritis. Semin Arthritis Rheum 18:198-224, 1989

12. Gejyo F, Brancaccio D, Bardin T: Dialysis Amyloidosis. Milan, 1989

13. Bardin T, Drüeke T, Kuntz D: β_2-microglobulin amyloidosis. Rev Rheum (Engl Ed), 61 (suppl): 1S-104S, 1994

14. van Ypersele de Strihou C, Drüeke T: Dialysis Amyloidosis. Oxford University Press, 1996

15. Kay J, Benson CB, Lester S, Corson JM, Pinkus G, Lazarus M, Owen WF: Utility of high resolution ultrasound for the diagnosis of dialysis-related amyloidosis. Arthritis Rheum 35:926-932, 1992

16. Muñoz-Gomex J, Gomez-Pérez R, Solé-Arques M, et al: Synovial fluid examinatioin for the diagnosis of synovial amyloidosis in patients with chronic renal failure undergoing haemodilysis. Ann Rheum Dis 46:324-326, 1987

17. Miyata T, Inagi R, Lida Y, Sato M, Yamada N, Oda O, Maeda K, Seo H: Involvement of β_2-microglobulin modified with advanced glycation end products in the pathogenesis of hemodialysis-associated amyloidosis. J Clin Invest 93:521-528, 1994

18. Zingraff J, Noel LH, Bardin T, et al: Beta-2 microglobulin amyloidosis as a complication of chronic renal failure (letter). N Engl J Med 323:1070-1071, 1990

19. Bardin T, Lebail-Darné JL, Zingraff J, Laredo JD, Voisin MC, Kreis H, Kuntz D: Dialysis arthropathy: outcome after renal transplantation. Am J Med 99:243-248, 1995

HERITABLE DISORDERS OF CONNECTIVE TISSUE

39

The molecular composition and organization of connective tissue (the extracellular matrix) are extraordinarily complex, and much remains unknown about the genes — their number, structure, map location, and regulation — that control synthesis, organization, and metabolism of this ubiquitous tissue. Thus far, the genes that specify more than 50 proteins involved in connective tissue metabolism have been mapped (1) (see Appendix IV). Mutations in the genes for these proteins cause a variety of disorders. The heritable disorders of connective tissue (HDCT) follow Mendel's laws, but like many such disorders, show both considerable variability within and among families and genetic heterogeneity (2,3).

Some common disorders, such as osteoarthritis, osteoporosis, and aortic aneurysms, involve predominantly connective tissue and are Mendelian in occasional families. However, multiple genes and other factors are likely important in cause and pathogenesis for the majority of cases.

The phenotypic characterization of HDCT, crude as it sometimes is, still outstrips biochemical or genetic understanding (4). More than 200 conditions are called HDCT. The more familiar ones have prevalences of 1/3000–4000 to 1/50,000; many are less prevalent. The subclassification of HDCT is unsatisfactory and must ultimately be based on pathobiology. But several phenotypic groupings are traditionally employed: 1) disorders of fibrous elements, such as osteogenesis imperfecta; 2) disorders of proteoglycan metabolism, including the mucopolysaccharidoses; 3) osteochondrodysplasias and dysostoses, such as achondroplasia; and 4) inborn errors of metabolism that secondarily affect connective tissue, such as homocystinuria and alkaptonuria.

MARFAN SYNDROME

Patients with the Marfan syndrome have abnormalities in multiple organs and tissues, especially the skeletal, ocular, cardiovascular, pulmonary, and central nervous systems. Diagnosis is based primarily on clinical features and the autosomal dominant inheritance pattern. The basic defect in all cases studied thus far is in fibrillin, the principal constituent of extracellular microfibrils (5). The locus (*FBN1*) for this protein maps to 15q21. Microfibrils are ubiquitous, 10–14 nm structures that form the substructure for deposition of tropoelastin during formation of elastic fibers. Thus, fibrillin is a functionally important molecule in any organ containing elastic fibers, such as arteries, ligaments, and lung parenchyma. In other tissues, such as the zonular fibers of the eye, at the epidermal–dermal junction, and in the perichondrium, microfibrils are not associated with elastin. Thus, defective fibrillin neatly explains the pleiotropic manifestations of Marfan syndrome. The current challenges are to understand the molecular and cellular pathogenesis of each clinical manifestation and the range of expression of fibrillin mutations, including those in disorders distinct from the Marfan syndrome. Autosomal dominant ectopia

lentis, autosomal dominant aortic aneurysm, and even autosomal dominant tall stature, all in the absence of the Marfan syndrome, are caused by mutations in *FBN1* (6). Some patients with the Shprintzen–Goldberg syndrome have mutations in *FBN1*. Congenital contractual arachnodactyly is linked to a locus (*FBN2*) on chromosome 5 that specifies another member of the fibrillin family of proteins, and recently a few mutations have been found in that gene.

Skeletal manifestations of Marfan syndrome include excessive stature; abnormal body proportions with a long arm span and an abnormally low ratio of the upper segment to the lower segment (dolichostenomelia); elongated digits (arachnodactyly); anterior thoracic deformity (pectus excavatum, carinatum, or an asymmetric combination); abnormal vertebral column curvature (loss of thoracic kyphos, resulting in a "straight back," and scoliosis); hyperextensibility or, less often, congenital contractures of appendicular joints; protrusio acetabula; and pes planus with a long, narrow foot. Most patients have myopia, and about one-half have subluxation of the lenses (ectopia lentis). Beginning in the sinuses of Valsalva, the ascending aorta gradually dilates, which is associated with fragmentation of the medial elastic fibers; aortic regurgitation and dissection result and are the main causes of death. Mitral valve prolapse occurs in a majority of patients and leads to severe mitral regurgitation in some, occasionally in childhood. Hernias are frequent. Apical bullae lead to pneumothorax in 5% of patients, and striae distensae over the pectoral, deltoid, and lumbar areas are a helpful diagnostic sign. Dural ectasia producing erosion of lower lumbar and sacral vertebrae is usually an incidental finding on computed tomography or magnetic resonance imaging, but this manifestation may lead to pelvic meningoceles or radicular problems.

Management of Marfan syndrome is both palliative and preventive. The size of the ascending aorta should be followed by echocardiography, β-adrenergic blockade is advisable to reduce stress on the aortic wall, and composite graft replacement should be undertaken when the aortic diameter is greater than twice expected (about 55 mm in the adult). Scoliosis should be aggressively managed in children and adolescents with bracing; when spinal curvature exceeds about 40 degrees, surgical stabilization should be considered. Hormonal advancement of pubarche can modulate excessive stature and prevent worsening spinal curvature by reducing the growth period. Most patients do not dislocate joints (the patella is the most common dislocation). Patients may be predisposed to develop degenerative arthropathy and osteoporosis in middle age. Women with Marfan syndrome are at increased risk of aortic dissection and rupture during pregnancy; an aortic root diameter greater than 40 mm is a contraindication to pregnancy.

HOMOCYSTINURIA

Homocystinuria usually refers to an inborn error in the metabolism of methionine due to deficient activity of the enzyme cystathionine β-synthase. Clinical features are superficially similar to those of the Marfan syndrome and include ectopia lentis, tall stature, dolichostenomelia, arachnodactyly, and anterior chest and spinal deformity (7). Generalized osteoporosis, "tight" joints, arterial and venous thrombosis, malar flush, mental retardation, and autosomal recessive inheritance are features of homocystinuria that are not consistent with Marfan syndrome, whereas aortic aneurysm and mitral prolapse are not features of homocystinuria. Back pain and vertebral collapse due to osteoporosis occur in some patients; most have no specific arthropathy.

The pathogeneses of the three cardinal manifestations — mental retardation, connective tissue disorder, and thrombosis — are not understood. One hypothesis holds that sulfhydryl groups of homocysteine and methionine interfere with collagen cross-linking. If true, this is a form of thiolism such as occurs from prolonged administration of penicillamine, a compound structurally similar to homocysteine. Fibrillin is rich in cysteine, and intra- and interchain disulfide bonds are crucial to the formation and function of microfibrils. Some of the phenotypic resemblance of homocystinuria to Marfan syndrome may be due to disruption of microfibrils by the reactive sulfhydryl moiety of homocysteine.

About one half of patients respond biochemically and clinically to large doses of vitamin B_6 (usually more than 50 mg pyridoxine per day). Adequate levels of folate and vitamin B_{12} are required for therapeutic and biochemical response. Pre-existent mental retardation and ectopia lentis are not reversed by pyridoxine treatment in patients who show biochemical correction, emphasizing the need for early diagnosis and therapy. This is now feasible since many states include testing for elevated blood methionine as part of newborn screening. Unfortunately, some pyridoxine-responders may escape detection in the typical screening protocols. In pyridoxine-nonresponders, a low methionine diet and oral betaine therapy (to stimulate remethylation of homocysteine to methionine) are the usual treatments; this approach is successful if the diet and vitamin are started in infancy and are tolerated.

STICKLER SYNDROME

The Stickler syndrome is a relatively common autosomal dominant condition with severe, progressive myopia, vitreal degeneration, retinal detachment, progressive sensorineural hearing loss, cleft palate, mandibular hypoplasia, hyper- and hypomobility of joints, epiphyseal dysplasia, and potential disability from joint pain, dislocation, or degeneration (8). This condition, also called progressive arthro-ophthalmopathy, is underdiagnosed, partly because many patients do not have the full syndrome and partly because clinicians fail to obtain a detailed family history that might suggest a hereditary condition. The diagnosis should be strongly considered in the following patients: any infant with congenitally enlarged ("swollen") wrists, knees or ankles, particularly when associated with the Robin anomalad (hypognathia, cleft palate, and glossoptosis); any young adult with degenerative hip disease; and anyone suspected of Marfan syndrome who has hearing loss, degenerative arthritis, or retinal detachment. In some families, the Stickler syndrome is linked to the α1(II) procollagen locus (COL2A1) on chromosome 12. A number of mutations in type II collagen, the structural macromolecule of both cartilage and the vitreous, have been found. In other families, the condition is caused by mutations in a gene for type XI collagen at 6p22-p21.3.

EHLERS–DANLOS SYNDROMES

The Ehlers–Danlos syndromes are a group of disorders whose wide phenotypic variability is largely due to extensive genetic heterogeneity. The cardinal features relate to the joints and skin: hyperextensibility of skin, easy bruisability, increased joint mobility, and abnormal tissue fragility (9,10). Internal manifestations tend to occur only in specific types of Ehlers–Danlos syndrome. Nine types are now accepted on the basis of phenotypic and inheritance characteristics (Table 39-1). Within individual types, however, biochemical studies have demonstrated considerable heterogeneity. Extensive phenotypic and biochemical characterization nonetheless fails the clinician as often as it helps; about one-half of patients who have at least one "cardinal" feature defy categorization (2,4).

(Table 39-1)
*Ehlers–Danlos syndromes**

Type	Inheritance	Skeletal Features	Other Features	Basic Defect
I	AD	Marked joint hypermobility	Skin hyperextensibility and fragility	Some with abn type V collagen
II	AD	Less severe than type I		Some with abn type V collagen
III	AD	Marked joint mobility	Mild skin hyperextensibility	?
IV	AD, AR	Hypermobile digits	Thin skin; bowel and arterial rupture	↓ procollagen III
V	X-L	Similar to type II		?
VI	AR	Marked joint hypermobility	Rupture of ocular globe	↓ lysyl hydroxylase
VII	AD, AR	Marked joint hypermobility and dislocations, short stature	Minimal skin changes	↓ type I procollagen N-peptide clevage
VIII	AD	Variable joint hypermobility	Periodontitis	?; some with ↓ type III collagen
X	AD	Mild joint hypermobility	Mild skin changes; mitral valve prolapse	? ↓ serum fibronectin

*According to revised terminology (5), the condition once termed EDS type IX (or X-linked cutis laxa) has been reclassified as a disorder of copper metabolism. The condition once termed EDS type XI has been reclassified as a disorder of joint instability. According to convention, EDS types IX and XI will now be vacant. AD = autosomal dominant; AR = autosomal recessive; X-L = X-linked.

Ehlers–Danlos type I (gravis form) and type II (mitis form) cause generalized hyperextensibility of joints and of skin, bruisability and fragility of the skin with gaping wounds from minor trauma, and poor retention of sutures. Congenital dislocation of the hips in the newborn, habitual dislocation of joints in later life, joint effusions, clubfoot, and spondylolisthesis are all consequences of the loose-jointedness. Hemarthroses and "hemarthritic disability" have been described and are analogous to the bruisability of the skin in this syndrome. Scoliosis is sometimes severe. Both of these types are inherited as autosomal dominant traits and show wide variability; hence their differentiation is qualitative and subjective (type I is more severe). Fetuses with type I are prone to premature rupture of placental membranes. The biochemical defect(s) have not been characterized in either type. Management of both types I and II stresses prevention of trauma and great care in treating wounds. Some instances of types I and II are due to mutations in the gene that encodes the α1 chain of type V collagen (11).

Patients with Ehlers–Danlos type III (benign hypermobility form) have less marked skin involvement than occurs in types I and II. Joint hyperextensibility ranges from extreme to moderate. Many people with mild joint laxity without joint instability are often labeled as having type III, particularly if relatives show similar manifestations (12). In some cases, such labeling does more harm than good, unless it is made quite clear that little, if any, disability is likely.

Ehlers–Danlos type IV (arterial form) is by far the most serious form because of a propensity for spontaneous rupture of arteries and bowel. The unifying pathogenetic theme is abnormal production of type III collagen. A variety of mutations in the COL3A1 gene have been described. Skin involvement is variable; some patients have thin, nearly translucent skin while others have only mildly hyperextensible skin. Joint laxity is also variable and may be limited to the digits. Inheritance is usually autosomal dominant, but many cases are sporadic occurrences in a pedigree, suggesting these patients are heterozygous for a new mutation.

Ehlers–Danlos type VI (ocular–scoliotic form) is characterized by fragility of the ocular globe, marked joint and skin hyperextensibility, a propensity for severe scoliosis, and autosomal recessive inheritance. Collagen in the skin contains little hydroxylysine because these patients are deficient in the enzyme that hydroxylates selected lysyl residues in the nascent collagen chains. Since vitamin C is a necessary cofactor of lysyl hydroxylase, pharmacologic doses may be beneficial.

Ehlers–Danlos type VII (arthrochalasis multiplex congenita) is typified by profound loose-jointedness, congenital dislocations, moderately short stature, and variable skin involvement. The underlying defect is an inability to cleave the N-propeptide from type I procollagen, which is necessary for conversion to mature collagen. Mutations at the cleavage site of α1(I) and α(I) procollagens and in the N-propeptidase can cause this phenotype; the procollagen defects behave as dominant traits, while the enzymopathy is recessive.

JOINT INSTABILITY SYNDROMES

The cardinal manifestation of *familial joint instability,* which once was classified as an Ehlers–Danlos type, is instability of numerous appendicular joints; recurrent dislocation is the usual presenting complaint (13). Joint hyperextensibility is variable but usually mild, and skin involvement is uncommon. This syndrome is not rare and is often associated with considerable disability. Autosomal dominant inheritance with marked variability within a family is the rule, which emphasizes the need for a comprehensive family history, including examination of close relatives, if possible. The biochemical defect is unknown.

Larsen syndrome is characterized by congenital and recurrent joint dislocations, skeletal dysplasia, and facial features of prominent forehead, depressed nasal bridge, and widely spaced eyes (14). Dislocation occurs at the knees (characteristically anterior displacement of the tibia on the femur), hips, and elbows. The metacarpals are short with cylindrical fingers lacking the usual tapering. Some patients also have cleft palate, hydrocephalus, abnormalities of spinal segmentation, and moderate-to-severe short stature. Several instances of multiple affected siblings with normal parents are known, suggesting autosomal recessive inheritance, but parent–child involvement also occurs, which is consistent with dominant inheritance. Thus, two clinically indistinguishable forms of Larsen syndrome may exist.

OSTEOGENESIS IMPERFECTA SYNDROMES

Several phenotypically distinct osteogenesis imperfecta syndromes exist (2,3,10,15). The disorders share osseous, ocular, dental, aural, and cardiovascular involvement. The current system of classification is based on inheritance pattern and clinical criteria (Table 39-2).

Type I osteogenesis imperfecta, the most common form, is autosomal dominant and is associated with considerable intrafamilial variability. One patient might be markedly short in stature, with frequent fractures and much disability, whereas an affected relative leads an unencumbered, vigorous life. Defects in the genes for both α1(I) and α2(I) procollagen can cause this syndrome.

(Table 39-2)
*Osteogenesis imperfecta syndromes**

Type	Inheritance	Skeletal Features	Sclerae	Other Features
IA	AD	Variable bony fragility and short stature, Wormian bones	Blue	Opalescent teeth, hearing loss
IB	AD	Variable bony fragility and short stature, Wormian bones	Blue	Normal teeth, hearing loss
II	AD	In utero fractures, little calvarial calcium	Blue	Pulmonary hypertension, neonatal death usual
III	Most sporadic	Variable fragility, deformity, scoliosis, joint laxity	Variable	Some with opalescent teeth
IVA	AD	Variable bony fragility and short stature, Wormian bones	Normal	Opalescent teeth, hearing loss
IVB	AD	Variable bony fragility and short stature, Wormian bones	Normal	Normal teeth, hearing loss

* AD = autosomal dominant.

Type II osteogenesis imperfecta encompasses the classic congenital variants, nearly all of which are lethal in infancy, if not in utero. Most cases arise as the result of a new mutation (the phenotype thus being transmissible as autosomal dominant, if the patient could live and reproduce) in either α1(I) or α2(I) procollagen. A "dominant-negative" model explains the severe phenotype produced by a heterozygous mutation. Rare patients have affected siblings and normal parents; in some of these cases, a parent has been shown to have the mutation at low level (1% to 10%) in the gonads.

Type III osteogenesis imperfecta comprises severe skeletal deformity, kyphoscoliosis, short stature, and variable fractures, and usually occurs sporadically, which suggests new mutations or autosomal recessive inheritance. *Type IV osteogenesis imperfecta* is similar phenotypically and genetically to type I, but it is rarer and not associated with blue sclerae.

The natural histories of the skeletal involvement among these types bear similarities. "Brittle bones" are a unifying theme; sometimes fractures occur in utero, particularly in type II, and permit radiographic antenatal diagnosis. In such cases, the limbs are likely to be short and bent at birth, and multiple rib fractures give a characteristic "beaded" appearance on radiographs. Other patients with types I or IV have few fractures or may escape them entirely, although the presence of blue sclerae, opalescent teeth, or hearing loss indicates the presence of the mutant gene. Brittleness and deformability result from a defect in the collagenous matrix of bone. The skeletal aspect of osteogenesis imperfecta is, therefore, a hereditary form of osteoporosis. "Codfish vertebrae" (scalloping of the superior and inferior vertebral bodies by pressure from the expansible intervertebral disc) or flat vertebrae are observed, particularly in older patients whose defects are exaggerated by senile or postmenopausal bone changes and in young patients who are immobilized after fractures or orthopedic surgery.

Usually the frequency of fractures decreases at puberty for patients with types I, III, and IV. Because union of fractures sometimes fail, pseudo-arthrosis may occur. Hypertrophic callus is common and may be difficult to distinguish from osteosarcoma. Debate continues as to whether the risk of true osteosarcoma is increased in any form of osteogenesis imperfecta. Regardless, the risk is not great, but osteosarcoma should be considered whenever skeletal pain occurs in the absence of fracture, particularly in an older patient. Joint laxity is sometimes striking in type I; dislocation of joints can result from deformity secondary to repeated fractures, lax ligaments, or tendon rupture.

The differential diagnosis of osteogenesis imperfecta includes idiopathic juvenile osteoporosis, Cheney syndrome (osteoporosis, multiple wormian bones, acro-osteolysis), pyknodysostosis (dwarfism, brittle bones, absent mandibular ramus, persistent cranial fontanelles, acro-osteolysis), and hypophosphatasia (14). In one family with a susceptibility to osteoporosis, the culprit was a mutation in type I collagen. This finding emphasizes that the ability to identify mutations in a particular gene does not necessarily facilitate clinical diagnosis. Furthermore, patients with common problems that are not thought to be syndromes may result from defects in one or another of the components of the extracellular matrix.

PSEUDOXANTHOMA ELASTICUM

The cardinal features of pseudoxanthoma elasticum involve the eyes, blood vessels, and skin (16). Although the most easily recognized finding in the ocular fundus is the angioid streak, which is caused by a break in Bruch's membrane, progressive visual loss occurs from retinal hemorrhages. The elastic fibers in the media of muscular arteries degenerates and the arterial wall develops a histologic pattern similar to Mönckeberg arteriosclerosis. Peripheral pulses are gradually lost, and intermittent claudication is common. Myocardial infarction, stroke, and gastrointestinal hemorrhage are also complications of vascular involvement and are the leading causes of death. The name of this condition is derived from the characteristic skin lesions that develop in regions of flexural stress and resemble plucked chicken skin. The skeleton and joints are not usually involved. Elastic fibers throughout the body show calcification. The basic defect is unclear, but genetic heterogeneity is evident by both autosomal recessive (the most common form) and autosomal dominant inheritance.

FIBRODYSPLASIA OSSIFICANS PROGRESSIVA

Fibrodysplasia ossificans progressiva (FOP) is characterized by progressive ossification of ligaments, tendons, and aponeuroses (17). An inexorable course begins in the first year or so of life, usually with a seemingly inflammatory process and nodule formation on the back of the thorax, neck, or scalp. Local heat, leukocytosis, and elevated sedimentation rate are observed at this stage, and these children are sometimes diagnosed with acute rheumatic fever. A valuable clue to the correct diagnosis is a short great toe, with or without a short thumb. FOP is the leading cause of congenital hallux valgus. Most cases of this autosomal dominant disorder are the consequence of new mutation. Life expectancy is considerably reduced, with progressive restriction in lung capacity contributing to respiratory insufficiency and terminal pneumonia.

MUCOPOLYSACCHARIDOSES

The mucopolysaccharidoses (MPS) are the result of inborn errors of proteoglycan catabolism (18). While phenotypically diverse, the individual disorders share mucopolysacchariduria and deposition of catabolites of proteoglycan in various tissues. Numerous distinct types of MPS can be distinguished on the basis of combined phenotypic, genetic, and biochemical analysis (Table 39-3). Relative short stature is the rule in all forms of MPS and can be profound in types IH (Hurler syndrome), II (Hunter syndrome), IV (Morquio syndrome, the prototypic "short trunk" form of dwarfism), and VI (Maroteaux–Lamy syndrome). Radiologically, the skeletal dysplasia is quite similar in character in all but MPS IV, differing among the others largely in severity (14). Although the term *dysostosis multiplex* has been used, it is not specific for the MPS because similar changes occur in a variety of storage disorders. The chief radiologic features are a thick calvaria, an enlarged J-shaped sella turcica, a short and wide mandible, biconvex vertebral bodies, hypoplasia of the odontoid, broad ribs, short and thick clavicles, coxa valga, metacarpals with widened diaphyses and pointed proximal ends, and short phalanges.

Survival to adulthood without severe retardation occurs with types IS (Scheie syndrome), II mild, IV, and VI. In these forms, progressive arthropathy and transverse myelopathy secondary to C1-C2 subluxation account for considerable disability. Joint replacement, particularly of the hips, has

(Table 39-3)
The mucopolysaccharidoses

Type	Eponym	Clinical Findings	Enzyme Deficiency
MPS I H	Hurler	Clouding of cornea, grave manifestations, death usually before age 10	α-L-iduronidase
MPS I S	Scheie	Stiff joints, cloudy corneae aortic valve disease, normal intelligence	α-L-iduronidase
MPS I H/S	Hurler–Scheie	Intermediate phenotype	α-L-iduronidase
MPS II, severe	Hunter, severe	No corneal clouding, grave manifestations, death before 15 years	Iduronate sulfatase
MPS II, mild	Hunter, mild	Survival to 30s to 60s, fair-to-normal intelligence; obstruction of airways, sleep apnea	Iduronate sulfatase
MPS IIIA	Sanfilippo A	Mild coarse facies and short stature, severe mental retardation	Heparan N-sulfatase
MPS IIIB	Sanfilippo B	Same as IIIA	N-acetyl-α-D-glucosaminidase
MPS IIIC	Sanfilippo C	Same as IIIA	Acetyl-CoA:α-glucosaminide N-acetyltranferase
MPS IIID	Sanfilippo D	Same as IIIA	N-acetylglucosamine-6-sulfate sulfatase
MPS IVA	Morquio A	Severe, distinctive bone changes, cloudy cornea, aortic regurgitation, thin enamel	Galactosamine-6-sulfate sulfatase
MPS IVB	Morquio B	Mild bone changes, cloudy corneae, hypoplastic odontoid, normal enamel	β-galactosidase
MPS VI, severe	Maroteaux–Lamy classic severe	Severe osseous and corneal changes, valvular heart disease, striking WBC inclusions, normal intellect, survival to 20s or beyond	Arylsulfatase B (N-acetylgalactosamine 4-sulfatase)
MPS VI, milder forms	Maroteaux–Lamy	Mild-moderately severe changes	Arylsulfatase B (N-acetylgalactosamine 4-sulfatase)
MPS VII	Sly	Hepatosplenomegaly, dysostosis multiplex, mental retardation, WBC inclusions	β-glucuronidase

been beneficial in several forms, especially type IS. Cervical fusion should be considered whenever upper motor neuron signs appear, a particular concern in types IH, IV, and VI. Stiff joints are a more or less striking feature of all except type IV. Like other somatic features, such as coarse facies, reduced joint mobility is less striking in type III. In type IS, stiff hands, hip arthropathy, and clouding of the cornea produce the main disabilities. Carpal tunnel syndrome contributes to the disability in all types. The major life-threatening problems in types II mild, IV, and VI are valvular heart disease and progressive narrowing of the middle and lower airways. Narrowing of the lower airway frequently presents as obstructive sleep apnea or complications with general anesthesia.

Genetic disturbances of mucopolysaccharide metabolism without mucopolysacchariduria include the mucolipidoses (19). Type II, which is also called I-cell disease because of conspicuous inclusions in cultured cells, is a severe disorder similar to Hurler syndrome. Patients with type III, also called pseudo-Hurler polydystrophy, have stiff joints, cloudy cornea, carpal tunnel syndrome, short stature, coarse facies, and sometimes mild mental retardation; often they survive to adulthood. Neither type II nor type III produce mucopolysacchariduria despite lysosomal storage of mucopolysaccharide and a demonstrable defect in degradation of mucopolysaccharides. Both are autosomal recessive and genetically heterogeneous. The basic biochemical defect is an enzyme responsible for post-translational modification of lysosomal enzymes. This defect results in multiple enzyme deficiencies and accumulation of both mucopolysaccharides and mucolipids in tissues.

Mucopolysacchariduria can be identified by one of several standard screening tests, at least one of which is part of the standard battery performed when a metabolic screen is ordered. Fractionation and characterization of the urinary mucopolysaccharides are useful in separating the several types of disorders, but enzymatic assay may be needed for diagnostic confirmation. Prenatal diagnosis by biochemical or molecular genetic methods is possible (20).

Like other lysosomal disorders, the mucopolysaccharide and mucolipid disorders have the following distinctive characteristics: 1) intracellular storage occurs; 2) the storage material is heterogeneous because the degradative enzymes are not strictly specific; 3) deposition is vacuolar on electron microscopy; 4) many tissues are affected; and 5) the disorders are clinically progressive. Replacement of the deficient enzyme is possible but technically difficult and of transient benefit. Bone marrow transplant is clearly effective in the disorders lacking central nervous system involvement and is still being investigated in patients who are mentally retarded.

REED EDWIN PYERITZ, MD, PhD

1. McKusick VA: On-line Mendelian Inheritance in Man. Baltimore, Johns Hopkins University Press, 1996 ["help@gdb.org."]
2. Royce PM, Steinmann B (eds): Connective Tissue and Its Heritable Disorders: Molecular, Genetic and Medical Aspects. New York, Wiley-Liss, 1993
3. Beighton P (ed): McKusick's Heritable Disorders of Connective Tissue, 5th ed. St. Louis, CV Mosby, 1993
4. Beighton P, de Paepe A, Danks D, et al: International nosology of heritable disorders of connective tissue, Berlin, 1986. Am J Med Genet 29:581-594, 1988

5. Pyeritz RE: Disorders of fibrillins and microfibrilogenesis: marfan syndrome, MASS phenotype, contractural arachnodactyly and related conditions. In Rimoin DL, Connor JM, Pyeritz RE (eds): Principles and Practice of Medical Genetics, 3rd ed. New York, Churchill Livingstone, 1997

6. Dietz HC, Pyeritz RE: Mutations in the human gene for fibrillin-1 (*FBN1*) in the Marfan syndrome and related disorders. Hum Molec Genet 4:1799-1809, 1995

7. Pyeritz RE: Homocystinuria. In Beighton P (ed): McKusick's Heritable Disorders of Connective Tissue, 5th ed. St. Louis, CV Mosby, 1993, pp 137-178

8. Rai A, Wordsworth P, Cappock JS, Zaphiropoulos GC, Struthers GR: Hereditary arthro-ophthalmopathy (Stickler syndrome): a diagnosis to consider in familial premature osteoarthritis. Br J Rheumatol 33:1175-1180, 1994

9. Byers PH: The Ehlers-Danlos syndromes. In Rimoin DL, Connor JM, Pyeritz RE (eds): Principles and Practice of Medical Genetics, 3rd ed. New York, Churchill Livingstone, 1997, pp 1067-1081

10. Byers PH: Disorders of collagen biosynthesis and structure. In Scriver CR, Beaudet AL, Sly WS, Valle DZ (eds): Metabolic and Molecular Bases of Inherited Disease, 7th ed. New York, McGraw-Hill, 1995, pp 4029-4078

11. Loughlin J, Irven C, Hardwick LJ, Butcher S, Walsh S, Wordsworth P, Sykes B: Linkage of the gene that encodes the α1 chain of type V collagen (COL5A1) to type II Ehlers–Danlos syndrome (EDS II). Hum Molec Genet 9:1649-1651, 1995

12. Beighton P, Grahame R, Bird H: Hypermobility of Joints, 2nd ed. New York, Springer-Verlag, 1989

13. Horton WA, Collins DL, DeSmet AA, Kennedy JA, Schmike RN: Familial joint instability syndrome. Am J Med Genet 6:221-228, 1980

14. Wynne-Davies R, Hall CM, Apley AG: Atlas of Skeletal Dysplasias. Edinburgh, Livingstone, 1985

15. Byers PH: Brittle bones-fragile molecules: disorders of collagen gene structure and expression. Trends Genet 6:293-300, 1990

16. Pope FM: Inherited abnormalities of elastic tissue. In Rimoin DL, Connor JM, Pyeritz RE (eds): Principles and Practice of Medical Genetics, 3rd ed. New York, Churchill Livingstone, 1997, pp 1083-1119

17. Conner JM, Evans DAP: Fibrodysplasia ossificans progressiva: the clinical features and natural history of 34 patients. J Bone Joint Surg 64B:766-783, 1982

18. Neufeld EF, Muenzer J. The mucopolysaccharidoses. In Scriver CR, Beaudet AL, Sly WS, Valle D (eds): The Metabolic and Molecular Bases of Inherited Disease. 7th Edition. New York, McGraw-Hill, 1995, pp 2465-2494

19. Kornfield S, Sly WS: I-cell disease and pseudo-hurler polydystrophy: disorders of lysosomal enzyme phosphorylation. In: Scriver CR, Scriver CR, Beaudet AL, Valle D (eds): The Metabolic and Molecular Bases of Inherited Disease. New York, McGraw-Hill, 1995, pp 2495-2508

20. Pyeritz RE: Prenatal diagnosis of connective tissue disorders. In Milunsky A (ed): Genetic Disorders and the Fetus: Diagnosis, Prevention and Treatment, 3rd ed. Baltimore, Johns Hopkins University Press, 1992, pp 491-506

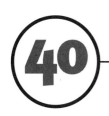

MISCELLANEOUS SYNDROMES INVOLVING SKIN AND JOINTS

40

LOBULAR PANNICULITIS

Several inflammatory diseases primarily affect cutaneous fat lobules. Two of these, Weber–Christian disease and pancreatic panniculitis, are associated with joint manifestations.

Weber–Christian disease is characterized by recurrent crops of erythematous nodules and plaques, particularly over the lower extremities but also on the arms, trunk, face, breasts, and buttocks. It is seen especially in young to middle-aged women. Systemic involvement of the mesentery, heart, lungs, kidneys, liver, spleen, adrenal glands, bone marrow, and central nervous system can occur. The development of skin lesions can be associated with fever, malaise, nausea, vomiting, abdominal pain, weight loss, hepatomegaly, and arthralgias. Painful osteolytic lesions have been reported (1). The prognosis is usually good, with gradual spontaneous resolution of the attacks, but the systemic form is occasionally fatal (2). The predominant causes of death are sepsis, hepatic failure, hemorrhage, and thrombosis.

Diagnosis of Weber–Christian disease requires a skin biopsy that includes fat. An α_1-antitrypsin level should be obtained to rule out a deficiency, although lesions seen in α_1-antitrypsin deficiency are clinically somewhat different, with frequent ulceration and oozing (3). Treatment includes nonsteroidal anti-inflammatory drugs (NSAIDs), corticosteroids, and antimalarial and immunosuppressive drugs.

Pancreatic panniculitis occurs in patients with either pancreatitis or pancreatic cancer of the acinar cells (4,5). The clinical appearance is tender red nodules, commonly in the pretibial region, but nodules may also occur on the thighs, buttocks, and other areas. If the fat necrosis is severe, the lesions can ulcerate, similar to that seen with α_1–antitrypsin deficiency. The skin lesions are often associated with arthralgias, especially in the ankles, which result from periarticular fat necrosis. Monarticular or oligoarticular arthritis affecting joints in the vicinity of skin lesions occurs in 60% of patients; fever, osteolytic bone lesions, pleuritis, pericarditis, or synovitis can also occur (6). The skin lesions frequently precede the diagnosis of pancreatic disease (5).

Skin biopsies of acute lesions show lobular and septal panniculitis with characteristic areas of fat necrosis consisting of ghost-like fat cells. Basophilic deposits of calcium may be seen. Chronic lesions show granulomatous and lipophagic panniculitis.

Pathogenesis may be related to the release of pancreatic enzymes such as trypsin, amylase, and lipase. Serum lipase or amylase levels are often increased, and increased levels have been found in fluid aspirated from skin lesions and pleural, pericardial, and ascitic fluid (4). Eosinophilia can occur. Cholecystectomy for gallstone-induced pancreatitis may be curative (5).

ERYTHEMA NODOSUM

Erythema nodosum is a syndrome of inflammatory cutaneous nodules, often found on the extensor lower legs. It can be acute, chronic, or migratory, it occurs three times more frequently in females, and it has a peak incidence between the ages of 20 and 30 years. Often the disease is self-limited and resolves in 3–6 weeks. Several conditions are associated with erythema nodosum (Table 40-1). The triad of bilateral hilar lymphadenopathy, erythema nodosum, and polyarthralgias is called Lofgren's syndrome. One-half of these patients have acute sarcoidosis, and the other half have an infection. The arthralgias can persist after resolution of skin lesions. Histology shows inflammation and thickening of the septae in the fat.

Diagnostic tests should usually include a full-thickness skin biopsy. Other tests that may be helpful on initial work-up include complete blood count with differential, antistreptolysin titer, chest x-ray, pharyngeal culture, and intradermal skin tests for tuberculosis, coccidioidomycosis, blastomycosis, and histoplasmosis. Virologic and yersinial titers may be helpful (7,8). Isolated cases have been seen with IgA nephropathy and cryoglobulinemia, both of which are associated with circulating immune complexes.

Treatment of any underlying condition is helpful. Bed rest, NSAIDs, potassium iodide, and occasionally oral glucocorticoids can be helpful.

ACNE SYNDROMES

Acne vulgaris is a common abnormality involving sebaceous follicles. The type of acne lesion depends on the depth

(Table 40-1)
Associations with erythema nodosum

Medications:	Sulfonamides, estrogen, oral contraceptives
Infections: Bacterial	*Streptococcus*, tuberculosis, *Yersinia*, leprosy, leptospirosis, tularemia, cat-scratch disease
Fungal	Coccidioidomycosis, blastomycosis, histoplasmosis, dermatophytes
Viruses	Paravaccina, infectious mononucleosis
Sarcoidosis	
Inflammatory bowel disease	
Malignancy:	Lymphoma and leukemia, postradiation therapy
Behçet's syndrome	
Pregnancy	

of inflammation into the dermis. More severe forms of acne have deeper subcutaneous invasion, leading to nodules and cysts. The more severe acne syndromes discussed below are associated with musculoskeletal abnormalities.

Acne Conglobata

This syndrome includes polyporous comedones, cysts, deep abscesses, draining sinuses, and bridging scars occurring on the buttocks, thighs, upper arms, face, posterior neck, back, and chest. Although most patients with acne conglobata are white, the associated musculoskeletal syndrome occurs mostly in black men over age 22. Musculoskeletal involvement is associated with skin flares and includes sacroiliitis with or without a peripheral arthropathy (9,10). Peripheral joint involvement is symmetric in 60% of patients. Arthralgias can be present. The disease is recurrent and episodic. The radiologic abnormalities include soft tissue swelling, periarticular osteoporosis, cartilage loss with joint space narrowing, erosions, periostitis, new bone formation, and alignment abnormalities. Coarse paravertebral ossifications, hyperostoses, smooth anterior syndesmophyte formations with corner erosions and sclerosis, and calcified tendons also have been reported. There are no constitutional symptoms. The triad of follicular occlusion includes acne conglobata, hidradenitis suppurativa, and dissecting cellulitis of the scalp, and has similar patient characteristics and musculoskeletal symptoms to acne conglobata alone.

Acne Fulminans

A rare form of acne seen mostly in white male adolescents, acne fulminans consists of a sudden onset of nodulocystic and ulcerated cysts on the face, back, chest, and shoulders. Acne vulgaris precedes this disorder, and exacerbation occurs with viral illness, stress, fatigue, or onset of isotretinoin treatment. Acne fulminans is associated with fever, weight loss, myalgia, myositis, elevated erythrocyte sedimentation rate (ESR), leukocytosis, anemia, osteoarthritis, and sterile osteolytic bone lesions. Circulating immune complexes have been detected in several cases. The bone lesions can be painful and occur most often in the clavicles and metaphyses of long bones. They tend to flare with the skin lesions and can be detected by bone scan. Arthritis is present in one-third of patients with the acne fulminans-associated musculoskeletal syndrome. Arthralgias and myalgias of the hips and shoulders are common. Myositis, associated with muscle weakness, normal muscle enzyme levels, and abnormalities on electromyelograms occur rarely. The arthritis is nondeforming, self-limited, and often involves the knees. Small-joint involvement and sacroiliitis are relatively uncommon. Sterile osteolytic bone lesions of the clavicles and metaphysis of long bones are commonly seen, a finding not typically found with acne conglobata (11). Radiographs of large joints often show diffuse areas of demineralization, periosteal new bone formation, and transverse bands of radiolucency. Biopsy of synovium has shown mild hyperplasia with moderate numbers of lymphocytes and plasma cells. Treatment includes isotretinoin, dapsone, oral corticosteroids, and azathioprine. Even with treatment, the prognosis is variable; some patients experience recurrent episodes of arthritis, arthralgias, and myalgias for years. Acne fulminans leaves cutaneous scars.

The pathogenesis of acne-associated musculoskeletal syndromes is unclear. Some patients with acne fulminans have an exaggerated response to intradermal *Propionibacterium acnes* antigen. Patients with acne conglobata have increased lymphocyte proliferation in response to *P. acnes,* but not to phytohemagglutinin, and some of these patients develop antibody against *P. acnes.*

Isotretinoin use for acne is associated in 27% of patients with mild transient myalgias and arthralgias that do not require stopping the treatment. About 10% of patients with these symptoms develop asymptomatic, small, hyperostotic lesions of the spine. Other isotretinoin-associated abnormalities include soft-tissue calcification of tendons and ligaments and arthritis (12). The musculoskeletal abnormalties of the various syndromes are summarized in Table 40-2.

PUSTULOSIS PALMARIS ET PLANTARIS

This disorder is a chronic, relapsing pustular eruption of the palms and soles. The pustules are seen mainly on the thenar eminence, mid-palm, heel, and instep. Pustulosis palmaris et plantaris has been associated with chronic recurrent multifocal osteomyelitis (CRMO) and sternocostoclavicular hyperostosis (SCCH). CRMO begins with an insidious pain and swelling of the affected bones, most commonly the medial ends of the clavicles and the distal metaphyses of long bones. It usually occurs in children and young adults, affecting females more than males, and 20% of those affected develop palmoplantar pustulosis. Diagnosis is based on the acute bone changes of lytic lesions with sclerotic rims adjacent to the growth plate and dense sclerosis in the chronic stage. Bone scan is more sensitive than radiographs. Laboratory tests show a mild leukocytosis and ESR. Rare complications include premature closure of the epiphyses, bony growth abnormalities, and thoracic outlet syndrome. The natural history of CRMO is recurrent exacerbations over months to years. Treatment with oral glucocorticoids is effective, but relapse after stopping the drug is common.

Most patients with SCCH have palmoplantar pustulosis. The SCCH causes pain and swelling in the upper anterior chest wall. Some patients have arthritis, ankylosing spondylitis, and sacroiliitis (13), and associated psoriatic skin lesions are common. SCCH appears to start in the soft tissue and secondarily involve bone. Complications rarely include subclavian compression and thrombophlebitis.

(Table 40-2)

Characteristics of musculoskelatal syndromes associated with acne*

Characteristic	AC	AF	Isotretinoin
Age (years)	>22	≤22	≤15
Gender (F:M)	1:4	1:37	1:1
Race	black	white	
Constitutional symptoms	–	+	–
Myalgias	–	+	–
Myositis	–	+	–
Arthralgias	+	+	+
Arthritis	+	+	–
Bone lesions	–	+	–
Skeletal hyperostoses	–	–	+

*Adapted from reference 9, with permission. AC = acne conglobata; AF = acne fulminans

SAPHO SYNDROME

Palmoplantar pustulosis, severe acne, and hidradenitis suppurativa are sometimes associated with aseptic skeletal conditions. The term SAPHO syndrome is an acronym for this cluster of findings, which includes synovitis, acne, palmoplantar pustulosis, hyperostosis, and osteitis (14). The upper anterior chest wall is most commonly involved, with osteosclerotic lesions, hyperostosis, and arthritis of adjacent joints. Osteosclerosis of vertebral bodies, hyperostosis, erosion of the vertebral plates, and unilateral sacroiliitis are frequently seen. Long bones can show osteosclerosis or osteolysis with periosteal new bone formation. Peripheral arthritis may be present but does not usually cause joint destruction. Awareness of this syndrome is important to avoid misdiagnosis of tumor or infection involving bone. A relationship between SAPHO syndrome and seronegative spondyloarthropathies is likely.

SWEET'S SYNDROME

Acute febrile neutrophilic dermatosis, or Sweet's syndrome, is usually seen in middle-aged women and presents with tender, red-blue papules and plaques on the face, neck, and arms (Fig. 40-1). Pustules and bullae may be present. Patients often have systemic symptoms, including fever, malaise, conjunctivitis, iridocyclitis, proteinuria, oral ulcerations, arthralgias, and arthritis (15). Approximately 20%–50% of patients have an acute self-limited polyarthritis involving the hands, wrists, ankles, and knees that occurs with the skin eruption (16). On rare occasions, pulmonary, renal, liver, pancreatic, or neurologic involvement has been reported (15). Elevated ESR and alkaline phosphatase are common. Sterile osteomyelitis is a rare development (15). Idiopathic Sweet's syndrome resolves spontaneously in 1–3 months if untreated, but 30% of patients have recurrences.

Skin pathology reveals a neutrophilic infiltrate with leukocytoclasis and edema of the papillary dermis. There is no evidence of vasculitis. Sweet's syndrome is associated with underlying malignancies in 10% of patients, particularly hematologic malignancies such as myeloid and myelomonocytic leukemia, but it has also been seen after respiratory illnesses, inflammatory bowel disease, pregnancy, and connective tissue disease. Approximately 50% of patients have a coexisting underlying condition (15).

The etiology of Sweet's syndrome is unknown, but some clinical aspects suggest that it is due to an immunologic reaction.

Orally administered glucocorticoids are usually effective. Other treatments include dapsone, aspirin, indomethacin, colchicine, doxycycline, clofazimine, potassium iodide, and cyclosporine.

PYODERMA GANGRENOSUM

Pyoderma gangrenosum is an uncommon ulcerative skin condition that is associated with underlying systemic diseases in about 50% of patients. The clinical appearance includes painful ulcers, commonly found on the legs, with well-defined, undermined borders with a surrounding erythema (Fig. 40-2). Lesions often begin as pustules. Healing of ulcers results in atrophic and cribriform scars. A superficial

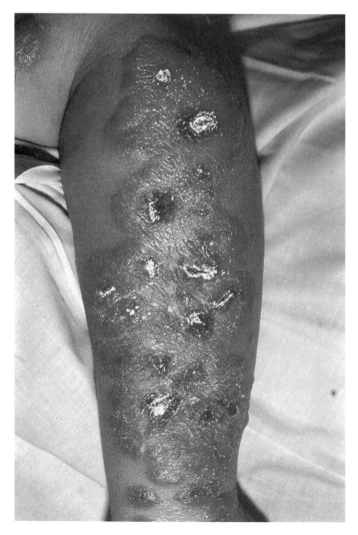

(Figure 40-1)
Typical cutaneous plaques of Sweet's sydrome.

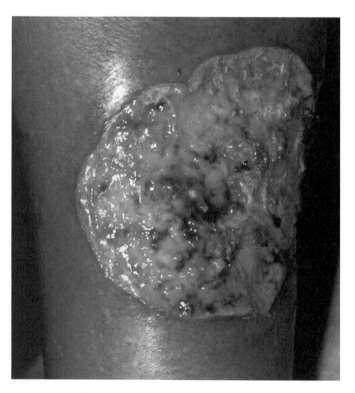

(Figure 40-2)
Typical leg ulcer of pyoderma gangrenosum in a patient with ulcerative colitis.

ulcer with bullous borders has been seen in association with preleukemic or leukemic conditions. Some patients with pyoderma gangrenosum develop arthralgias and a progressive erosive arthritis that is independent of an underlying rheumatoid arthritis condition.

Pyoderma gangrenosum is associated with inflammatory bowel disease (both Crohn's disease and ulcerative colitis), seronegative rheumatoid arthritis, and hematologic diseases (myelocytic leukemias, hairy cell leukemia, and myelofibrosis) (17). The inflammatory bowel disease can be asymptomatic and detected only by radiography. The course of the skin disease can be independent of the activity of the bowel disease or rheumatoid arthritis.

Histology in pyoderma gangrenosum is not diagnostic, but biopsies need to be done to rule out other causes of ulcers, such as vasculitis or infection. A monoclonal gammopathy, usually IgA but occasionally IgG or IgM, is seen in 10%–20% of cases. Work-up of suspected pyoderma gangrenosum should include a careful history and physical examination, skin biopsy for routine pathology and culture, gastrointestinal tract studies, complete blood cell count, and serum and immunoelectrophoresis. Immunofixation electrophoresis has been shown to be more sensitive in detecting the associated monoclonal gammopathies (18).

Pathogenesis of pyoderma gangrenosum is unknown, but numerous immunologic abnormalities have been described. Multiple granulocyte abnormalities involving chemotaxis, migration, defective bactericidal capacity, and oxidative burst have been identified. Abnormalities in cell-mediated immunity have also been noted. Treatment includes proper management of any underlying systemic disease, local therapy, sulfa and sulfones (dapsone, sulfasalazine, sulfapyridine), topical or intralesional glucocorticoids, oral and/or pulse intravenous prednisone, hyperbaric oxygen, clofazimine, minocycline, rifampin, cytotoxic drugs (azathioprine, cyclophosphamide, chlorambucil), and cyclosporine.

LICHEN MYXEDEMATOUS

This rare fibromucinous disorder consists of skin findings including waxy papules, sclerosis, and induration of the skin involving the hands, arms, face, trunk, and legs. There are some features of scleroderma, such as acrosclerosis, flexion contractures, and decreased oral orifice. On skin biopsy there is mucin in the dermis, diffusely thickened skin, and an increased number of large, stellate fibroblasts associated with irregular collagen bundles. Usually an associated monoclonal IgG lambda gammopathy is present. Other associations include multiple myeloma, Waldenstrom's macroglobulinemia, non-Hodgkins lymphoma, esophageal aperistalsis, inflammatory myopathy, erosive arthritis, median neuropathy, and sicca complex (19). The myopathy is commonly associated with dysphagia, and elevations in muscle enzymes and electromyelographic abnormalities are common. Raynaud's phenomenon, calcinosis cutis, telangiectasias, pulmonary diffusion abnormalities and hypertension, and digital ulcers are rare. Systemic disease with muscle weakness, dysphagia, and weight loss can occur. The course of the disease is variable, with reports of some patients having spontaneous resolution and others having a stable uncomplicated course. The etiology of scleromyxedema is unknown. Serum from patients with lichen myxedematous can stimulate proliferation of normal human skin fibroblasts in culture. It is possible that IgG lambda paraproteins activate the fibroblast.

Treatment has included retinoids, corticosteroids, PUVA (oral psoralen with UV radiation therapy), plasmapheresis, photopheresis, and chemotherapeutic agents. Treatment with melphalan, prednisone, and cyclophosphamide has been used. Melphalan carries a risk of sepsis and hematologic malignancies.

ERYTHEMA ELEVATUM DIUTINUM

Clinical features of erythema elevatum diutinum include multiple persistent erythematous plaques and nodules that are often located over extensor surfaces of joints on the hands, arms, and legs. The lesions can be pruritic or painful, especially after exposure to cold, and there are often arthralgias of the associated joint. Early lesions can be bullous or vesicular (Fig. 40-3). An association with rheumatoid arthritis has been reported (20).

Biopsy of early lesions shows a leukocytoclastic vasculitis with a dense neutrophilic dermal infiltrate, but later biopsies show fibrosis. Paraproteinemias, especially IgA, have been reported.

The etiology of erythema elevatum diutinum is unknown, but it is thought that immune complexes are involved in a similar mechanism seen in other forms of leukocytoclastic vasculitis. Intradermal injection of streptococcal antigen in patients with this disorder has induced characteristic lesions (21).

VICTORIA P. WERTH, MD

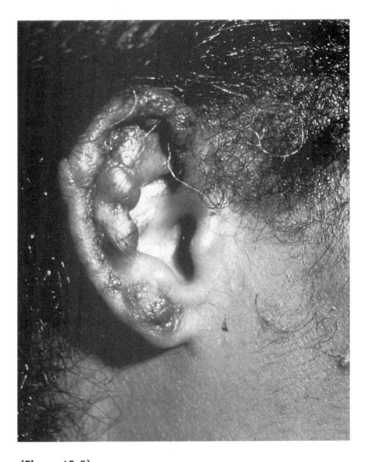

(Figure 40-3)
Tender skin nodules due to the cutaneous vasculitis of erythema elevatum diutinum.

1. Pinals RS: Nodular panniculitis associated with an inflammatory bone lesion. Arch Dermatol 101:359-363, 1970

2. Ciclitira PJ, Wight DGD, Dick AP: Systemic Weber-Christian disease. Br J Dermatol 103:685-692, 1980

3. Smith KC, Su WPD, Pitelkow MR, Winkelmann RK: Clinical and pathologic correlations in 96 patients with panniculitis, including 15 patients with deficient levels of alpha 1-antitrypsin. J Am Acad Dermatol 21:1192-1196, 1989

4. Mullen GT, Caperton EM Jr, Crespin Sr, Williams RC Jr: Arthritis and skin lesions resembling erythema nodosum in pancreatic disease. Ann Intern Med 68:75-87, 1968

5. Dahl PR, Su WPD, Cullimore KC, Dicken CH: Pancreatic panniculitis. J Am Acad Dermatol 33:413-417, 1995

6. van Klaveran RJ, de Mulder PHM, Boerbooms AMT, Van de Kaa CA, van Haelst UJGM, Wagener DJT, Hafkenscheid JCM: Pancreatic carcinoma with polyarthritis, fat necrosis, and high serum lipase and trypsin activity. Gut 31:953-955, 1990

7. Schorr-Lesnick B, Brandt LJ: Selected rheumatologic and dermatologic manifestations of inflammatory bowel disease. Am J Gastro 83:216-223, 1988

8. White JW: Erythema nodosum. Dermatol Clin 3:119-127, 1985

9. Knitzer RH, Needleman BW: Musculoskeletal syndromes associated with acne. Semin Arthritis Rheum 20:247-255, 1991

10. Rosner IA, Burg CG, Wisnieski JJ, Schacter BZ, Richter DE: The clinical spectrum of the arthropathy associated with hidradenitis suppurativa and acne conglobata. J Rheumatol 20:684-687, 1993

11. Laasonen LS, Karvonen S-L, Reunala TL: Bone disease in adolescents with acne fulminans and severe cystic acne: radiologic and scintigraphic findings. Am J Radiology 162:1161-1165, 1994

12. Pittsley RA, Yoder FW: Retinoid hyperostosis: skeletal toxicity associated with long-term administration of 13-cis-retinoic acid for refractory ichthyosis. N Engl J Med 308:1012-1014, 1983

13. Kasperczyk A, Freyschmidt J: Pustulotic arthroosteitis: spectrum of bone lesions with palmoplantar pustulosis. Radiology 191:207-211, 1994

14. Benhamou CL, Shamot AM, Kahn MF: Synovitis acne pustulosis hyperstosis osteomyletitis syndrome (SAPHO): a new syndrome among the spondyloarthropathies. Clin Exp Rheumatol 6:109-112, 1988

15. von den Driesch P: Sweet's syndrome (acute febrile neutrophilic dermatosis). J Am Acad Dermatol 31:535-556, 1994

16. Krauser RE, Schumacher HR: The arthritis of Sweet's syndrome. Arthritis Rheum 18:35-41, 1975

17. Callen JP: Pyoderma gangrenosum and related disorders. Med Clin N Am 73:1247-12261, 1989

18. Prystowsky JH, Kahn SN, Lazarus GS: Present status of pyoderma gangrenosum. Arch Dermatol 125:57-64, 1989

19. Dineen AM, Dicken CH: Scleromyxedema J Am Acad Dermatol 33:37-43, 1995

20. Yiannias JA, El-Azhary RA, Gibson LE: Erythema elevatum diutinum: a clinical and histopathologic study of 13 patients. J Am Acad Dermatol 26:38-44, 1992

21. Wolff HH, Scherer R, Maciejewski W, Braun-Falco O: Erythema elevatum diutinum. II. Immunoelectronmicroscopical study of leukocytoclastic vasculitis within the intracutaneous test reaction induced by streptococcal antigen. Arch Dermatol Res 261:17-26, 1978

41

HYPERTROPHIC OSTEOARTHROPATHY

Hypertrophic osteoarthropathy (HOA) or *acropachy* is a syndrome characterized by excessive proliferation of skin and bone at the distal parts of the extremities. Its most conspicuous feature is a unique bulbous deformity of the tips of the digits, conventionally known as clubbing. In advanced stages, periosteal proliferation of the tubular bones and synovial effusions become evident. The classification scheme of HOA is shown in Table 41-1 (1).

PATHOLOGY AND PATHOGENESIS

The bulbous deformity of the digits develops as a result of edema and excessive collagen deposition. In addition, endothelial cell activation and vascular hyperplasia are prominent features (2). Excessive fibroblast proliferation along the tubular bones elevates the periosteum, and new osteoid matrix is deposited.

Cyanotic heart diseases are an excellent model for studying the pathogenesis of HOA (3), because practically all these patients have lifelong clubbing, and more than one-third display the fully developed syndrome. Abnormalities of platelets, a feature of cardiogenic HOA, may provide a clue to pathogenesis. Patients with cardiogenic HOA frequently have circulating macrothrombocytes with disfigured volume distribution curves. Such abnormalities suggest that normally large platelets break up in the highly dichotomized pulmonary vascular bed. In patients with hemodynamics of right-to-left shunt, large platelets gain direct access to the systemic circulation, reach its most distal sites on axial streams, and interact with endothelial cells, which subsequently release fibroblast growth factor(s), thus inducing acropachy (4). This hypothesis is further supported by the finding of elevated levels of von Willebrand factor antigen in patients with cardiogenic HOA, as well as those with the primary form of HOA (5). Similar mechanisms may be operative in other conditions associated with HOA. Lesser degrees of right-to-left shunt are evident in lung cancer, intestinal polyposis, and the hepatopulmonary syndrome of liver cirrhosis. Moreover, endothelial cell activation is a prominent feature of endarteritis and endocarditis of infective etiology. More studies are needed to elucidate the pathogenesis of HOA.

CLINICAL FEATURES

Many patients are asymptomatic and unaware of the deformity of their digits (Fig. 41-1). However, other patients, particularly those with malignant lung tumors, may suffer incapacitating bone pain (6). Characteristically, this pain is deep-seated, and is often more prominent in the legs as a result of lower limb dependency.

Because the bulbous deformity of the digits is unique, diagnosis is based primarily on physical examination. The increased volume of soft tissue molds the fingernails into a "watch-crystal" convexity, and the nailbed rocks when palpated. Toes may also be affected, but early changes are more difficult to discern due to the normal splaying of the toes. The digital index is a practical bedside method to measure clubbing. With a non-elastic string, the circumference of each finger at the nailbed (NB) and at the distal interphalangeal joint (DIP) is measured. If the sum of the 10 NB/DIP ratios is more than 10, clubbing is most likely present (7).

(Table 41-1)
Classification of osteoarthropathy

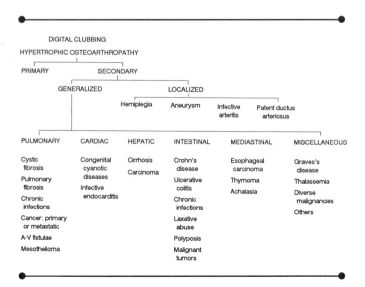

(Figure 41-1)
A clubbed finger on the left compared with a normal one on the right. The digital index is determined by measuring the circumference of each finger at the nailbed (NB) and the distal interphalangeal joint (DIP).

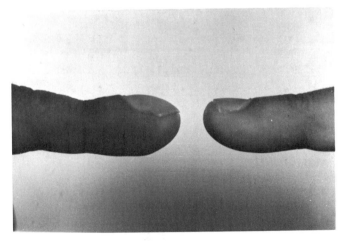

When the complete features of HOA are evident, thickening of the bones may be appreciated in areas of the extremities not covered by muscles, such as ankles and wrists. These areas can be tender to palpation. Effusions into large joints are a common, but by no means universal, finding. On examination, there is no detectable synovial hypertrophy. Range of motion of the affected joint may be slightly decreased. Arthrocentesis yields a clear viscous fluid with few inflammatory cells; the leukocyte count is typically less than 1000 cells/mm³. These findings indicate that HOA does not cause inflammatory or proliferative synovial disease, but rather the effusions are most likely a sympathetic reaction to the adjacent periostosis (8).

Particular types of HOA are associated with characteristic clinical findings. Thyroid acropachy is distinguished by an exuberant periosteal proliferation that involves mostly the small tubular bones of the hands and feet, and clubbing usually coexists with exophthalmos and pretibial myxedema. Primary HOA has a high male-to-female ratio (9:1) and appears to be associated with a familial predisposition; one-third of these patients report a close relative with the same illness. Patients with primary HOA may display a generalized skin hypertrophy called *pachydermoperiostosis.* This skin overgrowth roughens the facial features and can reach the extreme of *cutis verticis gyrata,* which is the most advanced stage of cutaneous hypertrophy. In addition, these patients often demonstrate glandular dysfunction of the skin that is manifested as hyperhidrosis, seborrhea, or acne (8).

Variant forms of HOA are localized to one or two extremities. Usually they occur as a response to prominent endothelial injury to the involved limb, such as damage caused by aneurysms or infective endarteritis, or they are associated with patent ductus arteriosus with reversal of blood flow (3).

LABORATORY TESTS AND IMAGING

There are no distinctive laboratory abnormalities associated with HOA. However, an array of biochemical alterations that reflect the underlying illness may be found.

Plain radiographs of the extremities may reveal abnormalities in an asymptomatic patient. Long-standing clubbing produces changes of the distal phalanx due to bone remodeling. Periostosis evolves in an orderly manner. When mild it involves few bones, usually tibias and fibulas; periosteal apposition is limited to the diaphysis and has a monolayer configuration. Severe periostosis affects all tubular bones, spreads to the metaphyses and epiphyses, and generates an irregular configuration (Fig. 41-2). Typically, the joint space is preserved, and there are no erosions or periarticular osteopenia. Bone changes are symmetric; initially periostosis affects the distal parts of the lower extremities and then evolves in a centripetal fashion (9). Radionuclide bone scanning is a sensitive method for demonstrating periosteal involvement.

DIAGNOSIS

When HOA is fully expressed, the "drumstick" fingers are so unique that recognition poses no dilemma. The symptoms of HOA can be subtle. Nevertheless in some patients with lung cancer, painful arthropathy may be the initial manifestation, occurring before clubbing is detectable. Such patients could be misdiagnosed as having an inflammatory arthritis (6). Patients with the exuberant skin hypertrophy of HOA may be misdiagnosed as having acromegaly.

Diagnostic criteria for HOA require the combined presence of clubbing and periostosis of the tubular bones (1). Synovial effusion is not essential for the diagnosis. Rheumatoid factor is usually absent, and very few inflammatory cells are present in the synovial fluid. An important clinical feature in the differential diagnosis is the location of pain: in HOA, pain involves not only the joint, but also the adjacent bone.

Patients should be classified as having the primary form of the syndrome only after a careful clinical scrutiny fails to disclose any underlying illness. If a previous healthy individual develops any of the manifestations of HOA, a thorough search for underlying illness should be undertaken. In a patient with a previous diagnosis of any of the secondary causes of HOA, clubbing is usually a poor prognostic sign. Clubbing in a patient with known rheumatic heart disease may indicate infective endocarditis. Similarly, a patient with history of prosthetic vascular surgery who develops periostosis of a limb may have a graft infection.

TREATMENT

Apart from the disfigurement, clubbing is usually asymptomatic and does not require therapy. Painful osteoarthropathy generally responds to analgesics or nonsteroidal anti-inflammatory drugs. Correction of a heart defect, removal of a lung tumor, or successful treatment of endocarditis produce rapid regression of the syndrome.

MANUEL MARTINEZ—LAVIN, MD

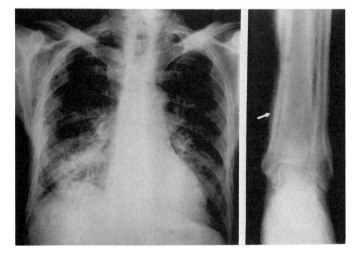

(Figure 41-2)
Radiographs of a 67-year old man with bronchogenic carcinoma. Periostosis of tibia and fibula is evident.

1. Martinez-Lavin M, Matucci-Cerinic M, Jajic I, Pineda C: Hypertrophic osteoarthropathy: consensus on its definition, classification, assessment and diagnostic criteria. J Rheumatol 20:1386-1387, 1993

2. Padula S, Broketa G, Sampieri A, Arakawa M, Matucci-Cerinic M, Downie E, Korn J: Increased collagen synthesis in skin fibroblast from patients with primary hypertrophic osteoarthropathy. Arthritis Rheum 37:1386-1394, 1994

3. Martinez-Lavin M: Elucidation of digital clubbing may help in understanding the pathogenesis of pulmonary hypertension associated to congenital heart defects. Cardiol Young 4:228-231, 1994

4. Vazquez-Abad D, Martinez-Lavin M: Macrothrombocytes in the peripheral circulation of patients with cardiogenic hypertrophic osteoarthropathy. Clin Exp Rheumatol 9:59-62, 1991

5. Matucci-Cerinic M, Martinez-Lavin M, Rojo F, Fonseca C, Kahaleh B: von Willebrand factor in hypertrophic osteoarthropathy. J Rheumatol 19:765-767, 1992

6. Schumacher HR: Articular manifestations of hypertrophic pulmonary osteoarthropathy in bronchogenic carcinoma. Arthritis Rheum 19:629-635, 1976

7. Vazquez-Abad D, Martinez-Lavin M: Digital clubbing: a numerical assessment of the deformity. J Rheumatol 16:518-520, 1989

8. Martinez-Lavin M, Pineda C, Valdez T, Cajigas JC, Weisman M, Gerber N, Steigler D: Primary hypertrophic osteoarthropathy. Semin Arthritis Rheum 17:156-162, 1988

9. Pineda C, Fonseca C, Martinez-Lavin M: The spectrum of soft tissue and skeletal abnormalities in hypertrophic osteoarthropathy. J Rheumatol 17:773-778, 1990

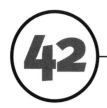

BONE AND JOINT DYSPLASIAS

Bone dysplasias are a broad group of conditions in which skeletal development and function are disturbed. They include the chondrodysplasias and osteochondroses discussed in this chapter, as well as osteodysplasias such as osteogenesis imperfecta syndromes (discussed in Chapter 39) and many others that are either extremely rare or of little relevance to rheumatology.

CHONDRODYSPLASIAS

The term chondrodysplasia—literally, abnormal (*dys*) cartilage (*chondro*) growth (*plasia*)—is used to designate inherited disorders of cartilage that affect its function as a template for bone growth (1). The clinical picture is typically dominated by varying degrees of dwarfism and bone and joint deformities. However, because the genes that harbor chondrodysplasia mutations are often not specific to bone growth, the clinical manifestations frequently extend to other cartilages, such as articular cartilage, and to other tissues (1-3).

Pathogenesis

Most bones develop and grow through the process of endochondral ossification, in which cartilage serves as a template for bone formation. In postembryonic growing bone, ossification occurs in the growth plate residing near the ends of bones (4). In essence, template cartilage is synthesized de novo in the distal growth plate and is replaced by an expanding front of bone in the proximal growth plate. Endochondral ossification accounts for linear bone growth from midgestation through the end of puberty.

The chondrodysplasias result from mutations in genes that encode the structural proteins of cartilage matrix and proteins that regulate growth plate function. These proteins, which contribute to different aspects of endochondral ossification, are required for bone growth to proceed in a normal fashion (5). Although poorly understood, the different types of chondrodysplasias reflect the functional consequences of disturbances in these proteins with regard to bone growth and other clinical manifestations.

Classification

Well over 100 clinical forms of chondrodysplasia are currently recognized. Based on their differences in clinical presentation, characteristic appearances of skeletal radiographs, growth plate histology, and pattern of inheritance, these disorders have been grouped into classes over the past decade (6). Originally, classification was based on qualitative similarities of radiographic skeletal features and the presumption that radiographic similarity reflected pathogenetic similarity. As the molecular genetic basis for many of the chondrodysplasias has begun to emerge, this presumption has held for the most part (5). Thus, a well-defined chondrodysplasia class typically contains a group of disorders ranging in severity from lethal at or around birth to very mild, often blending into the normal (nonchondrodysplasia) population. However, the classification system is in a state of flux due to the rapid pace at which the genetic basis of these disorders is being determined.

Diagnosis

A few conditions, such as achondroplasia, can be diagnosed simply by seeing a patient. However, the diagnosis is usually based on recognizing a unique combination of clinical, radiographic, and genetic features (1–3,7). Because the clinical features typically evolve over time, the natural history must be taken into account when patients are evaluated. The most useful information usually comes from skeletal radiographs; specific radiologic diagnostic criteria have been developed (7-10). Like the clinical picture, radiographic characteristics change with age. Films taken before puberty are usually more informative because the radiographic hallmarks of many disorders disappear after closure of the epiphyses. In fact, it is often difficult to make a specific diagnosis from postpubertal radiographs. Because many patients are the first and only known case in a family, a pedigree may be of little help as the inheritance pattern cannot be determined. Nevertheless, a family history sometimes provides critical clues toward a diagnosis.

Historically, laboratory tests have not been useful in diagnosing chondrodysplasia. However, as the mutations become better defined, genetic testing may be helpful in disorders caused by a recurrent mutation in the population, as is the case with achondroplasia. Although histologic evaluation of growth-plate specimens often reveal characteristic changes, biopsy is seldom warranted as the diagnosis can usually be made by other means.

Salient features of the more common chondrodysplasias are summarized in Table 42-1 (6), and additional information can be found in several recent reviews (1,2,5,7,11). The most up-to-date information is available through the Online Mendelian Inheritance in Man, developed by McKusick and colleagues (http://www3.ncbi.nlm.nih.gov/omim/).

CLASSIFICATION OF CHONDRODYSPLASIAS
Achondroplasias

This class of autosomal dominant disorders includes the following: thanatophoric dysplasia, the most common chondrodysplasia lethal in the perinatal period; achondroplasia, by far the most common nonlethal chondrodysplasia; and hypochondroplasia. Although the three differ substantially in severity, the features of each are qualitatively similar. Heterozygous mutations of the gene encoding fibroblast growth factor receptor 3 (FGFR3) have been identified in all three conditions.

Achondroplasia

The prototype of short-limb dwarfism, achondroplasia is recognizable at birth by a long narrow trunk, short limbs (especially proximally), and a large head with prominent forehead and hypoplasia of the midface. Most joints are hyperextensible, especially the knees, but elbow mobility is

(Table 42-1)

*Salient features of selected chondrodysplasias**

Class and Disorder	Inheritance	Gene Locus	Overall Severity	Rheumatologic Complications
Achondroplasia				
Thanatophoric dysplasia	AD	FGFR3	Lethal	—
Achondroplasia	AD	FGFR3	++/+++	Arthralgias
Hypochondroplasia	AD	FGFR3	+	
Spondyloephiphyseal dysplasia (SED)				
Achondrogenesis type II	AD	COL2A1	Lethal	—
Hypochondrogenesis	AD	COL2A1	Lethal	—
SED congenita	AD	COL2A1	+++	Precocious OA
Kniest dysplasia	AD	COL2A1	+++	Precocious OA, contractures
Stickler dysplasia	AD	COL2A1	++	Precocious OA
SED late onset	AD	COL2A1	+	Precocious OA
SED tarda	XLR	Unknown	+	Precocious OA
Multiple epiphyesal dysplasia				
Fairbank type	AD	COMP	+++	Arthralgias, precocious OA
Pseudoachondroplasia	AD	COMP	+++	Arthralgias, precocious OA
Diastrophic dysplasia				
Achondrogenesis type 1B	AR	DTDST	Lethal	—
Ateleosteogenesis type II	AR	DTDST	Lethal	—
Diastrophic dysplasia	AR	DTDST	+++	Precocious OA, contractures
Metaphyseal/chondrodysplasia				
Jansen type	AD	PTHrPR	+++	Contractures
Schmid type	AD	COL10A1	++	
McKusick type	AR	Unknown	+++	
Metatropic dysplasia	AD	Unknown	+++	Contractures
Chondrodysplasia punctata				
Rhizomelic type	AR	ACDPA	Lethal	Contractures
Conradi–Hünermann type	AD	Unknown	++/+++	Contractures
X-linked dominant type	XLD	ARSE	++/+++	Contractures
X-linked recessive type	XLR			
Brachyolmia				
Hobaek type	AR	Unknown	++	Arthralgia, stiffness in hip, back
Maroteaux type	AR	Unknown	++	Arthralgia, stiffness in hip, back
Autosomal dominant type	AD	Unknown	++	Arthralgia, stiffness in hip, back

* AD = autosomal dominant; AR = autosomal recessive; XLD = X-linked dominant; XLR = X-linked recessive; FGFR3 = fibroblast growth factor receptor 3; COL2A1 = type II collagen α1 chain; COMP = cartilage oligomeric matrix protein; DTDST = diastrophic dysplasia sulfate transporter; PTHrPR = parathyroid hormone-related protein receptor; COL10A1 = type X collagen α1 chain; ACDPA = acetyl-CoA:dihydroxyacetone phosphate acetyltransferase; ARSE = arylsulfatase E; OA = osteoarthritis.

limited. The most serious problems are related to a small spinal canal, especially at the foramen magnum level. This anomaly contributes to hypotonia, failure to thrive, developmental delay, apnea, and even quadriparesis and sudden death in infants. Common childhood problems include middle-ear infections, dental crowding, and bowing of the legs.

The lifespan is normal in the absence of life-threatening neurologic problems in early life. In adulthood, men reach an average height of 132 cm (about 45 inches) and women, 124 cm (about 40 inches). Pain is common in weight-bearing joints, probably due to misalignment of bones aggravated by physical activity and by obesity, which is common. However, people with achondroplasia rarely develop osteoarthritis. Stenosis of the lumbar spine may cause paresthesias, claudication and numbness of the legs, and bowel and bladder dysfunction.

Pregnant women with achondroplasia need to be monitored carefully and delivered by cesarean section. Because of the high prevalence of heterozygous achondroplasia in the short-stature community, people with this condition often marry; their offspring have a 25% risk for inheriting the much more severe homozygous achondroplasia.

Hypochondroplasia

Not usually recognized until late childhood, patients with hypochondroplasia appear to have "mild" achondroplasia with short limbs (mostly the proximal segments), a stocky build, and a normal or slightly enlarged head. The natural history is usually unremarkable other than for mild short (approximately 5 feet or less) stature. The true incidence of hypochondroplasia is unknown; because its features are mild, it may often escape detection.

Spondyloepiphyseal Dysplasias

Spondyloepiphyseal dysplasia (SED) is a large, diverse class of autosomal dominant disorders with clinical features that reflect varying degrees of dysfunction of type II collagen, the principal structural protein of cartilage. In severe forms, many types of cartilage and other tissues containing type II collagen are affected, whereas in milder forms, only articular cartilage is involved.

SED Congenita

This form of dysplasia is the prototype of short-trunk dwarfism. Neonates with SED congenita have a short neck, a short barrel-shaped trunk, and sometimes cleft palate and club foot. The proximal limbs are short, but the hands, feet, head, and face appear to be normal in size. The shortening becomes more prominent with time. Scoliosis commonly develops in childhood and may cause respiratory compromise. Odontoid hypoplasia may predispose to cervicomedullary instability and spinal cord compression, but sudden death is uncommon. Osteoarthritis, especially of the hips and knees, typically appears in the third decade. Severe myopia is common, and retinal detachment may occur in older children and adults. Adults range in height from 95 to 128 cm (about 35 to 50 inches).

Kniest Dysplasia

At birth, infants with Kniest dysplasia have a short trunk and limbs and a flat face with prominent eyes. Their fingers are long and knobby, and many have club foot and cleft palate. The most debilitating aspect is the progressive enlargement of joints during childhood, which is associated with painful contractures and, eventually, with osteoarthritis. Hearing loss is common, as is severe myopia that is often complicated by retinal detachment.

Stickler Dysplasia

The clinical picture of Stickler dysplasia is dominated by ocular problems. Severe myopia is usually present at birth, together with cleft palate and a small jaw. Retinal detachment may occur during childhood, as may choroidoretinal and vitreous degeneration. Sensorineural hearing loss often develops during adolescence. Osteoarthritis typically begins during the second or third decade of life. Short stature is not a feature of Stickler syndrome; indeed, some patients exhibit a Marfan-type habitus and joint laxity.

Late-Onset SEDs

Some type II collagen mutations manifest primarily as precocious osteoarthritis of weight-bearing joints. Radiographs usually reveal subtle changes of SED, but many of these patients are of normal stature and have no other abnormalities. The term familial (or autosomal dominant) osteoarthritis is sometimes used to describe this syndrome. Mutations of an unknown gene that maps to the X chromosome can produce a similar but distinct clinical picture in males, which is called SED tarda.

Multiple Epiphyseal Dysplasia and Pseudoachondroplasia

Multiple epiphyseal dysplasia (MED) and pseudoachondroplasia are classified together because mutations in the cartilage oligomeric matrix protein (COMP) gene have been found in both disorders.

The Fairbank type of MED is usually diagnosed in childhood because it is characterized by moderately short limbs, a waddling gait, and painful joints. Radiographs show generalized epiphyseal involvement. The Ribbing type of MED may not be detected until adolescence. Because involvement is typically restricted to the proximal femurs, the Ribbing type is often confused with bilateral Legg–Calvé–Perthes disease. Both types of MED are associated with moderately short stature (145 cm–170 cm) and osteoarthritis of weight-bearing joints.

Pseudoachondroplasia typically presents in the second or third year of life with a dramatic slowing of bone growth accompanied by a waddling gait and generalized joint laxity. The head and face appear normal, but the hands are short and broad, and ulnar deviation occurs. The growth deficiency worsens with age. Major complications are related to excessive joint mobility, most notably involving the knees, where it produces various deformities. Osteoarthritis of the hips and knees is common.

Diastrophic Dysplasia

Diastrophic dysplasia is usually apparent at birth. Infants display very short extremities and distinctive hands with short digits and proximal displacement of the thumb (hitchhiker thumb). There may be bony fusion of metacarpophalangeal joints producing symphalangism and ulnar deviation of the hands. Cleft palate and club foot are common. The external ears often become inflamed soon after birth; healing results in small, fibrotic ears (cauliflower deformity). Scoliosis and multiple joint contractures usually begin during childhood and are typically progressive and severe. Adult height varies from 105 to 130 cm (40 to 44 inches).

Metaphyseal Chondrodysplasias

The metaphyseal chondrodysplasias (MCDs) are a heterogeneous group of disorders that share radiographic involvement of the metaphyses. However, studies have shown that they do not share a common genetic basis.

Jansen's MCD

Severely shortened limbs, prominent forehead, and small jaw are present at birth. Some infants have club foot and hypercalcemia. Joints enlarge and become restricted during childhood. Flexion contractures at the hips and knees often result in a bent-over posture.

Schmid MCD

This disorder usually becomes apparent at age 2–3 years because of mild shortening of the limbs, especially the legs which are bowed, a waddling gait, and sometimes hip pain. Adults are of mildly short stature and have few problems.

McKusick MCD

Also called cartilage–hair hypoplasia, the McKusick type MCD manifests at age 2–3 years as growth deficiency. It is characterized by short limbs, bowed legs, and flaring of the lower rib cage. Hands and feet are short and broad, and fingers are short and stubby. Ligamentous laxity is marked. The hair tends to be blond and thin, and the skin is lightly pigmented. Some patients have associated problems, including immune deficiency, anemia, Hirschsprung's disease, and malabsorption. Adults exhibit marked dwarfism and are predisposed to certain infections and malignancies of the skin and lymphoid tissue.

Metatropic Dysplasia

Newborn infants with metatropic dysplasia have short limbs and a long narrow trunk. Kyphoscoliosis, which starts during late infancy or early childhood, may cause cardiorespiratory problems. Odontoid hypoplasia is common. Most joints become large and have restricted mobility, and contractures often develop at the hips and knees.

Chondrodysplasia Punctata

Disorders classified as chondrodysplasia punctata (CDP) share the radiographic finding of stippled epiphyses, but specific features differ substantially.

Rhizomelic CDP

At birth, rhizomelic CDP is evidenced by severe and symmetric shortening of limbs, multiple joint contractures, cataracts, ichthyosiform rash, absent hair, microcephaly, and flat face with hypoplasia of the nasal tip. These infants fail to thrive and usually die during the first year.

Conradi-Hünermann CDP

In contrast to the rhizomelic type, newborns with Conradi-Hünermann CDP have asymmetric and relatively mild limb shortening, distinctive facies, and varying degrees of contractures, cataracts, skin rash, and hair loss. The asymmetry may worsen and scoliosis may develop over time, but patients usually have a normal life span.

X-Linked CDP

CDP may be X-linked dominant or recessive. Both resemble Conradi-Hünermann CDP in clinical features, severity, and course. However, the recessive type is symmetric, in contrast to the dominant type.

Brachyolmia

Three types of brachyolmia are recognized, all of which have similar clinical features (Table 42-1). They present in early to mid-childhood with mildly short stature mainly involving the trunk. Back and hip pain typically arise during adolescence and continue into adulthood. Back stiffness is common and some patients develop scoliosis.

JUVENILE OSTEOCHONDROSES

The juvenile osteochondroses summarized in Table 42-2 are a heterogeneous group of disorders in which localized noninflammatory arthropathies result from regional disturbances of skeletal growth (12,13). Children may present with painless limitation of movement of affected joints (such as in Legg–Calvé–Perthes disease and Scheuermann's disease) or with local pain and sometimes tenderness and swelling (such as in Freiberg's disease, Osgood–Schlatter disease, and osteochondritis dissecans). Bone growth may be altered to produce deformities, such as bowing of the tibia in Blount's disease.

The diagnosis of juvenile osteochondrosis can usually be confirmed radiographically, and magnetic resonance imaging is sometimes useful to define the lesions. The pathogenesis is thought to involve ischemic necrosis of primary or secondary endochondral ossification centers. Some cases may be related to stress and injury. Most of these disorders occur sporadically, but familial forms have been described.

MANAGEMENT OF BONE AND JOINT DYSPLASIAS

No definitive treatment is available to counter defective bone growth for any of the bone and joint dysplasias. Consequently, management is directed at prevention and correction of skeletal deformities and preventing nonskeletal complications. Management is guided by knowledge of the natural history of these disorders, so that disorder-specific problems can be anticipated and treated early.

A number of problems are common to this group of disorders, including respiratory distress, osteoarthritis of weight-bearing joints, dental crowding, obesity, obstetrical difficulties, and psychologic problems related to short stature. General recommendations can be made to address these problems (1,3). For example, most patients with chondrodysplasia should avoid contact sports and other activities that traumatize or stress joints. Joint replacement is often necessary for progressive osteoarthritis. Dietary control should be instituted during childhood to prevent obesity in adulthood. Dental care should be started in early childhood

(Table 42-2)
Juvenile osteochondroses

Region Affected	Eponym(s)	Typical Age at Presentation	Sex Predilection
Capital femoral epiphysis	Legg–Calvé–Perthes disease, coxa plana	3–12 years	Male
Tibial tubercle	Osgood–Schlatter disease	10–16 years	None
Os calcis	Sever's disease	6–10 years	None
Head of second metatarsal	Freiberg's disease	10–14 years	None
Vertebral bodies	Scheuermann's disease	Adolescence	Male
Medial aspect of proximal tibial epiphysis	Blount's disease, tibia vara	Infancy or adolescence	None
Subchondral areas of diarthroidal joints (particularly knee, hip, elbow, and ankle)	Osteochondritis dissecans	10–20 years	Male

to manage crowding and misalignment effectively. Because of their small pelvic bones, pregnant women with most chondrodysplasias should be monitored in high-risk prenatal clinics and, in many instances, have their babies delivered by cesarean section. Intelligence is usually normal in the nonlethal chondrodysplasias, but since patients are so easily recognized as being "different" from their peers, they and their families often benefit from support provided by lay groups, such as the Little People of America and the Human Growth Foundation, and from publications directed to the lay population (11).

WILLIAM A. HORTON, MD

1. Horton WA, Hecht JT: The Chondrodysplasias. In Royce PM, Steinman B (eds): Extracellular Matrix and Heritable Disorders of Connective Tissue, New York, Alan R. Liss, 1993, pp 641-676

2. Rimoin DL, Lachman RS: Genetic disorders of the osseous skeleton. In Beighton P (ed): McKusick's Heritable Disorders of Connective Tissue, 5th ed. St Louis, Mosby, 1993, pp 557-690

3. Bassett GS, Scott CIJr: The Osteochondrodysplasias. In Morrissy RT (ed): Lovell & Winter's Pediatric Orthopaedics, 3rd ed. Philadelphia, J.B. Lippincott, 1990, pp 91-142

4. Horton WA: Morphology of connective tissue: cartilage. In Royce PM, Steinmann B (eds): Connective Tissue and Its Heritable Disorders. New York, Wiley-Liss, 1993, pp 73-84

5. Horton WA: Molecular genetics of the human chondrodysplasias—1995. Eur J Hum Genet 3:357-373, 1995

6. International Working Group on Constitutional Diseases of Bone/Spranger J: International classification of osteochondrodysplasias. Eur J Pediatr 151:407-415, 1992

7. Spranger J, Maroteaux P: The Lethal Osteochondrodysplasias. Adv Hum Genet 19:1-103, 1995

8. Spranger JW, Langer LO, Wiedemann H-R: Bone Dysplasias, An Atlas of Constitutional Disorders of Skeletal Development. Philadelphia, W.B. Saunders Co., 1974

9. Wynne-Davies R, Hall CM, Apley AG: Atlas of Skeletal Dysplasias. Edinburgh, Churchill Livingstone, 1985

10. Tabyi H, Lachman RS: Radiology of Syndromes, Metabolic Disorders, and Skeletal Dysplasias. 3rd ed. Chicago, Year Book Medical Publishers, 1990

11. Scott CI Jr, Mayeux N, Crandall R, Weiss J: Dwarfism, the Family and Professional Guide. Irvine, Short Stature Foundation & Information Center, Inc., 1994

12. Sharrard WJW: Abnormalities of the Epiphyses and Limb Inequality. In Paediatric Orthopaedics and Fracture, 3rd ed. Oxford, Blackwell Scientific Publications, 1993, pp 719-814

13. Tachdjian MO: Osteochondroses and Related Disorders. In Pediatric Orthopedics, 2nd ed. Philadelphia, W.B. Saunders, 1990, pp 932-1062

OSTEONECROSIS

Osteonecrosis is a generic term used to describe the death of all cellular elements of bone. Other synonyms for bone death are ischemic bone necrosis, avascular necrosis, aseptic necrosis, and osteochondritis dissecans, but osteonecrosis is the preferred term. Osteochondritis dissecans actually has a somewhat different meaning that implies the presence of a loose chip of dead bone in the articular cavity.

Osteonecrosis may occur in a variety of clinical settings associated with a disease (eg, Gaucher's disease), drug (eg, corticosteroids), physiologic process (eg, pregnancy), or pathologic process (eg, embolism), and it may occur in the absence of any apparent predisposing factor or condition (truly idiopathic) (1–7). The disorder affects individuals of both genders and in all age groups. For the most part, osteonecrosis involves the epiphysis of long bones such as the femoral and humeral heads, but other bones (eg, carpal, tarsal) can also be affected. More than one bone may be involved, either sequentially or simultaneously.

PATHOGENESIS

Bone death is the result of diminished arterial blood supply, an easily understood mechanism that can be reproduced in experimental animals. If blood flow is completely interrupted and not promptly restored, bone death inevitably ensues. The final outcome depends on the size of the affected area and the magnitude of the reparative process in which viable bone cells replace necrotic or nonviable bone. Failure to revitalize the involved area leads to bone collapse followed by some degree of joint incongruity and secondary osteoarthritis.

Prolonged ischemia may occur as a result of intra- or extravascular pathology within the bone itself. Small-vessel vasculitis, intravascular arteriolar thrombosis, venous occlusion, and microembolism are well-recognized causes of ischemia. Infiltrative processes such as Gaucher's disease indirectly alter the vascular supply by compressing the sinusoids. The direct toxic effect of some substances on different cell populations of the bone can also lead to osteonecrosis. For example, even moderate amounts of alcohol are toxic to osteocytes, and corticosteroids, both endogenous and exogenous, are toxic to lipocytes.

Intraosseous pressure (IOP), either as a primary (eg, infiltrative) process or a secondary (eg, altered blood supply) event, has been postulated as the common pathway of osteonecrosis (8). Increased pressure in bone—an organ that is essentially incapable of expanding—results in reduction (or further reduction) of blood supply, ischemia, and cell damage. The presence of increased IOP has been used in the past as a tool for early diagnosis of osteonecrosis.

Although it is likely that increased IOP plays an important role in the pathogenesis of osteonecrosis, other factors such as cytotoxicity may be equally important. Moreover, increased IOP is not the *sine qua non* of this disorder because it may occur in other pathologic processes such as osteoarthritis (9). Likewise, increased IOP has not been found in histo-logically proven experimentally induced osteonecrosis in rabbits (10). The pathogenesis will likely be better understood as histopathologic and imaging studies are performed in early disease, before radiologic evidence or even clinical signs emerge.

CLINICAL FEATURES

The first clinical manifestation of osteonecrosis is the relatively abrupt onset of severe pain. Initially, pain is elicited only with movement (in hip involvement, during weight-bearing activities), but later escalates to pain at rest. In the early stages, decreased range of motion is related primarily to pain (1,2). Some patients experience unbearable pain as the disease progresses, whereas other patients with similar radiographs do not. A certain degree of bone remodeling may allow a patient to remain functional despite decreased range of motion. However, a significant proportion of patients have persistent and worsening pain, progressive loss of range of motion, and significant loss of function. The time from onset of symptoms to incapacitation varies from months to years.

The most common clinical presentation encountered by rheumatologists is that of a young woman with systemic lupus erythematosus and Cushingoid features who has received high doses of corticosteroids. The average dose, cumulative dose, duration of corticosteroid use, and route of administration appear to be of less importance in the development of osteonecrosis. Other less common conditions associated with osteonecrosis are listed in Table 43-1.

A pre-clinical stage has been demonstrated in magnetic resonance imaging (MRI) studies comparing the symptomatic and nonsymptomatic contralateral joints. Abnormalities were found in the asymptomatic joint that predated clinical symptoms by a few weeks (1–3,8,11).

DIAGNOSIS

For years, the diagnosis of osteonecrosis has been based on plain radiographs, which identify advanced disease but do not detect early stages (1,2,11). Plain radiographs (such as neutral anteroposterior and frog leg views for detecting hip disease) are still useful. However, MRI is the diagnostic tool of choice for identifying preradiologic and even preclinical disease (2–4,11).

Although several classification systems for osteonecrosis have been developed, the one most commonly used describes five stages of disease (Table 43-2). Stages I through IV were originally described by Arlet and Ficat (12). Recently a fifth stage, 0, was added to include asymptomatic patients whose radiographs showed no abnormalities, but for whom MRI studies confirmed the presence of disease (11). However, it is likely that an improved staging system will be developed, now that MRI is available in most medical centers. Potentially, MRI could demonstrate the extent of bone involvement, which could be used to predict a patient's outcome (13,14).

(Table 43-1)
Diseases or conditions associated with osteonecrosis

Trauma
  Hip dislocation
  Hip fracture
  Postarthroscopy
Connective tissue disorders (CTDs)*
  Systemic lupus erythematosus
  Rheumatoid arthritis
  Vasculitis
  Other CTDs
Hematologic disorders
  Sickle cell disease
  Sickle cell-C disease
  Thalassemia minor
Infiltrative disorders
  Gaucher's disease
  Solid tumors
Metabolic disorders
  Gout
Disorders associated with fat necrosis
  Pancreatitis
  Pancreatic carcinoma
Embolism
  Decompression sickness

Corticosteroids (exogenous and endogenous)
  Asthma
  Aplastic anemia
  Leukemias and lymphomas
  Celiac disease
  Inflammatory bowel disease
  Cushing syndrome
  Organ transplantation
  Intra-articular and pulse intravenous administration
Cytotoxic agents
  Vinblastine
  Vincristine
  Cisplatin (intra-arterial)
  Cyclophosphamide
  Methotrexate
  Bleomycin
  5-Fluorouracil
Alcohol
Radiation
Pregnancy
Idiopathic[†]

* Almost all CTDs have been reported to be associated with osteonecrosis; corticosteroids have been used in the majority, but not in all, patients.
[†] No associated disorders.

Other tools for diagnosing osteonecrosis are seldom used now. These tests include invasive studies such as the so-called stress test, which measures IOP at baseline and after injection of 5 ml of saline (an IOP >30 mm Hg at baseline coupled with 10 mm Hg increase during stress testing indicated osteonecrosis). Venography was done usually in conjunction with the IOP stress test (blood flow abnormalities were found in early stages of disease). While conventional tomograms were useful for staging, they were not sensitive enough to detect early disease (1,2,8). Similarly, neither qualitative nor quantitative bone scintigraphy proved sensitive. Single-photon emission computerized tomography does not appear to offer any advantage over MRI.

Bone biopsies are not recommended for diagnosis, but histopathologic studies are useful to confirm the diagnosis of osteonecrosis before surgery. Characteristic findings include marrow fibrosis, fat cell necrosis, necrotic bone, and some evidence of reparative process.

There are no clear data on the sensitivity, specificity, or predictive values (positive and negative) of diagnostic procedures for osteonecrosis. Comparison of these procedures is unlikely because some are no longer in use. Moreover, because histologically proven dead bone (the "gold standard" for diagnosis) is not obtained in all patients (nor should it be), these data are not available in all cases. MRI appears to be both sensitive and specific for the diagnosis of osteonecrosis. MRI makes it possible to distinguish differences between normal bone and marrow, unrepaired dead bone and marrow, unrepaired dead bone with marrow replaced by debris, and zones of repair (3,4,11). Necrotic marrow and necrotic bone produce a high-signal intensity in both T1 and T2 images, whereas subchondral bone appears as dark striations. The combined appearance of these signals gives the characteristic, well-described serpiginous pattern (Fig. 43-1).

TREATMENT

Outcome criteria for the treatment of osteonecrosis have been developed by Stulberg et al (15) and are shown in Table 43-3.

Stages 0, I, and II may be treated by conservative measures or by core decompression. Conservative treatment in-

(Table 43-2)
*Staging in osteonecrosis**

Stage 0	Clinical manifestations absent; normal radiographs[†]
Stage I	Clinical manifestations present; normal radiographs[‡]
Stage II	Areas of osteopenia and osteosclerosis in radiographs
Stage III	Early bone collapse manifested as the "crescent sign" (translucent subcortical bone delineates the area of dead bone)
Stage IV	Late bone collapse manifested as flattening of the femoral head, with or without joint incongruity

* After Arlet and Ficat (12).
[†] Diagnosis made by magnetic resonance imaging.
[‡] Diagnosis made by invasive physiologic studies in published literature.

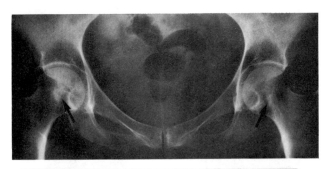

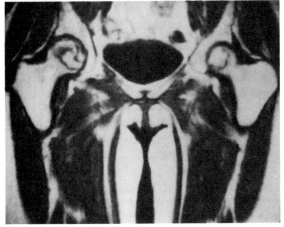

(Figure 43-1)

Stage II osteonecrosis of both femoral heads. **Top:** *Plain film of the pelvis and both hips shows patchy foci of increased density (arrows) characteristic of stage II osteonecrosis. The femoral heads are not collapsed.* **Bottom:** *T1-weighted coronal MRI shows curvilinear areas of low signal in both femoral heads typical of osteonecrosis. Courtesy of Wanda K. Bernreuter, MD.*

cludes the following elements: 1) judicious use of analgesics, 2) maintaining muscle strength and preventing contractures, and 3) assistive devices to facilitate ambulation for patients with osteonecrosis of the lower extremities. Patients with persistent, intractable pain and progressive functional loss should be considered for arthroplasty. Ideally, patients with hip involvement should have arthroplasty before total collapse of the femoral head occurs. Osteotomies have been considered of value in some patients, but prolonged nonweight bearing is essential for the success of this treatment. Patients with osteonecrosis of nonweight-bearing joints may not require any intervention, because they may have little pain and limited (but tolerable) functional loss.

The rationale for core decompression is to reduce IOP, reestablish blood supply, and allow living bone adjacent to dead bone to contribute to the reparative process (16). Good

(Table 43-3)

Recommended criteria in determining treatment outcome in osteonecrosis[*]

1. Clinical improvement as determined by a valid instrument (eg, Harris hip scale)
2. Radiographic stabilization
3. Bone survival (eg, femoral head survival)

[*] After Stulberg et al (15).

to excellent results have been obtained in the majority of patients with stages I and II osteonecrosis and even in a significant proportion of patients with stage III disease (15–19). The most convincing evidence of efficacy comes from a study by Stulberg et al. Fifty cases of stages I through III osteonecrosis of the hip (31 patients) were randomized to receive either conservative (nonweight bearing) or surgical (core decompression) treatment. Decompression more predictably reduced pain and changed the indications for further surgery than did conservative treatment in stage I and II patients. Clinical stabilization was achieved in 90% of stage I and II cases (15). In a study by Chan et al, core decompression and bone grafting halted disease progression in patients with early disease. In contrast, patients with advanced disease and a large area of bone involvement showed clinical and radiographic evidence of disease progression (17). Smith et al reported on 114 hips in 92 patients with osteonecrosis due to different causes (corticosteroid use, alcohol, trauma). Clinical failure, which was defined as the need for further surgery, occurred in 16% of the hips in stage I, 53% in stage IIA, 80% in stage IIB and 100% in stage IV (18). Finally, Warner et al studied 39 hips in 25 patients and found that 70% of those with stage I and II experienced stabilization, compared with 13% at stage III and IV (18). From the combined experience reviewed, core decompression should be considered as a reasonable treatment alternative for patients in early stages of osteonecrosis, primarily stage I.

In contrast to these positive results, Camp and Colwell (20) and Hopson and Siverhus (21) reported the failure of core decompression, even in patients in early stages of osteonecrosis. These investigators were impressed by the morbidity of the procedure, particularly the incidence of postsurgical subtrochanteric fractures. They strongly recommended abandoning this procedure, arguing that there is no evidence that core decompression actually decreases IOP for any length of time. They further recommended conservative treatment (nonweight bearing) for stages 0–II and arthroplasty or osteotomy for stages III and IV. However, most recent literature does not include osteotomy as a preferred procedure, but rather, supports bone grafting (*vide infra*) and joint arthroplasty. Whether to implant a cemented or an uncemented prosthesis is a matter of controversy. Uncemented prostheses are recommended for younger patients, but long-term data are not yet available to be dogmatic on this issue (22). The indications for a surgical procedure, namely arthroplasty, include not only evidence of radiographic progression but worsening pain and incapacitation.

Over the past few years, significant data have accumulated about bone grafting as an alternative for the treatment of osteonecrosis. Urbaniak et al conducted a follow-up study of 89 patients (103 affected hips), some with idiopathic osteonecrosis and some with histories of corticosteroids use, alcohol use, or trauma. The probability of failure within 5 years (defined as the need for arthroplasty) varied from 11% for patients in early-stage disease to nearly 30% for those with advanced osteonecrosis. All patients improved significantly, as measured by the standardized Harris questionnaire (23). Therefore, bone grafting may be a reasonable means of delaying arthroplasty in relatively young patients.

Electrical stimulation and exposure to pulse electromagnetic fields are of questionable value in the management of stages 0–II. Arthroscopy can be considered for removing loose bodies in patients with osteonecrosis involving the knee or shoulder.

PROGNOSIS

Diagnosing very early osteonecrosis using available technology should result in better outcomes. It is conceivable that purely conservative treatment may prove to be all that is required for patients with stages 0 and I disease, although core decompression appears to offer distinctive advantages in early disease. In more advanced disease, bone grafting may delay the need for arthroplasty and allow the patient to remain functional and relatively pain-free. A combination of factors (eg, size of the necrotic area, degree of bone collapse, underlying disorder) likely explains the lower success rate of arthroplasty in osteonecrosis than in other disorders, particularly osteoarthritis. Adequate follow up increases the likelihood of making proper and prompt management decisions.

GRACIELA S. ALARCÓN, MD, MPH

1. Steinberg ME, Steinberg DR: Osteonecrosis. In Kelley WN, Harris ED, Ruddy S, Sledge CB, (eds): Textbook of Rheumatology, 4th ed. Philadelphia, WB Saunders, 1993, pp 1628-1650

2. Mankin HJ: Nontraumatic necrosis of bone (osteonecrosis). N Engl J Med 326:1473-1479, 1992

3. Jergesen HE, Heller M, Genant HK: Magnetic resonance imaging in osteonecrosis of the femoral head. Ortho Clin N Am 16:705-716, 1985

4. Jergesen HE, Lang P, Moseley M, Genant HK: Histologic correlation in magnetic resonance imaging of femoral head osteonecrosis. Clin Orthop Related Res 253:150-163, 1990

5. Stulberg BN, Bauer TW, Belhobek GH, Levine M, Davis A: A diagnostic algorithm for osteonecrosis of the femoral head. Clin Orthop 249:176-182, 1989

6. Hungerford DS, Zizic TM: Alcoholism associated ischemic necrosis of the femoral head. Early diagnosis and treatment. Clin Orthop 130:144-153, 1978

7. Zizic TM, Marcoux C, Hungerford DS, Dansereau J-V, Stevens MB: Corticosteroid therapy associated with ischemic necrosis of bone in systemic lupus erythematosus. Am J Med 79:596-604, 1985

8. Zizic TM, Marcoux C, Hungerford DS, Stevens MB: The early diagnosis of ischemic necrosis of bone. Arthritis Rheum 29:1177-1186, 1986

9. Colwell CW Jr: The controversy of core decompression of the femoral head for osteonecrosis. Arthritis Rheum 32:797-800, 1989

10. Warner JJP, Philip JH, Brodsky GL, Thornhill TS: Studies of nontraumatic osteonecrosis. Manometric and histologic studies of the femoral head after chronic steroid treatment: an experimental study in rabbits. Clin Orthop 225:128-140, 1987

11. Lee MJ, Corrigan J, Stack JP, Ennis JT: A comparison of modern imaging modalities in osteonecrosis of the femoral head. Clin Radiol 42:427-432, 1990

12. Arlet J, Ficat P: Diagnostic de l'osteonecrose femorocapitale primitive au stade I (stade preradiologic): [The diagnosis of stage I (pre-radiologic) primary osteonecrosis of the femoral head]. Rev Chir Orthop 54:637-648, 1968

13. Sugano N, Ohzono K, Masuhara K, Takaoka K, Ono K: Prognostication of osteonecrosis of the femoral head in patients with systemic lupus erythematosus of magnetic resonance imaging. Clin Orthop Related Res 305:190-199, 1994

14. Lafforgue P, Dahan E, Chagnaud C, Schiano A, Kasbarian M, Acquaviva PC: Early-stage avascular necrosis of the femoral head: MR imaging for prognosis in 31 cases with a least 2 years of follow-up. Radiology 187:199-204, 1993

15. Stulberg BN, Bauer TW, Belhobek GH: Making core decompression work. Clin Orthop 261:186-195, 1990

16. Hungerford DS: Response: the role of core decompression in the treatment of ischemic necrosis of the femoral head. Arthritis Rheum 32:801-806, 1989

17. Chan TW, Dalinka MK, Steinberg ME, Kressel HY: Magnetic resonance imaging appearance of femoral head osteonecrosis following core decompression and bone grafting. Skeletal Radiol 20:103-107, 1991

18. Smith SW, Fehring TK, Griffin WL, Beaver WB: Core decompression of the osteonecrotic femoral head. J Bone Joint Surg 77:674-680, 1991

19. Warner JJP, Philip JH, Brodsky GL, Thornhill TS: Studies of nontraumatic osteonecrosis of the femoral head. Clin Orthop 225:104-127, 1987

20. Camp JF, Colwell CWJ: Core decompression of the femoral head for osteonecrosis. J Bone Joint Surg 68-A:1313-1319, 1986

21. Hopson CN, Siverhus SW: Ischemic necrosis of the femoral head: treatment by core decompression. J Bone Joint Surg 70-A:1048-1051, 1988

22. Piston RW, Engh CA, De Carvalho PI, Suthers K: Osteonecrosis of the femoral head treated with total hip arthroplasty without cement. J Bone Joint Surg 76:202-214, 1994

23. Urbaniak JR, Coogan PG, Gunneson EB, Nunley JA: Treatment of osteonecrosis of the femoral head with free vascularized fibular grafting: a long-term follow-up study of one hundred and three hips. J Bone Joint Surg 77:681-694, 1995

44 PAGET'S DISEASE OF BONE

Paget's disease of bone (osteitis deformans) is a focal disorder of bone remodeling that typically begins with excessive bone resorption followed by excessive bone formation. The primary disturbance is an exaggeration of osteoclastic bone resorption, initially producing a localized bone loss. The disorder is usually not recognized until the subsequent bone formation response is so pronounced that enlarged and deformed bones result. This excessive resorption and formation culminates at the tissue level in an abnormal mosaic pattern of lamellar bone associated with extensive vascularity and increased fibrous tissue deposition in adjacent marrow spaces.

EPIDEMIOLOGY

The prevalence of Paget's disease is high in the United States, Australia, and New Zealand, but the disease is rare in Asia. In the United States, Paget's disease is estimated to occur in 1%–3% of individuals over age 45, whereas in Japan, fewer than 200 patients have been reported. Paget's disease is rare before age 20; the estimated incidence among individuals older than 80 years of age is about 10% (1).

ETIOLOGY

The etiology of Paget's disease remains unknown, although some data suggest a significant genetic component. Reportedly, 15%–30% of patients with Paget's disease have a family history of the disorder with some indication of an autosomal dominant pattern of inheritance (2). One study reported an increased frequency of HLA-DQW1 antigens (3). Family studies suggest that a person with a first-degree relative has a 7 times higher risk of developing the condition than someone who does not have an affected relative. In families with early onset or severe Paget's disease, the risk is even greater (4).

Strong data suggest a viral etiology for Paget's disease (5). The changes in bone remodeling are thought to occur as a result of viral infection of osteoclasts. Inclusions resembling viral nucleocapsids have been identified in the nuclei and cytoplasm of osteoclasts at pagetic sites, but not in osteoclasts in normal bone from the same patient or from normal subjects. These virus particles resemble those of the paramyxovirus family. In vitro studies have demonstrated that these viruses promote the fusion of infected cells and, thus, the formation of multinucleated giant cells. It is possible that interleukin-6 may play a role in regulating the behavior of the osteoclast line in Paget's disease (6). Thus, the functionally hyperactive multinucleated osteoclasts in Paget's disease may result from a viral infection early in life that stimulates cell fusion between osteoclasts and the osteoclastic progenitor cells, which migrate to the pagetic site.

HISTOPATHOLOGY

Early in the disease process, osteolysis (loss of bone) is accompanied by some level of repair. The repair usually occurs in local areas near the regions of excessive resorption. Newly deposited bone is both woven and lamellar bone. The hematopoietic marrow, which is closely opposed to the area of increased resorption, is replaced by a hypervascular loose fibrous connective tissue. These changes occur in both cancellous and cortical bone. The typical mosaic pattern of Paget's disease results from the abnormal deposition of lamellar bone. In some circumstances, the rate of resorption decreases, but new bone formation may continue, resulting in an increased mass of bone per unit volume, which is termed the osteoblastic or sclerotic phase. Bone formation and resorption are closely coupled, even though formation appears excessive and involved bones may be larger than normal (5).

Overall, large increases in the rates of resorption and formation involve the increased movement of mineral ions from resorbing bone into newly forming bone. With resorption of bone matrix, there is increased urinary excretion of biochemical markers such as hydroxyproline-containing peptides; at times, these biochemical markers may be very elevated. The increased bone formation and increased local vascularity accounts for the rapid uptake of isotopes by the pagetic lesion, which is usually detected by bone scans.

Biochemical evidence of increased bone turnover include both osteoblastic and osteoclastic markers (7–15). Markers for both typically rise in proportion to each other, suggesting the preserved coupling of bone formation and resorption even in this abnormal state. The degree of elevation of the resorption and formation indices reflect the extent or severity of abnormal bone turnover. Active monostotic disease other than the skull has lower biochemical values as compared to involvement of multiple sites. The levels of these biochemical markers may be useful in monitoring the disorder over time and especially useful for measuring the effects of therapy.

Biochemical markers for new bone synthesis that may be useful include serum alkaline phosphatase, bone-specific alkaline phosphatase, type I procollagen carboxyterminal peptide, and osteocalcin. Urinary markers of resorption include hydroxyproline-containing peptides or pyridinium cross-linked peptides, but, as yet, no urinary markers for new bone formation have been identified. Elevated levels of serum alkaline phosphatase activity in patients with active disease reflect the increased osteoblastic activity, which is considered essential for bone formation and generally correlates with the extent and activity of the pagetic process. Of note, serum alkaline phosphatase levels may be normal at times, but this is rarely the case with skull involvement. An explosive increase in serum alkaline phosphatase levels occurs in patients who develop sarcoma at the site of pagetic involvement. Neither the newly available bone-specific serum alkaline phosphatase assays nor serum osteocalcin measurements appear to be as useful as the serum alkaline phosphatase. The most commonly used urinary marker is

24-hour hydroxyproline excretion corrected for milligrams of creatinine excreted. Since hydroxyproline is predominantly metabolized in the liver once released from collagen and is not unique to bone collagen, it is not a perfect measurement for monitoring bone resorption. The newer pyridinium crosslink markers are remarkably reproducible and are primarily directly related predominantly to bone collagen resorption, particularly in active disease states (16).

Serum calcium levels are typically normal in patients with Paget's disease unless prolonged bed rest is required. If an otherwise healthy ambulatory patient with Paget's disease has elevated serum calcium, other coexistent diseases should be considered, including primary hyperparathyroidism or cancer. Other biochemical abnormalities that have been described include elevations in serum uric acid and serum citrate.

CLINICAL FEATURES

The clinical presentation of Paget's disease totally depends on which bone is involved. The most common sites of involvement include the spine, pelvis, skull, femur, and tibia. In individuals with widespread disease, part of every bone may be involved. Typically, Paget's disease of bone is asymptomatic. It may be discovered on a screening x-ray for other purposes. However, the disorder may become clinically evident when bone involvement results in pain, gross deformity, compression of nerve roots or spinal cord, fracture of an involved bone, or alteration of joint structure and function leading to osteoarthritis or locally increased vascularity. When Paget's disease affects the long bones, the overlying skin may be warm and hyperemic, possibly due to increased blood flow to the entire region. The excessive circulation to the hypervascular bone may contribute to the development of high-output cardiac failure in some patients.

Skull involvement may produce enlargement of the head characterized by more-evident frontal bossing and dilated superficial cranial vessels. If the facial bones are involved as well, a typical leonine appearance may be noted. Deafness may result from disease of the temporal bone or ossicles. Compression of nerve or nerve roots may also occur. Pagetic involvement at the base of the skull may lead to basilar invagination or platybasia with consequent compression of structures in the posterior fossa, spinal cord, or more rarely, cerebellar tonsilar herniation. Symptoms of such a process may manifest as ataxia, weakness, or respiratory compromise.

Paget's disease affecting the spine may produce pain directly or as a result of nerve root irritation or compression. Pressure of the spinal cord is unusual. Limb pain may be due to the lesion itself or result from nerve root compression. If the pagetic lesion is near a joint, mechanical changes can lead to osteoarthritis; for example, arthritis in the knees may stem from disease of the distal femur or patella. Hip disease due to involvement of the femoral head or acetabulum is common and may be associated with protrusio acetabuli (17) (Fig. 44-1).

The radiographic appearance of pagetic bone reflects the underlying process. The initial pathologic lesion, which is osteolysis, appears as radiolucency on x-ray film and is particularly evident in the skull, where it is termed osteoporosis circumscripta. The advancing wedge of radiolucency in the long bones is called a flame-shaped radiolucency. The

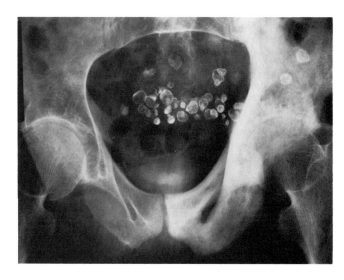

(Figure 44-1)

Pelvis of an 82-year-old man who had Paget's disease of bone for at least 10 years. The joint (cartilage) space of the left hip joint is severely narrowed and the iliopectineal line is thickened (brim sign), as evidenced by comparison with the opposite side.

apparent attempts to repair these areas are seen as areas of increased density or as coarsened trabecula. In some circumstances, the dimensions of the involved bone may increase along with thickening of the cortex, which results in an overt sclerotic appearance. Involvement of the iliopectineal line (brim sign) with thickening of the pelvic brim can be very helpful in distinguishing Paget's disease from the sclerotic lesions of metastatic carcinoma (Fig. 44-1).

In rare instances, tumors may develop in pagetic bone. Osteosarcomas develop in fewer than 1% of patients; a sudden rise in the serum alkaline phosphatase may be an early sign of this unfortunate event. Occasionally, other neoplasms such as giant cell tumors may also develop. Large non-neoplastic reparative granulomas consisting of a giant cell reaction may develop, particularly when the facial bones or skull are involved. These lesions are typically nonmetastatic but may be locally destructive (18). Metastatic tumors to these areas of increased blood flow have also been described.

THERAPY

Usually, Paget's disease is entirely asymptomatic and diagnosed on radiographs ordered for other reasons. Therapy is appropriate in symptomatic patients but should be withheld until a diagnosis is confirmed and other diseases such as metastatic cancer are ruled out. Indications for therapy include the presence of bone pain, impending surgery to correct a mechanical bone abnormality causing a neurologic deficit, and high-output cardiac failure. Nonsteroidal anti-inflammatory drugs suppress pain and inflammation but do not alter the natural history of the disease or the underlying biochemical abnormalities. Antiresorptive agents, including salmon calcitonin (available in both a parenteral solution and a nasal spray), human calcitonin (available as an injectable agent), and the bisphosphonates decrease bone resorption and bone formation and may decrease pain and improve function. In patients with high-output cardiac failure, antiresorptive agents are used to decrease cardiac demand. The use of antiresorptive agents may decrease the hypervascularity of bone and thus improve the outcome and decrease the complications associated with orthopedic surgery. Mithramycin (or plicamycin) is no longer considered to be appropriate therapy for Paget's disease.

Synthetic salmon calcitonin is significantly more potent than human calcitonin. Side effects of salmon calcitonin are a transient fall in serum calcium associated with clinically evident flushing. Subcutaneous doses every other day result in clinical improvement, usually within several weeks. Unfortunately, when therapy is discontinued, symptoms usually recur, and, over time, some patients seem to experience a plateau in therapeutic response. Except for patients with very active disease, daily doses seem to have no increased benefit over alternate-day dose. Some evidence suggests that salmon calcitonin may also be helpful as an analgesic through modulation of beta endorphins. Serum alkaline phosphatase as a marker of continued bone osteoblastic function decreases over time with continued therapy.

The bisphosphonates, which are analogs of inorganic pyrophosphate, are very potent drugs that inhibit osteoclast function (19). Disodium etidronate is administered orally in dosages of 5–10 mg/kg/day for no longer than 6 months. Because it is poorly absorbed and poorly bioavailable, disodium etidronate should be taken on an empty stomach. The known mineralization defect with etidronate may cause some patients to experience a temporary paradoxical increase in bone pain. The bisphosphonate pamidronate, although approved only for treatment of hypercalcemia of malignancy, has been used in Europe for Paget's disease. This agent has been associated with prolonged remissions, but the optimal therapeutic dose remains controversial and the agent requires parenteral administration (1). Alendronate, another new biphosphonate, may be successful as an oral drug in treating Paget's disease (20).

Once irreversible joint damage takes place, particularly in weight-bearing joints, little can be done, other than consider joint replacement if appropriate. Most patients do quite well with this intervention, although the surgery may cause extensive hemorrhage unless antiresorptive agents are used preoperatively.

LEE S. SIMON, MD

1. Singer FR: Paget's disease of bone. In DeGroot LJ (ed): Endocrinology. Philadelphia, 1995, pp 1259-1273
2. Foldes J, Shamir S, Brautbar C, Schermann L, Menczel J: HLA-D antigens and Paget's disease of bone. Clin Orthop 266:301-303, 1991
3. Singer FR, Mills BG, Park MS, et al: Increased HLA-DQWI antigen pattern in Paget's disease of bone. Clin Res 33:547A, 1985
4. Siris ES, Ottman R, Flaster E, Kelsey JL: Familial aggregation of Paget's disease of bone. J Bone Miner Res 6:495-500, 1991
5. Kanis JA: Pathophysiology and treatment of Paget's disease of bone. Durham [NC] Academic Press, 1991
6. Roodman GD, Kurihara N, Ohsaki Y, Kukita A, Hosking D, Demulder A, Smith FJ, Singer FR: Interleukin-6: a potential autocrine/paracrine factor in Paget's disease of bone. J Clin Invest 89:46-52, 1992
7. Taylor AK, Lueken SA, Libanati C, Baylink DJ: Biochemical markers of bone turnover for the clinical assessment of bone metabolism. Clin Rheum Dis 20:589-607, 1994
8. Charles P, Hasling C, Risteli L, Risteli J, Mosekilde L, Eriksin EF: Assessment of bone formation by biochemical markers in metabolic bone disease: separation between osteoblastic activity at the cell and tissue level. Calcif Tiss Int 51:406-411, 1992
9. Eriksen EF, Charles P, Melsen F, Mosekilde L, Risteli L, Risteli J: Serum markers of type I collagen formation and degradation in metabolic bone disease: correlation to bone histomorphometry. J Bone Min Res 8:127-132, 1993
10. Hassager AC, Risteli J, Risteli L, Jensen SB, Christiansen C: Diurnal variation in serum markers of type I collagen synthesis and degradation in healthy premenopausal women. J Bone Min Res 7:1307-1311, 1992
11. Delmas PD: Biochemical markers of bone turnover: methodology and clinical use in osteoporosis. Am J Med S5B:64s-68s, 1992
12. Delmas PD: Biochemical markers of bone turnover. J Bone Min Res 8(suppl 2):s549-s555, 1993
13. Simon LS, Krane SM, Wortman PD, Krane IM, Kovitz KL: Serum levels of type I and type III procollagen fragments in Paget's disease of bone. J Clin Endocrinol Metab 58:110-120, 1984
14. Robins SP, Black D, Paterson CR, Reid DM, Duncan A, Seibel MJ: Evaluation of urinary hydroxypyridinium crosslink measurements as resorption markers in metabolic bone diseases. Eur J Clin Invest 21:310-315, 1991
15. Delmas P, Gineyts E, Bertholin A, Garnero P, Marchand F: Immunoassay of pyridinoline crosslink excretion in normal adults and in Paget's disease. J Bone Min Res 8:643-648, 1993
16. Kushida K, Takahashi M, Kawana K, Inoue T: Comparison of markers for bone formation and resorption in premenopausal and postmenopausal subjects, and osteoporosis patients. J Clin Endocrinol Metab 80:2447-2550, 1995
17. Franck WA, Bress NM, Singer FR, Krane SM: Rheumatic manifestations of Paget's disease of bone. Am J Med 56:592-603, 1974
18. Upchurch KS, Simon LS, Schiller AL, Rosenthal DI, Campion EW, Krane SM: Giant cell reparative granuloma of Paget's disease of bone: a unique clinical entity. Ann Intern Med 98:35-40, 1983
19. Singer FR, Minoofar PN: Bisphosphonates in the treatment of disorders of mineral metabolism. Adv Endocrinol Metab 6:259-288, 1995
20. Adami S, Mian M, Gatti P, Rossini M, Zanberlan N, Bertoldof, LoCascio V: Effects of two oral doses of alendronate in the treatment of Paget's disease of bone. Bone 15:415-417, 1994

OSTEOPOROSIS AND METABOLIC BONE DISEASES

OSTEOPOROSIS

Osteoporosis is a systemic skeletal disease characterized by low bone mass and microarchitectural deterioration of bone tissue, with a consequent increase in bone fragility and susceptibility to fracture (1). The clinical significance of osteoporosis lies in the fractures that occur, including vertebral compression fractures, Colles' fractures of the forearm, and hip fractures (1,2). Women at the age of 50 have nearly a 40% chance of having an osteoporotic fracture.

Epidemiology

The prevalence of vertebral compression fractures is about 20% in postmenopausal white women. The incidence of hip fractures increases exponentially after age 50 in women and after age 60 in men. For white women aged 50, the overall lifetime risk for any fracture is 40%: 18% for hip fracture, 16% for vertebral fracture, and 16% for distal forearm fracture (2). For white men aged 50, the overall lifetime risk for fracture is about 15%: 6% for hip fracture, 6% for vertebral fracture, and 3% for forearm fracture. With the population trend toward aging and a slight trend toward increased fracture rate, the number of patients with osteoporotic fractures is steadily increasing. Although osteoporosis is a worldwide problem that affects every population and occurs in all geographic areas studied thus far, the fracture incidence differs markedly among different populations and ethnic groups; the incidence is greatest in whites and Asians and least in blacks.

Physiology

Bone is made up of two types: cortical and trabecular. Cortical bone comprises 80% of all bone, contains haversian systems, and is found mainly in long bones. Trabecular bone is found in flat bones (vertebrae, sternum, and pelvis) and the metaphyses of long bones.

Bone is constantly remodeled through the process of active formation and resorption. Resorption and formation occur in close temporal sequences, both in quantitative and qualitative balance—a phenomenon known as "coupling." Because osteoblasts replace virtually the same amount and type of bone tissue that has been resorbed, the amount of bone tissue at each remodeling locus does not change appreciably. In adults, 25% of trabecular bone is resorbed and replaced every year, compared with 3% of cortical bone, which indicates the rate of remodeling is controlled by local factors. Trabecular bone has a high surface-to-volume ratio, 70%–85% of which is in contact with the bone marrow.

The hallmark of osteoporosis is a reduction in skeletal mass caused by an imbalance between bone resorption and bone formation. Loss of gonadal function and aging are the two most important elements contributing to this imbalance.

Postmenopausal (type I) bone loss follows estrogen depletion (loss of ovarian function in women or castration in men). It is associated with increased rates of both bone resorption and formation, with the former exceeding the latter, and increased numbers of osteoclasts in trabecular bone. Thus, trabecular bone is the most affected by bone loss, and vertebral and Colles' fractures of the forearm are part of this syndrome (3).

Age-associated (type II) osteoporosis occurs because the amount of bone formed during each remodeling cycle decreases with age in both genders, most likely because the supply of osteoblasts is reduced in proportion to the demand for them. The demand for osteoblasts is determined by the frequency with which new multicellular units are created and new cycles of remodeling are initiated. Age-associated bone loss occurs primarily in cortical bone and results in fractures of the hip, proximal femur, humerus, ribs, pelvis, and vertebral bodies (3).

Risk Factors

Bone mass is the major measurable determinant of an individual's risk of osteoporotic fractures (Table 45-1). Bone mass increases during childhood and adolescence, peaks in

(Table 45-1)
Risk factors for osteoporosis and fractures*

Genetic
- Low bone mass
- Advanced age
- Female gender
- White or Asian
- Familial prevalence
- Early menopause
- Thinness or weight loss
- Abnormal hip axis length

Lifestyle and nutrition
- Smoking
- Heavy alcohol intake
- Low physical activity
- Low calcium intake

Medical conditions and medications
- Thiazide diuretics (+)
- Gastrectomy
- Corticosteroids
- Hyperthyroidism

Balance and gait impairment
- Sensory loss
- Muscle weakness
- Sedative use
- Cognitive impairment

*Adapted from Cummings et al (4), with permission.

the third or early fourth decade of life, and declines progressively thereafter. Women have less bone than men at all ages and experience a sharp acceleration of bone loss during the 5 years following menopause. Age-associated bone loss approximates 1% per year, but annual losses of 3%–5% are not uncommon in early menopause. Lifetime bone loss may reach 30%–40% of peak bone mass in women and 20%–30% in men. The magnitude of peak bone mass and the rate and duration of postmenopausal and age-associated bone loss determine the likelihood of developing osteoporosis. Falls, age, and existing fractures are all predictors of fracture incidence independent of bone mass.

At greatest risk for osteoporosis are white and Asian postmenopausal women who are thin or small, have a family history of the disease, experience premature menopause, lose a substantial amount of weight during adulthood, or have an abnormal hip axis length (4). Lifestyle factors that enhance the likelihood of osteoporosis include smoking cigarettes, abusing alcohol, being sedentary, and consuming too little calcium. Strong evidence indicates that genetic and lifestyle factors are important determinants of peak bone mass. Vitamin D deficiency may contribute to fracture risk in the elderly. Osteoporosis can develop from diseases such as multiple myeloma, severe primary hyperparathyroidism, surgical gastrectomy, and hyperthyroidism. Drugs that increase the risk of disease include corticosteroids (long-term use or high doses), gonadotropin-releasing hormone agonists and antagonists, and thyroid hormone replacement associated with subclinical or clinical hyperthyroidism. Estrogen deficiency in premenopausal women (caused by, for example, anorexia nervosa, excessive exercise, or hyperprolactinemia) induce bone loss and may reduce peak bone mass. Osteoporosis in middle-aged and elderly men is commonly associated with decreased testosterone levels, alcohol abuse, smoking, immobilization, and medications.

Falls are essential precipitating events in hip and other types of non-vertebral osteoporotic fractures in the elderly.

Risk factors for falls include balance and gait impairments that result from sensory loss, muscle weakness, sedative use, and cognitive impairments.

Diagnosis and Prediction of Risk

The only way to ascertain bone mineral density is by direct measurement (Table 45-2). Technology is now available to determine bone mass (or density) safely, conveniently, at a relatively low cost, and with an accuracy exceeding 95% and a precision error less than 1%. Single-photon absorptiometry (SPA) and single x-ray absorptiometry (SPX) are used to measure peripheral appendicular bones such as the forearm and calcaneus. Dual x-ray absorptiometry (DXA) has essentially replaced dual photon absorptiometry (DPA) for estimating axial, proximal appendicular (hip), and total body bone mass. Quantitative computed tomography (QCT) has been adapted to bone densitometry, but limited accessibility, relatively high radiation doses, and high cost have precluded its widespread use. Lower-cost methods such as ultrasound, x-ray photodensitometry, and others remain to be validated by careful clinical studies.

Bone mass measurement at any site is a reasonable predictor of fracture at all sites, although DXA of the proximal femur predicts hip fractures better than measurements at other sites. Recently, the World Health Organization (WHO) developed criteria for the diagnosis of osteoporosis by bone mineral density. The criteria use peak bone mass and assess risk of osteoporosis by the number of standard deviations between bone mineral density (BMD) and peak bone mass (T score). The BMD from any skeletal site can be used to assess risk of osteoporosis. Normal bone density is defined as a T score of 0–1, osteopenia as –1–2, osteoporosis as <–2, and severe osteoporosis as <–2.5 + fragility fractures (5). The WHO criteria are useful guidelines to help clinicians determine an individual patient's risk and severity of osteoporosis. Bone mass measurements are indicated as a guide for treating osteoporosis, as well as other bone-threatening con-

(Table 45-2)
Comparison of current techniques for measuring bone mineral density

Technique [*]	Cortical/Trabecular Ratio	Precision in Vivo (%)	Effective Accuracy Error (%)	Dose Equivalent (μSv)
SPA and SPX				
Distal third radius	95/5			
Ultradistal radius	60/40	1–2	4–6	<1
Os calcis	5/95			
DXA				
Lumbar spine				
Posterioanterior	50/50	1–3	4–8	1
Lateral	10/90		5–10	3
Proximal femur	60/40		4–8	1
Total body	80/20		1–2	3
QCT				
Single energy spine	0/100	2–4	5–15	50
Dual energy spine	0/100	4–6	3–6	100
pQCT	0/100	0.5–1	2–4	<1
Quantitative ultrasound				
UTV		0.25	2–4	0
BUA		1.3–3.8	?	0

[*] SPA = single-photon absorptiometry; SPX = single x-ray absorptiometry; DXA = dual X-ray absorptiometry; QCT = quantitative computed tomography; PQCT = peripheral QCT; UTV = ultrasound transmission attenuation; BUA = broad band ultrasound attenuation.

ditions, such as primary hyperparathyroidism and hypercortisolism.

In addition to the classic biochemical markers of bone metabolism (eg, urinary hydroxyproline, calcium excretion, and serum alkaline phosphatase and osteocalcin), new methods that estimate bone resorption (eg, serum and urine deoxypyridinoline) and bone formation (eg, serum bone-specific alkaline phosphatase and cross-links of type I collagen, N-telopeptide) have been developed and more are on the horizon. These tests, alone and in combination, may become useful in risk prediction, choice of therapy, and monitoring the time course of bone loss and the efficacy of therapy in combination with BMD measurements.

Prevention and Treatment

Because no effective, safe methods are available for restoring high-quality bone to the osteoporotic skeleton, prevention of osteoporosis is of the utmost importance. Approaches to prevention include maximizing peak bone mass and reducing postmenopausal and age-associated bone loss.

Calcium and Nutritional Requirements

Adequate calcium nutrition is essential for developing and maintaining a normal skeleton. A low calcium intake impairs peak bone mass and accelerates age-associated bone loss. Calcium supplementation at higher levels than the typical American intake of 600–800 mg/day has been shown to increase bone mass in children and adolescents and to retard the bone loss of aging (6). However, high calcium intake has a minimal-to-no protective effect against bone loss in the immediate postmenopausal period. Recommended calcium intakes for white females are 800 mg/day until age 10, 1500 mg/day during adolescence, 1200 mg/day in adulthood, and 1500 mg/day during pregnancy, lactation, and if at increased risk for osteoporosis. It is usually necessary to resort to calcium supplementation, although most individuals require only 500–1000 mg/day as a supplement to dietary sources to achieve these levels. Many forms of calcium supplements are available. Both calcium carbonate and citrate offer the highest calcium content per unit tablet weight (40% and 30%, respectively). Because calcium carbonate absorption is better in an acid environment, these supplements should be taken with food. Absorption of calcium citrate is slightly more efficient than calcium carbonate, and is not dependent on gastric acidity. However, calcium citrate is more expensive. At the recommended dietary intakes, calcium supplements are almost free of side effects. If constipation or intestinal colic occur with calcium carbonate, calcium citrate is a useful alternative. Care should be taken in prescribing calcium supplements to patients with renal stones, but if urine calcium excretion is not increased, the citrate salt can be used.

Physical Exercise

Stresses on the skeleton enhance bone development, while immobilization (eg, prolonged bedrest, weightlessness in space flight) causes significant bone loss. Vigorous exercise augments bone mineral density in the adult as long as it is continued. The main benefits of exercise in the elderly are to prevent bone loss from disuse and to promote mobility, agility, and muscle strength (7). However, sedentary individuals should consult their physicians before initiating an exercise program.

Estrogen

Hormone replacement therapy in postmenopausal women is effective in reducing skeletal turnover and slowing the rate of bone loss. Its use is also associated with a reduction in the risk of fracture, especially of the hip, wrist (Colles' fracture), and vertebrae (8). Several regimens for using estrogen to prevent bone loss have been recommended. Because estrogen primarily reduces the rate of bone loss, the earlier therapy is started, the more bone mass and structure will be maintained. Estrogen does reduce the rate of bone loss in estrogen-deficient women regardless of age, however; a reduction in bone loss has been observed among older women up to the eighth decade. The minimum dose required to prevent bone loss is 0.625 mg of conjugated estrogens (Premarin) or 1–2 mg of 17β-estradiol. Estrogen may also be delivered by epidermal patch, gel, or cream, and subcutaneous preparations are also effective. The benefits of estrogen continue for as long as treatment is provided, but when treatment is discontinued bone loss ensues at a rate comparable to that occurring immediately after menopause or ovariectomy. Both retrospective and prospective studies have confirmed that long-term protection against fractures requires estrogen treatment for 10 years after menopause (8).

The individual patient must make the decision to take estrogen, however, and the skeletal system is only one aspect of a postmenopausal woman's health. Estrogens are associated with an increased risk of uterine and breast cancer. The increased risk of uterine cancer with estrogen alone is essentially eliminated when progestogen is taken concurrently. Cyclic or continuous therapy with progestational agents is therefore recommended for women with an intact uterus. Although long-term estrogen therapy slightly increases the risk of breast cancer, estrogen decreases the risk of cardiovascular disease, which is the most common cause of mortality (9). Currently, large-scale studies are in progress to better define the benefits and risks of estrogen therapy.

Calcitonin

In women who cannot or choose not to take estrogens, other antiresorptive therapies can be used. Calcitonin (injectable and intranasal) inhibits bone resorption and can prevent perimenopausal trabecular bone loss. It is approved for this indication and for the treatment of postmenopausal and age-associated bone loss. Calcitonin may be most useful for osteoporosis characterized by high bone turnover. Retrospective and prospective studies have demonstrated that calcitonin reduces the incidence of osteoporotic fractures. The drug is safe and has analgesic properties. A reasonable and effective analgesic dose range is 50–100 units given subcutaneously, three times a week. To date, the use of this agent has been constrained by the route of administration and the cost, but the nasal formulation of salmon calcitonin has become available, and at a daily dose of 100–200 units it is effective in preventing bone loss associated with estrogen deficiency (10). Calcitonin is a useful medication for preventing steroid-induced osteoporosis and for osteoporosis in men. The absence of side effects is a major advantage to using this agent for primary prevention and established disease.

Bisphosphonates

Bisphosphonates are stable, active analogs of pyrophosphate that bind avidly to calcium apatite. These agents are potent inhibitors of bone remodeling, which lower both bone resorption and formation. However, the mode of action of these drugs is still not entirely clear, and each analog may affect remodeling with subtle but important differences. The agents are tolerated well and have no significant side effects. Etidronate, the first bisphosphonate available in the United States, increases the bone density in established osteoporosis by about 5% (11) and, over a 4-year period, was shown to decrease the incidence of new vertebral fractures (12). Continuous etidronate therapy can result in impaired bone mineralization and osteomalacia, however. The dose for treating or preventing postmenopausal osteoporosis is 400 mg/day for 2 weeks, repeated every 3 months. Etidronate, although an effective treatment, is not at this time approved by the United States Food and Drug Administration (FDA) for these indications.

Alendronate, which has been approved by the FDA for treating osteoporosis, is a second-generation biphosphonate. It is a potent inhibitor of bone turnover but has almost no impact on bone mineralization. Alendronate at doses of 10 mg/day has been found to prevent postmenopausal bone loss and to increase bone mineral density of the spine by about 6% over a 2–3 year period in patients with established osteoporosis. It has also been effective in reducing vertebral fractures, but the effect of alendronate on hip fractures is unknown. Several other bisphosphonates are currently in development (13).

Bisphosphonates are poorly absorbed from the gastrointestinal tract, and calcium or caffeine impairs absorption even more. These agents should therefore be taken on an empty stomach, and the patient should be instructed to remain upright for at least an hour after ingestion to improve absorption. Because of the low incidence of side effects, bisphosphonates may become important in the prevention of osteoporosis of all types.

Vitamin D and Its Analogs

Adequate vitamin D intake is particularly important in elderly individuals, who may be house-bound, sunlight-deprived, nutritionally deficient, or resistant to vitamin D. These considerations may explain the efficacy of vitamin D 800 IU/day and calcium supplements in reducing hip fractures in elderly institutionalized patients (14). A total of 400–800 IU/day of vitamin D is recommended for older individuals, which can be obtained by taking two multivitamins daily.

Some studies have found that large doses of 1,25-dihydroxyvitamin D3 (calcitriol) or its analogs increase bone mass (but not bone density) and reduce fracture frequency in subjects with established osteoporosis (15), causing only minimal serum and urine calcium elevations. However, calcitriol is an active form of vitamin D, and it can easily increase serum or urine calcium to dangerous levels. Because of the potential dangers of hypercalcemia and hypercalciuria from high doses of vitamin D, without consistent evidence that it increases bone mass or decreases fracture risk, calcitriol cannot be recommended at this time.

Agents that Stimulate Bone Formation

A therapeutic rationale for the use of sodium fluoride in osteoporosis is based on the ability of this compound to stimulate osteoblasts to make new bone, although bone made under the auspices of fluoride produces a fluorapatite crystal instead of hydroxyapatite. Studies show improvement in vertebral bone mass and a decreased incidence of spinal fractures when slow-release sodium fluoride is administered in doses of 25 mg twice a day in four 14-month cycles (12 months of fluoride, 2 months off of fluoride), along with calcium citrate 400 mg twice a day for 4 years (16). Unfortunately, in studies involving higher doses (75 mg a day), subjects experienced an increase in both spinal bone mass and apparent cortical fractures. Therefore, although bone mass may increase with fluoride, the bone quality was impaired. Side effects of high-dose fluoride include gastric upset, possible ulceration, possible increase in stress fractures, and plantar fasciitis. Although low doses of sustained-release sodium fluoride show promise in the treatment of osteoporosis, larger randomized controlled studies must be completed before this agent can be recommended.

Anabolic steroids are sometimes prescribed for elderly patients with advanced disease, although these agents are not FDA-approved for osteoporosis. These drugs appear to stimulate osteoblasts to form new bone, and, indeed, bone mass does increase. The side effects of anabolic steroids include masculinization, potential liver toxicity, and hyperlipidemia (possibly predisposing to an increased risk of cardiovascular disease); as a result, the use of these agents is restricted.

There is growing interest in the anabolic effect of parathyroid hormone (PTH). Both preclinical and clinical studies indicate that intermittent pharmacologic doses of PTH stimulate bone formation and increase bone mass. It restores bone to trabecular regions of the estrogen-depleted osteoporotic skeleton in both animals and humans (17,18). The bone-forming effects of PTH are predominantly at bone surfaces adjacent to bone marrow. Preliminary results from a 3-year study in postmenopausal women with established osteoporosis indicate that daily treatment with estrogen and a subcutaneous injection of human PTH (hPTH) amino acid fragment (1–34) significantly increases trabecular bone mass (18). Currently, PTH must be administered subcutaneously, but work in developing easier routes of administration is in progress.

CORTICOSTEROID-INDUCED BONE LOSS

Corticosteroids have several unfortunate effects on bone metabolism: decreased calcium absorption, increased urinary calcium excretion, decreased bone formation, and bone resorption that may remain normal or increase. In addition, corticosteroids reduce sex hormone production by reducing ACTH (adrenocorticotropic hormone) levels, affecting adrenal androgen production, and affecting gonad function directly. The use of corticosteroids is associated with rapid bone loss, especially in high-turnover trabecular bone, and increased fractures in predominantly trabecular sites such as the vertebrae and ribs. Bone loss is rapid; prednisone at doses higher than 7.5 mg/day for 6 months may decrease trabecular bone volume by as much as 20%, followed by a slow but continuous bone loss with longer use. Bone density measurements can be helpful in monitoring patients who must receive long-term corticosteroid therapy. Guidelines for the treatment and prevention of steroid-induced bone loss have recently been published (19) (see Appendix II). The defect in calcium absorption may be treated with daily doses of 1500-mg calcium supplements and 800 IU of vitamin D (two multivitamins/day). Treatment of low gonadotropin levels includes estrogen replacement for postmenopausal women (if not contraindicated) and testosterone (if found to be low) for men. Premenopausal women who experience menstrual irregularities can be treated with birth control pills or conjugated estrogen at 0.3 mg/day. Hypercalciuria, if present, can be treated with thiazide diuretics. Patients who are not receiving hormone replacement or who continue to lose bone mass despite hormone replacement can be treated with other antiresorptive agents, such as calcitonin or bisphosphonates (etidronate, alendronate). Unfortunately, no drugs that stimulate bone formation and increase bone mass in the presence of corticosteroids have been carefully studied, but patients who discontinue therapy can recover bone mass. Therefore, the dosage should be tapered to the lowest possible corticosteroid dose, and the drug stopped as soon as is possible. It is important to remember that alternate-day steroids do not impair calcium absorption, although they do not prevent bone loss in adults (20).

PRIMARY HYPERPARATHYROIDISM

Primary hyperparathyroidism is not a rare disorder; about 28 new cases per 100,000 population are diagnosed each year. A solitary parathyroid adenoma is usually the cause of excess secretion of PTH. Symptoms of primary hyperparathyroidism include abdominal pain, bone pain, renal stones, and psychiatric disorders. In its advanced state, the disease causes pathologic bone fractures, and the bone histology shows osteitis fibrosis with excessive resorption and formation. Bone loss seems to be more marked in cortical bone than in trabecular bone. Kidney stones result from hypercalcemia. Gastric ulcers and depression are also associated with the disease. Laboratory abnormalities include elevated serum PTH levels (the intact hormone should be measured), hypercalcemia, increased urinary calcium, cyclic adenosine monophosphate, and low serum phosphate. Often calcitriol levels are increased. Mild primary hyperparathyroidism is asymptomatic and is discovered during routine laboratory screening. Thus many cases are now discovered that would have previously been undetected. Physicians usually monitor these patients' calcium levels and bone mineral densities. Whether asymptomatic patients should undergo parathyroidectomy is unresolved.

OSTEOMALACIA

Osteomalacia (called rickets in children), caused by vitamin D deficiency, is characterized by excessive amounts of unmineralized osteoid material. While osteoid comprises less than 5% of normal bone, it can account for 40%–50% of bone in osteomalacia. Consequently, bone strength is reduced, which results in fractures and bone pain. The growth plate of bones are particularly affected in children, causing bowed legs and deformed skulls and ribs. The causes of vitamin D deficiency are multiple, but most cases result from decreased serum mineral levels due to toxins or poor dietary intake (Table 45-3).

In the presence of ultraviolet light, vitamin D is manufactured in skin from cholesterol precursors. The liver hydrox-

(Table 45-3)
*Osteomalacia**

Vitamin D Abnormalities	Laboratory Findings				
	Ca	PO$_4$	25-D	Calcitriol	Other Tests
Nutritional deficiency	D	D	D	D	I PTH and alkaline phosphatase
Secondary					
Liver disease	D	D	D	D	I PTH and alkaline phosphatase
Renal disease	D	I	N	D	I PTH and alkaline phosphatase
1α hydroxylase deficiency (vitamin D-dependent rickets type I)	D	D	N	D	I PTH and alkaline phosphatase
Resistance due to abnormal receptor	D	D	N	I	I PTH and alkaline phosphatse
(vitamin D-dependent rickets type II)	±D	D	N	N	
X-linked hypophosphatemic rickets (vitamin D-resistant rickets)	±D	D	N	N	Calcitriol is inappropriately normal
Hypophosphatemia					
Renal phosphate loss	N	D	N	N	
Excessive antacid intake	N	D	N	±I	
Hereditary hypophosphatemia with hypercalciuria	N	D	N	I	I urinary calcium
Toxicities					
Fluoride	N	N	N	N	
Etidronate	N	±I	N	N	
Parenteral aluminum	N	N	N	±D	D PTH
Other					
Hypophosphatasia	N	N	N	N	D alkaline phosphatase
Acidosis	N	N	N	N	
Oncogenic osteomalacia	±D	D	N	D	I PTH and alkaline phosphatase

* Ca = calcium; PO$_4$ = phosphate; 25-D = vitamin D precursor; PTH = parathyroid hormone. I = increased; N = normal; D = decreased.

ylates at the 25 position and then the kidney at the 1 position to form 1,25-dihydroxyvitamin D, which is the active metabolite. It is a steroid hormone with cellular receptors, and genetic defects have been described in the receptor number and function in some families.

RENAL OSTEODYSTROPHY

Patients with end-stage renal disease who need dialysis rarely have normal bones. Several patterns of bone disease may occur in these patients, but the most common is secondary hyperparathyroidism, which results from damaged kidneys that do not produce adequate amounts of calcitriol. The serum calcium is low, and because renal excretion is impaired, serum phosphorus levels are high. The excess serum phosphorus further suppresses renal hydroxylation of vitamin D. In response, PTH levels increase and bone resorption ensues in an effort to normalize serum calcium levels. In addition, the parathyroid gland is not as sensitive to serum calcium in patients with renal failure as it is in normal subjects, which further encourages excessive PTH production. Increases in PTH stimulate both bone formation and resorption; bone mass varies from patient to patient.

If serum phosphorus levels become too high, metastatic calcifications occur. Oral doses of aluminum-containing antacids are given to prevent intestinal absorption of phosphorus, but some aluminum is absorbed. Since aluminum is toxic to both osteoblasts and parathyroid cells, these patients may develop osteomalacia with low PTH levels (21). Other complications seen in dialysis patients include acidosis, hypogonadism, iron accumulation, amyloidosis from β_2-microglobulin accumulation, deficiencies in growth factors, and hypercortisolism from corticosteroid therapy. Therefore, the spectrum of bone disease in these patients may be multifactorial and complex. A bone biopsy is often the only way to determine the correct diagnosis.

NANCY E. LANE, MD

1. Riggs B, Melton LJ: The prevention and treatment of osteoporosis. N Engl J Med 327: 620-627, 1992

2. Melton LJ, Chrischilles EA, Cooper C, Lane AW, Riggs BL: How many people have osteoporosis ? J Bone Mineral Res 7:1005-1010, 1992

3. Manolagas S, Jilka R: Bone marrow, cytokines, and bone remodeling. N Engl J Med 332:305-310, 1995

4. Cummings SR, Nevitt MC, Browner WS, et al: Risk factors for hip fractures in white women. N Engl J Med 332:767-773, 1995

5. Kanis JA, Melton LJ, Christiansen C, Johnston CC, Khaltaev N: The diagnosis of osteoporosis. J Bone Min Res 9:1137-1140, 1994

6. Reid IR, Ames RW, Evans MC, Gamble GD, Sharpe SJ: Effect of calcium supplementation on bone loss in postmenopausal women. N Engl J Med 328:460-464, 1993

7. Province MA, Hadley EC, Hornbrook MC, et al: The effects of exercise on falls in elderly patients: a preplanned meta-analysis of the FICSIT Trials. JAMA 273:1341-1347, 1995

8. Cauley JA, Seeley DG, Ensrud K, et al: Fracture protection provided by long-term estrogen treatment. Ost Int 5:23-29, 1995

9. Grady D, Rubin SM, Pettite DB, Fox C, Black D, Ettinger B, Ernster VL, Cummings SR: Hormone replacement therapy to prevent disease and prolong life in postmenopausal women. Ann Intern Med 117:1016-1041, 1992

10. Reginster JY, Deroisy R, Lecart MP, Sarlet N, Zeqels B, Jupsin I, deLonqueville M, Franchimont P: A double-blind, dose flinding trial of intermittent nasal calcitonin for prevention of postmenopausal lumbar bone loss. Am J Med 98:452-458, 1995

11. Watts NB, Harris ST, Genant HK, et al: Intermittent cyclical treatment of postmenopausal osteoporosis. N Engl J Med 323:73-79, 1990

12. Harris ST, Watts NB, Jackson RD, et al: Effects of four years of intermittent cyclical etidronte treatment for postmenopausal osteoporosis. Am J Med 95:557-567, 1993

13. Kanis JA, Gertz BJ, Singer F, Ortolani S: Rationale use of alendronate in osteoporosis. Ost Int 5:1-13, 1995

14. Chapuy MC, Arlot ME, Duboeuf F, Brun J, Crouzet B, Arnaud S, Delmas P, Meinier PJ: Vitamin D3 and calcium to prevent hip fractures. N Engl J Med 327:1637-1642, 1992

15. Tilyard MW, Spears GFS, Thompson J, Dovey S: Treatment of postmenopausal osteoporosis with calcitriol or calcium. N Engl J Med 326:357-362, 1992

16. Pak CY, Saghaee K, Adams-Huet B, Piziak V, Peterson RD, Pointdexter JR: Treatment of postmenopausal osteoporosis with slow-release sodium fluoride. Ann Intern Med 12:401-408. 1995

17. Lane NE, Thompson JM, Strewler GJ, Kinney JH: Intermittent treatment with human parathyroid hormone (hPTH 1-34) increased trabecular bone volume but not connectivity in osteopenic rats. J Bone Min Res 10:1470-1477, 1995

18. Lindsay R, Cosman F, Nieves J, Dempster D, Shen V: A controlled trial of the effect of the effect of 1-34 hPTH n estrogen treated with osteoporotic women J Bone Min Res 851:S130, 1994

19. American College of Rheumatology Task Force on Osteoporosis Guidelines: Recommendations for the prevention and treatment of glucocorticoid-induced osteoporosis. Arthritis Rheum 39:1791-1801, 1996

20. Lukert BP, Raisz LG: Glucocorticoid-induced osteoporosis. Rheumatic Dis Clin North Am 20:629-669, 1994

21. Slatopolsky E: The interaction of parathyroid hormine and aluminum in renal osteodystrophy. Kidney Internat 31:842-854, 1987

Foreign bodies introduced into joints, tendon sheaths, or periarticular tissues may induce a chronic noninfectious monarthritis, tenosynovitis, or dactylitis (1-5). The most common types of material associated with synovitis are plant thorns, wood splinters, and sea urchin spines. Many types of plant thorns have been described in foreign body synovitis including date palm, sentinel palm, blackthorn, rose thorn, and cactus (6). Other materials such as glass (7), plastic (7), lead (8), and starch (9) introduced by penetrating injury may cause chronic inflammation. Metal (10), silicone (11), and polyethylene (12) detritus from the breakdown of joint prostheses may also induce chronic granulomatous synovitis.

CLINICAL FEATURES

When evaluating monarticular synovitis or tenosynovitis, a key question in obtaining a patient's history is how recently the joint or surrounding tissue was injured. Although most patients experience local pain and inflammation at the time of a penetrating injury, an asymptomatic period lasting days, weeks, or months often follows (3). The intensity and duration of the initial inflammatory reaction depend on the type of foreign body, toxic protein coating or charge, degree of bacterial contamination, and concomitant treatment with antibiotics and anti-inflammatory agents. As a result of the time lapse between injury and developing chronic synovitis, patients and physicians might not associate the current problem with a past injury, leading to delayed diagnosis. After a latent period, the synovitis often becomes subacute or chronic with variable degrees of inflammation, synovial thickening, and effusion. Fever is characteristically absent, except when the foreign body is a sea urchin spine (2), which may cause fever, myalgias, regional lymph node enlargement, and even synovitis of surrounding joints.

Although any joint can be involved, the most common ones are those unprotected by clothing, such as the hands, wrists, and knees. Children are most often affected (4), followed by adults with an occupational proclivity toward trauma, such as construction workers, farmers, and gardeners (3). Swimmers and those involved in other marine recreational activities are at risk for penetrating injury to the feet and hands from sea urchins (2).

Differential diagnosis includes other forms of acute and chronic monarticular arthritis such as septic arthritis, tuberculous or fungal arthritis, osteomyelitis, and juvenile rheumatoid arthritis. The differential diagnosis of dactylitis includes sarcoidosis, psoriasis, erysipelas, sporotrichosis, and atypical mycobacteria.

LABORATORY, RADIOLOGIC, AND PATHOLOGIC FINDINGS

Results of blood tests such as white cell count, differential, and erythrocyte sedimentation rate are usually normal; thus they may be helpful in differentiating foreign body synovitis from acute bacterial infection. Synovial fluid obtained by aspiration contains inflammatory cells with variable white cell counts ranging up to $100,000/mm^3$ (3) and a predominance of polymorphonuclear leukocytes. Bacterial and fungal cultures are sterile, except in the rare instances when a contaminating agent was introduced along with the foreign body. Plant thorns and other particulate matter are most often embedded in the synovium and not visible in synovial fluid. The exception is detritic synovitis, in which fragments of metal, polyethylene, or methylmethacrylate may be found in synovial fluid (11).

Radiographs may detect metallic foreign bodies, sea urchin spines (Fig. 46-1), and glass, especially leaded or pigmented glass. Plant thorns and wood are not visible on radiographs. Nonspecific radiographic findings in nonarticular lesions include soft tissue swelling and periostitis; joint effusion may be present in articular involvement. In primary bone involvement, a well-circumscribed osteolytic lesion or pseudotumor may be found. For the purpose of both diagnosis and perioperative localization, ultrasound may be useful for detecting wood and plastic (13), and computerized tomography may help identify wood and plant thorns (14). The role of magnetic resonance imaging in the detection of foreign bodies is not yet delineated.

Accurate diagnosis requires surgical removal of the foreign body followed by pathologic and microbiologic studies of synovial tissue. Pathologic examination reveals proliferation of synovial lining cells, hyperemia, and cellular infiltration (4). The predominant cells in the synovium are lymphocytes with focal collections of polymorphonuclear cells. Variable numbers of plasma cells and eosinophils have also been described. These features contrast with the marked diffuse polymorphonuclear infiltrates seen in acute septic arthritis. Giant cell formation is prominent in patients with foreign body synovitis (3), which is another distinguishing feature

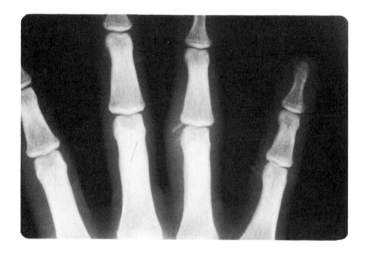

(Figure 46-1)
Soft tissue swelling surrounding a radiopaque sea urchin spine (composed of calcium carbonate) in a patient with foreign body synovitis.

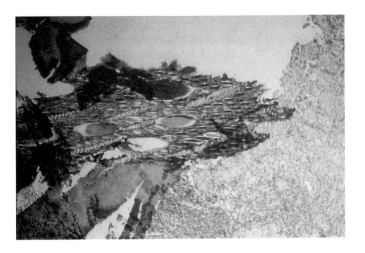

(Figure 46-2)

Photomicrograph of synovium revealing a wood fragment surrounded by a diffuse chronic mononuclear cell infiltrate. The birefringent multiple cell walls separated by thin fibrous septae are characteristic of vegetable material such as wood and plant thorns. This patient's knee was punctured by a toothpick. Reprinted from the Revised Clinical Slide Collection on the Rheumatic Diseases, with permission of the American College of Rheumatology.

not seen in acute septic arthritis. Synovial tissue should be examined with polarized light microscopy to detect birefringent plant thorn material (Fig. 46-2).

TREATMENT

Although anti-inflammatory agents may provide symptomatic relief, excisional biopsy with synovectomy is usually necessary for definitive treatment of chronic foreign body synovitis (3,5). This procedure can be performed through an arthroscope, but only if the joint is amenable to arthroscopy, if preoperative localization of the foreign body was accomplished by radiologic study, and if adequate arthroscopic synovectomy is possible. However, an open biopsy and extensive synovectomy are usually required because foreign bodies are often fragmented and poorly detectable by radiologic means.

MICHAEL J. MARICIC, MD

1. Sugarman M, Stobie DG, Quismorio FP, et al: Plant thorn synovitis. Arthritis Rheum 20:1125-1128, 1977
2. Cracchiolo A, Goldberg L: Local and systemic reactions to puncture injuries by the sea urchin spine and date palm thorn. Arthritis Rheum 20:1206-1212, 1977
3. Reginato AJ, Ferreiro JL, O'Connor CR, et al: Clinical and pathologic studies of twenty-six patients with penetrating foreign body injury to the joint, bursae, and tendon sheaths. Arthritis Rheum 33:1753-1762, 1990
4. Yousefzadeh DK, Jackson JH: Organic foreign body reaction: report of two cases of thorn-induced granuloma and review of the literature. Skeletal Radiol 3:167-176, 1978
5. Olengenginski TP, Bush DC, Harrington TM: Plant thorn synovitis: an uncommon cause of monoarthritis. Sem Arthritis Rheum 21:40-46, 1991
6. Zoltan JD: Cactus Thorn Synovitis. Arthroscopy 7:244-245, 1991
7. Goodnough CP, Frymore JW: Synovitis secondary to non-metallic foreign bodies. J Trauma 15:960-965, 1975
8. Farber JM, Rafii M, Schwartz D: Lead arthropathy and elevated serum levels of lead after gunshot wound of the shoulder. Am J Roentgenol 162:385-386, 1994
9. Freemont AJ, Porter ML, Tomlinson I, Clague RB, Jayson MIV: Starch synovitis. J Clin Pathol 37:990-992, 1984
10. Kitridou RC, Schumacher HR Jr, Sbarbaro JL, Hollander JL: Recurrent hemarthrosis after prosthetic knee arthroplasty: identification of metal particles in the synovial fluid. Arthritis Rheum 12:520-528, 1969
11. Christie AJ, Pierret G, Levitan J: Silicone synovitis. Sem Arthritis Rheum 19:166-171, 1989
12. Kaufman RL, Tong I, Beardmore TD: Prosthetic synovitis: clinical and histologic characteristics. J Rheumatol 12:1066-1074, 1985
13. Little CL, Parker MG, Callowich MC, Sartori JC: The ultrasonic detection of soft tissue foreign bodies. Invest Radiol 21:275-277, 1986
14. Bauer AR, Yutani D: Computer tomography localization of wooden foreign bodies in children's extremities. Arch Surg 118:1084-1086, 1983

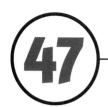

PEDIATRIC RHEUMATIC DISEASES

A. JUVENILE RHEUMATOID ARTHRITIS AND JUVENILE SPONDYLOARTHROPATHIES

JUVENILE RHEUMATOID ARTHRITIS

Juvenile rheumatoid arthritis (JRA) is the most common form of childhood arthritis and one of the more common chronic childhood illnesses. The cause is unknown. Diagnosis requires a combination of data from history, physical examination, and laboratory testing. For the vast majority of patients, the immunogenetic associations, clinical course, and functional outcome are quite different from adult-onset rheumatoid arthritis (RA). However, approximately 5%–10% of JRA patients who have rheumatoid factor-positive polyarticular arthritis beginning during adolescence have a disease that resembles adult-onset RA much more than JRA.

Epidemiology

The prevalence of JRA has been estimated to be between 57 and 113 per 100,000 children younger than 16 years old in the United States (1). The overall prevalence rate on January 1, 1980, for this age group in the Mayo Clinic population was estimated to be 113/100,000 (95% confidence intervals: 69.1, 196.3); the population studied was almost exclusively white and predominately of Northern European ancestry (2). Hochberg et al reported that the prevalence of JRA among urban blacks was 26/100,000 (95% confidence intervals: 7, 66) (3). In a recent population-based study from Sweden, Gère estimated the prevalence of JRA to be 86/100,000 (4). In addition, she reported that 50% of JRA patients have active disease that persists into adulthood (5). Neither the Mayo Clinic study nor Hochberg et al included adult-age JRA patients, resulting in an underestimation. All prevalence estimates have wide confidence intervals because of the relative rarity of JRA and the small number of actual cases detected in even the largest studies. This leads to enormous differences between the lower and upper estimates of actual JRA cases. The most commonly cited figure is 70,000 to 100,000 cases (active and inactive) of JRA in the US population under age 16 (1). Using Gère's report on disease persisting into adulthood, an estimated 35,000 to 50,000 people over age 16 have active JRA in the United States (5).

JRA affects a much smaller portion of the US population than adult-onset RA or osteoarthritis. However, compared to other pediatric-onset chronic illnesses, JRA is relatively common. JRA affects approximately the same number of children as juvenile diabetes, at least 4 times more than sickle cell anemia or cystic fibrosis, and at least 10 times more than hemophilia, acute lymphocytic leukemia, chronic renal failure, or muscular dystrophy (6).

Clinical Aspects

The diagnostic criteria for JRA are onset at less than 16 years of age, persistent arthritis in one or more joints for at least 6 weeks, and exclusion of other types of childhood arthritis (7). Four key points are often missed, resulting in misdiagnosis. 1) Arthritis must be present and is defined as swelling, effusion, or the presence of two or more of the following signs: limitation of motion, tenderness, pain on motion, or joint warmth. Arthralgia alone is not sufficient to satisfy this definition. 2) The arthritis must persist for at least 6 weeks. (Many European criteria require at least 12 weeks.) 3) More than 100 other causes of chronic arthritis in children must be excluded. 4) No specific laboratory or other test can establish the diagnosis of JRA.

JRA is subdivided into three types: systemic, polyarticular, and pauciarticular. These subtypes demonstrate unique clinical presentations, immunogenetic associations, and clinical courses (Table 47A-1). In fact, within the polyarticular and pauciarticular subtypes, further clinical grouping can be done, supporting the concept that JRA represents different forms of chronic arthritis.

Systemic Onset JRA (sJRA)

Approximately 10% of children with JRA have systemic onset characterized by daily or twice daily intermittent fever spikes >101° F and the presence of a characteristic JRA rash. The rash is pale pink, blanching, characterized by small macules or maculopapules, transient (minutes to a few hours), nonpruritic in 95% of cases, and most commonly seen on the trunk. Children with sJRA often have growth delay, osteopenia, diffuse lymphadenopathy, hepatosplenomegaly, pericarditis, pleuritis, anemia, leukocytosis, thrombocytosis, and elevated acute-phase reactants. Positive rheumatoid factor (RF) and uveitis are rare. The extra-articular features are almost always self-limited, are mild to moderate in severity, and most symptoms resolve when the fevers resolve. However, sJRA patients can develop pericardial tamponade or severe vasculitis with secondary consumptive coagulopathy, both of which are responsive to intense steroid therapy. The prognosis for sJRA is determined by the severity of the arthritis, which usually develops concurrently with the fever and rash, but in some patients does not develop for weeks or months after the onset of the fever. sJRA may develop at any age but the peak age of onset is 1 to 6 years old. Boys and girls are equally affected.

Polyarticular Onset (poJRA)

To be characterized as poJRA requires the presence of arthritis in five or more joints (Table 47A-1). Approximately 40% of JRA patients have polyarticular involvement. At least two distinct disease groups comprise poJRA and are most easily distinguished by the presence or absence of RF. RF-positive patients are almost always girls with later disease onset (at least 8 years old) who are usually HLA-DR4-positive, have symmetric small-joint arthritis, and are at greater

(Table 47A-1)
*JRA subtype characteristics**

	Systemic	Polyarticular	Pauciarticular
Frequency of cases	10%	40%	50%
Number of joints with arthritis at onset	Variable	≥5	≤4
Sex ratio (F:M)	1:1	3:1	5:1
Frequency of uveitis	1%	5%	20%
Frequency of rheumatoid factor positivity	<2%	5%–10%	<2%
Frequency of ANA positivity	5%–10%	40%–50%	75%–85%
Frequency of ≥5 joints involved any time during course of JRA	50%–60%	100%	40%
Frequency of active disease >10 years follow-up	42%	45%	41%
Frequency of erosions or joint space narrowing on radiographs	45%	54%	28%
Median time to develop erosions or joint space narrowing on radiographs (years after disease onset)	2.2	2.4	5.4
Frequency of adult height <5th percentile	50%	16%	11%

* JRA = juvenile rheumatoid arthritis; ANA = antinuclear antibody.

risk for developing erosions, nodules, and poor functional outcome, compared with RF-negative patients. RF-positive polyarticular JRA more closely resembles adult-onset RA more than any other subset. Clinical manifestations and outcome are highly variable, and include fatigue, anorexia, protein–caloric malnutrition, anemia, growth retardation, delay in sexual maturation, and osteopenia. poJRA may develop at any age, and girls outnumber boys 3 to 1.

Pauciarticular JRA (paJRA)

To be characterized as paJRA requires that the arthritis be present in four or fewer joints. Patients are subdivided into at least two distinct clinical groups: early onset and late onset. Early-onset paJRA patients are typically very young (1–5 years old) girls (girls outnumber boys 4 to 1), are often antinuclear antibody positive, have the greatest risk for developing chronic eye inflammation, and have the best overall articular outcome. Eye involvement occurs in 30%–50% of early-onset paJRA patients. The inflammatory process primarily involves the anterior chamber of the eye and is associated with no or minimal symptoms in more than 80% of affected children. Severe, irreversible eye changes can occur including corneal clouding, cataracts, glaucoma, and partial or total visual loss. Patients should be screened at regular intervals and treated by experienced eye specialists (8) (Table 47A-2). Late-onset paJRA is more common in boys; 50% are HLA-B27 positive, and patients are more likely to have enthesitis or tendinitis, with the arthritis often affecting large joints (shoulders, hips, knees) or the spine. If the eyes become involved in this older onset group, it is usually a very sudden onset of painful red eyes, but chronic complications are less likely to occur than in early-onset pauciarticular JRA.

Treatment

The standard of care for JRA incorporates the comprehensive, coordinated efforts of an interdisciplinary team of health care professionals and the family. Comprehensive means addressing all facets of an individual's life that may be affected by a chronic illness such as education, peer relations, self-esteem, social adjustment, family dynamics, vocational planning, and financial concerns. In clinical settings that have used this approach, young adult JRA patients have been shown to surpass both community standards and even their own siblings in level of post-secondary schooling and professional degree attainment (9).

The treatment of JRA begins with diagnosis. The patient, parents, influential extended family members (for example, grandparents) as well as the health-care team must be comfortable that the patient really does have JRA. The family shoulders the largest responsibility for the child's ongoing treatment. It is family members who will or will not give medications, put on splints, assist with prescribed exercises, adapt the family schedule to facilitate regular school attendance, maintain normal academic and vocational expectations, and so on. The therapeutic goals for JRA patients are relieving symptoms, maintaining joint motion and muscle strength, preventing or minimizing anatomic joint damage, maximizing functional status, promoting positive self-image, and encouraging productive family dynamics. Studies have shown that the negative psychologic impact of JRA is greater on the siblings than on the patient (9).

The treatment program can be divided into physical, social, and pharmacologic components. Physical (PT) and occupational (OT) therapists oversee the physical component, which consists of performing range-of-motion exercises for the involved joints two or three times per day. Splints are fabricated to minimize joint deformity or mechanical stress, or to correct contractures. In addition, joint protection techniques are taught to minimize joint trauma while the young person participates in activities of daily living (ADL). The PT and OT often consult with school personnel about physical education and classroom adaptations.

The social program relates to psychosocial adjustments, school adaptations, and vocational issues. The social worker and rheumatology nurse are deeply involved in this area. Patients and families often feel quite isolated and benefit from introduction to other families with children with JRA. The Arthritis Foundation sponsors national and regional activities of the American Juvenile Arthritis Organization (AJAO). The AJAO is a membership organization for children with juvenile-onset rheumatic diseases and their families. Early involvement of families with the AJAO can greatly facilitate productive adjustment to the challenges of a rheumatic disease. JRA does not affect intellectual capacity but can significantly impair educational achievement. However, most roadblocks to educational progress can be avoided or corrected with minor adaptations in the school environment. Teachers seldom have experience with students with JRA and will need specific recommendations, which will need to be repeated each school year. The AJAO has developed written materials and training workshops to aid parents and health care professionals in this area. In addition, a number of federal laws support the rights of children with chronic illness (including JRA) to receive education in the "least restrictive environment."

The pharmacologic management encompasses treatment of articular, ocular, and other manifestations of JRA. In many patients, the articular manifestations can be treated with nonsteroidal anti-inflammatory drugs (NSAIDs). NSAIDs are the first step of treatment for JRA. Achieving an anti-inflammatory effect requires larger doses than are needed for pain control (up to twice the analgesic dose) and consistent ingestion over a longer period of time. Approximately one-half of children with JRA who will respond to a particular NSAID have done so by 2 weeks of regular therapy, but up to 25% do not demonstrate clinical response until 8–12 weeks of continued therapy. The average time to demonstrate clinical response to a particular NSAID in JRA patients is 1 month (10). Many NSAIDs have been prospectively evaluated in patients with JRA, and overall efficacy rates are similar. However, individual patient response is idiosyncratic. A favorable response to the first NSAID used occurs in 50%–60% of JRA patients. About 50% of those demonstrating inadequate clinical response to the first NSAID improve with the next NSAID tried (11). In general, the selection of NSAID is driven more by logistics than scientific concerns. Liquid NSAIDs are often necessary in young patients, and four-times-a-day preparations are

avoided in school-aged children, if at all possible. Most children tolerate NSAID therapy well. The most frequent side effects are abdominal pain and anorexia. H2 blockers, sucralfate, misoprostol, or antacids are often given to minimize these complaints. The actual prevalence of gastritis or gastrointestinal ulceration with NSAID use in JRA patients is unknown, but it seems to be less common in children than adults (11). NSAIDs should be taken with food.

NSAIDs also may adversely affect coagulation, the liver, or renal function, or may cause central nervous system (CNS) symptoms. Increased bruising associated with daily activities is common, but significantly increased bleeding with trauma or surgery is rare. However, with most elective surgeries, especially those involving the mouth or throat, surgeons recommend temporary termination of NSAID therapy. Although elevated liver enzymes occur in 3%–5% of JRA patients treated with nonsalicylate NSAIDs and 15%–30% treated with salicylates, very few patients demonstrate clinical or laboratory evidence of functional liver impairment. Fewer than 5% demonstrate proteinuria or hematuria. CNS symptoms generally develop soon after starting treatment and are primarily mood changes (drowsiness or irritability), headaches, and tinnitus. Mood changes occur in 3%-5%, headaches are much more common with indomethacin, and tinnitus occurs primarily with salicylate use. The general practice is to perform complete blood cell count, serum glutamic-oxaloacetic transaminase, serum glutamate pyruvate transaminase, blood urea nitrogen, creatinine, and routine urinalysis every 3–4 months in JRA patients taking NSAIDs regularly.

Approximately two thirds of children with JRA are inadequately treated with NSAIDs alone (11). In a prospective blinded trial, oral methotrexate given once weekly at 10 mg/m^2 body surface area (BSA) was well tolerated and significantly more effective than placebo (12). Methotrexate is used primarily for sJRA or poJRA patients. Overall, approximately 70%–80% of JRA patients demonstrate clinical improvement on methotrexate therapy, although the rate of response may be lower in sJRA patients still demonstrating systemic features (12). In patients with significant arthritis despite methotrexate therapy at 10 mg/m^2 BSA, higher doses (up to 1 mg/kg/week, maximum of 50 mg/week) have been shown to be beneficial and generally well tolerated in short-term uncontrolled trials (11,13). At doses

(Table 47A-2)

American Academy of Pediatrics guidelines for frequency of screening eye exams in JRA patients

JRA Onset Subtype*	Age at Onset	
	7 Years	≥7 Years
Systemic	Annual	Annual
Polyarticular		
ANA positive	Every 3–4 months × 4 years, then every 6 months × 3 years, then yearly	Every 6 months × 4 years, then yearly
ANA negative	Every 6 months × 4 years, then yearly	Every 6 months × 4 years, then yearly
Pauciarticular		
ANA positive	Every 3–4 months × 4 years, then every 6 months × 3 years, then yearly	Every 6 months × 4 years, then yearly
ANA negative	Every 6 months × 4 years, then yearly	Every 6 months × 4 years, then yearly

* JRA = juvenile rheumatoid arthritis; ANA = antinuclear antibody.
Adapted with permission from Yancey and Gross (8).

greater than 20 mg/m² BSA per week, oral absorption is unpredictable, and parenteral administration results in more reliable dosing and generally fewer gastrointestinal side effects. The pharmacokinetics of subcutaneous and intramuscular administration are similar, with the former causing less patient discomfort. Folic acid (1 mg orally daily) is often given to decrease the frequency and severity of side effects. Therapeutic benefits do not usually become evident for at least 3–4 weeks, and maximal response is not reached until 3–6 months. Methotrexate not uncommonly causes oral ulcers, nausea, decreased appetite, and abdominal pain, but these side effects are generally mild and do not require alteration in dosage. Pulmonary complications from methotrexate are very rare in JRA patients, and reports of liver biopsies have been reassuring (14). At the current time, most pediatric rheumatologists follow the American College of Rheumatology monitoring guidelines for methotrexate toxicity developed for adult RA patients (15) (see Appendix II), even though the guidelines have not been evaluated or validated in patients with JRA.

Prospective controlled trials of oral gold (16), D-penicillamine, and hydroxychloroquine (17) in JRA patients documented no greater efficacy than placebo, and, accordingly, these drugs are infrequently used. Injectable gold has never been evaluated in JRA patients in a controlled trial, but significant clinical improvement is seen in 50%–60% of patients on injectable gold therapy (11). Injectable gold therapy requires painful intramuscular injections, is associated with a high frequency of side effects, and has been largely replaced by methotrexate in the treatment of JRA.

Sulfasalazine has shown encouraging results in open trials (11), and a placebo-controlled trial in JRA patients is currently underway in Holland. A phase I study of intravenous gamma globulin (IVGG) has shown promising results in patients with poJRA (11). However, given the expense of IVGG therapy, clear-cut efficacy first should be established in controlled trials. Glucocorticosteroids have been and will continue to be used for severe life-threatening complications of sJRA. The high frequency of significant side effects and lack of evidence that these drugs alter the natural history of articular manifestations strongly weigh against routine use in JRA.

Intra-articular steroids are indicated for patients with limited joint involvement. In paJRA patients with active arthritis in the knees, intra-articular triamcinolone resulted in suppression of the arthritis for ≥6 months in 70% of patients in one study and ≥12 months in 50% in another study (11). Recently, magnetic resonance imaging demonstrated that intra-articular steroid therapy resulted in significant long-lasting suppression of inflammation and pannus formation without evidence of toxic effects on cartilage (18).

Treatment of ocular inflammation in JRA patients should be directed by an ophthalmologist experienced in treating inflammatory eye disorders. Early detection, topical corticosteroids, dilating agents, and frequent follow-up are critical and effective in the majority of JRA children with uveitis. If not effective, then systemic or subtenons injections of corticosteroids are utilized. In severe cases, chlorambucil and cyclophosphamide have been used (7). An open trial suggested that NSAIDs may also be beneficial in decreasing the severity of inflammation in JRA patients with uveitis (7).

Several other extra-articular complications in JRA patients occur with sufficient frequency or severity to warrant mention. A significant number of patients demonstrate general-

ized retardation of linear growth, despite being of normal height at baseline and demonstrated normal baseline and stimulated secretion of growth hormone. Studies have demonstrated that up to 50% of JRA patients may be below the third percentile for height 5 years after disease onset. This risk for poor linear growth tends to be worse in sJRA and poJRA patients — especially those with persistent disease and those requiring corticosteroid treatment. Adult height below the fifth percentile was seen in 50% of systemic-onset, 16% of polyarticular-onset, and 11% of pauci-articular-onset JRA patients. Only 50% of the JRA patients with adult height below the fifth percentile had ever taken corticosteroids (7). Uncontrolled studies of growth hormone therapy in JRA demonstrated increased linear growth rates in approximately 60%–75% of the patients (7). In the absence of controlled trials and lack of clear evidence for growth hormone abnormalities in JRA patients, the appropriate role for growth hormone therapy is unclear. Approximately 30%–40% of JRA patients demonstrate chronic protein–calorie malnutrition. Despite normal fat stores in most instances, JRA patients demonstrate depletion of both visceral and somatic protein stores. This may result from a combination of factors—poor appetite, catabolic drugs such as corticosteroids, physical inactivity, and inflammatory medications leading to depletion of protein stores, for example. JRA patients should be monitored closely for both linear height and lean body mass growth. Dietary intervention may be necessary to maintain adequate caloric and protein intake. Nocturnal enteral nasogastric supplemental feedings have been well tolerated and successful in replenishing lean body mass and improving linear growth rates in JRA patients with severe protein–calorie malnutrition that did not improve with oral supplementation (7).

Outcome

In a summary of published outcome studies, more than 30% of JRA patients had significant functional limitations after 10 or more years of follow-up (19). Laaksonen demonstrated that 12% of JRA patients were in Steinbrocker classes III (limited self-care) or IV (bed or wheelchair bound) 3–7 years after disease onset, but 48% were classified in class III or IV 16 or more years after disease onset (7). Active synovitis can be detected in 30%–55% of JRA patients 10 years after disease onset (19). In a longitudinal study of JRA patients referred to a pediatric rheumatologist within the first 6 months of disease onset, 28% of the paJRA, 54% of the poJRA, and 45% of the sJRA patients demonstrated either erosions or joint-space narrowing on standard radiographs (19). Mortality rate estimates in JRA patients have ranged from 0.29–1.1/100 patients. These estimates represent a mortality rate 3–14 times greater than the standardized mortality rate for a similarly aged US population (19).

The outcome for JRA patients with uveitis has significantly improved over the past several decades. In the most recent study of ocular outcomes, at a mean follow-up of 9.4 years since onset of eye disease, 85% of patients had normal visual acuity and 15% had significant visual loss, including 10% who were blind in at least one eye (7).

JUVENILE SPONDYLOARTHROPATHIES

The spondyloarthropathies in childhood encompass four discrete clinical entities: juvenile ankylosing spondylitis, Reiter's syndrome, psoriatic arthritis, and arthropathies associated with inflammatory bowel disease. However, since these diseases often take many years to fully evolve and satisfy existing diagnostic criteria, it is not uncommon for children to have symptoms suggestive of spondyloarthropathy but not satisfy full criteria for diagnosis. For that reason, it has been suggested that spondyloarthropathies in children include another syndrome–seronegative enthesopathy and arthropathy (SEA syndrome). The SEA syndrome is applied to patients who are negative for RF, negative for antinuclear antibodies (ANA), and have enthesitis and either arthritis or arthralgia (7). SEA syndrome is designed to distinguish those children who may have symptoms consistent with other rheumatic diseases, such as JRA, but actually are more likely to develop spondyloarthropathy over time. In one series, 69% of children characterized as having the SEA syndrome developed probable or definite spondyloarthropathy at a mean follow up of 11 years. Children with a much higher risk for developing definite spondyloarthropathy were B27-positive, had a family history of spondyloarthropathy, or had definite arthritis and not just arthralgia (20).

The incidence and prevalence of the spondyloarthropathies in childhood is much less well studied than the epidemiology of JRA. In general, spondyloarthropathies are less common in children than JRA. Juvenile ankylosing spondylitis is reported to have a prevalence of 2–10 per 100,000 and an incidence of 0.3–0.4 per 100,000. The prevalence for psoriatic arthritis is 2–12 per 100,000 and for the arthritis associated with inflammatory bowel disease 0.5–1 per 100,000 (20).

Juvenile Ankylosing Spondylitis

Most published reports of juvenile ankylosing spondylitis use the same diagnostic criteria as for diagnosing ankylosing spondylitis in adults. However, to have juvenile ankylosing spondylitis, the patient's onset of the disease must occur at age 16 or younger. The adult criteria for ankylosing spondylitis require plain radiographic evidence of sacroiliitis. Since radiographic changes are known to occur years after the onset of clinical symptoms in many cases, establishing a definite diagnosis of juvenile ankylosing spondylitis may be delayed for many years. Of the patients who satisfy the diagnostic criteria, there is a male-to-female ratio of 6:1, and 82%–95% are HLA-B27–positive (20). The arthritis is usually episodic rather than chronic, and large joints of the lower extremities and the tarsal bones are much more commonly affected than the upper extremities or small joints of the hands. Enthesitis is common, as is lower back or buttock pain. In following patients with probable juvenile ankylosing spondylitis, it is important to monitor the lumbar spine motion and chest expansion very closely. The primary extra-articular manifestation of juvenile ankylosing spondylitis is acute iritis, which occurs in 5%–10% of patients. Tests for ANA and RF are characteristically positive, and plain radiographs often do not show the characteristic changes in the sacroiliac or lumbosacral spine for many years. Bone scans are seldom helpful because radioisotope uptake is typically increased in sacroiliac joints and the lumbar spine as a consequence of skeletal growth. Computed tomography and magnetic resonance imaging scans are difficult to interpret, because experience with normal findings in sacroiliac joints in children is limited. There are no pathognomonic laboratory tests. The treatment for juvenile ankylosing spondylitis is primarily NSAIDs; sulfasalazine has been shown to be potentially useful in a few open studies. Patients with severe

enthesis unresponsive to NSAIDs may benefit from low-dose prednisone (21).

Reiter's Syndrome

Reiter's syndrome is a form of reactive arthritis following genitourinary or gastrointestinal infection in association with conjunctivitis and urethritis. Reiter's syndrome does occur in children. The vast majority of cases are associated with dysenteric infection. Genitourinary infection as an initiating event is seen primarily in adolescents but also in sexually abused children. The articular involvement in children with Reiter's syndrome is usually large weight-bearing joints. These patients often have enthesitis, and the onset of the musculoskeletal symptoms can be quite acute. Urethritis is frequently asymptomatic and detected only as sterile pyuria, while conjunctivitis is almost always acute in onset. The patient may have oral ulcers and a characteristic (but relatively uncommon) skin rash, keratoderma blennorrhagicum, which starts as a papular eruption on the soles or palms that becomes pustular within a matter of days and then later becomes scaly. Often the clinical manifestations appear in an asynchronous fashion. The arthritis and conjunctivitis, although they may be acute, are usually self-limited and associated with excellent clinical outcomes. Treatment with NSAIDs is usually sufficient for musculoskeletal symptoms.

Arthritis Associated with Inflammatory Bowel Disease

Significant peripheral or axial arthritis may occur with either Crohn's disease or ulcerative colitis. Overall, 7%–20% of patients with inflammatory bowel disease develop arthritis. In the vast majority of instances, it is a peripheral arthritis involving primarily the large joints of the lower extremities. The male-to-female ratio is essentially equal, and there is no obvious association with HLA-B27. But a small subset of patients with inflammatory bowel disease develop axial arthritis; the male-to-female ratio is 4:1 in these patients, and HLA-B27 is positive in approximately 80%. In most instances, the arthritis is episodic and occurs with worsening of the bowel symptoms. In some cases, arthritis precedes the onset of gastrointestinal symptoms by months or rarely years. The association with underlying bowel disease may be suspected in these patients by the presence of frequent subclinical gastrointestinal symptoms and intermittent nocturnal diarrhea, as well as in patients who have severe systemic symptoms and signs (such as fatigue, weight loss, or fever) that seem excessive relative to the severity of the arthritis. In addition, the presence of erythema nodosum, frequent oral ulcers, pyoderma gangrenosum, digital clubbing, significant anemia, or significant hypoalbuminemia suggest the presence of inflammatory bowel disease. In most instances, the arthritis improves dramatically with treatment of the underlying bowel disease. The musculoskeletal manifestations are frequently episodic and last for 1–2 months.

Psoriatic Arthritis

Patients manifesting chronic arthritis in association with psoriasis with an onset at or before the age of 16 are said to have juvenile psoriatic arthritis. However, the classic psoriatic rash may not appear for many years. According to diagnostic criteria for childhood psoriatic arthritis developed in Vancouver, patients with "definite psoriatic arthritis" have arthritis and psoriasis or arthritis in association with any three of the following clinical characteristics: 1) dactylitis, 2) nail pitting or onycholysis, 3) history of psoriasis in first or second degree relatives, or 4) an atypical psoriatic rash. Patients are said to have "probable psoriatic arthritis" if arthritis and two of these four clinical characteristics are present. In the vast majority of cases, the arthritis is peripheral and may be associated with asymptomatic chronic uveitis in some patients. In studies of pediatric psoriatic arthritis, the association with B27 positivity is mixed in patients who have axial arthritis. About 50% of children have arthritis before the psoriatic rash appears. Flexor tenosynovitis in fingers or toes ("sausage digits") is not uncommon in psoriatic arthritis. The treatment for psoriatic arthritis is essentially the same as for JRA. A comprehensive physical program should be instituted. NSAIDs are the first line of treatment, but patients with more severe disease may require methotrexate (21). Monitoring for asymptomatic uveitis by slit-lamp examination should be done at the same frequency as for patients with JRA (Table 47A-2).

DANIEL J. LOVELL, MD, MPH

1. Singsen BH: Rheumatic diseases of childhood. Rheum Dis Clin North Am 16:581-599, 1990
2. Towner SR, Michet CJJ, O'Fallen WM, Nelson AM: The epidemiology of juvenile arthritis in Rochester, Minnesota. Arthritis Rheum 26:1208-1213, 1983
3. Hochberg MC, Linet MS, Sills EM: The prevalence and incidence of juvenile rheumatoid arthritis in an urban black population. Am J Public Health 73:1202-1203, 1983
4. Andersson Gère BA, Fasth A: Epidemiology of juvenile chronic arthritis in Southwestern Sweden—five year prospective population study. Pediatrics 90:950-958, 1992
5. Andersson Gère BA, Fasth A: The natural history of juvenile chronic arthritis: a population based cohort study. II. Outcome. J Rheumatol 22:308-319, 1995
6. Gortmaker S: Chronic childhood disorders: prevalence and impact. Ped Clin North Am 31:3-18, 1984
7. Cassidy JT, Petty RE: Textbook of Pediatric Rheumatology, 3rd ed. Philadelphia, WB Saunders, 1995
8. Yancey C, Gross R: Guidelines for ophthalmologic examinations in children with juvenile rheumatoid arthritis. Peds 92:295-296, 1993
9. White PH, Shear ES: Transition/job readiness for adolescents with juvenile arthritis and other chronic illness. J Rheumatol 19:28-31, 1992
10. Lovell DJ, Giannini EH, Brewer EJ: Time course of response to nonsteroidal antiinflammatory drugs in juvenile rheumatoid arthritis. Arthritis Rheum 27:1433-1437, 1984
11. Giannini EH, Cawkwell GD: Drug treatment in children with juvenile rheumatoid arthritis past, present and future. Ped Clin North Am 42:1099-1125, 1995
12. Giannini EH, Brewer EJ, Kuzmina N: Methotrexate in resistant juvenile rheumatoid arthritis: results of the USA-USSR double-blind, placebo controlled cooperative trial. N Engl J Med 326:1043-1049, 1992
13. Wallace CA, Sherry DD: Preliminary report of higher dose methotrexate and treatment in juvenile rheumatoid arthritis. J Rheumatol 19:1604-1607, 1992
14. Kugathasan S, Newman AJ, Dahms BB, Boyle JT: Liver biopsy findings in patients with juvenile rheumatoid arthritis receiving long-term, weekly methotrexate therapy. J Pediatr 128:149-151, 1996
15. Kremer JM, Alarcón GS, Lightfoot RW, Willkens RF, Furst DE, Williams HJ, Dent PB, Weinblatt ME: Methotrexate for rheumatoid arthritis: suggested guidelines for monitoring liver toxicity. Arthritis Rheum 37:316-328, 1994
16. Giannini EH, Brewer EJ, Kuzmina N: Auranofin in the treatment of juvenile rheumatoid arthritis: results of the USA-USSR double blind, placebo controlled cooperative trial. Arthritis Rheum 33:466-476, 1990
17. Brewer EJ, Giannini EH, Kuzmina N: D-penicillamine and hydroxychloroquine in the treatment of severe juvenile rheumatoid arthritis: results of the USA-USSR double-blind, placebo controlled trial. N Engl J Med 314:1269-1276, 1986
18. Huppertz H-I, Tschammler A, Horwitz A, Schwab O: Intraarticular corticosteroids for chronic arthritis in children: efficacy and effects on cartilage and growth. J Pediatr 127:317-321, 1995
19. Levinson JE, Wallace CA: Dismantling the pyramid. J Rheumatol 19:6-10, 1992
20. Cabral DA, Malleson PN, Petty RE: Spondylarthropathies of childhood. Ped Clin North Am 42:1051-1070, 1995
21. Burgos-Vargas R, Petty RE: Juvenile ankylosing spondylitis. Rheum Clin North Am 18:123-142, 1992

B. CONNECTIVE TISSUE DISEASES AND NONARTICULAR RHEUMATISM

The connective tissue diseases occur infrequently in childhood (Table 47B-1). However, the diversity of their manifestations makes them integral to the differential diagnosis of every child or adolescent who appears systemically ill. Each disease may initially present with diffuse aches and pains, prolonged fever of unknown origin, chronic anemia, recurrent infections, or unexplained fatigue and weight loss.

Children and adolescents with nonarticular rheumatism also present with fatigue, aches, pains, or stiffness. However, in contrast to the children with connective tissue diseases, they often appear well and lack systemic inflammatory changes. Nonarticular rheumatism includes both benign entities (eg, "growing pains") and disabling illnesses such as fibromyalgia and reflex sympathetic dystrophy, which produce significant morbidity.

SYSTEMIC LUPUS ERYTHEMATOSUS

Systemic lupus erythematosus (SLE) is the most common major connective tissue disease of childhood, with an estimated prevalence 5–10 per 100,000 (1). SLE predominantly affects adolescent females but may affect males and younger children. It is more common in African Americans, Asians, and Hispanics, but it may affect children of any age, race, and gender. Antinuclear antibodies (ANA) are found in virtually all cases of SLE, but this does not establish the diagnosis. ANA testing has high sensitivity (virtually all children with SLE are ANA-positive) but low specificity (many children who are ANA-positive do not have SLE).

The American College of Rheumatology criteria for the classification of definite SLE (2) apply to children (see Appendix I). However, it is important to recognize that the disease may evolve over time in childhood. Children may initially be diagnosed with idiopathic thrombocytopenic purpura because they do not fulfill four or more of the recognized criteria, only to develop renal involvement and hypocomplementemia typical of SLE months or even years later.

The onset of SLE in children is often gradual, and the malar rash seen in textbooks is not reliably present. In children and adolescents with fatigue and malaise, evidence of multisystem involvement should be actively sought. Pleural

Juvenile rheumatoid arthritis	189
Spondyloarthropathies	161
Nonarticular rheumatism (eg, fibromyalgia)	160
Systemic lupus erythematosus	53
Mechanical syndromes	49
Vasculitic diseases	37
Lyme disease	25
Rheumatic manifestations of endocrine disease	11
Scleroderma	10
Skeletal dysplasias	7
Disorders of collagen metabolism (eg, Marfans, Ehlers–Danlos)	6
Acute rheumatic fever	5
Infections of bones and joints	2
Malignancies (leukemia, neuroblastoma)	2
Other	5

*722 individual patients seen in a single calendar year for new or follow-up appointments; all initially referred for rheumatic disease evaluation by other physicians.

effusions, synovitis affecting the small joints of the hands or feet, hemolytic anemia, proteinuria, and hematuria are common manifestations of SLE that may not be detected during a routine office evaluation.

Less frequently, the onset is dramatic. Fever and rash may be accompanied by polyserositis (abdominal pain, pleural effusions), neurologic manifestations (seizures, hallucinations, depression, or coma), renal involvement (hematuria, proteinuria, hypertension, nephrotic syndrome), or pulmonary disease (effusions, hemorrhage, respiratory failure) occurring in any combination. Sudden overwhelming sepsis (resulting from neutropenia, functional asplenia, or hypocomplementemia) may also be present. Frequently, both antibiotics and corticosteroids are required in this setting since active SLE and infection may present simultaneously.

Renal involvement is common, occurring in up to two-thirds of children with SLE (3). There may be only mild glomerulitis, but many children suffer from diffuse proliferative glomerulonephritis or membranous nephritis that may ultimately lead to renal failure. Central nervous system involvement is also a common cause of morbidity. Dramatic manifestations such as transverse myelitis, seizures, coma, and psychosis are less common than subtle findings such as chronic depression, poor judgment, and impaired short-term memory. These changes result in poor school performance and family disruptions that contribute significantly to the morbidity of SLE.

Corticosteroids are extremely effective in reducing the inflammatory manifestations of SLE, but in children and adolescents the use of these drugs is associated with substantial morbidity. Cushingoid facies, short stature, acne, osteonecrosis, cataracts, pancreatitis, and accelerated atherosclerosis are well-recognized complications. For patients with severe disease, immunosuppressive drug regimens (such as periodic intravenous cyclophosphamide) have been associated with a dramatic reduction in both disease and steroid-related morbidity without excessive toxicity (4). The key to high-quality survival for children with SLE is early recognition and comprehensive management of both their medical and psychosocial needs.

MIXED CONNECTIVE TISSUE DISEASE

Mixed connective tissue disease (MCTD) is a variant of SLE with a greater frequency of Raynaud's phenomenon and hypergammaglobulinemia but a lower frequency of hypocomplementemia. Children with MCTD are also less likely to develop severe nephritis or require immunosuppressive therapy (5). A significant proportion of children with MCTD ultimately develop systemic sclerosis (6). Childhood MCTD should be suspected when both ANA and rheumatoid factor are found in a child with what appears to be SLE or dermatomyositis. Antibodies to Sm are typically absent, while those to U_1RNP are typically present; however, some patients with characteristic clinical features lack the expected serologic findings. Interestingly, MCTD shares with systemic sclerosis and juvenile dermatomyositis the frequent occurrence of nailfold capillary changes and Gottren's papules, suggesting an etiopathogenetic association.

ANTIPHOSPHOLIPID ANTIBODY SYNDROMES

Antiphospholipid antibodies (APL) occur in children and adolescents with SLE, but also in many children with a positive ANA without SLE (7,8). In addition, APL are found in a high percentage of children with unexplained strokes, and have also been reported in children with multiple pulmonary emboli. Proper therapy is uncertain. The risks of anticoagulation with warfarin seem greater than the risk of thrombosis in unselected APL-positive children and adolescents. Some physicians observe conservatively, others treat with a small daily dose of aspirin. Children with a history of stroke or embolic phenomena should be appropriately anticoagulated.

NEONATAL LUPUS SYNDROME

Neonatal lupus syndrome (NSLE) was initially recognized as the constellation of skin rash, hematologic abnormalities, and hepatitis in newborn children of mothers with SLE. NSLE includes children with congenital heart block with or without the other manifestations. The mothers of these children have serologic abnormalities (ANA and antibodies to SS-A/Ro and/or SS-B/La) but may not have other manifestations of SLE. The rash, hepatitis, and hematologic abnormalities result from passively transferred maternal autoantibodies and rarely require treatment with corticosteroids. The pathogenesis of complete heart block is unclear. Twins can be discordant, and the rate of recurrence is low with subsequent pregnancies. There is no specific therapy. Most of these children do well, although some ultimately require a pacemaker. However, rare neonates with NSLE develop congestive heart failure, which may be related to intrauterine infection (9).

JUVENILE DERMATOMYOSITIS

Juvenile dermatomyositis (JDMS) affects both genders with a slight female predominance. Most often the onset is slow, and the initial symptoms are not recognized. Parents of small children usually first notice a reluctance to go up or down stairs and an increased desire to be carried. With time, the child becomes "clumsy." Ultimately, medical intervention is sought because of rash, progressive weakness, or constitutional symptoms such as fever or weight loss.

The rash of JDMS is an erythematous discoloration most prominent on the face and the extensor surfaces of the elbows and knees. It is often ascribed by parents to the child's frequent falling. The heliotropic rash characteristic of this condition is a violaceous discoloration over the eyelids. Gottren's papules are inflammatory vasculitic lesions overlying the interphalangeal joints. They may be an early clue to the diagnosis, but are not always present. Proximal muscle weakness may be overlooked if testing for weakness is limited to evaluating grip strength, which tests distal muscle function. Frequently the diagnosis of JDMS is first considered when laboratory evaluation demonstrates muscle enzyme abnormalities (creatine phosphokinase, aspartate aminotransferase, or aldolase). All of these enzymes may be abnormal, but in some children, only the aldolase is elevated. The diagnosis is confirmed by characteristic electromyographic abnormalities, muscle biopsy, or the typical clinical picture. Arthritis may be present, but it usually resolves promptly after therapy is initiated. MCTD should be considered in those with persistent arthritis and muscle inflammation.

There are several distinct subsets of JDMS. The most common subset consists of proximal muscle weakness and mild heliotropic rash in children who have no evidence of vasculitis. The illness often resolves over a 6-month period with corticosteroid therapy alone. Children with a vasculitic rash or nailfold capillary abnormalities are more likely to have a chronic course and internal organ involvement. This subset includes those with Gottren's papules. Children with severe rash and markedly elevated muscle enzymes but only moderate weakness are in another, less common subset, which may be a distinct illness.

Special care must be taken to evaluate swallowing function and the gag reflex of children with dermatomyositis. A more nasal voice or frequent coughing when eating should be regarded with extreme concern. Aspiration due to weakness of the voluntary muscles that initiate swallowing is a prominent hazard. Chronic abdominal pain also must be regarded with concern. Although it may be benign, it sometimes results from small-vessel vasculitis. Small areas of bowel involvement may initially produce nonspecific abdominal pain, but progressive involvement may lead to perforation with catastrophic consequences. Cerebritis, which may be associated with hallucinations and dementia, or retinal vasculitis is also sometimes present. Other major internal organ complications include pulmonary fibrosis and cardiac damage with scarring, poor contractility, and possible conduction abnormalities.

Chronic weakness in childhood may also be the result of genetic conditions such as muscular dystrophy or metabolic conditions such as hyperthyroidism. Although some of these conditions are accompanied by an elevated level of muscle enzymes, they lack the characteristic rash and other evidence of vasculitis that commonly accompanies JDMS. Isolated polymyositis is very rare in childhood.

The majority of children with JDMS recover completely with corticosteroids alone. However, some have persistent active disease or develop unacceptable corticosteroid side effects (10). Low-dose oral methotrexate is often effective for mild disease. There are reported experiences with larger doses of methotrexate administered intramuscularly or intravenously, cyclophosphamide, and intravenous gammaglobulin or cyclosporine (11–13).

Diffuse calcification of subcutaneous tissues or muscle groups may be a debilitating complication of JDMS. Small areas of discrete calcification do not warrant surgical intervention unless they are causing discomfort. Rare patients develop severe, diffuse calcification (calcinosis universalis) following the acute phase of their illness. No satisfactory treatment exists. Regimens that interfere with calcification have greater effects on normal bone than on ectopic bone. Secondary infection of calcium deposits is a constant concern. Fortunately, severe complications are infrequent in children who are promptly diagnosed and appropriately treated.

SYSTEMIC SCLEROSIS

In children scleroderma is often present for a prolonged period before clinicians recognize the progressive thickening and hardening of the skin. Children suffer from the focal forms (morphea and linear scleroderma) more often than the systemic forms of systemic sclerosis (SS) and CREST syndrome (calcinosis, Raynaud's phenomenon, esophageal dysmotility, sclerodactyly, telangiectasia).

Linear scleroderma (LS) in childhood is a tight band-like constriction of the skin over the extremities or trunk. If involvement is limited and does not cross a joint, the condition is benign. However, thickening of the skin may be associated with atrophy of the underlying muscle and bone, as well as synovitis. LS crossing a joint or involving a large proportion of a limb in childhood often produces contractures and stunted growth. These cases may warrant therapy.

Some children develop lesions of both morphea and LS. There are also cases in which the skin lesions are associated with an inflammatory myopathy (sclerodermatomyositis) or other inflammatory lesions including uveitis. LS *en coup de sabre* is a special case involving the scalp and face. Typically, there is an area of thickening of the scalp that may extend down onto to the face. This condition is often confused with Parry–Romberg syndrome of progressive facial hemiatrophy. Parry–Romberg syndrome is associated with inflammation and atrophy of the deeper underlying tissues and often involves the central nervous system and tongue. Although typical cases of linear scleroderma *en coup de sabre* and Parry–Romberg syndrome are easily distinguished, there are cases that do not clearly fall into either category. The two diseases may be related (14).

In contrast to LS, systemic sclerosis in childhood may be life-threatening. Diffuse tightening of the skin is accompanied by inflammation and fibrosis of the internal organs (heart, lungs, and kidneys). The onset of SS is usually gradual. Often patients first seek care because of worsening Raynaud's phenomenon. On careful inspection, skin tightening is evident proximal to the forearm. Facial skin tightening results in a characteristic appearance with a sharp nose, almond-shaped eyes, and difficulty opening the mouth fully. Distal fingertip lesions, nailfold capillary abnormalities, or Gottren's papules also suggest scleroderma in a child with Raynaud's phenomenon. In rare instances, the first indication of illness is swallowing difficulties, malabsorption, or restrictive pulmonary disease (15).

The diagnosis of CREST syndrome in childhood is usually first suggested by the prominent telangiectasias. Induration and skin thickening are much less striking than in SS. Both SS and CREST may have life-threatening pulmonary involvement with fibrosis and decreased diffusion capacity. Swallowing dysfunction and widespread internal organ involvement resulting in malabsorption, cardiorespiratory failure, or renal disease are common late in the disease course in both conditions. Catastrophic hypertension secondary to renal involvement (scleroderma renal crisis) is described, but is infrequent in childhood.

The laboratory abnormalities associated with both SS and CREST syndrome are primarily those of chronic inflammation and those appropriate to the internal organ involvement. Most patients have ANA, and antibodies to Scl-70 are found in some but not all children with SS. Similarly, anti-centromere antibodies are considered characteristic of the CREST syndrome, but they are not always present.

There is no uniformly satisfactory treatment for childhood scleroderma. Localized forms that are only cosmetically disturbing are best treated topically. The systemic forms of scleroderma are traditionally treated with D-penicillamine, but while this drug has been beneficial for some patients, it has been ineffective for others. Trials involving methotrexate, cyclosporine, and a variety of biologic agents are underway (16,17). The long-term prognosis for children with SS or CREST is highly variable. In some, the disease relentlessly progresses, but others survive well into adulthood despite internal organ involvement.

Gottren's papules and nailfold capillary abnormalities are found in JDMS, SS, and MCTD but in no other conditions. This suggests that despite their highly varied clinical expression and prognosis, there is a fundamental relationship between these diseases. The explanation for this association and its etiopathogenic basis are not yet clear.

HENÖCH–SCHÖNLEIN PURPURA

Henöch–Schönlein purpura (HSP) is a common form of small-vessel vasculitis seen almost exclusively in childhood. The typical child with HSP presents with abdominal pain following an upper respiratory infection. This is followed by petechiae that are predominantly present over dependent areas such as the lower extremities, the buttocks, and the extensor surface of the upper extremities (Fig. 47B-1). Widespread immune complex deposition results in arthritis, abdominal pain, and nephritis in some patients. These manifestations may be severe, with varying degrees of skin rash and edema in dependent areas. Intestinal inflammation may lead to edema and bleeding with potential complications of intussusception, infarction, or perforation. Renal involvement may be chronic but rarely leads to renal failure (18).

There are no distinguishing laboratory abnormalities in HSP. The diagnosis is established by the characteristic clinical picture. Most children recover without therapy as the immune complexes are cleared from their sites of deposition. Typically, the illness is resolved within 2 weeks. Occasionally, recurrent immune complex deposition causes the illness to be prolonged or recurrent, a development of great concern in patients who develop nephritis, which may be severe. For children with severe abdominal pain or possible intussusception, steroids may be helpful. There is no clear evidence that steroids are beneficial for renal involvement (18). The arthritis associated with HSP is typically transient, but if it persists, nonsteroidal anti-inflammatory drugs usually provide relief. If a child appears to have unusually chronic or severe HSP, polyarteritis nodosa should be excluded.

MEDIUM- AND LARGE-VESSEL VASCULITIS

The presenting manifestations of polyarteritis nodosa (PAN) in childhood are highly variable. PAN often involves

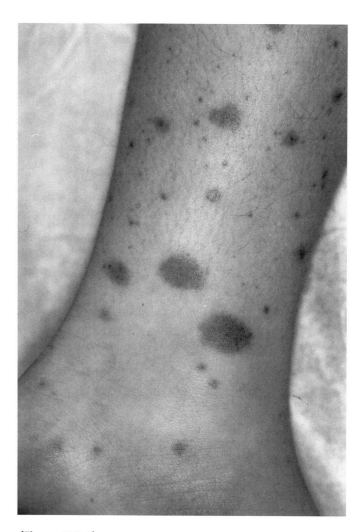

(Figure 47B-1)
Evolving rash of Henöch–Schönlein purpura on the left lower extremity.

the renal vessels, producing hematuria and hypertension; it may affect the mesenteric vessels, causing abdominal pain. If it affects more superficial vessels, rash or unexplained extremity pain can result. It may begin as a fever of unknown origin. PAN should be suspected in children with chronic fever and abdominal pain if infections, neoplasia, and inflammatory bowel disease have been excluded. When PAN presents with fever, rash, and joint pains, it may be confused with systemic-onset JRA. In other instances, the renal involvement and abdominal pain can be confused with HSP. PAN is distinguished by the presence of arterial inflammation, which may be demonstrated by biopsy of involved tissues or angiographic studies. In patients with hematuria or hypertension, renal angiography is useful to rapidly establish the correct diagnosis (Fig. 47B-2).

Like Kawasaki disease, PAN may produce coronary artery lesions. Nonspecific thickening of the coronary arteries is found in many inflammatory conditions. Whenever children with suspected Kawasaki disease fail to respond rapidly to the administration of intravenous gamma globulin, alternative diagnoses such as PAN must be carefully considered. Although corticosteroids may be relatively contraindicated in Kawasaki disease, they are the treatment of choice for children with PAN.

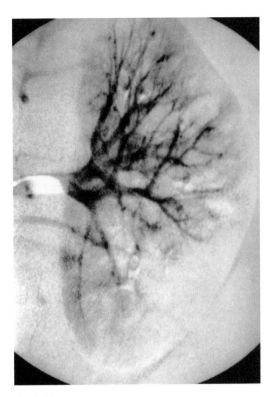

(Figure 47B-2)
Renal angiogram demonstrating small aneurysms of polyarteritis nodosa.

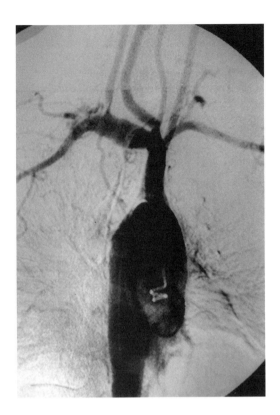

(Figure 47B-3)
Angiogram of the aortic arch demonstrating both aneurysmal dilation and stenosis of proximal vessels in a patient with Takayasu's arteritis.

Cutaneous PAN in childhood presents with tender subcutaneous nodules associated with markedly elevated erthyrocyte sedimentation rate and, in some cases, fever or malaise. All children should be investigated for evidence of internal organ involvement. Similar lesions may be seen in erythema nodosum, in the panniculitis of Weber–Christian disease, and in patients abusing intravenous drugs, but each has a different pathologic appearance.

Other forms of medium- and large-vessel vasculitis are rare in children and adolescents. Takayasu's arteritis frequently has its onset in adolescence (Fig. 47B-3) and is more common in females. The presenting complaints are fever, anemia, and elevated acute-phase reactants without apparent explanation. Involvement of the abdominal branches of the aorta may produce abdominal pain. The diagnosis is made only if it is actively sought. Most often, the left radial pulse is reduced or absent, but carotid, femoral, and renal arteries may be selectively involved. The diagnosis is suggested by the presence of asymmetric pulses, widening of the aortic arch on chest roentgenogram, or arterial bruits.

Wegener's granulomatosis and lymphomatoid granulomatosis are uncommon in adolescents. Their manifestations in childhood do not differ significantly from the findings in adults.

NONARTICULAR RHEUMATISM

Nonarticular rheumatism represents a diverse group of conditions of widely varied etiology. They are linked not by a common pathogenesis, but by the presence of pain and stiffness without arthritis or laboratory evidence of inflammation. Their importance arises from the frequency with which they are misdiagnosed. The most common is "growing pains." Growing pains typically occur in young children during the night. Young children often awaken during the night complaining of pain behind their knees. The pain responds to gentle massage or acetaminophen, but it may recur. These pains are never present during the day and do not interfere with activities. Typical growing pains do not require investigation. However, pains that occur on awakening or during the day require investigation, even though most are found to be mechanical in origin.

REFLEX SYMPATHETIC DYSTROPHY

Reflex sympathetic dystrophy (RSD) in children differs from that seen in adults. In the typical case, a child or adolescent suffers a significant injury that prevents normal activity. In many cases, the injury restricts the performance of specific activities such as dance, ice skating, or athletics, but in other cases the illness may interfere with the activities of daily living. Following injury, the child fails to recover in the expected manner and the disability becomes unusually prolonged. In severe cases, the affected extremity may be discolored and exceedingly sensitive to touch. Laboratory results are usually normal, but there may be osteoporosis on radiographic evaluation and even increased uptake on Tc99 bone scans.

Medical treatment of RSD is unsatisfactory. Despite the well documented initial injury, the origin of the problem is most often related to unrealistic expectations placed on the child or adolescent (19). Although some children respond to a program of vigorous physical therapy and pain management, unless attention is directed at seeking and correcting the psychologic stress, successful therapy is unlikely. RSD should be viewed as a family problem, not a problem of the child in isolation. With appropriate intervention, complete recovery may be expected (20).

MUSCULOSKELETAL PAIN AS A MANIFESTATION OF OTHER DISEASES

Many childhood malignancies that affect the bones or bone marrow may present with musculoskeletal pain. A child with excessive bone pain should always be evaluated for leukemia, even if definite synovitis is present. Leukemia, lymphoma, rhabdomyosarcoma, and neuroblastoma all may initially present with musculoskeletal pain or synovitis. With the exception of SLE, arthritis in childhood is commonly associated with an elevation of the platelet count. Musculoskeletal pain, a decreased platelet count, and arthritis suggest bone marrow infiltration and can be seen with both malignancies and storage diseases such as histiocytosis X.

Endocrine disorders including hypo- or hyperthyroidism, diabetes mellitus, hypo- and hyperparathyroidism, and pituitary tumors producing excessive amounts of growth hormone all may be complicated by musculoskeletal complaints. Musculoskeletal problems are also a major component of many genetic disorders of collagen metabolism including Marfan syndrome, Ehlers–Danlos syndrome, and the epiphyseal dysplasias.

In benign hypermobile joint syndrome, a possible genetic disorder of collagen metabolism, the ligaments supporting the joints are relatively lax. The child can typically hyperextend the fingers parallel to the forearm and hyperextend both the elbows and knees. Because these children have exceptional range of motion, they often exacerbate the condition by participating in gymnastics or other activities that place increased stress on their joints. The laxity results in repeated episodes of minor trauma to the joint, which produces pain and stiffness, sometimes with synovitis.

It is also important to note that gout does not occur in children except as a complication of malignancy, other causes of accelerated cell lysis, or renal compromise. Even under these circumstances, gouty arthritis in childhood is extremely rare (20).

THOMAS J. A. LEHMAN, MD

1. Lehman TJA: Systemic lupus erythematosus in childhood and adolescence. In Wallace DJ, Hahn BH (eds): Dubois' Lupus Erythematosus, 5th ed. Baltimore, Williams & Wilkins, 1997

2. Tan EM, Cohen AS, Fries JF, et al: The 1982 revised criteria for the classification of systemic lupus erythematosus. Arthritis Rheum 25:1271-1277, 1982

3. Lehman TJA, Mouradian JA: Systemic lupus erythematosus. In Holliday MA, Barratt TM, Avner ED (eds): Pediatric Nephrology, 3rd ed. Baltimore, Williams and Wilkins, 1993

4. Lehman TJ, Sherry DD, Wagner-Weiner L, McCurdy DK, Emery HM, Magilavy DB, Kovalesky A: Intermittent intravenous cyclophosphamide therapy for lupus nephritis. J Pediatr 114:1055-1060, 1989

5. Singsen BH, Bernstein BH, Kornreich HK, King KK, Hanson V, Tan EM: Mixed connective tissue disease in childhood. J Pediatr 90:893-900, 1977

6. Nimelstein SH, Brody S. McShane D, Holman HR: Mixed connective tissue disease: a subsequent evaluation of the original 25 patients. Medicine 59:239-248, 1980

7. Toren A, Toren P, Many A, et al: Spectrum of clinical manifestations of antiphospholipid antibodies in childhood and adolescence. Pediatr Hematol Oncol 10:311-315, 1993

8. Tucker LB: Antiphospholipid syndrome in childhood the great unknown. Lupus 3:367-369, 1994

9. Buyon JP: Neonatal lupus syndromes. Curr Opin Rheumatol 6:523-529, 1994

10. Spencer CH, Hanson V Singsen BH, Bernstein BH, Kornreich HK, King KK: Course of treated juvenile dermatomyositis. J Pediatr 105:399-408, 1984

11. Ansell BM: Management of polymyositis and dermatomyositis. Clin Rheum Dis 10:205-213, 1984

12. Lang BA, Laxer RM, Murphy G, Silverman ED, Roifman CM: Treatment of dermatomyositis with intravenous gammaglobulin. Am J Med 91:169-172, 1991

13. Girardin E, Dayer JM, Paunier L: Cyclosporine for juvenile dermatomyositis. J Pediatr 112:165-166, 1988

14. Lehman TJA: The Parry Romberg syndrome of progressive facial hemiatrophy and linear scleroderma en coup de sabre: mistaken diagnosis or overlapping conditions? J Rheumatol 19:844-845, 1992

15. Garty BZ, Athreya BH, Wilmott RR, Scarpa N, Doughty R, Douglas SD: Pulmonary functions in children with progressive systemic sclerosis. Pediatrics 88:1161-1167, 1991

16. Lehman TJA: Systemic and localized scleroderma in children. Curr Opin Rheumatol 8:576-579, 1996

17. Foldevari I, Lehman TJA: Is methotrexate a new perspective in the treatment of juvenile progressive systemic scleroderma? Arthritis Rheum 36:S218, 1993

18. Steward M, Savage JM, Bell B, McCord B: Long term renal prognosis of Henoch-Schoenlien purpura in an unselected childhood population. Eur J Pediatr 147:113-115, 1988

19. Sherry DD, Weisman R: Psychological aspects of childhood reflex neurovascular dystrophy. Pediatr 81:572-578, 1988

20. Cassidy J, Petty R: Musculoskeletal manifestations of systemic disease. In: Textbook of Pediatric Rheumatology, 3rd ed. Philadelphia, W.B. Saunders, 1995

C. KAWASAKI SYNDROME

In 1967, Dr. Tomasaku Kawasaki described a new clinical entity in Japanese infants and young children, which he designated mucocutaneous lymph node syndrome (1). Now called Kawasaki syndrome (KS) or Kawasaki disease, the illness has become the leading cause of acquired heart disease in children. Cardiovascular sequelae, which occur in up to 25% of patients with KS, vary in severity from asymptomatic coronary artery ectasia to giant coronary artery aneurysm with thrombosis, myocardial infarction, and death. As a result of both improved therapy and recognition of milder cases, the mortality of KS has fallen from 1%–2% to 0.08%.

DIAGNOSTIC CRITERIA

The Japanese Kawasaki Research Committee established diagnostic criteria for KS based on Dr. Kawasaki's first report and subsequent nationwide surveys. The Centers for Disease Control and Prevention adopted these same criteria for case definition in the United States (2) (Table 47C-1). Fever lasting 5 days plus four of five criteria must be present, or three of the five criteria if coronary artery aneurysms are demonstrated by two-dimensional echocardiography or angiography. Other illnesses that may present with similar symptoms and signs must be excluded (Table 47C-2). The diagnostic criteria alone are insufficient to exclude these illnesses without consideration of other clinical and laboratory data (3). When sufficient criteria are not present, the diagnosis is difficult. Symptoms and signs are particularly subtle in infants less than 6 months of age (4). Even without the required number of criteria, children can have coronary artery involvement (5).

CLINICAL MANIFESTATIONS

Kawasaki syndrome begins acutely with fever that is remittent, high (100–104°F), and prolonged (1–2 weeks) in untreated patients. Within 1 to 3 days, a rash, conjunctival injection, and oral mucosal changes typically appear. The rash does not have a distinct morphologic pattern. It has been described as macular, maculopapular (morbilliform), urticarial, erythema multiforme-like, and scarlatiniform. A confluence of the rash in the perineal region is seen in up to 60% of patients. The conjunctival injection is bilateral and more prominent on the bulbar than the palpebral conjunctiva. There is no corneal ulceration or exudate. Slit-lamp examination may reveal uveitis. Oral mucosal findings of ulcers, petechiae, and exudates typical of other febrile exanthems are not features of KS. The changes of the peripheral extremities usually begin 3–5 days after the onset of fever. The swelling may be painful and must be distinguished from the arthritis that also occurs in patients with KS. Later, at about 10–14 days after the onset of fever, the distinctive desquamation begins in the subungual region of the fingertips and/or toes (Fig. 47C-1).

Ninety percent or more of patients with KS experience a rash, conjunctival injection, and changes of the peripheral

(Table 47C-1)
*Diagnostic guidelines for Kawasaki syndrome**

Fever lasting >5 days plus four of the following five criteria:
1. Polymorphous rash
2. Bilateral conjunctival injection
3. One or more of the following mucous membrane changes:
   - Diffuse injection of oral and pharyngeal mucosa
   - Erythema or fissuring of the lips
   - Strawberry tongue
4. Acute, nonpurulent cervical lymphadenopathy (one lymph node must be > 1.5 cm)
5. One or more of the following extremity changes:
   - Erythema of palms and/or soles
   - Indurative edema of hands and/or feet
   - Membranous desquamation of the fingertips

Other illnesses with similar clinical signs must be excluded

* Based on the Centers for Disease Control and Prevention case definition.

(Table 47C-2)
Kawasaki syndrome: differential diagnosis

Bacterial
  Streptococcal scarlet fever
  Toxic shock syndrome
  Staphylococcal scalded skin syndrome
  Mycoplasma infection
Viral
  Rubeola
  Epstein–Barr virus infection
  Enterovirus infection
  Adenovirus infection
  Roseola
  Rubella
Spirochetal
  Leptospirosis
  Lyme disease
Parasitic
  Toxoplasmosis
Rickettsial
  Rocky mountain spotted fever
  Typhus
Allergic/autoimmune
  Stevens–Johnson syndrome
  Drug reactions
  Juvenile rheumatoid arthritis (systemic onset)
  Reiter's syndrome
Toxin
  Acrodynia (mercury)

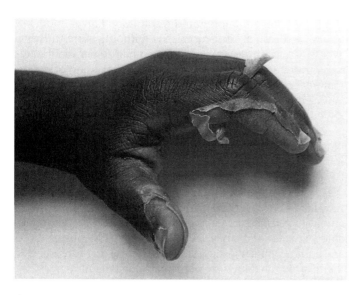

(Figure 47C-1)
Distinctive desquamation of the fingertips in Kawasaki syndrome.

extremities. Cervical adenopathy occurs in 50%–75% of patients. It may be unilateral or bilateral and involves one or more nodes that form a mass, sometimes as large as 5 cm. The nodes are firm, variably tender, and nonpurulent.

Most children with KS do not have cardiovascular symptoms. Cardiac examination, however, reveals tachycardia and gallop rhythms that are disproportionate to the degree of fever and anemia. These findings are secondary to myocarditis, which is present in at least 50% of patients. Arrhythmias are rare. New heart murmurs, from valvulitis or transient papillary muscle dysfunction, are heard in 1% of children with KS. Pericarditis occurs in 25% of patients with KS, but distant heart tones, a pericardial friction rub, or tamponade are unusual. Symptomatic congestive heart failure occurs infrequently (6).

Other clinical manifestations may include irritability, aseptic meningitis, seizures, transient paralysis, transient sensorineural hearing loss, upper respiratory congestion, cough, pneumonia, vomiting, diarrhea, hepatic dysfunction, noncalculous distention (hydrops) of the gallbladder, pancreatitis, urethritis, meatitis, and arthritis.

Because these clinical manifestations resolve spontaneously without specific treatment, the cardiovascular sequelae of KS were not initially appreciated until children died during or after recovery from the illness. Autopsies revealed a systemic vasculitis with a predilection for the coronary arteries. It is now well established by angiographic and echocardiographic data that up to 50% of untreated children with KS have coronary artery abnormalities and 15%–25% have aneurysms. Boys, children less than 1 year old, and children with a prolonged fever or a persistently elevated erythrocyte sedimentation rate are more likely to develop aneurysms, which are seen most often at 3–4 weeks. Approximately 50% of these aneurysms resolve. Factors positively associated with regression are smaller size and fusiform morphology of the aneurysm, female gender, and age less than 1 year. Children with giant aneurysms (>8 mm) have the worst prognosis. Myocardial infarctions, which are the principal cause of death in KS, occur most often in the first year. The majority of the infarctions occur while the child is at rest or asleep, and approximately one-third of the

children are asymptomatic. The mortality in children with myocardial infarctions is 32%.

Pathologic examination of regressed aneurysms reveals intimal thickening with proliferation of smooth muscle cells despite the normal caliber of the coronary artery. Results of exercise stress testing in these patients are normal. However, results of studies of coronary artery distensibility and vascular reactivity to isosorbide dinitrate are abnormal. Prolonged abnormalities of left ventricular function, even in children without aneurysms, have also been noted. Long-term follow-up is necessary to establish whether children who have recovered from KS are at risk for accelerated atherosclerosis or myocardial dysfunction (6).

LABORATORY STUDIES

Laboratory studies are not diagnostic in KS. In the initial 1–2 weeks of illness, there is a leukocytosis with a left shift, anemia, and increased acute-phase reactants. Thrombocytosis appears in the second week and may be marked. Urinalysis may reveal mild proteinuria or sterile pyuria from urethritis. In children with meningeal signs, cerebrospinal fluid may reveal a nonspecific pleocytosis. Liver function studies and pancreatic enzymes may be elevated. Complement levels are normal or increased. Tests for antinuclear antibodies and rheumatoid factor are negative. Antineutrophil cytoplasmic antibodies and antiendothelial cell antibodies have been detected but are of no diagnostic significance (7).

An electrocardiogram is recommended in the first week of illness. A two-dimensional echocardiogram with careful attention to the coronary arteries should be obtained at diagnosis, in the 2–3 weeks of illness, and about 1 month later. If results of these studies are abnormal, additional studies may be needed (8).

EPIDEMIOLOGY

KS is an illness of infants and young children. In Japan, where the most comprehensive data are available, 80% of cases involve children younger than 4 years old, and the male-to-female ratio is 1.4 to 1. Although KS has been reported throughout the world and in all racial groups, it is clearly more prevalent in children of Japanese ancestry and in Japan, where 116,848 cases have been reported since 1970 (9).

There is seasonal variation of KS, with more cases seen during the winter and spring. From 1979 to 1986, outbreaks occurred at 3–4 year intervals both in Japan and the United States. Temporal geographic spread from region to region was observed in Japan. A similar pattern has not been observed in the United States, where outbreaks have been limited to single communities. It is rare to see more than one patient with KS from the same family, neighborhood, school, or day care center, making person-to-person transmission unlikely. Epidemiologic studies have attempted to determine risk factors, which might provide insight into the cause of KS. Three associations have been identified: antecedent respiratory illness, carpet cleaning, and proximity to water. Subsequent data have been conflicting, however, and the significance of these associations remains unclear (10).

ETIOLOGY

The age-restricted susceptible population, the seasonal variation, the well-defined epidemics, and the acute self-limited clinical illness all suggest an infectious agent that is widespread and produces disease or immunity early in life. When a sufficient number of susceptible children have been added to the population, outbreaks occur. Extensive research, however, has failed to identify a causative agent (10). Numerous microorganisms have been implicated in individual cases or clinical series, but no unique or consistent association with the illness has been demonstrated. Initially promising studies for *Propionibacterium acnes* could not be confirmed by other investigators. A proposed retroviral cause has been disproved. Recent attention has focused on a superantigenic bacterial toxin, but again data are conflicting (11).

PATHOGENESIS

It is likely that immune activation and cytokine production are important in the pathogenesis of the vascular lesions in KS. Alterations in T cells, B cells, monocytes, and macrophages provide evidence of marked immune activation. Production of cytokines, which may predispose endothelial cells to injury, is elevated. Antibodies found in the sera of patients with KS have been shown to cause lysis of endothelial cells pretreated with interleukin-1, tumor necrosis factor, or interferon-gamma. Proposed triggers for the immune activation are conventional antigens of an infectious agent, superantigens, and heat-shock proteins. Genetic susceptibility may also play an important role. The exact mechanism of this immune-mediated injury remains to be determined (12).

TREATMENT

Intravenous fluids are indicated for many children who have high fever and inadequate oral intake. More aggressive support with diuretics, inotropic agents, or pacemakers may be needed for a few patients with myocarditis. Antibiotics are of no benefit, but may be administered until bacterial infection has been excluded. Steroids are not recommended. In the past, patients treated with corticosteroids had a higher incidence of aneurysms, and patients with aneurysms who received corticosteroids were more likely to develop ischemic heart disease (13,14).

Aspirin has been the most widely used therapeutic agent for KS. Doses of 80–100 mg/kg/day theoretically suppress inflammation, and doses of 3–10 mg/kg/day inhibit platelet aggregation. An intermediate, antipyretic dose of 30–50 mg/kg/day has been used by Japanese physicians. The optimum dosage regimen is still controversial and inadequately studied. When used alone, there is no convincing evidence that aspirin affects the incidence of coronary artery abnormalities (CAA) (15).

A beneficial effect from intravenous immunoglobulin (IVIG) was first reported by Japanese investigators. A multicenter prospective trial in the United States has demonstrated a significant reduction of CAA in patients treated during the first 10 days of illness with IVIG plus aspirin compared with aspirin alone (16). A second study by the same investigators compared IVIG 400 mg/kg/day for 4 consecutive days to a single dose of 2 gm/kg (17). Both treatment groups received aspirin 100 mg/kg/day for 14 days followed by 3–5 mg/kg/day. Children receiving the

single infusion had more rapid resolution of fever and laboratory indices of inflammation without more adverse events. Children receiving IVIG also had fewer giant coronary artery aneurysms and more rapid resolution of abnormalities of myocardial function (18,19). A single infusion of IVIG 2 gm/kg plus aspirin 100 mg/kg/day for 14 days followed by acetylsalicylic acid 3–5 mg/kg/day for 6–8 weeks is now the treatment of choice for KS in the first 10 days of illness (20). Guidelines for long-term management, based on the presence or absence of CAA, have been proposed by the American Heart Association (8).

The mechanism of action of IVIG in KS is unknown. The recommended dose and duration of treatment for both IVIG and aspirin may change as additional studies become available. Whether all commercially available IVIG preparations are equally effective has not been studied. More specific therapy awaits discovery of the causative agent.

DOROTHY WOODWARD WORTMANN, MD

1. Kawasaki T, Kosaki F, Okawa S, Shigematsu I, Yanagawa H: A new infantile acute febrile mucocutaneous lymph node syndrome (MLNS) prevailing in Japan. Pediatr 54:271-276, 1974
2. Morens D, O-Brien R: Kawasaki disease in the United States. J Infect Dis 137:91-93, 1978
3. Burns JC, Mason WH, Glode MP, et al: Clinical and epidemiologic characteristics of patients referred for evaluation of possible Kawasaki disease. J Pediatr 118:680-686, 1991
4. Burns JC, Wiggins JW, Toews WH, Newburger JW, Leung DYM, Wilson H, Grode MP: Clinical spectrum of Kawasaki disease in infants younger than 6 months of age. J Pediatr 109:759-763, 1986
5. Levy M, Koren G: Atypical Kawasaki disease: analysis of clinical presentation and diagnostic clues. Pediatr Infect Dis J 9:122-126, 1990
6. Wortmann DW: Kawasaki syndrome and the heart. In Hurst JW (ed): New Types of Cardiovascular Diseases: Topics in Clinical Cardiology. New York, IgaKu-Shoin, 1994, pp 141-163
7. Guzman J, Fung M, Petty RE: Diagnostic value of anti-neutrophil cytoplasmic antibodies and anti-endothelial cell antibodies in early Kawasaki disease. J Pediatr 124: 917-920, 1994
8. Dajani AS, Taubert KA, Takahashi M, et al: Guidelines for long-term management of patients with Kawasaki disease. Circulation 89:916-922, 1994
9. Yanagawa H, Yashiro M, Nakamura Y, Kawaski T, Kato H: Epidemiologic pictures of Kawasaki disease in Japan: from the nationwide survey in 1991 and 1992. Pediatr 95:475-479, 1995
10. Mason WH, Schneider T, Takahashi M: The epidemiology and etiology of Kawasaki disease. Cardiol Young 1:196-205, 1991
11. Terai M, Miwa K, Williams T, et al: The absence of evidence of staphylococcal toxin involvement in the pathogenesis of Kawasaki disease. J Infect Dis 172:558-561, 1995
12. Shulman ST, DeInocencio J, Hirsch R: Kawasaki disease. Pediatr Clin North Am 42:1205-1222, 1995
13. Kato H, Koike S, Yokoyama T: Kawasaki disease: effect of treatment on coronary artery involvement. Pediatr 62:175-179, 1979
14. Kato H, Inoue O, Akagi T: Kawasaki disease: cardiac problems and management. Pediatr Rev 9:209-217, 1988
15. Duronpisitkul K, Gururaj VJ, Park JM, Martin CF: The prevention of coronary artery aneurysm in Kawasaki disease: a meta-analysis on the efficacy of aspirin and immunoglobulin treatment. Pediatrics 96:1057-1061, 1995
16. Newburger JW, Takahashi M, Burn J, et al: The treatment of Kawasaki syndrome with intravenous gamma globulin. N Engl J Med 315:341-347, 1986
17. Newburger JW, Takahasi M, Beiser AS, et al: A single infusion of gamma globulin as compared with four infusions in the treatment of acute Kawasaki syndrome. N Engl J Med 324:1633-1639, 1991
18. Rowley AH, Shulman ST: Prevention of giant coronary artery aneurysms in Kawasaki disease by intravenous gamma globulin therapy. J Pediatr 113:290-294, 1988
19. Newburger JW, Sanders SP, Burns JC, Parness IA, Beiser AS, Colan SD: Left ventricular contractility and function in Kawasaki syndrome: effect of intravenous gammaglobulin. Circulation 79:1237-1246, 1989
20. Dajani AS, Taubert KA, Gerber MA et al: Diagnosis and therapy of Kawasaki disease in children. Circulation 87:1776-1780, 1993

REHABILITATION OF PATIENTS WITH RHEUMATIC DISEASE

Rheumatology rehabilitation is function oriented, which represents a paradigm shift from the disease- or illness-oriented model of rheumatology care. Rehabilitation of patients with rheumatic disease requires analysis of the functional effects of the pathologic changes produced. Rehabilitation-related terms have been defined by the World Health Organization (1). *Disease* is the process that causes a change in the structure or function of the body usually evidenced as the "signs and symptoms." *Impairment* occurs at the organ level and refers to the pathophysiologic consequences of disease, such as the anatomic damage and functional changes (loss of motion, deformity, pain, stiffness, or fatigue). *Functional limitations* or deficit (functional disability) refers to the loss of ability to perform the tasks in activities of daily living (ADL), work, and recreation, which is caused by an impairment (occurs at an individual level). Currently the term *disability* (previously called handicap) refers to an individual's limited physical ability that does not meet his or her needs. The functional limitation or extent of disability from an impairment is specific to an individual. (2) *Handicap* is the disadvantage due to impairment or disability that prevents fulfillment of the individual's normal role in society. The nature and severity of the handicap is largely determined by society's constraints.

Determination of rehabilitation treatment is based on assessment of functional deficits and evaluation of potential for improvement. Joint inflammation alters the structure and function of joints causing pain, reduced motion arc, decreased strength, and loss of endurance for motor tasks. In the early stages of arthritis, patients adapt and change the way physical tasks are performed to avoid pain and compensate for loss of strength and endurance. However, these adaptive changes may stress and irritate other joints. The rehabilitation goals in these early stages are to maintain, preserve, and improve function of involved joints. After extensive joint damage has occurred, rehabilitation goals include pain management and maximizing function through adaptive techniques and equipment. Following orthopedic surgical procedures rehabilitation programs are designed to promote increased motion, strength, and endurance.

INTERVENTIONAL APPROACH

Rheumatology rehabilitation may be in an outpatient setting, or more intensive inpatient therapy may be required in an acute or subacute rehabilitation unit (2). Medicare guidelines exist for treatment on an acute rehabilitation unit. Services must be "reasonable and necessary," and require close medical supervision by a physician with specialized training or experience in rehabilitation and 24-hour rehabilitation nursing services. The patient must need and receive at least three hours of physical therapy, occupational therapy, and other rehabilitative services each day. Patient impairment and functional disability must be sufficiently severe and complicated to require multidisciplinary team delivery of a coordinated care program. Substantial practical improvement must be expected, and therapeutic goals must be realistic. The rehabilitation program should be re-evaluated and adjusted periodically, because patients may fail to meet or may exceed the initial goals.

There are four key elements of the successful rheumatology rehabilitation program. First, goals should be realistic, measurable, and precisely defined after discussion with the patient. Type and site of rehabilitation is based on the patient's level of independence and degree of disability. Needs for adaptive equipment and modifications of home setting and work environment can be evaluated in a home or work site visit by a physical or occupational therapist. Availability of home assistance from spouse, relatives, or friends should be determined. Second, a realistic time-frame for goals should be determined. Rehabilitation goals should be adjusted according to patient performance and needs. Patients must have realistic expectations of results to avoid discouragement and improve adherence.

Third, preventive measures should be undertaken. These may include halting deterioration of function, anticipating or avoiding complications of disease, and making adjustments in lifestyle such as regular exercise, joint protection, and pacing of activities. Medical treatment should be optimized for maximum control of disease activity to reduce impairment. *Deconditioning*, the physiologic changes induced by inactivity, should be prevented with active range of motion exercises, strengthening exercises, and resumption of daily activities as soon as possible. Finally, enhancement or supplementation becomes necessary when prevention fails and functional limitations develop. One must distinguish between the patient's report of capabilities and actual performance to accurately identify the impairments, functional limitations, disabilities, and handicaps.

THE RHEUMATOLOGY REHABILITATION TEAM

The concept of an interdisciplinary team approach encourages active communication and cooperation among the various disciplines. The rheumatology rehabilitation team usually consists of a physician, a rehabilitation nurse with rheumatology expertise, a physical therapist (PT), an occupational therapist (OT), a psychologist, a medical social worker, a vocational rehabilitation counselor, a recreational therapist, and occasionally a speech therapist. The physician may be a rehabilitation specialist with rheumatology experience, a rheumatologist with rehabilitation experience, or a primary care physician with rehabilitation and rheumatology experience.

In a team meeting, the patient's status is reviewed briefly by each team member, and the goals and plans for the treatment program are discussed. Group evaluation of problems promotes consistency of purpose and efficient planning of therapies and follow-up.

Rehabilitation nurses integrate the knowledge and skills learned by the patient during the therapies to achieve self-care goals and independence; and provide patient education regarding medications and the disease process.

Physical therapists focus on improving the level of function by designing, together with the patients, an exercise program to increase range of motion, strength, coordination, and endurance. They teach patients how to transfer safely from bed to chair or wheelchair and how to get into and out of the bathtub, shower, and car. Physical therapists evaluate gait and ambulation safety and train patients to use canes, crutches, or wheelchairs. In addition, they may evaluate the patient for splints or braces, fabricate orthoses, and teach patients to use various modalities (heat, cold) to control pain. Physical therapists also perform home and worksite evaluations for accessibility, safety, and modifications.

Occupational therapists typically focus on upper extremity function, including ways to increase range of motion, strength, coordination, and endurance. They assess and train patients for independent and safe self-care skills, activities of daily living (bathing, grooming, dressing, toileting, personal hygiene, eating), and community skills. When problems occur, the OT develops education and training for compensatory or adaptive skills and recommends adaptive equipment. They can provide instruction in principles of joint protection and energy conservation, fabricate upper extremity orthoses, and perform home evaluations for accessibility and safety. They often instruct patients on the appropriate application of modalities for pain control.

Vocational rehabilitation counselors assist with reassessing vocational goals according to the patient's aptitude, interests, and functional abilities. They serve as resources for information about training programs, assistance for additional education, and workplace modifications.

Recreation therapists evaluate the patient's desired recreational activities and educate the patient about adapted recreations, new leisure activities, and social interests. They are often a valuable resource for adaptations and modifications that enable patients to continue to enjoy recreational activities.

Rehabilitation psychologists identify psychosocial issues through clinical interviews, personality inventories, and cognitive testing. They can provide insight into unique needs and goals of the patient. They often counsel patients and families to help with their adjustment to various impairments, disabilities, or handicaps, and other mental health needs. They also assist in understanding and managing behavioral issues.

Medical social workers often serve as communicators between the rehabilitation team and the family; coordinate planning for home care needs, work site needs, and financial concerns; and coordinate continued outpatient therapies.

ARTHRITIS REHABILITATION

In the broadest sense, rheumatology rehabilitation aims to maximize functional independence within the constraints imposed by the type of arthritis, its severity, and duration. A carefully designed rehabilitation program is an important part of the total management of patients with chronic arthri-

tis. The first step in planning a rheumatology rehabilitation program is assessment of function and disease status.

The function of all joints should be systematically measured once or twice a year to provide suitable monitoring of response to therapy and progression of disease. The concept of functional independence for the patient with arthritis involves personal activities of daily living as well as vocational, family, and social functioning. Therefore, it must be evaluated on an individual basis (Table 48-1). Typical impairments and functional deficits for individual joints with useful rehabilitation therapies will be discussed in the following section.

The multidimensional health status measurement tools provide important information about the patient's functional ability that would not likely be discussed in the standard clinical interview. Patient self-reports of physical, social, and emotional functional status may reveal difficulties with coping and ability to participate in social roles. The Arthritis Impact Measurement Scale (AIMS) (3) consists of nine scales of mobility, physical activity, dexterity, ADL, social activity, anxiety, depression, pain, and household activities. The AIMS II includes lower extremity function, satisfaction, patient preference, work status, income level, and comorbidity. The Health Assessment Questionnaire (HAQ) measures discomfort, disability, drug toxicity, disability index, dollar cost, and mortality. The HAQ disability index as-

(Table 48-1)
*Functional assessment screen**

Joint Region	Functional Assessment Maneuver
Upper extremity function	Able to comb hair, feed self, cut meat, buttoning, toilet hygiene.
Hand	Ability to grip 6-8 cm diameter plastic tube. Ability to bend fingers 2 through 5 around a pencil. Ability to manage round pincer grip with thumb and index finger. Ability to oppose thumb tip to base of 5th finger.
Wrist	Flexion extension +90°–80°
Elbow	With elbow at side, pronate and supinate hand so that thumb rests on table. Full extension of forearm, flex to touch mouth with fingers.
Shoulder	Grasp hand behind head and behind low back. Identify descrepancy between active and passive ROM to differentiate glenohumeral joint and rotator cuff disorders.
Lower extremity function	Arise from chair without using arms, ascend and descend stairs without handrail, cross intersection during green light.
Hip	Cross legs while sitting.
Knee	Full extension, place heel on opposite knee while seated. Carefully differentiate effusion, painful inflamed synovium from tissue contractures.
Ankles and feet	Able to walk on heels and toes.

* ROM = range of motion.

sesses dressing, arising, eating, walking, grooming, upper and lower extremity mobility, sexual activity, and psychological functioning. It includes a visual analog scale for pain (4). The modified HAQ includes questions on perceived satisfaction or perceived change in performance.

Self-reported functional abilities and limitations must be verified by direct observation and further in-depth interview. The Functional Independence Measure (FIM) is a standardized tool for observer-determined functional independence assessment used in most rehabilitation programs (5) (Table 48-2).

The most simple and affordable rehabilitation program that is effective will have the greatest adherence. Pain controlling modalities that have been advocated for patients with arthritis (6) include superficial and deep heat, superfi-

(Table 48-2)

The functional independence measure was developed by the American Congress of Rehabilitation Medicine and the American Academy of Physical Medicine and Rehabilitation Task Force for a National Uniform Data System for Medical Rehabilitation to rate severity of disability and the outcomes of medical rehabilitation treatments. Two measures are derived, Motor Function (first 13 items) and Cognitive Function (last 5 items) and are scaled from 0 to 100. Each item is rated on a 1 to 7 scale of level of functioning independently. Evidence for improvement in function is identified by increasing level number in each item, with Motor items and Cognitive items totaled separately.

Classification	Item
Self-care	Eating
	Grooming
	Bathing
	Dressing—upper body
	Dressing—lower body
	Toileting
Sphincter control	Bladder management
	Bowel management
Mobility	Bed, chair, wheelchair transfers
	Transfer to toilet
	Transfer to tub, shower
Locomotion	Walk or wheelchair
	Stair climbing
Communication	Comprehension
	Expression
Social cognition	Social interaction
	Problem solving
	Memory

Function levels

No helper
    7—Complete independence
    6—Modified independence
Modified dependence
    5—Supervision
    4—Minimal assistance (75% independent)
    3—Moderate assistance (50% independent)
Dependent on helper
    2—Maximal assistance (25% independent)
    1—Total assistance (<25% independent)

cial cold, mechanical modalities (massage, compression, and traction), transcutaneous electrical nerve stimulation (TENS), acupuncture, and topical treatments. Modalities are not curative therapies for arthritis but transiently decrease pain and stiffness in some patients.

Joint pain may be decreased with either heat or cold, but there are no predictable changes in range of motion or function. The normal knee has an intra-articular temperature of ±33°C, and the rheumatoid knee of ±36°C. Collagenase activity and hyaluronate synthesis cause increases up to 39°C, ligamentous laxity increases with rising temperatures, and irreversible tissue damage occurs above 41–42°C (7) Thermotherapy is administered superficially at 36–43°C with moist warm towels, infra-red radiation, hot packs, paraffin baths, and hydrotherapy. Deeper heating is administered with microwave and short-wave diathermy and ultrasound. With diathermy, high frequency magnetic waves create heat in tissues to a depth of 3–5 cm. Ultrasound produces high frequency acoustical energy to heat tissue 1–2°C up to 10 cm deep.

Application of superficial moist heat to joints with rheumatoid arthritis decreases joint pain by unknown mechanisms. Effects of superficial heat on intra-articular joint temperature are controversial (9). Superficial heating for less than 5 minutes decreases joint temperature, but increases joint temperature after 20 to 30 minutes' application. Application of moist hot packs, paraffin baths, and immersion in water (32–38°C) for 10–20 minutes, once or twice a day is advised. In patients with reduced sensation, fragile skin, or reduced circulation in the hands and feet, heat therapy should be avoided because of burn risk (10). Mineral baths and spa therapy are often advocated for patients with arthritis, but controlled studies have failed to demonstrate benefits (8).

Deep heating modalities such as short-wave or microwave diathermy and ultrasound increase intra-articular temperature and may increase cartilage damage. Deep heating is not recommended for joints, but may be helpful for muscle spasm, tendinitis, and bursitis. Microwave diathermy, which heats up more than soft tissues, should not be used over prosthetic joints.

Application of superficial cold to joints or muscles reduces swelling, raises the pain threshold, and decreases muscle spasm. Cryotherapy is most commonly used as initial treatment in acute musculoskeletal and soft tissue injuries. Cold may be applied with ice packs or vapocoolant sprays but should not be used in patients with Raynaud's phenomenon or cryoglobulinemia.

Topical treatment with liniments and ointments that contain methylsalicylate causes a feeling of warmth and a temporary decrease in pain. Capsaicin, a natural alkaloid from the hot pepper plant, excites polymodal C and A-delta fibers, causing a release of substance P, calcitonin gene-related peptide, and neurokinin A. Release of these substances causes an initial neurogenic inflammatory flare and transiently blocks nerve conduction when peptides are depleted. Capsaicin (0.075%) applied four times per day has been shown to decrease pain in patients with osteoarthritis or rheumatoid arthritis (9).

Transcutaneous electrical nerve stimulation of large myelinated nerve fibers at 70 hz causes release of endorphins in the spinal cord that diminish nociceptive input from unmyelinated C fibers and small myelinated A-delta fibers. This modality is more effective in relieving bony pain and neuralgic pain than pain from peripheral joints. Pain relief lasts from 6 to 24 hours after treatment. In patients with rheumatoid arthritis, placement of electrodes proximal to the wrist on the volar and palmar aspect of the forearm can reduce hand and wrist pain when gripping. For knee arthritis, TENS treatment 30–60 minutes 3 times per day (70 hz) via 4 electrodes placed around the knee can decrease pain but has not been shown to alter walking. Reports of pain relief with TENS are similar to relief reported with acupuncture. In controlled studies, results are much less impressive.

Fatigue is a debilitating problem for some patients with rheumatoid arthritis or other inflammatory joint diseases. The patient may be using the term *fatigue* to describe muscle weakness, lack of endurance for daily activities, excessive daytime sleepiness related to a specific sleep disorder, or sedating medication side effects. Sleep quality and alertness during the day should be assessed routinely. Persistent daytime sleepiness indicates need for evaluation of a specific sleep disorder. Dissatisfaction with sleep quality or insomnia should prompt attention to possible depression, nocturnal joint pain, pain from carpal tunnel syndrome, or excessive use of stimulants or depressants (alcohol or caffeine). Depression may make a patient feel fatigued during the day, representing lack of initiative and motivation. Medications may cause daytime fatigue or actual sedation as side effects. Almost all patients with chronic rheumatoid arthritis become deconditioned, with reduced maximal oxygen uptake or consumption during physical activity. Submaximal conditioning exercise improves endurance time and produces a lower perceived exertion at specific levels of work intensity.

THERAPEUTIC EXERCISE

Stretching is a good warm-up for strengthening and conditioning exercises. Stretching exercises can be done passively by a therapist or actively by the patient contracting opposing muscle groups to preserve or increase range of motion. Several routines for upper and lower extremity groups have been described and are suitable for home or group participation (10-12).

Strengthening exercises may be *isometric* (muscle contraction but no joint motion), *isotonic* (muscle contraction and joint motion), or *isokinetic* (muscle contraction with joint movement against moving resistance). In isotonic exercises, if the muscle is shortening during contraction, it is a concentric contraction; if the muscle is lengthened, it is a eccentric contraction. Muscle contractions against high resistance for a few repetitions increases strength and size of Type II muscle fibers. Muscle contractions against low resistance with many repetitions increases endurance. Isometric exercises are useful in preparation for joint replacement surgery. Patients can be taught to monitor symptoms safely and to limit exercises to avoid injury. High-resistance exercises taken through a full range of motion may further damage diseased periarticular tissues and ligaments and increase pain. If pain is induced by the motion, muscle contraction is reflexly inhibited so there will be no strengthening effect and additional tissue damage may occur. Low-intensity isokinetic strength training (50% of maximal voluntary contraction) can increase knee extensor muscle strength without adversely affecting knee synovitis (13).

Protracted bed rest should be avoided. Rather, the therapeutic exercise program should include stretching, strengthening, and aerobic conditioning exercises; routine activities; and one or two mid-day rest periods. Exercise training programs have been shown to increase muscle strength and improve aerobic condition without worsening joint disease in rheumatoid arthritis. Conditioning exercises may be carried out using a stationary bicycle, walking program, swimming program, or aerobic dancing with low-impact gliding steps (10-12). Aerobic conditioning with low-impact exercises (walking, rowing, cycling, swimming) should be carried out with a day of rest between exercise days. The training heart rate should be 60% to 80% of the maximum heart rate achieved on a baseline graded exercise stress test. The exercise activity is prescribed at the work intensity that achieves the training heart rate 5 to 10 minutes at that workload. Duration should be increased by 5-minute increments per week. Thereafter, exercise intensity can be increased as the heart rate response decreases with conditioning.

PATIENT EDUCATION

Patient education programs can help teach patients to reduce the effort required for routine daily tasks. Patients may be taught alternative body positioning, organization, sequencing, and simplification of individual tasks. Pacing of daily activities is a critical skill; analyzing tasks to plan stages for carrying them out will permit success in independent functioning. Occupational therapists and physical therapists are skilled at teaching patients ways to simplify tasks and use specialized tools or assistive devices. They can also make suggestions for modifying the work environment (11).

ASSISTIVE DEVICES

Assistive devices and adaptive aids compensate for functional deficits, reduce pain, and promote maintenance of independence for patients with arthritis. Most assistive devices recommended with arthritis were actually developed for patients with neuromuscular deficits and may not accommodate joint deformities or impaired finger dexterity. Axillary or forearm crutches and canes are effective in reducing weight on an affected leg. Grips for canes and crutches can be modified to accommodate problems with wrist and hand arthritis. Elevated chair and toilet seats compensate for lower extremity weakness. Enlarged hand grips in cars, bathtubs, and showers facilitate transfers and prevent falls. A variety of assistive devices for hand functions can be suggested by the occupational therapist to maintain independence in meal preparation, self-care, housekeeping, and vocational tasks.

SPECIFIC REHABILITATION TREATMENTS

In rheumatoid arthritis, C1–C2 involvement with synovitis in the apophyseal joints and transverse ligament causes pain and instability of the atlantoaxial segment. Avoidance of prolonged positions and use of exercises to stretch cervical paraspinal muscles during the workday decrease pain. Exercises include shoulder rolls and shrugging, together with range of motion stretching of the neck in all planes. Superficial heat may decrease pain. Cervical isometric strengthening exercises are performed by pushing the head against the hand placed on the sides of the head with exertion of maximal force held for 10 seconds. Repetitions of this maneuver are done several times daily with both sides of the head, the forehead and the occiput. Cervical traction should not be used for patients with rheumatoid neck disease. A soft collar, worn constantly for up to 6 weeks may result in stabilization and usually provides some symptomatic relief without inconvenience. The Philadelphia collar provides more support and limitation of extension but is less well-tolerated.

Shoulder

Goals of managing shoulder pain are to control pain and maintain normal motion. Active range of motion exercises using Codman exercise (pendular arm exercise) adds traction to the glenohumeral joint by stretching the capsule and avoiding active abduction, which would produce pain. Codman exercises involve grasping a 5-lb weight while dangling the arm and swinging it in a forward and backward lateral plane and circumduction arc. These exercises may be active or passive. Finger wall climbing while the patient faces the wall, ranges with a wand or broom handle, hangs from an overhead chinning bar, or reaches for the ceiling or top of a door frame are good stretching exercises. Patients should work toward being able to clasp their hands behind the head with the elbows back.

Elbow

Elbow flexion of at least 90° is needed to get the hand to the mouth and for self care. Loss of extension and forearm supination/pronation results in loss of upper extremity function. Active range of motion stretching can be employed to increase extension and forearm supination as well as to strengthen the extensor muscles. Stretching a piece of elastic during elbow extension exercises also helps strengthen the triceps.

Wrist and Hand

Protection of wrist and hand joints that have been weakened by chronic inflammation is extremely important. An occupational therapist specializing in hand and wrist evaluation can provide important instruction to patients to prevent physical injury to the fragile joint tissues. Proper mechanics and positioning, together with adaptive equipment, may prevent further deformity and loss of function. As a general rule, all hand movements that result in force exerted against the radial side of each finger should be avoided. Abrupt force may contribute to subluxation and ulnar deviation of the metacarpophalangeal joints. Strong grasp plus twisting motion should be avoided.

In early rheumatoid arthritis, rehabilitation goals are to preserve function, reduce pain, and prevent deformity. Joint protection techniques, splinting, and selective exercises are designed to balance forces, but there are no data that they prevent deformity. A *resting splint* is designed to help reduce pain by immobilizing the hand and wrist. A *functional* or *static working splint* (extends to mid-palmar crease) is designed to support the wrist protectively in a position for use during activities (14).

Active range of motion and balanced resistive exercises are thought to prevent contractures in patients who have reducible deformities and active synovitis by stretching intrinsic muscles and reducing ulnar deviation forces. (15,16). Exercises for the wrists involve stretching in extension, flexion, pronation, and supination. Proximal interphalangeal ring splints minimize swan neck and boutonnière deformities. If the tendon mechanism is intact, strengthening of muscles that oppose the direction of the contractures may be beneficial. However, contractures at metacarpophalangeal and proximal interphalangeal joints, if related to subluxation, cannot be corrected by exercise.

Hip

Patients with a painful hip have a shortened stride length and lean toward the painful side during single leg support to minimize contraction of the hip abductors and reduce reactive forces on the hip joint. Hip flexors gradually shorten, resulting in pain with forced extension of the hip while walking. If hamstrings are tight, lumbar lordosis adds painful back symptoms. Patients with rheumatoid arthritis involvement of hip or knee have a typical gait characterized by the pelvis moving towards the involved hip and ipsilateral knee flexion. A cane in the opposite hand decreases the need for this antalgic lean and reduces hip joint forces by 60%. The cane should be long enough to reach the greater trochanter, and the elbow should be flexed about 20°. If the patient bends forward, the cane is too short. The tip of the cane should be placed about 8 inches ahead of and lateral to the toes of the unaffected leg. If a load is to be carried, it should be carried on the side of the involved hip to decrease the force of abductors required during single leg support. Hip contractures are due to tight hip flexor muscles and/or a tight joint capsule. Active and passive range of motion stretching exercises should be carried out bearing in the supine position (non-weight bearing) to loosen tight muscles, reduce spasm, and increase motion. Non-weight bearing, strengthening exercises should also be performed, raising the leg in prone, supine, and side-lying to strengthen flexors, extensors, abductors, and adductors. If the hip is too painful to raise the leg, strengthening by isometric contractions is produced by "pressing" the leg into the bed in prone, supine, and side-lying positions. Abductors can be strengthened by gluteal isometric contractions.

Knee

Flexion contractures greater than 5°–10° cause a limp, alter the biomechanics of gait inducing symptoms in hips and ankles, increase energy expenditure of walking, and impair balance (17). Quadriceps and hamstring weakness are common in RA. Atrophy of the vastus medialis, the muscle used in the last few degrees of extension to lock the knee in place, occurs early in RA. Normal quadriceps strength is important for knee stability. Quadriceps strengthening exercises should begin with isometric contractions. Resistive extension exercises will provide progressive quadriceps strengthening, reduce pain, and improve walk time and endurance. (18) Braces for knee pain and instability are bulky and poorly tolerated by patients with arthritis (19). A Swedish knee cage or hinged knee brace to limit extension may reduce pain. A knee–ankle–foot orthosis or Lennox Hill brace provides some medial lateral stability.

Foot and Ankle

Tibio-talar and subtalar arthritis-related heel pain can be decreased with a weight bearing ankle–foot orthosis or ankle immobilizer with a cushioned heel shoe. Talonavicular joint damage and subtalar joint damage results in midfoot instability and pain. Instability in the hind foot leads to collapse of the medial longitudinal arch and outward rotation of calcaneus (valgus deformity of the heel). A hindfoot orthosis can re-align the calcaneus and reduce pronation of the foot. A heel cup can relieve pressure on calcaneal spur or rheumatoid nodules in the heel pad. Arch supports distribute weight over a larger surface area and reduce localized pain. Midfoot pain can often be relieved with a good quality high-top athletic shoe that has a firm longitudinal arch support and generous width.

Forefoot pain and tenderness cause the patient to keep body weight back over the heels during walking and result in a shuffling gait. Relief of forefoot pain can be obtained with shoes that have an impact-absorbing sole and an extra-deep toe box with generous width to prevent squeezing of the metatarsal row during walking. Metatarsal head pain can be diminished by metatarsal bars, metatarsal pads, or molded inserts. For those with marked metatarsophalangeal subluxation and toe flexion deformities complicated by calluses and skin breakdown, custom-made orthopedic shoes must be prescribed.

MAREN L. MAHOWALD, MD
DENNIS DYKSTRA, MD, PhD

1. International classification of impairments, disabilities and handicaps: A manual of classifications relating to the consequences of disease. World Health Organization, Geneva, Switzerland, 1990

2. Commission on Accreditation of Rehabilitation Facilities: Section 2.II.A: Medical rehabilitation programs; comprehensive inpatient categories one through three. In: Supplement to the 1994 Standards Manual and Interpretive Guidelines for Organizations Serving People With Disabilities, pp 1-4, 1994

3. Meenan RF, Anderson JJ, Kagis LE, et al: Outcome Assessment in Clinical Trials. Arthritis Rheum 27: 1344-1352, 1984

4. Fries JF, Spitz P, Kraines RG, Holman HR: Measurement of patient outcome in arthritis. Arthritis Rheum 23:137-145, 1980

5. Granger GV, Hamilton BB: The uniform data system for medical rehabilitation: report of first admissions for 1990. Am J Phys Med Rehabil 71:10-16, 1992

6. Nicholas JJ: Physical modalities in rheumatological rehabilitation. Arch Phys Med Rehabil, 75:994-1011, 1994.

7. Oosterveld FGJ and Rasker JJ: Treating arthritis with locally applied heat or cold. Semin Arth Rheum 24:82-90, 1994

8. Elkayam O, Wigler I, Tishler M, et al: Effect of spa therapy on tibias in patients with rheumatoid arthritis and osteoarthritis. J Rheumatol 18:1799-1803, 1991

9. McCarty GM and Mc Carty DJ, Effect of topical capsaicin in therapy of painful osteoarthritis of the hands. J Rheumatol 19:604-607, 1992

10. Ytterberg SR, Mahowald ML, and Krug HE, Exercise for arthritis. Balliere's Clin Rheumatol 8:161-187, 1994

11. Minor, MA, et al: Efficacy of physical conditioning exercise in patients with rheumatoid arthritis and osteoarthritis. Arthritis Rheum 32:1396-1405, 1989

12. Kovar PA, Allegrante JP, Mackenzie CR, et al: Supervised fitness walking in patients with osteoarthritis of the knee. Ann Intern Med 116:529-534, 1992

13. Lyngberg KK, Ramsing BU, Nawrockie A, et al: Safe and effective isokinetic knee extension training in rheumatoid arthritis. Arth Rheum 37:623-628, 1994

14. Stern EB, Ytterberg SR, Krug HE, Mullen G, Mahowald ML: Immediate and short-term effects of three commercial wrist extensor orthoses on grip strength and function in patients with rheumatoid arthritis. Arthritis Care Res 9:42-50, 1996

15. Hoenig H, Groff G, Pratt K, et al: A randomized controlled trial of home exercise on the rheumatoid hand. J Rheumatol 20:785-789, 1993

16. Brighton SE, Lubbe JE, and Van Der Merwe CA: The effect of a long-term exercise programme on the rheumatoid hand. Brit J Rheumatol 32: 392-395,1993

17. Potter PJ, Kirby RL,MacLeod DA: The effects of simulated knee-flexion contractures on standing balance. Am J Phys Med Rehabil 69:144-147,1990

18. Fisher NM, Pendergast DR: Effects of a muscle exercise program on exercise capacity in subjects with osteoarthritis. Arch Phys Med Rehabil 75: 792-197, 1994

19. Merritt JL: Advances in orthotics for the patient with rheumatoid arthritis. J Rheumatol 14 (Suppl 15): 62-67,1987

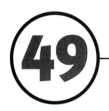# PSYCHOSOCIAL FACTORS

A variety of psychosocial factors may influence the health status of patients with arthritis. Although most studies of the psychosocial dimensions of arthritis have focused on patients with rheumatoid arthritis (RA), psychosocial factors are important in all rheumatic conditions and disorders of the musculoskeletal system.

ENVIRONMENTAL STRESS

Arthritis and related musculoskeletal disorders (ARMD) are frequently associated with multiple stressors, including depression and other psychologic disorders, work disability, and loss of highly valued social, leisure, and nurturant activities. In a population-based study of Ontario residents, ARMD ranked first as the cause of chronic health problems, long-term disabilities, and visits with health professionals, and ranked second as the cause of restricted activity days and use of medication (1).

Patients with RA frequently report that increases in stress tend to precede flares in disease activity. Frequent daily stresses are associated with altered immune function. Increases in interpersonal stress appear to be causally related to increases in objective and subjective markers of disease activity, including physician's global ratings, degree of total T-cell activation, interleukin-2 receptor expression, and higher proportion of circulating B cells relative to T cells (2). These findings are consistent with patients' beliefs in an association between stress and disease flares and suggest that stress management interventions may be helpful adjuncts to medical management of RA (3, 4).

DEPRESSION

Depression is common in patients with ARMD. The National Health and Nutrition Epidemiologic Follow-Up Study in the United States showed that 16% of all persons with chronic musculoskeletal pain had scores indicative of depression on the Center for Epidemiologic Studies-Depression scale (5). A study of 6153 patients seen at one treatment center for 12 years found that the frequency of probable depression was 37% in patients with RA (6). The frequency of probable depression was 33% in patients with osteoarthritis of the knee or hip and 49% in patients with fibromyalgia (6).

The relationships between depression and health status variables in patients with ARMD are complex. In general, the relationships between depression and pain, disability, and loss of valued activities are independent of disease activity. The National Health and Nutrition Survey of the United States suggested that depression amplifies pain and also is influenced by pain (7). Among patients with RA, the most important predictors of depression scores are patients' ratings of pain intensity and scores on the Health Assessment Questionnaire (HAQ) Disability Index (8). Loss of valued activities may be a better predictor of depression among women with RA than is increased disability.

Most studies of emotional states in patients with ARMD have focused on negative states such as depression. There has been a tendency to assume that a negative affect or emotional state is simply the opposite of a positive affect (for example, an absence of feelings of excitement). Recent evidence suggests that an evaluation of affect, both positive and negative, is useful in patients with ARMD. For example, activity limitation measured by the HAQ among patients with RA is associated with frequent use of maladaptive pain coping strategies and relatively infrequent use of adaptive strategies (9). There are important differences in the determinants of these coping strategies. Maladaptive coping is associated with low positive affect and high negative affect, whereas adaptive coping is associated with high positive affect. Thus, both positive and negative affect contribute to the relationships between pain coping strategies and activity limitation.

COGNITIVE FACTORS AND COPING STRATEGIES

The health-related beliefs and coping strategies used by individuals tend to be highly associated with their health status. Two important beliefs involve perceptions of learned helplessness and self-efficacy.

Learned helplessness is the perception that no viable solutions are available to eliminate or reduce the source of a stressful situation. Learned helplessness is associated with specific emotional, motivational, and cognitive deficits in adaptive coping with stress and may underlie a portion of the psychologic distress and functional disability in patients with ARMD. Many patients may develop the belief that their disease is beyond their control because the disease is of unknown cause, has no cure, and is predicted to have a chronic or generally unpredictable course. This perception of uncontrollability may cause the patient to experience anxiety and depression (emotional deficits) that, in turn, may lead to increased pain and reduced attempts to either engage in activities of daily living (motivational deficits) or to develop new means of adapting to disabilities and distress (cognitive deficits).

The importance of perceptions of helplessness in adapting to arthritis has been confirmed in many studies. High levels of helplessness among patients with RA are associated with low self-esteem, use of maladaptive coping strategies, high levels of pain and depression, and high levels of functional impairment. In addition, a high level of helplessness at baseline predicts greater flare activity among patients with RA after a 3-month trial of a disease-modifying drug (10). Therefore, improving perceptions of control over arthritis symptoms may be desirable. Nevertheless, patients who believe they can control their symptoms suffer psychologic distress in response to increased pain unless they cognitively restructure their pain experiences, such as adopting the belief that pain has made life more precious.

Another cognitive factor closely related to perceptions of symptom control is *self-efficacy*. In contrast to perceptions of control over multiple arthritis symptoms, self-efficacy represents a belief that one can perform specific behaviors or tasks to achieve specific health-related goals. Any individual may exhibit great variation in self-efficacy for different behaviors. For example, an individual may have high self-efficacy for pacing daily activities with scheduled rest periods, whereas self-efficacy for performing exercises prescribed in physical therapy may be low.

Self-efficacy tends to predict health status if individuals believe that the relevant behaviors will lead to improved health and if they value improved health status. High baseline levels of self-efficacy for pain and functional ability among patients with RA and osteoarthritis are strongly associated with low levels of pain, disability, and depression at the time of initial assessment as well as at a 4-month follow-up evaluation (11). High self-efficacy for pain is significantly correlated with low frequencies of observable pain behaviors among persons with RA and fibromyalgia, even after controlling for demographic factors and measures of disease severity (12). In addition, improvements in self-efficacy produced by stress management training are associated with improvements in ratings of depression, pain, and walking speed made by patients with RA at 15 month follow-up (13). Two measures of self-efficacy are currently available: an instrument developed by Lorig and colleagues for patients with arthritis (11) and a questionnaire produced for patients with various chronic pain syndromes (14). No comparative studies have been performed with these two measures. Moreover, it recently has been suggested that these measures actually assess self-efficacy for specific behaviors as well as more global beliefs regarding control (15). It is expected that future work will resolve the measurement issues in this area.

The coping process comprises several stages that include: appraisal of the threat associated with a particular stressor; performing motor and cognitive actions (coping strategies) that may control the impact of the stressor; and evaluating the outcomes produced by these actions and, if necessary, performing alternative coping responses.

Studies of coping among patients with ARMD have used primarily three instruments: the Ways of Coping Scale, the Coping Strategies Questionnaire, and the Vanderbilt Pain Management Inventory. Passive coping strategies, such as catastrophizing (believing that no coping strategy will effectively control symptoms), are associated with high levels of pain among patients with RA. Conversely, psychologic adjustment and relatively low levels of pain and functional impairment have been found to be associated with strategies such as focusing on positive thoughts during pain episodes and infrequent use of catastrophizing. Similar results have been seen in studies of patients with osteoarthritis and fibromyalgia (16,17).

PSYCHOSOCIAL INTERVENTIONS

Given the relationships between health status and psychosocial factors, great effort has been devoted to testing psychosocial interventions that may improve patients' pain, emotional states, or function. Recent investigations also have assessed the extent to which these interventions help patients reduce health care utilization and costs.

The major psychosocial interventions can be classified according to the factors that the interventions were intended to modify in order to improve patient health status. Nevertheless, many of the interventions share common treatment components. These interventions do not include protocols that are intended only to increase patient knowledge, exercise, or adherence with treatment regimens.

Several investigators have examined the effects of group psychologic therapies on patients' symptom control and health status. A biofeedback-assisted group therapy intervention that trained patients with RA and their family members in relaxation and behavioral problem-solving skills has been evaluated. This intervention, relative to attention-placebo and no adjunct treatment conditions, produced significant reductions in pain behavior and disease activity after treatment ended (18). A 1-year follow-up showed that patients who received the psychologic intervention reported lower levels of pain and depression than those who received no adjunct treatment. This intervention was also associated with significantly lower use of health care resources and lower medical service costs compared with no adjunct treatment and attention-placebo conditions (19). Similar interventions have produced reductions in pain and psychologic distress over periods ranging from 15 to 30 months in patients with RA and fibromyalgia (4,20,21).

The Arthritis Self-Management Program is an intervention that focuses on enhancing perceptions of self-efficacy. This program produces significant increases in self-efficacy for pain and other symptoms, as well as significant reductions in pain ratings and arthritis-related physician visits among patients with RA and osteoarthritis that persist for 4 years after treatment initiation (22). Estimated net 4-year savings in health care costs are $648 for each patient with RA and $189 for each patient with osteoarthritis. However, the Arthritis Self-Management Program does not alter functional ability among the patients.

The effects of coping skills training on patients with osteoarthritis of the knee have been investigated (23). This training, relative to arthritis education and standard care, produced significant reductions in patients' ratings of pain and psychologic disability that generally were maintained at 6-month follow-up. In addition, patients who received coping skills training reported significant reductions in physical disability from post-treatment to follow-up.

Two recent innovations in coping skills training are telephone intervention by trained lay personnel to deliver training and the development of preventive interventions. The telephone interventions produce significant improvements in pain and disability among patients with osteoarthritis (24), as well as significant improvements in psychologic status among patients with systemic lupus erythematosus (25). Preventive interventions provide training in self-help activities (eg, exercise, maintenance of adaptive daily activities) to persons with acute musculoskeletal pain to reduce the risk of developing chronic pain syndrome (26). For example, a brief preventive intervention for patients with first episodes of musculoskeletal pain has been evaluated (27). The intervention, delivered by a physician and physical therapist, reinforced to patients the importance of maintaining daily activities and rapid return to work. It was found that this intervention, relative to usual medical treatment (ie, analgesic medication and advice to rest as needed) produced significantly lower incidence of disability and episodes of work absenteeism due to musculoskeletal pain at a one year follow-up assessment. Moreover, the preventive intervention reduced the risk of developing a chronic pain syndrome by more than 8 times. It is expected that preventive and other forms of early interventions will be developed by patients with ARMD in the future.

LAURENCE A. BRADLEY, PhD

1. Badley EM, Rasooly I, Webster GK: Relative importance of musculoskeletal disorders as a cause of chronic health problems, disability, and health care utilization: findings from the 1990 Ontario Health Survey. J Rheumatol 21:505-514, 1994

2. Harrington L, Affleck G, Urrows S, et al: Temporal covariation of soluble interleukin-2 receptor levels, daily stress, and disease activity in rheumatoid arthritis. Arthritis Rheum 36:199-203, 1993

3. Bellamy N, Bradley LA: Workshop on chronic pain, pain control, and patient outcomes in rheumatoid arthritis and osteoarthritis. Arthritis Rheum 39:357-362, 1996

4. Parker JC, Smarr KL, Buckelew SP, et al: Effects of stress management on clinical outcomes in rheumatoid arthritis. Arthritis Rheum 38:1807-1818, 1995

5. Magni G, Marchetti M, Moreschi C, et al: Chronic musculoskeletal pain and depressive symptoms in the National Health and Nutrition Examination. I. Epidemiologic follow-up study. Pain 53:163-168, 1993

6. Hawley DJ, Wolfe F: Depression is not more common in rheumatoid arthritis: a 10-year longitudinal study of 6,153 patients with rheumatic disease. J Rheumatol 20:2025-2031, 1993

7. Magni G, Moreschi C, Rigatti-Luchini S, et al: Prospective study on the relationship between depressive symptoms and chronic musculoskeletal pain. Pain 56:289-297, 1994

8. Wolfe F, Hawley DJ: The relationship between clinical activity and depression in rheumatoid arthritis. J Rheumatol 20:2032-2037, 1993

9. Zautra AJ, Burleson MH, Smith CA, et al: Arthritis and perceptions of quality of life: an examination of positive and negative affect in rheumatoid arthritis patients. Health Psychol 14:399-408, 1995

10. Nicassio PM, Radojevic V, Weisman MH, et al: The role of helplessness in the response to disease modifying drugs in rheumatoid arthritis. J Rheumatol 20:1114-1120, 1993

11. Lorig K, Chastain RL, Ung E, et al: Development and evaluation of a scale to measure perceived self-efficacy in people with arthritis. Arthritis Rheum 31:37-44, 1989

12. Buckelew SP, Parker JC, Keefe FJ, et al: Self-efficacy and pain behavior among subjects with fibromyalgia. Pain 59:377-384, 1994

13. Swan KL, Parker JC, Wright GE, et al: The importance of enhancing self-efficacy in rheumatoid arthritis. Arthritis Care Res 10:18-26, 1997

14. Anderson KO, Dowds BN, Pelletz RE, et al: Development and initial validation of a scale to measure self-efficacy beliefs in patients with chronic pain. Pain 63:77-84, 1995

15. Brady TJ: Do common arthritis self-efficacy measures really measure self-efficacy? Arthritis Care Res 10:1-8, 1997

16. Blalock SJ, DeVellis BM, Giorgino KB: The relationship between coping and psychological well-being among people with osteoarthritis: a problem-specific approach. Ann Behav Med 17:107-115, 1995

17. Martin MY, Bradley LA, Alexander RW, et al: Coping strategies predict disability in fibromyalgia. Pain 68:45-53, 1996

18. Bradley LA, Young LD, Anderson KO, et al: Effects of psychological therapy on pain behavior of rheumatoid arthritis patients: treatment outcome and six-month follow-up. Arthritis Rheum 30:1105-1114, 1987

19. Young LD, Bradley LA, Turner RA: Decreases in health care resource utilization in patients with rheumatoid arthritis following a cognitive-behavioral intervention. Biofeed Self-Regulat 20:259-268, 1995

20. White KP, Nielson WR: Cognitive-behavioral treatment of fibromyalgia syndrome: a follow-up assessment. J Rheumatol 22:717-721, 1995

21. Keefe FJ, Van Horn Y: Cognitive-behavioral treatment of rheumatoid arthritis pain: maintaining treatment gains. Arthritis Care Res 6:213-222, 1993

22. Lorig KR, Mazanson PD, Holman HR: Evidence suggesting that health education for self-management in patients with chronic arthritis has sustained health benefits while reducing health care costs. Arthritis Rheum 36:439-446, 1993

23. Keefe FJ, Caldwell DS, Williams DA, et al: Pain coping skills training in the management of osteoarthritic knee pain. II: Follow-up results. Behav Ther 21:435-437, 1990

24. Weinberger M, Tierney WM, Cowper PA, et al: Cost-effectiveness of increased telephone contact for patient with osteoarthritis: a randomized, controlled trial. Arthritis Rheum 36:243-246, 1993

25. Maisiak R, Austin JS, West SG, et al: The effect of person-centered counseling on the psychological status of persons with systemic lupus erythematosus or rheumatoid arthritis. Arthritis Care Res 9:60-66, 1996

26. Linton SJ, Bradley LA: Strategies for the prevention of chronic pain. In: Gatchel RJ, Turk DC, eds. Psychological approaches to pain management: a practitioner's handbook. New York, Guilford Press, 1996, pp 438-457

27. Linton SJ, Hellsing AL, Anderson D: A controlled study of the effects of an early intervention on acute musculoskeletal pain problems. Pain 54:353-359, 1993

50

PATIENT EDUCATION

Over the past two decades, the community of rheumatology health professionals has made tremendous contributions to patient care through the discovery of diagnostic tools and the development of effective treatment modalities. Various forms of arthritis are now diagnosed earlier and treated aggressively with a number of disease-modifying drugs. Complimenting these advances have been a score of education programs and health services that have been demonstrated efficacious in assisting patients to cope with their chronic disease.

These rheumatology education programs have become a model for outcomes-based research in other areas of chronic illness. Literature reviews from 1983 through 1991 provide a historical context for the progress in patient education, from theoretical advances, successes in changing knowledge, behaviors, psychosocial, and health status toward outcomes studies and areas for future programs (1–4). Most importantly, arthritis patient education programs have been shown to alter health status and improve quality of life (2,3).

DEFINITION OF PATIENT EDUCATION

Patient education has been defined as "planned, organized learning experiences designed to facilitate voluntary adaptation of behaviors or beliefs conducive to health" (5). Education programs are most effective when they are planned and designed with defined goals and learning objectives targeted toward specific groups of people with similar forms of arthritis. During office visits, it is hoped that physicians will increase patient knowledge that will result in a change in patient behaviors. However, these exchanges are more likely to enhance disease management. This differs significantly from the education class or lecture designed specifically to provide information aimed at affecting the patient's health behaviors.

Patient education is interpreted to cover a broad spectrum of human factors. While the focus is primarily on behaviors and beliefs, the scope of patient education also incorporates additional elements that influence human behaviors. These factors encompass knowledge, communication abilities, and sense of control, all of which affect health outcomes (6). Moreover, people all learn differently, which makes it more challenging to develop educational programs that meet individuals needs. For example, a newly diagnosed rheumatoid arthritis patient who has good communication skills, extended family and social supports, and adequate health insurance may require additional educational information about the disease. Thus, the major goal of an education program for this patient may be to increase the patient's knowledge about the disease. A single mother diagnosed with systemic lupus erythematosus who has limited health insurance, Spanish as a primary language, and works two jobs to support her family may also require educational information about her disease. However, in addition to a program to increase knowledge about the disease, she may also require psychosocial support, skill development such as time management skills, and information on stress techniques. Thus, the nature of the disease and the individual's learning method, psychosocial needs, and socioeconomic factors dictate that some patient education programs concentrate on behaviors and beliefs, while other programs focus on acquisition of knowledge, skills development, and enhancement of control over illness.

GOALS OF PATIENT EDUCATION

The goals of patient education programs for patients with rheumatic diseases are as varied as the theoretical framework that shape them. Daltroy and Liang (2) have emphasized that patient education goals are similar to those of traditional medical care: to improve function, relieve pain, enhance psychologic well-being, maintain satisfactory social interaction and employment, and control disease activity. Lorig (7) has demonstrated that additional aims of patient education are to maintain or improve health and to slow deterioration. Currently more than 75 patient education programs cited in the literature encompass these goals and demonstrate that patient education can affect functional and psychosocial health status (5).

Research has effectively demonstrated the value of planned, goal-oriented programs. Patient education programs should always be evaluated to be certain that the desired goals are achieved. Evaluation tools developed to measure educational outcomes, psychologic function, social function, and quality of life should be used when developing new programs.

THEORETICAL FRAMEWORKS

The contributions of health educators, behavioral psychologists, and social psychologists have resulted in numerous modifications in the types of arthritis education programs that are available. The capacious definition of patient education has resulted in the concentration of programs designed to increase or change knowledge, behavior and beliefs, psychosocial function, and health status.

Traditionally, health education programs have emphasized increase in knowledge about disease as the main outcome (8). In studies developed to enhance knowledge, 94% were successful in reaching their desired goals (9). This is not surprising, because people diagnosed with chronic disease often seek out information of various sorts during the course of their illness. Transfer of knowledge is essential in any learning process. However, many variables can interfere with a patient's quest for information. Culturally determined health beliefs and behaviors, as well as generation gaps, may prohibit some patients from seeking information about their disease. Physicians also may not have effective communication skills or teaching capabilities. Moreover, acquisition of knowledge alone does not result in changing health beliefs or health behaviors.

There is universal agreement that contributing to patients' knowledge about their illness is an important aspect of the overall treatment plan. The focus over recent years has not been whether there should be patient education programs but rather *which* programs to offer, to *whom,* and through *what* educational modality. Patient education classes, peer telephone information and counseling lines, video conferences, and educational support groups are just a few of the programs available to patients. The focus of educational planning presently centers on identifying the specific factors that cause patients to learn new information and subsequently alter their behavior. Perhaps the greatest contribution to the field of patient education has been the research findings that have influenced education programs towards effecting positive health outcomes.

Self-efficacy, an extension of social learning theory, refers to an individual's belief in his or her capability to mobilize the motivation, cognitive resources, and courses of action needed to meet situation demands (10). Lorig and colleagues have used the concept of self-efficacy to help patients live their lives with the chronic symptoms of their illness. The emphasis is on behavior and one's belief that a behavior can be carried out in a specific situation. Work in this area has led to further research demonstrating that a sense of control over one's illness is a precursor to resulting behaviors. In arthritis education programs, the aim is to develop interventions that increase self-efficacy and self-confidence to enable patients to meet the physical and emotional challenges posed by their illness. Examples of the types of interventions used to enhance a patient's self-efficacy are mastery of skills, role modeling, reinterpreting symptoms, and persuasion. In recent years, social support has emerged as a concept vital to the success of patient education programs.

Patient education programs have also been shown to have a significant effect on patients' health status. Bradley et al (11) demonstrated reduced pain behavior using a psychologic intervention, while Parker et al (12) have shown that a cognitive–behavioral pain management program can increase coping behaviors and one's confidence in the ability to control pain. These studies on educational interventions address the most common concerns reported by patients: pain, depression, and disability.

CHALLENGES IN PATIENT EDUCATION

Perhaps the major challenge for patient educators is to develop programs that effectively reach diverse patient populations. Some forms of rheumatic disease are disproportionately prevalent in the Latino, African American, and Asian communities. Yet, most education programs to date have been designed and attended by mostly white, middle-class patients. Little is known about the adaptability of current programs for patients from various cultural backgrounds who adhere to culture-specific health beliefs and behaviors, and for whom English is not the primary oral and written language. Robbins and colleagues (13) piloted a culturally sensitive Spanish version of the Systemic Lupus Erythematosus Self-Help (SLESH) course, but there was no evidence of pre- and post-test change in depression, self-efficacy, or functional status. These findings raise questions about the adaptability of standardized programs and the reliability of outcome measures for culturally diverse populations. There is a need to further understand how culturally determined health beliefs and behaviors affect health status so that appropriate programs can be developed.

As more people use on-line technology, the opportunities for patient education programs via the Internet are unlimited. Programs are already available that can be accessed by patients from their homes and have similar effects on health status as the more traditional face-to-face program formats. Horton's LupusLine (14), a peer-counseling telephone service, and its Spanish counterpart Charle de Lupus, can be accessed by lupus patients from their homes. These programs have been developed to enhance coping ability, increase knowledge about lupus, and reduce isolation. Maishiak's arthritis information telephone line also allows patients access to information via telephone (15). Building upon interventions such as these home-to-home education programs through computers are an untapped source for new programs targeted at specific patient populations.

PRACTICAL APPLICATIONS

Patient education is a mutual responsibility of the patient and the physician. Physicians must recognize that educational information is a vital component of the treatment plan that empowers patients to manage their disease and ultimately alter their functional and social status. Through education, patients who become experts about their disease contribute to the treatment plan and enhance their own quality of life.

With the changing role of physicians in the current health care environment, it is unrealistic for the primary health care provider to also be the health educator. The physician's role is to recognize the patient's educational needs and, as part of the treatment plan, to make a referral to the appropriate health care provider. The office practice nurse, physical therapist, and other health care providers are excellent sources of information on education programs. The most comprehensive references for education programs are available from the Arthritis Foundation, the American College of Rheumatology (ACR), and the Association of Rheumatology Health Professionals, a division of ACR composed of nurses, physical and occupational therapists, psychologists, social workers, and health educators.

EXAMPLES OF PATIENT PROGRAMS

The Arthritis Foundation offers a variety of programs disseminated through its regional and state-wide chapters. The Education and Services department and the American Juvenile Arthritis Organization, a section of the foundation, coordinates programs with the assistance of volunteers, many of whom are health professionals in clinical practice and research centers. Two examples of nationally disseminated programs are the Arthritis Self-Management Program (ASMP) and the Systemic Lupus Erythematosus Self-Help (SLESH) course.

The ASMP program developed by Lorig and her colleagues is a 6-week, 2 hour per session program offered to lay persons who are taught, and in turn teach the course to other arthritis patients. The original goals of ASMP were to provide knowledge about chronic illness and teach skills to assist patients in coping with their illness. The theoretical assumption is that enhanced knowledge and adoption of self-management behaviors will result in improved functional outcomes (16). Many of the program activities teach people new behaviors that lead to increased function. Randomized research trials of the program have found that people who participate in the program improve health behaviors, self-efficacy, and health status (17).

The Systemic Lupus Erythematosus Self-Help (SLESH) course is similar to ASMP but is designed specifically for lupus patients and their family members. SLESH is a 7-week, $2^1/_2$ hour per session course designed to teach patients how to take a more active role in their health care. The course not only provides educational information but also empowers patients with the necessary skills and emotional support to better cope with the crises that result from the disease (18).

Other sources of patient education programs are available to both patients and professionals. Disease-specific organizations such as the Lupus Foundation, the Scleroderma Society, and the Fibromyalgia Association offer programs for patients and their families. These organizations have national offices with regional or state-wide local chapters. In addition, hospitals often offer programs through departments of community education, nursing, or social services. Academic institutions with rheumatology research centers have education programs that are part of the overall services offered. Currently there are 14 multipurpose Musculoskeletal and Arthritis Disease Centers funded by the National Institutes of Health that are located at 14 academic centers around the country. These centers are engaged in arthritis studies, some of which include education programs that are available to the patient population.

LAURA ROBBINS, DSW, MSW

1. Lorig K, Visser: Arthritis patient education standards: a model for the future. Patient Educ Counsel 24:3-7,1994

2. Daltroy L, Liang M: Advances in patient education in rheumatic disease. Ann Rheum Dis 50:415-417,1991

3. Daltroy L, Goeppinger J: Arthritis health education: 15 years of research. Health Educ Q 20:1-16,1993

4. Hiran P, Laurant D, Lorig K: Arthritis patient education studies, 1987-1991: a review of the literature. Patient Ed Counsel 24:9-54, 1992

5. Burckhardt C: Arthritis and musculoskeletal patient education standards. Arthritis Care Res 7:1-4,1994

6. Daltroy L, Liang M: Arthritis education: opportunities and state of the art. Health Educ Q 20:3-16, 1993

7. Lorig K: Common Sense Patient Education. Victoria, Fraser Publication, 1992

8. Breckon D, Harvey J, Lancaster R: Community health education: settings, roles, and skills for the 21st century, Maryland, Aspen Publication, 1994

9. Lorig K, Konkol L, Gonzalez V: Arthritis patient education: a review of the literature. Patient Ed Counsel 10:207-252, 1987

10. Gonzalez V, Goeppinger J, Lorig K: Four psychosocial theories and their application to patient education and clinical practice. Arthritis Care Res 3:132-143,1990

11. Bradley LA, Young LD, Anderson KO, et al: Effects of psychological therapy on pain behavior of rheumatoid arthritis patients: treatment outcome and six-month follow-up. Arthritis Rheum 30;1105-1114,1987

12. Parker JC, Frank RG, Beck NC, et al: Pain management in rheumatoid arthritis patients: a cognitive-behavioral approach. Arthritis Rheum 31:593-601,1988

13. Robbins L, Allegrante JP, Paget SA: Adapting the systemic lupus erythematosus self-help (SLESH) for Latino SLE patients. Arthritis Care Res 6:97-103,1993

14. Horton R, Steiner-Grossman P: LupusLine Leader's Manual: a step-by-step guide to starting a peer counseling service. New York, Hospital for Special Surgery, 1993

15. Maisiak R, Koplon S, Heck L: User evaluation of an arthritis information telephone service. Arthritis Care Res 2:75-79, 1989

16. Lorig K, Seleznick M, Lubeck D, Ung E, Chastain R, Holman H: The beneficial outcomes of the arthritis self-management course are not adequately explained by behavior change. Arthritis Rheum 32:91-95,1989

17. Lorig D, Holman H: Arthritis self-management studies: a twelve-year review. Health Educ Q 20:17-28,1993

18. Braden C, McGlone K, Pennington F: Specific psychosocial and behavioral outcomes from the systemic lupus erythematosus self-help course. Health Educ Q 20:29-41,1993

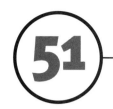

THERAPEUTIC INJECTION OF JOINTS AND SOFT TISSUES

51

Treatment of joint inflammation by local injection has been an important facet of arthritis care ever since Hollander demonstrated that hydrocortisone salts could be effective for this purpose (1). The major objectives of local injection are to enter a painful structure, remove any excess fluid that might be present, and instill the corticosteroid suspension likely to provide the longest duration of relief. Salutary results may ensue from temporary relief of pain by the local anesthetic, distention of a contracted joint space, and the systemic effects of corticosteroids absorbed from synovium and adjacent soft tissues. Local injection minimizes the hazards inherent in systemic corticosteroid therapy, while assuring the direct application of potent medication to the active site of disease.

The indications for local injection are listed in Table 51-1. Injections should never be the sole intervention—even for isolated regional disorders—and other aspects of each treatment program should be respected and continued. Joint injection is relatively contraindicated when the process causing the regional problem is obscure, especially if infection may be present. Established infections, either regional (cellulitis) or systemic (bacteremia), constitute absolute contraindication to therapeutic injections, although swollen joints or bursae should definitely be entered if involvement as source or seed of infection is suspected. Previous failure to respond to local injection should preclude a repeat attempt, unless technical features of the last treatment (including strict adherence to a postinjection rest regimen) were suboptimal. Bleeding diatheses, whether endogenous or pharmaceutically induced, dictate caution when induction of hemarthrosis seems possible. However, this should not avert decompression of established joint swelling that might be due to bleeding.

The most common complication after a single injection is a transient increase in pain, often accompanied by local inflammatory signs. This effect, most likely from a local reaction to corticosteroid crystals, was seen following 6% of injections in a large series of patients with rheumatoid arthritis (RA) (2), but generally subsides within 4–24 hours with rest, analgesia, and cold packs. Since such flares tend to be provoked by the less-soluble corticosteroid preparations, patients with a history of post-injection flare should be given one of the more soluble corticosteroids. Rarely, skin and subcutaneous tissue atrophy at the site of injection; darker-skinned patients should be forewarned about potential loss of pigmented cells, which can be distressing. Systemic effects from single injections are common, although usually mild and transient, and include flushing, slight agitation, and exacerbation of diabetic symptoms. Patients who have received repeated injections can show signs of exogenous hypercortisolism. Adrenal suppression is possible when injections are given more than once or twice a month; thus, frequently injected patients facing major physiologic stress (eg, abdominal surgery) should have adrenal reserve tested to determine whether supplemental corticosteroids should be given.

Concerns that cartilage and supporting structures might be weakened by repeated corticosteroid injections, with accelerated destruction of a joint as a consequence, have not been supported by clinical observations or studies of primate models. The commonly stated limit of 3–4 injections/year for large weight-bearing joints should be observed for nearly normal joints, but patients with established arthritis for which few therapeutic alternatives exist can be injected more frequently. Tendons, ligaments, and their attachments to bone can be disrupted by corticosteroid when directly injected; thus, care must be taken to confine injections to adjacent synovial sheaths and bursae. Chances for directly inducing infection are extremely slim, with incidence rates from 1:1000 to 1:16,000 in experienced hands; however, in several series examining risk factors for septic arthritis, up to 20% of infected joints had been injected within the previous 3 months (3).

INJECTION TECHNIQUE

Success at therapeutic injection derives from familiarity with the regional anatomy of the structure to be entered; techniques for certain specific joints and bursae are described in Chapter 7. Before other preparations take place, the clinician should have a clear mental image of the site to be entered (emphasized by pinpoint or fingernail indentation) and the path to be taken by the needle. The patient should be positioned so that structures on either side of the injection target are relaxed. Skin cleansing and use of sterile gloves provide sufficient asepsis; sterile drapings are needed only for the immunocompromised patient or if the procedure is anticipated to be lengthy or difficult. Measures to reduce the sensation of needle puncture (eg, spraying the site with ethyl chloride solution or infiltrating skin and subcutaneous tissues with lidocaine delivered through an ultra-

(Table 51-1)
Indications for therapeutic injection of musculoskeletal structures

1. When only one or a few joints are inflamed, provided infection has been excluded
2. In systemic polyarthritis syndromes (eg, rheumatoid arthritis, psoriatic arthritis) as adjunct to systemic drug therapy
3. To assist in rehabilitation and prevent deformity
4. To relieve pain in osteoarthritis exhibiting local inflammatory signs
5. In soft tissue regional disorders (eg, bursitis, tenosynovitis, periarthritis, rheumatoid nodules, epicondylitis, ganglia)

thin needle) are generally appreciated by the patient; when lidocaine is used, the track to the structure of interest can be found with certainty and marked by leaving the needle in place pending puncture of the same site with a larger needle. Even when delivery of medication is the sole purpose, the clinician should attempt to remove fluid from the structure to ensure that the needle has indeed entered a synovial space (4); obtainable synovial fluid should be evacuated to remove phlogistic material and to minimize dilution of the injected compound.

Of the corticosteroid preparations available (Table 51-2), the less-soluble compounds tend to be preferred for joint space injections, although some physicians avoid the fluorinated compounds for peritenon and bursal injections because of their propensity to cause soft tissue atrophy (2). The optimal dose and volume to be injected to any specific structure has never been rigorously determined, but most clinicians deliver 1–2 ml of corticosteroid to large joints (knees, hips, shoulders), half that to medium joints (wrists, elbow, ankles), and half again that (or less) to small joints and soft tissue sites. Dilution with lidocaine provides some immediate temporary relief to the patient, assures the clinician that the desired structure was entered, and provides a vehicle to deliver corticosteroid to all areas of the joint space. To promote this latter effect, some clinicians inject a 10-ml steroid–lidocaine mixture into larger joints (5). Moving an injected joint through its physiologic range and gentle massage of an injected soft tissue structure also promote drug delivery. Some limitation on joint use following injection can prolong therapeutic benefit, but the optimum duration has yet to be determined; mandated rest (enforced with a sling, splint, or crutches) as long as 3 weeks for upper extremity joints and 6 weeks for lower extremity joints has been described. The only controlled trial published thus far found that 6 months after injection, triamcinolone-injected knees rested 24 hours after injection fared significantly better than injected knees that had not been rested (6).

INJECTIONS IN SPECIFIC DISORDERS

The often dramatic effects of corticosteroid injections in RA can sometimes lead to an unfortunate overdependence on this modality and neglect of other forms of therapy. For the RA patient who receives more than an occasional injection, keeping track on a dedicated log in the outpatient record can spot trends to overreliance on intra-articular therapy. Certain extra-articular features of RA respond well to local injections, particularly entrapment neuropathies due to synovial proliferation at the volar aspect of the wrist (carpal tunnel, median nerve), medial aspect of the elbow (cubital tunnel, ulnar nerve), and medial aspect of the ankle (tarsal tunnel, posterior tibial nerve). Rheumatoid nodules usually shrink in response to corticosteroid injection nearby (7).

The role of local corticosteroids in osteoarthritis remains relatively controversial. An older study of knee OA showing no additional benefit from cortisone when compared to injections of inert compounds or placebo puncture (8) has not stemmed the popularity of intra-articular corticosteroids for painful knee OA, and has been partly controverted by subsequent studies (9,10). Although inflammation in OA is considered a secondary phenomenon, features of local inflammation are often present and predict responsiveness to injection (10). However, pain often arises from structures exterior to the joint capsule. Experienced clinicians inject the irritated pes anserine bursa in patients with knee pain and OA (11) (Fig. 51-1). A study that compared periarticular delivery of corticosteroids to the traditional intra-articular route found pain relief to be greater and longer lasting in patients given soft tissue injection (12).

(Table 51-2)
Corticosteroid preparations for therapeutic injection

Compound (In Order of Relative Solubility)	Concentration (mg/ml)	Glucocorticoid Potency (Hydrocortisone Equivalents/mg)
Triamcinolone hexacetonide*	20	5
Triamcinolone acetonide*	40	5
Prednisolone tebutate	20	4
Methylprednisolone acetate	20,40,80	5
Dexamethosone acetate*	8	25
Hydrocortisone acetate	25,50	1
Triamicinolone diacetate*	40	5
Betamethasone sodium phosphate and acetate*	6	25
Dexamethasone sodium phosphate*	4	25
Prednisolone sodium phosphate	20	4

* Fluorinated compounds.

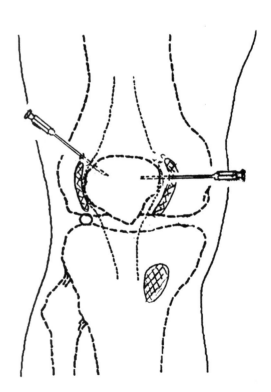

(Figure 51-1)
Aspiration and injection sites for the painful knee. Circle lateral to patellar tendon at joint line can be entered to deliver corticosterioids into flexed knee. Hatched areas on either side of patella correspond to soft tissue sites described by Sambrook et al (12). Hatched area medial and inferior to joint line represents region of pes anserine bursa.

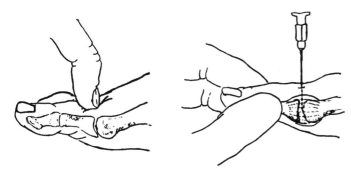

(Figure 51-2)

*Arthrocentesis/injection of first metatarsophalangeal joint. Joint line is palpated, then marked with imprint of thumbnail **(left)**. Gentle distraction of phalanx widens joint space, easing entry into capsule by needle oriented perpendicularly to phalanx, penetrating skin at the marked joint line just medial to extensor tendon **(right)**. Modified from McCarty DJ: A basic guide to arthrocentesis. Hospital Medicine 4:77-97, 1968, with permission.*

Joint entry is important for diagnosis of crystalline arthropathy and can also be employed for treatment, often at the same setting. Intra-articular injection avoids the potential toxicities of systemic nonsteroidal anti-inflammatory drugs, colchicine, or steroids and is safe, provided that in-

fection is unlikely. With concomitant gout and infection a negligible possibility when a typical joint flares without systemic features (13), local injection immediately after obtaining synovial fluid may be the treatment of choice (Fig. 51-2).

Numerous regional disorders respond to local injection. Certain common entities, such as trochanteric bursitis, require only that the tender site be pinpointed before being entered. Injections for tendinitis and entrapment neuropathies require additional skill and should not be attempted without an experienced guide (14). Only a few disorders affect the true shoulder joint (glenohumeral joint) in isolation, notably primary osteoarthritis, infection, and adhesive capsulitis. The latter process can be treated by injection with a large volume of dilute corticosteroid–anesthetic mixture (15) but requires definite joint entry (Fig. 51-3).

ROBERT W. IKE, MD

1. Hollander JL, Brown EM, Jessar RA, Brown CY: Hydrocortisone and cortisone injected into arthritic joints: comparative effects of and use of hydrocortisone as a local antiarthritic agent. JAMA 147:1629-1635, 1951

2. McCarty DJ, Harman JG, Grassanovich JL, Qian C: Treatment of rheumatoid joint inflammation with intrasynovial triamcinolone hexacetonide. J Rheumatol 22:1631-1635, 1995

3. von Essen R, Savolainen HA: Bacterial infection following intra-articular injection. Scand J Rheumatol 18:7-12, 1989

4. Jones A, Regan M, Ledingham J, Pattricj M, Manhire A, Doherty M: Importance of placement of intra-articular steroid injections. BMJ 307:1329-1330, 1993

5. Schaffer TC: Joint and soft-tissue arthrocentesis. Primary Care 20:757-770, 1993

6. Chakravarty K, Pharoah PDP, Scott DGI: A randomized controlled study of post-injection rest following intra-articular steroid therapy for knee synovitis. Br J Rheumatol 33:464-468, 1994

7. Ching DW, Petrie JP, Klemp P, Jones JG: Injection therapy of superficial rheumatoid nodules. Br J Rheumatol 31:775-777, 1992

8. Miller JH, White J, Norton TH: The value of intra-articular injections in osteoarthritis of the knee. J Bone Joint Surg 40B:636-643, 1958

9. Dieppe PA, Sathapatayavongs B, Jones HE, Bacon PA, Ring EFJ: Intra-articular steroids in osteoarthritis. Rheumatol Rehab 19:212-217, 1980

10. Gaffney K, Ledingham J, Perry JD: Intra-articular triamcinolone hexacetonide on knee osteoarthritis: factors influencing the clinical response. Ann Rheum Dis 54:379-381, 1995

11. Larsson L-G, Baum J: The syndrome of anserina bursitis: an overlooked diagnosis. Arthritis Rheum 28:1062-1065, 1985

12. Sambrook PN, Champion GD, Browne CD, Cairns D, Cohen ML, Day RO: Corticosteroid injection for osteoarthritis of the knee: peripatellar compared to intra-articular route. Clin Exp Rheum 7:609-613, 1989

13. Ike RW: Bacterial Arthritis. In Koopman WJ (ed): Arthritis and Allied Conditions, 13th ed. Baltimore, Williams & Wilkins, 1996, pp 2267-2295

14. Doherty M, Hazelman B, Hutton CW, Maddison PJ, Perry JD: Rheumatology Examination and Injection Techniques. London, WB Saunders, 1992

15. Jacobs LG, Barton MA, Wallace WA, Ferrousis J, Dunn NA, Bossingham DH: Intra-articular distension and steroids in the management of capsulitis of the shoulder. BMJ 302:1498-1501, 1991

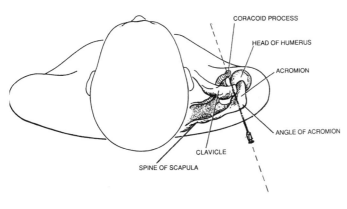

(Figure 51-3)

Posterior approach for entry in the glenohumeral joint. Line drawn from point 1 cm medial to the angle of acromion through tip of the coracoid process passes directly through the glenohumeral joint. Optimal site for entry is located 1 cm inferior and 1 cm medial to the bend of acromial angle, found by palpating the spine of scapula. Keeping the index finger of opposite hand on the coracoid process during procedure provides mental target for the aspirating/injecting needle.

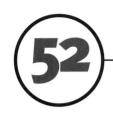

NONSTEROIDAL ANTI-INFLAMMATORY DRUGS

The rheumatic diseases are characterized by varying degrees of tissue damage, inflammation, and loss of normal function, and some are associated with annoying rashes, disabling arthritis, or lethal nephritis or cerebritis. Although scores of distinct rheumatic diseases and syndromes exist, only a few classes of drugs are available to treat them. This chapter discusses the extensively used nonsteroidal anti-inflammatory drugs (NSAIDs), including aspirin and other salicylates.

Inflammation is essentially a local response to tissue injury and normally consists of a sequence of events that results in elimination of the injurious agent, healing of the damaged tissue, and restoration of normal function. With a chronic inflammatory disease such as rheumatoid arthritis (RA), the normal homeostatic capacity of the microenvironment is exceeded, resulting in amplification of the inflammatory process by the products of injured tissue and possibly by the loss of inhibitory mechanisms, continued inflammation, progressive tissue injury, disease manifestations, and increasing loss of function (1).

By impairing the activity of various natural mediators of inflammation, NSAIDs partially prevent the final expression of inflammation. Because they act on terminal events in the inflammatory cascade (see Chapter 5, Mediators of Inflammation), the benefits of NSAIDs are quickly evident. Since they do not prevent tissue injury, it is not surprising that joint damage and other evidence of organ damage may progress during therapy. Sustained drug-induced remission is not expected with the short-acting anti-inflammatory agents.

POSSIBLE MECHANISMS OF ACTION

Under appropriate laboratory conditions, NSAIDs have been demonstrated to uncouple oxidative phosphorylation, inhibit lysomal enzyme release, inhibit complement activation, antagonize the generation or activity of kinins, inhibit cyclooxygenase, inhibit lipoxygenase, inhibit phosphodiesterase, inhibit free radicals, alter lymphocyte responses, and decrease granulocyte and monocyte migration and phagocytosis (2).

The structural identification of arachidonic acid, its metabolites, and the pertinent metabolic enzymes beginning in 1964 provided the chemical tools with which to study inter-relationships of these substances with inflammation, and to characterize the effects of NSAIDs upon this metabolic process (3). Arachidonic acid is cleaved from membrane phospholipids by specific phospholipases, oxidized and cyclized by the enzyme cyclooxygenase to form a cyclic endoperoxide, prostaglandin G_2 (PGG_2), which is converted to PGH_2 by peroxidation, with concomitant production of unstable toxic oxygen radicals. The cyclic endoperoxides have a half-life of about 5 minutes and promote the aggregation of platelets. PGH_2 is then converted to the stable prostaglandins E_2 and $F_{2\alpha}$, thromboxane, or prostacyclin, depending on the enzymes in its microenvironment. Thromboxane A2 is synthesized by platelets and promotes their aggregation, but it has a half-life of only about 30 seconds before being rapidly hydrolyzed to inactive thromboxane B_2. Prostacyclin (PGI_2), which is synthesized within arterial walls, opposes the effects of thromboxane A_2 by inhibiting aggregation of platelets and is a potent vasodilator (2,3).

Some of the biologic actions of the cyclic endoperoxides and their metabolites reproduce many of the signs of acute inflammation. Erythema is associated with the vasodilating activities of PGE_1, PGE_2, PGD_2, and PGI_2. Edema formation is promoted by increased vascular permeability induced by prostaglandins of the E series and their potentiation of bradykinin and histamine. Injection of PGE has also been demonstrated to cause pain and fever and to promote local bone resorption and cartilage destruction, depending on the sites of application. Elevated levels of prostaglandins have been demonstrated in synovial effusions from untreated patients with inflammatory arthritis (2).

The recent discovery and characterization of two isoenzymes of cyclo-oxygenase have helped explain the linkage between the anti-inflammatory benefits and the gastrointestinal (GI) adverse effects of the present NSAIDs (4). Cyclooxygenase-1 (COX_1) is constitutively present in many tissues, and is responsible for the physiologic production of homeostatic and cytoprotective prostanoids in the gastric mucosa, endothelium, platelets, and kidney. Its inhibition is linked to many of the familiar adverse effects of NSAIDs. Cyclooxygenase-2 (COX_2) is not produced by unstimulated cells. Its production in leukocytes, vascular smooth muscle cells, human rheumatoid synoviocytes, and brain neurons is induced by stimuli such as mitogens, cytokines, and endotoxin, thus catalyzing the synthesis of pro-inflammatory prostaglandins. COX_2 is associated with carrageenan-induced inflammation in experimental animals, certain aspects of inflammatory pain, and perhaps fever (4–6). Human COX_1 and COX_2 show only 60% homology of their nucleic acid and amino acid structures. The availability of pure COX_1 and COX_2 makes it possible to rapidly determine the relative inhibitory potency of available and potential NSAIDs for each isoenzyme.

Various laboratories have published the results of in vitro studies of the relative ratios of COX_1/COX_2 inhibition by a number of NSAIDs (7–9). In general, aspirin, indomethacin, tolmetin, naproxen, piroxicam, and ibuprofen inhibit the homeostatic COX_1 isoenzyme at much lower concentrations than those required to inhibit the pro-inflammatory COX_2 isoenzyme. Diclofenac and nonacetylated salicylate inhibit both approximately equally, and etodolac inhibits COX-2 at somewhat lower concentrations than those needed to inhibit COX_1. Investigational agents are being developed that have COX_2/COX_1 inhibition ratios of 1000 or more. These highly selective COX_2 inhibitors should cause little or no gastric adverse effects (due to COX_1 inhibition) at doses that completely inhibit COX_2 and the pro-inflammatory prostaglandins.

NSAIDS reduce, but do not completely eliminate, the signs and symptoms of established inflammation. The presence of drug in the blood is associated with a rapid onset of benefit, but exacerbation of signs and symptoms occurs quickly after metabolism or excretion of the drug. NSAIDs have no major effect on the underlying disease process. In addition to their anti-inflammatory effects, NSAIDs decrease pain, suppress fever, and decrease platelet adhesiveness, leading to a multitude of short-term and long-term, prescribed and nonprescribed uses. In the United States, available NSAIDs include aspirin, salicyl salicylate, magnesium choline salicylate, other salicylates, ibuprofen, phenyl-

butazone, indomethacin, sulindac, naproxen, tolmetin, fenoprofen, meclofenamate sodium, diflunisal, piroxicam, ketoprofen, diclofenac, flurbiprofen, etodolac, ketorolac, nabumetone, and oxaprozin (Table 52-1). Others are under development or available elsewhere (1). Although ketorolac is given parenterally and indomethacin is also marketed in a rectal suppository form, all other available NSAIDs are administered orally. Aspirin, the salicylates, ibuprofen, naproxen sodium, and ketoprofen are available without prescription in the United States.

NSAIDs (including the active acidic metabolite of nabumetone) are organic acids and are highly bound to plasma proteins, properties that may enhance drug concentrations in inflamed tissues that are more permeable to plasma proteins and tend to have a low pH. They may be classified by their chemical structure, but it is more useful to remember their plasma half-life, which is related to the frequency of administration and in some instances to the occurrence of adverse reactions, especially in elderly persons (Table 52-1). Traditionally, NSAIDs have been developed in

(Table 52-1)
Some nonsteroidal anti-inflammatory drugs

Drug	Dose Range (mg/Day)	Half-life (Hours)	Doses per Day	Gastrointestinal Adverse Effects*
Hetero carboxylic acids				
Aspirin (acetylsalicylic acid)	1000–6000	4–15	2–4	+++
Magnesium choline salicylate	1500–4000	4–15	2–4	+
Salsalate	1500–5000	4–15	2–4	+
Diflunisal	500–1500	7–15	2	+++
Meclofenamate sodium	200–400	2–3	4	++
Phenylacetic acids				
Ibuprofen	1200–3200	2	3–6	++
Fenoprofen	1200–3200	2	3–4	++
Ketoprofen	100–400	2	3–4	++
Diclofenac	75–150	1–2	2–3	++
Flurbiprofen	100–300	3–4	2–3	++
Naphthaleneacetic acids				
Naproxen	250–1500	13	2	++
Indoleacetic acids				
Indomethacin	50–200	3–11	2–4	+++
Sulindac	300–400	16	2	+++
Etodolac	600–1200	7	3–4	+
Pyrrolealkanoic acids				
Tolmetin	800–1600	1	4–6	++
Pyrazolidinediones				
Phenylbutazone	200–800	40–80	1–4	++
Oxicams				
Piroxicam	20	30–86	1	+++
Pyrrolo-pyrrole				
Ketorolac (oral and parenteral)†	15–150	4–6	4	+++
Naphthylalkanone				
Nabumetone	1000–2000	24	1–2	+
Oxazolepropionic acid				
Oxaprozin	600–1200	49–60	1	++

* + = mild, no change in drug regimen required; ++ = frequent, may need to add gastroprotective agent; +++ = more frequent and/or severe, often requires withdrawal of the drug.
† Not recommended for long-term use.

the pharmaceutical industry by screening molecular modifications of known active compounds for their ability to suppress the swelling induced by injecting carrageenan into the paw of a rat immediately after drug administration. Advances in knowledge now permit the selection of compounds for their ability to suppress specific elements of the inflammatory process.

ADVERSE EFFECTS OF NSAIDS

Although NSAIDs are generally well-tolerated, they are associated with a wide spectrum of potential clinical toxicities. None is completely safe. Aspirin is the most difficult to use effectively, has more frequent side effects, and is more dangerous if overdoses are taken. The major toxicities of NSAIDs occur in the gastrointestinal (GI) tract, central nervous system, hematopoietic system, kidney, skin, and liver. Generally, side effects tend to be dose related (2).

Gastrointestinal Effects

NSAIDs as a group tend to cause gastric irritation and to exacerbate peptic ulcers (10). NSAID-induced suppression of COX-1 increases gastric acid production, decreases the production of gastric mucus and bicarbonate, and decreases the rate of cellular proliferation of the gastric mucosa, which impairs the normal protective mechanisms of the stomach. NSAIDs worsen gastrointestinal bleeding, both by increasing acid production in the stomach and by decreasing platelet adhesiveness. Indomethacin, sulindac, and meclofenamate sodium have an extensive enterohepatic recirculation, which increases gastrointestinal exposure to these drugs and enhances their gastrointestinal toxicity. Firmly compressed regular aspirin tablets may dissolve slowly in the stomach, causing irritation and superficial ulceration of gastric mucosa directly under the undissolved tablet. Ion-trapping of weak organic acids such as NSAIDs in mucosal cells leads to back diffusion of hydrogen ions and may result in mucosal damage (10).

The US Food and Drug Administration estimates that gastrointestinal ulcers, bleeding, and perforation occur in approximately 1%–2% of patients using NSAIDs for 3 months and approximately 2%–5% of those using them for 1 year. In a meta-analysis of nine case-control and seven cohort studies, Gabriel and colleagues (11) reported an overall odds ratio of the risk of serious adverse GI events associated with NSAID use (compared with controls) to be 2.74. The risk was higher for patients aged 60 and older (5.52) and when concomitant corticosteroids were used (1.83). In large prospective, placebo-controlled, long-term clinical trials of low-dose aspirin (75–1300 mg/day) for treatment or prevention of myocardial infarction or strokes, between 10 and 74 excess cases of severe GI events per 10,000 person years occurred in the aspirin-treated patients compared with the placebo-treated control patients (12). Soll et al (13) noted that half of NSAID-associated ulcers are also associated with *Helicobacter pylori*, an independent risk factor for peptic ulcer disease that has not been systematically evaluated in epidemiologic studies. The effect of coexisting *H. pylori* infection and its eradication on the effectiveness of prophylaxis against NSAID-associated ulcer complications has not been determined as yet.

Peptic symptoms in patients taking NSAIDs are often treated with antacids, administration with a meal, H_2 blockers, omeprazole, the synthetic prostaglandin misoprostol, or carafete. A double-blind, randomized, placebo-controlled study prospectively evaluated serious upper GI clinical events in 8843 rheumatoid arthritis patients (52 years of age or older; mean age 68) who were taking one or more of 10 specified NSAIDs, but who did not have active peptic ulcer disease and were not taking anti-ulcer medications (14). During the 6-month study, 25 serious upper GI events (0.5% rate of complication) occurred in the group randomized to misoprostol 200 mcg four times a day (n = 4404) and 42 (0.95% rate of complication) in the placebo group (n = 4439), a statistically significant difference ($P = 0.049$). Risk factors for NSAID-associated upper GI complications were similar to those found in case-control and cohort studies: older age, previous peptic ulcer disease (odds ratio twice that of baseline patients), previous GI bleeding (odds ratio 2.5), and history of cardiovascular disease (1.84). There was a relatively uniform occurrence of GI adverse events over the time course of the 6-month trial in both groups. Other suspected risk factors include concomitant corticosteroid use, degree of disability, and presence of comorbidity. Misoprostol appeared to decrease the serious complications by 40% overall, but there was a higher protection in patients with risk factors (14).

Fatal outcomes are more likely in elderly or debilitated patients. Higher dosages of NSAIDs probably entail greater risk than lower dosages. The patient's disease, age, and degree of inflammation need to be considered in determining the optimal dosage for an individual patient, and every attempt should be made to use the lowest dose that adequately controls the patient's symptoms. Other strategies to minimize NSAID gastropathy include the substitution of a nonacetylated salicylate and supplemental gastroprotective agents as described above (1). Of even greater potential in preventing side effects is the recent discovery of cyclooxygenase isoforms, which may lead to developing clinically useful, potent, highly selective COX_2 inhibitors that will markedly reduce the incidence of upper GI risks with NSAID therapy and change the clinical paradigms for their use.

Anticoagulant Effects

NSAIDs may produce two types of anticoagulant effects. In the first type, platelet adhesiveness is decreased by inhibiting a prostaglandin-initiated sequence that is necessary for platelet activation. Because platelets lack mitochondria and are unable to synthesize additional cyclooxygenase, acetylation of this enzyme by aspirin irreversibly decreases platelet aggregation in response to various stimuli. This effect persists for about 10–12 days until the acetylated platelets are replaced by newly produced platelets that have not been exposed to aspirin (1). This property has led to the use of aspirin in doses as low as 80 mg daily to prevent platelet aggregation and emboli in patients prone to transient ischemic attacks, but it also enhances bleeding due to peptic ulcers or other causes. In contrast to aspirin, cyclooxygenase inhibition by the other NSAIDs is reversible. Their platelet effects also are reversible and persist only as long as the drug is present. A second type of anticoagulant effect occurs when protein-bound NSAIDs displace warfarin from plasma protein-binding sites, thus increasing warfarin's anticoagulant effect. This effect is clinically significant only for phenylbutazone and for salicylates in toxic concentrations.

To avoid excessive bleeding at surgery, aspirin should be stopped 2 weeks preoperatively, but other NSAIDs need be stopped only long enough to allow for their complete excretion. For example, because of their short half-lives, tolmetin and ibuprofen can be stopped 24 hours preoperatively, because they will be completely excreted and have no effect on platelet adhesiveness at the time of the surgery. Because the nonacetylated salicylates are poor inhibitors of cyclooxygenase, they have little or no effect on platelets and sometimes may be used when other NSAIDs are contraindicated by an excessive risk of bleeding (1).

Hepatic Effects

Reversible hepatocellular toxicity, characterized by elevations of one or more liver enzymes, has been observed in up to 15% of patients treated with NSAIDs and has been emphasized with diclofenac (15). Transaminase elevations usually revert to normal after the drug is discontinued, and levels sometimes become normal even when the drug is continued. Rarely, NSAID-induced hepatic dysfunction may be more severe, causing elevated bilirubin or prolonged prothrombin times, in which case discontinuing the drug is mandatory. Phenylbutazone-induced hepatocellular cholestasis and granulomatous hepatitis may be fatal in some patients. In the case of benoxaprofen, failure to recognize early evidence of hepatic toxicity led to fatal hepatorenal syndrome in some patients, and the drug was subsequently withdrawn from marketing. Fatal fulminant hepatitis has occurred on rare instances with other NSAIDs, emphasizing that serum transaminase levels should be checked on a regular basis during treatment with NSAIDs.

Renal Effects

NSAIDs may decrease creatinine clearance and increase creatinine concentrations in some patients predisposed by hypovolemia, impaired renal function, or decreased renal blood flow, probably by suppressing the vasodilatory function of renal prostaglandins (1). These creatinine elevations sometimes revert to normal even with continued use of the drug, but NSAIDs should be used cautiously in patients with conditions that may impair renal perfusion or function, in patients with decreased circulating blood volume, and in elderly persons who are predisposed to these conditions. Use of NSAIDs in rheumatic diseases associated with a high incidence of renal involvement, such as systemic sclerosis and systemic lupus erythematosus, also deserves caution. Acute interstitial nephritis and the nephrotic syndrome rarely occur with NSAIDs, but the greatest number of cases have been reported with fenoprofen. Most patients recover when the drug is discontinued, but occasionally dialysis or high-dose corticosteroid therapy has been needed to support patients until they recover renal function. Reversible acute renal failure or hyperkalemia may occur when indomethacin and triampterine are combined.

Other Adverse Effects

Other fairly common side effects include various types of skin reactions and rashes (2). Hypersensitivity responses include an aspirin-associated syndrome of rhinitis, nasal polyposis, and asthma. Anaphylaxis has been associated with tolmetin and zomepirac, but it occasionally has occurred with other NSAIDs. Agranulocytosis and aplastic anemia have been reported rarely with a number of NSAIDs but appear to be more frequent with phenylbutazone. These adverse effects have resulted in a number of deaths, particularly in women over the age of 60 years. Salicylates cause blood level-related tinnitus and hearing loss, and overdoses can cause numerous central nervous system manifestations including coma and death; overdoses of other NSAIDs are much less toxic than overdoses of salicylates or acetaminophen. Headaches occur with indomethacin, and confusion may appear in elderly patients treated with indomethacin, naproxen, or ibuprofen. Aseptic meningitis has occurred rarely in patients with systemic lupus erythematosus or mixed connective tissue disease who were treated with ibuprofen or other NSAIDs (2).

PHARMACOKINETICS

In general, currently available NSAIDs are rapidly and completely absorbed after oral administration, unless enteric coating (to decrease gastric irritation) or encapsulation (to produce sustained release) is used. Aspirin and sulindac have active metabolites with longer half-lives than the parent drugs. Indomethacin, meclofenamate sodium, and sulindac display enterohepatic recirculation. Salicylate and diflunisal exhibit Michalis–Menton kinetics; consequently, the plasma half-life of the drug increases as the plasma concentration increases. Thus, doses need be given less frequently when plasma concentrations are high, and toxic concentrations take longer to clear than would be anticipated. Nabumetone is a poor inhibitor of prostaglandin synthesis but is rapidly transformed by the liver to an acidic metabolite with potent inhibitory effects; its absorption is improved by concomitant food. Essentially all available NSAIDs ultimately are converted to inactive metabolites by the liver and are excreted predominantly in urine, although sulindac may also be converted to an inactive metabolite by the kidney. Biliary excretion occurs with some NSAIDs and their metabolites; moderate decreases in creatinine clearance prolong plasma clearance of active drug less markedly than would be the case if unmetabolized active drug or active metabolite were cleared only by renal excretion. Nevertheless, dosage reduction and extra care are advisable when NSAIDs are used in elderly patients or those with impaired renal function. Probenecid impairs the excretion of many NSAIDs. NSAIDs may increase the activity of oral hypoglycemics or warfarin by displacement from the protein binding sites (1,2).

ASPIRIN AND NSAID USE

It is important to individualize treatment with aspirin and NSAIDs. Substantial individual variability is present with respect to the pharmacology and pharmacokinetics of these drugs, which also vary in effectiveness in different disorders. In addition, the optimum dosage varies from one disorder to the next. Simple acute headaches or muscle aches, for example, can be treated with intermittent low or moderate doses of acetaminophen, aspirin, ibuprofen, ketoprofen, or naproxen sodium, which are available without prescription. Similar dosing with ibuprofen is particularly useful for menstrual cramps. Osteoarthritis may require more prolonged therapy, but generally moderate doses are sufficient. Patients with rheumatoid arthritis or other types of chronic inflammatory arthritis usually need prolonged treatment with maximum tolerated doses of NSAIDs and receive little or no benefit from acetaminophen.

The NSAIDs are usually more effective than the salicylates for acute gout, acute bursitis, and spondyloarthopathies such as ankylosing spondylitis and Reiter's syndrome. Indomethacin is often tried first in these conditions and is usually effective, although relatively high doses are needed and intolerance is fairly common. Other NSAIDs are also effective, but phenylbutazone is used only if the others fail, because of its greater risk of potentially fatal bone marrow suppression.

NSAIDs or aspirin are commonly used in the treatment of rheumatoid arthritis. The selection of a particular agent depends on a patient's medical history, such as a previous bleeding or gastrointestinal intolerance, and on the personal preference and experience of the prescribing physician. Enteric-coated aspirin and nonacetylated salicylates tend to be better tolerated than plain aspirin. When salicylates are used, the dose is adjusted to achieve a serum salicylate level of 20–30 mg/dl (200 to 300 µg/ml); however, serum drug levels of other NSAIDs are rarely used to determine therapeutic levels. If the patient has insufficient benefit or intolerable toxicity to a specific NSAID, another is often substituted, usually at a moderate dose to establish tolerance. The dose is then cautiously increased to the maximum recommended or tolerated level and continued for at least 2 weeks at that dose. Insufficient benefit or intolerance may prompt additional therapeutic trials of other NSAIDs until the patient has achieved satisfactory control of the inflammation with tolerable side effects (1).

There is little evidence to suggest that combinations of salicylate and NSAIDs or two NSAIDs are more beneficial than single drug therapy. Furthermore, toxicity is probably additive (2).

Caution is advised in prescribing NSAIDs to hospitalized patients, to elderly patients, to patients with peptic ulcer disease, impairment of renal or hepatic function, congestive heart failure, or hypertension, and to those being treated with anticoagulants, oral hypoglycemics, or other drugs that may interact with the NSAID. Patients should be followed especially closely (including monitoring of hematologic, renal, and hepatic status) during introduction of an NSAID, when doses are increased, or when the patient's condition changes (1).

Even optimal use of NSAIDs does not completely suppress all evidence of inflammation, particularly in chronic rheumatoid arthritis. If the patient with RA does not develop a spontaneous remission within a number of months, a disease-modifying antirheumatic drug should be added to the continuing NSAID therapy (see Chapter 54).

HAROLD E. PAULUS, MD
KEN J. BULPITT, MD

1. Clements PJ, Paulus HE: Nonsteroidal antirheumatic drugs. In Kelley WN, et al (eds): Textbook of Rheumatology, 5th edition. Philadelphia, WB Saunders, 1997, pp 707-740

2. Schlegel, SI: General characteristics of nonsteroidal antiinflammatory drugs. In Paulus HE, Furst DE, Dromgoole S (eds): Drugs for Rheumatic Disease. New York, Churchill Livingstone, 1987, p 203

3. Samuelsson, B: An elucidation of the arachidonic acid cascade: discovery of prostaglandins, thromboxane and leukotrienes. Drugs 33(Suppl 1):2, 1987

4. Vane JR: Toward a better aspirin. Nature 367:215-216, 1994

5. Crofford LJ, Wilder RL, Ristimaki AP, Sano H, Remmers EF, Epps HR, Hla T: Cyclooxygenase-1 and -2 expression in rheumatoid synovial tissues. J Clin Invest 93:1095-1101, 1994

6. Masferrer JL, Zweifel BS, Manning PT, et al: Selective inhibition of inducible cyclooxygenase 2 in vivo is anti-inflammatory and nonulcerogenic. Proc Natl Acad Sci USA 91:3228-3232, 1994

7. Gierse JK, Hauser SD, Creely DP, Koboldt C, Rangwala SH, Isakson PC, Seibert K: Expression and selective inhibition of the constitutive and inducible forms of human cyclooxygenase. J Biochem 305(Pt 2):479-484, 1995

8. Mitchell JA, Akarasereenont P, Thiemermann C, Flower RJ, Vane JR: Selectivity of nonsteroidal anti-inflammatory drugs as inhibitors of constitutive and inducible cyclooxygenase. Proc Natl Acad Sci USA 90:11693-11697, 1994

9. Glaser K, Sung ML, O'Neill K: Etodolac selectively inhibits human prostaglandin G/H synthase 2 (PGHS-2) versus human PGHS-1. Euro J Pharmacol 281:107-111, 1995

10. Schoen RT, Vender RJ: Mechanisms of nonsteroidal anti-inflammatory drug-induced gastric damage. Am J Med 86:449-458, 1989

11. Gabriel SE, Jaakkimainen L, Bombardier C: Risk for serious gastrointestinal complications related to use of nonsteroidal anti-inflammatory drugs: a meta-analysis. Ann Intern Med 115:787-96, 1991

12. Willet LR, Carson JL, Strom BL: Epidemiology of gastrointestinal damage associated with nonsteroidal anti-inflammatory drugs. Drug Safety 10:170-181, 1994

13. Soll AH, Weinstein, WM, Kurota J, McCarthy D: Nonsteroidal anti-inflammatory drugs and peptic ulcer disease. Ann Intern Med 114:307-319, 1991

14. Silverstein FE, Graham DY, Senior JR, Davies HW, Struthers BJ, Bittman RM, Geis S: Misoprostol reduces serious gastrointestinal complications in patients with rheumatoid arthritis receiving nonsteroidal anti-inflammatory drugs. Ann Intern Med 123:241-249, 1995

15. Katz LM, Love PY: NSAIDs and the liver. In Famaey JP, Paulus HE (eds): Clinical Applications of NSAIDs: Subpopulation Therapy and New Formulations. New York, Marcel Dekker, 1992, pp 247-263

53

CORTICOSTEROIDS

Corticosteroid use is one of the most important and controversial subjects in rheumatology. The dramatic anti-inflammatory effects of corticosteroids were first described in the setting of treating rheumatoid arthritis (RA). This unexpected discovery resulted in a Nobel prize in 1950 (1,2). The subsequent realization, however, that long-term supraphysiologic therapy produced devastating side effects led to polarized views of the role of corticosteroids in the pathogenesis and therapy of rheumatic diseases. Many of the major issues remain unresolved, and the controversies continue today (3–5). Nevertheless, corticosteroid therapy remains a prominent component of rheumatologic practice because the short-term efficacy of these powerful hormones remains unsurpassed.

CORTICOSTEROID PHYSIOLOGY

Corticosteroid hormones are essential for normal development and maintenance of homeostasis during both basal and stress conditions. They represent one of the most important products of the hypothalamic–pituitary–adrenal (HPA) axis and the central stress response system. In addition to their powerful anti-inflammatory actions, they regulate a broad array of metabolic and central nervous system (CNS) functions (Table 53-1). Under basal conditions, corticosteroid levels fluctuate with a circadian rhythm that follows the light–dark cycle. Under stressful conditions, however, the central stress response ("fight or flight") is stimulated and markedly enhances the production and secretion of adrenal corticosteroids. Inflammatory stress is associated with production of cytokines such as tumor necrosis factor α (TNF-α) and interleukins (IL) 1 and 6. These cytokines normally stimulate the HPA axis and corticosteroid production, which results in feedback suppression of cytokine production and the inflammatory response. Inadequate corticosteroid production facilitates unchecked amplification of inflammatory mechanisms and concomitant tissue injury (3,4,6,7). Defects in this bidirectional feedback loop between the CNS and peripheral inflammatory pathways are suspected to contribute to several rheumatic diseases, including RA (6,7). Tissue resistance to the actions of corticosteroids (Table 53-1) has also been postulated to play a role in the pathogenesis of several rheumatic diseases. It is these pathogenetic hypotheses, in the context of the potentially serious side effects of corticosteroid therapy, that drive the continuing interest and controversies on corticosteroids (3–6). Although corticosteroids are not a "cure" for any rheumatic disease, their involvement in the pathogenesis of many diseases, particularly RA, appears probable (6).

CELLULAR AND MOLECULAR EFFECTS OF CORTICOSTEROIDS

All of the effects of corticosteroids are mediated by receptors, designated as the type 1 or mineralocorticoid receptors and the type 2 or corticosteroid receptors. Type 1 receptors are located mainly in the kidneys and various parts of the CNS and are believed to be critical in the basal regulation of circadian variation of adrenocortical activity. Type 2 receptors are present in virtually all cells of the body and mediate the anti-inflammatory and metabolic actions of corticosteroids. In the absence of corticosteroid ligands, type 2 receptors normally exist in association with several classes of heat-shock proteins. Upon corticosteroid binding, the heat-shock proteins disassociate from the receptor, and the corticosteroid–receptor complex then migrates to the nucleus to regulate gene expression and other cellular activities. Major intracellular activities of the corticosteroid–receptor complex include competitive inactivation of c-fos:c-jun complexes and NF-κβ activity. The NF-κβ inhibition is mediated through the induction of an inhibitory factor, I-κβ (8,9). c-fos:c-jun and NF-κβ are important transcriptional activating factors and have prominent roles in driving the cellular production of most proinflammatory cytokines and other mediators. Corticosteroids also enhance production of cyclic adenosine monophosphate and destabilize several classes of mRNAs, including cytokine mRNAs. Recent data demonstrate that type 2 receptors are produced in two alternatively spliced forms: alpha and beta. The alpha form mediates the classic anti-inflammatory activities of the corticosteroid receptor. The beta form, interestingly, inhibits corticosteroid action and competes with the alpha form (10). Thus, the ratio of alpha to beta type 2 receptors in a cell is hypothesized to modulate the cellular actions of corticosteroids. If beta forms predominate in a cell, they confer "resistance" in that cell to corticosteroid action (10).

The primary outcome of corticosteroid action at the cellular level is inhibition of the cascade of inflammatory and immune mechanisms at virtually all levels (Table 53-1). Neutrophil and monocyte migration into the inflammatory site, antigen processing and presentation to lymphocytes, and cellular activation and differentiation are all suppressed. Corticosteroids are particularly active on immature T lymphocytes, activated T-effector lymphocytes, natural killer cells, and immature B cells, but they have minimal suppressive effects on mature antibody-producing B cells. Normally, they potently suppress production of proinflammatory cytokines such as TNF-α and IL-1 and related mediators such as gamma interferon, prostaglandin E₂, and leukotrienes. Importantly, suppressive effects are minimal on the production of anti-inflammatory cytokines such as IL-4 and IL-10. As a consequence, corticosteroids tend to skew or bias immune responses toward humoral immunity (or type 2 immune responses) and to suppress cellular immunity (or type 1 immune responses). These differential immunologic effects may play a role in determining the therapeutic response to corticosteroids, or lack thereof, in various rheumatic diseases. Diseases mediated primarily by type 1 cell-ular immunity, such as RA, tend to respond dramatically to corticosteroid therapy, whereas diseases that probably involve type 2 humoral immune mechanisms, such as lupus

(Table 53-1)

Major physiologic, cellular, and molecular effects of corticosteroids relevant to rheumatic diseases

Physiologic Effects

    Enhance behavioral arousal and euphoria

    Increase blood glucose and liver glycogen

    Promote insulin resistance

    Depress thyroid function

    Depress reproductive function and reproductive hormone synthesis

    Increase muscle catabolic activity

    Enhance activity of detoxifying enzymes

    Impair wound healing

    Suppress acute inflammation

    Suppress type 1 (cell-mediated/delayed hypersensitivity type) immune responsiveness relative to type 2 (humoral)

Cellular Effects

    Alter neuronal activities in many parts of brain resulting in changes in neuropeptide and neurotransmitter synthesis, release, and actions (particularly catecholamines, γ-aminobutyric acid, and prostaglandins)

    Suppress synthesis and release of corticotropin and gonadotropin-releasing hormones from hypothalamus

    Suppress synthesis and release of adrenocorticotropic, thyroid-stimulating, and growth hormone by the pituitary

    Suppress synthesis and release of cortisol and androgens by the adrenal gland

    Suppress estrogen synthesis by ovary and testosterone synthesis by testes, and decrease the action of these hormones on target cells

    Suppress osteoblast growth

    Promote type IIb skeletal muscle fiber atrophy

    Alter adipocyte activity resulting in changes in adipose tissue distribution

    Decrease fibroblast proliferation, DNA, and collagen synthesis

    Suppress fibroblast production of phospholipase A_2, cyclooxygenase-2, prostaglandins, and metalloproteinases

    Depress endothelial cell functions including expression of adhesion molecules involved in inflammatory cell recruitment to inflammatory sites

    Suppress neutrophil, eosinophil, and monocyte migration

    Inhibit macrophage antigen presentation to lymphocytes

    Suppress immune/inflammatory effector cell activation and differentiation (macrophages, T cells, mast cells, natural killer cells, and immature B cells)

    Increase apoptosis of immature and activated T lymphocytes

    Suppress proinflammatory mediator production (eg, tumor necrosis factor α, interleukin-1, γ interferon, prostaglandins, leukotrienes)

Molecular Effects

    Bind plasma cortisol-binding globulin and cellular type 1 or type 2 corticosteroid receptors

    Stimulate disassociation of corticosteroid receptor from heat-shock protein-90, 70, 56, and 26, translocation to nucleus, and binding to glucocorticoid responsive genes

    Enhance transcriptional activity of genes to which cortisol-receptor complexes bind, although overall effect may be inhibitory

    Inactivate c-jun:c-fos transcriptional activator proteins

    Enhance I-κβ production and suppress NF-κβ activity

    Destabilize mRNA for many proinflammatory cytokine genes

    Enhance beta-adrenergic receptor expression

    Enhance cyclic adenosine monophosphate production

glomerulonephritis, require therapy with supraphysiologic levels of corticosteroids for disease suppression.

CORTICOSTEROID PHARMACOLOGY

Corticosteroids are 17-hydroxy, 21-carbon steroid molecules whose principal, naturally occurring form is cortisol (hydrocortisone). Numerous synthetic derivatives have been produced for systemic therapy (Table 53-2), but prednisone, prednisolone, and methylprednisolone are the most widely used. One of the most potent synthetic corticosteroids is dexamethasone, but it is not commonly used for anti-inflammatory therapy because of its long half-life. The biologic effects of these preparations are influenced by multiple factors including dose, scheduling, route of administration, and patient, disease, and tissue variables. For exam-

ple, corticosteroid availability is influenced by its binding to cortisol-binding globulin (transcortin), which is not only present in plasma but is also expressed at different levels in various tissues.

Corticosteroid therapy is not rigorously standardized. Therapeutic dosing regimens are usually individualized for each disease state and patient in a manner that attempts to maximize therapeutic effects and to minimize side effects. To achieve these goals, a variety of approaches have evolved. In general, increasing doses and frequency of administration enhance anti-inflammatory activity and increase side effects, and high-dose schedules tend to be used when urgent control of the disease process is required. For example, intermittent high-dose supraphysiologic intravenous bolus treatment (eg, 1000 mg of methylprednisolone daily for 3 days)

(Table 53-2)
Corticosteroid formulations used for systemic therapy

Form	Relative Anti-inflammatory Potency	Equivalent Dose (mg)	Biologic Half-life (Hours)
Hydrocortisone	1	20	8–12
Cortisone	0.8	25	8–12
Prednisone	4	5	12–26
Methylprednisolone	5	4	12–36
Prednisolone	5	4	12–36
Dexamethasone	20–30	0.75	36–54

may be used to treat acute glomerulonephritis in systemic lupus erythematosus (SLE) or vasculitis in RA. Although this regimen has pronounced effects on lymphocyte function and numbers, it often produces sustained clinical effects for weeks and even months. Daily or alternate day high-dose oral treatment (eg, 60 mg of prednisone daily for up to 1 month, followed by tapering to the lowest possible dose that maintains disease control) is often employed in the setting of acute, severe, but less threatening disease such as thrombocytopenia or pleurisy in SLE. Intermittent low oral doses in the physiologic range (eg, <7 mg of prednisone daily on an as-needed basis) can be used for symptomatic control in RA. With this regimen, rapid development of side effects is unlikely, and it gives the patient control over withdrawing from corticosteroid therapy. Alternate-day therapy is usually preferred, but in many conditions such as RA, patients cannot tolerate alternate-day schedules. Local injections or topical therapy are also very useful approaches for many conditions and are preferred when possible because they target the area specifically involved. Side effects are also minimized. Several corticosteroid formulations are available for these indications (eg, triamcinolone acetonide or hexacetonide) (3,4).

SIDE EFFECTS OF CORTICOSTEROID THERAPY

The pharmacologic side effects of corticosteroids are not distinct from their normal physiologic effects, but reflect the same underlying biologic actions. The likelihood of developing side effects depends on the type of corticosteroid, dose, duration of exposure, and a multitude of host, tissue, and cell variables. It needs to be emphasized that corticosteroids are not merely powerful anti-inflammatory drugs, but rather are essential hormones involved in maintaining homeostasis of numerous physiologic functions. Not surprisingly, both corticosteroid deficiency and excess have pathophysiologic consequences. Therapeutic administration that supplements an endogenous deficiency is less likely to produce side effects. In contrast, therapy that exceeds physiologic need will produce a syndrome that resembles Cushing syndrome, except that adrenal production of corticosteroids and androgens is suppressed in iatrogenic Cushing syndrome (Table 53-3). Several side effects deserve particular emphasis: osteoporosis, infection, adrenal insufficiency, and corticosteroid withdrawal syndromes (3,4).

Osteoporosis

All corticosteroid preparations currently used clinically inhibit bone formation and promote the development of os-

teoporosis. As a consequence, vertebral compression fractures are a frequent and devastating complication, and active prevention measures should be employed. The likelihood of developing osteoporosis is closely linked to the maximum dose and cumulative duration of therapy, but it should always be anticipated with any extended period of therapy regardless of dose. Men and postmenopausal women are most sensitive, and patients in whom the disease process itself causes bone loss, such as those with RA, are at high risk. Corticosteroids induce osteoporosis through inhibiting ovarian and testicular sex hormones, as well as adrenal androgens. They also inhibit intestinal calcium absorption and promote secondary hyperparathyroidism, which leads to osteoclast activation and osteoblast inhibition. Thus, therapeutic preventive measures should emphasize adequate calcium intake and vitamin D. Estrogen replacement therapy should be considered for postmenopausal women, and androgen replacement therapy should possibly be considered for men. Bisphosphonate therapy is also possibly indicated (3–5). Deflazacort is a corticosteroid preparation in clinical evaluation that has less inhibitory effects on bone, but it is not yet available in the United States.

Infections

Corticosteroid deficiency renders patients susceptible to severe, even life-threatening, tissue injury in response to infection because of the unrestrained inflammatory response. Conversely, corticosteroid excess leads to impaired inflammatory and immune responses and an increased incidence and severity of infections (ie, impaired host defense). As expected, the likelihood of developing infection in the course of corticosteroid treatment depends on the maximum dose and cumulative duration of therapy. Doses of prednisone around 2–10 mg/day are rarely associated with infectious complications, whereas doses of prednisone in the range of 20–60 mg/day have pronounced suppressive effects on host defense mechanisms and lead to a progressive increase in infection risk after 14 days of treatment. Cumulative doses greater than 700 mg are associated with progressively increased risk of infection. The primary risk is for infections with facultative intracellular microbes such as mycobacteria, *Pneumocystis carinii*, and fungi. Patients also develop more severe cases of acute pyogenic infections. It is important to note that high-dose corticosteroids can mask the symptoms of infectious diseases such as abscesses and bowel perforation. Thus, unusual degrees of suspicion are required to make these diagnoses. Except for herpes, viral infections are generally not a major problem during corticosteroid treatment (3–5).

Adrenal Insufficiency

Administration of corticosteroids suppresses endogenous HPA axis function and may produce secondary adrenal deficiency. The development of this side effect can occur with as little as 5 days of prednisone treatment with 20–30 mg/day, although, in this setting, pituitary–adrenal function normally returns rapidly after stopping corticosteroids. In contrast, patients treated for more prolonged periods of time (weeks to months) may require up to 12 months for HPA axis function to return to normal after corticosteroid therapy, and it should be assumed that all patients treated with more than 20 mg of prednisone per day for 1 month have some degree of HPA axis deficiency. The risk to the patient is dur-

(Table 53-3)
*Side effects of long-term corticosteroid therapy**

Common

    Hypertension

    Negative balance of calcium and secondary hyperparathyroidism

    Negative balance of nitrogen

    Truncal obesity; moon facies; supraclavicular fat deposition; posterior cervical fat deposition (buffalo hump); mediastinal widening (lipomatosis); weight gain

    Impaired wound healing; facial erythema; thin, fragile skin; violaceous striae; petechiae and ecchymoses

    Acne

    Suppression of growth in children

    Adrenal insufficiency secondary to hypothalamic–pituitary–adrenal axis suppression

    Hyperglycemia; diabetes mellitus

    Hyperlipoproteinemia; atherosclerosis

    Sodium retention; hypokalemia

    Increased risk of infection; neutrophilia; monocytopenia; lymphopenia; suppressed delayed-type hypersensitivity reactions

    Myopathy

    Osteoporosis; vertebral compression fractures

    Osteonecrosis (aseptic necrosis of bone) of femoral heads and other bones

    Alterations in mood or behavior, such as euphoria, emotional lability, insomnia, depression, increased appetite

    Posterior subcapsular cataracts

Uncommon

    Metabolic alkalosis

    Diabetic ketoacidosis, hyperosmolar nonketotic diabetic coma

    Peptic ulcer disease (usually gastric), gastric hemorrhage

    "Silent" intestinal perforation

    Increased intraocular pressure and glaucoma

    Benign intracranial hypertension or pseudotumor cerebri

    Spontaneous fractures

    Psychosis

Rare

    Sudden death with rapid administration of high-dose pulse therapy

    Cardiac valvular lesions in patients with systemic lupus erythematosus

    Congestive heart failure in predisposed patients

    Panniculitis (following withdrawal)

    Hirsutism or virilism, impotence, secondary amenorrhea

    Hepatomegaly due to fatty liver

    Pancreatitis

    Convulsions

    Epidural lipomatosis

    Exophthalmos

    Allergy to synthetic corticosteroids resulting in urticaria, angioedema

*Reprinted with permission from Sternberg EM, Wilder RL: Corticosteroids. In McCarty DJ, Koopman WJ (eds): Arthritis and Allied Conditions: A Textbook of Rheumatology, 12th ed. Philadelphia, Lea & Febiger, 1993, pp 665-682.

ing periods of corticosteroid taper and warrants close follow-up and attention to symptoms of deficiency. The major concern is the development of acute adrenal insufficiency during general anesthesia, surgery, trauma, or an acute infectious disease. Patients may require supplemental corticosteroid therapy in these settings. If doubt exists about the existence of adrenal insufficiency, an adrenocorticotropic hormone stimulation test may be indicated (3,4).

Withdrawal Syndromes

Corticosteroid deficiency classically presents in Addisonian crisis with fever, nausea, vomiting, hypotension, hypoglycemia, hyperkalemia, and hyponatremia, but other syndromes are also noted. Most often, patients develop an exacerbation of their underlying inflammatory disease. Some patients develop a symptom complex consisting of diffuse muscle and joint pains, weight loss, fever, and headache. In this setting, plasma cortisol levels do not correlate with symptoms and are frequently higher than "normal." Withdrawal syndromes require increased dosages of corticosteroid administration and careful slow taper over a period of weeks to months. In general, at doses >40 mg/day, prednisone can be tapered at a rate of about 10 mg/week. At doses between 20 and 40 mg/day, one can usually taper about 5 mg/week. Below 20 mg/day, and especially less than 5 mg/day, withdrawal symptoms are common, because the dosage changes are occurring within the normal physiologic range of corticosteroids. For example, a rapid reduction of prednisone from 5 to 2.5 mg/day represents a 50% reduction in available corticosteroid and, not surprisingly, is often associated with severe withdrawal symptoms. Reductions in these situations can often be best managed by a patient-dictated schedule. Close follow up is indicated in all cases. Occasionally, a switch to alternate-day schedule is done as the first step before reducing the average daily dose. This therapeutic strategy frequently works well in conditions such as SLE, but it is rarely tolerated by patients with RA, who report marked worsening of symptoms on the "off" day of therapy.

In general, considering the broad spectrum of rheumatic diseases and patient variables, corticosteroid therapy must be individualized with attention directed at avoiding or preventing the side effects associated with both corticosteroid excess and deficiency.

RONALD L. WILDER, MD, PhD

1. Hench PS, Kendall EC, Slocumb CH, Polley HF: The effect of a hormone of the adrenal cortex (17-hydroxy-11-dehydrocorticosterone:compound E) and of pituitary adrenocorticotropic hormone on rheumatoid arthritis. Proc Staff Meet Mayo Clin 24:181-197, 1949

2. Hench PS, Kendall EC, Slocumb CH, Polley HF: Effects of cortisone acetate and pituitary ACTH on rheumatoid arthritis, rheumatic fever and certain other conditions. Arch Intern Med 85:545-666, 1950

3. Sternberg EM, Wilder RL: Corticosteroids. In McCarty DJ, Koopman WJ (eds): Arthritis and Allied Conditions: A Textbook of Rheumatology, 12th ed. Philadelphia, Lea & Febiger, 1993, pp 665-682.

4. Wilder RL: Corticosteroids. In Koopman WJ (ed): Arthritis and Allied Conditions: A Textbook of Rheumatology, 13th ed. Baltimore, Williams & Wilkins, 1996

5. Boumpas DT, Chrousos GP, Wilder RL, Cupps TR, Balow JE: Glucocorticoid therapy for immune-mediated diseases: basic and clinical correlates. Ann Intern Med 119:1198-1208, 1993

6. Wilder RL: Neuroendocrine-immune interactions in autoimmunity. Annu Rev Immunol 13:307-38, 1995

7. Chrousos GP: The hypothalamic–pituitary–adrenal axis and immune-mediated inflammation. N Engl J Med 332:1351-1362, 1995

8. Auhan N, DiDonato JA, Rosette C, Helmberg A, Karin M: Immunosuppression by glucocorticoids: inhibition of NF-kappa B activity through induction of I kappa B synthesis. Science 13:232-233, 1995

9. Scheinman RI, Cogswell PC, Lofquist AK, Baldwin AS Jr: Role of transcriptional activation of I kappa B alpha in mediation of immunosuppression by glucocorticoids. Science 13:283-286, 1995

10. Bamberger CM, Bamberger A-M, de Castro M, Chrousos GP: Glucocorticoid receptor beta: a potential inhibitor of glucocorticoid action in humans. J Clin Invest 95:2435-2441, 1995

DISEASE-MODIFYING ANTIRHEUMATIC DRUGS

The treatment of rheumatoid arthritis (RA) and other systemic rheumatic diseases has changed significantly over the past 20 years. The variety of drugs available has increased dramatically, and there is greater acceptance of treating early RA much more aggressively. The appreciation that cartilage erosions occur early in the disease has led to the early use of disease-modifying antirheumatic drugs (DMARDs), also known as slow-acting antirheumatic drugs. It is important, however, to consider the potential adverse effects of these drugs and to choose treatment that provides maximum benefit to the patient with a minimum of risk. In using these agents, it is important to try to answer three questions: What drugs are available? Is there a rationale for choosing one drug over another? How do we tell whether the drug is working or producing adverse reactions?

The question of which drug to select for an individual is influenced by a number of factors. For example, rheumatoid patients with low-grade early synovitis are often started on antimalarial agents or sulfasalazine, while those with more aggressive disease (such as synovitis plus extra-articular manifestations) might be started on low-dose methotrexate or gold. However, a meta-analysis of randomized controlled trials on RA demonstrated little difference in efficacy between methotrexate, injectable gold, penicillamine, and sulfasalazine (2). Auranofin and hydroxychloroquine, on the other hand, were significantly less effective.

The combination of DMARDs and corticosteroids is often begun early in RA with the intent to reduce or to cease the corticosteroids once the synovitis is controlled. Although these approaches seem theoretically sensible, efficacy and safety of these regimens remain unproven because of the lack of controlled studies.

CLINICAL PHARMACOLOGY OF DMARDS

The DMARDs have complex mechanisms of action, and all have multiple effects (Table 54-1).

Antimalarial Agents

Hydroxychloroquine and chloroquine have been used in the treatment of connective tissue diseases since the early 1950s. The pharmacokinetics of both are characterized by extensive accumulation in tissues and large volumes of distribution leading to very long half-lives. It might take 3 to 4 months before steady-state plasma concentrations are reached, which may explain some of the delayed action (3). The optimal therapeutic concentration for hydroxychloroquine has not yet been established, although concentrations in RA of 700–2100 ng/ml (blood) have been proposed. Antimalarial drugs have been shown to be effective in RA and to suppress both musculoskeletal and systemic manifestations of systemic lupus erythematosus (SLE) (4). Chloroquine seems to be no different from hydroxychloroquine in reducing symptoms, but it is associated with a higher incidence of

side effects. The major adverse reactions are indigestion, skin rash, visual disturbance, and retinopathy, although retinal toxicity is extremely rare at currently recommended doses (5 mg/kg/day chloroquine diphosphate and 7.5 mg/kg/day hydroxychloroquine sulfate). Fundoscopic examination and visual field testing are recommended every 6 months (Table 54-2), although there are no data to support the cost effectiveness of this intensive monitoring. Quinacrine is another antimalarial most often used for cutaneous SLE.

Penicillamine

Penicillamine forms disulfides and acts as a metal chelator. Its multiple mechanisms of action include reduction in immunoglobulin synthesis by monocytes and lymphocytes, inhibition of polymorphonuclear leukocyte and T-lymphocyte function, and possibly, protection of tissues from damage by free radicals (5). Penicillamine is rapidly absorbed and con-

(Table 54-1)

*Mechanism of action of disease-modifying antirheumatic drugs**

Antimalarial agents	Inhibit lysosomal enzymes
	Inhibit PMN and lymphocyte responses (in vitro)
	Inhibit IL-1 release (in vivo)
	Cartilage protection (in vitro)
	Down-regulate autoantigen responses
Sulfasalazine	Inhibits PMN migration
	Reduces lymphocyte responses
	Inhibits angiogenesis
Penicillamine	Inhibits neovascularization (in vitro)
	Inhibits PMN myeloperoxidase
	Scavenges free radicals
	Inhibits T cell function
	Impairs antigen presentation
Gold	Inhibits PMN function
	Inhibits T and B cell activity
	Inhibits macrophage activation (in vitro)
Methotrexate	Decreases thymidilate synthetase activity and subsequent DNA synthesis
	Diminishes PMN chemotaxis
	Reduces soluble IL-2 receptor
Azathioprine	Interferes with DNA synthesis
	Inhibits lymphocyte proliferation
Cyclophosphamide	Crosslinks DNA, leading to cell death
	Decreases circulating T and B cells
Chlorambucil	Similar to cyclophosphamide
Cyclosporine	Blocks synthesis/release of IL-1 and IL-2

* PMN = polymorphonuclear leukocytes; IL = interleukin.

(Table 54-2)

*Monitoring disease-modifying antirheumatic drug therapy**

Antimalarial agents	Regular vision assessment (fundoscopic examination, visual field evaluation, or use of AMSLER grid)
Sulfasalazine	CBC and LFTs biweekly for first 3 months, then monthly
Penicillamine	CBC and urinalysis biweekly on initiating or changing dose, then 1–3 monthly
Gold compounds	
Injectable	CBC and urinalysis before each injection initially, then before every second or third injection. Urinalysis monitored by patient
Oral	CBC and urinalysis 2–4 weeks
Methotrexate	CBC and LFTs biweekly, then 1–3 monthly
Cyclophosphamide	CBC and urinalysis monthly after initial weekly tests
Azathioprine	CBC 1–2 weekly initially, then 1–3 monthly; LFTs 1–3 monthly
Chlorambucil	CBC monthly initially, then 3 monthly
Cyclosporine	CBC, serum creatinine, blood pressure weekly, then 2–4 weekly on maintenance dose

* None of these monitoring schemes has been assessed from a perspective of cost effectiveness. Also see Appendix II for American College of Rheumatology guidelines for drug monitoring.
CBC = complete blood count; LFTs = liver function tests.

verted into disulfides or inorganic sulfates. Its bioavailability is decreased by food, antacids, and iron supplements. The drug has a relatively short half-life of between 2 and 7 hours. Penicillamine is effective in RA in doses of 600–1500 mg daily, although the higher dose is associated with a significant increase in side effects. There are conflicting data as to whether penicillamine prevents joint erosions in RA.

More than 25% of patients taking penicillamine have to discontinue the drug because of side effects within the first 12 months. The major adverse reactions are skin rashes, proteinuria, hematuria, neutropenia, thrombocytopenia, and a variety of autoimmune phenomena including the induction of antinuclear antibodies and drug-induced lupus, Goodpasture's syndrome, and myasthenia gravis (Table 54-3).

Some of these adverse reactions occur more frequently in patients who demonstrate slow sulfoxidation, and there may also be an association with HLA-DR3 and B8. Penicillamine should be started in doses between 125 and 250 mg/day and increased to a maximum of 750 mg/day over a period of a few months. When disease is controlled the dose can be reduced, but most patients suffer an exacerbation of their symptoms if the drug is stopped. While taking penicillamine patients need to have regular blood and urine tests, as outlined in Table 54-2.

Sulfasalazine

Although sulfasalazine was initially developed as an antirheumatic drug, only in the past 15 years was its efficacy in RA and the seronegative spondyloarthropathies recognized (6). Sulfasalazine interferes with a variety of cellular and mediator aspects of inflammation. The drug is split by colonic bacteria into its two component parts, sulfapyridine and 5-amino salicylic acid (5-ASA). 5-ASA is poorly absorbed, while sulfapyridine (the active component) is metabolized in the liver by acetylation. Sulfasalazine is significantly better for treating RA than placebo, and there is some suggestion that it slows the development of bony erosions. It seems to have similar efficacy to gold and penicillamine, although comparative clinical trials have not been of sufficient power to demonstrate differences. Up to 50% of patients develop side effects within the first 4 months of treatment, but for the majority, these reactions are mild (7). Side effects include skin rashes, nausea and abdominal pain, hepatic enzyme abnormalities, central nervous system disturbances, and blood dyscrasias, particularly in patients who have glucose-6 phosphate dehydrogenase deficiency (Table 54-3). Oligospermia also occurs, as does discoloration of urine and sweat. Liver function tests and blood cell counts need to be vigilantly monitored during the first 3–4 months of therapy (Table 54-2).

Gold

The sulfhydryl-containing organic gold compounds have been used since the early 1920s for treating RA. They are also effective in juvenile chronic arthritis and psoriatic arthritis. The gold complexes fall into two major groups: water-soluble thiolates and the fat-soluble phosphine derivative (7). The chemistry of gold compounds is complex; it is

(Table 54-3)

*Toxicities associated with disease-modifying antirheumatic drugs**

	Mucocutaneous	Hematologic	Gastrointestinal	Hepatic	Renal
Hydroxycholoroquine	+	+	++	–	–
Sulfasalazine	++	++	++	++	–
D-penicillamine	+++	++	++	+	++
Oral gold	+	+	+++	+	+
Parenteral gold	+++	++	+	+	++
Azathioprine	+	++	++	++	–
Methotrexate	–	+	+++	++	–
Cyclophosphamide	–	+++	++	–	–
Chlorambucil	–	+++	+	–	–
Cyclosporine	–	+	+++	+	++

* Toxicities range from – = no association to +++ = strong association.

still not quite clear in what form gold circulates in the body. Gold compounds interfere with lymphocyte, monocyte, and neutrophil function, as well as with immunoglobulin and antibody production. The metabolites of gold compounds that circulate in the blood are bound primarily to plasma proteins, but significant concentrations of gold are found within the red cells. Gold is eliminated very slowly from the body, with significant tissue concentrations found 20 years after the last dose.

Plasma concentrations of gold vary significantly among patients but are of the order of 300 µg/100 ml when patients are stabilized on a 50 mg/week regimen. Injectable gold complexes are used in doses of 10–50 mg/week. The frequency of injections is reduced once a total dose of 1 g has been given. Aurothioglucose (an oily complex) is absorbed slightly more slowly than aurothiomalate following intramuscular injection. Doses of auranofin are 3–6 mg/day; side effects are dose-related. Gold is taken up more quickly by inflamed tissues, particularly the macrophage. The half-life of both oral and intramuscular gold compounds is long, but accumulation of gold in patients on auranofin is slightly less than in those on intramuscular gold. Injectable gold complexes have been shown to be significantly better than placebo in patients with RA, although the relative change in measures of disease activity, such as functional capacity, grip strength, and active joint count, are relatively modest (8). Injectable gold compounds are of similar efficacy to other DMARDs, including penicillamine, sulfasalazine, azathioprine, and methotrexate (2). Few patients remain on gold therapy for longer than 5 years because of loss of efficacy or adverse reactions.

Adverse reactions to gold complexes are the major reasons for discontinuing therapy. Auranofin has few serious adverse reactions, although dose-related diarrhea is common. Mucocutaneous reactions, proteinuria, and thrombocytopenia are also seen. Skin rashes and mouth ulcers are also common with intramuscular gold, while blood dyscrasias, proteinuria, and pulmonary complications are rare but potentially lethal (Table 54-3). Eosinophilia may predict adverse reactions. A significant number of patients who develop severe blood dyscrasias on gold therapy have a progressive fall in their white blood cell (WBC) or platelet count prior to developing a significant problem. There is still a wide variation in monitoring strategies, but Liang and Fries (9) have suggested the following. 1) Have patient fill out a questionnaire on side effects before each injection. 2) Order WBC and platelet counts weekly and complete blood count monthly. 3) Have patient perform dip-stick urinalysis for blood and protein before each injection. 4) Review patient's chart monthly.

In a recent review of the efficacy of gold compounds, Champion et al (7) concluded that doses in the range of 10–50 mg/week for 1–2 years are more effective than placebo and that dose–response relationships in the range of 10–150 mg/week have not been established. The most commonly used regimen after test doses is 50 mg/week until the patient has received a total of 1000 mg or has dramatically improved. Doses are spread out when apparent maximum improvement is achieved. Excellent clinical response occurs in 20%–35% of patients and peaks at 6–12 months, but only one-half of these patients maintain this response after 12 months. Intramuscular methylprednisolone given during the induction of intramuscular gold therapy significantly improves the rapidity and degree of response to treatment (10).

Methotrexate

Methotrexate is an analog of folic acid and aminopterin and inhibits dihydrofolate reductase impairing DNA synthesis (11). Low doses are rapidly absorbed after oral administration. The parent compound and metabolites circulate bound to serum albumin. Methotrexate is oxidized to an active metabolite, 7-hydroxy methotrexate, and metabolites and parent drug accumulate in the liver as polyglutamates. The drug is eliminated from the body by the kidneys and by biliary excretion in the feces. In doses of 7.5–20 mg/week, methotrexate has been shown to be better than placebo and equal to or slightly better than azathioprine, penicillamine, antimalarials, and gold. Tugwell et al (12) performed a meta-analysis of clinical trials that showed the drug works relatively rapidly (within 1–2 months) with efficacy peaking at 6 months. RA patients remain on methotrexate longer than on other DMARDs.

Adverse effects are the major concern with long-term use (Table 54-4). Anorexia and nausea, particularly in the 24 hours after dosing, are quite common but can be reduced or eliminated by administering folic acid, which does not affect the anti-inflammatory activity of methotrexate. Liver enzymes become transiently elevated in up to 60% of patients, but this does not correlate with the development of hepatic fibrosis. Although the incidence of moderate fibrosis is very low, there is still some concern about long-term use, since fibrosis does seem to correlate with the concentration of methotrexate and its metabolites in hepatic tissues. The American College of Rheumatology has issued guidelines for monitoring hepatotoxicity of methotrexate (Table 54-5)

(Table 54-4)
Side effects of methotrexate

	Frequency*	Management
Gastrointestinal		
Abdominal pain	+++	Temporary withdrawal
Nausea	+++	Usually allows tolerance at a lower dose in addition to folate therapy
Diarrhea	+	
Stomatitis	+++	
Hepatotoxicity		
Abnormal enzymes	+++	Temporary withdrawal
Hepatic fibrosis	+	
Hematologic		
Macrocytosis	+++	
Neutropenia	+	Cease
Pancytopenia	+	Cease
Skin		
Alopecia rash	++	Dose modification
Respiratory		
Pneumonitis	+	Withdraw (opportunistic infection)
Risk of infection		
Herpes zoster	+	

* + = <5%; ++ = 5%–15%; +++ = >15%.

(Table 54-5)
American College of Rheumatology guidelines for monitoring hepatotoxicity during methotrexate therapy[*]

Before intitiating treatment
  Baseline tests: complete blood cell count, serum creatinine, liver chemistry tests, serum albumin, hepatitis B and C serology
  Liver biopsy if transaminases are elevated or patient has history of high alcohol intake or hepatitis
During treatment
  Liver function tests every 4–8 weeks
  Liver biopsy during treatment if aspartate aminotransferase levels are elevated in five of nine or six of twelve readings over a period of 12 months or if there is a fall in serum albumin

---

[*] Condensed from Kremer JM et al (13).

(13). Particular caution should be taken in all patients with known risk factors or previous liver damage, such as alcohol abuse, hepatic viral infection, obesity, and diabetes. Methotrexate-associated pulmonary disease has been reported in up to 10% of patients and includes infections (usually opportunistic) and noninfectious causes (14).

Azathioprine

Azathioprine is an oral purine analog that interferes with the synthesis of adenosine and guanine. Approximately one-half of the oral dose is absorbed. Azathioprine has a plasma half-life of approximately 60–90 minutes resulting from re-nal excretion, cellular uptake, and metabolism. Controlled clinical trials have demonstrated azathioprine to be better than placebo and to have a significant steroid-sparing effect. It has been shown to be beneficial in the treatment of RA, SLE, and a variety of other connective tissue diseases. Comparative studies against hydroxychloroquine, penicillamine, intramuscular gold, and cyclophosphamide in RA have shown azathioprine to be no different from these DMARDs, but slightly more likely to produce side effects (15). Nausea, vomiting, and diarrhea are relatively common but do not usually necessitate cessation of treatment. Bone marrow suppression and hepatitis can also occur, but the real risk with azathioprine is an increase in the incidence of lymphoproliferative malignancies after long-term treatment (16).

Alkylating Agents

Nitrogen mustard alkylating agents substitute alkyl radicals into other molecules such as DNA and RNA. The most commonly used alkylating agents in the treatment of rheumatic diseases are chlorambucil and cyclophosphamide. Chlorambucil is rapidly absorbed and has a half-life of approximately 2 hours (15). It has been used in doses of 0.1–0.3 mg/kg/day for the treatment of RA, juvenile chronic arthritis, vasculitis, and systemic sclerosis. Chlorambucil is particularly beneficial for reducing the severity and incidence of amyloidosis that may complicate RA, juvenile chronic arthritis, and ankylosing spondylitis (15). The drug can induce chromosomal damage, and the major adverse reaction is an increased risk of leukemia and other malignancies (Table 54-3).

Cyclophosphamide is a derivative of nitrogen mustard and can be taken orally or intravenously. The drug has a plasma half-life between 2 and 10 hours and is metabolized primarily by the liver, with small contributions by kidney and lung (15). Cyclophosphamide itself is inactive, but it is converted into the active metabolite, which produces the immunosuppressive effect and also causes bladder toxicity. It has been shown to be effective in the treatment of severe RA, SLE, and systemic vasculitis. The usual oral dose of cyclophosphamide is 50–150 mg/day (0.7–3 mg/kg/day). In many clinical situations, however, it is now possible to substitute lower (and, therefore, less toxic) total dose regimens of intermittent intravenous bolus (0.5–1 g/meter^2 body surface area) every 4–6 weeks. Adverse events are frequent with cyclophosphamide and include hemorrhagic cystitis with the potential for bladder carcinoma, immunosuppression leading to increased risk of infection (particularly herpes zoster), suppression of gonadal function in both females and males, and an increased incidence of lymphoma and other hematologic malignancies that may appear long after the drug is ceased (17).

Cyclosporine

Cyclosporine is an immunomodulating agent that selectively blocks the synthesis and release of interleukin-1 from monocytes and interleukin-2 from helper T cells. Absorption of cyclosporine is slow, often incomplete, and reduced by food. The drug is highly bound to plasma protein, particularly the lipoproteins. Cyclosporine undergoes extensive metabolism, primarily in the liver, and has a terminal elimination half-life between 6 hours (in healthy volunteers) and 20 hours (in patients with severe liver disease) (18). Cyclosporine has been shown to be effective in comparison to placebo in patients with RA and to have similar efficacy to azathioprine and penicillamine. The major problem with cyclosporine is that the majority of patients have a significant decrease in renal function and increase in blood pressure while on the drug. Usually this occurs with the higher doses (>7 mg/kg/day), but occasionally even with low doses (<5 mg/kg/day). Renal function returns to normal once the drug is ceased (19).

COMBINATION THERAPY

The majority of patients with RA are currently treated with a variety of agents prescribed concurrently, typically a nonsteroidal anti-inflammatory drug (NSAID), DMARD, and corticosteroid. Although combinations of two or more DMARDs are commonly used, there are few well-designed randomized controlled trials of sufficient duration that have demonstrated that combination DMARD therapy works (20). What does seem clear is that combinations of DMARDs are not associated with increased toxicity.

With the increasing number of DMARDs available for treating RA, it is important to individualize treatment and maximize response. DMARDs suppress disease activity in the short term, but few patients achieve a complete remission. Fries (21) has enunciated the following six principles as a treatment strategy for rheumatoid arthritis: 1) start DMARDs early before joint damage occurs; 2) use one or multiple DMARDs continuously through the disease; 3) monitor disability and other outcome measures regularly so that disease progression can be plotted serially; 4) set goals for response in terms of reduction of disease activity a priori so that decisions to change therapy can be planned; 5) change DMARD therapy serially to new agents, alone or in combination, at each decision point; 6) use analgesics and NSAIDs as adjunctive therapy for symptomatic relief as required. These principles should be applied to the management of any rheumatic disease, with patients being assessed for disease activity at frequent intervals and treatment adjusted accordingly. In this way, we should be in a position to continually reassess therapy and maximally suppress disease activity.

PETER BROOKS, MD

1. Emery P: The optimal management of early rheumatoid disease: the key to preventing disability. Brit J Rheumatol 33:765-768, 1991

2. Felson DT, Anderson JJ, Meenan RF: The comparative efficacy and toxicity of second line drugs in rheumatoid arthritis. Arthritis Rheum 33:1449-1461, 1990

3. Tett S, Cutler D, Day RO: Antimalarials in rheumatic diseases. Baillieres Clin Rheumatol 4:467-489, 1990

4. The Canadian Hydroxychloroquine Study Group: a randomised study of the effect of withdrawing hydroxychloroquine sulphate in systemic lupus erythematosus. N Engl J Med 324:150-154, 1991

5. Joyce DA: D-penicillamine. Clin Rheumatol 4:553-574, 1990

6. Porter DR, Capell HA: The use of sulphasalazine as a disease modifying antirheumatic drug. Baillieres Clin Rheumatol 4:535-551, 1990

7. Champion GD, Graham GG, Ziegler JB: The gold complexes. Baillieres Clin Rheumatol 4:491-534, 1990

8. Clark P, Tugwell P, Bennett K, Bombardier C: Meta analysis of injectable gold in rheumatoid arthritis. J Rheumatol 6:442-447, 1989

9. Liang MH, Fries JF: Containing costs in chronic disease: monitoring strategies in the gold therapy of rheumatoid arthritis. J Rheumatol 5:241-244, 1978

10. Choy EHS, Kingsley GH, Corkhill MM, Panayi GS: Intramuscular methylprednisolone during the induction of chrysotherapy. Br J Rheumatol 31:734-739, 1993

11. Songsiride JN, Furst DE: Methotrexate: a rapidly acting drug. Baillieres Clin Rheumatol 4:575-593, 1990

12. Tugwell P, Bennett K, Ghent M: Methotrexate in rheumatoid arthritis. Ann Intern Med 107:358-366, 1987

13. Kremer JM, Alarcon GS, Lightfoot RW, et al: Methotrexate for rheumatoid arthritis: suggested guidelines for monitoring liver toxicity. Arthritis Rheum 37:316-328, 1994

14. Berrera P, Laan RFJM, Van Riel PLCM, et al Methotrexate related pulmonary complications in rheumatoid arthritis. Ann Rheum Dis 53:434-439, 1994

15. Luqmani RA, Palmer RG, Bacon PA: Azathioprine, cyclophosphamide and chlorambucil. Baillieres Clin Rheumatol 4:595-619, 1990

16. Matteson EL, Hickey AR, Maguire L, Tilson HH, Urowitz MB: Occurrence of neoplasia in patients with rheumatoid arthritis enrolled in a DMARD registry. J Rheumatol 18:809-814, 1991

17. Radis CD, Kahl LE, Baker GL, et al: Effects of cyclophosphamide on the development of malignancy and long-term survival in patients with rheumatoid arthritis. Arthritis Rheum 38:1120-1127, 1995

18. Kahan BD: Drug therapy: cyclosporin. N Engl J Med 321:1725-1738, 1989

19. Tugwell P, Bombardier C, Gent M, et al: Low dose cyclosporine versus placebo in patients with rheumatoid arthritis. Lancet 335:1051-1056, 1990

20. Brogigni M, Paulus HE: Combination therapy. Baillieres Clin Rheumatol 9:689-710, 1995

21. Fries JF: Re-evaluating the therapeutic approach to rheumatoid arthritis: the sawtooth strategy. J Rheumatol 17(suppl)12-15, 1990

BIOLOGIC AGENTS AS POTENTIAL NEW THERAPIES FOR RHEUMATIC DISEASES

Considerable clinical and basic research activity is being directed at the potential use of biologic agents as therapies for rheumatic diseases. Biologic agents can be broadly defined and generally include monoclonal antibodies (MAb) directed against selected cell-surface markers (ie, CD4, CD5, etc), and recombinant forms of molecules such as interleukin-1 receptor antagonist (IL-1ra), recombinant soluble tumor necrosis factor (TNF) receptor fusion protein, and interleukin-10 (IL-10). Therapies with MAb directed against several cell-surface constituents and cytokine inhibitors have been shown to be safe and possibly efficacious in early clinical trials. However, it is important to emphasize that biologic agents tested to date generally have been evaluated in patients with refractory and long-standing disease. Moreover, most of these trials have been of short duration and aimed at defining the pharmacokinetics and safety profiles of these new agents.

Although the etiology of rheumatoid arthritis (RA) remains unknown, several immune and inflammatory pathways that likely contribute to cartilage and bone destruction have been elucidated (1). Recent advances in molecular technology have made it possible to identify distinct cell subsets, cell-surface markers, and cell products that contribute to the pathologic immune-mediated inflammatory responses of RA. The major cellular and humoral pathways currently implicated in the pathogenesis of RA are presented in Figure 55-1.

CELLULAR TARGETS

T lymphocytes play a pivotal role in initiating and modulating humoral and cellular immune responses. Considerable evidence supports the view that T cells contribute importantly to the pathogenesis of animal models of RA (2). Previous experimental therapies to suppress T-cell function in humans with RA include lymphapheresis, thoracic duct drainage, total lymphoid irradiation, and more recently cyclosporine. Each of these methods has been reported to have some beneficial effect. More recent therapeutic approaches have employed MAb directed against T-cell antigens such as CD4, CD7, CD5, and CD52, as well as agents directed at interleukin-2 receptors (CD25) expressed on activated T cells (Fig. 55-1). T-cell receptor (TCR) peptides and DR4-derived peptides also are being investigated as potential immunomodulating vaccines.

Anti-CD4 Monoclonal Antibodies

Anti-CD4 MAb therapy in several animal models of human autoimmune disease, including collagen-induced arthritis, systemic lupus erythematosus, myasthenia gravis, experimental allergic encephalomyelitis (EAE), diabetes mellitus, thyroiditis, and uveitis in mice, further supports CD4 T cells as playing a role in the pathogenesis of these disorders. Anti-CD4 MAb may exert an effect in autoimmune disorders through several mechanisms. For example, CD4 cell depletion may be accomplished either by directly killing the cells (complement-mediated or by inducing apoptosis) or by antibody-mediated clearance of CD4 T cells (by complement- and Fc receptor-mediated mechanisms). Other

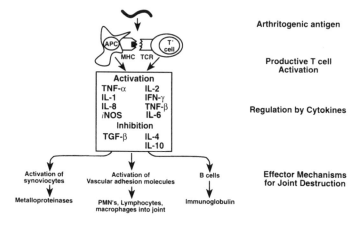

(Figure 55-1)

Schematic diagram illustrating the major cells and cellular products implicated in the immune-mediated inflammatory process of rheumatoid arthritis. APC = antigen-presenting cell; MHC = major histocompatibility complex; TCR = T cell receptor; TNF = tumor necrosis factor; IL = interleukin; iNOS = inducible nitric oxide synthase; IFN = interferon; TGF = transforming growth factor; PMN = polymorphonuclear leukocytes.

(Table 55-1)

Cellular targets of biologic agents tested in RA*

Biologic Agent	Target
Murine anti-CD4 MAb	CD4 antigen
Chimeric anti-CD4 MAb	CD4 antigen
Humanized anti-CD4 MAb	CD4 antigen
Murine anti-CD7 MAb	CD7 antigen
Anti-Campath 1H MAb	CD52 antigen
Murine-anti CD5 ricin fusion toxin	CD5 antigen
Anti-IL-2R monoclonal antibodies	IL-2 receptor (CD25)
Diphtheria IL-2 fusion protein	IL-2 receptor (CD25)
T-cell receptor peptide vaccines	T-cell receptors
DR4/DR1 peptide vaccines	MHC molecules

* RA = rheumatoid arthritis; MAb = monoclonal antibody; IL = interleukin; MHC = major histocompatibility complex.

possible mechanisms of anti-CD4 MAb include inducing antibody-dependent cellular toxicity; blocking the interaction of CD4 T cells with antigen-presenting cells; or transmitting an inhibitory signal to the CD4 T cells. The fact that F(ab')$_2$ fragments of anti-CD4 MAb are effective argues against the need for physical depletion (3).

Chimeric and humanized anti-CD4 MAb exhibit lower immunogenicity than the parent murine MAb. Uncontrolled studies in refractory RA using cM-T412, which is a depleting anti-CD4 MAb, provided early safety data (4); however, subsequent placebo-controlled trials evaluating cM-T412 demonstrated no clinical benefit in the treated groups compared with placebo (5, 6). A biologic response was noted with depletion of peripheral CD4 T cells. However, there was prolonged depletion of CD4 T cells for several months. This effect was enhanced by the administration of multiple doses. The etiology of the prolonged CD4 depletion is not known. This property limits the dosage and the frequency of administering cM-T412. In addition, the degree of depletion in these trials did not correlate with clinical responses to cM-T412. This lack of correlation is consistent with animal models of autoimmune disease in which the efficacy of anti-CD4 MAb is not dependent upon physical depletion of T cells. These data are in agreement with the view that modulation of T-cell function (ie, tolerance induction) is more likely responsible for the effectiveness of anti-CD4 MAb therapy in animal models (3).

There are at least two possible explanations for the failure of cM-T412 to exert significant beneficial effects. At safe dosages, the quantity of this depleting MAb is inadequate for modulating T-cell function at local sites of inflammation. Alternatively, T cells may not be important in the perpetuation of RA. Studies in progress with nondepleting humanized and primatized anti-CD4 MAb may help resolve these important issues.

Anti-CD52 Monoclonal Antibody

CD52 (Campath antigen) is present on all lymphocytes and some monocytes. The function of the CD52 antigen is unknown. Campath-1H, a humanized IgG1 rat MAb, has been evaluated in patients with RA in uncontrolled trials (7). Marked depletion of peripheral lymphocytes, primarily CD4 T cells, was observed. The prolonged depletion of peripheral CD4 cells probably precludes using adequate doses of this antibody to control disease. Despite the profound peripheral CD4 depletion, patients still had active disease, and, in some cases, numerous lymphocytes still remained in the synovial tissue.

Anti-CD7 Monoclonal Antibody

CD7 is a cell-surface antigen present on helper and suppressor T cells. Murine and chimeric anti-CD7 MAb have been evaluated in uncontrolled trials in a small number of patients with refractory RA. Although significant T lymphopenia occurred, no significant clinical improvement was noted.

Anti-CD5 Ricin Toxin Conjugate

CD5 is an antigen found on all T cells (helper and cytotoxic) and on a subset of B cells. A murine MAb to CD5 was linked to the A chain of ricin (a potent plant toxin that inhibits protein synthesis and directly kills cells) to create an anti-CD5 immunoconjugate with enhanced potency. This immunoconjugant has been evaluated in patients with refractory and early RA. The agent reversibly depleted circulating T cells and reversibly inhibited T-cell proliferative responses to antigens and mitogens. Side effects were common and included rash, fatigue, fever, nausea, vomiting, hypoalbuminemia, and myalgias. In addition, immune responses to the murine anti-CD5 MAb were often observed. Although the initial uncontrolled trials offered encouraging results, a placebo-controlled trial did not demonstrate significant clinical improvement in the treated groups compared with the placebo group.

Interleukin-2 Receptor-Directed Immunotherapy

To more specifically target T cells involved in the perpetuation of potentially pathogenetic immune responses, MAbs directed against cell-surface antigens expressed on activated T cells have been developed. Specifically, activated T cells express high-affinity IL-2 receptors (IL-2R or CD25), which are not expressed on resting T cells. IL-2R is also expressed on activated B cells. Activation antigens such as IL-2R represent attractive targets for selectively abrogating active immune responses without interfering with resting T cells. MAb to IL-2R has been shown to suppress rodent allograft rejection, murine lupus nephritis, and collagen-induced arthritis. Limited studies of a MAb to the IL-2 receptor in patients with RA showed modest benefit, however no controlled trials have been conducted.

Diphtheria interleukin-2 fusion protein (DAB-486 IL-2) is encoded by a chimeric gene that consists of the nucleotide sequence for the enzymatically active fragment A of diphtheria toxin DT and the membrane translocating portion of DT fragment B fused to the coding sequence for human IL-2. DAB-486 IL-2 binds avidly to IL-2R, is rapidly internalized, and then inhibits protein synthesis, which results in death of the targeted cells. In a placebo-controlled 1-month trial, five daily intravenous infusions of DAB-486 IL-2 were associated with modest but statistically significant clinical improvement (8). A subset of patients who received three monthly treatment courses in an open-label phase had significant improvements in clinical parameters. Toxicity associated with DAB-486 IL-2 included nausea, fever, and transient elevated transaminases. No significant decreases in peripheral CD25 T cells occurred, and therefore, the mechanism of action of this agent is unknown. A truncated version, DAB-389 IL-2 fusion protein, has also been evaluated in a refractory RA cohort. Again, a subset of patients improved. Agents that selectively inhibit activated T cells need to be evaluated further in RA patients with earlier disease to elucidate factors that may predict clinical response and define the mechanism(s) of action of such agents.

T-Cell Receptor Peptide Vaccine

More specific approaches to T-cell–directed immunotherapy of autoimmune diseases include identification of TCR gene products expressed by activated T-cell clones. This approach is based on the hypothesis that receptors on T cells specific for an inciting or perpetuating autoantigen share variable region determinants that are not expressed by most T cells. The majority of T cells express the αβ form of TCR on their surface. The individuality of T-cell clones is based on distinct amino acid sequences in the variable regions of the constituent TCR α and β chains. Analysis of T-cell repertoires in autoimmune diseases is an area of intense scientific interest, because MAb to specific autoreactive T cells or use of TCR peptides as vaccines potentially could be therapeutic.

In adjuvant arthritis, the disease can be transferred with T-cell clones specific for the inciting antigen. Small numbers of T cells are required, illustrating that very few antigen-specific T cells can initiate and maintain chronic arthritis. In type II collagen-induced arthritis, TCR Vβ families have been identified that appear to contribute to the pathogenesis of this disease. Administration of MAb to these TCRs suppressed the arthritis, whereas the administration of MAb to other Vβ regions was ineffective.

Vaccination using autoreactive T cells is effective in preventing arthritis in the rat adjuvant arthritis model and murine collagen-induced arthritis. T-cell vaccination in rat adjuvant arthritis not only protects animals from developing the disease, but it also induced remission of established disease. Vaccination with disease-associated TCR variable region peptides in an EAE model is also effective in preventing neurologic disease in these animal models. Synthetic TCR V-region peptides have been safely administered intradermally to patients with multiple sclerosis, and an immune response to these peptides was induced in some patients.

There is considerable interest in identifying disease-related TCR variable regions in patients with RA. At this time, a major problem with vaccination with TCR-derived peptides in human RA is the lack of definitive information concerning the nature of putative pathogenic T cells in RA and no clear evidence of an inciting agent. Nonetheless, analysis of activated synovial T cells in some patients indicates oligoclonal expansion of T cells bearing $V\beta_{14}$ and $V\beta_{17}$ TCR. Preliminary studies using recombinant $V\beta_{14}$ and $V\beta_{17}$ TCR peptides have been initiated to evaluate the safety of using this approach (9). No untoward adverse events have been noted. Placebo-controlled trials currently in progress using these peptides will provide further insight into their clinical usefulness.

B-Cell Receptors

The antigen receptor on B cells is the immunoglobulin molecule itself. Immunoglobulins consist of constant regions that are shared by several antibodies of a particular isotype and variable regions that include unique determinants called *idiotypes*. Immunoglobulins that react with the same antigenic epitope may express shared idiotypes. Therefore, B cells bearing the relevant cell-surface idiotype may be targeted with an anti-idiotype MAb and their function modulated. The potential therapeutic usefulness of anti-idiotypic MAb is suggested by studies in which a MAb directed against an idiotype shared by pathologic anti-DNA antibodies was used to successfully suppress nephritis in New Zealand B/W mice.

Antigen-Presenting Cells

Activation of specific T cells by antigen-presenting cells can also be prevented by agents that block recognition structures on the antigen-presenting cells. A reasonable target for this approach in RA would be major histocompatibility complex (MHC) class II antigens that are associated with disease (eg, HLA-DR1 and relevant HLA-DR4 subtypes). The recognition of antigen by CD4 T cells requires that antigens be presented as peptides to T cells in a complex with

self MHC class II gene products on antigen-presenting cells. MAb directed against appropriate disease-related MHC class II allelic products have been tested in several animal models of human autoimmune diseases. The mechanism underlying the apparent therapeutic effectiveness is unclear, but it seems unlikely that the effect can be entirely ascribed to physical blockade of the MHC class II molecule targeted, because effects are observed long after the antibody has been administered. MAb directed against MHC class II molecules might also deplete B cells (and perhaps other MHC class II–bearing cells) that could result in generalized, rather than selective, immunosuppression. An alternative approach is the construction of "designer pep-tides" that block antigen presentation–specific, disease-related MHC alleles without depleting B cells. Such an approach has successfully prevented EAE. Recently, DR4/DR1 peptides have been evaluated in a phase I study as a vaccine for treating RA, and these same peptides are now being tested in a larger phase II trial.

CYTOKINE TARGETS

The precise role(s) of cytokines in autoimmune diseases is still under investigation. The cytokines found in high quantities in RA synovial tissue and fluid, such as tumor necrosis factor α (TNF-α), IL-1, and IL-6, are pleiotropic in their biologic effects, and many of their biologic effects overlap (10). These cytokines have been targeted in clinical trials in RA patients (Table 55-2).

IL-1 likely plays a role in the pathogenesis of RA by virtue of its capacity to induce the release of metalloproteinases from chondrocytes and trigger prostaglandin E_2 (PGE_2) and collagenase production by synovial cells. In addition, IL-1 stimulates bone resorption, T-cell activation, the expression of adhesion molecules, and hepatic acute-phase protein synthesis. Therefore, inhibition of IL-1 activity is a logical strategy in an attempt to down-regulate the inflammatory process of RA.

Evidence supporting a role for TNF-α in the pathogenesis of RA includes the presence of TNF-α at the cartilage pannus junction and increased levels of TNF-α in RA synovial fluid. Furthermore, TNF-α production by synovial cells is increased in patients with active RA but not in patients with inactive RA. Several pro-inflammatory actions of TNF-α may contribute to its role in the pathogenesis of RA. In addition to stimulating the release of other pro-inflammatory cytokines including IL-6, IL-8, IL-1β, and leukemia in-

(Table 55-2)

Cytokine and adhesion molecule biologic agents tested in patients with rheumatoid arthritis*

Biologic Agent	Target
IL-1 receptor antagonist	IL-1
Soluble IL-1 receptor	IL-1
Soluble TNF receptor fusion proteins	TNF-α
Humanized anti-TNF MAb	TNF-α
Chimeric anti-TNF MAb	TNF-α
Murine anti-ICAM-1 MAb	ICAM-1
Murine anti-IL-6 MAb	IL-6

IL = interleukin; TNF = tumor necrosis factor.

hibitory factor (LIF), TNF-α also induces the release of proteases from neutrophils, fibroblasts, and chondrocytes. Furthermore, TNF-α induces expression of endothelial adhesion molecules, which leads to rapid transmigration of leukocytes into extravascular sites.

While IL-1 shares many activities with TNF-α, TNF-α appears to represent a more attractive therapeutic target because it may be a pivotal cytokine in regulating the expression of other inflammatory mediators in RA. This view is supported by observations that inhibition of TNF-α suppresses spontaneous production of IL-1, IL-6, and granulocyte–macrophage colony-stimulating factor (GM-CSF) by synovial cells, whereas inhibition of IL-1 does not diminish expression of TNF-α. As a result of these observations, there is increased interest in inhibiting TNF as a strategy to modulate TNF-α activity in patients with RA.

IL-1 Inhibition

Potential approaches to preventing the pathogenic effects of IL-1 in RA include blocking its production, binding IL-1, inhibiting receptor binding of IL-1, or altering intracellular responses triggered by IL-1. Two naturally occurring inhibitors of IL-1—interleukin-1 receptor antagonist (IL-1ra) and soluble IL-1 receptor (sIL-1R)—have been identified. Although these natural inhibitors of IL-1 are present at inflammatory sites, there is an imbalance toward IL-1 that favors the proinflammatory activities of IL-1.

IL-1ra is a specific inhibitor of IL-1 activity that functions by blocking the binding of IL-1 to its cell-surface receptors, but it does not possess agonist activity. Recombinant IL-1ra (rIL-1ra) blocks IL-1–induced degradation of proteoglycans and inhibition of glycosaminoglycan synthesis in bovine nasal cartilage explants. It prevents IL-1–induced synovial cell PGE_2 and collagenase secretion by chondrocytes. In addition, it reduces the severity of joint lesions in rat adjuvant arthritis, streptococcal cell-wall arthritis, and collagen-induced arthritis.

rIL-1ra has been evaluated in phase I and phase II trials in patients with RA. In the phase II multicenter double-blind trial, rIL-1ra was given for three weeks subcutaneously in various doses and frequencies. Clinical and biochemical responses (C-reactive protein [CRP]) were noted. Continued improvement occurred over the subsequent month with once-a-week injections. More recently, in a large double-blind, placebo-controlled trial of 6 months duration, there was significant improvement as defined by the American College of Rheumatology clinical response criteria. Further placebo-controlled trials are underway to evaluate the long-term efficacy and safety of this agent.

It is important to note two key issues regarding rIL-1ra as a therapy for RA. First, excess levels of IL-1ra—up to 100 times more than IL-1 levels—are required to inhibit the activities of IL-1. Essentially, all IL-1 receptors on cells must be occupied by IL-1ra if the functions of IL-1 are to be inhibited. Second, IL-1ra does not block the activities of TNF-α, and the ongoing proinflammatory activities of TNF can occur despite blocking IL-1.

Another approach being evaluated to inhibit IL-1 is using one of the two types of sIL-Rs, designated type I and type II. Recombinant sIL-1R type I (rhu sIL-1RI) has been shown to suppress the late-phase response of cutaneous allergy in humans and inflammation in animal models of arthritis, and it reduces the severity of paralysis and shortens the duration

of disease in a rat model of EAE. Recent data suggest that sIL-1R type I binds more avidly to IL-1ra than to IL-1β or IL-1α, whereas sIL-1R type II binds more avidly to IL-1α and IL-1β than it does to IL-1ra. Therefore, treatment with rhu sIL-1R1 potentially may shift the inflammatory balance toward an increased availability of IL-1, thus exacerbating an inflammatory response. However, clinical trials with rhu sIL-1R1 in RA, administered either intra-articularly or subcutaneously, have not demonstrated an exacerbation of disease (11). Results from a large placebo-controlled trial using rhu sIL-1R1 in patients with active RA did not demonstrate any improved clinical benefits in the treated patients versus those who received placebo.

TNF-α Inhibition

A chimeric anti-TNF MAb, cA2, has been tested in patients with RA. In an uncontrolled trial, 20 patients with active RA were treated with 20 mg/kg of cA2. Significant improvement in joint counts as well as decreases in serum CRP and IL-6 levels occurred within 6 weeks after treatment. These encouraging results were reproduced in a double-blind, placebo-controlled trial in which 19 of 24 patients treated with 10 mg/kg of cA2 and 11 of 25 patients treated with 1 mg/kg of cA2 achieved a 20% Paulus clinical response (ie, 20% improvement in painful and swollen joint counts plus improvement in at least 4 of 6 other disease activity parameters) at week 4 (12). More than 50% of the patients treated with 10 mg/kg of cA2 had greater than 50% Paulus clinical responses. Although retreatment with cA2 has been effective, development of antibodies to cA2 may incrementally limit the duration of subsequent treatment responses. A humanized anti-TNF MAb is being evaluated in patients with RA, and results from the phase I trial are also encouraging.

Another approach to inhibit the action of TNF-α is soluble TNF receptor (sTNFR) fusion proteins. There are two known membrane receptors for TNF-α, designated type I (p55/60) and type II (p75/80). sTNFR fusion proteins have been isolated and demonstrated to arise from the shed extracellular portion of the membrane-bound type I and type II molecules. Both p60 and p80 sTNFRs, as well as TNF-α have been detected in the synovial lining layers, and in the subsynovium.

The role of sTNFR in modulating inflammatory immune reactions is currently being investigated. Like the natural inhibitors of IL-1 (sIL-1R or IL-1ra), sTNFRs are thought to be natural inhibitors of TNF activity. There appears to be an imbalance of the sTNFRs and TNF-α at inflammatory sites (in favor of TNF-α). Therefore, one approach for treating RA is to administer recombinant sTNFR fusion proteins to inhibit the activities of TNF-α. Two recombinant sTNFR fusion protein products (p60 and p80) have been evaluated as potential therapies for RA. To increase the half-life, affinity, and bioavailability of the sTNFRs, the monomeric sTNFRs are fused to the Fc region of an immunoglobulin, forming a divalent recombinant TNFR fusion protein (rhu TNFR:Fc).

In animal model studies, the rhu TNFR:Fc p80 fusion protein was shown to reduce both the incidence and severity of collagen-induced arthritis. In a phase I dose escalation study of 16 refractory RA patients, rhu TNFR:Fc p80 was associated with a 44% mean improvement in total pain and total joint scores in patients receiving the active drug compared with 22% improvement in patients receiving placebo (13). In addition, biochemical markers of CRP significantly decreased in the patients receiving the highest dose of this fusion protein. A large placebo-controlled trial has confirmed these initial results. RA patients who received the highest dose had more than 60% improvement in swollen and tender joint counts after 3 months of treatment. Further placebo-controlled trials are in progress to evaluate the long-term efficacy and safety of sTNFR fusion proteins as potential therapies for RA.

Interleukin-6 Inhibition

Interleukin-6 induces B-cell differentiation, activates T cells, and induces acute-phase protein synthesis in hepatocytes. However, there is evidence that IL-6 also has anti-inflammatory properties that include induction of IL-1ra and sTNFR (p55) and inhibition of lipopolysaccharide-induced TNF-α and IL-1β production in cultured human monocytes. In an uncontrolled trial, an anti-IL-6 MAb was given to five patients with RA who had also received a murine anti-CD4 MAb. Serum IL-6 levels unexpectedly increased in four of these patients who improved clinically. Therefore, the role of IL-6 in inflammatory disorders such as RA is not clear.

Interferon Therapy

Recombinant interferons have been evaluated in a variety of autoimmune disorders. Interferon gamma (IFN-γ) was the first biologic agent evaluated for the treatment of RA. IFN-γ has several potential relevant properties including its ability to inhibit B-cell activation and cytokine production by macrophages and monocytes, as well as its antiproliferative effects. However, IFN-γ can induce and enhance the expression of MHC class II antigens on cells, which might be anticipated to aggravate autoimmune disorders such as RA. In addition, there are conflicting reports from studies of animal models of arthritis regarding whether treatment with IFN-γ resulted in worsening or improvement of disease.

Several uncontrolled clinical trials and double-blind placebo-controlled trials to determine the efficacy of recombinant IFN-γ for the treatment of RA have been completed (14). Overall, minimal clinical improvement was noted except in one study. Administration of recombinant IFN-γ resulted in disease exacerbation in several patients with multiple sclerosis and in one patient with systemic lupus erythematosus (SLE). In addition, in the NZB/NZW F1 animal model of lupus nephritis, treatment with recombinant IFN-γ accelerated the development of glomerulonephritis, whereas administration of an anti-IFN-γ MAb resulted in substantial clinical improvement characterized by marked decreases in proteinuria, delay in DNA antibody production, and increased survival rate.

Interferon alpha (IFN-α) has also been evaluated as a potential therapeutic agent for the treatment of both hepatitis B and C. Double-blind placebo-controlled trials have now confirmed the usefulness of recombinant IFN-α for the treatment of hepatitis C. However, relapses after completion of the trials occurred in more than 50% of the patients treated with 3 million units three times a week for 6 months. Evidence suggests that treatment with recombinant IFN-α has beneficial effects in patients with hepatitis C-related cryoglobulinemia. The efficacy of IFN-α in treating cryoglobulinemia is probably attributable to its antiviral activity, rather than immunomodulatory characteristics. Small uncontrolled trials have been conducted with IFN-α in Beh-

çet's syndrome, RA, hepatitis B-related arthritis, and hepatitis B-related polyarteritis nodosa. Encouraging results from these pilot studies will need to be confirmed in larger controlled trials.

Recombinant interferon beta (IFN-β) is approved by the Food and Drug Administration for the treatment of remitting/relapsing multiple sclerosis. This agent was shown to significantly reduce both the rate of exacerbations and the number of new lesions, as detected by serial magnetic resonance imaging in patients with relapsing/remitting forms of multiple sclerosis. Potential mechanisms by which IFN-β may work in multiple sclerosis include inhibition of viral replication, antiproliferative mechanisms, and immunomodulatory activities, such as up-regulation of IL-4.

ADHESION MOLECULES

The pattern of expression of cell adhesion molecules on endothelial cells and their respective ligands on the surfaces of circulating leukocytes appears to determine the site of leukocyte emigration from the intravascular space and the nature of the leukocyte populations attracted into the inflammatory lesion. Selectins appear to play a central role in promoting the initial interaction between activated endothelial cells and circulating leukocytes, a phenomenon referred to as "rolling." Regarding lymphocytes, the precise sequence of events involved in endothelial cell binding and transmigration has not been precisely established. There is evidence that interaction of the β integrin leukocyte function antigen-1 (LFA-1) with its ligand, intercellular adhesion molecule-1 (ICAM-1), can mediate transendothelial migration of T cells.

Several animal models have provided insights regarding the importance of adhesion molecules in inflammatory responses. Murine MAb to LFA-1 β chain (anti-CD18) and to ICAM-1 (anti-CD54) inhibited neutrophil migration into the lungs in rabbits with phorbol myristic acetate-induced lung inflammation. Anti-CD18 has also been shown to inhibit inflammation in a rabbit model of antigen-induced arthritis. In addition, treatment with anti-CD54 MAb resulted in significant amelioration of chronic inflammation in this animal model.

In an open-label study, 32 patients with RA were treated with varying doses of a murine anti-ICAM-1 MAb (15). Clinical improvement of disease activity was noted in approximately one-half of the patients receiving high doses of the MAb. Side effects were common and included headache, fever, nausea and vomiting, and skin reactions. Human antimouse antibody responses were common and precluded retreatment with this murine MAb. Treatment with anti-ICAM-1 MAb induced T-cell hyporesponsiveness that correlated with the therapeutic benefit. Further trials are warranted to determine the usefulness of other (ie, nonmurine) types of anti-adhesion molecules as potential therapies for RA.

ORAL TOLERIZATION

Oral administration of putative autoantigens such as collagen, myelin basic protein, insulin, and protein S is effective in blocking the induction of disease or ameliorating established disease in animal models of autoimmune disease including collagen-induced arthritis, EAE, diabetes mellitus, and autoimmune uveitis. The mechanisms underlying oral tolerance, or "antigen-driven bystander suppression," may involve clonal anergy or deletion, or it may involve induction of regulatory cells at the site of inflammation that are capable of producing anti-inflammatory cytokines such as IL-4, IL-10, or transforming growth factor beta (TGF-β). The encouraging results in animal models have prompted an interest in the oral administration of autoantigens as a therapy for human autoimmune diseases including multiple sclerosis, RA, uveitis, and diabetes mellitus. In a controlled trial with 60 RA patients, small doses of solubilized chicken type II collagen or placebo were given for 3 months. Statistically significant improvements were noted in the treated group in several disease activity parameters (16). A larger placebo-controlled trial evaluating the efficacy of oral administration of type II collagen as a therapy for RA is underway. Biologic effects of oral collagen have not yet been demonstrated in humans.

OTHER POTENTIAL THERAPIES

Ongoing efforts to evaluate nondepleting anti-CD4 MAb will be important to determine whether these antibodies can induce tolerance or can be given in high enough doses to produce clinical efficacy. Other potential cellular and cytokine therapies that have been tested in animal models of autoimmune diseases include anti-gp39 antibodies, anti-B7 antibodies, CTLA-4 immunoglobulin fusion protein, recombinant IL-4, and recombinant IL-10.

IL-10 and IL-4 are regulatory cytokines that have the potential for modulating autoimmune diseases. Specifically, IL-10 inhibits many functions of macrophages, including release of IL-1, IL-6, IL-8, TNF-α, and other proinflammatory cytokines, while stimulating production of anti-inflammatory cytokines IL-1ra and sTNFRs. Recombinant IL-10 is currently being evaluated in humans with inflammatory bowel disease and RA.

CONCLUSION

Thus far, biologic therapies aimed at cellular targets have not provided significant clinical benefit in patients with RA in the trials completed to date. Nondepleting anti-CD4 MAbs that perhaps can induce tolerance and can be given at higher doses have the potential of inducing immunosuppression. Other cellular targets, including B7 and gp39 antigens, offer potential therapeutic approaches.

The recent encouraging results with TNF-α and IL-1 inhibitors using Mab, rhu TNFR:Fc p80, and IL-1ra in short-term clinical trials need to be evaluated for their ability to provide long-term disease modification. Gene therapy provides another potential approach to treating autoimmune disorders. The goal is to target expression of anti-inflammatory molecules to involved synovial tissue. Candidate molecules include cytokine antagonists such as rIL-1ra and sTNFR. The feasibility of this approach has been tested in animal models using rIL-1ra (17). Combinations of anti-CD4 and anti-TNF MAb have yielded synergistic benefit in animal models of autoimmune disease, and using combinations of biologic agents in humans with RA will be of considerable interest in the future. Other recombinant cytokines

such as IL-10 and IL-4 are now being evaluated in early phase I trials in RA.

LARRY W. MORELAND, MD
WILLIAM J. KOOPMAN, MD

1. Koopman WJ, Gay S: Do nonimmunologically mediated pathways play a role in the pathogenesis of rheumatoid arthritis? Rheum Dis Clin North Am 19:107-122, 1993

2. Ranges GE, Sriram S, Cooper SM: Prevention of type II collagen-induced arthritis by in vivo treatment with anti-L3T4. J Exp Med 162:1105-1110, 1985

3. Carteron NL, Schimenti CL, Wofsy D: Treatment of murine lupus with F(ab')2 fragments of monoclonal antibody to L3T4: suppression of autoimmunity does not depend on T-helper cell depletion. J Immunol 142:1470-1475, 1989

4. Moreland LW, Bucy RP, Pratt PW, Tilden A, LoBuglio AF, Khazaeli M, Everson M, Sanders ME, Allen E, Kilgariff C, Khrayeb I, Daddona P, Koopman WJ: Use of a chimeric monoclonal anti-CD4 antibody in patients with refractory rheumatoid arthritis. Arthritis Rheum 36:307-318, 1993

5. Moreland LW, Pratt PW, Mayes M, Postlethwaits A, Weisman M, Schnitzer T, Lightfoot R, Calabrese L, Woody JN, Koopman WJ: Double-blind, placebo controlled multicenter trial using chimeric monoclonal anti-CD4 antibody in rheumatoid arthritis patients receiving concomitant methotrexate. Arthritis Rheum 38:1581-1588, 1995

6. van der Lubbe PA, Dijkmans BAC, Markusse HM, Nassander U, Breedveld FC: A randomized, double-blind, placebo-controlled study of CD4 monoclonal antibody therapy in early rheumatoid arthritis. Arthritis Rheum 38:1097-1106, 1995

7. Weinblatt ME, Maddison PJ, Bulpitt KJ, Hazleman BL, Urowitz MB, Sturrock RD, Coblyn JS, Maier AL, Spreen WR, Manna VK, Johnston JM: Campath-1H: a humanized monoclonal antibody, in refractory rheumatoid arthritis. An intravenous dose-escalation study. Arthritis Rheum 38:1589-1594, 1995

8. Moreland LW, Sewell KL, Trentham DE, Sullivan WF, Shmerling RH, Bucy RP, Parker KC, Swartz WG, Woodworth TG, Koopman WJ: Diphtheria-interleukin-2 fusion protein (DAB486IL-2) in refractory rheumatoid arthritis: a double-blind placebo-controlled trial with open label extension. Arthritis Rheum 38:1177-1186, 1995

9. Moreland LW, Heck LW, Koopman WJ, Saway PA, Adamson TC, Fronek Z, O'Connor RD, Morgan EE, Dively JD, Chieffo NM, Freeman TD, Richieri SP, Carlo DJ, Brostoff SW: Vβ17 T cell receptor peptide vaccine: results of a phase I dose finding study in patients with rheumatoid arthritis. Ann NY Acad Sci 756:211-214, 1995

10. Arend WP, Dayer JM: Inhibition of the production and effects of interleukin-1 and tumor necrosis factor α in rheumatoid arthritis. Arthritis Rheum 38:151-160, 1995

11. Drevlow BE, Lovis R, Haag MA, Sinacore JM, Jacobs C, Blosch C, Beck C, Landay A, Moreland LW, Pope RM: Recombinant human interleukin-1 receptor, type 1 (rhu IL-1R1) in the treatment of patients with active rheumatoid arthritis. Arthritis Rheum 39:257-265, 1996

12. Elliott MJ, Maini RN, Feldman M, Kalden JR, Antoni C, Smolen JS, Leeb B, Breedveld FC, MacFarlane JD, Bijl H, Woody JN: Randomized double-blind comparison of chimeric monoclonal antibody to tumor necrosis factor alpha (cA2) versus placebo in rheumatoid arthritis. Lancet 344:1105-1110, 1994

13. Moreland LW, Margolies GR, Heck LW, Saway A, Blosch C, Hanna R, Koopman WJ: Recombinant soluble tumor necrosis factor receptor (p80) fusimprotein: toxicity and dose finding trial in refractory rheumatoid arthritis. J Rheumatol 23:1849-1855, 1996

14. Cannon GW, Pincus SH, Emkey RD, Denes A, Cohen SA, Wolfe F, Saway PA, Jaffer TM, Weaver AL, Cogen L, Schindler JD: Double-blind trial of recombinant gamma-interferon versus placebo in the treatment of rheumatoid arthritis. Arthritis Rheum 32:966-973, 1989

15. Kavanaugh AF, Davis LS, Nichols LA, Norris SH, Rothlein R, Scharschmidt LA, Lipsky PE: Treatment of refractory rheumatoid arthritis with a monoclonal antibody to intercellular adhesion molecule 1. Arthritis Rheum 37:992-999, 1994

16. Trentham DE, Dynesius-Trentham RA, Orav EJ, Combitchi D, Lorenzo C, Sewell KL, Hafler DA, Weiner HL: Effects of oral administration of type II collagen on rheumatoid arthritis. Science 261:1727-1730, 1993

17. Evans C, Robbins PD: Prospects for treating arthritis by gene therapy. J Rheumatol 21:779-782, 1994

56

OPERATIVE TREATMENT OF RHEUMATIC DISEASE

Operative treatments that can effectively relieve pain and improve function in patients with arthritis include joint debridement, synovectomy, osteotomy, soft tissue arthroplasty, resection arthroplasty, fusion, and joint replacement (1–3). In addition, patients with rheumatoid arthritis (RA) may benefit from tenosynovectomy and repair or reconstruction of tendons. Patients with arthritis should be evaluated for possible surgical treatment before they develop advanced deformity, joint disability, contractures, or muscle atrophy that might compromise the results of operative treatment and increase the risks of complications. Although operative treatments of arthritis can dramatically improve the quality of life for many individuals, they also expose patients to serious risks. Potential operative and perioperative complications include blood loss, cardiac arrhythmia and arrest, nerve and blood vessel injury, infection, venous thrombosis, and pulmonary embolism. Late postoperative complications include delayed infection and loosening and wear of implants. Furthermore, the benefits of surgical procedures, including synovectomies, joint debridement, and osteotomies, may deteriorate with time. For these reasons, the potential risks and expected short-term and long-term outcomes of operative treatment must be carefully evaluated for each patient.

PREOPERATIVE EVALUATION

With the exception of patients in whom arthritic disorders have caused or may cause spinal instability and neurologic damage, operative treatment of patients with arthritis is elective. Thus, patients should have an extensive preoperative evaluation and should understand the full range of therapeutic options. Consideration of surgical intervention requires a thorough understanding of the degree of pain and functional limitation, as perceived by the patient, as well as an understanding of the patient's social and occupational needs and expectations. Before planning surgery, patients should understand the potential benefits and risks of operative treatment. In general, the patients most likely to derive lasting benefit from operative treatment are those with joint pain unrelieved by nonsurgical treatment. The patient's age, overall health status, and capacity to comply with postoperative rehabilitation and precautions also help determine the outcome of operative treatment.

Failure to carefully evaluate the cause of the symptoms can lead to disappointing results, despite technically excellent operative treatment. Common diagnostic dilemmas include differentiating hip joint pain from lumbar radicular pain and shoulder joint pain from cervical radicular pain. Patients with RA may have a septic joint that is not readily apparent because of the inflammatory nature of the disease and the use of medications that suppress the inflammatory response. A careful history, physical examination, and plain radiographs are sufficient to define the cause of symptoms for most patients, but joint aspiration, electrodiagnostic studies, and additional imaging studies are needed to clarify the cause of pain and loss of function in some patients.

Before being considered for surgical intervention, patients should complete a regimen of nonoperative treatments including drug therapy, ambulatory aides, activity modification, physical therapy, and orthoses. Braces may control instability and decrease pain in the spine, knee, ankle, wrist, or thumb. A cane may be considered for patients with lower extremity arthritis. Weight reduction often decreases obese patients' symptoms and increases the probability of successful operative treatment. Some evidence suggests that obese patients have an increased incidence of infection and increased intraoperative blood loss following total joint arthroplasty (4,5). However, some overweight patients find that the pain and loss of mobility caused by arthritis make it more difficult to reduce weight or avoid gaining weight. In these individuals, surgeons may recommend proceeding with operative treatment, despite the increased risks associated with obesity.

The importance of a thorough preoperative history and physical examination, as well as careful perioperative medical management, cannot be overemphasized. Patients may have serious cardiac, pulmonary, renal, or peripheral vascular disorders that require evaluation and treatment before they undergo surgery. Carious teeth, pharyngitis, cystitis, and other potential sources of infection should be treated before surgery. Men with symptoms of prostatic hypertrophy need a urologic evaluation before surgery, and women should be evaluated for asymptomatic urinary tract infections. All patients should receive instructions about the planned procedure, the risks and common complications, the type and extent of postoperative rehabilitation, and expectations for postoperative pain relief and function.

DISEASE-RELATED FACTORS

Operative treatment options, indications for surgical treatment, preoperative evaluation and preparation, complications and outcomes vary considerably among rheumatic diseases. Thus, the physician must consider the unique features of each disease in making decisions or advising patients about operative treatment.

Osteoarthritis

A number of current surgical procedures can decrease symptoms for patients with osteoarthritis (OA) while preserving or restoring a cartilaginous articular surface. These procedures include arthroscopic joint debridement, resection or perforation of subchondral bone to stimulate formation of cartilaginous tissue, and use of grafts to replace degenerated articular cartilage (1). By removing loose fragments of cartilage, bone, meniscus, and, in some instances, osteophytes, joint debridement may improve joint mechanical function and may decrease pain in some patients.

Osteotomies realign joints and thereby redistribute joint loads. Surgeons plan these procedures to correct malalignment and shift loads from severely degenerated regions of the articular surface to regions that have remaining articular cartilage. In selected patients with OA, osteotomies of the hip and knee decrease pain, but, in general, the results from this procedure are less predictable than from joint replacement. For these reasons, surgeons most commonly recommend osteotomies for young active people who have a stable joint with a functional range of motion, good muscle function, and some remaining articular cartilage.

Joint fusion (arthrodesis) can relieve pain and restore skeletal stability and alignment in patients with advanced OA. Because this procedure eliminates joint motion, it has limited application. Furthermore, fusion of one joint increases the loading and motion of other joints and may thereby accelerate degeneration of these joints. For example, fusion of the hip increases the probability of developing degenerative disease in the lumbar spine and ipsilateral knee joint. Currently, most arthrodeses are performed for degeneration of cervical and lumbar spine, wrist and ankle, inter-

phalangeal and metatarsophalangeal joints of the hands and feet.

For selected joints, resection of degenerated articular surfaces and replacement with implants fabricated from polyethylene, metal, or other synthetic materials can relieve pain and allow the patient to maintain joint mobility (Fig. 56-1). Over the past several decades, replacement of the hip and knee have proved to be effective methods of relieving pain and maintaining or improving function. Joint replacements, however, have limitations. None of the currently available synthetic materials duplicates the ability of articular cartilage to provide a painless, low-friction gliding surface and to distribute loads across the joint, nor do current implants create a bond as stable and durable as that between articular cartilage and bone. Thus, the wear on implants limits their lifespan, and loosening can lead to failure.

Rheumatoid Arthritis

Patients with RA require careful evaluation to prevent operative and perioperative neurologic injury, establish the sequence and timing of joints to be treated surgically, and reduce the risks of infection and other complications.

Cervical spine involvement, especially atlantoaxial subluxation, is common in RA and can lead to spinal instability

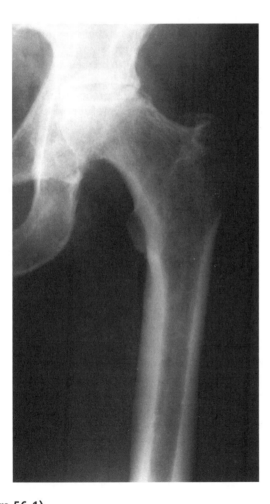
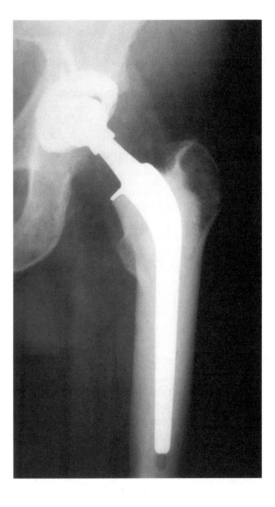

(Figure 56-1)
*Left: Radiograph of the left hip of a 52-year-old man with osteonecrosis and advanced osteoarthritis. Loss of articular cartilage has reduced the joint space to a thin line. The patient has severe hip pain and minimal hip motion. **Right:** Radiograph after the joint has been resected and replaced with a metal femoral component fixed with methylmethacrylate cement and an uncemented metal acetabular component containing a polyethylene liner. The patient no longer has hip pain and lacks only a few degrees of normal hip motion.*

and increased risk of neurologic deficits. Neurologic changes may be difficult to recognize because of limited joint motion and associated disuse muscle atrophy. To evaluate the risk of neurologic injury, patients should have active flexion and extension lateral cervical radiographs within a year before surgery. In a retrospective review of 113 patients with RA who underwent total hip or knee arthroplasty, Collins et al (6) reported significant atlantoaxial subluxation, atlantoaxial impaction, and/or subaxial subluxation in 69 patients (61%). Thirty-five of these 69 patients (50%) had no clinical signs or symptoms of instability at the time of admission for joint replacement arthroplasty. Instability of greater than 7–10 mm at the atlantoaxial joint or greater than 4 mm at subaxial levels on flexion and extension lateral radiographs generally requires stabilization before other elective surgery is performed. Patients with lesser degrees of atlantoaxial and subaxial involvement should be evaluated by the anesthesiologist preoperatively and consideration given to an awake intubation.

Patients with involvement of several joints require careful planning and timing of various joint procedures in order to allow optimal rehabilitation. For example, patients scheduled for lower extremity surgery may require surgical stabilization of the upper extremity first to allow crutch ambulation and use of the upper extremities to assist with transfers, rising from a chair, and stair climbing. The patient with multiple lower extremity joint involvement may benefit from having joints treated sequentially or simultaneously, depending on the joints involved and the severity of the disease. The patient with severe disease and contractures of both knees may benefit from having both knees replaced at the same time. If only one knee is replaced, a flexion contracture in the untreated knee will cause the patient to keep the operatively treated knee flexed when standing and thereby compromise rehabilitation following surgery. Foot and ankle disease are generally addressed before hip and knee arthroplasty to provide the patient with a stable lower extremity on which to stand and rehabilitate the hip and knee.

Long-term use of corticosteroids increases the complexity of surgical treatment. Patients may require "stress dose" steroids perioperatively because their adrenal function is inhibited. Long-term corticosteroid use combined with the effects of the disease can cause connective tissue changes that make the skin and superficial blood vessels friable. Extreme caution must be used in physically handling such a patient, because even mild pressure can cause a hematoma or skin ulceration, and adhesive tape can tear the skin. In addition, patients with RA treated with total joint arthroplasties have a higher incidence of infection than patients with OA (4). Whether these infections are due to corticosteroids or immunologic complications of the disease itself is unclear. Patients with RA frequently have more than one joint arthroplasty, and infection of one arthroplasty is associated with an increased incidence of subsequent infection of another total joint (7).

Juvenile Rheumatoid Arthritis

Most patients with juvenile rheumatoid arthritis (JRA) are skeletally immature and therefore can develop growth disturbances. Limb-length discrepancy is not uncommon, particularly in younger patients who have growth acceleration around an involved joint. Moreover, functional limb-length

may be compromised by joint contractures. Fortunately, the great majority of limb length discrepancies stabilize by adulthood and do not require equalizing procedures. Joint replacement arthroplasty, reserved for patients who are debilitated by pain or decreased function, is generally delayed until patients are skeletally mature. Joint replacement is also delayed because the life expectancy of a young patient is greater than that of current prostheses. Moreover, each subsequent revision surgery necessarily involves greater periprosthetic bone loss and less predictable long-term results. Patients with juvenile RA may benefit from tendon lengthening to correct contractures and prophylactic procedures, such as synovectomy, to alleviate symptoms and possibly delay articular destruction.

Osteonecrosis

Most surgical treatments of osteonecrosis have been developed for treatment of the hip. Core decompression (ie, drilling a channel from the lateral surface of the femur into the necrotic region of the femoral head), with or without bone grafting, has been advocated for patients who have femoral osteonecrosis without collapse or acetabular changes. In most series, these procedures have decreased pain in a high percentage of patients. This treatment is generally considered ineffective in patients whose femoral head shows any signs of collapse. Less commonly used treatments include femoral osteotomies, designed to place an intact segment of the femoral head in a weight-bearing position, and hip arthrodesis. Total hip replacement has produced excellent results in patients with osteonecrosis, but durability of the prosthesis is a concern, particularly for young patients.

Ankylosing Spondylitis

Joint replacements decrease pain and improve function for patients with advanced joint disease due to ankylosing spondylitis, and some patients can benefit from osteotomies that correct spinal deformities. Patients with ankylosing spondylitis present operative and perioperative challenges. Spinal involvement can lead to extensive ligamentous calcification and heterotopic ossification, which make regional anesthesia difficult, if not impossible. Patients with prolonged disease also develop severe kyphotic deformities of the cervical, thoracic, and lumbar spine, which can impede endotracheal intubation. Restricted chest excursion may further complicate intraoperative and postoperative care.

Patients with ankylosing spondylitis, as well as those with diffuse idiopathic skeletal hyperostosis and post-traumatic osteoarthrosis, are at increased risk for postoperative heterotopic ossification. Gains in total range of motion are often limited by periarticular heterotopic ossification, long-standing soft tissue contractures, and muscle atrophy. Prospective evaluations have proved the efficacy of fractionated and single low-dose radiation therapy to the hip and abductor musculature when begun early in the postoperative period.

Psoriatic Arthritis

A unique perioperative risk in patients with psoriatic arthritis is the development of a flare of psoriasis at the operative site as a result of the physiologic and/or psychologic stress of surgery. In addition, these patients may have an increased incidence of postoperative infections. Menon and Wroblewski (8) reported superficial wound infection in 9.1% and deep-wound infections in 5.5% of their 38 patients with psoriatic arthritis treated with total hip arthroplasty.

Hemophilic Arthropathy

Despite the risk of excessive bleeding, operative treatment can produce good results in patients with hemophilic arthropathy. Synovectomy, commonly performed in the knee and elbow, improves range of motion and decreases pain in most patients. Total knee and total hip replacements can improve function and relieve pain in patients with advanced joint degeneration (9,10).

Patients with hemophilic arthropathy may be particularly difficult to manage perioperatively. Factor replacement has risks and must be carefully monitored. A thrombotic event may be precipitated by repeated factor infusions, and disseminated intravascular coagulation after elective surgery has been reported. A subgroup of patients with high levels of factor antibody are generally contraindicated for major elective surgery.

It is unclear whether well-controlled hemophilic patients who are not infected with human immunodeficiency virus (HIV) are at increased risk for nontransfusion-related infection. Septic arthritis has been reported as a rare complication of hemophilia, but one that must be promptly distinguish from an acute hemarthrosis and definitively treated.

Enteropathic Arthropathy

Patients with inflammatory bowel disease are at increased risk of perioperative and late infections, particularly when orthopedic implants are used. Infection may occur by hematogenous seeding or direct contamination via a fistula or colostomy.

Pigmented Villonodular Synovitis

This disorder most commonly involves the knee and has been reported in patients ranging in age from the second to the ninth decade. Synovectomy, by arthrotomy or arthroscopy, usually provides symptomatic relief, and may be curative in patients with the localized form of disease. The diffuse form of pigmented villonodular synovitis responds less favorably to synovectomy, with recurrences in more than one-third of patients.

Synovial Chondromatosis

This rare condition results in the formation of cartilaginous fragments that may lie in synovial joint cavities, the synovium, or, in some instances, in the periarticular soft tissues. Synovial chondromatosis causes joint pain, joint catching and locking, loss of motion, and can lead to degeneration of the articular surfaces. Removal of intra-articular loose bodies and, in some instances, synovectomy can relieve symptoms and improve motion in patients who have not developed degenerative joint disease (11). However, in many joints the cartilage fragments re-accumulate. In patients with degenerative joint disease, joint replacement combined with synovectomy can cure the disease.

SITES OF SURGICAL INTERVENTION

The operative treatments that provide the best results vary not only among rheumatic diseases and patients, but also among anatomic sites. Thus, the most appropriate procedure should be chosen based on the joint involved, as well as the type of disorder, the patient's age, and other social and medical factors.

Hip

The most common operative treatments for arthritis of the hip are cemented (ie, inserted with polymethylmethacrylate cement) and uncemented total hip arthroplasty. More than 120,000 hip prostheses are implanted in the United States each year (12) (Fig. 56-1). Nearly 30 years of clinical studies now document the success of total hip replacement for the treatment of disabling pain and impairment in a wide variety of hip disease (13). Initially, surgeons limited hip replacement to patients between 60 and 75 years of age, but over the past decade, studies have shown that younger and more elderly patients also can benefit from this procedure (2,3).

The risk of postoperative venous thrombosis and infection after hip replacement has significantly decreased in the past two decades (14). Loosening of the joint remains the predominant cause of long-term failure (Fig. 56-2). Improvements in cement techniques have decreased the incidence of aseptic femoral loosening from as high as 40% to less than 5% 10 years after the procedure for many groups of patients (15). In contrast, cemented acetabular components continue to have a high rate of loosening, despite improved cement techniques. Preliminary reviews of the results with uncemented acetabular components suggest that they may have better results.

Despite its great success, total hip arthroplasty has important limitations, particularly for a young patient who is likely to outlive the prosthesis. Alternatives to arthroplasty include osteotomy, arthrodesis, and resection arthroplasty. Femoral and pelvic osteotomies have been shown to be effective in relieving pain in young patients with acetabular dysplasia and minimal or no radiographic degenerative change. Results are less favorable in patients over 40 years of age and in those with significant degenerative changes. Arthrodesis of the hip offers young patients with hip arthritis a dependable, durable, pain-free hip. Once fusion is obtained, the patient may return to vigorous physical activity without the limitations imposed on arthroplasty patients. Resection arthroplasty is seldom performed as a primary procedure today. It is generally reserved for salvage of a failed hip arthroplasty that is not amenable to revision.

Knee

Arthroscopy has advanced the treatment of many forms of knee arthritis. It is particularly useful for patients whose symptoms may be attributed to a specific mechanical etiology, such as a meniscus tear or loose body. Arthroscopic synovectomy can decrease pain and swelling for patients with hemophilia, pigmented villonodular synovitis, synovial chondromatosis, and early RA without significant cartilage erosion. Arthroscopic debridement or chondroplasty for degenerative knee arthritis, unless complicated by a degenerative meniscal tear or intra-articular loose bodies,

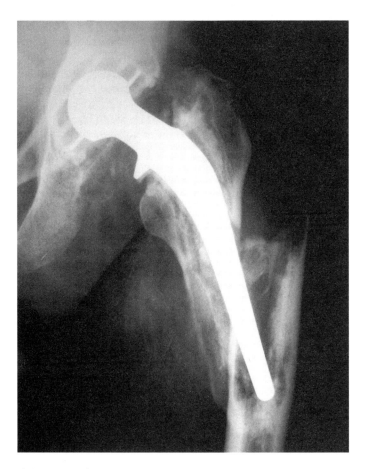

(Figure 56-2)
Radiograph showing a left hip replacement with bone resorption around the femoral bone cement, loosening of the prosthesis, and a fracture through the proximal femur. This 67-year-old man had a hip replacement 14 years ago, but was not evaluated for the past 7 years. Despite the development of severe periprosthetic osteolysis, he did not notice any problems with his hip until he tripped on an electrical cord and sustained the fracture. Earlier detection of the asymptomatic osteolysis followed by surgical revision would have prevented the fracture and extensive loss of bone.

may provide short-term relief of symptoms in selected patients (11).

Osteotomy about the knee is intended to redirect the weight-bearing axis away from a degenerative portion of the tibiofemoral joint and may also stimulate development of fibrocartilage in the unloaded degenerative compartment (1). Most of these procedures are valgus osteotomies of the proximal tibia, performed to redirect weight-bearing forces from a degenerative medial tibiofemoral articulation through a better-preserved lateral compartment. Femoral osteotomies are preferred for valgus and excessive varus deformities of the knee. Osteotomies are generally chosen over total knee arthroplasties for young, heavy, active patients and should be reserved for patients with noninflammatory disease (16).

Total knee or hip arthroplasties may be performed with cement or bone ingrowth as the means of fixation. Several large series have demonstrated that tibial and femoral results are excellent regardless of the type of fixation (17). Patellar problems are the leading cause of failure after total knee arthroplasty.

Knee arthrodesis is an option for patients with recalcitrant infection or for failed total knee arthroplasty that cannot be effectively revised. Despite loss of knee motion, a functional lower extremity that permits painless weight bearing can be expected with the use of current techniques.

Foot and Ankle

Surgical options for the foot and ankle include cheilectomy (resection of an osteophyte), arthroscopic debridement, osteotomy, arthrodesis, and replacement arthroplasty.

Osteophytes may develop at the periphery of a joint and cause symptoms related to impingement during normal walking. The osteophytes occur on the dorsum of the first metatarsophalangeal joint and the anterior aspect of the tibiotalar joint. Cheilectomy often provides relief of mechanical symptoms and associated pain. Loose bodies may also be a source of mechanical symptoms and are amenable to arthroscopic removal.

Arthrodeses of the foot and ankle offer pain relief and stability for patients with severe arthritis. Fusions of these joints are well tolerated, even by children, despite some restriction of stressful activities such as hill climbing and running. Infection and delayed wound healing have been reported in 25%–40% of patients with RA who undergo tibiotalar arthrodesis, yet most patients have excellent long-term results.

Unlike total replacement arthroplasty of the hip and knee, ankle replacement arthroplasties have not produced predictable results. Most surgeons now limit the use of this procedure to treatment of inflammatory arthritis in minimally active elderly patients who have multiple joint involvement.

Hand and Wrist

When considering surgical interventions of the hand and wrist, clinicians should obtain a history of the patient's functional abilities, carefully noting any recent changes. Inability to actively flex or extend interphalangeal (IP) or metacarpophalangeal joints (MCP) when passive motion is preserved usually signals a ruptured tendon. Tenosynovectomy not only decreases pain and increases range of motion and grip strength, but also appears to protect the tendons, particularly when combined with resection of abnormal bony prominences. Acute tendon ruptures should be evaluated promptly by a surgeon before fibrosis and contractures develop. In the rheumatoid hand, the MCP joints are frequently reconstructed with silicone implants that function as flexible spacers.

Arthrodesis is commonly performed in the IP joints, carpus, and wrist for end-stage joint degeneration in most rheumatic disorders. Interphalangeal joints are best managed with arthrodesis in a partially flexed position. Surgeons rarely recommend arthrodesis of arthritic thumb carpometacarpal joints, because motion of these joints is particularly important for overall hand function. The degenerative thumb carpometacarpal joint is amenable to interposition arthroplasty, which yields excellent pain relief and increased grip strength.

Experience with arthroplasty of the wrist is limited, partially because the predictable results can be obtained with wrist fusion. Wrist arthroplasty designs have yielded improved clinical outcome, but component failure remains a problem (18).

Elbow

Arthritis involving primarily the radiohumeral articulation is not uncommon in RA and post-traumatic joint disease. Radial head resection offers increased range of motion and decreased pain in appropriately selected patients (19). Synovectomy may be performed alone or in conjunction with other procedures, such as radial head resection. Arthroscopy has been used effectively to perform synovectomies as well as to remove loose bodies and osteophytes from arthritic elbows. Elbow joint replacement arthroplasty, while newer than hip and knee arthroplasty, has developed rapidly (20).

Shoulder

Arthrodesis of the shoulder yields excellent pain relief and provides a stable upper extremity with long-term durability for young patients with severe glenohumeral arthritis. Fusion is reliably obtained in the majority of patients with relatively few complications. Despite rigid fusion of the glenohumeral joint, abduction of 50 degrees and flexion of 40 degrees in the shoulder girdle are possible via scapulothoracic motion.

Total shoulder arthroplasties provide effective pain relief and improved general functions of daily living for a high proportion of patients. The most common long-term complication reported is glenoid component loosening (21). To this end, recent studies have explored the use of hemiarthroplasty, which is replacement of the humeral head without resurfacing the glenoid. This method has proved effective in selected patients, including those with cuff tear arthropathy.

Cervical Spine

The clinical problems caused by rheumatic disorders of the cervical spine are pain, compromised neurologic function, and mechanical instability that causes or has the potential to cause pain and neurologic deficits. Spinal fusion can decrease pain, restore stability, and, in some instances, prevent neurologic deficits. Surgical decompression of the spinal cord and nerve roots can relieve pain and improve neurologic function in selected patients.

Generally accepted indications for surgical intervention in RA patients with cervical spine involvement are pain refractory to nonoperative modalities, neurologic deterioration, and radiographic evidence of impending spinal cord compression (22). Whereas the anterior atlantodental interval has been traditionally used to determine the degree of atlantoaxial instability, the posterior atlantodental interval has recently been shown to be an important predictor of the potential for postoperative neurologic improvement (23). Evidence also suggests that patients who undergo cervical arthrodesis earlier in the course of their disease have more satisfactory results than those for whom arthrodesis is delayed (22). Pain is relieved in most patients, but neurologic improvement is variable and closely related to preoperative radiographic instability and neurologic status (23).

POSTOPERATIVE COMPLICATIONS

Serious complications of operative treatment of arthritis surgery include infection, nerve and blood vessel injury, pulmonary embolus, and joint dislocation. Although most complications occur during surgery or within the first postoperative weeks, they may arise at any time after surgery. Arthroplasty patients in particular must be monitored indefinitely for subtle radiographic evidence of periprosthetic osteolysis, which, if treated early, may halt progression to massive bone loss and catastrophic failure (12) (Fig. 56-2). The vast majority of failures among lower extremity total joint prostheses occur after the first decade (13), and most patients remain asymptomatic until substantial bone loss, subsidence, and even fracture have occurred. Therefore, routine follow-up, including careful standardized clinical and comparative radiographic evaluation, is imperative on a regular basis throughout the patient's life.

In addition, patients must be carefully monitored for early signs of infection. Early detection of infection in a prosthetic joint may make it possible to save the implants. However, it is rare to successfully treat chronic joint infections without removing the implants. Patients with several joint arthroplasties who develop sepsis in one prosthetic joint should be treated aggressively and observed closely, because they have a substantial risk of developing a metachronous infection in another artificial joint.

W. TIMOTHY BALLARD, MD
JOSEPH A. BUCKWALTER, MD

1. Buckwalter JA, Lohmander S: Operative treatment of osteoarthrosis: current practice and future development. J Bone Joint Surg 76A:1405-1418, 1994
2. Ballard WT, Callaghan JJ, Sullivan PM, Johnston RC: The results of improved cementing techniques for total hip arthroplasty in patients less than fifty years old. A ten year follow-up study. J Bone Joint Surg 76A:959-964, 1994
3. Ballard WT, Callaghan JJ, Johnston RC: Revision of total hip arthroplasty in octogenarians. J Bone Joint Surg 77-A:585-589, 1995
4. Wymenga AB, Horn JR, Theeuwes A, Muytjens HL, Slooff TJ: Perioperative factors associated with septic arthritis after arthroplasty: prospective multicenter study of 362 knee and 2,651 hip operations. Acta Orthop Scand 63:665-671, 1992
5. Lehman DE, Capello WN, Feinberg JR: Total hip arthroplasty without cement in obese patients. J Bone Joint Surg 76A:854-862, 1994
6. Collins DN, Barnes CL, FitzRandolph RL: Cervical spine instability in rheumatoid patients having total hip or knee arthroplasty. Clin Orthop Rel Res 272:127-135, 1991
7. Murray RP, Bourne MH, Fitzgerald RH: Metachronous infections in patients who have had more than one total joint arthroplasty. J Bone Joint Surg 73A:1469-1474, 1991
8. Menon TJ, Wroblewski BM: Charnley low-friction arthroplasty in patients with psoriasis. Clin Orthop Rel Res 300:127-128, 1983
9. Kelly SS, Lachiewicz PF, Gilbert MS, Bolander ME, Jankiewicz JJ: Hip arthroplasty in hemophilic arthropathy. J Bone Joint Surg 67A:828-834,1995
10. Lachiewicz PR, Inglis AE, Insall JN, Sculco TP, Hilgartner MW, Bussel JB: Total knee arthroplasty in hemophilia. J Bone Joint Surg 76A:1361-1366, 1985
11. Ogilvie-Harris DJ, Saleh K: Generalized synovial chondromatosis of the knee: a comparison of removal of the loose bodies alone with arthroscopic synovectomy. Arthroscopy 10:166-170, 1994
12. Total Hip Replacement. NIH Concensus Statement 12:1-31, 1994
13. Schulte KR, Callaghan JJ, Kelley SS, Johnston RC: The outcome of Charnley total hip arthroplasty with cement after a minimum twenty-year follow-up: the results of one surgeon. J Bone Joint Surg 75-A:959-975, 1993
14. Fitzgerald RH: Total hip arthroplasty sepsis: prevention and diagnosis. Orthop Clin North Am 23:259-264, 1992
15. Sullivan PM, MacKenzie JR, Callaghan JJ, Johnston RC: Total hip arthroplasty with cement in patients who are less than fifty years old. J Bone Joint Surg 76A:863-869, 1994
16. Insall JN, Joseph DM, Msika C: High tibial osteotomy for varus gonarthrosis: a long-term follow-up study. J Bone Joint Surg 66A:1040-1048, 1984
17. Rand JA, Ilstrup DM: Survivorship analysis of total knee arthroplasty. Cumulative rates of survival of 9200 total knee arthroplasties. J Bone Joint Surg 73A:397-409, 1991
18. Bosco JA, Bynum DK, Bowers WH: Long-term outcome of Volz total wrist arthroplasties. J Arthroplasty 9:25-31, 1994
19. Summers GD, Talor AR, Webley M: Elbow synovectomy and excision of the radial head in rheumatoid arthritis: a short term palliative procedure. J Rheumatol 15:566-569, 1988

20. Kraay MJ, Figgie MP, Inglis AE, Wolfe SW, Ranawat CS: Primary semi-constrained total elbow arthroplasty: survival analysis of 113 consecutive cases. J Bone Joint Surg 76B:636-640, 1994

21. Brostrom LA, Wallensten R, Olsson E, Anderson D: The Kessel prosthesis in total shoulder arthroplasty: a five-year experience. Clin Orthop Rel Res 277:155-160, 1992

22. Ranawat CS, O'Leary P, Pellici P, Tsairis P, Marchisello P, Dorr L: Cervical spine fusion in rheumatoid arthrits. J Bone Joint Surg 61A:1003-1010, 1979

23. Boden SD, Dodge LD, Bohlman HH, Rechtine GR: Rheumatoid arthritis of the cervical spine. J Bone Joint Surg 75A:1282-1297, 1993

57

QUESTIONABLE REMEDIES

"Alternative" medicine has gained widespread public attention and has received governmental endorsement, as indicated by the establishment of the National Institutes of Health Office of Alternative Medicine. To be able to communicate effectively with patients with rheumatic diseases, it is essential that clinicians become familiar with some of the questionable remedies available for arthritis (1–4). In 1993 the American College of Rheumatology formed a committee on questionable remedies to address certain pertinent issues. The committee deliberately selected the term *questionable* (following the approaches of the National Council Against Health Fraud and the American Cancer Society), which serves to avoid euphemisms for other forms of therapy. There are three types of therapies: genuine (those proven acceptably safe and effective), questionable, and ineffective. These designations are preferable to terms such as unapproved (which suggests that the Food and Drug Administration approval is either pending or has been denied), false (disproven), unproven (experimental), dubious (very doubtful), nonstandard (falling short of practice standards), irregular (not used by mainstream medicine), or alternative or complementary (which reflect treatment options either questionable or conventional) (1,3).

The use of questionable remedies among patients with rheumatic diseases is widespread. The appeal of questionable medicine is clear: It offers hope. Many patients with rheumatic diseases suffer greatly, struggling to cope with their illness and with the limitations of science and medical practices. The essence of medicine is the reduction of uncertainty. Unfortunately, both health-care providers and patients must learn to live with considerable uncertainty—not always an easy task. Patients continue to hope and may turn away from science to seek understanding, relief, and empowerment from questionable sources.

The traditional response of the medical profession has been to dismiss, disdain, and sometimes ridicule questionable remedies. There are several explanations for this attitude. Questionable remedies often evoke discomfort and prejudice in traditionally trained physicians. Often the remedy seems to defy rational explanation, and is purveyed by practitioners whom physicians consider unsavory or intellectually inferior. Because practitioners of questionable remedies sometimes have a different belief system, physicians may be reluctant to consider their notions. Yet dismissing questionable remedies without first conducting scientific studies risks missing potentially beneficial therapies (3,4).

Efforts to combat the public's misperceptions through education and communication about questionable remedies have met with limited success. The fact is that "Doctor's diet cures arthritis" has instant appeal for the media, whereas "Doctor's diet doesn't cure arthritis" takes years of research, writing, and revision before appearing in the medical literature (3).

The contemporary view of science asserts that human problems can be understood and solved by science and that science epitomizes rationality, integrity, progress, and open-mindedness. But medical science has embraced superstition (tonsillectomies and adenoidectomies in the recent past and perhaps some current practices such as coronary artery bypass surgery), perpetuated fraud, committed errors, and fallen prey to conservatism, pigheadedness, fashion, and trends (3,4).

THE HAZARDS OF QUESTIONABLE REMEDIES

Some questionable therapies are not merely innocuous but are harmful. There are documented instances of patients receiving therapies other than those advertised or promised with such adverse results as bone marrow aplasia, serious infections from contaminants, and death (3-5). Patients seeking questionable remedies may also inappropriately neglect their illness. Moreover, expenditures on questionable remedies divert scarce health care resources.

SELECTED QUESTIONABLE REMEDIES

Prominent remedies used to treat arthritis include diet, vitamin and mineral supplements, fish oils, antimicrobial drugs (nitroimidazole, rifamycin, ceftriaxone, ampicillin, and amantadine), biologic agents (thymopoietin, transfer factor, placenta-derived factors, venoms, and herbal remedies), pharmacologic agents (cis-retinoic acid, isoprinoside, amiprolose, thalidomide, and dapsone), topical preparations (dimethyl sulfoxide), mechanical/instrumental approaches (hyperbaric oxygen, laser irradiation, acupuncture, photophoresis, electromagnetic radiation), chiropractic manipulation, homeopathy, biofeedback, exercise, and miscellaneous others (eg, sitting in abandoned uranium mines).

Antimicrobial Agents

A microbial etiology for rheumatoid arthritis (RA) has long been an attractive but unproven hypothesis. If true, then antimicrobial agents could be useful therapy. Levamisole, an imidazole derivative, has proved effective in treating RA. Based on this experience and the possibility that RA may be caused by *Amoeba limax*, nitroimidazole antimicrobial drugs have been tried, but results have not been impressive (1). Rifamycin, an antibiotic that blocks DNA-dependent RNA polymerase and inhibits cellular protein synthesis, has been claimed to be beneficial for knee synovitis in RA patients (6).

Tetracycline therapy was initially proposed as a potential therapy for RA, based on a putative mycoplasma etiology. Recent studies have shown that the tetracyclines, particularly minocycline, reduce collagenase activity, limit bone resorption, affect T-cell function, perturb neutrophil function, and appear to be antiproliferative, anti-inflammatory, and antiarthritic in animals and possibly in humans. Recent prospective randomized, double-blind, placebo-controlled trials have shown statistically significant but clinically modest benefits of minocycline for RA (7,8). Other antimicrobials have been considered for arthritis therapy. Patients with chronic inflammatory arthritis and antibody titers to *Borrelia burgdorferi* of 1:64 or greater have shown encouraging responses to ceftriaxone (9). Ampicillin has been claimed to be beneficial in RA patients under certain conditions (10). Amantadine, an antiviral agent, was reported to be useful in a group of patients with teenage-onset juvenile RA who had elevated antibody titers to influenza A and who were born during an influenza epidemic (11). These are provocative observations. If confirmed, they could be interpreted to mean that chronic arthritis in some patients results from bacterial, spirochete, or viral infection and that antimicrobials have important antirheumatic properties.

Exercise

Little is known about potentially therapeutic exercises for arthritis patients or about the long-term consequences of exercise on the musculoskeletal system (12). Reports have suggested that patients with arthritis improve with aerobic dance, water aerobics, treadmill exercise, stationary cycling, and Nautilus-type training. Several investigators examined a possible relationship between running and osteoarthritis. Most studies reported that runners without underlying biomechanical problems did not develop arthritis at a rate detectably different from nonrunning healthy populations. Runners also had reduced disability and mortality rates (13,14). These observations seemed to be valid for many other sports activities as well. People who have no underlying joint abnormality and engage in recreational exercise that puts joints through normal motions, carried out within the limits of comfort, do not inevitably develop joint injury problems, even after many years. Moreover, certain physical exercises for selected patients may provide important psychological and clinical benefits.

Foods, Diet, and Nutritional Supplements

For years, special diets for arthritis have been relegated to quackery. It has generally been reasoned that if there was a relationship between diet and arthritis, it would have been discovered long ago. This position has been revisited in recent years, and it appears that food may affect arthritis, at least in some cases, in two ways. First, some patients are allergic to certain foods and their rheumatologic symptoms may be a manifestation of food allergy. Second, certain types of diets with particular amounts of calories, protein, and fatty acids may affect the immune system and thus modify the inflammation that occurs with arthritis (15).

Physicians and patients are intrigued that arthritis may occasionally be the result of hypersensitivity to foods. Palindromic rheumatism has been associated with sodium nitrate, Behçet's syndrome with black walnuts, systemic lupus erythematosus (SLE) with canavanine in alfalfa (which may cross-react with native DNA or activate B lymphocytes) and with hydralazine, and RA with many substances including house dust, tobacco, smoke, petrochemicals, tartrazine, dairy products, wheat, corn, and beef. In addition, rheumatoid-like synovitis in rabbits can be induced by cows' milk (15). Recent careful, prospective, placebo-controlled, double-blind studies confirmed that, for selected patients, inflammatory arthritis may be associated with foods. Some of these patients had evidence of immunologic reactivity to these food antigens (15).

However, there is no compelling evidence that any diet, other than a healthful balanced one, is consistently helpful for arthritis patients. Studies of a popular diet (eliminating red meat, additives, preservatives, fruit, dairy products, herbs, spices, and alcohol) for arthritis patients have found no consistent effect on disease (2).

Nutritional status exerts a profound influence on immune responsiveness and disease expression. For example, mice with SLE and arthritic rats fed diets rich in eicosapentaenoic acid (a naturally occurring polyunsaturated fatty acid analog) fare better than control animals. Clinical trials of fish oils and plant seed oils indicate modest decreases in certain symptoms for patients with RA but not for those with SLE. These observations suggest that dietary factors that modify arachidonic acid-derived prostaglandin or leukotriene generation affect inflammatory and immunologic responses and may, therefore, ameliorate symptoms of rheumatic diseases (1,2,15).

Various nutritional substances, including copper, zinc, and vitamin B, are claimed to be helpful for arthritis patients. In general, the evidence supporting such claims is scant. Copper salts have been shown to be antirheumatic in clinical trials, but they are associated with many adverse effects and have never evolved as important therapeutic agents. In one study, some patients with RA benefited from oral zinc; however, improvement was not great or consistent and was not confirmed by other studies. L-histidine helped a small subgroup of patients with RA but is not an important therapeutic agent. Evidence to support the efficacy of vitamin C for arthritis patients is lacking (1,2,15).

Biologic Agents

Some of the newer biological agents, such as monoclonal antibodies, interleukins, cytokines, and similar products, have exciting potential (see Chapter 55). Although their therapeutic roles are not yet established, these biologic agents are not usually considered "alternative" remedies. Venoms affect inflammatory and immune responses in vitro but have no documented clinical utility.

Other Questionable Remedies

Laser therapy, homeopathy, and biofeedback appear to show varying degrees of promise in certain situations, but these therapies require more confirmatory data before being considered for general use in rheumatology (1). Recent reports have suggested the possible efficacy of thalidomide, manipulation (16), electromagnetic radiation (17), photo- or chemopheresis (18), yoga (19), *Tripterygium wilfordii Hook* F (20), acupuncture (21), and mud (22). These, however, should still be considered questionable or investigational approaches. Dimethyl sulfoxide and hyperbaric oxygen are not of proven value. It should be stressed in this context that placebo effects can be quite powerful in arthritis patients, with a substantial improvement in symptoms in a high percentage of patients.

PERSPECTIVE

There is no reason to conclude that questionable therapies have an important role in the routine management of rheumatic diseases. Nonetheless, it is essential to critically re-examine prevailing notions regarding antimicrobials, diet, and exercise because new insights about pathogenesis and therapy of rheumatic diseases have been and will be gained. At the same time, healthy skepticism must be balanced with willingness to consider nontraditional concepts. It is important to recognize the current limitations of science in enabling an understanding of rheumatic diseases. There is a need to be cautious about being dogmatic in interpreting those notions not thoughtfully scrutinized, while resolute against those notions that are false. Ultimately, the goal is a better understanding of illness and care for patients.

RICHARD S. PANUSH, MD

1. Panush RS: Is there a role for diet or other questionable therapies in managing rheumatic diseases? Bull Rheum Dis 42:1-4, 1993

2. Panush RS: Diet and other questionable remedies for arthritis. In Koopman WS (ed): Arthritis and Allied Coditions. Baltimore, MD, Williams & Wilkins, 1997, pp 857-870

3. Panush RS: Alternative medicine: science or superstition? [editorial] J Rheumatal 21:8-9, 1994

4. Panush RS: Reflections on unproven remedies. Rheum Dis Clin North Am 19:201-206, 1993

5. Kraus A, Guerra-Bautista G, Alarcon-Segovia D: *Salmonella arizona* arthritis and septicemia associated with rattlesnake ingestion by patients with connective tissue diseases:a dangerous compilation of folk medicine. J Rheumatol 18:1328-1331, 1991

6. Gabriel SE, Conn DL, Luthra H: Rifampin therapy in rheumatoid arthritis. J Rheumatol 17:163-166, 1990

7. Kloppenburg M, Breedveld FC, Terwiel J, Maller C, Dijkmans BAC: Minocycline in active rheumatoid arthritis: a double-blind controlled trial. Arthritis Rheum 37:629-636, 1994

8. Tilley BC, Alarcon GS, Heyse SP, et al: Minocycline in rheumatoid arthritis: a 48 week, double-blind, placebo-controlled trial. Ann Intern Med 122:81-89, 1995

9. Caperton EM, Heim-Duthoy K, Matzke GR, Peterson PK, Johnson RC: Ceftriazone therapy of chronic inflammatory arthritis. Arch Intern Med 150:1677-1682, 1990

10. Wawrzynska-Pagowska J, Brzezinska B: A trial of ampicillin in the treatment of rheumatoid arthritis: results of long-term observations indicating the possibility of inhibiting the progression of bone deformity. Rheumatologia 22:1-10, 1984

11. Pritchard MH, Munro J: Preliminary report: successful treatment of juvenile chronic arthritis with a specific antiviral agent. Br J Rheumatol 28:521-524, 1989

12. Panush RS, Lane N (eds): Exercise and Rheumatic Disease. Bailliere's Clinical Rheumatology 8:XI-XII, 1-239, 1994

13. Panush RS, Hanson CS, Caldwell JR, Longley S, Stork J, Thoburn R: Is running associated with osteoarthritis? An eight-year follow up study. J Clin Rheumatol, 1:35-39, 1995

14. Fries JF, Singh G, Morfeld D, Hubert HB, Lane NE, Brown BW: Running and the development of disability with age. Ann Intern Med 121:502-9, 1994

15. Panush RS (Ed): Nutrition and rheumatic diseases. Rheum Dis Clin North Am 17:i-XIII, 197-447, 1991

16. Shekelle PG, Adams AH, Chassin MR, Hurwitz EL, Brook RH: Spinal manipulation for low-back pain. Ann Intern Med 117:590-597, 1992

17. Trock DH, Bollet AJ, Markoll R: The effect of pulsed electromagnetic fields in the treatment of osteoarthritis of the knee and cervical spine. Report of randomized, double-blind, placebo-controlled trials. J Rheumatol 21:1903-11, 1994

18. Laing TJ, Ike RW, Griffiths CEM, et al: A pilot study of the effect of oral 8-methoxypsoralen and intraarticular ultraviolet light on rheumatoid synovitis. J Rheumatol 22:29-33, 1995

19. Garfinkel MS, Schumacher HR, Husain A, Levy M, Reshetar RA: Evaluation of a yoga-based regimen for treatment of osteoarthritis of the hands. J Rheumatol 21:2341-3, 1994

20. Tao X, Davis LS, Lipsky PE: Effect of the chinese herbal remedy *Tripterygium Wilfordii Hook* F on human immune responsiveness. Arthritis Rheum 34:1274-1281, 1991

21. Berman BM, Lao L, Greene M, Anderson RW, Wong RH, Langenberg P, Hochberg MC: Efficacy of traditional Chinese acupuncture in the treatment of symptomatic knee osteoarthritis: a pilot study. Osteoarthritis Cartilage 3:139-142, 1995

22. Sukenik S, Giryes H, Hlaevy S, Neumann L, Flusser D, Buskila D: Treatment of psoriatic arthritis at the Dead Sea. J Rheumatol 21:1305-9, 1994

APPENDIX I

Criteria for the Classification and Diagnosis of the Rheumatic Diseases

The criteria presented in the following section have been developed with several different purposes in mind. For a given disorder, one may have criteria for: 1) classification of groups of patients (eg, from population surveys, selection of patients for therapeutic trials, or analysis of results of interinstitutional patient comparisons), 2) diagnosis of individual patients, 3) estimations of disease frequency and/or severity (epidemiologic surveys) including remission, and 4) assistance in determination of prognosis.

The original intention was to propose criteria as guidelines for *classification* of disease syndromes for the purpose of assuring correctness of diagnosis in patients taking part in clinical investigation rather than for individual patient diagnosis. However, the proposed criteria have in fact been used as guidelines for patient diagnosis as well as for research classification. One must be cautious in such application because the various criteria are derived from the use of analytic techniques that allow the minimum number of variables to achieve the best group discrimination, rather than to attempt to arrive at a diagnosis in each patient, regardless of the amount of information needed.

The proposed criteria are empiric and not intended to include or exclude a particular diagnosis in any individual patient. They are valuable in offering a standard to permit comparison of groups of patients from different centers that take part in various clinical investigations including therapeutic trials.

The ideal criterion is absolutely sensitive, ie, all patients with the disorder show this physical finding or the positive laboratory test, and absolutely specific, ie, the positive finding or test is never present in any other disease. Unfortunately, few such criteria or sets of criteria exist. Usually the greater the sensitivity of a finding, the lower its specificity, and vice versa. When criteria are established empirically, as in the modified Jones criteria for rheumatic fever or the American College of Rheumatology criteria for rheumatoid arthritis, attempts are made to select reasonable combinations of sensitivity and specificity.

Existing criteria derive from an incomplete concept of disease and imperfect diagnostic technology and will require many years for full refinement and accuracy. Thus, criteria are expected to change as improved knowledge and techniques become available in the different disease areas and as concepts of pathophysiology change. This is a vital and dynamic area of research in which rheumatology leads other disciplines in medicines.

Criteria for the Classification of Rheumatoid Arthritis*

CRITERION	DEFINITION
1. Morning stiffness	Morning stiffness in and around the joints, lasting at least 1 hour before maximal improvement
2. Arthritis of three or more joint areas	At least three joint areas simultaneously have had soft tissue swelling or fluid (not bony overgrowth alone) observed by a physician. The 14 possible areas are right or left PIP, MCP, wrist, elbow, knee, ankle, and MTP joints
3. Arthritis of hand joints	At least one area swollen (as defined above) in a wrist, MCP, or PIP joint
4. Symmetric arthritis	Simultaneous involvement of the same joint areas (as defined in 2) on both sides of the body (bilateral involvement of PIPs, MCPs, or MTPs is acceptable without absolute symmetry)
5. Rheumatoid nodules	Subcutaneous nodules, over bony prominences, or extensor surfaces, or in juxtaarticular regions, observed by a physician
6. Serum rheumatoid factor	Demonstration of abnormal amounts of serum rheumatoid factor by any method for which the result has been positive in <5% of normal control subjects
7. Radiographic changes	Radiographic changes typical of rheumatoid arthritis on posteroanterior hand and wrist radiographs, which must include erosions or unequivocal bony decalcification localized in or most marked adjacent to the involved joints (osteoarthritis changes alone do not qualify)

* For classification purposes, a patient shall be said to have rheumatoid arthritis if he/she has satisfied at least four of these seven criteria. Criteria 1 through 4 must have been present for at least 6 weeks. Patients with two clinical diagnoses are not excluded. Designation as classic, definite, or probable rheumatoid arthritis is *not* to be made.

Reprinted from Arnett FC, Edworthy SM, Bloch DA, et al: The American Rheumatism Association 1987 revised criteria for the classification of rheumatoid arthritis. Arthritis Rheum 31:315–324, 1988, with permission of the American College of Rheumatology.

Criteria for Determining Progression, Remission, and Functional Status of Rheumatoid Arthritis

Classification of Progression of Rheumatoid Arthritis

Stage I, Early

* 1. No destructive changes on roentgenographic examination

2. Radiographic evidence of osteoporosis may be present

Stage II, Moderate

* 1. Radiographic evidence of osteoporosis, with or without slight subchondral bone destruction; slight cartilage destruction may be present

* 2. No joint deformities, although limitation of joint mobility may be present

3. Adjacent muscle atrophy

4. Extraarticular soft tissue lesions, such as nodules and tenosynovitis may be present

Stage III, Severe

* 1. Radiographic evidence of cartilage and bone destruction, in addition to osteoporosis

* 2. Joint deformity, such as subluxation, ulnar deviation, or hyperextension, without fibrous or bony ankylosis

3. Extensive muscle atrophy

4. Extraarticular soft tissue lesions, such as nodules and tenosynovitis may be present

Stage IV, Terminal

* 1. Fibrous or bony ankylosis

2. Criteria of stage III

* The criteria prefaced by an asterisk are those that must be present to permit classification of a patient in any particular stage or grade.

Reprinted from Steinbrocker O, Traeger CH, Batterman RC: Therapeutic criteria in rheumatoid arthritis. JAMA 140:659-662, 1949, with permission.

Criteria for Clinical Remission in Rheumatoid Arthritis*

Five or more of the following requirements must be fulfilled for at least two consecutive months:

1. Duration of morning stiffness not exceeding 15 minutes
2. No fatigue
3. No joint pain (by history)
4. No joint tenderness or pain on motion
5. No soft tissue swelling in joints or tendon sheaths
6. Erythrocyte sedimentation rate (Westergren method) less than 30 mm/hour for a female or 20 mm/hour for a male

* These criteria are intended to describe either spontaneous remission or a state of drug-induced disease suppression, which simulates spontaneous remission.
No alternative explanation may be invoked to account for the failure to meet a particular requirement. For instance, in the presence of knee pain, which might be related to degenerative arthritis, a point for "no joint pain" may not be awarded.
Exclusions: Clinical manifestations of active vasculitis, pericarditis, pleuritis or myositis, and unexplained recent weight loss or fever attributable to rheumatoid arthritis will prohibit a designation of complete clinical remission.

Reprinted from Pinals RS, Masi AT, Larsen RA, et al: Preliminary criteria for clinical remission in rheumatoid arthritis. Arthritis Rheum 24:1308-1315, 1981, with permission of the American College of Rheumatology.

Criteria for classification of functional status in rheumatoid arthritis*

Class I:	Completely able to perform usual activities of daily living (self-care, vocational, and avocational)
Class II:	Able to perform usual self-care and vocational activities, but limited in avocational activities
Class III:	Able to perform usual self-care activities, but limited in vocational and avocational activities
Class IV:	Limited in ability to perform usual self-care, vocational, and avocational activities

* Usual self-care activities include dressing, feeding, bathing, grooming, and toileting. Avocational (recreational and/or leisure) and vocational (work, school, homemaking) activities are patient-desired and age- and sex-specific.

Reprinted from Hochberg MC, Chang RW, Dwosh I, et al: The American College of Rheumatology 1991 revised criteria for the classification of global functional status in rheumatoid arthritis. Arthritis Rheum 35:498-502, 1992, with permission of the American College of Rheumatology.

Criteria for the Diagnosis of Juvenile Rheumatoid Arthritis

I. General

The JRA Criteria Subcommittee in 1982 reviewed the 1977 Criteria (1) and recommended that *juvenile rheumatoid arthritis* be the name for the principal form of chronic arthritic disease in children and that this general class should be classified into three onset subtypes: systemic, polyarticular, and pauciarticular. The onset subtypes may be further subclassified into subsets as indicated below. The following classification enumerates the requirements for the diagnosis of JRA and the three clinical onset subtypes and lists subsets of each subtype that may be useful in further classification.

II. General criteria for the diagnosis of juvenile rheumatoid arthritis:

A. Persistent arthritis of at least six weeks duration in one or more joints

B. Exclusion of other causes of arthritis (see list of exclusions)

III. JRA onset subtypes

The onset subtype is determined by manifestations during the first six months of disease and remains the principal classification, although manifestations more closely resembling another subtype may appear later.

A. Systemic onset JRA: This subtype is defined as JRA with persistent intermittent fever (daily intermittent temperatures to 103°F or more) with or without rheumatoid rash or other organ involvement. Typical fever and rash will be considered probable systemic onset JRA if not associated with arthritis. Before a definite diagnosis can be made, arthritis, as defined, must be present.

B. Pauciarticular onset JRA: This subtype is defined as JRA with arthritis in four or fewer joints during the first six months of disease. Patients with systemic onset JRA are excluded from this onset subtype.

C. Polyarticular JRA: This subtype is defined as JRA with arthritis in five or more joints during the first six months of disease. Patients with systemic JRA onset are excluded from this subtype.

D. The onset subtypes may include the following subsets:

1. Systemic onset
   a. Polyarthritis
   b. Oligoarthritis
2. Oligoarthritis (Pauciarticular onset)
   a. Antinuclear antibody (ANA) positive-chronic uveitis
   b. Rheumatoid factor (RF) positive
   c. Seronegative, B27 positive
   d. Not otherwise classified
3. Polyarthritis
   a. RF positivity
   b. Not otherwise classified

IV. Exclusions

A. Other rheumatic diseases
   1. Rheumatic fever
   2. Systemic lupus erythematosus
   3. Ankylosing spondylitis
   4. Polymyositis or dermatomyositis
   5. Vasculitic syndromes
   6. Scleroderma
   7. Psoriatic arthritis
   8. Reiter's syndrome
   9. Sjögren's syndrome
   10. Mixed connective tissue disease
   11. Behçet's syndrome
B. Infectious arthritis
C. Inflammatory bowel disease
D. Neoplastic diseases including leukemia
E. Nonrheumatic conditions of bones and joints
F. Hematologic diseases
G. Psychogenic arthralgia
H. Miscellaneous
   1. Sarcoidosis
   2. Hypertrophic osteoarthropathy
   3. Villonodular synovitis
   4. Chronic active hepatitis
   5. Familial Mediterranean fever

V. Other proposed terminology

Juvenile chronic arthritis (JCA) and juvenile arthritis (JA) are new diagnostic terms currently in use in some places for the arthritides of childhood. The diagnoses of JCA and JA are not equivalent to each other, nor to the older diagnosis of juvenile rheumatoid arthritis or Still's disease. Hence reports of studies of JCA or JA cannot be directly compared with one another nor to reports of JRA or Still's disease. Juvenile chronic arthritis is described in more detail in a report of the European Conference on the Rheumatic Diseases of Children (2) and juvenile arthritis in the report of the Ross Conference (3).

1. JRA Criteria Subcommittee of the Diagnostic and Therapeutic Criteria Committee of the American Rheumatism Association: Current proposed revisions of the JRA criteria. Arthritis Rheum 20(Suppl)195-199, 1977
2. Ansell BW: Chronic arthritis in childhood. Ann Rheum Dis 37:107-120, 1978
3. Fink CW: Keynote address: Arthritis in childhood, Report of the 80th Ross Conference in Pediatric Research. Columbus, Ross Laboratories, 1979, pp 1-2

Criteria for the Classification of Spondyloarthropathy*

Inflammatory spinal pain
or
Synovitis
>Asymmetric or
>Predominantly in the lower limbs

and one or more of the following
Positive family history
Psoriasis
Inflammatory bowel disease
Urethritis, cervicitis, or acute diarrhea within 1 month before arthritis
Buttock pain alternating between right and left gluteal areas
Enthesopathy
Sacroiliitis

* This classification method yields a sensitivity of 78.4% and a specificity of 89.6%. When radiographic evidence of sacroiliitis was included, the sensitivity improved to 87.0% with a minor decrease in specificity to 86.7%. Definition of the variables used in classification criteria follow.

VARBLE	DEFINITION
Inflammatory spinal pain	History or present symptoms of spinal pain in back, dorsal, or cervical region, with at least four of the following: (a) onset before age 45, (b) insidious onset, (c) improved by exercise, (d) associated with morning stiffness, (e) at least 3 months' duration
Synovitis	Past or present asymmetric arthritis or arthritis predominantly in the lower limbs
Family history	Presence in first-degree or second-degree relatives of any of the following: (a) ankylosing spondylitis, (b) psoriasis, (c) acute uveitis, (d) reactive arthritis, (e) inflammatory bowel disease
Psoriasis	Past or present psoriasis diagnosed by a physician
Inflammatory bowel disease	Past or present Crohn's disease or ulcerative colitis diagnosed by a physician and confirmed by radiographic examination or endoscopy
Alternating buttock pain	Past or present pain alternating between the right left gluteal regions
Enthesopathy	Past or present spontaneous pain or tenderness at examination of the site of the insertion of the Achilles tendon or plantar fascia
Acute diarrhea	Episode of diarrhea occurring within one month before arthritis
Urethritis	Nongonococcal urethritis or cervicitis occurring within one month before arthritis
Sacroiliitis	Bilateral grade 2–4 or unilateral grade 3–4, according to the following radiographic grading system: 0 = normal, 1 = possible, 2 = minimal, 3 = moderate, and 4 = ankylosis

Reprinted from Dougados M, Van Der Linden S, Juhlin R, et al: The European Spondylarthropathy Study Group preliminary criteria for the classification of spondylarthropathy. Arthritis Rheum 34:1218–1227, 1991, with permission of the American College of Rheumatology.

Criteria for the Classification of Systemic Sclerosis (Scleroderma)*

A. Major criterion

Proximal scleroderma: Symmetric thickening, tightening, and induration of the skin of the fingers and the skin proximal to the metacarpophalangeal or metatarsophalangeal joints. The changes may affect the entire extremity, face, neck, and trunk (thorax and abdomen).

B. Minor criteria

1. *Sclerodactyly:* Above-indicated skin changes limited to the fingers

2. *Digital pitting scars or loss of substance from the finger pad:* Depressed areas at tips of fingers or loss of digital pad tissue as a result of ischemia

3. *Bibasilar pulmonary fibrosis:* Bilateral reticular pattern of linear or lineonodular densities most pronounced in basilar portions of the lungs on standard chest roentgenogram; may assume appearance of diffuse mottling or "honeycomb lung." These changes should not be attributable to primary lung disease.

* For the purposes of classifying patients in clinical trials, population surveys, and other studies, a person shall be said to have systemic sclerosis (scleroderma) if the one major or two or more minor criteria are present. Localized forms of scleroderma, eosinophilic fasciitis, and the various forms of pseudoscleroderma are excluded from these criteria.

Adapted from Subcommittee for Scleroderma Criteria of the American Rheumatism Association Diagnostic and Therapeutic Criteria Committee: Preliminary criteria for the classification of systemic sclerosis (scleroderma). Arthritis Rheum 23:581–590, 1980, with permission of the American College of Rheumatology.

Criteria for the Classification of Acute Gouty Arthritis

A. The presence of characteristic urate crystals in the joint fluid, or

B. A tophus proved to contain urate crystals by chemical means or polarized light microscopy, or

C. The presence of six of the following 12 clinical, laboratory, and x-ray phenomena listed below:

    1. More than one attack of acute arthritis

    2. Maximal inflammation developed within 1 day

    3. Attack of monarticular arthritis

    4. Joint redness observed

    5. First metatarsophalangeal joint painful or swollen

    6. Unilateral attack involving first metatarsophalangeal joint

    7. Unilateral attack involving tarsal joint

    8. Suspected tophus

    9. Hyperuricemia

    10. Asymmetric swelling within a joint (radiograph)

    11. Subcortical cysts without erosions (radiograph)

    12. Negative culture of joint fluid for microorganisms during attack of joint inflammation

Adapted from Wallace SL, Robinson H, Masi AT, et al: Preliminary criteria for the classification of the acute arthritis of primary gout. Arthritis Rheum 20:895–900, 1977, with permission of the American College of Rheumatology.

Criteria for the Classification of Fibromyalgia*

1. History of widespread pain

    Definition. Pain is considered widespread when all of the following are present: pain in the left side of the body, pain in the right side of the body, pain above the waist, and pain below the waist. In addition, axial skeletal pain (cervical spine or anterior chest or thoracic spine or low back) must be present. In this definition, shoulder and buttock pain is considered as pain for each involved side. "Low back" pain is considered lower segment pain.

2. Pain in 11 of 18 tender point sites on digital palpation.[†]

    Definition. Pain, on digital palpation, must be present in at least 11 of the following 18 tender point sites:

    Occiput: bilateral, at the suboccipital muscle insertions.

    Low cervical: bilateral, at the anterior aspects of the intertransverse spaces at C5-C7.

    Trapezius: bilateral, at the midpoint of the upper border.

    Supraspinatus: bilateral, at origins, above the scapula spine near the medial border.

    Second rib: bilateral, at the second costochondral junctions, just lateral to the junctions on upper surfaces.

    Lateral epicondyle: bilateral, 2 cm distal to the epicondyles.

    Gluteal: bilateral, in upper outer quadrants of buttocks in anterior fold of muscle.

    Greater trochanter: bilateral, posterior to the trochanteric prominence.

    Knee: bilateral, at the medial fat pad proximal to the joint line.

* For classification purposes, patients will be said to have fibromyalgia if both criteria are satisfied. Widespread pain must have been present at least 3 months. The presence of a second clinical disorder does not exclude the diagnosis of fibromyalgia.
† Digital palpation should be performed with an approximate force of 4 kg. For a tender point to be considered "positive" the subject must state that the palpation was painful. "Tender" is not to be considered "painful."

Adapted from Wolfe F, Smythe HA, Yunus MB, et al: The American College of Rheumatology 1990 criteria for the classification of fibromyalgia. Report of the multicenter criteria committee. Arthritis Rheum 33:160–172, 1990, with permission of the American College of Rheumatology.

Diagnostic Guidelines for Kawasaki Syndrome*

Fever lasting >5 days plus four of the following criteria

1. Polymorphous rash
2. Bilateral conjunctival injection
3. One or more of the following mucous membrane changes:
   Diffuse injection of oral and pharyngeal mucosa
   Erythema or fissuring of the lips
   Strawberry tongue
4. Acute, nonpurulent cervical lymphadenopathy (one lymph node must be >1.5 cm)
5. One or more of the following extremity changes:
   Erythema of palms and/or soles
   Indurative edema of hands and/or feet
   Membranous desquamation of the fingertips

* Other illnesses with similar clinical signs must be excluded.

Reprinted from Kawasaki T, Kosaki T, Okawa S, et al: A new infantile acute febrile mucocutaneous lymph node syndrome (MLNS) prevailing in Japan. Pediatrics 54:271–276, 1974, with permission.

Criteria for the Classification of Sjögren's Syndrome*

1. Ocular symptoms
   Definition. A positive response to at least one of the following three questions:
   (a) Have you had daily, persistent, troublesome dry eyes for more than 3 months?
   (b) Do you have a recurrent sensation of sand or gravel in the eyes?
   (c) Do you use tear substitutes more than three times a day?
2. Oral symptoms
   Definition. A positive response to at least one of the following three questions:
   (a) Have you had a daily feeling of dry mouth for more than 3 months?
   (b) Have you had recurrent or persistently swollen salivary glands as an adult?
   (c) Do you frequently drink liquids to aid in swallowing dry foods?
3. Ocular signs
   Definition. Objective evidence of ocular involvement, determined on the basis of a positive result on at least one of the following two tests:
   (a) Schirmer-I test (≤5 mm in 5 minutes)
   (b) Rose bengal score (≥4, according to the van Bijsterveld scoring system)
4. Histopathologic features
   Definition. Focus score ≥1 on minor salivary gland biopsy (focus defined as an agglomeration of at least 50 mononuclear cells; focus score defined as the number of foci per 4 mm^2 of glandular tissue)
5. Salivary gland involvement
   Definition. Objective evidence of salivary gland involvement, determined on the basis of a positive result on at least one of the following three tests:
   (a) Salivary scintigraphy
   (b) Parotid sialography
   (c) Unstimulated salivary flow (≤1.5 ml in 15 minutes)
6. Autoantibodies
   Definition. Presence of at least one of the following serum autoantibodies:
   (a) Antibodies to Ro/SS-A or La/SS-B antigens
   (b) Antinuclear antibodies
   (c) Rheumatoid factor
   Exclusion criteria: preexisting lymphoma, acquired immunodeficiency syndrome, sarcoidosis, or graft-versus-host disease

* For primary Sjögren's syndrome, the presence of three of six items showed a very high sensitivity (99.1%), but insufficient specificity (57.8%). Thus, this combination could be accepted as the basis for a diagnosis of probable primary Sjögren's syndrome. However, the presence of four of six items (accepting as serologic parameters only positive anti-Ro/SS-A and anti-La/SS-B antibodies) had a good sensitivity (93.5%) and specificity (94.0%), and therefore may be used to establish a definitive diagnosis of primary Sjögren's syndrome.

Reprinted from Vitali C, Bombardieri S, Moutsopoulos HM, et al: Preliminary criteria for the classification of Sjögren's syndrome. Arthritis Rheum 36:340–347, 1993, with permission of the American College of Rheumatology.

Criteria for the Diagnosis of Rheumatic Fever*

MAJOR MANIFESTATIONS	MINOR MANIFESTATIONS	SUPPORTING EVIDENCE OF PRECEDING STREPTOCOCCAL INFECTION
Carditis	Clinical findings	Positive throat culture or rapid streptococcal antigen test
Polyarthritis	Arthralgia	Elevated or rising streptococcal antibody titer
Chorea	Fever	
Erythema marginatum	Laboratory findings	
Subcutaneous nodules	Elevated acute phase reactants	
	Erythrocyte sedimentation rate	
	C-reactive protein	
	Prolonged PR interval	

* If supported by evidence of preceding group A streptococcal infection, the presence of two major manifestations, or of one major and two minor manifestations indicates a high probability of acute rheumatic fever.

Reprinted from Special Writing Group of the Committee on Rheumatic Fever, Endocarditis, and Kawasaki Disease of the Council on Cardiovascular Disease in the Young, American Heart Association: Guidelines for the diagnosis of rheumatic fever: Jones criteria, updated 1992. JAMA 268:2069-2073, 1992, with permission.

Criteria for the Classification of Polyarteritis Nodosa*

CRITERION	DEFINITION
1. Weight loss ≥4 kg	Loss of 4 kg or more of body weight since illness began, not due to dieting or other factors
2. Livedo reticularis	Mottled reticular pattern over the skin of portions of the extremities or torso
3. Testicular pain or tenderness	Pain or tenderness of the testicles, not due to infection, trauma, or other causes
4. Myalgias, weakness, or leg tenderness	Diffuse myalgias (excluding shoulder and hip girdle) or weakness of muscles or tenderness of leg muscles
5. Mononeuropathy or polyneuropathy	Development of mononeuropathy, multiple mononeuropathies, or polyneuropathy
6. Diastolic BP >90 mm Hg	Development of hypertension with the diastolic BP higher than 90 mm Hg
7. Elevated BUN or creatinine	Elevation of BUN >40 mg/dl or creatinine >1.5 mg/dl, not due to dehydration or obstruction
8. Hepatitis B virus	Presence of hepatitis B surface antigen or antibody in serum
9. Arteriographic abnormality	Arteriogram showing aneurysms or occlusions of the visceral arteries, not due to arteriosclerosis, fibromuscular dysplasia, or other noninflammatory causes
10. Biopsy of small or medium-sized artery containing PMN	Histologic changes showing the presence of granulocytes or granulocytes and mononuclear leukocytes in the artery wall

* For classification purposes, a patient shall be said to have polyarteritis nodosa if at least three of these 10 criteria are present. The presence of any three or more criteria yields a sensitivity of 82.2% and a specificity of 86.6%. BP = blood pressure; BUN = blood urea nitrogen; PMN = polymorphonuclear neutrophils.

Reprinted from Lightfoot RW Jr, Michel BA, Bloch DA, et al: The American College of Rheumatology 1990 criteria for the classification of polyarteritis nodosa. Arthritis Rheum 33:1088–1093, 1990, with permission of the American College of Rheumatology.

Criteria for the Classification of Giant Cell Arteritis*

CRITERION	DEFINITION
1. Age at disease onset ≥50 years	Development of symptoms or findings beginning at age 50 or older
2. New headache	New onset of or new type of localized pain in the head
3. Temporal artery abnormality	Temporal artery tenderness to palpation or decreased pulsation, unrelated to arteriosclerosis of cervical arteries
4. Elevated erythrocyte sedimentation rate	Erythrocyte sedimentation rate ≥50 mm/hour by the Westergren method
5. Abnormal artery biopsy	Biopsy specimen with artery showing vasculitis characterized by a predominance of mononuclear cell infiltration or granulomatous inflammation, usually with multinucleated giant cells

* For purposes of classification, a patient shall be said to have giant cell (temporal) arteritis if at least three of these five criteria are present. The presence of any three or more criteria yields a sensitivity of 93.5% and a specificity of 91.2%.

Reprinted from Hunder GG, Bloch DA, Michel BA, et al: The American College of Rheumatology 1990 criteria for the classification of giant cell arteritis. Arthritis Rheum 33:1122–1128, 1990, with permission of the American College of Rheumatology.

Criteria for the Classification of Wegener's Granulomatosis*

CRITERION	DEFINITION
1. Nasal or oral inflammation	Development of painful or painless oral ulcers or purulent or bloody nasal discharge
2. Abnormal chest radiograph	Chest radiograph showing the presence of nodules, fixed infiltrates, or cavities
3. Urinary sediment	Microhematuria (>5 red blood cells per high power field) or red cell casts in urine sediment
4. Granulomatous inflammation on biopsy	Histologic changes showing granulomatous inflammation within the wall of an artery or in the perivascular or extravascular area (artery or arteriole)

* For purposes of classification, a patient shall be said to have Wegener's granulomatosis if at least two of these four criteria are present. The presence of any two or more criteria yields a sensitivity of 88.2% and a specificity of 92.0%.

Reprinted from Leavitt RY, Fauci AS, Bloch DA, et al: The American College of Rheumatology 1990 criteria for the classification of Wegener's granulomatosis. Arthritis Rheum 33:1101–1107, 1990, with permission of the American College of Rheumatology.

Criteria for the Classification of Takayasu Arteritis*

CRITERION	DEFINITION
Age at disease onset ≤40 years	Development of symptoms or findings related to Takayasu arteritis at age ≤40 years
Claudication of extremities	Development and worsening of fatigue and discomfort in muscles of one or more extremity while in use, especially the upper extremities
Decreased brachial artery pulse	Decreased pulsation of one or both brachial arteries
BP difference >10 mm Hg	Difference of >10 mm Hg in systolic blood pressure between arms
Bruit over subclavian arteries or aorta	Bruit audible on auscultation over one or both subclavian arteries or abdominal aorta
Arteriogram abnormality	Arteriographic narrowing or occlusion of the entire aorta, its primary branches, or large arteries in the proximal upper or lower extremities, not due to arteriosclerosis, fibromuscular dysplasia, or similar causes; changes usually focal or segmental

* For purposes of classification, a patient shall be said to have Takayasu arteritis if at least three of these six criteria are present. The presence of any three or more criteria yields a sensitivity of 90.5% and a specificity of 97.8%. BP = blood pressure (systolic; difference between arms).

Reprinted from Arend WP, Michel BA, Bloch DA, et al: The American College of Rheumatology 1990 criteria for the classification of Takayasu arteritis. Arthritis Rheum 33:1129–1132, 1990, with permission of the American College of Rheumatology.

Criteria for the Classification of Henoch-Schönlein Purpura*

CRITERION	DEFINITION
1. Palpable purpura	Slightly raised "palpable" hemorrhagic skin lesions, not related to thrombocytopenia
2. Age ≤20 at disease onset	Patient 20 years or younger at onset of first symptoms
3. Bowel angina	Diffuse abdominal pain, worse after meals, or the diagnosis of bowel ischemia, usually including bloody diarrhea
4. Wall granulocytes on biopsy	Histologic changes showing granulocytes in the walls of arterioles or venules

* For purposes of classification, a patient shall be said to have Henoch-Schönlein purpura if at least two of these four criteria are present. The presence of any two or more criteria yields a sensitivity of 87.1% and a specificity of 87.7%.

Reprinted from Mills JA, Michel BA, Bloch DA, et al: The American College of Rheumatology 1990 criteria for the classification of Henoch-Schönlein purpura. Arthritis Rheum 33:1114–1121, 1990, with permission of the American College of Rheumatology.

Criteria for the Classification of Hypersensitivity Vasculitis*

CRITERION	DEFINITION
Age at disease onset >16 years	Development of symptoms after age 16
Medication at disease onset	Medication was taken at the onset of symptoms that may have been a precipitating factor
Palpable purpura	Slightly elevated purpuric rash over one or more areas of the skin; does not blanch with pressure and is not related to thrombocytopenia
Maculopapular rash	Flat and raised lesions of various sizes over one or more areas of the skin
Biopsy including arteriole and venule	Histologic changes showing granulocytes in a perivascular or extravascular location

* For purposes of classification, a patient shall be said to have hypersensitivity vasculitis if at least three of these five criteria are present. The presence of any three or more criteria yields a sensitivity of 71.0% and a specificity of 83.9%.

Reprinted from Calabrese LH, Michel BA, Bloch DA, et al: The American College of Rheumatology 1990 criteria for the classification of hypersensitivity vasculitis. Arthritis Rheum 33:1108–1113, 1990, with permission of the American College of Rheumatology.

Criteria for the Classification of Churg-Strauss Syndrome*

CRITERION	DEFINITION
Asthma	History of wheezing or diffuse high-pitched rales on expiration
Eosinophilia	Eosinophilia >10% on white blood cell differential count
Mononeuropathy or polyneuropathy	Development of mononeuropathy, multiple mononeuropathies, or polyneuropathy (ie, glove/stocking distribution) attributable to a systemic vasculitis
Pulmonary infiltrates, non-fixed	Migratory or transitory pulmonary infiltrates on radiographs (not including fixed infiltrates), attributable to a systemic vasculitis
Paranasal sinus abnormality	History of acute or chronic paranasal sinus pain or tenderness or radiographic opacification of the paranasal sinuses
Extravascular eosinophils	Biopsy including artery, arteriole, or venule, showing accumulations of eosinophils in extravascular areas

* For classification purposes, a patient shall be said to have Churg-Strauss syndrome if at least four of these six criteria are positive. The presence of any four or more of the six criteria yields a sensitivity of 85% and a specificity of 99.7%.

Adapted from Masi AT, Hunder GG, Lie JT, et al: The American College of Rheumatology 1990 criteria for the classification of Churg-Strauss syndrome (allergic granulomatosis and angiitis). Arthritis Rheum 33:1094–1100, 1990, with permission of the American College of Rheumatology.

Criteria for the Diagnosis of Behçet's Disease*

CRITERION	DEFINITION
Recurrent oral ulceration	Minor aphthous, major aphthous, or herpetiform ulceration observed by physician or patient, which recurred at least three times in one 12-month period
Plus two of	
Recurrent genital ulceration	Aphthous ulceration or scarring, observed by physician or patient
Eye lesions	Anterior uveitis, posterior uveitis, or cells in vitreous on slit lamp examination; or retinal vasculitis observed by ophthalmologist
Skin lesions	Erythema nodosum observed by physician or patient, pseudofolliculitis, or papulopustular lesions; or acneiform nodules observed by physician in postadolescent patients not on corticosteroid treatment
Positive pathergy test	Read by physician at 24–48 hours

* Findings applicable only in the absence of other clinical explanations. The presence of recurrent oral ulceration and any two of the remaining criteria yields a sensitivity of 91% and a specificity of 96%.

Reprinted from International Study Group for Behçet's Disease: Criteria for diagnosis of Behçet's disease. Lancet 335:1078–1080, 1990, with permission.

Criteria for the Classification of Systemic Lupus Erythematosus*

CRITERION	DEFINITION
1. Malar rash	Fixed erythema, flat or raised, over the malar eminences, tending to spare the nasolabial folds
2. Discoid rash	Erythematous raised patches with adherent keratotic scaling and follicular plugging; atrophic scarring may occur in older lesions
3. Photosensitivity	Skin rash as a result of unusual reaction to sunlight, by patient history or physician observation
4. Oral ulcers	Oral or nasopharyngeal ulceration, usually painless, observed by a physician
5. Arthritis	Nonerosive arthritis involving two or more peripheral joints, characterized by tenderness, swelling, or effusion
6. Serositis	a) Pleuritis—convincing history of pleuritic pain or rub heard by a physician or evidence of pleural effusion OR b) Pericarditis—documented by ECG or rub or evidence of pericardial effusion
7. Renal disorder	a) Persistent proteinuria greater than 0.5 grams per day or greater than 3+ if quantitation not performed OR b) Cellular casts—may be red cell, hemoglobin, granular, tubular, or mixed
8. Neurologic disorder	a) Seizures—in the absence of offending drugs or known metabolic derangements; eg, uremia, ketoacidosis, or electrolyte imbalance OR b) Psychosis—in the absence of offending drugs or known metabolic derangements; eg, uremia, ketoacidosis, or electrolyte imbalance
9. Hematologic disorder	a) Hemolytic anemia—with reticulocytosis OR b) Leukopenia—less than $4000/mm^3$ total on two or more occasions OR c) Lymphopenia—less than $1500/mm^3$ on two or more occasions OR d) Thrombocytopenia—less than $100,000/mm^3$ in the absence of offending drugs
10. Immunologic disorder	a) Positive LE cell preparation OR b) Anti-DNA: antibody to native DNA in abnormal titer OR c) Anti-Sm: presence of antibody to Sm nuclear antigen OR d) False positive serologic test for syphilis known to be positive for at least 6 months and confirmed by *Treponema pallidum* immobilization or fluorescent treponemal antibody absorption test
11. Antinuclear antibody	An abnormal titer of antinuclear antibody by immunofluorescence or an equivalent assay at any point in time and in the absence of drugs known to be associated with "drug-induced lupus" syndrome

* The proposed classification is based on 11 criteria. For the purpose of identifying patients in clinical studies, a person shall be said to have systemic lupus erythematosus if any four or more of the 11 criteria are present, serially or simultaneously, during any interval of observation.

Reprinted from Tan EM, Cohen AS, Fries JF, et al: The 1982 revised criteria for the classification of systematic lupus erythematosus (SLE). Arthritis Rheum 25: 1271–1277, 1982, with permission of the American College of Rheumatology.

Criteria for the Diagnosis of Polymyositis and Dermatomyositis*

CRITERION	DEFINITION
Symmetrical weakness	Weakness of limb-girdle muscles and anterior neck flexors, progressing over weeks to months, with or without dysphagia or respiratory muscle involvement
Muscle biopsy evidence	Evidence of necrosis of Type I and II fibers, phagocytosis, regeneration with basophilia, large vesicular sarcolemmal nuclei and prominent nucleoli, atrophy in a perifascicular distribution, variation in fiber size, and an inflammatory exudate, often perivascular
Elevation of muscle enzymes	Elevation in serum of skeletal muscle enzymes, particularly creatine phosphokinase and often aldolase, serum glutamate oxaloacetate, and pyruvate transaminases, and lactate dehydrogenase
Electromyographic evidence	Electromyographic triad of short, small, polyphasic motor units, fibrillations, positive sharp waves, and insertional irritability, and bizarre, high-frequency repetitive discharges
Dermatologic features	A lilac discoloration of the eyelids (heliotrope) with periorbital edema, a scaly, erythematous dermatitis over the dorsum of the hands (especially the metacarpophalangeal and proximal interphalangeal joints, Gottron's sign), and involvement of the knees, elbows, and medial malleoli, as well as the face, neck, and upper torso

* Confidence limits can be defined as follows. For a definite diagnosis of dermatomyositis, three of four criteria plus the rash must be present; for a definite diagnosis of polymyositis, four criteria must be present without the rash. For a probable diagnosis of dermatomyositis, two criteria plus the rash must be present; for a probable diagnosis of polymyositis, three criteria must be present without the rash. For a possible diagnosis of dermatomyositis, one criterion plus the rash must be present; for a possible diagnosis of polymyositis, two criteria must be present without the rash.

The following findings exclude a diagnosis of dermatomyositis or polymyositis.
- Evidence of central or peripheral neurologic disease, including motor-neuron disorders with fasciculations or long-tract signs, sensory changes, decreased nerve conduction times, and fiber-type atrophy and grouping on muscle biopsy.
- Muscle weakness with a slowly progressive, unremitting course and a positive family history or calf enlargement to suggest a muscular dystrophy.
- Biopsy evidence of granulomatous myositis such as with sarcoidosis.
- Infections, including trichinosis, schistosomiasis, trypanosomiasis, staphylococcosis, and toxoplasmosis.
- Recent use of various drugs and toxins, such as clofibrate and alcohol.
- Rhabdomyolysis as manifested by gross myoglobinuria related to strenuous exercise, infections, crush injuries, occlusions of major limb arteries, prolonged coma or convulsions, high-voltage accidents, heat stroke, the malignant-hyperpyrexia syndrome, and envenomation by certain sea snakes.
- Metabolic disorders such as McArdle's syndrome.
- Endocrinopathies such as thyrotoxicosis, myxedema, hyperparathyroidism, hypoparathyroidism, diabetes mellitus, or Cushing's syndrome.
- Myasthenia gravis with response to cholinergics, sensitivity to d-tubocurarine, and decremental response to repetitive nerve stimulation.

Adapted from Bohan A, Peter JB: Polymyositis and dermatomyositis (first of two parts). N Engl J Med 292:344–347, 1975, with permission.

Criteria for the Classification and Reporting of Osteoarthritis of the Hand, Hip, and Knee

Classification criteria for osteoarthritis of the hand, traditional format*

Hand pain, aching, or stiffness
  and
Three or four of the following features:
  Hard tissue enlargement of two or more of 10 selected joints
  Hard tissue enlargement of two or more DIP joints
  Fewer than three swollen MCP joints
  Deformity of at least one of 10 selected joints

---

* The 10 selected joints are the second and third distal interphalangeal (DIP), the second and third proximal interphalangeal, and the first carpometacarpal joints of both hands. This classification method yields a sensitivity of 94% and a specificity of 87%. MCP = metacarpophalangeal.

Reprinted from Altman R, Alarcón G, Appelrouth D, et al: The American College of Rheumatology criteria for the classification and reporting of osteoarthritis of the hand. Arthritis Rheum 33:1601–1610, 1990, with permission of the American College of Rheumatology.

Classification criteria for osteoarthritis of the hip, traditional format*

Hip pain
  and
At least two of the following three features:
  ESR <20 mm/hour
  Radiographic femoral or acetabular osteophytes
  Radiographic joint space narrowing (superior, axial, and/or medial)

---

* This classification method yields a sensitivity of 89% and a specificity of 91%. ESR = erythrocyte sedimentation rate (Westergren).

Reprinted from Altman R, Alarcón G, Appelrouth D, et al: The American College of Rheumatology criteria for the classification and reporting of osteoarthritis of the hip. Arthritis Rheum 34:505–514, 1991, with permission of the American College of Rheumatology.

Criteria for classification of idiopathic osteoarthritis (OA) of the knee*

CLINICAL AND LABORATORY	CLINICAL AND RADIOGRAPHIC	CLINICAL†
Knee pain plus at least five of nine:	Knee pain plus at least one of three:	Knee pain plus at least three of six:
Age >50 years	Age >50 years	Age >50 years
Stiffness <30 minutes	Stiffness <30 minutes	Stiffness <30 minutes
Crepitus	Crepitus	Crepitus
Bony tenderness	+	Bony tenderness
Bony enlargement	Osteophytes	Bony enlargement
No palpable warmth		No palpable warmth
ESR <40 mm/hr		
RF <1:40		
SF OA		
92% sensitive	91% sensitive	95% sensitive
75% specific	86% specific	69% specific

* ESR = erythrocyte sedimentation rate (Westergren); RF = rheumatoid factor; SF OA = synovial fluid signs of OA (clear, viscous, or white blood cell count <2,000/mm³).
† Alternative for the clinical category would be four of six, which is 84% sensitive and 89% specific.

Reprinted from Altman R, Asch E, Bloch G, et al: Development of criteria for the classification and reporting of osteoarthritis: classification of osteoarthritis of the knee. Arthritis Rheum 29:1039–1049, 1986, with permission of the American College of Rheumatology.

APPENDIX II

Guidelines for the Management of Rheumatic Diseases

Practice guidelines represent a recent and important development in rheumatology. Guidelines, which are developed by a panel of experts, address a broad range of clinical issues from the approach to diagnosis of musculoskeletal signs and symptoms to patient management. Guidelines provide a framework for clinical practice and serve a valuable educational function for students of the rheumatic diseases. Moreover, because in very few instances have guidelines been tested in clinical settings, they present an opportunity to study whether they result in efficiencies or improvements in diagnosis and patient management. This appendix lists guidelines published by the American College of Rheumatology as of July, 1997 with the recognition that additional guidelines are forthcoming.

Initial Evaluation of the Adult Patient with Acute Musculoskeletal Symptoms

"Red flags" suggesting the need for urgent evaluation and management of the patient with musculoskeletal symptoms

FEATURE	DIFFERENTIAL DIAGNOSIS
History of significant trauma	Soft tissue injury, internal derangement, or fracture
Hot, swollen joint	Infection, systemic rheumatic disease, gout, pseudogout
Constitutional signs and symptoms (eg, fever, weight loss, malaise)	Infection, sepsis, systemic rheumatic disease
Weakness	
Focal	Focal nerve lesion (compartment syndrome, entrapment neuropathy, mononeuritis multiplex, motor neuron disease, radiculopathy*)
Diffuse	Myositis, metabolic myopathy, paraneoplastic syndrome, degenerative neuromuscular disorder, toxin, myelopathy,* transverse myelitis
Neurogenic pain (burning, numbness, paresthesia)	
Asymmetric	Radiculopathy,* reflex sympathetic dystrophy, entrapment neuropathy
Symmetric	Myelopathy,* peripheral neuropathy
Claudication pain pattern	Peripheral vascular disease, giant cell arteritis (jaw pain), lumbar spinal stenosis

* Radiculopathy and myelopathy may be due to infectious, neoplastic, or mechanical processes.

Reprinted from American College of Rheumatology Ad Hoc Committee on Clinical Guidelines: Guidelines for the initial evaluation of the adult patient with acute musculoskeletal symptoms. Arthritis Rheum 39:1–8, 1996, with permission of the American College of Rheumatology.

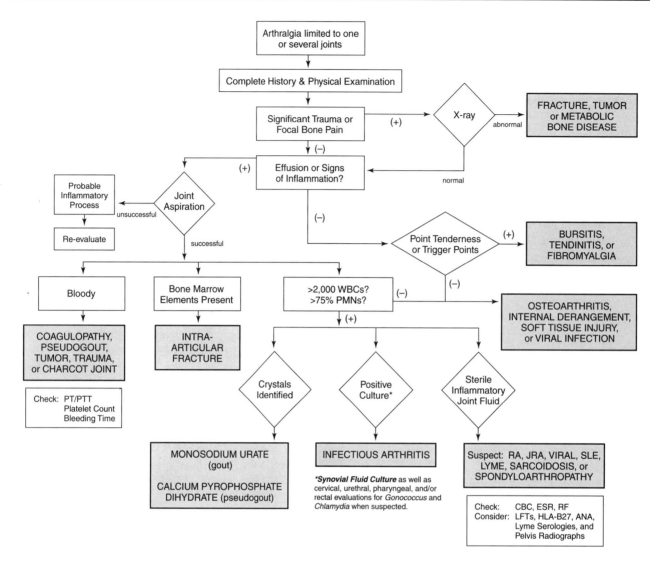

* WBCs = white blood cells; PMNs = polymorphonuclear neutrophils; PT = prothrombin time; PTT = partial thromboplastin time; RA = rheumatoid arthritis; JRA = juvenile rheumatoid arthritis; SLE = systemic lupus erythematosus; CBC = complete blood cell count; ESR = erythrocyte sedimentation rate; RF = rheumatoid factor; LFTs = liver function tests; ANA = antinuclear antibodies.

Reprinted from American College of Rheumatology Ad Hoc Committee on Clinical Guidelines: Guidelines for the initial evaluation of the adult patient with acute musculoskeletal symptoms. Arthritis Rheum 39:1–8, 1996, with permission of the American College of Rheumatology.

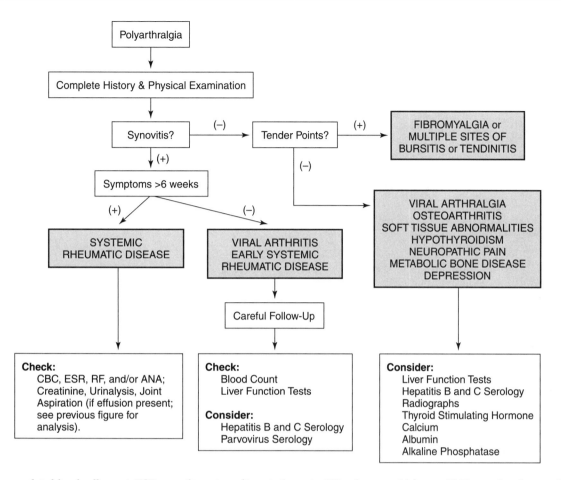

* CBC = complete blood cell count; ESR = erythrocyte sedimentation rate; RF = rheumatoid factor; ANA = antinuclear antibodies.

Reprinted from American College of Rheumatology Ad Hoc Committee on Clinical Guidelines: Guidelines for the initial evaluation of the adult patient with acute musculoskeletal symptoms. Arthritis Rheum 39:1–8, 1996, with permission of the American College of Rheumatology.

Management of Rheumatoid Arthritis

Baseline evaluation of patients with rheumatoid arthritis

Subjective
  Degree of joint pain
  Duration of morning stiffness
  Presence or absence of fatigue
  Limitation of function
Physical examination
  Documentation of actively inflamed joints
  Documentation of mechanical joint problems: loss of motion, crepitus, instability, malalignment and/or deformity
  Documentation of extraarticular manifestations
Laboratory
  Erythrocyte sedimentation rate/C-reactive protein
  Rheumatoid factor*
  Complete blood cell count†
  Electrolytes†
  Creatinine†
  Hepatic panel†
  Urinalysis†
  Synovial fluid analysis‡
  Stool guaiac†
Radiography
  Radiography of selected involved joints§

---

* Performed only at baseline to establish the diagnosis; may be repeated 6–12 months after disease onset if negative initially.
† Performed at baseline to assess organ dysfunction due to comorbid diseases, before starting medications.
‡ Performed at baseline if necessary, to rule out other diseases; may be repeated during disease flares to rule out septic arthritis.
§ May have limited diagnostic value early in the disease, but helps to establish a baseline for periodically monitoring disease progression and response to treatment.

Reprinted from American College of Rheumatology Ad Hoc Committee on Clinical Guidelines: Guidelines for the management of rheumatoid arthritis. Arthritis Rheum 39:713–722, 1996, with permission of the American College of Rheumatology.

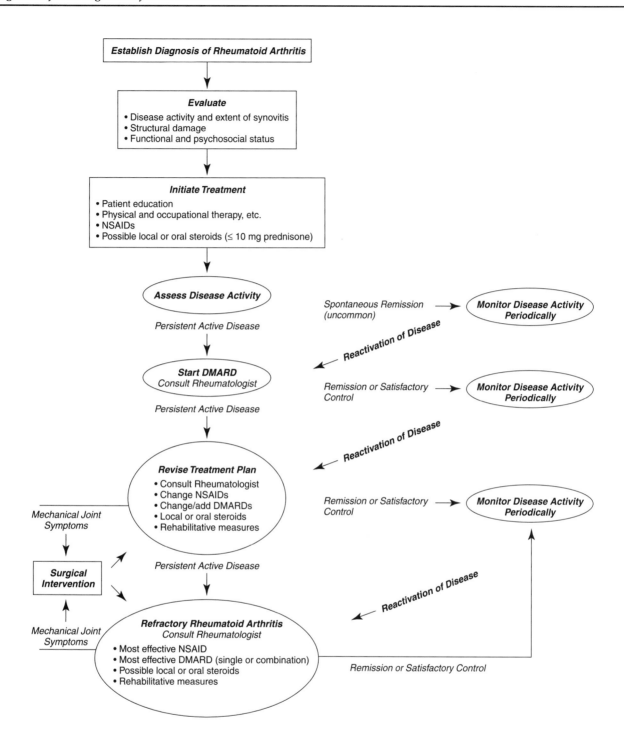

Reprinted from American College of Rheumatology Ad Hoc Committee on Clinical Guidelines: Guidelines for the management of rheumatoid arthritis. Arthritis Rheum 39:713–722, 1996, with permission of the American College of Rheumatology.

Monitoring Drug Therapy in Rheumatoid Arthritis

Recommended monitoring strategies for drug treatment of rheumatoid arthritis*

DRUGS	TOXICITIES REQUIRING MONITORING†	BASELINE EVALUATION	MONITORING — SYSTEM REVIEW/EXAMINATION	MONITORING — LABORATORY
Salicylates, nonsteroidal anti-inflammatory drugs	Gastrointestinal ulceration and bleeding	CBC, creatinine, AST, ALT	Dark/black stool, dyspepsia, nausea or vomiting, abdominal pain, edema, shortness of breath	CBC yearly, LFTs, creatinine testing may be required‡
Hydroxychloroquine	Macular damage	None unless patient is over age 40 or has previous eye disease	Visual changes, funduscopic and visual fields every 6–12 months	—
Sulfasalazine	Myelosuppression	CBC, and AST or ALT in patients at risk, G6PD	Symptoms of myelosuppression§, photosensitivity, rash	CBC every 2–4 weeks for first 3 months, then every 3 months
Methotrexate	Myelosuppression, hepatic fibrosis, cirrhosis, pulmonary infiltrates or fibrosis	CBC, chest radiography within past year, hepatitis B and C serology in high-risk patients, AST or ALT, albumin, alkaline phosphatase, and creatinine	Symptoms of myelosuppression§, shortness of breath, nausea/vomiting, lymph node swelling	CBC, platelet count, AST, albumin, creatinine every 4–8 weeks
Gold, intramuscular	Myelosuppression, proteinuria	CBC, platelet count, creatinine, urine dipstick for protein	Symptoms of myelosuppression§, edema, rash, oral ulcers, diarrhea	CBC, platelet count, urine dipstick every 1–2 weeks for first 20 weeks, then at the time of each (or every other) injection
Gold, oral	Myelosuppression, proteinuria	CBC, platelet count, urine dipstick for protein	Symptoms of myelosuppression§, edema, rash, diarrhea	CBC platelet count, urine dipstick for protein every 4–12 weeks
D-penicillamine	Myelosuppression, proteinuria	CBC, platelet count, creatinine, urine dipstick for protein	Symptoms of myelosuppression§, edema, rash	CBC, urine dipstick for protein every 2 weeks until dosage stable, then every 1–3 months
Azathioprine	Myelosuppression, hepatotoxicity, lymphoproliferative disorders	CBC, platelet count, creatinine, AST or ALT	Symptoms of myelosuppression§	CBC and platelet count every 1–2 weeks with changes in dosage, and every 1–3 months thereafter
Corticosteroids (oral ≤ 10 mg of prednisone or equivalent)	Hypertension, hyperglycemia	BP, chemistry panel, bone densitometry in high-risk patients	BP at each visit, polyuria, polydipsia, edema, shortness of breath, visual changes, weight gain	Urinalysis for glucose yearly
Agents for refractory RA or severe extraarticular complications				
Cyclophosphamide	Myelosuppression, myeloproliferative disorders, malignancy, hemorrhagic cystitis	CBC, platelet count, urinalysis, creatinine, AST or ALT	Symptoms of myelosuppression§, hematuria	CBC and platelet count every 1–2 weeks with changes in dosage, and every 1–3 months thereafter, urinalysis and urine cytology every 6–12 months after cessation
Chlorambucil	Myelosuppression, myeloproliferative disorders, malignancy	CBC, urinalysis, creatinine, AST or ALT	Symptoms of myelosuppression§	CBC and platelet count every 1–2 weeks with changes in dosage, and every 1–3 months thereafter
Cyclosporin A	Renal insufficiency, anemia, hypertension	CBC, creatinine, uric acid, LFTs, BP	Edema, BP every 2 weeks until dosage stable, then monthly	Creatinine every 2 weeks until dose is stable, then monthly; periodic CBC, potassium, and LFTs

* CBC = complete blood cell count (hematocrit, hemoglobin, white blood cell count) including differential cell and platelet counts; ALT = alanine aminotransferase; AST = aspartate aminotransferase; LFTs = liver function tests; BP = blood pressure.

† Potential serious toxicities that may be detected by monitoring before they have become clinically apparent or harmful to the patient. This list mentions toxicities that occur frequently enough to justify monitoring. Patients with comorbidity, concurrent medications, and other specific risk factors may need further studies to monitor for specific toxicity.

‡ Package insert for diclofenac (Voltaren) recommends that AST and ALT be monitored within the first 8 weeks of treatment and periodically thereafter. Monitoring of serum creatinine should be performed weekly for at least 3 weeks in patients receiving concomitant angiotensin-converting enzyme inhibitors or diuretics.

§ Symptoms of myelosuppression include fever, symptoms of infection, easily bruisability, and bleeding.

Reprinted from American College of Rheumatology Ad Hoc Committee on Clinical Guidelines: Guidelines for monitoring drug therapy in rheumatoid arthritis. Arthritis Rheum 39:723–731, 1996, with permission of the American College of Rheumatology.

*Antirheumatic drug therapy in pregnancy and lactation, and effects on fertility**

DRUG	FDA USE-IN-PREGNANCY RATING†	CROSSES PLACENTA	MAJOR MATERNAL TOXICITIES	FETAL TOXICITIES	LACTATION	FERTILITY
Aspirin	C; D in third trimester	Yes	Anemia, peripartum hemorrhage, prolonged labor	Premature closure of ductus, pulmonary hypertension, ICH	Use cautiously; excreted at low concentration; doses > 1 tablet (325 mg) result in high concentration in infant plasma	No data
NSAIDs	B; D in third trimester	Yes	As for aspirin	As for aspirin	Compatible according to AAP	No data
Corticosteroids						
Prednisone	B	Dexamethasone and betamethasone	Exacerbation of diabetes and hypertension, PROM	IUGR	5–20% of maternal dose excreted in breast milk; compatible, but wait 4 hours if dose > 20 mg	No data
Dexamethasone	C					
Hydroxychloroquine	C	Yes: fetal concentration 50% of maternal	Few	Few	Contraindicated (slow elimination rate, potential for accumulation)	No data
Gold	C	Yes	No data	1 report of cleft palate and severe CNS abnormalities	Excreted into breast milk (20% of maternal dose); rash, hepatitis, and hematologic abnormalities reported, but AAP considers it compatible	No data
D-penicillamine	D	Yes	No data	Cutis laxa connective tissue abnormalities	No data	No data
Sulfasalazine	B; D if near term	Yes	No data	No increase in congenital malformations, kernicterus if administered near term	Excreted into breast milk (40–60% maternal dose); bloody diarrhea in 1 infant; AAP recommends caution	Females: no effect; males: significant oligospermia (2 months to return to normal)
Azathioprine	D	Yes	No data	IUGR (rate up to 40%) and prematurity, transient immunosuppression in neonate, possible effect on germlines of offspring	No data; hypothetical risk of immunosuppression outweighs benefit	Not studied; can interfere with effectiveness of IUD
Chlorambucil	D	Teratogenic effects potentiated by caffeine	No data	Renal angiogenesis	Contraindicated	No data
Methotrexate	X	No data	Spontaneous abortion	Fetal abnormalities (including cleft palate and hydrocephalus)	Contraindicated; small amounts excreted with potential to accumulate in fetal tissues	Females: infrequent long-term effect; males: reversible oligospermia
Cyclophosphamide	D	Yes; 25% of maternal level	No data	Severe abnormalities; case report: male twin developed thyroid papillary cancer at 11 years and neuroblastoma at 14 years	Contraindicated; has caused bone marrow depression	Females: age > 25 years, concurrent radiation, and prolonged exposure increase risk of infertility; males: dose-dependent oligospermia and azoospermia regardless of age or exposure
Cyclosporin A	C	Yes	No data	IUGR and prematurity; 1 case report: hypoplasia of rightleg; not an animal teratogen and unlikely to be a human one	Contraindicated due to potential for immunosuppression	No data

* ICH = intracranial hemorrhage; AAP = American Academy of Pediatrics; PROM = premature rupture of membranes; IUGR = intrauterine growth retardation; CNS = central nervous system; IUD = intrauterine device.

† Food and Drug Administration (FDA) use-in-pregnancy ratings are as follows: A = Controlled studies show no risk. Adequate, well-controlled studies in pregnant women have failed to demonstrate risk to the fetus. B = No evidence of risk in humans. Either animal findings show risk but human findings do not, or, if no adequate human studies have been performed, animal findings are negative. C = Risk cannot be ruled out. Human studies are lacking and results of animal studies are either positive for fetal risk or lacking as well. However, potential benefits may justify the potential risk. D = Positive evidence of risk. Investigational or post-marketing data show risk to the fetus. Nevertheless, potential benefits may outweigh the potential risk. X = Contraindicated in pregnancy. Studies in animals or humans, or investigational or post-marketing reports, have shown fetal risk which clearly outweighs any possible benefit to the patient.

Reprinted from American College of Rheumatology Ad Hoc Committee on Clinical Guidelines: Guidelines for monitoring drug therapy in rheumatoid arthritis. Arthritis Rheum 39:723–731, 1996, with permission of the American College of Rheumatology.

Recommendations for monitoring for hepatic safety in rheumatoid arthritis (RA) patients receiving methotrexate (MTX)

A. Baseline
   1. Tests for all patients
      a. Liver blood tests (aspartate aminotransferase [AST], alanine aminotransferase [ALT], alkaline phosphatase, albumin, bilirubin), hepatitis B and C serologic studies
      b. Other standard tests, including complete blood cell count and serum creatinine
   2. Pretreatment liver biopsy (Menghini suction-type needle) only for patients with:
      a. Prior excessive alcohol consumption
      b. Persistently abnormal baseline AST values
      c. Chronic hepatitis B or C infection
B. Monitor AST, ALT, albumin at 4–8-week intervals
C. Perform liver biopsy if:
   1. Five of 9 determinations of AST within a given 12-month interval (six of 12 if tests are performed monthly) are abnormal (defined as an elevation above the upper limit of normal)
   2. There is a decrease in serum albumin below the normal range (in the setting of well-controlled RA)
D. If results of liver biopsy are:
   1. Roenigk grade I, II, or IIIA, resume MTX and monitor as in B, C1, and C2 above
   2. Roenigk grade IIIB or IV, discontinue MTX
E. Discontinue MTX in patient with persistent liver test abnormalities, as defined in C1 and C2 above, who refuses liver biopsy

Reprinted from Kremer JM, Alarcón GS, Lightfoot RW Jr, et al: Methotrexate for rheumatoid arthritis: suggested guidelines for monitoring liver toxicity. Arthritis Rheum 37:316–328, 1994, with permission of the American College of Rheumatology.

Osteoarthritis of the Hip

Nonpharmacologic therapy*

Patient education
   Self-management programs (eg, Arthritis Self-Help Course)
Health professional social support via telephone contact
Weight loss (if overweight)
Physical therapy
   Range of motion exercises
   Strengthening exercises
   Assistive devices for ambulation
Occupational therapy
   Joint protection and energy conservation
   Assistive devices for ADLs and IADLs
Aerobic aquatic exercise programs

* ADLs = activities of daily living; IADLs = instrumental ADLs.

Medical management of symptomatic osteoarthritis of the hip

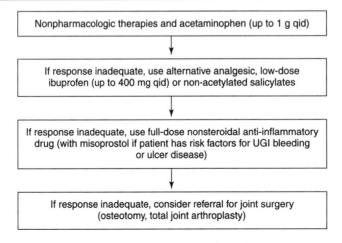

Reprinted from Hochberg MD, Altman RD, Brandt KD, et al: Guidelines for the medical management of osteoarthritis: part I. Osteoarthritis of the hip. Arthritis Rheum 38:1535–1540, 1995, with permission of the American College of Rheumatology.

Osteoarthritis of the Knee

*Nonpharmacologic therapy**

Patient education
   Self-management programs (eg, Arthritis Self-Help Course)
Health professional social support via telephone contact
Weight loss (if overweight)
Physical therapy
   Range of motion exercises
   Quadriceps strengthening exercises
   Assistive devices for ambulation
Occupational therapy
   Joint protection and energy conservation
   Assistive devices for ADLs and IADLs
Aerobic exercise programs

* ADLs = activities of daily living; IADLs = instrumental ADLs.

Medical management of symptomatic osteoarthritis of the knee

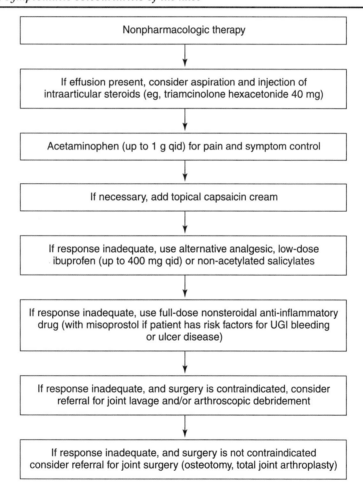

Reprinted from Hochberg MD, Altman RD, Brandt KD, et al: Guidelines for the medical management of osteoarthritis: part II. Osteoarthritis of the knee. Arthritis Rheum 38:1541–1546, 1995, with permission of the American College of Rheumatology.

Prevention and Treatment of Glucocorticoid-induced Osteoporosis

Initial evaluation

History and physical
- Documentation of height, weight, muscle strength, balance, vision
- Documentation of medication history
- Documentation of menstrual history in menstruating women/infertility in men
- Family history (mother and father) of fractures

Lifestyle modification
- Documentation of modifiable influences
  - Calcium and vitamin D intake
  - Smoking
  - Medications
  - Prevention of falling
  - Alcohol intake

Patient education
- Prevention of falling
- Physical therapy
  - Back extension exercises
  - Posture training
  - Balance
  - Gait evaluation
  - Assistive devices
  - Kypho-orthosis (as needed)

Pain control
- Nonpharmacologic strategies
- Calcitonin (intranasal or injectable)
- Muscle relaxants
- Analgesics; narcotics when necessary

Laboratory
- Complete blood cell count
- Erythrocyte sedimentation rate
- Serum creatinine
- 24-hour urinary calcium
- Serum calcium
- Serum phosphorus
- Serum alkaline phosphatase
- Serum electrolytes
- Serum 25-hydroxyvitamin D
- Serum testosterone (male)
- Serum luteinizing hormone (female)
- Serum albumin
- Serum levels of liver enzyme

Dual-energy x-ray absorptiometry
- Hip (all patients)
- Spine (patients below age 60)

Follow-up for abnormal laboratory findings

ABNORMAL FINDING	FOLLOW UP EVALUATION
High serum calcium, low serum phosphorus, low urinary calcium	Measure intact parathyroid hormone
Low serum calcium, low serum phosphorus, low urinary calcium	Measure 25-hydroxy-vitamin D
Taking thyroid replacement	Measure thyroid-stimulating hormone
High serum creatinine	Evaluate for renal osteo-dystrophy
Elevated 24-hour urinary calcium	Add thiazide diuretic with potassium supplement
Elevated total protein or serum globulin	Obtain serum protein electrophoresis and serum and urine immunoelectrophoresis

Approach to the patient starting long-term glucocorticoid treatment

A. Calcium and vitamin D supplementation
B. Patient education
C. Treatment based on dual-energy x-ray absorptiometry
  T score ≥ -1
    hormone replacement therapy
  T score < -1
    hormone replacement therapy only in postmenopausal women

Modified from American College of Rheumatology Task Force on Osteoporosis Guidelines: Recommendations for the prevention and treatment of glucocorticoid-induced osteoporosis. Arthritis Rheum 39:1791–1801, 1996.

Approach to a patient receiving long-term corticosteroids who has osteoporosis

A. Physical therapy
B. Patient Education
C. Treatment based on dual-energy x-ray absorptiometry findings and laboratory results

   T score ≥ – 1 and normal lab results

   Calcium and vitamin D supplementation
   Hormone replacement therapy
   Reinforce physical therapy

   T score ≥ –1 and abnormal lab results

   Reinforce physical therapy
   Treat underlying causes
   Calcium and vitamin D supplementation
   Hormone replacement therapy

   T score < –1 and normal lab results

   Calcium and vitamin D supplementation
   Reinforce physical therapy
   Hormone replacement therapy

   T score < –1 and abnormal lab results

   Reinforce physical therapy
   Treat underlying conditions
   Calcium and vitamin D supplementation

Modified from American College of Rheumatology Task Force on Osteoporosis Guidelines: Recommendations for the prevention and treatment of glucocorticoid-induced osteoporosis. Arthritis Rheum 39:1791–1801, 1996.

*Hormone replacement therapy**

May elect to initiate immediately or after results of DEXA reveal a BMD T score ≥ –1. (Adjustment of testosterone levels in men should be considered only after results of DEXA reveal a BMD T score ≥ –1.)

Postmenopausal women

Estrogen replacement therapy: A progestin must be added for any woman with an intact uterus. If refused or contraindicated, prescribe calcitonin or bisphosphonates.

Premenopausal women with intact ovarian function (ages 13–50)

Estrogen-containing oral contraceptives (minimum of 50 μg of estradiol or equivalent). If refused or contraindicated, prescribe calcitonin.

Men

Testosterone (if serum testosterone abnormally low). If refused or contraindicated, prescribe calcitonin or bisphosphonates.

* DEXA = dual-energy x-ray absorptiometry; BMD = bone mineral density.

Reprinted from American College of Rheumatology Task Force on Osteoporosis Guidelines: Recommendations for the prevention and treatment of glucocorticoid-induced osteoporosis. Arthritis Rheum 39:1791–1801, 1996.

APPENDIX III

CD Markers Associated with Rheumatic Diseases

Lymphocytes are composed of distinct subsets that are phenotypically and functionally diverse. Initially, polyclonal and later, monoclonal antibodies were used to isolate lymphocyte subsets. Differences in the expression of membrane proteins were associated with differences in function, providing the opportunity to study the role of lymphocyte subpopulations in normal and pathologic immune responses. Studies were greatly enhanced by the availability of monoclonal antibodies and the development of the CD (cluster of differentiation) nomenclature. International consensus conferences are held to assign CD numbers to cell surface markers expressed on particular lineages or differentiation stages which have defined biochemical structures and are recognized by groups ("clusters") of monoclonal antibodies. CD markers on lymphocytes have been frequently associated with two functions, facilitating adhesion and cell–cell interaction or transmitting signals across the cell membrane thereby regulating lymphocyte activation.

This list is adapted from the results of the 6th International Workshop on Human Leukocyte Differentiation Antigens held in Kobe, Japan in 1996. Information provided in a table of human CD antigens from Research Diagnostics (http://www.researchd.com/rdicdabs/cdindex.htm) has been incorporated. CD guides are also available at http://www.ncbi.nlm.nih.gov./prow.

CD ANTIGEN	OTHER NAMES	CELLULAR EXPRESSION	FUNCTIONS
CD1a-d		Cortical thymocytes, Langerhans cells, dendritic cells, B cells, intestinal epithelium	MHC class I-like molecules Possible role in antigen presentation
CD2	LFA-2 (leukocyte function-associated antigen-2)	T cells, thymocytes, NK cells	Adhesion Binds CD58 T cell activation
CD3		Thymocytes, T cells	Associated with the T cell antigen receptor-signal transduction
CD4		MHC class II restricted T cells	Co-receptor for MHCclass II molecules-signal transduction Receptor for HIV-1 and HIV-2 gp120
CD5		Thymocytes, T cells, B cell subset	Binds CD72
CD6		Thymocytes, T cells, B cell subset	Binds ALCAM
CD7		Pleuripotent hematopoietic cells, thymocytes, T cells	?
CD8		MHC class I restricted T cells	Co-receptor for MHC class I molecules-signal transduction
CD11a	LFA-1 (leukocyte function-associated antigen-1)	Leukocytes	α^L subunit of integrin (associated with CD18) Binds CD50, CD54, and CD102
CD11b	Mac-1 CR3 (α chain)	Myeloid cells, NK cells	α^M subunit of integrin (associated with CD18) Binds CD54, complement component iC3b, and extracellular matrix proteins
CD11c	CR4 (α chain)	Monocytes, granulocytes, NK cells	α^X subunit of integrin CR4 (associated with CD18) Binds fibrinogen

CD ANTIGEN	OTHER NAMES	CELLULAR EXPRESSION	FUNCTIONS
CD14		Myelomonocytic cells	LPS receptor
CD15	FcγRIII	Granulocytes	Sialyl form is a ligand for selectin
CD16 a-b		Neutrophils, NK cells, macrophages	Low affinity Fc receptor Phagocytosis ADCC
CD18		Leukocytes	Integrin β2 subunit - associates with CD11a, b, and c
CD19		B cells	Forms complex with CD21 and CD81 Co-receptor for B cells
CD20		B cells	Role in regulating B cell activation
CD21	CR2	Mature B cells, FDC	Receptor for C3d and EBV Co-receptor for B cells
CD22		Mature B cells	Adhesion of B cells to monocytes and T cells
CD23	FcεRII	Mature B cells, activated macrophages, eosinophils, FDC, platelets	Low affinity IgE receptor Ligand for CD19: CD21: CD81 co-receptor
CD25	Tac, IL-2R	Activated T cells, B cells, monocytes	IL-2 receptor (α-chain)
CD26	Dipeptdyl peptidase IV	Activated B and T cells, macrophages	Protease-possibly implicated in HIV entry into cells
CD27		Medullary thymocytes, T cells	
CD28		T cell subset, Activated B cells	Activation of naive T cells Receptor for costimulatory signal (signal 2) Binds CD80 and CD86
CD29		Leukocytes	Integrin β1 subunit Associates with CD49a in VLA-1 integrin
CD30	Ki-1	Activated B and T cells	Possible marker for TH$_2$ cells
CD31	PECAM-1	Monocytes, platelets, granulocytes, B cells, endothelial cells	Adhesion
CDw32	FcγRII	Monocytes, granulocytes, B cells, eosinophils	Low affinity Fc receptor for aggregated Ig/immune complexes
CD34		Hematopoietic precursors, capillary endothelium	Ligand for CD62
CD35	CR1	Erythrocytes, B cells, monocytes, neutrophils, eosinophils, FDC	Complement receptor 1 Binds C3b and C4b Mediates phagocytosis

CD ANTIGEN	OTHER NAMES	CELLULAR EXPRESSION	FUNCTIONS
CD40		B cells, monocytes, dendritic cells	Binds to CD40 ligand Costimulatory signal to B cells
CD43	Leukosialin, Sialophorin	Leukocytes except resting B cells	Binds CD54
CD44	Pgp-1	Leukocytes, erythrocytes	Binds hyaluronic acid Mediates adhesion of leukocytes
CD45	Leukocyte common antigen (LCA), T200, B220	Leukocytes	Tyrosine phosphatase Augments signalling through antigen receptor of B and T cells Multiple isoforms result from alternative splicing
CD45RA		B cells, naive T cells, monocytes	Isoform of CD45 containing A exon
CD45RB		B and T cell subsets, monocytes, macrophages, granulocytes	Isoform of CD45 containing B exon
CD45RO		B and T cell subsets, monocytes, macrophages	Isoform of CD45 containing none of the A,B, or C exons
CD46		Hematopoietic cells, nonhematopoietic cells	Membrane cofactor protein Binds to C3b and C4b to permit their degradation by Factor I
CD47		All cells	Possibly costimulation of T cells
CD49a	VLA-1	Activated T cells, monocytes	α1 integrin Associates with CD29 Binds collagen and laminin
CD49b	VLA-2	B cells, monocytes, platelets	α2 integrin Associates with CD29 Binds collagen and laminin
CD49c	VLA-3	B cells	α3 integrin Associates with CD29 Binds laminin and fibronectin
CD49d	VLA-4	B cells, thymocytes	α4 integrin Associates with CD29 Binds fibronectin, Peyerís Patch homing receptor, and VCAM-1
CD49e	VLA-5	Memory T cells, monocytes, platelets	α5 integrin Associates with CD29 Binds fibronectin
CD49f	VLA-6	Memory T cells, thymocytes, monocytes	α6 integrin Associates with CD29 Binds laminin
CD50	ICAM-3 (intracelluar adhesion molecule-3)	Thymocytes, B cells, T cells, monocytes, granulocytes	Adhesion

CD ANTIGEN	OTHER NAMES	CELLULAR EXPRESSION	FUNCTIONS
CD51	Vitronectin receptor	Platelets, megakaryocytes	Integrin - associates with CD61 Binds vitronectin, von Willebrand factor, fibrinogen and thrombospondin
CD54	ICAM-1 (intracelluar adhesion molecule-1)	Hematopoietic cells, nonhematopoietic cells	Binds CD11a/Cd18 and CD11b/CD18 integrins Receptor for rhinovirus
CD55	DAF (decay accelerating factor)	Hemopoietic cells, nonhemopoietic cells	Binds C3b Disassembles C3 convertase
CD56	NKH-1	NK cells	Isoform of Neural Cell Adhesion Molecule (NCAM) Adhesion
CD57	HNK-1, Leu-7	NK cells, T cell subset, B cells, monocytes	Oligosaccharide - expressed on cell surface glycoproteins
CD58	LFA-3 (leukocyte function-associated antigen-3)	Hemopoietic cells, nonhemopoietic cells	Adhesion Binds CD2
CD59		Hemopoietic cells, nonhemopoietic cells	Binds complement components C8 and C9 Blocks assembly of membrane attack complex
CD60		T cell subset, platelets, monocytes	
CD61		Platelets, megakaryocytes, macrophages	Integrin β3 subunit Associates with CD41 or CD51
CD62E	ELAM-1 (endothelium leukocyte adhesion molecule-1), E-selectin	Endothelium	Binds sialyl-Lewis x Mediates rolling interaction of neutrophils on endothelium
CD62L	L-selectin, LECAM-1, LAM-1 (leukocyte adhesion molecule -1)	B cells, T cells, monocytes, NK cells	Binds CD34 and GlyCAM Mediates rolling interactions with endothelium
CD62P	P-selectin	Platelets, megakaryocytes, endothelium	Adhesion Binds sialyl-Lewis x Mediates interaction of platelets with neutrophils and monocytes Rolling interaction of neutrophils on endothelium
CD64	FcγRI	Monocytes, macrophages	High affinity receptor for IgG
CD66		Neutrophils	Unknown Member of carcino-embryonic antigen (CEA) family
CD68	Macrosialin	Monocytes, macrophages	Early activation antigen

CD ANTIGEN	OTHER NAMES	CELLULAR EXPRESSION	FUNCTIONS
CD69		Activated B and T cells, macrophages, NK cells	Early activation antigen
CD70	Ki-24	Activated B and T cells, macrophages	Costimulation
CD71		Activated leukocytes	Transferrin receptor
CD72		B cells	Ligand for CD5
CD73		B and T cell subsets	Ecto-5'-nucleotidase-dephosphorylates nucleotides to allow nucleoside uptake
CD74		MHC class II positive cells	MHC class II associated invariant chain
CD77		Germinal center B cells	
CD79a-b	Igα, Igβ	B cells	Components of B cell antigen receptor (analogous to CD3) Cell surface expression and signal transduction
CD80	B7-1	B cell subset	Costimulator Ligand for CD28 and CTLA-4
CD81		Lymphocytes	Associates with CD19 and CD21 to form B cell co-receptor
CD86	B7-2	Monocytes, activated B cells	Costimulation
CD87		Granulocytes, monocytes, macrophages, activated T cells	Urokinase plasminogen activator receptor
CD88	C5aR	Polymorphonuclear leukocytes, macrophages, mast cells	Receptor for complement component C5a
CD89	FcαR	Monocytes, macrophages, granulocytes, neutrophils, B and T cell subsets	IgA receptor
CD91		Monocytes	α2 macroglobulin receptor
CD94		T cell subsets, NK cells	Inhibits killing
CD95	Apo-1, Fas	Many cells	Binds Fas ligand induces apoptosis
CD102	ICAM-2 (intracelluar adhesion molecule-2)	Resting lymphocytes, monocytes, vascular endothelial cells	Binds CD11a/CD18 but not CD11b/CD18
CD103	αE integrin	Intraepithelial lymphocytes, few circulating lymphocytes	αE integrin
CD104	β4 integrin	Epithelia, Schwann cells, tumor cell subset	β4 integrin

CD ANTIGEN	OTHER NAMES	CELLULAR EXPRESSION	FUNCTIONS
CD105	Endoglin	Endothelial cells, bone marrow cell subset, activated macrophages	
CD106	VCAM-1	Endothelial cells	Adhesion Ligand for VLA-4
CD114		Granulocytes	G-CSF receptor
CD115	M-CSFR	monocytes, macrophages	Macrophage Colony Stimulating Factor (M-CSF) receptor
CD116	GM-CSFRα	Monocytes, neutrophils, eosinophils, endothelium	Granulocyte Macrophage Colony Stimulating Factor (GM-CSF) receptor (α chain)
CD117	c-kit	Hematopoietic progenitors	Stem Cell Factor (SCF) receptor
CD118	IFNα, βR	Many cells	Interferon α, β receptor
CD119	IFNγR	Macrophages, monocytes, B cells, endothelium	Interferon γ receptor
CD120a	TNFR-I (p55)	Hematopoietic cells nonhematopoietic cells, epithelial cells (high)	TNF receptor - type I
CD120b	TNFR-II (p75)	Hematopoietic cells nonhematopoietic cells, myeloid cells (high)	TNFα, β receptor - type II
CD121a	IL-1R, type I	Thymocytes, T cells	IL-1 receptor - type I Signal transduction
CDw121b	IL-1R, type II	B cells, macrophages, monocytes	IL-1 receptor - type II Unknown function
CD122	IL-2Rβ	NK cells, resting T cell subset, B cell subset	IL-2 receptor (β chain)
CDw123	IL-3R	Bone marrow stem cells, granulocytes, monocytes, megakaryocytes	IL-3 receptor (α chain)
CD124	IL-4R	Mature B and T cells, hematopoietic precursor cells	IL-4 receptor
CDw125	IL-5R	Eosinophils, basopohils	IL-5 receptor
CD126	IL-6R	Activated B cells, plasma cells	IL-6 receptor (α chain)
CD127	IL-7R	Bone marrow lymphoid precursors, pro-B cells, mature T cells, monocytes	IL-7 receptor
CDw128	IL-8R	Neutrophils, basophils, T cell subset	IL-8 receptor

CD ANTIGEN	OTHER NAMES	CELLULAR EXPRESSION	FUNCTIONS
CDw130	IL-6R β	Activated B cells, plasma cells, endothelial cells	IL-6 receptor (β subunit)
CDw131			IL-3R (common β chain)
CD132			Common γ chain
CD134	Ox40		Costimulation
CDw137	4-1BB		Costimulation
CD138	Syndecan 1	Plasma cells	
CD140a		Endothelial cells	PDGF receptor (α chain)
CD140b		Endothelial cells	PDGF receptor (β chain)
CD141		Endothelial cells	Thrombomodulin
CD142	Tissue factor	Endothelial cells	
CD143	ACE (angiotensin converting enzyme)	Endothelial cells	
CD144	Cadherin		
CDw150	SLAM (surface lymphocyte activation marker)		Costimulation
CD152	CTLA-4	T cells	Costimulation-negative signal
CD153		T cells	Ligand for CD30
CD154		Activated T cells	Ligand for CD40
CD155			Polio Virus receptor (PVR)
CD158a	p58.1	NK cells	MHC class I specific NK receptor
CD158b	p58.2	NK cells	MHC class I specific NK receptor
CD161	NKRP-1A	NK cells	
CD162	P-selectin glycoprotein ligand-1 (PSGL-1)		Adhesion
CD164			Adhesion
CD165			Adhesion
CD166	ALCAM		Adhesion

APPENDIX IV

Human Genome Maps for the Rheumatic Diseases

In order to understand the genetic basis of disease, researchers have set the goal of constructing a complete genetic and physical map of the human genome. A selection of genes relevant for rheumatic diseases is shown here.

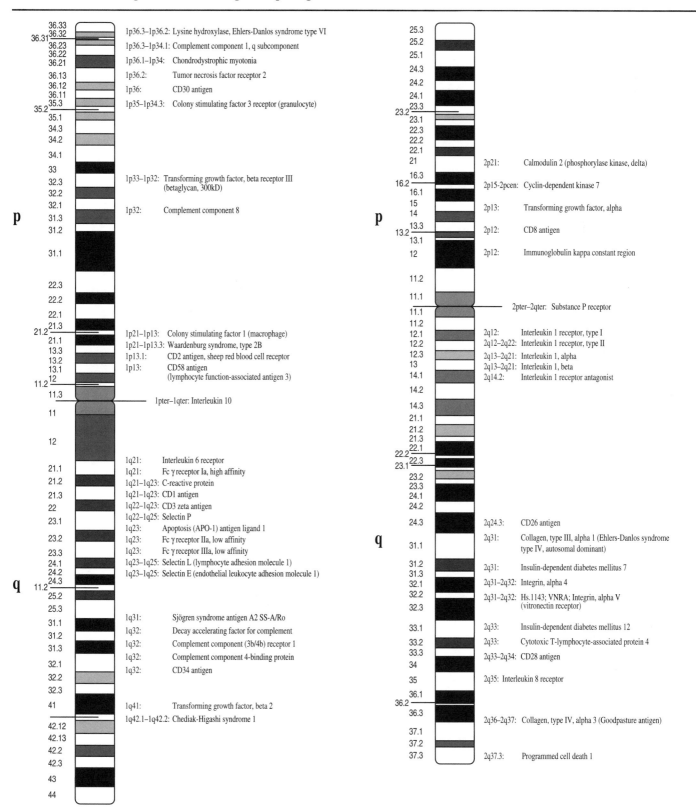

Chromosome 1

1p36.3–1p36.2: Lysine hydroxylase, Ehlers-Danlos syndrome type VI
1p36.3–1p34.1: Complement component 1, q subcomponent
1p36.1–1p34:   Chondrodystrophic myotonia
1p36.2:   Tumor necrosis factor receptor 2
1p36:   CD30 antigen
1p35–1p34.3:   Colony stimulating factor 3 receptor (granulocyte)

1p33–1p32:   Transforming growth factor, beta receptor III
               (betaglycan, 300kD)
1p32:   Complement component 8

1p21–1p13:   Colony stimulating factor 1 (macrophage)
1p21–1p13.3:   Waardenburg syndrome, type 2B
1p13.1:   CD2 antigen, sheep red blood cell receptor
1p13:   CD58 antigen
               (lymphocyte function-associated antigen 3)

1pter–1qter: Interleukin 10

1q21:   Interleukin 6 receptor
1q21:   Fc γ receptor Ia, high affinity
1q21–1q23:   C-reactive protein
1q21–1q23:   CD1 antigen
1q22–1q23:   CD3 zeta antigen
1q22–1q25:   Selectin P
1q23:   Apoptosis (APO-1) antigen ligand 1
1q23:   Fc γ receptor IIa, low affinity
1q23:   Fc γ receptor IIIa, low affinity
1q23–1q25:   Selectin L (lymphocyte adhesion molecule 1)
1q23–1q25:   Selectin E (endothelial leukocyte adhesion molecule 1)

1q31:   Sjögren syndrome antigen A2 SS-A/Ro
1q32:   Decay accelerating factor for complement
1q32:   Complement component (3b/4b) receptor 1
1q32:   Complement component 4-binding protein
1q32:   CD34 antigen

1q41:   Transforming growth factor, beta 2
1q42.1–1q42.2: Chediak-Higashi syndrome 1

Chromosome 2

2p21:   Calmodulin 2 (phosphorylase kinase, delta)
2p15-2pcen: Cyclin-dependent kinase 7
2p13:   Transforming growth factor, alpha
2p12:   CD8 antigen
2p12:   Immunoglobulin kappa constant region

2pter–2qter: Substance P receptor

2q12:   Interleukin 1 receptor, type I
2q12–2q22:   Interleukin 1 receptor, type II
2q13–2q21:   Interleukin 1, alpha
2q13–2q21:   Interleukin 1, beta
2q14.2:   Interleukin 1 receptor antagonist

2q24.3:   CD26 antigen
2q31:   Collagen, type III, alpha 1 (Ehlers-Danlos syndrome
               type IV, autosomal dominant)
2q31:   Insulin-dependent diabetes mellitus 7
2q31–2q32:   Integrin, alpha 4
2q31–2q32:   Hs.1143; VNRA; Integrin, alpha V
               (vitronectin receptor)
2q33:   Insulin-dependent diabetes mellitus 12
2q33:   Cytotoxic T-lymphocyte-associated protein 4
2q33–2q34:   CD28 antigen
2q35:   Interleukin 8 receptor

2q36–2q37:   Collagen, type IV, alpha 3 (Goodpasture antigen)

2q37.3:   Programmed cell death 1

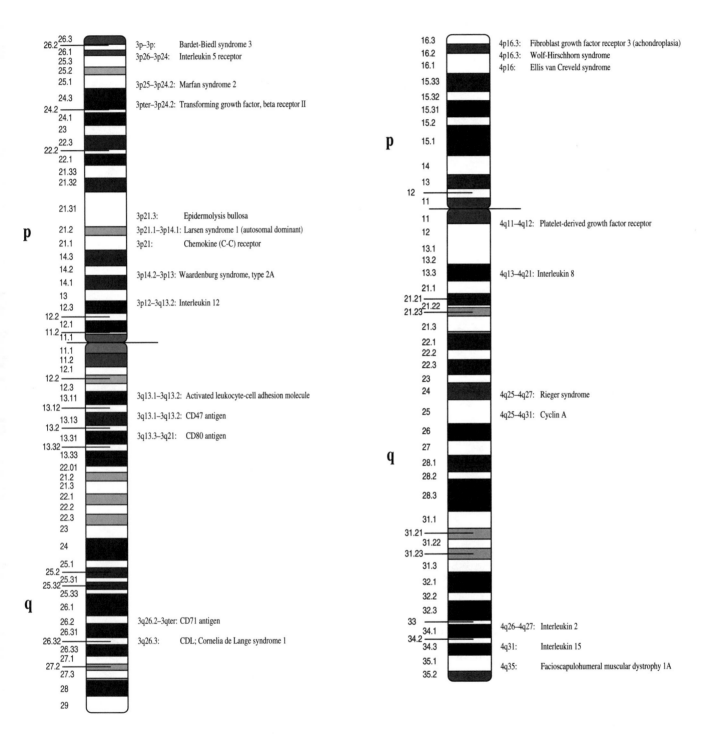

Chromosome 3

3p–3p:	Bardet-Biedl syndrome 3
3p26–3p24:	Interleukin 5 receptor
3p25–3p24.2:	Marfan syndrome 2
3pter–3p24.2:	Transforming growth factor, beta receptor II
3p21.3:	Epidermolysis bullosa
3p21.1–3p14.1:	Larsen syndrome 1 (autosomal dominant)
3p21:	Chemokine (C-C) receptor
3p14.2–3p13:	Waardenburg syndrome, type 2A
3p12–3q13.2:	Interleukin 12
3q13.1–3q13.2:	Activated leukocyte-cell adhesion molecule
3q13.1–3q13.2:	CD47 antigen
3q13.3–3q21:	CD80 antigen
3q26.2–3qter:	CD71 antigen
3q26.3:	CDL; Cornelia de Lange syndrome 1

Chromosome 4

4p16.3:	Fibroblast growth factor receptor 3 (achondroplasia)
4p16.3:	Wolf-Hirschhorn syndrome
4p16:	Ellis van Creveld syndrome
4q11–4q12:	Platelet-derived growth factor receptor
4q13–4q21:	Interleukin 8
4q25–4q27:	Rieger syndrome
4q25–4q31:	Cyclin A
4q26–4q27:	Interleukin 2
4q31:	Interleukin 15
4q35:	Facioscapulohumeral muscular dystrophy 1A

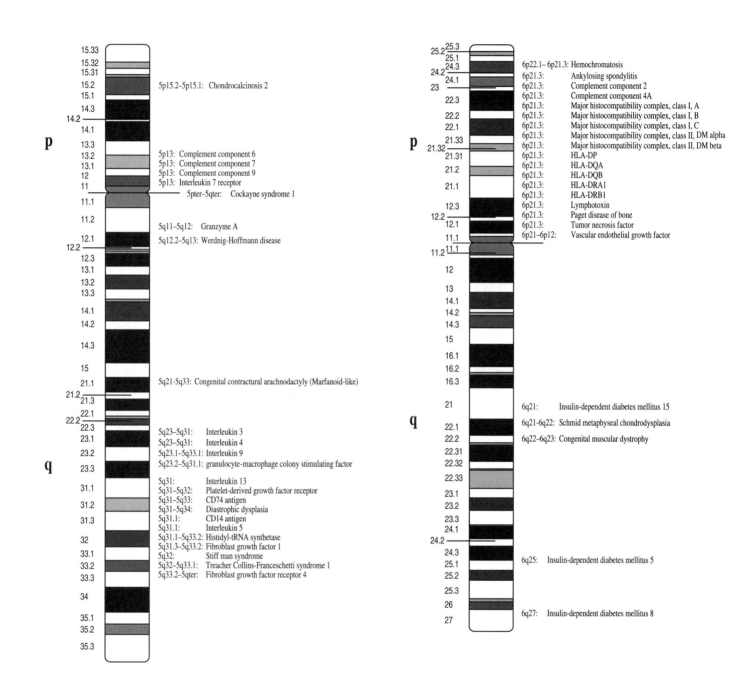

Chromosome 5

5p15.2–5p15.1: Chondrocalcinosis 2

5p13: Complement component 6
5p13: Complement component 7
5p13: Complement component 9
5p13: Interleukin 7 receptor
5pter–5qter: Cockayne syndrome 1

5q11–5q12: Granzyme A
5q12.2–5q13: Werdnig-Hoffmann disease

5q21-5q33: Congenital contractural arachnodactyly (Marfanoid-like)

5q23–5q31: Interleukin 3
5q23–5q31: Interleukin 4
5q23.1–5q33.1: Interleukin 9
5q23.2–5q31.1: granulocyte-macrophage colony stimulating factor

5q31: Interleukin 13
5q31–5q32: Platelet-derived growth factor receptor
5q31–5q33: CD74 antigen
5q31–5q34: Diastrophic dysplasia
5q31.1: CD14 antigen
5q31.1: Interleukin 5
5q31.1–5q33.2: Histidyl-tRNA synthetase
5q31.3–5q33.2: Fibroblast growth factor 1
5q32: Stiff man syndrome
5q32–5q33.1: Treacher Collins-Franceschetti syndrome 1
5q33.2–5qter: Fibroblast growth factor receptor 4

Chromosome 6

6p22.1– 6p21.3: Hemochromatosis
6p21.3: Ankylosing spondylitis
6p21.3: Complement component 2
6p21.3: Complement component 4A
6p21.3: Major histocompatibility complex, class I, A
6p21.3: Major histocompatibility complex, class I, B
6p21.3: Major histocompatibility complex, class I, C
6p21.3: Major histocompatibility complex, class II, DM alpha
6p21.3: Major histocompatibility complex, class II, DM beta
6p21.3: HLA-DP
6p21.3: HLA-DQA
6p21.3: HLA-DQB
6p21.3: HLA-DRA1
6p21.3: HLA-DRB1
6p21.3: Lymphotoxin
6p21.3: Paget disease of bone
6p21.3: Tumor necrosis factor
6p21–6p12: Vascular endothelial growth factor

6q21: Insulin-dependent diabetes mellitus 15
6q21-6q22: Schmid metaphyseal chondrodysplasia
6q22–6q23: Congenital muscular dystrophy

6q25: Insulin-dependent diabetes mellitus 5

6q27: Insulin-dependent diabetes mellitus 8

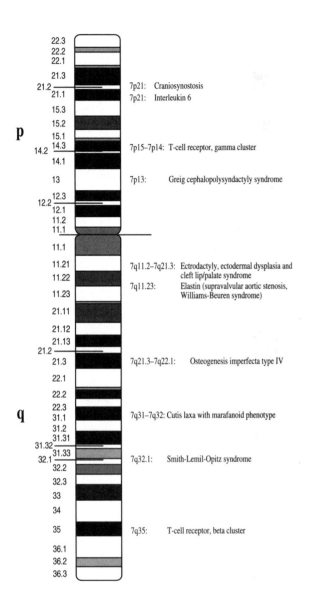

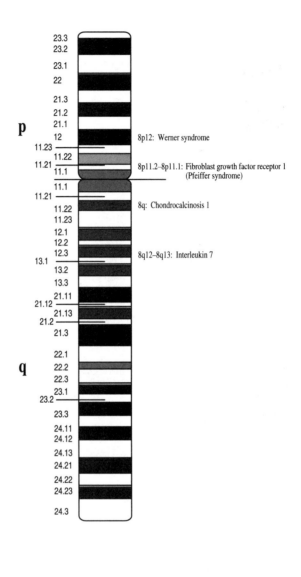

Chromosome 7

Chromosome 8

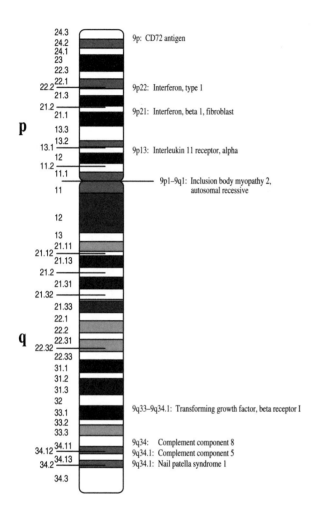

Chromosome 9

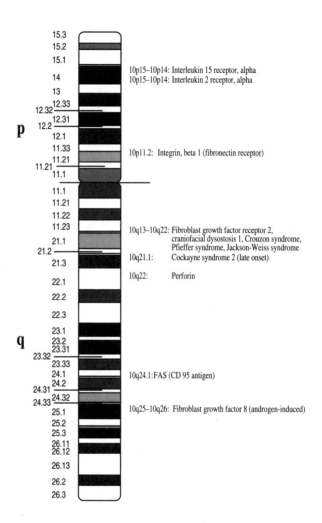

Chromosome 10

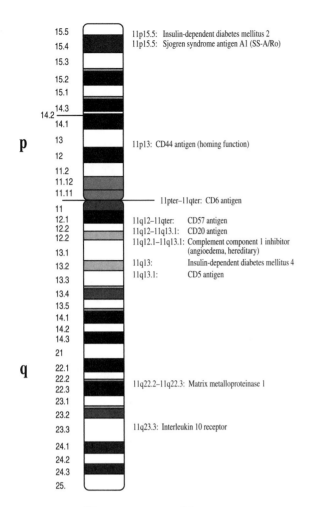

15.5	11p15.5: Insulin-dependent diabetes mellitus 2
15.4	11p15.5: Sjogren syndrome antigen A1 (SS-A/Ro)
15.3	
15.2	
15.1	
14.3	
14.2 14.1	
p 13	11p13: CD44 antigen (homing function)
12	
11.2	
11.12	
11.11	11pter–11qter: CD6 antigen
11	
12.1	11q12–11qter: CD57 antigen
12.2	11q12–11q13.1: CD20 antigen
12.2	11q12.1–11q13.1: Complement component 1 inhibitor
13.1	(angioedema, hereditary)
13.2	11q13: Insulin-dependent diabetes mellitus 4
13.3	11q13.1: CD5 antigen
13.4	
13.5	
14.1	
14.2	
14.3	
21	
q 22.1	
22.2	
22.3	11q22.2–11q22.3: Matrix metalloproteinase 1
23.1	
23.2	
23.3	11q23.3: Interleukin 10 receptor
24.1	
24.2	
24.3	
25.	

Chromosome 11

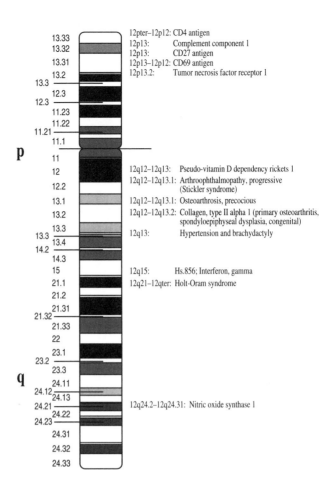

13.33	12pter–12p12: CD4 antigen
13.32	12p13: Complement component 1
13.31	12p13: CD27 antigen
13.2	12p13–12p12: CD69 antigen
12.3	12p13.2: Tumor necrosis factor receptor 1
11.23	
11.22	
11.21	
11.1	
p 11	
12	12q12–12q13: Pseudo-vitamin D dependency rickets 1
12.2	12q12–12q13.1: Arthroophthalmopathy, progressive
13.1	(Stickler syndrome)
13.2	12q12–12q13.1: Osteoarthrosis, precocious
13.3	12q12–12q13.2: Collagen, type II alpha 1 (primary osteoarthritis,
13.4	spondyloepiphyseal dysplasia, congenital)
14.2	12q13: Hypertension and brachydactyly
14.3	
15	12q15: Hs.856; Interferon, gamma
21.1	12q21–12qter: Holt-Oram syndrome
21.2	
21.31	
21.32	
21.33	
22	
23.1	
23.2	
23.3	
q 24.11	
24.12	
24.13	12q24.2–12q24.31: Nitric oxide synthase 1
24.21	
24.22	
24.23	
24.31	
24.32	
24.33	

Chromosome 12

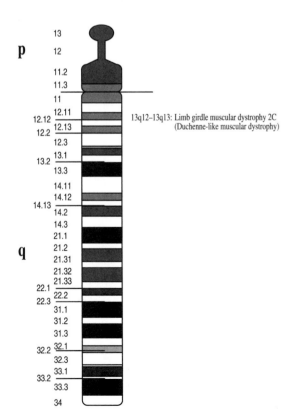

13	
p 12	
11.2	
11.3	
11	
12.11	13q12–13q13: Limb girdle muscular dystrophy 2C
12.12 12.13	(Duchenne-like muscular dystrophy)
12.2 12.3	
13.1	
13.2 13.3	
14.11	
14.12	
14.13 14.2	
14.3	
21.1	
q 21.2	
21.31	
21.32	
21.33	
22.1 22.2	
22.3	
31.1	
31.2	
31.3	
32.2 32.1	
32.3	
33.1	
33.2	
33.3	
34	

Chromosome 13

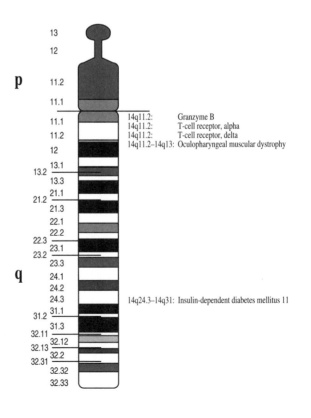

13	
12	
p 11.2	
11.1	
11.1	14q11.2: Granzyme B
11.2	14q11.2: T-cell receptor, alpha
11.2	14q11.2: T-cell receptor, delta
12	14q11.2–14q13: Oculopharyngeal muscular dystrophy
13.1	
13.2 13.3	
21.1	
21.2 21.3	
22.1	
22.2	
22.3	
23.1	
23.2 23.3	
24.1	
q 24.2	
24.3	14q24.3–14q31: Insulin-dependent diabetes mellitus 11
31.1	
31.2 31.3	
32.11	
32.12	
32.13 32.2	
32.31	
32.32	
32.33	

Chromosome 14

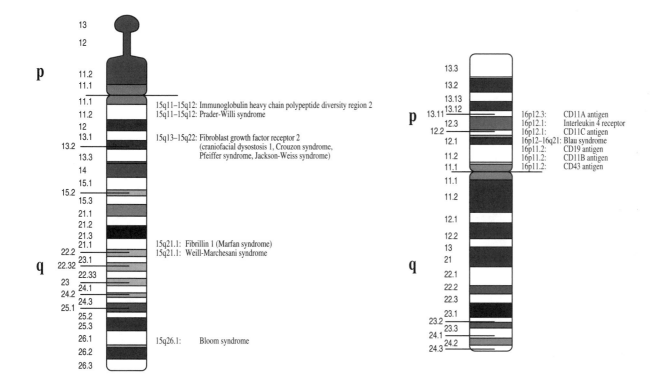

15q11–15q12: Immunoglobulin heavy chain polypeptide diversity region 2
15q11–15q12: Prader-Willi syndrome

15q13–15q22: Fibroblast growth factor receptor 2
(craniofacial dysostosis 1, Crouzon syndrome,
Pfeiffer syndrome, Jackson-Weiss syndrome)

15q21.1: Fibrillin 1 (Marfan syndrome)
15q21.1: Weill-Marchesani syndrome

15q26.1: Bloom syndrome

Chromosome 15

16p12.3: CD11A antigen
16p12.1: Interleukin 4 receptor
16p12.1: CD11C antigen
16p12–16q21: Blau syndrome
16p11.2: CD19 antigen
16p11.2: CD11B antigen
16p11.2: CD43 antigen

Chromosome 16

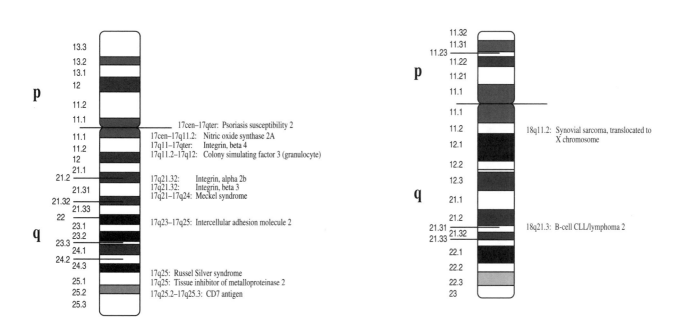

17cen–17qter: Psoriasis susceptibility 2
17cen–17q11.2: Nitric oxide synthase 2A
17q11–17qter: Integrin, beta 4
17q11.2–17q12: Colony simulating factor 3 (granulocyte)

17q21.32: Integrin, alpha 2b
17q21.32: Integrin, beta 3
17q21–17q24: Meckel syndrome

17q23–17q25: Intercellular adhesion molecule 2

17q25: Russel Silver syndrome
17q25: Tissue inhibitor of metalloproteinase 2
17q25.2–17q25.3: CD7 antigen

Chromosome 17

18q11.2: Synovial sarcoma, translocated to
X chromosome

18q21.3: B-cell CLL/lymphoma 2

Chromosome 18

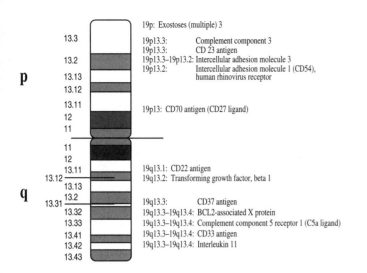

19p: Exostoses (multiple) 3

19p13.3: Complement component 3

19p13.3: CD 23 antigen

19p13.3–19p13.2: Intercellular adhesion molecule 3

19p13.2: Intercellular adhesion molecule 1 (CD54), human rhinovirus receptor

19p13: CD70 antigen (CD27 ligand)

19q13.1: CD22 antigen

19q13.2: Transforming growth factor, beta 1

19q13.3: CD37 antigen

19q13.3–19q13.4: BCL2-associated X protein

19q13.3–19q13.4: Complement component 5 receptor 1 (C5a ligand)

19q13.3–19q13.4: CD33 antigen

19q13.3–19q13.4: Interleukin 11

Chromosome 19

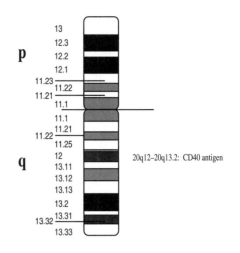

20q12–20q13.2: CD40 antigen

Chromosome 20

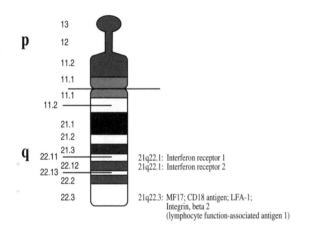

21q22.1: Interferon receptor 1

21q22.1: Interferon receptor 2

21q22.3: MF17; CD18 antigen; LFA-1; Integrin, beta 2 (lymphocyte function-associated antigen 1)

Chromosome 21

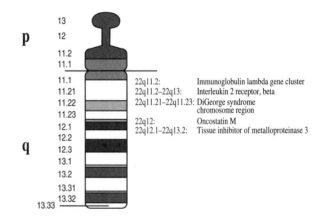

22q11.2: Immunoglobulin lambda gene cluster

22q11.2–22q13: Interleukin 2 receptor, beta

22q11.21–22q11.23: DiGeorge syndrome chromosome region

22q12: Oncostatin M

22q12.1–22q13.2: Tissue inhibitor of metalloproteinase 3

Chromosome 22

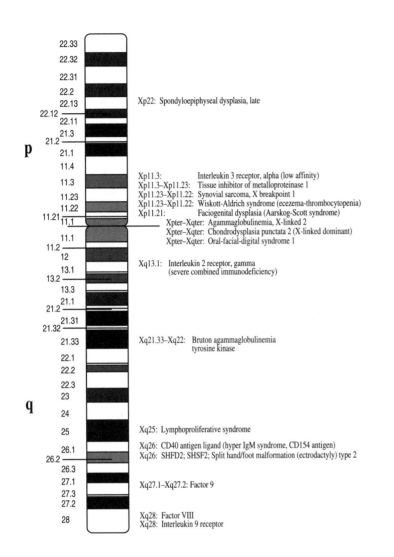

Chromosome X

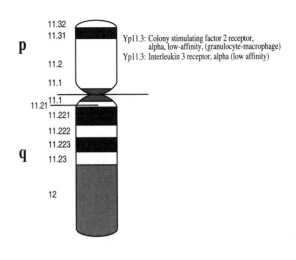

Chromosome Y

*An updated map of the human genome can be found at the following internet address http://gdbwww.gdb.org/gdb/report.html

APPENDIX V

Drugs Used in Treating Rheumatic Diseases

This appendix provides basic, practical information on the drugs most commonly used to treat patients with rheumatic disorders. The drugs are listed alphabetically by the clinical category that best describes their pharmacologic class or action or primary indication in rheumatology. It is not intended to be all inclusive nor to provide comparative information helpful for the selection of individual drugs. Chapters within the *Primer* that provide a more detailed description of the drug are indicated, and the prescribing physician is strongly encouraged to consult these chapters or other similar text reference material for drug indications and comparisons of drug efficacy or toxicity. In addition, it is recommended that the prescribing physician be familiar with the package insert provided by the manufacturer as well as the *Physician's Desk Reference* (PDR) or similar information prior to prescribing these drugs.

ANALGESICS (SEE PRIMER CHAPTER 14B)

DRUG	BRAND NAME(S)	DOSAGE	SIDE EFFECTS	CAUTIONS AND CONTRAINDICATIONS
Acetaminophen	*Anacin* (aspirin-free), *Excedrin caplets, Panadol, Tylenol*	1,000 to 4,000 mg per day in 3 or 4 doses	When taken as prescribed, acetaminophen is usually free of side effects. Fasting, drinking alcohol, and/or taking excessive amounts of acetaminophen may result in liver or kidney damage.	A history of alcohol abuse, kidney disease, hepatitis, or other liver disease
Acetaminophen with codeine*	*Fioricet, Phenaphen with Codeine, Tylenol with Codeine*	1,200 to 2,400 mg acetaminophen combined with 60 to 480 mg of codeine per day in 2 to 4 doses. Take with food.	Constipation, dizziness or light-headedness, drowsiness, nausea, fatigue or weakness, vomiting	A history of drug or alcohol abuse; asthma; head injury; prostate or gastric problems; liver, kidney or thyroid disease; sensitivities to acetaminophen, codeine or sulfites
Propoxyphene hydrochloride	*Darvon, PC-Cap, Wygesic*	65 mg every 3 to 4 hours as needed, no more than 390 mg per day	Dizziness or lightheadedness, drowsiness, nausea, vomiting	Current or previous serious depression, use of tranquilizers or antidepressants
Tramadol	*Ultram*	50 to 400 mg per day in 2 to 4 doses	Dizziness, nausea, constipation, headache, sleepiness	Liver disease, asthma, kidney disease, history of drug or alcohol abuse

*Chronic use may cause psychological and physical dependence.

CORTICOSTEROIDS (SEE PRIMER CHAPTER 53)

DRUG	BRAND NAME(S)	DOSAGE	SIDE EFFECTS	CAUTIONS AND CONTRAINDICATIONS
Cortisone	Cortone Acetate	Dosages of corticosteroids are highly variable and determined by the rheumatic disease to be treated. In general, the lowest dose that successfully controls the condition should be used. Corticosteroids should be taken with food or an antacid. A single daily dose should be taken with breakfast. It is very important that corticosteroids, when used long-term, not be stopped abruptly; dosage must be tapered gradually. For discussion of diseases in which corticosteroids are commonly used see the following *Primer* chapters: 9C – Rheumatoid arthritis 19C – Systemic lupus erythematosus 21 – Myositis 23C – Vasculitis 24 – Polymyalgia rheumatica	Cushing's syndrome (weight gain, moon-face, thin skin, muscle weakness), osteoporosis, cataracts, hypertension, increased appetite, elevated blood sugar, indigestion, insomnia, mood changes, nervousness or restlessness, cramps, immune suppression/infection	Active infection (or inactive tuberculosis), hypothyroidism, herpes simplex of the eye, hypertension, osteoporosis, gastric ulcer, diabetes
Dexamethasone	Decadron, Hexadrol			
Hydrocortisone	Cortef, Hydrocortone			
Methylprednisolone	Medrol			
Prednisolone	Prelone			
Prednisolone sodium phosphate (liquid only)	Pediapred			
Prednisone	Deltasone, Orasone, Prednicen-M, Sterapred			
Triamcinolone	Aristocort			

DISEASE-MODIFYING ANTIRHEUMATIC DRUGS (DMARDS) (SEE PRIMER CHAPTER 9C AND 54)

DRUG	BRAND NAME(S)	DOSAGE	SIDE EFFECTS	CAUTIONS AND CONTRAINDICATIONS
Auranofin (oral gold)	Ridaura	3 to 9 mg per day in a single dose or in 2 or 3 doses	Abdominal or stomach cramps or pain, bloated feeling, decrease in or loss of appetite, diarrhea or loose stools, gas or indigestion, mouth sores, nausea or vomiting, skin rash or itching, photosensitivity	Adverse reaction to gold-containing drugs, inflammatory bowel disease, kidney or liver disease
Azathioprine	Imuran	50 to 150 mg per day in 1 to 3 doses, based on body weight. Take with food.	Loss of appetite, nausea or vomiting, skin rash, bone marrow suppression, infection, malignancy, pancreatitis	Kidney or liver disease, concomitant use of allopurinol, pregnancy
Cyclophos- phamide	Cytoxan	50 to 150 mg per day orally in a single morning dose. Fluid intake (2-3 L per day) and emptying bladder before bedtime is important.	Infertility in men and women, loss of appetite, bone marrow supression, infection, hemorrhagic cystitis, malignancy	Kidney or liver disease, any active infection, pregnancy
Cyclosporine	Sandimmune Neoral	2.5 to 5 mg per kg per day in 1 or 2 doses	Bleeding, tender or enlarged gums; fluid retention; hypertension; increase in hair growth; loss of renal function; loss of appetite; trembling or shaking of hands; tremors	Sensitivity to castor oil (if receiving drug by injection), liver or kidney disease, active infection, hypertension
Hydroxychloro- quine sulfate	Plaquenil	200 to 600 mg per day in 1 or 2 doses. Take with food.	Diarrhea, loss of appetite, nausea, stomach cramps or pain, skin rash, retinopathy, neuromyopathy	Allergy to any antimalarial drug, retinal abnormality, G6PD deficiency, pregnancy
Methotrexate	Rheumatrex	7.5 to 25 mg p.o. or IM per week in a single dose	Cough, diarrhea, hair loss, loss of appetite, unusual bleeding or bruising, fever, pneumonitis, infection, stomatitis	Bone marrow suppression, liver and lung disease, alcoholism, immune- system deficiency, active infection, pregnancy
Minocycline	Minocin	200 mg per day in 2 doses. Take on an empty stomach.	Dizziness, vaginal infections, nausea, headache, skin rash, hyperpigmentation	Sensitivity to tetracyline medications, sun sensitivity
Penicillamine	Cuprimine, Depen	125 to 250 mg per day in a single dose to start, increased to not more than 1,500 mg per day in 3 doses. Take on an empty stomach.	Diarrhea, joint pain, lessening or loss of sense of taste, loss of appetite, fever, hives or itching, mouth sores, nausea or vomiting, skin rash, stomach pain, lymphadenopathy, bone marrow suppression, unusual bleeding or bruising, weakness	Penicillin allergy, blood disease, kidney disease
Sulfasalazine	Azulfidine	2 to 3 grams per day in 2 to 4 doses	Stomach pain, achiness, diarrhea, dizziness, headache, light sensitivity, itching, appetite loss, liver abnormalities, lowered blood count, nausea or vomiting, rash	Allergy to sulfa drugs or aspirin, kidney or liver disease, blood disease, bronchial asthma
Gold sodium thiomalate (injectable)	Myochrysine	10 mg in a single dose the first week, 25 mg the following week, then 25 to 50 mg per week thereafter. Frequency may be reduced after 1 g total dose	Photosensitivity; irritation or soreness of tongue; metallic taste; skin rash or itching; soreness, swelling or bleeding of gums; unusual bleeding or bruising; white spots on lips or in mouth or throat, oral ulcers, proteinuria, bone marrow suppression	Kidney disease, bone marrow suppression, colitis
Aurothioglucose (injectable)	Solganol			

DRUG	BRAND NAME(S)	DOSAGE	SIDE EFFECTS	CAUTIONS AND CONTRAINDICATIONS
ANTIDEPRESSANTS: Tricyclics				
Amitriptyline hydrochloride	*Elavil, Endep*	10 to 100 mg per day in a single dose at bedtime	Difficulty concentrating, dizziness, drowsiness, dry mouth, headache, increased appetite (including craving for sweets), nausea, sleep disturbances, unpleasant taste, urinary retention, weakness or tiredness, weight gain	A history of seizures, urinary retention, heart problems, glaucoma or other chronic eye conditions; use of thyroid medication or another antidepressant
Doxepin	*Adapin, Sinequan*	10 to 100 mg per day in a single dose at bedtime		
Nortriptyline	*Aventyl, Pamelor*	10 to 100 mg per day in a single dose at bedtime		
MUSCLE RELAXANTS				
Cyclobenz-aprine	*Cycloflex, Flexeril*	10 to 30 mg per day in 1 to 3 doses	Dizziness or lightheadedness, drowsiness, dry mouth. Alcohol, other antidepressants or monoamine oxidase (MAO) inhibitors may increase risk of side effects.	Glaucoma, urinary retention, cardiac or peripheral vascular disease, hyperthyroidism.

DRUG	BRAND NAME(S)	DOSAGE	SIDE EFFECTS	CAUTIONS AND CONTRAINDICATIONS
Allopurinol	*Lopurin, Zyloprim*	100 to 400 mg per day in a single dose with food.*	Hives, itching, liver-function abnormalities, bone marrow suppression, nausea, skin rash or sores. Acute attacks of gout are a common initial reaction to medication, but can be minimized if taken along with colchicine.	Kidney disease concomitant, use of azathioprine or mercaptopurine. Discontinue medication at the first sign of a rash, which may indicate an allergic reaction.
Colchicine	*Only available as generic*	0.6 to 1.2 mg per day in 1 to 3 doses for prevention. 0.5 or 0.6 mg every one to two hours (no more than 8 doses per day) to stop acute attacks. Take with food and encourage fluid intake.	Diarrhea, nausea and vomiting, stomach pain	History of alcohol abuse, intestinal disease, kidney or liver disease, low white blood cell count or low platelet count
Probenecid and Colchicine	*ColBenemid, Proben-C*	1 tablet (500 mg probenicid and 0.5 mg colchicine) 2 or 3 times per day. Take with food and encourage fluid intake.*	Diarrhea, nausea and vomiting, stomach pain, headache, joint pain and swelling, loss of appetite, nausea, skin rash, vomiting. Drug may interfere with urine glucose tests.	History of alcohol abuse, intestinal disease, kidney or liver disease, low white blood cell count or low platelet count, blood disease, use of antineoplastics, heparin, NSAIDs, nitrofurantoin or zidovudine
Probenecid	*Benemid, Probalan*	500 to 3,000 mg per day in 2-3 doses. Take with food.*	Headache, joint pain and swelling, loss of appetite, nausea, skin rash, vomiting. Drug may interfere with urine glucose tests.	Blood disease, kidney disease, kidney stones, use of antineoplastics, heparin, NSAIDs, nitrofurantoin or zidovudine
Sulfinpyrazone	*Anturane*	200 to 800 mg per day in 2-4 doses. Take with food.*	Bone marrow suppression, rash, abdominal pain	Ulcers, anemia, low white blood cell count, use of other sulfa drugs, insulin or anticoagulants.

*The dosage of a urate–lowering agent should be that which gets the serum urate concentration to 5.0 mg/d or less.

DRUG	BRAND NAME(S)	DOSAGE	SIDE EFFECTS	CAUTIONS AND CONTRAINDICATIONS
Diclofenac potassium	*Cataflam*	75 to 100 mg per day in a single dose[‡]	Abdominal pain, diarrhea, dizziness, drowsiness, fluid retention, gastric ulcers and bleeding, greater susceptibility to bruising or bleeding, heartburn, indigestion, lightheadedness, nausea, nightmares, rash, ringing in ears

Side effects may be more pronounced for people with pre-existing heart or kidney disease. May cause confusion in elderly people with kidney impairment. | Sensitivity or allergy to aspirin, nonacetylated salicylates, or similar drugs; kidney or liver disease; heart disease; high blood pressure; asthma; peptic ulcers; use of anticoagulants |
Diclofenac sodium	*Voltaren*	100 to 150 mg per day in 2 doses		
Etodolac	*Lodine*	400 to 1,200 mg per day in 1 to 4 doses		
Fenoprofen calcium	*Nalfon*	900 to 2,400 mg per day in 3 or 4 doses; never more than 3,200 mg per day		
Flurbiprofen	*Ansaid*	200 to 300 mg per day in 2 or 3 doses		
Ibuprofen[$]	**Prescription:** *Motrin* **Non-prescription:** *Advil, Motrin IB, Nuprin*	Adults: 1,200 to 3,200 mg per day in 3 or 4 doses; Children: 35-45 mg/kg/day in divided doses		
Indomethacin	*Indocin*	50 to 200 mg per day in 2 to 4 doses		
Ketoprofen	**Prescription:** *Orudis, Oruvail* **Non-prescription:** *Actron, Orudis KT*	150 to 300 mg per day in 3 or 4 doses		
Ketorolac[*]	*Toradol*	**Oral:** Up to 40 mg per day in 4 to 6 doses **Injected:** Up to 120 mg per day in 4 doses		
Meclofenamate sodium	*Meclomen*	200 to 400 mg per day in 3 or 4 doses		
Mefenamic acid[†]	*Ponstel*	1,000 mg per day in 4 doses		
Nabumetone	*Relafen*	500 to 2,000 mg per day in 1 or 2 doses		
Naproxen[$]	*Naprosyn*	Adults: 500 to 1,500 mg per day in 2 or 3 doses; Children: 15-20 mg/kg/day in divided doses		
Naproxen sodium	**Prescription:** *Anaprox* **Non-prescription:** *Aleve*	550 to 1,650 mg per day in 2 or 3 doses		
Oxaprozin	*Daypro*	1,200 to 1,800 mg per day in a single dose		
Piroxicam	*Feldene*	20 mg per day in a single dose		
Sulindac	*Clinoril*	300 to 400 mg per day in 2 doses		
Tolmetin sodium[$]	*Tolectin*	Adults: 1,200 to 1,800 mg per day in 3 doses; Children: 25-30 mg/kg/day in divided doses		

*This medication is for short-term relief of pain and should not be used for more than 5 days. Dosage should be adjusted for people who weigh less than 110 pounds and used with caution in elderly patients.

† This medication is for short-term relief of pain and should not be used for more than 7 days.

‡ NSAIDs should be taken with food.

$Approved for use in children.

DRUG	BRAND NAME(S)	DOSAGE	SIDE EFFECTS	CAUTIONS AND CONTRAINDICATIONS
Alendronate	*Fosamax*	10 mg per day in a single dose. Take with a full glass of water first thing in the morning. Do not eat or drink anything else, take any other medications or lie down for at least 30 minutes after taking the drug.	Irritation and ulcers of the throat and esophagus, bone pain or tenderness, diarrhea, difficulty swallowing, nausea, taste changes	Swallowing or gastric emptying difficulties, hypercalcemia, pregnancy, kidney disease, intestinal or bowel disease
Calcitonin (injection)	*Calcimar, Miacalcin*	100 IUs per day in a single dose	Diarrhea, flushing of skin, local inflammation at injection site, loss of appetite, nausea, stomach pain, vomiting, allergic reaction	
Calcitonin (nasal spray)	*Miacalcin*	200 IUs per day, in a single dose. Alternate nostrils daily. It is necessary to activate the pump prior to each dose.	Nasal irritation, diarrhea, flushing of the skin, loss of appetite, nausea, stomach pain, vomiting, allergic reaction	
Calcium		Females: Children: 800 mg/day; Adolescents: 1,500 mg/day; Adults: 1,200 mg/day; Pregnancy: 1,500 mg/day Males: Children: 800 mg/day Adolescents: 1000 mg/day Adults: 500-1000 mg/day	At recommended doses, free of side effects. Rare constipation, intestinal colic, or kidney stones	Kidney stones
Conjugated estrogens	*Premarin, Premphase, Prempro*	Taken daily or in four-week cycles of 0.625 mg per day for 3 weeks followed by 1 week of rest from drug. Women who have not had a hysterectomy should take this drug in conjunction with progestin.	Abdominal cramps, breast swelling and tenderness, loss of appetite, nausea, rapid weight gain, stomach bloating, edema	Undiagnosed vaginal bleeding; breast cancer or other estrogen-dependent cancer; a family history of breast cancer; problems related to circulation or blood clotting
Vitamin D		400-800 IUs per day		

SALICYLATES (SEE PRIMER CHAPTER 52)

DRUG	BRAND NAME(S)	DOSAGE	SIDE EFFECTS	CAUTIONS AND CONTRAINDICATIONS
ACETYLATED SALICYLATES				
Aspirin	Anacin, Ascriptin, Bayer, Bufferin, Ecotrin, Excedrin Tablets	Adults: 1,300 to 4,000 mg per day in 4 doses; Children: 75-90 mg/kg/day in divided doses*	Abdominal cramps and pain, deafness, gastric ulcers, heartburn or indigestion, increased bleeding tendency, nausea or vomiting, ringing in ears	Sensitivity or allergy to aspirin or nonacetylated salicylates, kidney or liver disease, heart disease, high blood pressure, asthma, peptic ulcers, use of anticoagulants
NONACETYLATED SALICYLATES				
Choline magnesium trisalicylate	CMT, Tricosal, Trilisate	3,000 mg per day in 2 or 3 doses	Use of alcohol may increase the risk of gastric ulcers and bleeding, as well as kidney and liver damage. Side effects may be more pronounced for people with pre-existing heart or kidney disease. May cause confusion in elderly people with kidney impairment.	
Choline salicylate	Arthropan	3,480 to 6,960 mg per day in 3 or 4 doses		
Diflunisal	Dolobid	500 to 1,000 mg per day in 2 doses		
Magnesium salicylate	Magan, Doan's Pills, Mobidin	2,600 to 4,800 mg per day in 3 to 6 doses		
Salsalate	Disalcid, Mono-Gesic, Salflex, Salsitab, Amigesic, Anaflex 750, Marthritic	1,500 to 3,000 mg per day in 2 or 3 doses		
Sodium salicylate	(Available as generic only)	1,950 to 3,900 mg per day in 3 or 4 doses		

*Salicylates should be taken with food.

Adapted from Mary Anne Dunkin: Drug guide. **Arthritis Today** *11(4):28-46, 1997*

SUBJECT INDEX

Page numbers followed by "t" refer to information found in tables, and page numbers followed by "f" refer to information found in figures.

A

AA amyloid, 342
Achilles tendinitis, 145–46
Achilles tendon, rupture of, 146
Achondroplasias, 373–75
Acne conglobata, 366
Acne fulminans, 366
Acne syndromes, 365–66, 366t
Acquired immunodeficiency syndrome (AIDS). *See also* Human immunodeficiency virus (HIV) infection
  and hemophilia, 335
  and reactive arthritis, 186
Acrolein, in systemic lupus erythematosus, 260
Acromegaly, 122, 352
Acro-osteolysis, 271
Actinomycosis, and arthritis, 211
Activation-induced cell death (AICD), 85–86
Acute articular inflammation, 223
Acute calcific periarthritis, 223
Acute gouty arthritis, 235f
Acute intermittent gout, 234–35
Acute neuropathic arthropathy, 322–23
Acute-phase reactants
  in ankylosing spondylitis, 191
  laboratory assessment for, 94, 186, 188
  in rheumatic fever, 214
Adams, Robert, 2
Adhesion molecules, role in inflammation, 17, 24, 40, 40f, 439t, 441
Adhesive capsulitis (frozen shoulder), 91–92, 139, 163
Adrenocorticotropic hormone (ACTH), 80
  in acute gout, 241
Adson test, 140
Adynamic bone disease, 357
Aggrecan, 16, 16f, 20, 34–35, 37–38
Alcohol consumption, effects of on gout, 232
AL disease, 340–42
  amyloid neuropathy in, 340–41
  cardiomyopathy in, 341
  carpal tunnel syndrome in, 341
  and deficiency of clotting factor X, 341

Algodystrophy. *See* Reflex sympathetic dystrophy
Alkaptonuria (ochronosis), 122, 329–30, 330f
Alkylating agents, 435
Allergic granulomatosis angiitis, 4–5
Allodynia, 319
Allopurinol, in treatment of gout, 241–42
Alopecia, in systemic lupus erythematosus, 251, 260
Alphaviruses, and arthritis, 202–3
Aluminum-induced bone disease, 356–57, 390
Alzheimer's disease, amyloid deposits in, 340
American Association for the Study and Control of Rheumatic Diseases, 5
American College of Rheumatology (ACR), 5, 417
  classification algorithms for osteoarthritis, 219
  criteria for diagnosis of reactive arthritis, 187
  criteria for diagnosis of rheumatoid arthritis, 161
  on liver biopsies, 171
  term selection by, 2, 3
  treatment guidelines for methotrexate, 396, 434–35
American Committee for the Control of Rheumatism, 5
American Juvenile Arthritis Organization (AJAO), 395, 417
American Rheumatism Association (ARA). *See* American College of Rheumatology
Amitriptyline, 126
Amniocentesis, in Gaucher's disease, 332
Amphiarthroses, 10
Amputation, in osteosarcoma, 348
Amyloidoses, 122, 339–43
  AA amyloid, 342
  and aging, 342
  in AL disease, 340–42
  amyloids, 339–40
  in ankylosing spondylitis, 191
  in Behçet's disease, 308
  biopsy in, 340
  chemical classification of, 339t
  clinical features of, 339
  familial amyloidosis, 342
  in familial Mediterranean fever, 128
  genetic factors in, 342

Amyloidoses (cont'd)
  β-microglobulin amyloid, 342
  in myeloma-associated disorders, 337
    Ostertag, 342–43
    in reactive arthritis, 186
    renal, 342–43
Amyopathic dermatomyositis, 277
Anaphylatoxins, 48
Anemia, 214, 328
Angiography, 113
Angioimmunoblastic lymphadenopathy, 338
Angiotensin-converting enzyme (ACE), 62, 275
Ankles
  arthrocentesis of, 99f
  disorders of, 145–48
  operative treatments for, 447
  pannus of, 156f
  in physical examination, 93–94
  rehabilitation for, 411–12
  in rheumatoid arthritis, 164
Ankylosing spondylitis (AS), 120–21, 189–93
  in circulatory system, 191
  clinical features of, 189t, 189–91
  comparison with related disorders, 181t
  disease course of, 192
  extraskeletal manifestations of, 190–91
  history of, 3
  laboratory assessment for, 191
  neurologic involvement in, 190
  operative treatments for, 445–46
  pregnancy in, 193
  principles of management of, 192t
  radiography in, 191, 191f
  skeletal manifestations of, 189–91
  treatment of, 192–93
Ankylosis, in neuropathic arthropathy, 323
Anserine bursitis, 144
Anterior interosseous nerve syndrome, 141
Anthracycline compounds, 341
Antibiotics, 173, 194–95, 200
  in Lyme disease, 206, 206t
  in rheumatic fever, 214
  in systemic sclerosis, 274
Antibodies. *See also* Antinuclear antibodies; Autoantibodies; Immunoglobulins
  anti-DNA, 248, 255
  to cytokines, 47
  diseases caused by, 74–75

Antibodies (cont'd)
  as immunologic markers, 17–18
  monoclonal, 437–38
  role in development of vasculitis, 291
Anti-CD4 monoclonal antibodies, 437–38
Anti-CD7 monoclonal antibody, 438
Anti-CD52 monoclonal antibody, 438
Anti-CD5 ricin toxin conjugate, 438
Anticholinergic side effects, medications with, 286t
Anti-DNA antibodies, in systemic lupus erythematosus, 248, 255
Antigen-presenting cells (APC), 68–70, 69f, 75, 292, 439
Antimalarial drugs, 170, 259, 279, 287, 432
Antineutrophil cytoplasmic antibodies (ANCA), 54, 95–96, 188, 291, 291f, 302
Antinuclear antibodies (ANA), 244
  diseases associated with positive test for, 95
  in systemic lupus erythematosus, 247, 248t, 250
  in systemic sclerosis, 264
Antiphospholipid antibody syndrome (APS), 246, 313–15, 399
  clinical features of, 313–14
  differential diagnosis of, 314
  etiology of, 313
  laboratory assessment for, 314
  pathogenesis of, 313
  pregnancy loss in, 314
  prognosis for, 315
  treatment of, 314–15
Anti-RNA polymerase, 267–68, 270
Antisignal recognition protein (SRP), 96
Aortitis, 186, 190
Apatite crystals, 222–25, 357. *See also* Crystal-induced arthritis; Deposition diseases
Apoptosis, 86, 86f
Arachidonic acid, 41–42
  and leukotrienes, 60–61
  and lipoxins, 61
  metabolism activation of, 196
  and prostaglandins, 58–60, 59f
  and thromboxane, 59f
Arthritis. *See also names of specific conditions and diseases*
  fungal, 118, 120, 209
  infectious, 118 (*see also* Septic arthritis)

Cardiovascular manifestations (cont'd)
in Lyme disease, 205
in reactive arthritis, 186
in relapsing polychondritis, 310
in rheumatoid arthritis, 166
in sarcoidosis, 326
in systemic lupus erythematosus, 246–47, 254, 255, 261
in systemic sclerosis, 270, 274
Carnitine, 22, 280
Carpal tunnel syndrome (CTS), 357
in AL disease, 341
in bacterial arthritis, 209
causes of, 142, 154
and endocrine disease, 351
in mucopolysaccharidoses, 363
in physical examination, 91
in rheumatoid arthritis, 163–64
symptoms of, 142
Cartilage oligomeric matrix protein (COMP), 17, 18
Cathepsin D, 52
Cathepsin E, 52
Cathepsin G, 54
Cathepsin L, 52
Cathepsin N, 52
Cazenave, Pierre A., 4
CD44, as lymphocyte homing receptor, 35–36
CD4 (helper T cells), 69, 73–74, 159, 292
CD markers, appendix, 476
Cecil, Russell L., 2–3
Cell-mediated glandular destruction, 284
Central nervous system (CNS), 80, 285
Central nervous system (CNS) vasculitis, 297–98. See also Vasculitis
clinical features of, 297–98
diagnosis of, 298
laboratory assessment for, 298
treatment of, 303
Cervical disc herniation, 135
Cervical spine, 163, 166, 445, 448
Cervical spondylitic myelopathy, 135
Cervical spondylosis, 135
Cervicitis, 198
Champion, G. D., 434
Chan, T. W., 380
Charcot, Jean-Martin, 2
Charcot joints, 26, 209
Charcot Marie-Tooth disease, 26
Chauffard, Anatole M., 5
Chemotaxis, 39
Chest wall, disorders of anterior, 148
Chikungunya fever virus, and arthritis, 202–3
Children. See Pediatric rheumatic diseases

Chlamydia trachomatis, 182, 184, 194–95
Chlorambucil, in Behçet's syndrome, 309
Cholesterol, in synovial fluid, 224. See also Deposition diseases
Chondrocalcinosis, 328, 330. See also Calcium pyrophosphate dihydrate (CPPD) deposition disease
Chondrocytes, 14. See also Articular cartilage
in bone formation, 19
in osteoarthritis, 217
and proteinase activity, 196
regulation of cartilage proteoglycans by, 37
Chondrodysplasias
achondroplasia, 373–75
chondrodysplasia punctata, 376
classification of, 373–76
clinical features of, 374t
diagnosis of, 373
diastrophic dysplasia, 375
metaphyseal chondrodysplasia, 375–76
metatropic dysplasia, 376
multiple epiphyseal dysplasia and pseudoachondroplasia, 375
pathogenesis of, 373
spondyloepiphyseal dysplasias, 375
Chondromatosis, 345
Chorea minor, 1, 2, 213, 253
Chowne, W. D., 4
Chronic calcific periarthritis, 223
Chronic fatigue syndrome, 125
Chronic overuse syndrome, 151t
Chronic recurrent multifocal osteomyelitis (CRMO), 366
Chronic tophaceous gout, 235–36, 236f, 238f
Churg, Jacob, 5
Churg-Strauss syndrome, 296–97
classification criteria, 461
clinical features of, 296
diagnosis of, 297
laboratory assessment for, 296–97
treatment of, 302
Circinate balanitis, 185, 186f
Circulating immune complexes, laboratory assessment for, 97
Circulatory system. See Cardiovascular manifestations
Coagulation system, 62, 118, 196
Cobb's method, for measuring spinal curvature, 134f
Coburn, Alvin F., 2
Coccidioidomycosis, 209–10

Cogan's syndrome, 298
COL2A1 gene, in collagen, 16f
Colchicine
in acute gout, 240
in Behçet's syndrome, 309
in calcium pyrophosphate dihydrate (CPPD) deposition disease, 227, 228
in familial Mediterranean fever, 128
in hyperimmunoglobulin D and periodic fever, 129
in intermittent gout, 241
in transplant gout, 242
Collagen, 28–32. See also Articular cartilage
assembly of, 30f
biosynthesis of, 31t, 31–32
classification of, 28–31, 29f
and collagen gene expression, 32
degradation of, 32
effect of defects of, 19
extracellular matrix components of, 15–17, 16t
and genes, 29, 31–32
interactions with proteoglycans, 36
structure of, 28
types of, 15t, 15–16, 28–31
and vascular endothelium, 24
Collagenases, 55
Collagen vascular disease, 277–78
Collins, D. N., 445
Collis, William R., 2
Colony-stimulating factors (CSF), 43–44
Colwell, C. W. J., 380
Combination protocols, in drug treatment, 173, 178, 435–36
Complement system, 48–51
activation of, 48, 49f
alternative pathway of, 48–49
classical activation pathway of, 48–49, 49f
control of, 49–50
deficiencies of, 50, 50f, 249
discovery of, 48
functions of, 48, 48f
and immune complex diseases, 50
laboratory assessment of, 96–97
measurement of, 50–51, 51t
nomenclature of, 48
receptors of, 49–50
therapeutic implications of, 51
Computed radiography, 106, 107f, 282
Computed tomography (CT), 107–9, 108f, 112, 191
Comroe, Bernard, 1
Conjunctivitis, 286
in Kawasaki syndrome, 404
in reactive arthritis, 184
in rheumatoid arthritis, 165

Connective tissue diseases, 244–45
and heritable disorders of, 359–64
hormonal therapy for, 353
mixed, 121, 399t
and nonarticular rheumatism, 398–403
origin of term for, 4
undifferentiated, 244–45
Coombs' test
in antiphospholipid antibody syndrome, 314
in systemic lupus erythematosus, 255
Coping Strategies Questionnaire, 414
Copper, in Wilson's disease, 330
Corticosteroids, 427–31
in acute gout, 241
in adrenal insufficiency, 429–30
in ankylosing spondylitis, 192
in Behçet's syndrome, 309
and bone loss, 388–89
cellular and molecular effects of, 427–28
effects of relevant to rheumatic diseases, 428t
formulations of for systemic therapy, 429t
and infections, 429
and modulation of immune and inflammatory responses, 81
and operative treatments for arthritis, 445
in osteoporosis, 429
pharmacology of, 428–29
physiology of, 427
in polymyalgia rheumatica, 306
in reflex sympathetic dystrophy, 321
in relapsing polychondritis, 311
in rheumatic fever, 214
in rheumatoid arthritis, 163, 169, 431
in RS3PE, 129
in sarcoidosis, 327
side effects of, 429–31, 430t
in Still's disease, 318
in systemic lupus erythematosus, 258–59, 259t
and T cells, 81, 427–28
in Wegener's granulomatosis, 302
withdrawal syndromes of, 430–31
Costochondritis, 148
CPPD disease. See Calcium pyrophosphate dihydrate (CPPD) deposition disease
CR1, 51
Cranial arteritis. See Giant cell arteritis
C-reactive protein (CRP), 94, 162

Creatine phosphokinase (CPK), 22

CREST (calcinosis, Raynaud's phenomenon, esophageal disability, sclerodactyly, telangiectasia), 4, 224, 267f, 269, 400–1

Crohn's disease, 182–83, 308–9

Crowned dens syndrome, 226

Cryoglobulinemia, 299–300
 classification of, 299–300
 clinical features of, 299t, 300
 diagnosis of, 300
 laboratory assessment for, 300
 pathophysiology of, 300
 treatment of, 303

Cryptococcosis, 210

Crystal-induced arthritis, 117–18, 120, 199. See also Deposition diseases; Gout; Osteoarthritis

Cumulative trauma disorder (CTD), 153

Cush, J. J., 316

Cushing's disease, 352

Cutis verticis gyrata, 371

Cyclobenzaprine, 126

Cyclooxygenase (COX), 58–59, 422, 424

Cyclophosphamide, 172–73, 304
 in relapsing polychondritis, 311
 in Sjögren's syndrome, 287
 in Still's disease, 318
 in systemic lupus erythematosus, 259–60
 in systemic sclerosis, 274
 in Wegener's granulomatosis, 302

Cyclosporin A, 195, 260–61, 311

Cyclosporine, 172, 242, 287, 309, 435

Cysticercosis, 211

Cytokines, 43–47
 antibodies to, 47
 and biologic agents tested in rheumatoid arthritis, 439t
 in collagen gene expression, 32, 293
 colony-stimulating factors, 43–44
 and endothelial cells, 292
 functional classification of, 44t
 growth and differentiation factors, 43–47
 immunoregulatory, 45–46, 73–74
 in osteoarthritis, 217
 pathogenic mechanisms in articular infection, 196
 production of, 41–42
 proinflammatory, 446–47
 regulation of effects of, 47
 stimulation of, 80
 in systemic sclerosis, 265–66
 in vasculitis, 293

Cytopenias, in systemic lupus erythematosus, 255, 261

Cytotoxic agents, 302

D

Daltroy, L., 416

Danazol, in systemic lupus erythematosus, 260–61

Dapsone, in systemic lupus erythematosus, 261

Dawson, Martin H., 3

Decorin, 17, 36

Deep Koebner effect, 176

Deep vein phlebitis, 308

Dehydroepiandrosterone (DHEA), 83, 261

Delayed-type hypersensitivity, 74

Deposition diseases, 328–34. See also Amyloidoses; Calcium pyrophosphate dihydrate (CPPD) deposition disease; Crystal-induced arthritis; Gout

Depression, 126–27, 413. See also Psychosocial factors, and arthritis

De Quervain's tenosynovitis, 141

Dermatomyositis, 245, 282f
 in adults, 277
 classification critera, 463
 history of, 4
 juvenile, 277, 278, 399–400

Descemet's membrane, 31

Detritic synovitis, 324

DHEA sulfate (DHEAS), 83

Diabetes mellitus
 as cause of neuropathic arthropathy, 322, 352
 computed tomography in, 108f
 and DISH, 351
 foot in, 322, 323f
 scleroderma-like disorders in, 272

Diagnostic tests, characteristics of, 94. See also names of individual diseases, laboratory assessment for

Dialysis, musculoskeletal problems in, 356–58
 and bone and joint infections, 357
 and dialysis arthropathy and β microglobulin amyloid, 357
 and disorders of microcrystalline origin, 357
 muscular involvement in, 357
 renal osteodystrophy, 356
 in systemic lupus erythematosus, 261

Diarrheal illness, and reactive arthritis, 187. See also Septic arthritis

Diarthroses, 10

Diffuse collagen disease, 4

Diffuse fasciitis with eosinophilia (DFE), 271

Diffuse idiopathic skeletal hyperstosis (DISH), 351–52

Dipeptidases, 62

Discoid lupus lesions, 251, 252f. See also Systemic lupus erythematosus

Disease-modifying antirheumatic drugs. See DMARDS

Dislocations, of joints, 153

Disseminated gonococcal infection (DGI), 198f, 198–99

DMARDS (disease-modifying antirheumatic drugs), 169–70, 170t, 280, 432–36
 alkylating agents, 435
 antimalarials, 170, 259, 279, 287, 432
 azathioprine, 172, 194, 195, 260, 309, 435
 and combination therapy, 173, 178, 435–36
 cyclosporine, 172, 242, 287, 309, 435
 gold, 171, 395–96, 433–34
 mechanism of action of, 432t
 methotrexate (see Methotrexate)
 monitoring of, 433t
 penicillamine, 172, 432–33
 sulfasalazine, 170–71, 178, 192, 194, 395, 433
 toxicities of (see Toxicity index scores, for drugs)

Dolorimeter, 124

Dracunculosis, and arthritis, 211

Drug abusers, 197

Drugs, appendix, 492 See also DMARDS; names of individual drugs and drug types; Toxicity index scores, for drugs

Drummond, P. D., 320

Dual-energy x-ray absorptiometry (DEXA), 112–13

Dundas, David, 2

Dupuytren's contracture, 143

Dynamic stenosis, 135

Dysautonomia, 25

Dysostosis multiplex. See Mucopolysaccharidoses

Dysphagia, 269, 278, 400

Dysplasias, 373–77

Dyspnea, 269, 270

E

Early-onset gout. See Gout

Eccentric contraction, 11

Edema, pitting, 93, 128–29

Ehlers-Danlos syndrome, 360–61

Ehrich, William E., 4

Ehrmann, Salomon, 4

Elastin, 32

Elbows, 163
 arthrocentesis of, 99f
 disorders of, 140–41
 operative treatments for, 448
 rehabilitation for, 411

ELISA tests, 206

Endocarditis, bacterial, 120

Endocrine diseases, arthropathies associated with

Endocrine diseases (cont'd)
 musculoskeletal disorders, 351t, 351–52
 musculoskeletal sequelae of, 352
 sex hormones and autoimmune diseases, 352–53

Endothelial cells, 24, 32, 291–92

Endothelium-derived relaxation factor (EDRF) (nitric oxide). See Nitric oxide

Enteropathic arthropathy, operative treatments for, 446

Eosinophilia-myalgia syndrome (EMS), 271–72

Epidermal growth factor (EGF), 44

Eppinger, Hans, 4

Epstein-Barr virus infection, 125

Erythema elevatum diutinum, 368

Erythema infectiosum rash, 201f

Erythema marginatum, 213–14

Erythema nodosum, 365, 365t

Erythrocyte sedimentation rate (ESR), 94, 127, 162, 255, 295

Estrogen
 deficiency of, 352
 and immunity, 83
 therapy in osteoporosis, 387

Evaluation, of rheumatic patient, 89–115, 465
 arthrocentesis, 98–100
 arthroscopy, 105f, 105–6
 imaging techniques, 106–15
 laboratory assessment for, 94–97
 medical history, 89
 physical examination, 90–94
 symptoms of rheumatic disorders, 89–90

Exercise, 126, 192, 193, 387, 410, 451

Exudative erythema. See Systemic lupus erythematosus

F

Fabry's disease, 332

Factor VIII deficiency, and hemophilia A, 335

Familial amyloidosis, 342

Familial Mediterranean fever (FMF), 120, 128, 340

Farber's disease, 332

Fast twitch oxidative glycolytic (FOG) fibers, 21. See also Skeletal muscles

Fatigue, 125, 410

Fauconnet, M., 4

Feet
 bones of, 147f
 diabetic, 322, 323f
 disorders of, 145–48
 operative treatments for, 447
 in physical examination, 93–94

Lymphomas, 284–85, 338. *See also* Neoplasms, of joints
Lysosomal lipid storage disease, 332

α₂-macroglobulin, 55
Macrophages, 41–42
Maduromycosis, and arthritis, 211
Magnetic resonance imaging (MRI), 109f, 109–11, 110f, 113, 114f, 134f, 282
Maier, Rudolf, 4
Major histocompatibility complex (MHC), 68–69. *See also* HLA alleles; Immunity
  and peripheral tolerance, 84–85
  in rheumatoid arthritis, 155
  in systemic lupus erythematosus, 248–49
  in vasculitis, 292
Malar rash, in systemic lupus erythematosus, 251, 252f
Malignant soft tissue tumors
  fibrosarcoma, 346
  liposarcoma, 345
  malignant fibrous histiocytoma, 345
  rhabdomyosarcoma, 346
  synovial sarcoma, 345–46
Malignant tumors, of bone
  chondrosarcoma, 348
  osteosarcoma, 347–48, 348f
  parosteal osteosarcoma, 348
Marfan syndrome, 32, 359
Maroteaux-Lamy syndrome. *See* Mucopolysaccharidoses
Mast cells, 45
Matrilysin (Pump-1), 55
Matrix metalloproteinases. *See* Metalloproteinases (MMP), matrix
Mayaro virus, and arthritis, 203
McAdam, L. P., 311
McArdle's disease (myophosphorylase deficiency), 279
McCarty, Daniel J., 1
McKusick MCD, 375–76
McMurray's sign, 152
Medial epicondylitis, 140
Medial plica syndrome, 145
Mediators, of inflammation. *See* Inflammation, mediators of
Medical history, aspects of patient, 89
Melphalan, in AL disease, 341
Meningococcal arthritis, 119
Meralgia paresthetica, 144
Meselamine, 194
Mesenteric vasculitis, in systemic lupus erythematosus, 254
Metabolic bone diseases, 385–90
Metalloelastase (MMP-12), 55

Metalloproteinases (MMP), matrix, 54–56
  membrane-type, 56
  production of, 60
  and tissue destruction in rheumatoid arthritis, 160
  tissue inhibitors of, 54–56
  types of, 54–56
Metatarsalgia, 147
Metatropic dysplasia, 376
Methotrexate, 195, 434–35
  in ankylosing spondylitis, 192
  in idiopathic inflammatory myopathies, 279
  in juvenile rheumatoid arthritis, 395
  monitoring of, 435t, 472
  in psoriatic arthritis, 178
  in rheumatoid arthritis, 165, 171–72
  in sarcoidosis, 327
  in seronegative spondyloarthropathies, 194
  side effects of, 434, 434t
  in Still's disease, 318
  in systemic lupus erythematosus, 259
  in Wegener's granulomatosis, 302
Michet, C., 311–12
β-microglobulin amyloid, 342
Microscopic polyangiitis, 299
  clinical features of, 299
  diagnosis of, 299
  laboratory assessment for, 299
  treatment of, 302
Miescher, Peter A., 4
Minerals, deposition in joints, 222–25. *See also* Deposition diseases
Mithramycin, in Paget's disease, 384
Mitochondrial myopathies, 280
Mixed connective tissue disease (MCTD), 121, 399t
Monarticular arthritis. *See also* Osteoarthritis; Osteonecrosis; Septic arthritis
  causes of, 116t
  evaluation, 466
  history of, 116
  laboratory assessment for, 117
  physical examination in, 116–17
  radiography in, 117
  synovial biopsy in, 117
  synovial fluid analysis in, 117
  treatment of, 117–18
  types of, 118
Monarticular joint disease, 116–18
  diagnosis of, 116–18
  inflammatory causes of, 116t
  noninflammatory causes of, 116t
  physical examination in, 116–17
  types of, 116–18

Money, Angle, 2
Monoclonal antibodies, 17–18
Mononeuropathies, 26
Monosodium urate monohydrate (MSUM) crystals, 222
Morquio syndrome. *See* Mucopolysaccharidoses
Morton's neuroma, 93, 147
MTP synovitis, 93
Mucin clot, in synovial fluid, 103
Mucopolysaccharidoses, 362–63, 363t
Mucopolysacchariduria, 363
Multicentric reticulohistiocytosis, 332–33, 333f
Multiple epiphyseal dysplasia (MED), 375
Multiple sclerosis (MS), 286
Muscles. *See* Skeletal muscles
Musculoskeletal and Arthritis Disease Centers, 418
Musculoskeletal system
  and bone (*see* Bone)
  evaluation of pain in, 123t, 123–24
  and joints, 10–14
  pain in as manifestation of other diseases, 403
  and peripheral nerves, 25–27
  and skeletal muscle (*see* Skeletal muscles)
  treatment of in systemic sclerosis, 274
  and vascular endothelium, 23–25
Mycobacteria, atypical, 209
Mycobacterial arthritis, 118, 120, 207–9
Mycobacterium bovis, 209
Mycobacterium leprae, 209
Mycobacterium marinum, 143, 209
Mycobacterium tuberculosis, 207
Myeloma-associated disorders, 337
Myelopathy, 135–36
Myoadenylate deaminase deficiency, 280
Myofascial pain syndrome, 125t
Myofilaments, in skeletal muscles, 21f. *See also* Skeletal muscles
Myopathies, idiopathic inflammatory, 276–82
  and causes of muscle weakness, 279–80
  classifications of, 276, 276t
  clinical features of, 276–78
  diagnosis of, 281t
  epidemiology of, 276
  genetic factors in, 278
  pathogenesis of, 278–79
  primary metabolic, 279
  testing for, 280–81
  treatment of, 279
  triggering events for, 278
Myophosphorylase deficiency (McArdle's disease), 279

Myositis, and malignancy, 278
Myositis-specific antibodies (MSA), 96

Nails (finger), 177, 185, 264f
Neck strain. *See* Low back and neck disorders
Neisser, Albert, 5
Neisseria gonorrhoeae, arthritis induced by, 118, 119, 184, 197, 198f, 198–99
Neisseria meningitidis, arthritis induced by, 198–99
Neonatal lupus syndrome (NSLE), 399. *See also* Systemic lupus erythematosus
Neoplasms, of joints, 344–50
  benign bone, 346–47
  benign soft tissue, 344–45
  diagnosis of, 346
  malignant bone, 347–48
  malignant soft tissue, 345–46
  management of, 346
  and tumor simulators, 348–49
Nephelometric immunoassays, 50–51
Nephritis, 247f, 247t, 247–48, 253t, 287. *See also* Renal manifestations
Nephrosclerosis, 233
Nerve action potential (NAP), 25
Nerve entrapments, 140–44, 154
Nerves, peripheral, 25–27
  degeneration and regeneration of, 25–26
  demyelination and remyelination of, 26
  membrane excitability in, 26
  role of, 25
Neurapraxia, 25
Neuroendocrine system
  and immunity, 80–83
  and Lyme disease, 205, 206
Neuropathic arthropathy, 322–24, 323f
  clinical features of, 322
  diagnosis of, 323
  epidemiology of, 322
  hepatic effects of, 425
  management of, 324
  neurologic conditions associated with, 322t
  pathology of, 323–24
  pathophysiology, 324
  prevention in, 324
  radiography in, 323
  renal effects of, 425
  surgery in, 324
  synovial fluid in, 323
Neutrophils, 39–41, 46, 160, 233, 265
Nichols, Edward, 2
Nitric oxide (endothelium-derived relaxation factor (EDRF)), 23, 42, 62–63, 63f
Nitric oxide synthase (NOS), 63f

Tietze's syndrome, 148
Tinel's sign, 91, 140, 141, 142, 146, 154
Tissue inhibitors of metalloproteinases (TIMPs), 217
Todd, Edgar W., 2
Tolerization, 441–42
Total hemolytic complement assay (THC, CH50), 50
Toxicity index scores, for drugs, 170, 171t, 172t, 259, 260, 280, 433t
Toxic oil syndrome (TOS), 271–72
Toxin-induced disorders, 123, 271–72
Transcutaneous electrical nerve stimulation (TENS), 409
Transforming growth factor beta (TGF-β), 32, 44, 160, 265
Transient regional osteoporosis, 321
Transplantation
  gout in, 236–37, 242–43
  and systemic lupus erythematosus, 261
Trauma, and psoriatic arthritis, 176
Trendelenburg gait, 93
Trochanteric bursitis, 93, 143
Tropheryma whippelii, 188
T-tubule system, 21. See also Skeletal muscle
Tuberculin skin tests, 207, 333
Tuberculous arthritis, 208–9
Tuberculous spondylitis. See Pott's disease
Tumor-necrosis factor alpha (TNF-α), 37, 44, 158, 265
  inhibition, 440–41
  role in pathogenesis of rheumatoid arthritis, 439–40
Tumor-necrosis factor beta (TNF-β), 44, 46
Tumor simulators, 348–49

Tumor simulators (cont'd)
  aneurysms, 349
  myositis ossificans, 349
  pigmented villonodular synovitis, 349, 349f
  synovial cysts, 348–49
  Type I procollagen, 28f

Ulcerative colitis, 367f
Ulnar nerve entrapment
  elbow, 140–41
  wrist, 142–43
Ultrasound, 111
Undifferentiated connective tissue syndromes (UCTS), 244–45
Unverricht, Heinrich, 4
Urbaniak, J. R., 380
Urethritis, 184, 198
Uric acid, 1, 230. See also Gout; Hyperuricemia
Uveitis
  in ankylosing spondylitis, 190, 192
  in Behçet's disease, 307
  in Kawasaki syndrome, 404
  in reactive arthritis, 185–86
  in sarcoidosis, 326
  in seronegative spondyloarthropathies, 195

Vanderbilt Pain Management Inventory, 414
Van der Meer, J. W. M., 129
Vascular endothelium, 23–25
  activated, 24, 24f
  anatomy of, 23–24
  as endocrine organ, 23–24
  function of, 23–24
Vasculitis, 201, 289–304. See also Behçet's disease; Central nervous system (CNS) Vasculitis

Vasculitis (cont'd)
Hypersensitivity vasculitis
  antibodies in, 291
  associated with rheumatic diseases, 297
  clinical features of, 291–92, 294–300
  epidemiology of, 289, 289t
  immune complexes in, 291
  laboratory assessment for, 294–300
  long-term therapy of, 303–4
  medium and large-vessel, 401–2
  mesenteric, 254
  pathogenesis of, 291–92
  pathology of, 289–91, 290t
  retinal, 309
  rheumatoid, 173
  in rheumatoid arthritis, 295
  in systemic lupus erythematosus, 295
  treatment of, 301–4
Vasoactive amines, 62
Vidal, Emil, 5
Viral arthritis, 120, 201–4
Virchow, Rudolf, 2
Vitamin D
  deficiencies of, 386
  derivatives of, 357
  therapy, 315, 388
Volar flexor tenosynovitis, 143
Von Willebrand factor, 23, 42
Vossius, Adolf, 5

Waaler, Erik, 3
Wagner, Ernst L., 4
Waldenström's macroglobulinemia, 337–38
Ways of Coping Scale, 414
Weber-Christian disease, 365
Wegener, Friedrich, 4
Wegener's granulomatosis, 4
  classification criteria, 460
  clinical features of, 297
  cytokine expression in, 293

Wegener's granulomatosis (cont'd)
  diagnosis of, 297
  laboratory assessment for, 95–96, 297
  treatment of, 302–3
Weight loss, in osteoarthritis, 220
Weiss, Soma, 4
Weissenbach, Raymond J., 4
Wells, William C., 2
Western blot tests, 206
Westphal, Carl F., 4
Whateley, Thomas, 5
Whiplash, 136. See also Low back and neck disorders
Whipple's disease, 121, 188
Wiedmann, 5
Wilson's disease, 330–31
Winterbauer, Richard H., 4
Wollaston, William H., 1
Wollf's law, 20
Work disability, due to rheumatic diseases, 6–7
World Health Organization (WHO), 407
Wrists
  arthrocentesis of, 100f
  disorders of, 141–43, 199f
  operative treatments for, 447–48
  in physical examination, 91
  rehabilitation for, 411
  and tendon rupture, 164

Xenotransplantation, 51
Xerostomia, 286–87
Xiphodynia. See Xiphoid cartilage syndrome
Xiphoid cartilage syndrome (xiphoidalgia), 148

Yergason's sign, 139
Yersinia enterocolitica, 182

BULLETIN:
a brief public report intended for immediate release on a matter of public interest

BULLETIN ON THE RHEUMATIC DISEASES:

a FREE brief report intended for bimonthly release on the matter of rheumatic diseases

It's as simply defined as that – a free subscription to the *Bulletin on the Rheumatic Diseases*, available to medical and health practitioners by the Arthritis Foundation. Published eight times per year, each eight-page newsletter summarizes current rheumatology research and raises compelling questions about the future of caring for people with rheumatic diseases. Each issue contains several articles written by distinguished authorities working in the field of rheumatology. Join the thousands of informed *Bulletin* readers. Order your free subscription today!

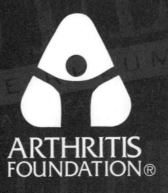

ARTHRITIS FOUNDATION®

FREE SUBSCRIPTION
TO *Bulletin on the Rheumatic Diseases*

8 issues FREE!

YES! I would like to receive my personal copy of *Bulletin on the Rheumatic Diseases*.

Please check one:

- ○ a) Family Practitioner
- ○ b) Pediatrician
- ○ c) General Internist
- ○ d) Subspecialty Internist
- ○ e) Orthopedic Surgeon
- ○ f) Rheumatologist
- ○ j) Podiatrist
- ○ k) Medical Library
- ○ l) Physiatrist
- ○ m) Medical Student
- ○ n) Nurse
- ○ o) Occupational Therapist
- ○ p) Physical Therapist
- ○ q) Other Health Professional

How many patients with joint or musculoskeletal disorders do you see each week?

- ○ a) None
- ○ b) 1-5
- ○ c) 6-10
- ○ d) 11-20
- ○ e) more than 20

Name		
Address		
City	Zip	State
Country		

※ PLEASE SEND $20 SHIPPING AND HANDLING FOR FOREIGN SUBSCRIPTIONS

FREE SUBSCRIPTION
TO *Bulletin on the Rheumatic Diseases*

8 issues FREE!

YES! I would like to receive my personal copy of *Bulletin on the Rheumatic Diseases*.

Please check one:

- ○ a) Family Practitioner
- ○ b) Pediatrician
- ○ c) General Internist
- ○ d) Subspecialty Internist
- ○ e) Orthopedic Surgeon
- ○ f) Rheumatologist
- ○ j) Podiatrist
- ○ k) Medical Library
- ○ l) Physiatrist
- ○ m) Medical Student
- ○ n) Nurse
- ○ o) Occupational Therapist
- ○ p) Physical Therapist
- ○ q) Other Health Professional

How many patients with joint or musculoskeletal disorders do you see each week?

- ○ a) None
- ○ b) 1-5
- ○ c) 6-10
- ○ d) 11-20
- ○ e) more than 20

Name		
Address		
City	Zip	State
Country		

※ PLEASE SEND $20 SHIPPING AND HANDLING FOR FOREIGN SUBSCRIPTIONS

The mission
of the Arthritis
Foundation
is to support
research to
find the cure
for and prevention
of arthritis and
to improve the
quality of life
for those affected
by arthritis.

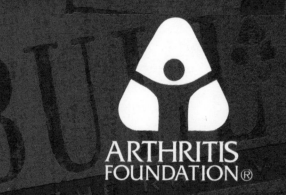

ARTHRITIS
FOUNDATION®

Your first class stamp
on this card helps us
find more research to
find cures for arthritis.
Thank you!

BUSINESS REPLY MAIL
FIRST CLASS MAIL   PERMIT # 11125   ATLANTA, GA

POSTAGE WILL BE PAID BY ADDRESSEE

Bulletin on the Rheumatic Diseases
Arthritis Foundation
1330 West Peachtree Street
Atlanta, Georgia 30309

NO POSTAGE
NECESSARY IF
MAILED IN THE
UNITED STATES

Your first class stamp
on this card helps us
find more research to
find cures for arthritis.
Thank you!

BUSINESS REPLY MAIL
FIRST CLASS MAIL   PERMIT # 11125   ATLANTA, GA

POSTAGE WILL BE PAID BY ADDRESSEE

Bulletin on the Rheumatic Diseases
Arthritis Foundation
1330 West Peachtree Street
Atlanta, Georgia 30309

NO POSTAGE
NECESSARY IF
MAILED IN THE
UNITED STATES